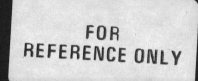

Companion to psychiatric studies

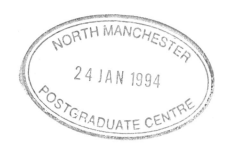

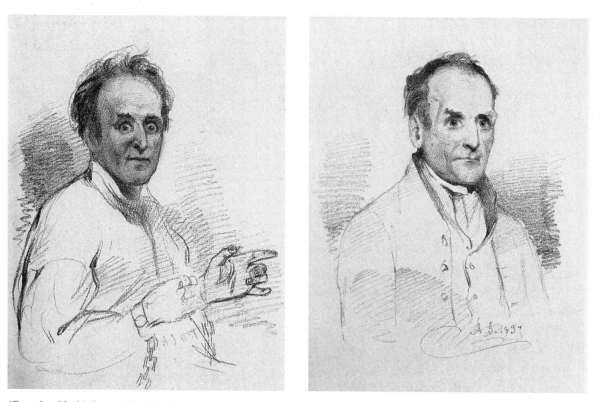

(Reproduced by kind permission of the Royal College of Physicians of Edinburgh)

These drawings by the Scottish portraitist Charles Gow were originally commissioned by Sir Alexander Morison (1779–1866) for his book *The Physiognomy of Mental Diseases*. The originals are in a large folio of similar drawings, presented by Morison to the library of the Royal College of Physicians of Edinburgh. Most of the subjects were his own patients in the Bethlehem Hospital (now the Bethlem Royal Hospital) or other asylums in London, but some were from the Salpetrière in Paris.

The sketches are labelled 'mania-excited' and 'mania-lucid interval' respectively, and were drawn at Bethlem.

Alexander Morison is a figure of some importance in British psychiatry as the course of public lectures on Diseases of the Mind which he delivered annually in Edinburgh from 1823 onwards, and for many years in London also, constituted what was probably the first formal teaching of psychiatry in Britain. Although he was President of the Edinburgh College of Physicians in 1827–28, he spent most of his professional life in London as visiting physician to the Bethlem Hospital and to other private and public asylums. He was knighted in 1838 and in 1864 he endowed an annual lectureship in mental disease for the Edinburgh College of Physicians, which still survives. The introduction to his *Outlines of Lectures on Mental Diseases*, published in 1825, might well serve as an introduction to any contemporary textbook of psychiatry:

> The subject of mental derangement is generally allowed to be the most difficult branch of medical science; at the same time it must be admitted, that much may be done to improve our knowledge of it, and that too little attention has hitherto been paid to mental diseases in the education of those destined for the medical profession.

Companion to psychiatric studies

Edited by

R. E. Kendell CBE MD FRCP FRCPsych
Chief Medical Officer,
Scottish Office Home and Health Department,
Edinburgh;
Formerly Professor of Psychiatry,
University of Edinburgh

A. K. Zealley FRCP(Edin) FRCPsych
Medical Director and Consultant Psychiatrist,
Royal Edinburgh Hospital;
Honorary Senior Lecturer, Department of Psychiatry,
University of Edinburgh,
Edinburgh

FIFTH EDITION

CHURCHILL LIVINGSTONE
EDINBURGH LONDON MADRID MELBOURNE NEW YORK AND TOKYO 1993

CHURCHILL LIVINGSTONE
Medical Division of Longman Group UK Limited

Distributed in the United States of America by Churchill Livingstone Inc., 650 Avenue of the Americas, New York, N. Y. 10011, and by associated companies, branches and representatives throughout the world.

First edition 1973
Second edition 1978
Third edition 1983
Fourth edition 1988
Fifth edition 1993

ISBN 0-443-04668-9

British Library Cataloguing in Publication Data
A catalogue record for this book is available from the British Library.

Library of Congress Cataloging in Publication Data
Companion to psychiatric studies / edited by R.E.Kendell,
    A.K.Zealley—5th ed.
        p. cm.
    Includes bibliographical references and index.
    ISBN 0-443-04668-9
    1.Psychiatry.   I. Kendell, R. E. (Robert evan)
II. Zealley, A. K. (Andrew K.)
    DNLM: 1. Mental Disorders. 2. Psychiatry.WM 100
C735] RC454.C635   1992
616.89—dc20
DLM / DLC
for Library of Congress   92-4934
                                              CIP

For Churchill Livingstone

Publisher: Peter Richardson
Project Editor: Lucy Gardner
Copy Editor: Rich Cutler
Indexer: Nina Boyd
Production Controllers: Nancy Henry, Mark Sanderson
Sales Promotion Executive: Douglas McNaughton

The
publisher's
policy is to use
**paper manufactured
from sustainable forests**

Printed and bound in Great Britain by
Butler & Tanner Ltd, Frome and London

Contents

Preface to the Fifth Edition

The first edition of this textbook was edited by Dr Alistair Forrest and published in 1973. Since then, the pace of new developments in psychiatry and demand for the book have, between them, made it necessary for a new edition to be produced every five years. We have edited the last three of these — the third in 1983, the fourth in 1988 and now this fifth edition. Although the book has grown steadily from 719 pages in the third edition to 955 in this, our aims and the basic format have been the same throughout.

The *Companion to Psychiatric Studies* is intended as a general textbook for all postgraduate students of psychiatry, as comprehensive in scope and as catholic in orientation as the constraints of a single volume will allow. Unlike most psychiatric textbooks, it includes a series of chapters devoted to other academic disciplines — the social sciences, psychology, neuroanatomy, neuropharmacology, neurochemistry and statistics — as well as chapters on personality development, neurotoxicology, measurement in psychiatry, epidemiology and research design. This is because the relevance of these various disciplines to psychiatric practice is increasing steadily and because it is our impression that many clinicians are uncertain where to go for basic, up-to-date information about aspects of these disciplines with a direct bearing on their own. The main emphasis of the book, however, is on the phenomena of psychiatric illnesses and, above all, on their treatment. Six chapters are devoted entirely to therapy and a substantial part of most of the other clinical chapters is concerned with treatment.

Most textbooks are bought and read primarily by examination candidates and, of course, we welcome the fact that our *Companion to Psychiatric Studies* is widely used by candidates for both parts of the examination for Membership of the Royal College of Psychiatrists. We hope, though, that it will also be read by psychiatrists in other countries and by those who are no longer faced with the need to pass examinations, for the book is not concerned with examination tactics, nor has its content been restricted to an examination syllabus. We hope, too, that the *Companion* will be useful to a wider readership — to clinical psychologists, social workers, psychiatric nurses and, as a reference text, to medical students.

There are several changes in the detailed content of this new edition compared with the fourth. The introductory chapter on The Nature of Psychiatric Disorders by Dr Kendell and the chapter on Neuroimaging Techniques by Professor Eve Johnstone are entirely new and Mr McGuire's chapter on Statistics and Research Design, which was dropped from the last two editions through lack of space, has been revised and brought back in response to many requests. Five other chapters have been completely rewritten by new authors. They are: Psychiatric Disorders of Childhood and Adolescence by Dr P. Hoare and Professor W. Parry-Jones respectively, The Psychiatriy of Old Age by Dr A. Jacques, Disorders of Sleep by Professor C. Shapiro and Psychiatry in General Practice by Dr I. Pullen. The other 34 chapters have all been extensively revised and updated in response to developments in the last five years in our understanding of the biological basis of psychiatric disorders, the introduction of new classifications, major changes in the management of chronic illness and the structure of the National Health Service and a variety of other changes in professional attitudes and treatment policies.

There are references in many chapters to the successive editions of the American Psychiatric Association's Diagnostic and Statistical Manual of Mental Disorders (DSM III, DSM IIIR and DSM IV) and also to the new (tenth) revision of the International Classification of Diseases and Related Health Problems (ICD-10). To save space, detailed references to these various publications are not given at the end of every chapter. Instead, they are described and discussed in the chapter on Diagnosis and Classification and listed at the end of that chapter.

Throughout, where the male pronoun is used, this also refers to the female unless otherwise indicated.

R. E. K.

Edinburgh R. E. K. 1993

A. K. Z.

Preface to the Fourth Edition

Although it is only five years since the third edition of this book was published another is already needed. This is largely a reflection of the accelerating pace of change in psychiatry. Interest in and information about the biological basis of mental disorders are both expanding rapidly, attitudes are changing, old mental hospitals are being closed, community psychiatry is struggling to become a reality and the Mental Health Acts of 1983 and 1984 have created a new legal framework for psychiatric practice throughout the United Kingdom. These changes may be inconvenient for the editors and writers of textbooks but in most other respects they are very welcome.

Like its three predecessors this edition of the *Companion to Psychiatric Studies* is intended as a general textbook for all postgraduate students of psychiatry, as comprehensive in its scope and as catholic in its orientation as the confines of a single volume will allow. As with most textbooks it will, inevitably, be widely used by examination candidates, in this case mainly by candidates for the examination for Membership of the Royal College of Psychiatrists. We hope, though, that it will also be read by psychiatrists who are no longer faced with the need to pass examinations, and that it will be useful to a wider readership — to clinical psychologists, to social workers, to psychiatric nurses and, as a reference text, to medical students.

There are many changes in the detailed content of this edition. Two new chapters have been introduced — Psychiatric epidemiology by Professor Kreitman and Epilepsy by Professor Fenton. Seven other chapters — Social science in relation to — psychiatry, The biological determinants of personality, Organic disorders, Psychiatry in general medicine, Forensic psychiatry, Individual psychotherapies and Psychiatric rehabilitation — have been completely rewritten by new authors, most of them acknowledged experts in that field. Apart from the historical introduction all the other 32 chapters have been extensively revised and updated.

Much of the typing involved was done by Mrs Patricia Rose. We are extremely grateful to her for all the help she gave us, and for her patience.

Edinburgh, 1988

R. E. K.
A. K. Z.

Contributors

John Bancroft MD FRCP FRCP(Edin) FRCPsych
Clinical Consultant, MRC Reproductive Biology
Unit; Honorary Senior Lecturer, Department of
Psychiatry, University of Edinburgh, UK

Ivy-Marie Blackburn PhD MA DipClinPsychol
Consultant Clinical Psychologist, Cognitive Therapy
Centre, St Nicholas Hospital, Collingwood Clinic,
Newcastle upon Tyne, UK

D. H. R. Blackwood MB ChB PhD MRCP MRCPsych
Senior Lecturer, Department of Psychiatry, University
of Edinburgh, UK

M. R. Bond MD PhD FRCPsych FRCS(Edin) FRCP(Glas)
DPM
Professor of Psychological Medicine, University of
Glasgow, UK

Jonathan Chick MA MPhil FRCP(Edin) FRCPsych
Consultant Psychiatrist, Royal Edinburgh Hospital;
Senior Lecturer in Psychiatry, University of
Edinburgh, UK

Derek Chiswick MB ChB MPhil FRCPsych
Consultant Forensic Psychiatrist, Royal Edinburgh
Hospital; Honorary Senior Lecturer, Department of
Psychiatry, University of Edinburgh, UK

Anthony W. Clare MD FRCPI FRCPsych MPhil
Clinical Professor of Psychiatry, Trinity College
Dublin; Medical Director, St Patrick's Hospital,
Dublin, Eire

John L. Cox BM BCh(Oxon) MA DPM FRCPsych
FRCP(Edin) DM(Oxon)
Professor of Psychiatry, School of Postgraduate
Medicine, Keele University; Consultant Psychiatrist,
North Staffordshire Health Authority, Stoke-on-
Trent, UK

A. J. Dewar MA(Cantab) MSc DIC PhD
Head of Regulatory Affairs, Crop Protection Division,
Shell International Chemical Company Limited, Shell
Centre, London, UK

J. A. T. Dyer MB ChB FRCPsych
HM Medical Commissioner, Mental Welfare
Commission for Scotland; Honorary Senior Lecturer,
Department of Psychiatry, University of Edinburgh,
UK

Christopher G. Fairburn MA DM MPhil FRCPsych
Wellcome Trust Senior Lecturer, Department of
Psychiatry, Oxford University, Warneford Hospital,
Oxford, UK

George W. Fenton MB FRCP(Edin) FRCP(Lond)
FRCPsych DPM
Professor of Psychiatry, University of Dundee,
Ninewells Hospital and Medical School, Dundee, UK

Christopher P. L. Freeman MB ChB MPhil FRCPsych
Consultant Psychotherapist, Royal Edinburgh
Hospital; Senior Lecturer, Department of Psychiatry,
University of Edinburgh, UK

Judy Greenwood MB MRCPsych
Consultant Psychiatrist, Community Drug Problem
Service, Royal Edinburgh Hospital, Edinburgh, UK

J. D. Haldane FRCP(Edin) FRCPsych DPM
Formerly Senior Lecturer and Director, Unit for
Marital and Family Studies, Department of Mental
Health, University of Aberdeen, UK

Peter Hoare DM MA BM BCh MRCPsych
Senior Lecturer, Department of Child and Adolescent
Psychiatry, University of Edinburgh, Royal Hospital
for Sick Children, Edinburgh, UK

Alan Jacques MB BCh DPM FRCPsych
Consultant in Old Age Psychiatry, Royal Victoria
Hospital, Edinburgh, UK

Eve C. Johnstone MD FRCP FRCPsych DPM
Professor of Psychiatry, Department of Psychiatry,
University of Edinburgh, UK

Kathleen Jones BA PhD
Emeritus Professor, Department of Social Policy,
University of York, UK

R. E. Kendell CBE MD FRCP FRCPsych
Chief Medical Officer, Scottish Office Home and
Health Department, Edinburgh; Formerly Professor
of Psychiatry, University of Edinburgh, UK

N. Kreitman MD FRCP(Edin) FRCPsych
Formerly Director, Medical Research Council Unit for
Epidemiological Studies in Psychiatry; Honorary
Professor, Edinburgh University Department of
Psychiatry

G. G. Lloyd MD FRCP FRCPsych
Consultant Psychiatrist, Royal Free Hospital,
London, UK

John B. Loudon MB ChB FRCPsych DPM(Edin)
Consultant Psychiatrist and Honorary Senior Lecturer,
Royal Edinburgh Hospital; Honorary Senior Lecturer,
University of Edinburgh, UK

Una McCluskey BSocSc DipSW
Lecturer, Department of Social Policy and Social
Work, University of York, UK

Peter McGuffin MB PhD FRCP FRCPsych
Professor of Psychological Medicine, University of
Wales College of Medicine, Cardiff, UK

R. J. McGuire BSc MA MEd
Formerly Senior Lecturer in Clinical Psychology,
Departments of Psychology and Psychiatry, University
of Edinburgh, Edinburgh, UK

F. M. McPherson MA DCP PhD FRPsS CPsychol
Director, Tayside Area Clinical Psychology Department, Royal Dundee Liff Hospital, Dundee, UK

Peter Maguire FRCPsych DPM
Director, Cancer Research Campaign Psychological
Medicine Group, Christie Hospital, Manchester, UK

Robin M. Murray MD DSc FRCP FRCPsych
Professor of Psychological Medicine, Institute of
Psychiatry, London, UK

William Ll. Parry-Jones MA MD FRCP(Glas) FRCPsych
DPM
Professor of Child Health and Adolescent Psychiatry,
University of Glasgow, Royal Hospital for Sick
Children, Glasgow, UK

David F. Peck BA DAP FBPsS
Area Clinical Psychologist, Highland Health Board,
Inverness, UK

Ian M. Pullen FRCPsych
Consultant Psychiatrist, Royal Edinburgh Hospital;
Honorary Senior Lecturer, Department of Psychiatry,
University of Edinburgh, UK

Jean Reid MB ChB MRCPsych
Lecturer in Psychological Medicine, University of
Glasgow, UK

Bruce Ritson MD FRCPsych FRCP
Consultant, Alcohol Problem Clinic, Royal Edinburgh
Hospital; Senior Lecturer, Department of Psychiatry,
University of Edinburgh, UK

Colin M. Shapiro BSc(Hons) MB BCh MRCPsych FRCP(C)
Professor of Psychiatry, University of Toronto, The
Toronto Hospital, Toronto, Ontario, Canada

John Strang MB BS MRCPsych
Consultant Psychiatrist in Drug Dependence,
National Addiction Centre, Maudsley Hospital/
Institute of Psychiatry, London, UK

E. Szabadi MD PhD DSc DipNeurol FRCPsych
Professor of Psychiatry, University of Nottingham,
Queen's Medical Centre, Nottingham, UK

Lawrence J. Whalley MD FRCPsych
Professor of Mental Health, University of Aberdeen, UK

Sula Wolff MA FRCP FRCPsych
Honorary Fellow, Department of Psychiatry,
University of Edinburgh, UK

Andrew K. Zealley FRCP (Edin) FRCPsych
Medical Director and Consultant Psychiatrist,
Royal Edinburgh Hospital; Honorary Senior Lecturer,
Department of Psychiatry, University of Edinburgh,
UK

1. The nature of psychiatric disorders

R. E. Kendell

And little by little I can look upon madness as a disease like any other
Vincent van Gogh

HISTORICAL ASSUMPTIONS ABOUT MADNESS

Madness has a long history. Most cultures have recognised people who were either temporarily or permanently 'deranged' and most languages have a word for the phenomenon. The cause of this derangement was even more puzzling 2000 or 200 years ago than it is today and many different assumptions have been made about its origins. At one time or another madness has been attributed to divine intervention, evil spirits, fevers, heredity, unbridled passions, strong liquor, the influence of the moon and blows to the head. Madmen have been regarded with revulsion, pity, hilarity, reverence and indifference and their disordered proclamations treated with derision, mockery, horror, or, occasionally, with grave respect. But throughout this kaleidoscopic jumble of attitudes and opinions the dominant assumption has generally been that madness was a disease of some kind. Certainly, attempts to alleviate madness were usually made by the same people, and by the same means, as attempts to cure illnesses of other kinds. Whether he was priest, shaman, physician or apothecary, the appointed authority used much the same ceremonies, spells, potions or medicaments to treat madness as he did to treat a wide variety of other more obviously medical disorders.

In the 4th century BC Plato discussed madness in his *Phaedo* and distinguished 'madness given us by divine gift' from natural madness. The former was inspired by Apollo, Dionysus, Aphrodite or the Muses; the latter originated in physical disease. His contemporary Hippocrates, or the corpus of writings attributed to him, described at least five forms of madness — phrenitis (acute mental disturbance with fever), mania (acute mental disturbance without fever), melancholia (chronic mental disturbance), epilepsy (convulsions) and hysteria (paroxysmal conditions seen in women) and regarded all of them as medical conditions requir-

ing treatment (Menninger 1963). Both aetiological hypotheses, the supernatural and the medical, persisted for the next 2000 years. For Richard Burton in the 17th century and John Wesley in the 18th, religious melancholy was, quite literally, ensnarement by the Devil, but physicians — Greek, Roman, Arab and European — almost invariably accepted Hippocrates' assumptions. Celsus, Areteus and Galen, writing in the 1st and 2nd centuries AD, all regarded melancholia and other forms of madness as diseases and Galen's four humours provided an explanatory framework which was at least as plausible for melancholia (attributed, as the name implies, to an excess of black bile if the patient was sad and fearful, or of yellow bile if he was angry and agitated) as for illnesses of other kinds. In the 11th century AD the great Persian philosopher physician Avicenna incorporated Galen's teachings about madness and the four humours into his vastly influential *Canon of Medicine*. As a result, a coherent set of assumptions about the nature and causes of madness were shared by the Christian and Moslem worlds for several hundred years. Although by the 18th century respect for ancient authorities, and for Galen's humoral pathology, had finally crumbled, the central assumptions of Hippocrates, Galen and Avicenna about the nature of madness still held sway. When Lady Mary Wortley Montagu commented in a letter that 'madness is as much a corporeal distemper as the gout or asthma' she was simply voicing the commonplace views of her contemporaries, both educated and uneducated (Porter 1987).

Towards the end of that century, however, an important change took place. It slowly became clear that the armamentarium of 18th century medicine — the special diets, bleeding, purging, emetics and blistering — however valuable they might be for fashionable 'nervous disorders' like hypochondriasis and hysteria, had little effect on madness itself, a state of affairs emphasised in England by the impotence of George III's physicians to alleviate his recurrent bouts of insanity. At the same time the waning of religious fervour that accompanied this 'Age of Reason' meant that the theological assumptions of Burton and Wesley were no longer acceptable. An explanatory and therapeutic vacuum was thus developing and the managers of the new private madhouses moved into it. Francis Willis, the clergyman who was eventually called in to treat the mad king, was typical of this new breed. Willis was a charismatic healer with extensive personal experience of handling lunatics by virtue of having lived for years with several in his house. His therapeutic powers depended partly on this experience and partly on his personality, on what he would have called moral authority and we might regard as psychotherapy. The success of the York Retreat, which had been opened by the Quaker William Tuke in 1796, reinforced Willis' influence, for at least in its early days The Retreat was demonstrably more effective than other madhouses at calming and curing the insane, despite the fact that it used no medicaments and employed no physician.

The success of the novel regime of William Tuke's Retreat, together with a widespread revulsion against the brutal repressions of the 18th century, symbolised by Pinel's historic decision to unchain his patients in the Bicêtre, led in the first half of the 19th century to a widespread commitment to 'moral treatment' of the insane. Indeed, this provided the basic therapeutic regime of the new lunatic asylums which were fast replacing the private madhouses. Moral treatment assumed that kindness, an ordered regime with regular occupation, regular religious observance, wholesome food and an avoidance of passion and excess would lead to the recovery of most forms of insanity and that medications, and indeed physicians, were generally unnecessary. At the same time autopsies were making it increasingly clear that insanity was not accompanied by the visible pathologies that characterised so many other diseases.

Madness becomes mental disease

In this climate it became increasingly reasonable to assume that insanity was fundamentally different from other disease; that it was a manifestation of disease of the mind, not of the body, and required moral rather than somatic therapies. In the early years of the 19th century a new term, mental disease, began to replace the old terms madness and lunacy, and there was much debate about whether a mind could be diseased in the absence of any disease of the brain, and whether

philosophers might not be better fitted to treat diseased minds than physicians. Although it was eventually conceded that mental disease still lay within the province of medicine, and members of the emerging psychiatric profession like Benjamin Rush insisted that the fundamental pathology of diseases of the mind was somatic (Rush himself believed it lay 'primarily in the blood vessels of the brain') the new term had come to stay (Hunter & Macalpine 1963). Eminent 19th century alienists like Griesinger repeatedly emphasised their conviction that mental illnesses were diseases of the brain ('*Psychische Krankheiten sind Erkrankungen des Gehirns*') but the doubts remained, even within their own profession; and it remained the case throughout that century and the first third of the next that mental diseases were largely uninfluenced by the physician's pharmacopoeia and, apart from general paralysis, could not be shown to be accompanied by brain pathology, either macroscopic or microscopic.

The territory of psychiatry is still formally described as mental illness or mental disorder even though these terms now embrace a far broader range of conditions than they did when they were first introduced. (The American Psychiatric Association uses 'mental disorders' and the World Health Organization 'mental and behavioural disorders' as their main generic terms.) The implication still persists, therefore, that psychiatric disorders are disorders of the mind, and fundamentally different from disorders of the body. Although the philosophical problem of the relationship between mind and body remains unsolved, and may indeed be insoluble, we are far better informed than the early 19th century physicians who coined the term mental disease. We are aware of a wide range of situations in which alterations to the structure or functioning of the brain result in predictable changes in the subjective experience of the subject, or in his behaviour or cognitive performance. We can also demonstrate that mental activity is accompanied by increased metabolic activity in discrete areas of the brain.

THE CEREBRAL SUBSTRATE OF MENTAL PHENOMENA

Stimulating electrodes deep within the brains of conscious subjects can evoke sensory experiences, emotions or vivid memories which have the subjective characteristics of familiar mental phenomena and come and go as the stimulating electrode is switched on and off. Pharmacological agents of various kinds will induce mood states, improve or impair memory, alter perceptions or induce unconsciousness. Lesions in specific areas of the brain will produce predictable changes in the subject's ability to speak, to understand the speech of others, to remember past events, to recognise familiar people or objects, or to hear, see, taste or smell. Section of the corpus callosum creates a situation in which one side of the brain can be shown to know things of which the other hemisphere is ignorant. We can also demonstrate increased energy consumption (increased regional blood flow, oxygen uptake or glucose utilisation) by different parts of the brain as the subject thinks about different things — of the left hemisphere when a verbal problem is tackled and of the right hemisphere when an arithmetic or spatial problem is tackled. In short, we are increasingly able to control, restrict or enhance mental activity by manipulating the functioning or integrity of the brain, and to observe the biochemical events accompanying conscious mentation. We are not in a position to say, and perhaps never will be, that all mental activity has a neurophysiological substrate but we can observe, and influence, an increasingly wide range of close spatial and temporal relationships between mental activity and the structure or functioning of the brain. We can also build computers which can store memories, recognise familiar situations, solve problems, take decisions, plan ahead and even become confused in ways that closely mimic human mentation.

It is therefore reasonable for us to assume that all mental activity, normal or abnormal, is accompanied by, and could not take place without, transmission of nervous impulses within and energy consumption by particular neural networks in the brain. We cannot prove that all mental activity necessarily has a neurophysiological substrate and that all mental events are accompanied by matching somatic events, but in the absence of contrary evidence it is reasonable to assume that they do. Whether a mind can exist in the absence of a functioning brain is a theological question, not a scientific one.

If this philosophical position is accepted, as it is in one form or another by most contemporary neuroscientists, it follows that there is, strictly speaking, no such thing as disease of the mind or mental disorder and that Griesinger was right — mental illnesses are diseases of the brain, or at least involve disordered brain function — because all mental events are accompanied by and dependent on events in the brain. (Thomas Szasz was also right; mental illness is a myth, though not for the reasons he believed.) Acceptance of this argument does not, however, commit psychiatrists to a crude somaticism. It does not imply that we should ignore the role of social and psychological factors in the genesis of psychiatric disorders, still less that we should abandon psychological forms

of treatment, or discard concepts like grief, hostility and loneliness in favour of catecholamine and neuropeptide assays.

The functions of the cerebral hemispheres

Despite the impressive advances of the last two decades we know far less about the structure and functioning of the human brain than we do about any other organ in the body. That is why we understand so little about the aetiology of most psychiatric disorders. We know quite enough, though, to realise that the functions and physiology of the brain are far more complex than those of any other organ, probably by several orders of magnitude. So we should not be surprised if psychiatric disorders have characteristics which are not shared with other diseases. One of the most important distinguishing characteristics of psychiatric disorders is the contribution which the patient's previous experience and current psychological and social predicaments — his childhood upbringing, recent life events, the fact that he always feels unwanted, or is lonely or demoralised — make to their aetiology. This is hardly surprising, however, if one reflects that it is one of the brain's most important functions to keep a detailed record of past experience. Sensory perceptions can only be recognised and assessed in the light of a memory of the implications and sequelae of similar perceptions in the past; and appropriate decisions about future behaviour can only be made after reviewing the consequences of previous responses in similar situations. Moreover, because man is pre-eminently a social species with a uniquely long period of dependent immaturity, the most important information and the most important appraisals are almost bound to concern his relationships with other people, particularly his own family.

Stressful past experiences and the patient's appraisal of his current social environment play a part in the genesis of many illnesses. Asthma, migraine and acute myocardial infarction are obvious examples. They play a much greater role in the genesis of psychiatric disorders, however, and for good reasons. To remember what has happened in the past, to appraise current situations in the light of that memory, and to create moods and action plans appropriate to these appraisals are amongst the brain's most important functions. It should not surprise us, therefore, that psychiatric illnesses characteristically involve disorders of perception, memory, cognition, mood and volition. Memory is of central importance because it is involved in most of these activities. Information processing is the brain's most basic function and the means by which meaning, which is derived from the interrelationships between different items of information, is attributed to events and symbols. The brain's memory stores are as crucial to this role as the memory banks of a computer are to its functioning. It is no coincidence, therefore, that memories and meanings play a key role in most psychological theories of the aetiology of psychiatric disorders. Although the physical substrate of memory is still obscure it is apparent that the physical basis of short-term memory (up to 60 seconds) and long-term memory are different; that information storage is achieved by facilitating connectivity in neuronal pathways; and that both the hippocampus and long-term potentiation utilising N-methyl-D-aspartate receptors are involved in this process. For present purposes the detailed mechanisms are unimportant. What matters is that memory has a physical substrate in the brain and almost certainly cannot exist in the absence of that substrate.

MENTAL AND PHYSICAL ILLNESS

If psychiatric disorders generally involve disordered brain function, and there is, strictly speaking, no such thing as disease of the mind or mental disorder, a further question obviously arises: what is the difference between psychiatric disorders like schizophrenia and obsessional disorder and diseases of the brain like encephalitis and Parkinson's disease? Or indeed between psychiatric disorders and bodily disease in general?

The answer is that the difference is no more fundamental than the difference between, say, gastro-intestinal and cardiovascular disorders. Psychiatric disorders tend to involve the patient's whole personality, his social behaviour and his ability to make rational responses to both incoming sensory information and internal cognitive assessments because they involve dysfunctions of the cerebral mechanisms responsible for perception, memory, cognition and mood. Their effects are therefore more global, pervasive and subtle than those of disorders of, for example, the gall bladder or the hip joint. But this is a difference of degree, not a qualitative difference. In fact the classification of individual disorders as 'mental' or psychiatric is in large measure determined by the fact that, for historical reasons, they or related conditions have generally been treated by psychiatrists. If anorexia nervosa were still treated mainly by gynaecologists and endocrinologists it would be regarded, and classified, as a gynaecological or endocrine disorder. If alcoholism and other forms of drug dependence and abuse were usually treated by specialist 'alcohologists' with no

psychiatric training they would almost certainly be classified separately from mental or psychiatric disorders. The fact that multi-infarct dementia is regarded and classified as a psychiatric rather than as a vascular disorder well illustrates the utilitarian basis of disease classifications. What matters is not aetiology or pathology so much as which medical specialty has traditionally treated the disorder and possesses the requisite diagnostic and therapeutic expertise. The distinction between 'neurological' disorders of the brain like Parkinson's disease and psychiatric disorders like schizophrenia is particularly artificial and can only be understood in the light of the different historical origins of psychiatry and neurology, and the unfortunate 19th century dichotomy between mind and brain. Eventually the distinction is likely to be abandoned. For the time being, however, the skills required to diagnose and treat Parkinson's disease and multiple sclerosis on the one hand and schizophrenia and obsessional disorders on the other are probably sufficiently different to justify two different specialties.

The distinction between mental and physical illness, and the mind/body distinction from which it is derived, has encouraged patients and many doctors to believe that the two are fundamentally different. Both are apt to assume that mental illness is evidence of a certain lack of moral fibre, and that, if they really tried, psychiatric patients ought to be able to control their anxieties, their despondency and their strange preoccupations and 'snap out of it'. It is true, of course, that we all believe in 'freewill'; we believe that we ourselves and other people can exercise a certain amount of control over our feelings and behaviour. But why should we expect people suffering from phobic or depressive illnesses to be able to exercise more control over their symptoms than those suffering from, say, myxoedema or arthritis? In a similar vein, patients complaining of intense fatigue or abdominal pain are often dismayed to be told that they have a depressive illness, and interpret such a diagnosis as meaning that their doctor does not believe that they are really in pain, or are exhausted by the slightest exertion, and is dismissing their complaints as 'all in the mind'. All too often doctors make similar assumptions and perceive it as their job to decide whether such patients are ill, or 'just depressed'. They may even attempt to reassure them by saying 'There's nothing wrong, all the tests are negative, you're just depressed', or words to that effect.

In reality, depressive and other psychiatric illnesses do not differ in any material respect from so-called bodily illnesses. It has already been demonstrated that they are almost bound to involve cerebral dysfunction of some kind; and the evidence that there is an important genetic component to the aetiology of depressions and panic disorder implies that there must be biological differences, qualitative or quantitative, between people who are and are not liable to depressive illnesses and anxiety states. The symptoms of depression and phobic anxiety are just as 'real' and painful as those of other illnesses and can no more be overcome by an effort of will than the symptoms of myxoedema. They can, however, be treated effectively with antidepressant drugs which have no effect on mood in other people, and the panic attacks of phobic subjects can be precipitated by intravenous lactate infusions which are similarly without effect in other people. Again, these differences in response imply the existence of underlying biological differences.

The implications of the terms mental illness and mental disorder are therefore seriously misleading, and have had a baneful influence on medical and lay attitudes for nearly 200 years. In the words of those appointed by the American Psychiatric Association to draft DSM-IV, mental disorder 'could not be a more unfortunate term, preserving as it does an outdated mind–body duality. There is much that is physical in the so-called mental disorders, and much mental in the so-called physical disorders. The term organic disorder is an equal abomination...' (Frances et al 1991). For this reason the terms mental illness and mental disorder will be avoided in this book. They will be replaced by the terms psychiatric illness and psychiatric disorder, which imply simply that the conditions in question are usually treated by doctors with a psychiatric training. This does not imply, though, that members of other professions ought not to be involved in their treatment. It does not represent a covert bid for psychiatric hegemony. Clinical psychologists, social workers, psychiatric nurses and members of other professions too already make a substantial contribution to the care of the psychiatrically ill and it is likely that their roles will increase in the future. In any case, it is well known that in the UK most people with psychiatric disorders are treated, if they are treated by anybody, by their general practitioners.

The role of cerebral pathology

Insisting that psychiatric illnesses are not mental illnesses does not imply that they are illnesses of the brain, or bodily illnesses. Neither minds, nor brains nor bodies become ill in isolation. Only people, or in a wider context organisms, become ill or develop diseases. The most characteristic symptom of so-called bodily illness is pain, a purely subjective or mental phenomenon. The first symptom of most systemic illnesses, from the common cold to typhoid fever, is vague generalised malaise, another purely subjective experience. On the other hand, we know, or at least are justified in assuming, that psychiatric conditions like paranoid psychoses and obsessional illnesses whose manifestations may be entirely subjective must involve cerebral dysfunctions.

Many of these cerebral dysfunctions are genetic in origin. We already know, for example, that genetic factors contribute to the aetiology of schizophrenic and affective psychoses, Alzheimer's disease, most depressive illnesses, panic disorder, obsessional disorders, alcohol dependence, and many kinds of mental handicap. It is likely, too, that some life experiences result not merely in the registration of a memory but in enduring changes in brain morphology. It is well established that the richness and complexity of synaptic pathways in the developing brain and the thickness of the cerebral cortex are permanently influenced by the complexity and significance of incoming sensory information (Diamond 1988). A young animal kept in the dark throughout the early weeks of life, for example, does not develop normal visual association areas in its occipital cortex. The consistency and chronicity of the complex of symptoms developing after overwhelmingly terrifying experiences (post-traumatic stress disorder) strongly suggests that enduring changes in cerebral functioning have occurred, that the revealing phrase 'scarred for life' is more than a metaphor.

It must not be assumed, however, that all psychiatric disorders are necessarily based on cerebral dysfunctions of some kind. In the first place, what we regard as illness or disorder appears to shade insensibly into normality. Many studies of the distribution of psychiatric symptoms in the general population have failed to reveal any boundary or discontinuity between depressive or anxiety disorders and the temporary emotional disturbances of everyday life. More fundamentally, illness is itself a socially defined concept and involves value judgements which are liable to change from time to time and place to place. Someone who develops depression of mood, insomnia, anhedonia, impaired concentration and weight loss after losing his job or his reputation is regarded as having a psychiatric illness, namely a depressive disorder. Someone who develops identical symptoms after losing his parent or spouse, on the other hand, is not, probably because grief after bereavement is both expected and esteemed, and we are loath to label something we esteem as illness. It is unlikely, though, that there is any difference in the underlying mechanisms. Similarly, paedophilia is regarded as a psychiatric disorder but homosexuality is not, not because of any assumed difference in the underlying causes of the two phenomena, but because our culture strongly disapproves of the former but not of the latter. Because the concept of illness or disorder involves a value judgement, the phenomena we choose to label as psychiatric disorder and those which eventually prove to be rooted in a cerebral dysfunction of some kind will only be identical if we deliberately define the terms psychiatric disorder and cerebral dysfunction to achieve this end. All we can or need say at present is that we have strong presumptive evidence that most severely handicapping psychiatric disorders are probably rooted in cerebral dysfunctions, and that these may be either inborn or acquired, or a combination of the two.

ORGANIC AND FUNCTIONAL DISORDERS

The argument that most psychiatric disorders should be assumed to involve a cerebral pathology of some kind implies among other things that the distinction between 'organic' and 'functional' disorders is pointless. Indeed, in this context it implies that both these adjectives are inherently meaningless. The concept of functional illness was first introduced by neurologists like Reynolds (1855), whose classification of chronic diseases of the encephalon contained groups of disorders characterised by 'exaltation of function', by 'decrease of functional activity' and by 'excess of some functions and diminution of others'. Subsequently, the terms organic and functional came to be used to distinguish conditions such as general paralysis and hydrocephalus, in which there were overt pathological changes in the brain to account for the patient's symptoms, from those like chorea and epilepsy in which the consequences of disturbed cerebral function could be observed but no structural lesion could be detected. Gowers, for example, classified Parkinson's disease, chorea, torticollis, epilepsy and narcolepsy as functional in his *Manual of Diseases of the Nervous System*, because at the time there was no 'visible lesion' to justify regarding any of these conditions as organic (Gowers 1893). Although, as his contemporary Möbius observed, 'The differentiation is useless, because it is to a large extent dependent on the methods of investigation: the pathological findings are always being added to by advances in histology', the distinction was adopted by psychiatrists and has remained in use ever since (Lewis 1971). In a psychiatric context the term functional has been used mainly as a convenient epithet to distinguish affective,

schizophrenic and paranoid psychoses from dementias and confusional states. The fact that these two groupings tended to have different symptoms gave some credence to the distinction. Unfortunately, the inherent shortcomings of the functional label have been exacerbated by a widespread assumption that the term implies not merely that no overt pathology has yet been identified but that there is no pathology to be found; that the disorder is purely mental. Mayer-Gross and his colleagues commented 40 years ago in their textbook that they were 'aware of the semantic confusion due to vagueness and ambiguity in the application of these terms (organic and functional) and of the frequent criticisms of their use', but then pointed out that 'no-one has so far been able to suggest satisfactory alternatives' (Mayer-Gross et al 1954). That is still the case. However, the evidence that has accumulated in the last decade that a substantial proportion of schizophrenic illnesses — the prototype of functional psychoses — are accompanied by overt cerebral pathology, but do not differ in other respects from those that do not, has made the term functional increasingly inappropriate. Its implications are ambiguous and misleading and it probably delayed recognition of the substantial cognitive impairment exhibited by many chronic schizophrenics. It will therefore not be used in this book. The terms organic psychosis and organic disorder will be reluctantly retained, not because they are appropriate but for lack of any satisfactory alternative. Neither term, though, seems likely to be retained in DSM-IV.

ENDOGENOUS AND PSYCHOGENIC DISORDERS

The dichotomy between endogenous and psychogenic or reactive illnesses is equally objectionable. The term endogenous was introduced to psychiatry by Möbius in 1893, and has always been equated with heredity. Initially, it was contrasted with exogenous disorders, Bonhoeffer's term for confusional and toxic states whose causes were somatic but external to the brain (Lewis 1971). Subsequently, endogenous disorders were more commonly contrasted with psychogenic or reactive states. This terminology implied that the depressions or psychoses to which the dichotomy was applied were either endogenous or reactive, despite much evidence that hereditary factors and life experiences were both involved in the genesis of most depressions and many psychoses. To make matters worse, the meaning of psychogenic was rarely defined, and was expanded by Scandinavian psychiatrists to include disorders 'growing out of innate constitutional factors as, for example, the psychopathies' (Faergeman 1963). Because of this semantic chaos, and the unwarranted aetiological dichotomy they implied, the terms psychogenic and endogenous have been expunged from contemporary classifications and the concept of reactive illness survives only in the American Psychiatric Association's concept of brief reactive psychosis — shortlived psychotic episodes developing in the immediate aftermath of overwhelming stress.

THE FUTURE

It must be emphasised once more that the twin propositions that psychiatric illnesses do not differ in any fundamental way from other illnesses, and that all psychiatric disorders in which there is a substantial impairment of function almost certainly involve a cerebral malfunction of some kind, do not imply that psychological and social factors do not play a major aetiological role in many psychiatric disorders, or that psychological and social therapies are inappropriate or ineffective. To take just three examples, the evidence that recent life events play a major role in the genesis of depressive illnesses, that the emotional atmosphere within the family is a major determinant of early relapse in schizophrenia and that psychological treatments can be effective in depressive, phobic and obsessional disorders is beyond challenge, and in each case perfectly compatible with an assumption of cerebral dysfunction.

If we are convinced, however, that even neurotic illnesses and other so-called minor disorders probably involve a malfunctioning neuronal substrate we should be prepared to devote the main thrust of our research to exploring this neuronal substrate, and to elucidating the mechanisms by which stress of various kinds causes it to malfunction. Psychiatry already possesses a variety of highly effective pharmacological therapies. The most important of these — the neuroleptics, the tricyclic antidepressants and lithium — were all discovered by chance, without any prior understanding of the cerebral mechanisms they influenced. How much more effective then can we expect the new generation of neuropharmacological agents to be that are developed by design to correct identified neuronal dysfunctions. Yet even though the most important future developments in treatment and prevention are likely to be derived from the biological sciences, there is no reason in principle why psychological and social interventions should not continue to play a major and even an expanding role. The various disorders resulting from substance abuse illustrate this very well. We can look forward with confidence to a time when the means by which alcohol and other psychoactive substances produce intoxication, dependence and tissue damage are understood at a cellular and molecular level. Almost certainly this knowledge will bring with it new means of detecting, reducing and perhaps reversing intoxication, dependence and tissue damage, and of identifying high-risk individuals in advance. This does not mean, though, that it will no longer be important to understand the social forces and psychological pressures that lead people into careers of abuse and dependence, or that political, social and economic measures may not continue to be the most effective means of combating drug misuse on a national scale. However detailed our understanding of underlying neuronal mechanisms eventually becomes, and however potent the resulting pharmacological and other physical therapies may be, the understanding and treatment of psychiatric disorders is always going to require a rounded appreciation of the social setting in which they develop, and an empathic understanding of the patient's inner feelings.

REFERENCES

Diamond M C 1988 Enriching heredity: the impact of the environment on the anatomy of the brain. Free Press, New York

Faergeman P M 1963 Psychogenic psychoses. Butterworths, London

Frances A J, First M B, Widiger T A et al 1991 An A to Z guide to DSM-IV conundrums. Journal of Abnormal Psychology 100: 407–412

Gowers W R 1893 A manual of diseases of the nervous system, vol 1. Reprinted 1970 by Hafner, Darion

Hunter R, Macalpine I 1963 Three hundred years of psychiatry 1535–1860. Oxford University Press, London

Lewis A 1971 'Endogenous' and 'exogenous': a useful dichotomy? Psychological Medicine 1: 191–196

Mayer-Gross W, Slater E, Roth M 1954 Clinical psychiatry. Cassell, London

Menninger K 1963 The vital balance: the life process in mental health and illness. Viking Press, New York

Porter R 1987 Mind-forg'd manacles: a history of madness in England from the restoration to the regency. Athlone Press, London

Reynolds J R 1855 The diagnosis of diseases of the brain, spinal cord, nerves and their appendages. Churchill, London

2. Social science in relation to psychiatry

Kathleen Jones

Why should psychiatrists in training be concerned with the social sciences? Their training programmes are already packed with the hard data of a profession based on medical science. Why should they spend time and effort on what many regard as the more speculative and less precise work of sociologists and other social scientists?

The most fundamental reason is that a sense of personal identity, for psychiatrist and patient alike, derives from family relationships, work relationships, neighbourhood and community relationships. We are sons/daughters, husbands/wives, parents, colleagues, friends, citizens, members of associations, societies and clubs (social theorists dispose of this collection of relationships more neatly by talking about 'significant others'). For most of us, our network is defining and sustaining. Relationships specify 'the way one is pinpointed on the social map...to be located in society means to be at the intersection of social forces' (Berger 1974).

Psychiatric illness is typically accompanied by troubled or broken relationships, and the patient's illness cannot be treated with sensitivity unless the psychiatrist has some understanding of the social dynamics of the situation. John A and Mary B may both be diagnosed as suffering from schizophrenia; but if John is a wealthy Old Etonian stockbroker with a large circle of friends and relatives, while Mary is a Caribbean-born lone parent of five children, living a precarious inner-city existence, their life situations, and the resources available to them, may be very different.

The social sciences offer understanding of the social contexts in which patients live out their lives; they also help to explain some of the major crises of modern life, in which macro-events, like the Gulf War, the collapse of the housing market, the rise in unemployment or the current changes in the National Health Service, can have a sudden and sometimes devastating impact on the lives of individuals. Wright Mills developed a powerful argument against the view that patients could be treated in isolation from their environment:

> ...it is *not* true, as Ernest Jones asserted, that "man's chief enemy and danger is his own unruly nature and the dark forces pent up within him". On the contrary, "man's chief danger" lies in the unruly forces of contemporary society itself, with its alienating methods of production, its enveloping techniques of political domination, its international anarchy — in a word, its pervasive transformations of the very nature of man, and the conditions and aims of his life. (Wright Mills 1959)

The policy of community care requires that most people suffering from a psychiatric disorder, most of the time, will live in this increasingly complex, increasingly plural and increasingly fluid society. Before the run-down of psychiatric hospitals, patients often stayed in hospital for long periods, their community contacts effectively broken. Even as late as the 1950s, many hospitals kept to the practice of asking friends and relatives not to visit for the first month, to give the patient 'time to settle down'. The hospital culture provided a stable common background and a protection against outside pressures, and the role of 'patient' obscured other roles; but if community care is to be more than a convenient fiction, the great variety of social contexts in which patients have to find meaning and purpose have to be more clearly appreciated than in the past.

THE MEDICAL MODEL AND THE SOCIAL MODEL

The medical model of psychiatric disorder goes back to the Macmillan Committee of 1924–1926, which, in its anxiety to avoid the stigmatisation involved in such specialised terms as 'asylum' and 'lunatic', stressed the interaction of mind and body, and the view that any illness was an illness of the whole person. At that time, the best hope of securing more resources for the badly underfunded mental health services seemed to lie in stressing the links of psychiatry with the rest of medicine, in creating a new frame of reference with the terminology of 'doctors', 'patients' and 'hospitals'. This policy was successful in 1948, when psychiatry was finally included in the new National Health Service, rather than being left (as it was in the first two drafts of the new Health Service) in the hands of the local authorities (Jones 1972).

After World War II, interaction between the social sciences and psychiatry was very promising for a time. For about 20 years, each was able to learn from the other. Stanton & Schwarz (1954) examined the different perceptions of psychiatrists and patients, and argued that all aspects of the patient's daily life were relevant to the management of his illness. Caudill (1958) contributed an acutely observed study of inter-action processes on a psychiatric ward from an anthro-pological perspective. Belknap (1956) examined the culture of a large, impersonal hospital with a rapid turnover of doctors and a poor quality of care. The most comprehensive publication of the collaborative works was the Walter Reed Symposium (Greenblatt et al 1957). This contained 38 different papers in which psychiatrists, sociologists and psychologists examined such long-standing problems as custodial attitudes among staff, the depersonalising effect of hospital routine, and the administrative differences between psychiatric and general hospitals. Rapoport (1960) evaluated the work of Maxwell Jones at the Henderson Hospital, and Jones & Sidebotham (1962) attempted to find a workable measure of the efficiency of psychiatric care.

The approach of most of these writers was mildly psychodynamic and strongly humanitarian. Patients were to have their dignity preserved, administration was to serve therapy and not to block it, communica-tion was to flow in all directions; but the assumptions were liberal rather than radical. Though the psychiatrist might divest himself of his white coat and be on first-name terms with his patient, he was still ultimately in control of the process. Stanton & Schwarz argued strongly for psychiatrists to control all aspects of administration, even down to supplying soap for the wards.

For psychiatrists, the development of the phenothiazines changed the situation permanently and decisively. Psychiatry strengthened its links with general medicine. Psychopharmacology seemed to offer the possibility of precise, scientific and objective treat-ment, and greatly reduced psychiatrists' interest in what the social scientist had to offer in the way of

insight. They had a powerful new armoury of treatment which required careful observation and monitoring, but was not dependent on an understanding of the patient's social context or emotional reactions. They seemed no longer to have to concern themselves with individual or social problems, with human hopeless-ness and inadequacy and injustice.

The medical view which emerged from these changed circumstances can be summarised as follows:

- Psychiatric disorders are diseases with distinct pathologies, courses and outcomes
- Psychiatry is a branch of medicine
- The aetiology of psychiatric disorder is at present imperfectly understood, but the causes are primarily genetic and biochemical
- Diagnosis and prescription are reasonably exact sciences, and will become more so
- Hospital, clinic and general practitioner services are the appropriate agencies for treatment.

Psychiatrists who strongly support the medical model readily admit that as yet very little firm evidence exists about the aetiology of the functional psychoses, the neuroses and the psychosomatic disorders, i.e. about the great majority of conditions which they are accustomed to treat. Their view is based on the conviction that, before long, biological and biochemical research will clarify the morbid processes underlying these conditions, and that they will be conquered as completely as cholera, typhus and smallpox were conquered in the 19th century.

The difficulty with this tidy philosophy is that there is no guarantee that the highly successful medical conquest of the gross plagues will be repeated, or that research in the natural sciences will produce compar-able findings. It would be a great step forward if they did; but the hope of 'a cure for schizophrenia' may be simplistic. What we know of schizophrenia, which accounts for about two-thirds of all severe and chronic psychiatric disorder, suggests that the aetiology is complex, and probably includes both social and biological factors. The usefulness of a rigorously medical approach, both to psychiatrists and their patients, seems limited.

While psychiatry has drawn closer to medicine, many social scientists have developed a different model:

- 'Mental illness' and 'psychiatric disorder' are medical terms for what are basically problems in human relationships
- Psychiatry is (or ought to be) one of the helping professions

- Treatment is an art as well as a science
- Drugs and electroconvulsive therapy (ECT) merely suppress distress, and may be methods of social control
- Medical labels are stigmatising; most people diagnosed as psychiatric patients can manage to live in the community if they are accorded some human dignity, and reasonable conditions of life.

Supporters of the social model see what psychiatrists term 'psychiatric disorder' primarily as individual behaviour determined by social forces. The difficulty with this view, which received strong support from the 'antipsychiatry' school (Laing 1959, 1975, Szasz 1961, 1963, 1971, 1975, Laing & Esterson 1964, Basaglia 1980) is that it goes to the other extreme in entirely ignoring the physiology and biochemistry of psychiatric disorder.

Both perspectives have been subject to exaggeration and a rigidity of approach which amounts to tunnel vision. They now have differing frames of reference, different terminologies and different discourses. Common sense suggests that the time has come for a synthesis. It is to be hoped that psychiatrists and social scientists can bring themselves to admit that both medical factors and social factors have a bearing on what the Prince of Wales described as 'the whole of a person's needs, within the whole of the society in which that person lives' (Royal College of Psychiatrists 1991). The mental health services urgently need the strengths of both. A first step in the present context may be to attempt an outline of the state of the art from the social science side.

THE SCOPE OF THE SOCIAL SCIENCES

There is a persistent confusion in the public mind between sociology, which is one of the social sciences, and the full range of the social sciences. The range also includes economics, politics, social statistics, social policy, organisational theory and practice, social history, social psychology, aspects of law and medicine and planning and architecture, and social work — all subjects relating to the individual in his physical and social environment, and as different from one another as anatomy is from physiology or family therapy from psychosurgery. Some of these are developments from established disciplines with a long history; others are relatively new.

The general expansion in the social sciences which accompanied the expansion of the universities in the 1960s led to exaggerated expectations from some of the new disciplines. In the 1960s and 1970s, some major research projects were set up on government funding — Educational Priority Area Projects (Halsey 1972), Community Development Projects (Loney 1983) and the Transmitted Deprivation Project (Brown & Madge 1982). When social scientists reported at the end of 3–5 years that the problems were more complex than the government believed, that the government might not have asked the right questions, and that they were unable to produce clear plans for the immediate solution of major social problems, they were held to have 'failed', and the Social Science Research Council was reduced to its present status as the Economic and Social Research Council, with minimal funding.

'The early euphoria was breeding disillusionment' Sir Claus Moser commented in his presidential address (1991) to the British Association:

Their earlier high profile had led to an impression that the social sciences would solve the major problems of our time. Of course, much research did throw light on key issues. But inflation did not disappear, world economies, not least our own, proved increasingly hard to manage, the devastating problems of the third world remained devastating; even in developed countries like ours, social problems — such as crime, drugs, poverty — if anything became worse... So a backlash was inevitable, and led to the social sciences becoming grossly *under*-valued.

Sir Claus is concerned to point out that the distinction between 'hard data' and 'soft data' cannot be drawn with all the natural sciences on one side of the divide, and all the social sciences on the other. Some social sciences are 'harder' than others: he thinks that economics probably has the greatest theoretical strength and explanatory power at present; but he points out that the natural sciences also deal with 'hard' and 'soft' data — physics is notably 'harder' than biology.

Social scientists are often unable to carry out controlled experiments on human subjects; but research workers in astronomy and some branches of medicine may similarly have to operate without rigorous experimental controls. The natural scientist has the advantage of being able to rely (more or less) on certain constants, like the law of gravity or the speed of light; but the social scientist deals with 'shifting and complex phenomena', so that the most accurate observations may apply only to a particular time and place, and a particular set of circumstances. Nevertheless, the social sciences are 'every bit as important as their physical counterparts. The human problems of our time are so momentous that we should all have some understanding of the problems and the solutions' (Moser 1991).

Research methods in the social sciences are very varied, ranging from large-scale quantitative studies to very sensitive small-scale case studies, and from descriptive work to highly theoretical analyses. The influence of the natural sciences on the development of social science research has been a mixed blessing. It has fostered precision of thought and rigorous methodology; but precise methodologies may be inappropriately applied in this very different context. There are many examples in the psychiatric literature of methodologies which are 'more appropriate to clinical drug trials than (to) the study of human beings *in extremis*' (Korer 1991).

The natural sciences are primarily concerned with *convergent* problems — the kind of problems which permit of a right answer, e.g. 'What are the coordinates in space and time of a particular event?' The social sciences are primarily concerned with *divergent* problems, which require the exercise of a high quality of judgement, and rarely permit of a clear-cut and permanent solution:

> The true problems of living — in politics, economics, education, marriage, etc. — are always problems of overcoming or reconciling opposites. They...have no solution in the ordinary sense of the word. They demand of man not merely the employment of his reasoning powers, but the commitment of his whole personality. Naturally, spurious solutions, by way of a clever formula, are always being put forward; but they never work for long, because they invariably neglect one of the two opposites, and thus lose the very quality of human life. (Schumacher 1973)

Many avenues of work in the social sciences do require quantification; but (as in 19th century psychiatry) description and observation must come before the construction of scales and the formulation of hypotheses. There is no point in counting heads until the basic situation is sufficiently well understood to make the exercise meaningful. If the categories are unsound, or the items inappropriately weighted, the results will be worthless. It is not only the computer which suffers from the phenomenon of 'garbage in — garbage out'. The important point is that the demand that *all* work in the social sciences should be capable, here and now, of statistical verification, or that social scientists should find 'right answers' of universal applicability to enduring problems such as poverty, famine, crime and disability is simply not realistic.

Some aspects of work in the field of psychiatry which involve an understanding of social policy or social work are dealt with elsewhere in this book, particularly in Chapters 28–30, 31, 33 and 42. The choice of illustrations from the very wide field which remains must be limited. The remainder of this chapter is devoted to issues of particular importance to psychiatry: concepts of normality and deviance; the critique of institutional life; the theoretical basis of community care; and the problems of multi-disciplinary teamwork.

CONCEPTS OF NORMALITY

Social scientists are often concerned to test 'what everyone knows', and, having established the facts, to look for explanations and implications. The popular view of what is 'normal' in attitudes and behaviour is subject to at least three sources of distortion.

First, people derive much of their information from the press and television. Readers with a psychiatric training will be aware that popular presentations of psychiatric issues do not always match objectively ascertained fact. Similarly, media views of the world we live in (particularly those presented by advertisements, which have the hidden agenda of persuading us to buy this or that by pandering to our prejudices) may need factual correction (Leiss et al 1958, Goffman 1979, Browne 1981).

Second, the basic constructs by which people order their thoughts on such matters as marriage and family life, the respective roles of men and women, the significance of work and questions of law and order are formed in their early years, often largely on parental models, and are not easily shaken. Social theorists use the term 'cultural lag' to describe the gap between popular understanding of social processes, and the stage which those processes have actually reached (Bottomore 1962). An example can be seen in some of the Middle Eastern states, where advanced technology exists side by side with social repression and extremes of wealth and poverty; but readers may be able to find their own examples nearer home.

Third, there is a tendency to confuse 'normal' with 'desirable'. Social science findings on family life, for example, have met with considerable resistance from civil servants and administrators who have a clear image of a 'normal family'. It consists of a male breadwinner, a dependent wife and two or three children under the age of 16 years. In fact, only some 26% of households consist of a married couple with dependent children, and two out of three married women have paid employment (HMSO 1991). The Study Commission on the Family produced two reports (1980, 1983) on changing family patterns which establish and analyse the facts about the reduction in family size, the rise in cohabitation, the increased divorce rate and the four-generation family. The emphasis which psychiatrists, social workers and psychologists have placed on the traditional nuclear family and the early stages of parenthood may be due to a particular anxiety concerning the role of the mother. Following John Bowlby's major work in his report to the World Health Organization (Bowlby 1951), anxiety developed about the effects of 'maternal deprivation' on young children. Bowlby argued that a child needs a strong human bond in the early years, and this has been widely confirmed by subsequent research. However, Rutter (1972), who reviews this work, points out that Bowlby never advanced the thesis often credited to him, that this bond could only be made with the biological mother. Children need many kinds of support: love, stable relationships, food, care and protection, discipline, models of behaviour, play and conversation. To separate out some of these functions and to label them 'mothering' is an artificial categorisation.

Concentration on the family or household group as the norm also obscures the fact that very large numbers of people now live alone. A quarter of all households are now one-person households — and the greatest increase in recent years has been among the under-30s, not among the elderly (HMSO 1991).

Social scientists have investigated commonly held views of social class (Bottomore 1965, Rose 1968, Jowell & Airey 1984). Findings of particular importance to members of the medical profession are those of Newson & Newson (1970), Cartwright & Anderson (1981) and the *Black Report* (Department of Health and Social Security 1980). Newson & Newson pointed to social class differences in family life. The families of unskilled manual workers are more likely to have strong role segregation between husband and wife, to stereotype the children in terms of gender and to rely on 'non-verbal methods' (such as physical punishment) for controlling the children. It may be held 'normal' to subject children to threats that someone will 'take them away' if they fail to behave, and to indulge in quite painful teasing. Middle-class children are relatively protected in childhood, future oriented, and encouraged to learn communication skills. Cartwright & Anderson (1981) found that middle-class patients tended to have longer consultations with their doctors than did working-class patients, and that more information was communicated between doctor and patient — in both directions.

The *Black Report*, which came from the Office of the Chief Scientist at the then Department of Health and Social Security, was a major study on access to the health services. Taking the two extremes of the social class index as points of comparison, the committee found that the risk of death before retirement was two and a half times as great for social class V as for social class I, and the neonatal mortality rate

was twice as high. If the mortality rates for social class I had been applied to social class V in the 2 years 1970–1972 alone, 74 000 people under the age of 75 years would still have been alive at the time of publication, including 10 000 children and 32 000 men of working age. There was 'a consistency of class gradients in mortality throughout the life-time', and, though the evidence was less firm, this appeared to be paralleled in many mortality rates. Sickness rates were higher for unskilled and partly skilled workers; restricted activity was more common; rates of 'long-standing illness' as defined in the General Household Survey were twice as high as in the professional classes. This detailed and authoritative study came to the conclusion that the National Health Service had not in fact provided equality of access for all social classes.

Recent work suggests that, though sharp class distinctions remain a feature of British society, occupation is no longer the only or the main generator of wealth for large sections of the population. The rapid increase in home ownership and the uneven rise in house prices in the 1980s created a situation in which the most valid distinction was between those in the private housing sector and those in rented accommodation (Murie 1983). Even more strikingly, those who inherited houses (and already possessed homes of their own) acquired large sums of disposable capital (Lowe 1990). Another relatively new factor is that mass unemployment, spread across all social groups, has been equally decisive in breaking the link between education and employment. Traditionally, a good education was a passport to a secure occupation, but that is no longer the case, even for the medical profession.

Social scientists have also explored concepts of 'normality' in relation to race (Rex 1983, Rex & Mason 1986, Wrench & Reid 1990), gender (Mead 1962, Mitchell 1971, 1974, Oakley 1972, 1974, EOC 1981, Ortner & Whitehead 1981) and criminality (Walker & McCabe 1968, 1973, Cohen 1972, Hough & Mayhew 1983).

Psychiatrists who are interested in such fundamental questions as why (even excluding the excess of elderly women) there are more women than men in psychiatric hospitals, and 30 times more men than women in prison, or why the first admissions figures for schizophrenia in people of Afro-Caribbean origin are very much higher than those for the white population (Harrison et al 1988, Littlewood & Liversedge 1988, Knowles 1991) can find a useful basic literature in the social sciences for tackling some very complex questions.

CONCEPTS OF DEVIANCE

In the 1960s, when psychiatry was turning away from the social sciences to a more orthodox medical perspective, some social scientists developed a radical critique of psychiatry which was both abrasive and searing. The principal tenets of the 'deviance theory' approach are that people categorised as deviants, such as criminals or people suffering from psychiatric disorders — 'the bad and the mad' — may have their own rationale for their actions; that deviant acts are defined by society — not in response to immutable laws based on morality, but as a means of maintaining group equilibrium. It is notable that the debates centred on minor kinds of antisocial behaviour, such as petty theft or cannabis smoking, rather than on offences against the person, such as murder or aggravated assault. The argument was that such petty offences were permitted in one society and 'criminalised' in another. Social labelling, it is argued, is stigmatising, and may lead to 'secondary deviance' by reinforcing deviant behaviour. The psychiatric patient who is sent to hospital is more likely to develop bizarre symptoms; the boy who is sent to prison is more likely to become a persistent offender. The perspective of the so-called deviant is as valid as that of the professionals (doctors, police, magistrates, social workers) who are principally acting as 'agents of social control' (Lemert 1951, Becker 1964). In a short but lucid paper, Erikson (1962) takes the view that the deviant has a symbolic importance, showing us 'the difference between the inside of a group and the outside'. Deviants are not a threat to the stability of society, but rather a group whose existence demonstrates the boundaries of acceptable conduct, providing 'on-going drama at the edge of group space'. Gathering 'marginal people into tightly segregated groups' warns the rest of us about the consequences of unacceptable behaviour.

Deviance theorists do not seem to have noticed that in rejecting one set of social stereotypes — 'mentally ill', criminal', 'disabled' and so on — they were creating another by bringing all these groups together under the label of 'deviants'. Perhaps the limits of confusion were reached in a conference held in the mid 1970s in London on 'The Marginal Population': 'marginal' was defined as covering mentally ill, mentally handicapped and physically disabled people, the unemployed, women, pensioners, offenders, 'ethnic' groups and young people: in fact, considerably more than half the population — everybody except white male adults in employment who were both mentally and physically fit.

Deviance theory drew on a parallel movement in ethnomethodology, which involved the examination of the meanings and significance of everyday events without prior mental constructs (Garfinkel 1967) and symbolic interactionism, which focused on the content of human interaction rather than on the status of the interacting parties (Filmer et al 1972). To put the issues simply, we talk of a 'doctor' holding a 'consultation' with a 'patient' in his 'surgery' or 'consulting room'. All these terms involve preconceptions about what is taking place. What if we abandon the preconceptions? We are left with two people sitting in an enclosed space with some equipment. What assumptions does each make of the other's understanding of the situation? What is the actual significance of their verbal exchange and their actions? What currents of meaning and emotion are involved, but never brought into the open? How different are their perceptions of what occurs?

Useful elements from this critique have filtered into the medical field in the form of concepts of 'health behaviour' and 'sick role behaviour' (Parsons 1950, Balint 1957, Kasl & Cobb 1966, Bennett 1977, Davis 1978, Mechanic 1979). Most readers will be familiar with the material of the 'Balint Seminars' (Balint & Norell 1973) on the importance of listening to the patient rather than acting like a detective in pursuit of symptoms. Stimson & Webb (1975) offer a challenging view from the patient's perspective. During a consultation, a patient may use tact to dissuade the doctor from coming to what he thinks might be inappropriate conclusions, producing symptoms which it is hoped will steer the doctor in the right direction. While there is 'some semblance of formality', and the patient is at pains to appear complaisant and acquiescent, his role may not be as passive as it appears. 'People these days have many other sources of knowledge', and, after the consultation, the patient will evaluate the treatment decision and make his own decision on whether to accept it or not.

Social science findings sometimes confirm conventional wisdom — in which case the response tends to be: 'We knew that all the time: why spend time and money on finding out?' Sometimes they deny conventional wisdom — in which case the response is: 'Social scientists are subversive — they upset the established order'. Most social scientists try to keep to as much objectivity as human beings are capable of — recognising that individual value systems and individual experience may always lead to distortion. The testing of conventional wisdom is an important task — but it is understandable that it is not always a popular one.

INSTITUTIONAL LIFE

Social scientists have played a major part in two issues of particular concern to psychiatrists: the testing of 'therapeutic community' principles, and the analysis of the pathology of the psychiatric hospital culture.

The therapeutic community

The ideas which came to characterise the therapeutic community movement started within psychiatry. The seminal paper is a brief account by Main (1946) of his work as an army psychiatrist working with men suffering from battle fatigue. He found his military status (as a brigadier) a barrier to a therapeutic relationship. Usually only a brief contact was possible, which meant that there was no time to work through the status differences which separated him from junior officers or what the army calls 'other ranks' (sergeants, corporals and privates). His short cut was an attempt to abandon both military rank and medical status — to seek 'a sincere relationship' in which one-to-one human contact was possible. In this respect, he anticipated the work of the ethnomethodologists. The giving of respect and dignity to the patient was the essence of therapy.

Maxwell Jones (1952, 1962, 1968) developed his ideas from similar experiences with military patients and returned prisoners of war. His inspiration was to graft the new understanding of the importance of minimising status differences on to the developing theory and practice of group work. The essentials of his system were decentralisation in decision making (freeing patients and paramedical staff to take part in the running of the community, rather than leaving decisions exclusively to the doctor), the encouragement of free interaction without defensiveness or fear of reprisal, and the concept of the group as a microcosm of the outside world. Rather than offering 'asylum', the hospital offered a supportive environment in which pressures could be acknowledged, and problems could be worked through.

The movement was essentially psychodynamic and anti-authoritarian. Learning was seen as a two-way process, in which patients and staff came to share a network of values and expectations, a community culture. If the basic tenets were democratic and permissive (quite extreme behaviour being tolerated on the grounds that acting out was therapeutic), it was also analytical. Staff and patients were continuously faced with the group's interpretations of their words and action.

The therapeutic community system was widely publicised and widely experimented with. Phrases such as 'everything is treatment', 'collapsing the authority pyramid' and 'all treatment is rehabilitation' became common currency. Patients who had previously been treated as passive began to take an active part in their own progress, developing peer group support systems, and showing unexpected capacities to help each other through periods of crisis. Nurses and social workers found new and satisfying roles; but the movement had inherent limitations. It required a very high level of interpersonal skills in practitioners, together with the professional confidence necessary to abandon formal roles and claims to expertise. Therapists had to offer more, and to demand less in the way of professional respect. Some found this threatening; others found the demands contradictory. They had professional skills and professional responsibilities which could not be set aside in the interests of 'democratisation'.

Rapoport (1960), a sociologist who spent more than 2 years studying the system at the Henderson Hospital, pointed to these and other problems: the conflict which emerged periodically between the established ward culture and the actual demands of the changing ward population — a clear case of cultural lag which led to crises in the group; the fact that the system worked best with one type of patient (young male homosexual psychopaths) but was less appropriate for other patients. Rapoport found that successful participation required a very strong ego — yet the average ego strength of the group was equivalent to that of a child aged $2\frac{1}{2}$ years.

The application of the therapeutic community system in recent years has been in a much modified form and, in the psychiatric hospital world, it has been largely defeated by dwindling patient populations and much-shortened lengths of stay. However, the principles have been applied to a variety of other settings — schools, hostels, residential homes — to good effect.

The pathology of the psychiatric hospital

It was ironic that when the therapeutic community movement was at its strongest in the psychiatric hospital field, an iconoclastic attack came from a social psychologist and former anthropologist, Erving Goffman. In spite of its title, *Asylums* (Goffman 1961) was not primarily about psychiatric hospitals. Goffman was attempting a cross-service analysis of institutional life, arguing that psychiatric hospitals shared the pathological features of other institutions, such as homes for the blind or the aged, prisons, concentration camps, army barracks, boarding schools and monasteries or convents. His empirical base for the study was very limited, but he quoted effectively from many published sources, and the intellectual attack was sharp and powerful. He was concerned with 'total institutions' — places where 'a large number of like-situated individuals, cut off from the wider society for an appreciable period of time, together lead an enclosed, formally administered round of life'. More scholarly than some of his followers, he was careful not to claim that all psychiatric hospitals were 'total institutions'. He was concerned to set up an ideal type, i.e. to state an extreme case as a model against which real-life situations could be measured. The process, which derives from Max Weber's ideal type of bureaucracy (Weber 1922) is well enough known in the social sciences, but led to many misunderstandings. One edition of *Asylums* was actually advertised in Britain as 'the truth about mental hospitals'.

However, Goffman's analysis, which drew on the current insights of deviance theory and symbolic interactionism, went far beyond the therapeutic community movement in insisting on the validity of patients' experiences. Total institutions, he argued, had 'encompassing tendencies', characterised by four features: *batch living*, *binary management*, the *inmate role* and the *institutional perspective*. Goffman was particularly good at identifying and naming processes, and thus bringing them to public attention. Batch living was described as the antithesis of domestic living: in the normal circumstances of domestic life, people have three spheres of activity — home, work and play (or leisure). In institutional living, these three spheres are collapsed into one. Inmates live under 'an overall rational plan' with formal rules and regulations, with no freedom of movement, and no choice of companions. They live constantly under surveillance in 'large blocks of managed people'. Binary management means that staff and inmates live in different worlds. Staff tend to feel 'superior and righteous', while inmates are made to feel 'weak, inferior and guilty'. The two groups coexist with little understanding of each other, and may use a special tone of voice in talking to one another.

How does an ordinary citizen become an inmate? Goffman describes the 'betrayal funnel', through which relatives or professionals may send the individual if his presence or behaviour becomes inconvenient. An interview with a doctor is arranged, and then he is passed from hand to hand, to end 'in a psychiatric ward, stripped of almost everything' while the relative goes back to 'a world... incredibly thick with freedoms and privileges'. The patient is then taught the 'inmate role' through a process of 'mortification' or 'role stripping'. This involves a highly ritualised admission procedure, in which he is forced to give a life history (the events recorded being carefully selected to support the hypotheses that he is the kind of person the institution exists to treat), and to submit to being weighted, bathed, physically examined and possibly fingerprinted. The bath is of particular symbolic significance, since physical nakedness, cleansing and the substitution of institutional clothing for his own clothes represent something like a baptism into the new institutional life. He is 'shaped and coded' — no longer a person but a patient.

From this time on, he must adopt the 'institutional perspective' — a view of life which validates the institution's existence through such means as the house magazine, the open day and the sports day, which create an artificial sense of community, and deny his own individual experience. Thus the 'assault on the self' is pursued, and the patient may react in one of four ways: withdrawal into his own fantasy life; open rebellion; 'colonisation', in which he pretends to accept the official view, but saves his own views against the day of release; and (most pitiable of all) 'conversion', in which he genuinely comes to accept the official view of his status.

To Goffman, the patient's greatest loss is privacy, and psychodynamic approaches, such as that of the therapeutic community, may be the greatest threat to privacy, since they involve 'looping' — the collapse of the patient's defences on himself by using his own evidence against him. ECT, drugs, psychosurgery, and group and individual therapy are all seen as modes of attack rather than as sources of assistance.

Barton (1959) coined the term 'institutional neurosis', referring to the clinical effects of poor hospital care, which included low self-esteem, withdrawal of interest, and inability to plan for the future. He considered this a 'disease' which was independent of the illness responsible for the patient's admission to hospital, increasing in severity with the duration of stay in hospital, but preventable and treatable. The links between his thinking and Goffman's seem clear, but while Goffman was a theoretician, Barton was a practising psychiatrist concerned to produce a handbook for psychiatric hospital nurses.

Opinions differed as to whether Barton had discovered a new illness. Wing (1978) prefers the term 'secondary handicap' (a variant on Becker's term 'secondary adjustment'), and emphasises that individuals living outside institutions can also be affected by the negative attitudes of others to their primary handicap. Among chronic schizophrenic patients, it may be difficult to decide how far emotional flattening, poverty of ideas and social withdrawal are due to the original illness, and how far they result from other people's reactions.

While these and similar criticisms of psychiatric hospital life were recognised as relevant, and often acted upon in the psychiatric hospital setting, the movement against the hospitals gathered force. One major influence was the work of the revisionist social historians. Foucault (1961) reinterpreted the history of psychiatric hospitals, seeing what had previously been evaluated as a humanitarian reform movement as no more than an insidious form of repression. He argued that psychiatric hospitals exist to warn the rest of society against bizarre behaviour, not to treat patients. Later he was to argue (Foucault 1975) that prisons exist as a warning against breaking the law. In both works, he goes beyond the common Marxist assertion that humanitarianism is 'false consciousness' (in the sense that it delays the 'revolution') to assert that it is a deliberately chosen weapon of class control.

Foucault's analysis is complicated for English-speaking readers by the fact that he is writing in French, and translation can be misleading. Further, he writes from Paris, and in the context of a distinctively European set of philosophical arguments deriving from the works of such writers as Althusser, Sartre and Lévi-Strauss, and, further back in time, from Nietzsche, Marx and Hegel. His dazzling command of imagery, such as his description of the 'Ship of Fools' — 'made fast among things and men. Retained and maintained. No longer a ship but a hospital' — or his account of the early days of the York Retreat, owes little to historical research. He can be arrogant, rhetorical and grandiose. He can fly in the face of facts, dismissing them as superficial while he digs for 'underlying unities'; but he is always readable, and often thought-provoking. His own adverse experience in psychiatric hospitals in the early 1950s (when he studied for a diploma in psychopathology) is deeply felt. The recognition that apparent humanitarianism may be a cloak for social control, that closed institutions may provide an outlet for the sadistic instincts of some staff, and that repressive systems of management are an offence against human dignity is valuable, even to those of less extreme political views who do not share Foucault's despair (Jones & Fowles 1984).

The revisionist genre is now well established (Rothman 1971, 1980, Scull 1977, 1979, 1981, 1989, Skultans 1979, Bynum et al 1985, Digby 1985, Porter 1985). Such writers have focused largely on the evils, real or imagined, of the psychiatric hospital service. Their trademark is the use of the 18th century term

'madness' for psychiatric disorder. While their protest is basically against the psychiatric system, they seem to have little or nothing positive to suggest to replace hospital care.

COMMUNITY AND COMMUNITY CARE

What is meant by 'the community', and how does it care? Discussion of 'hospital and community' frequently overlooks one basic factor: *the community is not a place.* A hospital has a defined and recognisable territory, a staff, procedures, guidelines, standards, monitoring practices. 'The community' has none of these things: the term tends to mean 'everything except the hospital'.

'Community' was a popular term in the 1960s. Community work, community arts, community education, all started from the premise that there were positive strengths in society which could be utilised to help those in need. There were community programmes, and (in the USA) Community Mental Health Centers; but when the steam went out of the community movement, and society moved into a less caring and more commercial mode, we were left with 'community care', which was expected to work wonders with minimal resources. Professor R.M. Titmuss's prediction (Titmuss 1968) that community care would mean the transfer of patients from the care of the trained to the care of the untrained has been borne out in subsequent events.

Willmott & Thomas (1984) have shown that 'community policy' has been invoked in some 20 different areas of the national life, and has many different meanings. Bulmer (1987) suggests that the common thread in all these meanings is some sense of locality; but reliance on locality ignores the fact that locality is of decreasing importance in social activity in modern life. 'Therefore, to promulgate policies that are based upon activities which are supposed to take place in the locality may well be at odds with the patterns of social arrangement which exist in society' (Bulmer 1990).

One study (Jones 1988) found that a sample of 150 psychiatric patients followed up after discharge from hospital went to 14 different types of setting: living alone; living with their family; living with other relatives; sheltered housing; National Health Service hostel; local authority hostel; hostel for transients; local authority residential home; private sector home; lodging house; bed and breakfast; lodgings with landlady; general hospital; no fixed abode; return to psychiatric hospital. Each of these possibilities involves a different living situation: for instance, a hostel run by the health authority as long-term provision for previously institutionalised patients is very different from a Salvation Army hostel for transients, many of whom stay for no more than a few days. A lodging house run by a private proprietor for ten or 12 former patients is different from lodgings with a motherly landlady who cooks and does the washing. Official terms like 'own home' (a mansion; a cardboard box?), 'hostel' and 'lodgings' obscure important differences.

Care 'in the community' may involve many different people in different combinations: in the statutory sector, psychiatrists, community psychiatric nurses (CPNs), social workers, psychologists, general practitioners, health visitors, and others; in the private sector, homes and lodgings; in the voluntary sector, the work of MIND and the National Schizophrenia Fellowship is well known. Other organisations such as SANE (Schizophrenia — a National Emergency) and APCMI (the Association for the Pastoral Care of the Mentally Ill) are now developing services; but for many former patients the burden of care falls on relatives, and in particular on women (Parker 1981, Bulmer 1986, Perring et al 1990). Though it had been anticipated that neighbours and neighbourhood groups would be a major source of support, the contribution from locally based groups was very limited (Abrams et al 1981, Bulmer 1986).

After 30 years of community care policies, we have no adequate typology of the kinds of care available in the community and little information about the appropriateness of particular types of care for patients with particular constellations of need, or about the combinations of services actually available to patients. Some may be regularly visited by a CPN or a social worker (rarely by both, though their skills are very different). They may also make regular clinic visits, see their general practitioner regularly, go to a sheltered workshop or go to a club. Others fall through the gaps in uncoordinated services, and receive no care at all. It takes a good deal of social skill to be able to make personal contacts, to draw on the services available, and make the best of them; but people with severe psychiatric disorders often lack precisely that capacity because of their condition. There is at least a suspicion that the patients with the greatest needs may receive the least help.

While elderly long-term patients (some with as many as 30 or 40 years' hospital stay) are for the most part being carefully resettled, many others are being discharged to minimal bed and breakfast accommodation or squalid lodging houses as the hospitals run down (Wallace 1986). Some are left homeless or end up in prison after the commission of minor offences,

because there is nowhere else for them to go. Such people may simply have no contact with the medical services. They often do not have a general practitioner, and would not have the energy and initiative to consult one. They reach the mental health services only as casualties, in crisis conditions which could be avoided if they had somewhere to live, and someone to supervise their care.

The Mental Health Act (HMSO 1983) placed new responsibilities on social workers; but these were for the most part concerned with the compulsory admission of patients to hospital rather than with community care (Sheppard 1990). The Act 'appeared to imply an expansion of mental health resources to make it possible to prevent hospital admission and to provide after-care following discharge' but 'the social perspective on the use of compulsory powers suffers the severe handicap of resource starvation' (Barnes et al 1990). Adequate resources have not been forthcoming.

Bayley (1973) made a useful distinction between care *in* the community and care *by* the community. Many former psychiatric hospital patients are now 'in the community' (in the sense that they are not in hospital) but care 'by the community' may often be little more than rhetoric.

Community care now extends to many other groups in addition to patients with a psychiatric condition. Some of these are much easier to provide services for on a community basis. Community care seems to work best with people who have mild disabilities, who have good communication skills, who have an active social network of family and friends, and whose behaviour is stable and predictable. It is relatively successful for mentally handicapped people (now often termed 'people with learning difficulties') (Baldwin & Hattersley 1991), the infirm elderly (Challis et al 1988, Fennell et al 1988), and people with physical handicaps (Blaxter 1976, Stopford 1987). Visible handicaps attract sympathy. (For instance, the general public is more sympathetic to blindness than to deafness, and to people in wheelchairs than to those suffering from heart conditions or arthritis.) People with chronic psychiatric difficulties lose out on all these counts. They are severely affected in ways which often inhibit their ability to communicate; their social networks tend to be tenuous and fragmented (Erickson 1976); their behaviour can be both unstable and — to the lay eye — unpredictable and even threatening. Yet there is no equivalent to the white stick or the wheelchair to create public sympathy. Of all the groups who are now being transferred from hospital to community care, they may be the most difficult to provide services for.

Two commentators from the USA have suggested reasons why governments may have tolerated or even encouraged alarm about psychiatric hospital conditions, but may be more resistant to setting up good community services. Scull (1977) points out that psychiatric hospitals on both sides of the Atlantic were old, expensive to maintain, and largely unsuitable for modern methods of care and treatment. Building costs were too high for them to be replaced by new forms of residential care. Yet admission rates were rising steadily, and public pressure to improve conditions was mounting. If governments could not afford to replace the hospitals, or to improve them to an acceptable level, the best political option was to declare for abolition — thus turning public pressure *against the psychiatric hospital system*. Scull points out that, once health and welfare services began to develop in the community, the opportunity cost of not using hospital services rose sharply — 'segregative modes of social control became, in relative terms, far more costly and difficult to justify'. He argues that the rapid introduction of the new policy without consultation in the field, the lack of forward planning, and the failure to provide for appropriate methods of evaluation were deliberate acts of policy, designed to fragment opposition and to prevent demonstration of the hardships which would result.

Wildavsky (1970), in a broader analysis, points out that a number of countries moved in the 1960s to policies based on 'the five De's' — deinstitutionalisation, decriminalisation, de-education, demedicalisation and decentralisation. Psychiatric hospitals were not the only institutions to be reduced in population, and the whole movement, in Wildavsky's view, relates to a central issue of public policy: Western industrialised nations had introduced health and welfare provision on an unprecedented scale. Demand seemed to be unlimited; but as public expectations soared ahead of provision, politicians realised that they had to impose limits if they wanted to stay in power. Deinstitutionalisation and demedicalisation were primarily ways of saving public money.

Decentralisation has meant that the results of this process are impossible to quantify. There have been no published figures on UK psychiatric hospital populations since 1986, and no official attempts have been made to overcome the formidable problems of providing meaningful statistics for community care. Manpower in the Government Statistical Service has been cut from about 9000 in 1979 to 4200 (Moser 1991). While economic statistics have been maintained to their former level of sophistication, social statistics have suffered badly. The *Rayner Review* (HMSO 1981) not only encouraged the reduction of official statistical services, but laid it down as a matter of principle that the government had no obligation to provide statistics for the public use: it need only produce statistics for its own purposes. This view has been strongly opposed by the Royal Statistical Society.

The defects of current community care policy provide an excellent example of how the psychiatric services are affected by political and economic issues — and how useful social statistics and social research could be in enabling psychiatrists and other professionals to think clearly and plan coherently for the services of the future.

MULTIPROFESSIONAL TEAMWORK

The move from hospital to community services will increasingly involve psychiatrists in new kinds of teamwork, which some may not find wholly congenial. It is no accident that many psychiatrists have preferred to work with community psychiatric nurses, whose basic training is, like their own, hospital based, and part of an accepted framework of medical understanding, rather than with social workers; but the Department of Health's plans (Hansard 1990) for local authorities to take over community care services in mental health means that psychiatrists will need to learn to work with the varied personnel of the Social Services Department, whose knowledge-base is in the social sciences.

Social policy analysts can help in explaining why and how the organisational imperatives of Social Services Departments differ from those of the National Health Service. While there is much discussion of collaboration and cooperation, Social Services and the Health Services have different aims and purposes, different systems of decision-making and accountability, and different financial and planning procedures based on different time-scales (Thomas & Stoten 1974). In the past decade, when all services run by local authorities have been subject to many financial restrictions — including the ill-fated poll tax, which is reputed to have cost them £130 million in administrative expenses alone — there have been few if any opportunities for service development (Pinker 1985, Nellis 1989, Young 1989). As Bulmer (1987) makes clear, there have been many National Health Service/local authority meetings to discuss cooperation and collaboration, but what he terms 'the steel shutter' comes down between the two when financial issues are discussed. Two services which have existed in a state of mutual misunderstanding and lack of synchronisation since 1948 do not find it easy to work together when both are hard pressed.

Social theory can assist in the analysis of professions and professionalisation. Ever since Durkheim (1893) produced his seminal work on the division of labour, attention has been concentrated on the process of *structural differentiation*. As knowledge accumulates, the work of a single worker fragments into a number of specialisms. The medical practitioner has common origins with the magician and the priest: in less developed societies than our own, the three roles can still be found combined in the shaman or witch doctor. Even in the past 100 years, the process of structural differentiation has operated within medicine to produce many new specialisms, and this has been regarded as progress. But when specialisms develop outside medicine, in psychology, in social work, and to some extent in nursing, the adjustment may be harder to make.

Many aspects of social theory have a bearing on the present situation in which psychiatrists are required to work with people of different academic backgrounds and training. Such concepts as *status, reference groups, group formation, group membership and structure, conformity* and *ideology* are relevant, and may be found in any good sociology textbook. There is also a relevant specific literature on 'professionalisation', a term preferred to 'profession' because the situation is not static. Particular occupational groups may become more professional over time, for instance by increasing the length of the course leading to a qualification, or by adopting a code of ethics; they may also become less professional over time, by substituting routine measures for professional judgement, or by being prepared to take strike action which would harm their clients. Millerson (1964), in a survey of 21 studies of professionalisation, listed what were thought to be the essential elements of professional status. The elements included skill based on theoretical knowledge, the provision of training and education, tests of the competence of members, organisation, adherence to a code of conduct and altruistic service. Vollmer & Mills (1966) edited a rich collection of analyses of the processes of professionalisation, including a thoughtful paper by Sutherland (1966), who points out that professional burglars satisfy all the requirements except the last two. Elliott (1972), has a schema in which he sets down the main characteristics of the established and prestigious professions such as medicine and law, and draws a continuum from each to the opposite pole, which represents the characteristics of routine and non-professional work. Thus the 'decision-making' dimension runs from 'unprogrammed' — the professional using his own judgement — to 'programmed' — the non-professional obeying detailed instructions; the 'identity' dimension runs from a professional identity which is a central life interest, to an identity which has nothing to do with work. It is possible to plot any profession — or 'semi-profession' or 'sub-profession' — on his nine dimensions, and to chart changes over time.

Psychiatrists, like many professional groups, are subject to contradictory pressures. They derive their professional status from being medical practitioners, from membership of a Royal College, from a training which is still predominantly hospital based, and medically oriented, and from the exclusive power to prescribe pharmacological and other treatments. Yet, while the power-base of psychiatry is indisputably medical, the knowledge-base is becoming increasingly split. To work effectively for patients in the changing services, psychiatrists will need to keep one foot in medicine, and to plant the other firmly in the social sciences. It is perhaps an uncomfortable stance; but a re-engagement with the social view of their discipline may prove necessary to professional survival.

REFERENCES

Abrams P, Abrams S, Humphrey R, Snaith R 1981 Action for care: a review of Good Neighbour Schemes in England. The Volunteer Centre, London

Baldwin S, Hattersley J 1991 Mental handicap: social science perspectives. Tavistock/Routledge, London

Balint M 1957 The doctor, his patient and the illness. Tavistock, London

Balint E, Norell J S (eds) 1973 Six minutes for the patients. Tavistock, London

Barton W R 1959 Institutional neurosis. Wright, Bristol

Basaglia F 1980 Problems of law and psychiatry: the Italian experience. International Journal of Law and Psychiatry 3: 17–37

Bayley M J 1973 Mental handicap and community care. Routledge & Kegan Paul, London

Becker H S (ed) 1964 The other side: perspectives on deviance. Free Press, New York

Belknap I 1956 Human problems in a state mental hospital. McGraw Hill, New York

Bennett A E (ed) 1977 Communication between doctors and patients. Nuffield Provincial Hospitals Trust/Oxford University Press, London

Berger P L (1974) Man in society. In: Berger B (ed) Readings in sociology. Basic Books, New York

Blaxter M 1976 The meaning of disability. Heinemann, London

Bottomore T B 1962 Sociology: a guide to problems and literature. Allen & Unwin, London

Bottomore T B 1965 Classes in modern society. Allen & Unwin, London

Bowlby J 1951 Maternal care and mental health. World Health Organization, Geneva

Brown M, Madge N 1982 Despite the welfare state. Heinemann, London

Browne B W 1981 Images of family life in magazine advertisements. Praeger, New York

Bulmer M 1986 Neighbours: the work of Philip Abrams. Cambridge University Press, Cambridge

Bulmer M 1987 The social basis of community care. Allen & Unwin, London

Bulmer M 1990 Problems in community care. In: Jones K (ed) Community care and schizophrenia (report of conference held at Oxford, July 1990). In press

Bynum WF, Porter R, Shepherd M 1985-1988. The anatomy of madness. Tavistock, London. 3 vols

Cartwright A, Anderson R 1981 General practice revisited: a second study of patients and their doctors. Tavistock, London

Caudill 1958 The mental hospital as a small society. Harvard University Press, Cambridge, MA

Challis D, Lodge B, Woods R 1988 New approaches to the care of the elderly: a handbook for the caring professions. Hutchinson, London

Cohen S 1972 Folk devils and moral panics. McGibbon & Kee, London

Davis A (ed) 1978 Relationship between doctors and patients. Saxon House/Teakfield, Farnborough

Department of Health and Social Security 1980 Inequalities in health: report of a research working group. Subsequently published as the Black report. Penguin, London

Digby A 1985 Madness, morality and medicine. Cambridge University Press, Cambridge

Durkheim E 1893 The division of labour in society. English edn 1984 Halls W D (ed), Macmillan, Basingstoke

Elliott P 1972 The Sociology of the professions. Routledge & Kegan Paul, London

EOC 1981 Community care policy and women's lives. Equal Opportunities Commission, Manchester

Erickson G 1976 Personal networks and mental illness. Unpublished DPhil thesis, University of York

Erikson K 1962 Notes on the sociology of deviance. Social Problems 9: 307

Fennell G, Philippson C, Evers H 1988 The sociology of old age. Open University Press, Milton Keynes

Filmer P, Phillipson M, Silverman D, Walsh D 1972 New directions in sociological theory. Collier-Macmillan, London

Foucault M 1961 Folie et déraison: histoire de la folie â l'âge classique, Plon, Paris. Howard R (trans) 1975 Madness and civilisation. Pantheon, New York, and Tavistock, London

Foucault M 1975 Surveiller et punir. Sheridan A (trans) 1977 Discipline and punish. Tavistock, London

Garfinkel H 1967 Studies in ethnomethodology. Prentice-Hall, New Jersey

Goffman E 1961 Asylums: essays on the social situation of mental patients and other inmates. Anchor Books, Doubleday, New York

Goffman E 1979 Gender advertisements. Macmillan, London

Greenblatt D, Levinson D J, Williams R 1957 The patient and the mental hospital. Free Press, Glencoe, IL

Halsey A H (ed) 1972 Educational priority: report on a project sponsored by the Department of Education and Science and the Social Science Research Council, vol 1. EPA problems and policies. Her Majesty's Stationery Office, London

Hansard 1990 Parliamentary debates, House of Commons. Her Majesty's Stationery Office, London, No 1531, pp 999–1001

Harrison G, Owens D, Holton A, Neilson D, Boot D 1988 A prospective study of severe mental disorder in Afro-Caribbean patients. Psychological Medicine 18: 643–657

HMSO 1981 Rayner review. Government Statistical Services, Cmnd 8236. Her Majesty's Stationery Office, London, annexe 2, para 17

HMSO 1983 Mental Health Act. Her Majesty's Stationery Office, London, sections 4, 13, 14, 114, 115, 117, 135

HMSO 1991 Social trends. Her Majesty's Stationery Office, London, tables 2.1, 2.3, 4.2

Hough J M, Mayhew P 1983 The British crime survey: the first report. Home Office, London

Jones K 1972 A history of the mental health services. Routledge & Kegan Paul, London

Jones K 1988 Experience in mental health: community care and social policy. Sage Publications, London

Jones K, Sidebotham R 1962 Mental hospitals at work. Routledge & Kegan Paul, London

Jones M 1952 Social psychiatry. Tavistock, London

Jones M 1962 Social psychiatry in the community, in hospitals and in prisons. Charles C Thomas, Springfield, IL

Jones M 1968 Social psychiatry in practice. Pelican Books, London

Jones K, Fowles A J 1984 Ideas on institutions. Routledge & Kegan Paul, London

Jowell R, Airey C 1984 British social attitudes: the 1984 report. Gower, London

Kasl S V, Cobb S 1966 Health behaviour, illness behaviour and sick-role behaviour. Archives of Environmental Health 12: 246

Knowles C 1991 Afro-Caribbeans and schizophrenia: how does psychiatry deal with issues of race, colour and ethnicity? Journal of Social Policy 20: 173–190

Korer J 1991 Review of Perring, Twigg and Atkin (qv). Journal of Social Policy 20: 281

Laing R D 1959 The divided self. Tavistock, London

Laing R D 1975 The politics of experience and the bird of paradise. Penguin, London

Laing R D, Esterson A 1964 Sanity, madness and the family. Tavistock, London

Leiss W, Kline S, Jhally S 1958 Social communication in advertisements. Routledge & Kegan Paul, London

Lemert E 1951 Social pathology. McGraw Hill, New York

Littlewood R, Liversedge M 1988 Psychiatric illness among British Afro-Caribbeans. British Medical Journal 296: 950–951

Loney M 1983 Community against government. Heinemann, London

Lowe S G 1990 Home ownership and capital accumulation. In: Brenton M, Ungerson C (eds) Social policy review 1990. Longmans, Harlow

Main T F 1946 The hospital as a therapeutic community. Bulletin of the Menninger Clinic 10: 66

Mead M 1962 Male and female: a study of the sexes in a changing world. Penguin, London

Mechanic D 1979 Medical sociology, 2nd edn. Free Press, Glencoe, IL

Millerson G 1964 The qualifying associations. Routledge & Kegan Paul, London

Mitchell J 1971 Women's estate. Penguin, London

Mitchell J 1974 Psychoanalysis and feminism. Allen Lane, London

Moser C 1991 Our need for an informed society: presidential address to the British Association. Hamlyn Foundation, London

Murie A 1983 Housing inequality and deprivation. Heinemann, London

Nellis M 1989 Social work. In: Brown P, Sparks R (eds) Beyond Thatcherism. Open University Press, Milton Keynes, pp 104–120

Newson J, Newson E 1970 The family and its future. Churchill, London

Oakley A 1972 Sex, gender and society. Temple Smith, London

Oakley A 1974 Housewife. Allen Lane, London

Ortner S B, Whitehead H 1981 Sexual meanings: the cultural construction of gender and sexuality. Cambridge University Press, Cambridge

Parker G 1981 With due care and attention: the study of research on informal care. Family Policy Studies Centre, London

Parsons T 1950 Illness and the role of the physician. American Journal of Orthopsychiatry 21: 452

Perring C, Twigg J, Atkin K 1990 Families caring for people diagnosed as mentally ill: the literature re-examined. Her Majesty's Stationery Office, London

Pinker R A 1985 Social welfare and the Thatcher administration. In: Bean P, Ferris J, Whynes D (eds) In defence of welfare. Tavistock, London, pp 183–205

Porter R 1985 A social history of madness: stories of the insane. Weidenfeld and Nicolson, London

Rapoport R N 1960 Community as doctor. Tavistock, London

Rex J 1983 Race relations in sociological theory, 2nd edn. Routledge & Kegan Paul, London

Rex J, Mason J D 1986 Theories of race and ethnic relations. Cambridge University Press, Cambridge

Rose A G 1968 The working class. Longmans, Harlow

Rothman D J 1971 The discovery of the asylum: social order and disorder in the New Republic. Little Brown, Boston

Rothman D J 1980 Conscience and convenience: the asylum and its alternatives in progressive America. Little Brown, Boston

Royal College of Psychiatrists 1991 Address by HRH the Prince of Wales, Patron. Guardian, London, July 6

Rutter M 1972 Maternal deprivation reassessed. Penguin, London

Schumacher E F 1973 Small is beautiful: a study of economics as if people mattered. Sphere Books, London, pp 79–83

Scull A T 1977 Decarceration: community treatment and the deviant: a radical view. Prentice-Hall, Englewood Cliffs

Scull A T 1979 Museums of madness: the social organisation of insanity in the nineteenth century. Allen Lane, London

Scull A T (ed) 1981 Madhouses, mad-doctors and madmen: the social history of psychiatry in the Victorian era. University of Pennsylvania Press, Philadelphia

Scull A T 1989 Social order/mental disorder: Anglo–American society in historical perspective. Berkeley University Press. California.

Sheppard M 1990 The role of the approved social worker. Joint Unit for Social Services Research, Sheffield

Skultans V 1979 English madness: ideas on insanity 1580–1890. Routledge & Kegan Paul, London

Stanton A, Schwarz M 1954 The mental hospital. Basic Books, New York

Stimson G V, Webb B 1975 Going to see the doctor: the consultation process in general practice. Routledge & Kegan Paul, London

Stopford V 1987 Disability: causes, characteristics and coping. Edward Arnold, London

Study Commission on the Family 1980 Happy families. Family Policy Studies Centre, London

Study Commission on the Family 1983 Families in the future. Family Policy Studies Centre, London

Sutherland E 1966 Professionalism in illegitimate occupations. In: Vollmer H M, Mills D L (eds) Professionalization. Prentice-Hall, Englewood Cliffs, p 33

Szasz T S 1961 The myth of mental illness: foundations of a theory of personal conduct. Dell, New York

Szasz T S 1963 Law, liberty and psychiatry: an inquiry into the social uses of mental health practices. Macmillan, New York

Szasz T S 1971 The manufacture of madness: a comparative study of the Inquisition and the mental health movement. Routledge & Kegan Paul, London

Szasz T S (ed) 1975 The age of madness: history of involuntary mental hospitalisation. Routledge & Kegan Paul, London

Thomas N, Stoten B 1974 The NHS and local government: co-operation or conflict? In: Jones K (ed) The year book of social policy in Britain, 1973. Routledge & Kegan Paul, London

Titmuss R M 1968 Commitment to welfare. Allen and Unwin, London, pp 247–262 (reprint of speech to the Annual Conference of the National Association for Mental Health, 1961)

Vollmer H M, Mills D L (eds) 1966 Professionalization. Prentice-Hall, Englewood Cliffs

Walker N, McCabe S 1968, 1973 Crime and insanity in England, 2 vols. Edinburgh University Press, Edinburgh

Wallace M 1986 The forgotten illness. Times Newspapers, London (series of articles first published in The Times, 16, 17, 18 December 1985 and 3 March 1986)

Weber M 1922 Wirtschaft und Gesellschaft, Tübingen. English trans in Runciman W G (ed), Mathews E (trans) 1978 Max Weber: selections in translation. Cambridge University Press, Cambridge, pp 341–354

Wildavsky A 1970 The art and craft of policy analysis. Macmillan, New York

Willmott P, Thomas D 1984 Community in social policy. Policy Studies Institute, London

Wing J K 1978 Schizophrenia: towards a new synthesis. Academic Press, London

Wrench J, Reid E 1990 Race relations research in the 1990s: mapping out an agenda. Council for Racial Equality, London

Wright Mills C 1959 The sociological imagination. Oxford University Press, New York

Young H 1989 One of us. Macmillan, London, pp 538–589

3. Psychology in relation to psychiatry

F. M. McPherson

DEFINITION OF PSYCHOLOGY

One frequently used definition of psychology is 'the scientific study of the behaviour of humans and other animals'. 'Behaviour' refers not only to those actions which are overt and directly observable (potentially, at least) by other people, such as social interaction, speech and motor skills, but also to internal, 'private' processes such as thinking and the experience of emotion. The description of these private processes as 'behaviour' results from a long debate about the scientific basis of psychology. Science normally deals only in data which are public and reliable, i.e. which are capable of being observed in a similar way by everyone. However, our thoughts and feelings are known only to ourselves and cannot be observed directly by other people. At one time, many psychologists argued that, because these private phenomena could not be studied by the normal methods of science, they were thus outside the scope of psychology. Others argued that they should be studied, but by methods (e.g. 'introspection') which were different from those used in other sciences. The compromise position, which is now held by most psychologists, is that inner processes can be studied scientifically, but only indirectly, by way of their behavioural concomitants. Thus, we cannot observe Mr Smith's feelings of anxiety directly and so cannot study these feelings scientifically. However, we can observe his verbal reports (e.g. that he says that he feels anxious), his social behaviour (e.g. that he avoids certain situations), his physiological responses (e.g. that his heart rate is raised) and that he has a high score on an anxiety questionnaire. We can also compare these observations with those which we made of Mr Brown and conclude which of the two is the more anxious. In these ways, internal, 'private' processes and experiences become capable of being studied by the normal methods of science. The term 'behaviour' in the definition thus draws attention to how the subject matter of psychology should be studied. The main technical problem in psychology is therefore to devise behavioural indices of private experience such as thoughts and feelings.

SCOPE AND CONTENT OF THE CHAPTER

The descriptions and explanations of psychiatric disorders and their treatment make frequent use of psychological theories and findings. The aim of this chapter is to prepare the reader for these accounts by introducing some of the basic concepts of scientific psychology. Several other chapters also discuss psychological principles and findings — in particular, those on biological determinants of personality (Ch 4), personality development (Ch. 5), measurement (Ch. 9) and behavioural and cognitive therapies (Ch. 40) and this chapter should be read in conjunction with them. The first topics to be considered will be learning and cognition. These are given prominence for two reasons. They are particularly relevant to psychiatry. Also, each is the starting point of a general approach to psychology.

Faced with the task of explaining all human and animal behaviour, psychologists have adopted the strategy of concentrating on one limited area of behaviour and developing theories and methods which describe, predict and explain behaviour within that area. These theories and methods are then applied to other areas, in the hope that they will prove useful there also. Thus, the study of simple learning in animals gave rise to a set of ideas ('behaviourism') which has been widely used to explain highly complex human behaviour such as thinking, emotion and personality. Similarly, the study of human thinking has provided an alternative approach ('cognitive psychology') for the study of emotion, motivation, learning and personality.

The chapter will then deal with aspects of two other major areas of scientific psychology: social behaviour and emotion. In discussing all four topics — learning, cognition, social behaviour and emotion — reference will be made in passing to the findings of two other areas of psychology: psychophysiology, which is concerned with the relation between behaviour and physiological structures and processes; and animal behaviour, which is studied both in its natural setting (ethology) and in the laboratory.

Two topics will then be considered — intelligence and personality — which are examples of the 'individual differences' approach to psychology, in which the main interest is to identify and measure the ways in which people differ from one another.

In conclusion, brief reference will be made to the role of clinical pyschologists, the health profession with particular expertise in psychological assessment and treatment. This draws attention to the dual nature of psychology: it is a scientific discipline, concerned with investigating and developing systematic theories of behaviour; and also an applied profession, whose practitioners use the methods and findings of psychology not only in the health field but in a variety of other settings such as education and industry.

LEARNING AND CONDITIONING

Introduction

The study of learning has been a central issue in psychology for almost a century. This topic is important to psychiatrists for three main reasons. First, more than other human ability, it is our vastly greater capacity to adapt to the demands of the environment and to benefit from experience — in other words, to learn — that distinguishes humans from other animals. Secondly, various theories and methods have evolved from the study of learning which have proved to be of practical value in the understanding and treatment of some types of psychiatric illness. Thirdly, as noted above, the study has given rise to an approach — 'behaviourism' — which has been very influential in the scientific study of psychology in general.

Definition

Learning is 'any relatively permanent change in behaviour which is brought about as a result of past experience'. Note that the definition refers to any change in behaviour — not merely the rote learning of facts or the acquisition of skills such as driving, but also changes in social behaviour, language and other communication skills, feelings, and emotional expression, attitudes and beliefs. 'Experience' refers to 'events

in the social and physical environment of the learner' and is specified in order to exclude changes due to maturation, senility, injury or illness. Learning is not always intentional, nor is the learner always aware that it is taking place.

Classical and operant conditioning

'Conditioning' is a very simple form of learning. Classical and operant conditioning will be discussed separately because there are differences in how they are usually demonstrated, in their terminology and in the types of human behaviour which they are used to explain: classical conditioning is used mainly to account for the development of emotional responses and operant conditioning for the development of voluntary behaviour, such as social, language and motor skills. However, psychologists increasingly tend to group both under the heading 'learning by association'. This term draws attention to the view of the behaviourists that both types of learning occur because of the association of events — because of two events occurring at or about the same time.

Classical conditioning

Classical conditioning or 'respondent learning' was first studied in detail by the Russian psychologist Pavlov and is concerned primarily with automatic, involuntary behaviour such as a reflex response to a physical stimulus. The main effect of classical conditioning is to increase the number of different stimuli which can elicit a given reflex or response. When a reflex occurs 'naturally', without previous learning, it is described as an unconditional — usually mistranslated as unconditioned — reflex (UR) and the stimulus as an unconditional stimulus (US). Classical conditioning occurs when a stimulus which does not naturally produce a reflex is associated with (i.e. is made to occur at or about the same time as) a stimulus which does naturally elicit the reflex. After several such associations, the stimulus, when applied on its own without the US, will be found to elicit the reflex. When it does, it is referred to as the conditional stimulus (CS) because its power to elicit the reflex is conditional upon its having been associated with the US. The reflex when elicited by the US was termed the UR; when elicited by the CS, it is termed the conditional reflex (CR).

In Pavlov's best-known experiments, the UR was salivation by a dog to the stimulus of food (US) placed in its mouth. A stimulus which does not normally elicit salivation, such as the sound of a bell, was associated with the US and, after several such pairings, the bell when presented alone was able to produce salivation (the bell was the CS and the bell-induced salivation was the CR).

The behaviourist position is that classical conditioning occurs because of the association between the US and CS, i.e. because they occurred at the same time. Any stimulus occurring along with the US could acquire the power to evoke the US. It is also unnecessary for the learner to notice or understand the association between US and CS. In support of this view, classical conditioning has been demonstrated in primitive animals such as flatworms and even in decorticate specimens.

Operant conditioning

Sometimes termed 'instrumental learning', operant conditioning has been studied most comprehensively by the American psychologist Skinner. He was concerned with behaviour which is under the control of an individual and with which that person operates upon (hence 'operant') or influences his environment. The effect of operant conditioning is to change (increase or decrease) the frequency with which a behavioural act occurs in a given setting. This frequency is influenced by the consequences of the act. In a typical experiment, a rat is placed in a box in which there is a lever which, when pressed, sends a pellet of food into the box. After exploring the box for some time, the rat will accidentally press the lever and so obtain food. This may occur several times before there is any noticeable change in the rat's behaviour, but gradually the rat will begin to press the lever more frequently, until eventually it spends most of its time doing so. The frequency of occurrence of the lever-pressing behaviour has thus been altered, and from the whole range of activities which the rat could have performed in the box, it has learned to perform only one.

There are three main types of operant conditioning situation:

1. *Reward training.* Behaviour increases in frequency because its consequences are rewarding to the learner. For example, the rat pressed the lever more often because by doing so it obtained a reward of food.

2. *Escape training.* Behaviour is learned because its consequences are escape from, or removal of, something unpleasant. For example, a rat given an electric shock at one end of a box can quickly learn to escape the shock by running to the other end.

3. *Avoidance training.* Behaviour is learned because it enables the learner to avoid something unpleasant.

For example, if in the 'escape training' situation a bell is rung a few seconds before the shock is delivered, the rat may learn to run away at the sound of the bell, so avoiding the shock altogether.

With operant conditioning also, the behaviourist position is that learning occurs because of the association between a behavioural act and its consequences, e.g. lever pressing followed by food. The frequency of almost any behaviour can be modified in this way. It is also unnecessary for the learner to be aware of the association.

Basic principles and concepts

The following are some of the terms, concepts and principles which are used in the description and explanation of classical and operant conditioning.

Stimulus and response. Although in laboratory studies the stimulus and response are defined and quantified very precisely, when used clinically the terms tend to be employed loosely, with 'response' being used for any item of behaviour and 'stimulus' referring to any event in the environment which evokes a response.

Reinforcement. A reinforcing event is one which increases the frequency, or probability of occurrence, of the behaviour that immediately precedes it. Reinforcement is therefore the process of increasing the frequency of an item of behaviour by presenting or removing a reinforcing consequence ('reinforcer'). A distinction is made between behaviour occurring more often because of the addition of a reinforcer ('positive reinforcement' — as in reward training) and because of the removal of a reinforcer ('negative reinforcement' — as in avoidance and escape training).

It is important to distinguish between negative reinforcement, in which the aim is to establish a new response, and punishment, in which the aim is to suppress an existing item of behaviour by applying an aversive stimulus whenever it appears.

The principle of reinforcement (or 'law of effect'), stated non-technically, is that if an item of behaviour is followed by a reward, or by the removal of an aversive stimulus, then that behaviour will tend to increase in frequency.

Acquisition and extinction of learned behaviour. Learning typically occurs gradually and erratically, with periods of rapid improvement being interspersed with 'plateaux' when no change in performance is observable. It may occur as a result of a single reinforcement ('one-trial learning') but usually many reinforcements are necessary for stable learning.

Learned responses do not usually continue for ever and in the absence of reinforcement they tend to disappear ('extinction'). One measure of the strength of a response, i.e. of how well it has been learned, is its resistance to extinction; one index of this is the number of responses made after the withdrawal of reinforcement. Extinction, like learning, may not be permanent and, after a period during which an item of behaviour appears to have been completely extinguished, it may reappear ('spontaneous recovery').

Schedules of reinforcement. This term refers to the rules according to which reinforcement is delivered. Continuous reinforcement of an item of behaviour exists when every occurrence of the behaviour is followed by reinforcement. Intermittent reinforcement is when only some of the occurrences of the behaviour are reinforced.

Resistance to extinction. Schedules of reinforcement are important because they have a powerful effect on the strength of the learned behaviour. In general, behaviour learned under intermittent reinforcement conditions is more resistant to extinction, i.e. is learned 'better', than that learned under continuous reinforcement conditions. Other factors which affect the extent to which a learned item of behaviour will resist extinction include the type of behaviour, the characteristics of the learner, and the nature of the reinforcer.

Reinforcers. Any stimulus or event is potentially capable of acting as a reinforcer. Some — e.g. food, or escape from pain — influence behaviour because they appear to satisfy basic drives; these are termed 'primary reinforcers'. However, most reinforcers are not effective 'naturally' and acquire reinforcing properties only because they have been regularly associated with a primary reinforcer; these are termed 'secondary reinforcers'. For example, in a reward training situation, if food was given to the rat whenever a bell sounded, eventually (through classical conditioning) the rat would learn to press the lever to obtain the sound of the bell, even if no food followed.

Generalisation and discrimination. Stimulus generalisation occurs when a response which has been conditioned to one stimulus is produced by another stimulus without any additional learning having taken place, e.g. a baby which has learned to smile to its mother may then smile at all adults. The opposite is discrimination, shown when the learner responds to one stimulus but not to another.

Clinical aspects of conditioning

Classical and operant conditioning are relevant to psychiatric practice in two ways: they have been used in the explanation of several disorders and as the basis of some approaches to treatment and training. Some examples are given below.

Development of fears

Studies of babies have shown that very few specific fears are innate and that therefore the great majority of the fears which adults experience have been learned during their lives. Studies of adults show that fears typically persist for very long periods — someone afraid of spiders will often remain so throughout his life. Any theory of anxiety must explain how fears are acquired and how they are maintained.

Two-stage theory. Mowrer (1939) proposed that there are two stages in the development of fears. The first explains the acquisition of fears by classical conditioning. Generalised fear reactions (UR) can be produced 'naturally', by simple stimuli such as sudden movement (US) or those which cause pain. In classical conditioning theory, any stimulus which becomes associated with the US will subsequently function as a CS, giving rise to 'conditional fear'. The fear thus evoked by the CS might spread to other stimuli through generalisation and secondary conditioning. For example, a child might touch (US) a hot stove so experiencing fear (UR); thereafter, the sight of the stove (CS) will elicit fear (CR); stimulus generalisation and secondary reinforcement will then ensure that the child is afraid of other stoves and perhaps also of harmless objects which were in the kitchen at the time.

The maintenance of fear is explained by operant conditioning. A specific fear, once established, will serve as a 'drive', i.e. as a biological need whose reduction is reinforcing. Any behaviour which reduces the fear will therefore be reinforced and, according to operant conditioning principles, will tend to recur — as in the escape and avoidance examples described above. The escape from, and avoidance of, the CS thus has a crucial role in the maintenance of fears, because they prevent any possibility of the extinction which would occur if the CS was presented in the absence of the US.

For about 40 years, this theory formed the basis of influential accounts of the development of normal fears, of phobic avoidance and of socialisation — how children learn, through punishment, not to carry out certain behavioural acts. The two-stage theory was able to explain some features of phobias — the avoidance, their irrational nature and that they cannot often be reasoned away. However, it had some deficiencies, which were addressed by Eysenck (1976).

Eysenck's theory of the neuroses. In the several versions of his theory of the neuroses, Eysenck accepted the two-stage theory as the basis of the acquisition of normal anxiety and also of phobic symptoms, which he regarded as learned responses that, however, are maladaptive. The only difference between a phobia of cats and normal fear of fire is that the latter is adaptive, in that the fear helps the individual to survive, whereas avoidance of cats or other phobic objects serves no useful purpose.

Although it was originally held that phobias developed from the accidental pairing of a CS and US, the epidemiology of phobias does not reflect this randomness — phobias of cats are very much more common than phobias of electrical appliances, although (non-fatal) incidents resulting in pain and fear are probably more common with the latter. To account for this, Seligman's (1971) concept of 'preparedness' suggests that there are certain stimuli to which anxiety is very readily conditioned; once established to these stimuli, anxiety is very resistant to extinction. These 'prepared' stimuli are usually those such as insects, small animals, or heights which would have been dangerous to primitive man and which now frequently appear as phobias. In a typical experiment to illustrate 'preparedness', human subjects watched photographs (CS) of snakes (a 'prepared' stimulus) and of flowers, while being given electric shocks (US). Conditional anxiety (CR) which persisted long after the withdrawal of the shock was very quickly established to the snake photograph whereas it developed only slowly, and was quickly extinguished, when the CS was a photograph of flowers.

The notion of 'prepared conditioning' accounts for the non-random occurrence of phobias, their often very rapid onset and their resistance to extinction. However, it is difficult to demonstrate experimentally because it is often impossible to exclude alternative explanations of the results; for example, in the above illustration, the subjects' prior experience of snakes and flowers might have influenced the results. However, many psychologists accept that something similar to 'prepared conditioning' does occur.

The three pathways model. Rachman (1978) addressed another criticism of the two-stage theory; that fears often appear to develop without the individual ever having had direct contact with the feared stimulus. He proposed that direct conditioning is only one of three major 'pathways' to the acquisition of fear, and that it can also be acquired vicariously by observing someone else showing fear (observational learning — see below) or by being given information about the stimulus, e.g. by reading. A particular fear in a specific individual can be acquired via any one or any combination of these pathways. Although the evidence is not yet conclusive, it may be that the informational pathway is particularly important in the development of the mild fears commonly encountered in everyday life, while direct conditioning experiences are the most common cause of clinical phobias (e.g. see Ost 1985).

Acquisition of new responses

So far, the discussion of learning has concentrated on factors which affect the frequency with which an item of behaviour is performed. The crucial role of reinforcement has also been noted. However, before a response can be reinforced, it must first be made. The rat in the operant conditioning examples given above must first press the lever before these responses can be reinforced by food. In the experimental situation, it is easy to induce these responses — the basic movements are already in the rat's repertoire and the animal is quite likely to press the lever accidentally. On the other hand, when we consider how humans acquire complex skills, the rat and lever do not provide a very useful model; learner golfers do not usually swing the club randomly in the hope of hitting a long, straight drive which can then be reinforced. Most complex human skills are not in our natural repertoire and must first be acquired before they can be reinforced.

Observational learning. This is the process by which an individual can learn a response vicariously by observing an event and its consequences. This observational learning is particularly important in the acquisition of social behaviour, and many social skills are acquired merely by an individual observing them being performed by another person (the model) without the learner overtly practising the skills during the observation period (social modelling).

Observation can have other effects also. Emotion can be aroused in someone who observes another person showing a strong emotional response. This emotion might then be conditioned to stimuli present in the vicinity, so that these stimuli will subsequently elicit the emotion. This may be the basis of the 'vicarious learning' pathway for the acquisition of anxiety postulated by Rachman (see above). Conversely, the presence of a calm, confident model can reduce anxiety in an observer. Clinically, modelling is used in social skills training and in the treatment of phobias.

In clinical practice, psychologists have developed several techniques for establishing new responses; three of particular importance are shaping, prompting and chaining.

Shaping. Also called the 'method of successive approximations', this involves reinforcing behaviour which gradually becomes more similar to the final, required behaviour. Thus, in training a handicapped child to speak, a therapist might first reinforce any sound made by the child, e.g. a grunt; when the frequency of these grunts increases, the therapist might select the most 'speech-like' sounds and selectively reinforce them. Shaping would continue in this way with sounds being selected and reinforced which bear closer and closer resemblance to recognisable words. A similar, although less systematic, procedure occurs 'naturally' when mothers, by their selective attention, reinforce the 'speech-like' sounds made by their infants.

Prompting. This is a method of guiding the learner to make the required response. Prompts are often verbal, such as instructions, or physical, when the trainer guides the learner through the necessary movements. Once the behaviour has been well established, the prompts may be gradually withdrawn ('fading').

Chaining. This is a method of breaking down a complex pattern of behaviour into a sequence of simple acts, the first of which is then reinforced. When this act is occurring reliably, the contingencies are changed so that the first two acts in the sequence must be performed before reinforcement is given. Each next act is added until the entire sequence has been learned. For example, a programme to train a child to feed himself might begin with reinforcement of his grasping the spoon; when that had been achieved, the child might be reinforced only when he grasped the spoon and placed it in the dish, and so on.

Programmes which begin with reinforcement of the first act in the sequence, as in the above example, are known as forward chaining. In backward chaining the final act in the sequence is the first to be reinforced, with the programme working backwards through the sequence. Chaining is effective because each act in the sequence serves both as a reinforcer for the preceding act and as a stimulus for the succeeding act, indicating to the learner that reinforcement will occur.

The behavioural approach

The behavioural approach to psychology is based on these concepts of simple learning. It makes four assumptions: (1) that the same laws of learning apply in more or less the same form to all species (i.e. that what holds for rats holds also for humans); (2) that the concepts and laws of simple learning, such as those of reinforcement, are central to explanations of complex human behaviour such as language, social interaction, personality and emotions; (3) that what determines whether learning takes place is association (i.e. two stimuli occurring at about the same time, or an item of behaviour being followed by a reinforcer) and that it is unnecessary for the learner to have thought about what was happening or to have understood the connection between, for example, his behaviour and the reward; and (4) that these explanations should thus concentrate on factors in the external environment — stimuli, reinforcers, behavioural responses — rather than on 'internal' processes such as thoughts, motives or feelings.

COGNITIVE PROCESSES

Introduction

Cognitive processes are those which are concerned with our ability to identify, understand, retain and use information both from our external (physical and social) environment and from internal processes, such as memory.

Impaired cognitive processes are a prominent feature of many psychiatric disorders. In addition, the cognitive approach is currently the main psychological source of theories explaining the cause and nature of psychiatric disorders and of psychological methods for their treatment.

Unfortunately, the scientific study of cognitive processes is in a confused state because some models of cognitive processes which were accepted during the 1960s and 1970s have now been shown to be inadequate. No attempt will therefore be made to present an integrated account of cognitive processes; instead, several topics relevant to psychiatry will be discussed.

Information processing

To illustrate cognitive processes, consider what is involved in reading this paragraph and subsequently answering an exam question based on its content. From the mass of competing sights and sounds, the reader must be able to focus on the page (selective attention), organise the jumble of shapes into words (pattern recognition) and then interpret and make sense of them so that their precise meaning is understood (perception). The information thus obtained is encoded and held briefly in short-term memory before being again encoded and passed into long-term memory where it is retained. When required, it will be retrieved and recalled and communicated in some form.

Information processing is in fact considerably more complex that this, in at least three ways. First, the information does not pass through these stages in an orderly sequence. Instead, different processes interact and occur in parallel. In particular, memory interacts with many of the other processes. Secondly, the individual does not passively receive information but instead actively seeks out some information while rejecting other stimuli. The meaning given to incoming stimuli depends to a large extent on how these stimuli are interpreted by the individual on the basis of his past experience and expectations. Thirdly, it is seldom that someone is required merely to retrieve and repeat an item of information. More usually, it is necessary to 'manipulate' the information mentally, i.e. to think about how it could be used, perhaps to combine it with other information, and then use it so as to carry out a task or solve a problem.

Attention

Limited capacity

In our external and internal environments, at any one time there is obviously much more information potentially available to us than can be noticed, understood and retained by our brains; indeed, a great deal more information is transmitted through our sense organs than can be dealt with adequately. Because of this limited capacity of our information-processing system, it is essential that we are able to restrict the total input to a manageable amount and to ensure that only important information is allowed through for processing while the irrelevant and unimportant are screened out.

Selective attention

To some extent, the selection is done for us by the stimuli themselves. For example, our attention tends to be attracted by intense stimuli (loud noises, bright lights) and by variable stimuli (intermittent noise, flashing lights). However, we ourselves exercise much greater influence by choosing to attend to ('notice') certain sensory inputs while ignoring other potential sources of information; thus, the (safe) driver will deliberately look at the road rather than the scenery.

The 'shadowing' experiment. Our ability to concentrate on one source of input while ignorant ('rejecting') input from other sources has been demonstrated by the 'shadowing' task (Cherry 1953). In this, different messages are played simultaneously through headphones into the left and right ears of someone who has to repeat out loud the input to one ear while ignoring that to the other. That we are able to perform this task at all shows the selective nature of

attention. The limited capacity of our attention processes is illustrated by how little of the 'rejected' message is noticed — usually only its physical features (e.g. whether it is loud or soft) but not its content. The limit to what we can 'take in' at one time is set, not by the amount of sensory input, but by the ability of the brain to process the input. This is illustrated when the 'shadowing' task is changed so that the subject has to attend to, and repeat, a well-known nursery rhyme while ignoring the message played into the other ear. In this case, we notice much more of the message than in the original experiment; because the nursery rhyme is familiar and predictable, it can be processed by the brain with little effort, so freeing some capacity to deal with the other input.

The cocktail party phenomenon. It is a common experience that, when talking to one group of people at a party, we notice if our name is spoken by someone in another group, even if we were not deliberately listening for our name. This suggests that 'rejected' input is not entirely excluded, but that our information-processing system briefly retains and analyses a great deal of information of which we are unaware; only if this analysis indicates that the input is 'important' in some way is it allowed through into consciousness. There are various theories about how this is carried out. However, the important point is that, without being aware of doing so, we seem to be able constantly to monitor our environment for stimuli of particular 'importance' to us, upon which our full attention can then be focused.

Divided attention. Many real-life activities require us to attend to several sources of input simultaneously, e.g. driving while listening to the car radio. How we do this depends upon the nature of the input. The 'nursery rhyme' version of the shadowing task showed that if the inputs are familiar and predictable, e.g. if the road is traffic-free and the radio is playing a well-known tune, we have enough information-processing capacity to attend to both. However, if we have to attend fully to one, e.g. if traffic increases, we will reject the other input and so not notice the radio. Sometimes, we can attend to competing inputs by switching our full attention quickly from one to the other, although the time taken to switch attention — about a second — will reduce the efficiency with which we deal with each input.

Attention and past experience

The above account provides several examples of how our past experience influences what we attend to in any given situation. First, sensory input which is familiar and predictable can be processed with little conscious effort. One consequence of learning a skill thoroughly is that it becomes 'automatic' and so requires less attention. The skills which we have acquired will therefore influence what we are able to notice. Secondly, certain stimuli are 'important' to us and will therefore be more likely to be detected (as in the cocktail party phenomenon). Thirdly, our past experience often teaches us what to expect in any setting and hence what to 'look for'. This may lead us to concentrate on one source of input while ignoring other potential information; or we might search for particular stimuli (e.g. listen to hear if the baby is crying). The advantage of this is obvious, in that it enables us to use our limited capacity to best advantage. The dangers are that, if our attention is determined to some extent by our past experience and our expectations, we are less likely to attend to and notice unexpected events.

Our past experience therefore has a crucial effect on our future experience, because it influences our selection of input. Because people differ considerably in their past experience we are each likely to attend to different aspects of some situation or event and 'each of us literally chooses, by his way of attending to things, what sort of universe he shall appear to himself to inhabit' (William James 1890).

Perception

The functions of the processes of perception are to organise identify and impose meaning on sensory input.

Perceptual organisation

There has been a great deal of research into the primitive organisation of sensory data. When we look at something our sensory input is a pattern of light rays which are continually shifting and which bear little resemblance to the objects which give rise to them. However, we impose order on this pattern and are able to distinguish objects from their background, to detect whether they are stationary or moving, near or far, etc.

For 300 years the main controversy in this area has concerned the extent to which this organisation is innate or the result of experience. Experiments have been carried out on the ability of infants to perceive different shapes and sizes, on animals reared from birth in the dark and on those few humans who have attained sight in adulthood after having been blind from birth. The results are not entirely conclusive, but it appears that in lower organisms there is an innate tendency for the visual world to be organised. In humans, much more depends upon learning. While there is some innate basis for visual perception (e.g. infants tend to prefer looking at complex rather than at plain visual stimuli), perceptual organisation is largely built up through interaction between the individual and his immediate environment.

Psychological meaning

Less is known about the more complex interpretation of sensory data which is involved when we perceive not only that an object is distinct from its background but that it is, for example, a house or our uncle. Many psychologists emphasise that perception of this sort is similar to conceptualisation (see below). Thus, when we identify an object as a house we 'go beyond the information given' and attribute to it features which are not directly observable by our sense organs. Gregory (1968) suggests how this is done: 'Perception seems to be a matter of looking up information that has been stored about objects and how they behave in various situation... We can think of perception as being essentially the selection of the most appropriate stored hypothesis according to current sensory data.'

Personal influences on perception

Whatever the process, it is clear that how we perceive ourselves and our environment is influenced by three sets of personal factors. The first is our past experience of the stimulus being perceived. The more information we have about a stimulus, the fewer alternative meanings it can have and the faster and more accurately it will be perceived. Objects which are familiar and those which are expected are recognised more quickly and accurately than the unfamiliar and unexpected. Secondly, our attitudes and values, which also of course reflect past experience, have an important influence on perception. Valued objects and prestigious people are often perceived as larger than they are; obese and anorectic patients view themselves as, respectively, thinner and fatter than they really are. There is also some evidence for a mechanism of perceptual defence, which reduces our ability to perceive stimuli which we would find anxiety-provoking or threatening. Thirdly, current physical and emotional state can influence perception; hungry and thirsty people perceive stimuli related to food and drink more rapidly than other stimuli and there is some evidence that anxious and non-anxious patients perceive threatening stimuli differently (Brewin 1988).

These personal influences are greatest when the sensory input is ambiguous and so can be interpreted in different ways. This is the principle underlying projective tests (see below).

Memory

Although there is considerable controversy about how memory can best be understood, there is agreement that it is useful to distinguish short–term memory — when information is required to be stored for only a few seconds — from long–term memory — when it has to be retained for longer periods, from minutes to years. (The physical basis of memory is discussed in Chapter 8.)

Short–term memory

Capacity. The main feature of short-term memory is that is has very limited storage capacity. Miller (1956) argued that the average limit is seven items plus or minus two. This memory span can be determined by presenting (showing or saying) an unrelated list of words or numbers to people, at intervals of about 1 second, and asking them to recall them in order. The 'magic number' seven has proved to be remarkably constant in different studies and most people recall between five and nine items.

Functions. Short-term memory has two functions. One is to serve as a 'working memory', holding information for a few seconds while it is used in some other cognitive task before being forgotten. Many everyday tasks involving perception, problem solving and communication require information to be retained only for short periods while it is used. For example, when we look up a phone number, we must retain it for the few seconds necessary to dial; during this time, the number is held in short-term memory. Secondly, short-term memory serves as part of the process by which longer-term memories are formed. While being held in short-term memory, information is evaluated and a decision made whether it needs to be retained for longer than a few seconds. If it does, the necessary rehearsal and encoding can take place to enable the information to pass into long-term memory.

Retrieval and forgetting. For information to enter short-term memory, it must first be attended to. The discussion of attention (above) indicated the highly selective nature of the process; a great deal of information potentially available in the environment is not remembered because it was not selected for attention in the first place. We are usually aware of what is in our short-term memory — it is, in effect, what we are thinking about at any time. Retrieval of information from short–term memory seems to involve a serial search during which each item is examined in turn, although we are unaware of this process because it occurs so quickly.

The forgetting of short-term memories seems mainly to be due to its limited capacity, with newer items displacing older memories.

Long–term memory

Function. Long-term memory is 'memory' in the lay sense of the word. Its function is to retain — for periods of between minutes and a lifetime — verbal, and other types of record of personal experiences and of more formal information, such as facts, rules and the meaning of words and concepts.

Transfer from short-term memory. Most theories assume that information enters long-term memory via short-term memory. However, there are disagreements about how this transfer from short-term to long-term memory takes place. Some theories emphasise the importance of rehearsal, i.e. the repeating of information, either out loud or, more usually, silently. Mere repetition is probably not a very efficient method and it may be that rehearsal is effective because it enables us to 'work on' the information — attempting to relate it to other information, to devise associations or mnemonics for it, or to code it according to its meaning or other features. This process of rehearsal or encoding influences the length of time for which information is stored in long-term memory before being forgotten.

Storage. Information in long-term memory is stored in various ways. Much of it is catalogued or encoded verbally, according to its meaning and verbal associations. Some is stored according to the imagery which it evokes and some according to its physical properties — visual or, less commonly, auditory, tactile or olfactory. It is likely that there are different long-term memories for facts as opposed to skills and for general facts (such as the meaning of words) and personal facts.

Retrieval and forgetting. Retrieval of long-term memories can be demonstrated by recall (i.e. by recreating the information) or by recognition (i.e. by realising that information is familiar). Usually, more can be recognised than can be recalled. The retrieval process is clearly crucial, for there is little value in having an item of information stored away if it cannot be located, retrieved and used when required. There must be a sophisticated process which permits a search to be made very quickly through the vast number of stored memories, which decides which are required in any given situation, and which retrieves them, while inhibiting the recall of similar but unwanted memories. Unfortunately, little is known about this process.

Most theorists accept that retrieval failures are major causes of forgetting. The efficiency of retrieval depends in part upon the initial coding. If the information has been stored in a bizarre or unusual way, or in ways which are irrelevant to subsequent needs, the search process may take so long that the information will not be recalled when required and will, in effect, be forgotten. Possibly the most important factor which can impair the retrieval of a memory is interference by memories which are similar to it in some way (as when we recall the name Jane instead of Joan) or by the memory having previously been associated with another cue in some way (as when we recall a friend's previous rather than current address).

However, retrieval failures are not the only cause of forgetting from long-term memory. Presumably memory traces decay with time, although the process is not well understood psychologically.

Memory and emotion

Emotion interacts with memory in several ways. All examinees know that anxiety reduces the ability to recall information; what happens is probably that the thoughts which accompany anxiety ('I'm going to fail') interfere with the retrieval process.

Emotion can also affect forgetting by disrupting attention. When we are preoccupied with our thoughts, we have insufficient mental capacity unused to enable us to focus our attention upon external events; these will therefore not be noticed and will not pass into short-term memory. This happens to everyone on occasion, but the inattention and hence forgetting is clearly likely to be greater when the preoccupations are stronger and longer lasting, as in clinical anxiety and depression.

Under some circumstances, emotion can enhance recall. There is evidence that we tend to rehearse emotionally charged information more than unemotional information — this is true both for pleasant and unpleasant emotions. Because rehearsal influences subsequent retrieval, emotional material will therefore be remembered better. This may explain the vivid memories of many disaster survivors.

In addition, if when information was originally encoded and passed into long-term memory we were experiencing strong emotion, this will probably have influenced how the information was stored or catalogued. When we subsequently experience the same emotion, we are therefore more likely to retrieve that information than other information which had been associated with a different emotion or with none.

This aspect of memory is relevant to the cognitive theory of depression (see Ch. 41).

Concepts and schemata

A basic notion in cognition, which has had considerable influence clinically, is that information in memory is stored in an organised way, these organisations being referred to by different psychologists as concepts, personal constructs or schemata. These *schemata* develop through learning and are, in effect, ways of grouping memories according to their shared characteristics.

The role of schemata has already been referred to in connection with organising memory — they are the 'filing systems' which allow specific memories to be identified and retrieved more quickly than if a search had to be conducted through a mass of unconnected memories. Our schemata also affect selective attention and perception by indicating what is likely to be important and what can be expected in any setting, and how what is attended to can be interpreted.

There is an interactive relationship between incoming stimuli and stored schemata. The latter will constantly be modified by new information stored in memory (referred to as 'accommodation' by Piaget — see Ch. 5) but the incoming stimuli will also be interpreted and altered in the light of existing schemata ('assimilation').

Within any one individual, the organisation of schemata is likely to be relatively stable, so that there are consistencies in the sort of stimuli to which we pay attention and in how these stimuli are interpreted. There are, of course, big differences among individuals, based on our past experience, in what we attend to and in how we explain and interpret the same events. There are also differences in the extent to which individuals accommodate and assimilate.

Thus, someone who has developed, through experience, schemata which interpret the world as threatening, will be more likely to attend to and 'notice' threatening stimuli, will tend to interpret (perceive) ambiguous stimuli as threatening, and will be more likely to recall threatening memories — all of which will strengthen the original schemata. Notions of this sort are central to cognitive theories of psychiatric disorder (see Ch. 41) and to various attempts to study the personalities of people by analysing the structure and content of their schemata, e.g. the personal construct theory of Kelly (1955).

Clinical aspects of cognition

Cognitive processes are relevant to psychiatry in two main ways. First, cognitive disorders are prominent among the signs and symptoms of several psychiatric disorders. Secondly, cognitive theories have been developed to explain some disorders and to form the rationale of treatment methods. These latter will be described in Chapter 41 so this section will merely illustrate some cognitive disorders.

Unfortunately, although there is a vast literature reporting attempts to identify and explain cognitive disorders, much of this research is very poor, because experimenters have often made elementary methodological errors, such as ignoring the heterogeneity of certain clinical groups, failing to control confounding variables, such as motivation and drug effects, and using inappropriate measures. In addition, because of the variety of different patient groups, experimental procedures and theoretical concepts employed, it is almost impossible to summarise the findings of those studies which have been performed competently. Much of the best work has been on memory disorders.

Memory in dementia

The majority of studies of senile and presenile dementia and of the amnesic syndrome have used the verbal-learning:recall method in which patients are given verbal material, such as lists of words, to learn to a criterion of success. There is ample evidence that, on tasks of this sort, the learning ability of patients with dementia is worse than that of non-dementing people of the same age. This evidence led to the widely accepted conclusion that the main problem in dementia is in transforming information from short-term into long-term memory. Further research suggested that the deficit might result from short-term memory being able to *hold* less information because its capacity is reduced in dementia, so reducing the time available for rehearsal, or because the patient's ability to rehearse, or otherwise encode, incoming information has become less efficient.

A quite different explanation of the above findings, for which there is some evidence, is that the patient's ability to consolidate new material is unaffected and that the learning deficit results from a relative inability to *retrieve* newly learned information from long-term memory. In the classic experiment, Weiskrantz & Warrington (1970) showed that patients, who when

assessed by normal tests of recall and recognition had apparently learned few words from a list, were able to improve their performance to normal if they were given cues, such as the initial letters of the words. One explanation is that these patients are able to store information but only in such a way that it cannot be elicited by the normal processes of retrieval, possibly due to a failure to suppress or inhibit competing memories in long-term memory. The cue enabled the retrieval process to work normally, so indicating that the information had, after all, been stored in long-term memory.

Very long-term memories

The fate of very long-term memories in dementia and following traumatic head injury has been studied, in particular to test Ribot's law (1882), one implication of which is that retrograde amnesia tends to affect more recent, rather than more remote, memory. While clinically the law has been widely accepted, it is only quite recently that systematic investigations, employing questionnaires to assess public events, have confirmed that events nearest in time to the onset of dementia, or to the occurrence of head injury, are less likely than more remote events to be remembered.

Rehabilitation

Interesting possibilities for the rehabilitation of memory-disordered patients are suggested by some of these theoretical accounts of memory. For example, information appears to be retained in long-term memory in at least two independent stores, one of which retains a verbal trace of the information and the other a visual or spatial image. Memory might thus be improved by teaching such patients to use both simultaneously or, if only one has been affected by the brain disease or injury, by teaching them to use only the other, unaffected store. The suggestion that cues improve retrieval has also led to speculation that memory could be improved if the patient's environment was arranged so that cues were given for the recall both of facts and of sequences of behaviour. However, the clinical value of 'memory training' has yet to be demonstrated empirically.

Memory in anxiety and depression

Patients suffering from anxiety and depression often complain of 'poor memory' but clinical assessment and research studies have shown no deficits under controlled conditions. Often this occurs because the patient has exaggerated the frequency or severity of normal forgetfulness. Something similar seems also to occur in many elderly people who, because they expect to experience memory loss, notice and attach greater importance to lapses in memory than younger people do. In addition, as noted above, information might not have entered memory in the first place, because of inattention due to the patient's preoccupations. And memories already in long-term memory might not be recalled due to temporary disruption of the retrieval process by the patient's emotions.

Cognitive approach

In the past two decades, cognitive psychology has taken over from behaviourism as the dominant ideology of the scientific discipline of psychology. It has also taken over as the main psychological source of psychiatrically relevant theories and techniques. Examples include the cognitive appraisal approach to stress, the attribution accounts of emotion and social perception, the personal construct theory of personality and the various cognitive theories and therapies discussed in Chapter 41.

Many of the very wide range of theories and methods which are now referred to as 'cognitive' make little use of the detailed findings of cognitive psychology and it is difficult to characterise this approach with any precision. What most of the theories seem to have in common is that they describe and explain psychological phenomena in terms of how individuals acquire, interpret and use information.

SOCIAL AND EMOTIONAL BEHAVIOUR

Social behaviour

Like cognitive psychology, social psychology is a diffuse field, with large numbers of studies having been carried out whose results defy summary and without many general, explanatory principles. The following topics are among the best researched of those which are relevant to psychiatry.

Social learning

Social learning theory, developed by Bandura (1977), is a general approach to the explanation of a wide range of human activities, which derives from conditioning theory. It accounts for these activities in terms of the learning history of the individual. Secondary reinforcement, in particular acting through social

behaviour, is central to this approach. These social reinforcers (e.g. showing approval or giving attention) probably derive their effect from being associated with primary reinforcers (e.g. food, tactile stimulation, avoidance of punishment) in infancy and childhood. Once established, social reinforcers provide a powerful means by which one individual can alter, direct and maintain the behaviour of someone else. Effective social reinforcers include the giving or withholding of approval, affection and attention.

Social learning theory has been responsible for many practical innovations in the field of health, e.g. the use of 'near peers' as models to transmit desired attitudes and behaviour — such as 'saying no to drugs' — to young people.

Although not derived directly from social learning theory, there have been many examples of how analysing abnormal or deviant behaviour in terms of its history of social reinforcement can often make it more explicable. For example, studies of long-stay psychiatric and mental handicap wards, school classrooms and parent–child interactions have shown how staff and parents can inadvertently increase bizarre or disruptive behaviour by paying attention to it, while ignoring normal and adaptive behaviour. These studies in turn have led to treatment and management approaches which emphasise the selective social reinforcement of 'desirable' behaviour rather than the punishment of unwanted activities; there is ample evidence of the effectiveness of this approach in clinical, educational and family settings (see Ch. 41).

Social information processing

The cognitive approach to psychology has also influenced the study of social behaviour.

Stereotypes. Stereotypes are beliefs about a class of people which are then applied to individual members of the class to provide information about that person in the absence of specific knowledge ('fat people are jovial, John is fat, therefore John must be jovial').

Schemata were discussed earlier, with the point being made that, while they have the advantage of allowing us to process large amounts of information, their disadvantage is that they can produce bias by influencing what we attend to and how it is perceived.

If stereotypes are thought of as schemata about people, many of their features can be understood. They are resistant to change because, once the schema has been formed, we select information from our environment, and recall memories, which support the schema. The importance of first impressions (the primacy effect) comes about because, on the basis of our first judgements of someone we have met for the first time, we categorise that person (i.e. develop a schema), which influences the information which we obtain subsequently.

We also have self-schemata, or stereotypes about ourselves, and there is evidence that we spend more time seeking and attending to information which confirms rather than contradicts our stereotypes.

Attribution. Attribution is the process by which we attempt to explain our own behaviour and that of others — the explanations which we find for why someone was angry or why someone else was promoted at work. Heider (1958) who developed attribution theory suggested that Western society has a collective schema which gives too much weight to personal ('dispositional') explanations (e.g. 'aggressiveness', 'honesty' and 'industriousness') and too little to situational causes (e.g. 'conflicting demands', 'poverty' or 'lack or reinforcement').

More generally, attributions are now being implicated in the aetiology of some psychiatric disorders such as depression and as factors determining their course. Treatment approaches are being developed in which patients are taught to re–attribute their explanations of their own behaviour.

Social skills training

Perhaps the approach to social psychology which has had most impact on British psychiatry in recent years has been the social skills model of Argyle (1978). In this, social interaction is regarded as a skilled performance — like playing tennis — in which the individual pursues certain goals, continuously modifies his behaviour in response to feedback and performs skilled motor activities. Feedback is the process by which the individual obtains information with which to evaluate his performance so as to take any necessary corrective action. In social interaction, much feedback comes from non-verbal communication including voice (e.g. emphasis on certain words, loudness or intonation), facial cues (e.g. expression, eye contact, head nodding), proximity and touch (e.g. how close the other person stands to you, whether he touches you), and gestures and posture (e.g. sitting relaxed or tense, use of hands). These and other non-verbal aspects of communication serve: (1) to convey emotion and attitudes, often more vividly than speech; (2) to give emphasis to verbal communication; and (3) to convey social reinforcement by way of facial expression, attention and other non-verbal signs of approval.

Clinically, this approach has encouraged the development of social skills training methods in which individuals are trained by instruction, role playing and modelling to interpret and emit appropriate, non-verbal signals to be reinforcing to others, and to employ specific conversational skills, such as refusing an invitation. As well as having led to effective treatment methods, the approach encouraged a valuable re-attribution of the cause of social difficulties, so that they can now be seen not as representing personality deficits (which are unchangeable) but as resulting from lack of appropriate skills (which can be taught).

Emotional behaviour

For many years, the study of emotion had little relevance to clinical practice. The two developments which revitalised the field were the 'three systems' approach to anxiety and the introduction of a cognitive perspective.

Three systems of anxiety

It has long been recognised that an anxious person can show three different types of symptom — the physiological, the behavioural (e.g. avoidance) and the cognitive (e.g. 'anxious thoughts'). However, it was assumed that these were three indices of the same, unitary phenomenon, i.e. that there was something called 'anxiety' which showed itself in these different ways. However, it is now recognised, in the widely quoted words of Lang (1970), that 'fear is not some … lump that lives inside people'. Rather, it is a set of loosely related systems whose degree of association is possibly influenced by the intensity of the anxiety. At extreme levels (calmness and panic), the three systems are probably closely related, i.e. all three are very low or very high, respectively. Mostly, however, they are desynchronised, i.e. are partly independent of one another, so that changes in one are not necessarily paralleled by changes in the others.

There are obvious implications of this perspective both for assessment and treatment.

Increasingly, other emotions are being described in terms of these partly independent systems.

Cognitive determinants of emotion

One set of findings which probably has a considerable, although as yet largely unexplored, relevance to psychiatry derives from attribution theory (see above).

A question which has intrigued psychologists for a century (and philosophers for much longer) is: how do we come to experience different emotions? One theory is that each emotion is 'caused' by its own, unique patterns of autonomic arousal, and certainly Ax (1953) showed that anger and fear were each associated with different patterns. However, it is not certain that these patterns caused the different feelings and there is little evidence relating other patterns of autonomic activity to specific emotions. A more widely accepted view is that of Mandler (1975), who suggests that autonomic arousal provides an undifferentiated stimulus or feeling which demands explanation. The specific interpretation and labelling of the arousal — and hence which emotion we report — depends upon our cognitions, which are based on our past experience, expectations and present situation.

This role of cognitive factors in determining emotion was illustrated by Schachter & Singer (1962) in one of the classic psychological experiments. Sympathetic reactions were produced in volunteers by the injection of adrenaline. The social context was varied by placing one group with 'angry' and another group with 'euphoric' experimenters. Although the physiological bases were thus identical, those individuals in the 'angry' condition experienced anger while those in the 'euphoric' condition experienced euphoria. Confronted by undifferentiated sensations for which they had no other explanation, the individuals had thus interpreted them according to their social context. One obvious clinical implication is that some autonomic reactions may be described differently by different patients, according to their past experience, expectations and social context (Tyrer 1976).

Stress and coping

The role of cognitive factors in emotion is also seen in current accounts of stress.

Stress. The term 'stress' is widely used in conceptualising the relationship between an individual's social and physical environment, psychological characteristics and physical and psychological health.

Considerable research has gone into identifying stressors (the environmental causes of stress). The physical environment is a potent source of stress (e.g. levels of noise, temperature and illumination) as are some life events (e.g. bereavement, separation and unemployment) and several work-related factors (e.g. overload, role ambiguity, role conflict, poor promotion prospects). The various effects of stress include those related to work (e.g. absenteeism, low job satisfaction), many symptoms and signs of psychiatric and psychological disorder (e.g. increased consumption of alcohol and drugs, reduced self-esteem, anxiety and depression), and a variety of physical disorders (e.g. myocardial infarction, hypertension and gastrointestinal disturbances).

Cognitive appraisal. Psychological research into the differing responses of individuals to stressors has concentrated on the cognitive and behavioural efforts of an individual to manage environmental and personal demands. In an influential account, Lazarus (1966) conceptualised stress as an interaction between the demands of a situation and the individual's ability to cope. His reaction depends upon his cognitive appraisals, i.e. continuously re-evaluated judgements about these demands and the resources which he has available to meet them.

Primary appraisals assess whether the situation is irrelevant, benign or stressful — and, if stressful, whether it is potentially harmful, threatening or challenging. Secondary appraisal involves judgements about what coping methods are available and how successful they are likely to be.

In other words, an important determinant of how we react to, and cope with, a potentially stressful situation is how we interpret the situation and our own ability to deal with it effectively. If it is appraised as challenging, and if we regard ourselves as having the necessary skills to manage, we are likely to cope well. Stress (or, more accurately, strain) occurs when the situation is viewed negatively, as potentially dangerous, and when we regard our coping skills as being insufficient.

INDIVIDUAL DIFFERENCES

Introduction

The study of individual differences

Scientific psychology involves not only the study of those basic laws of behaviour which apply to everyone, but also the description and measurement of differences between people. There are four main reasons for studying these 'individual differences': (1) to identify the major ways in which people differ from one another psychologically; (2) to discover the reasons for such differences; (3) to determine the distribution of these differences in a particular community; and (4), in professional applied psychology, to compare one person with others, in order to arrive at a diagnosis, to select the most suitable candidate for a job or to make some other practical decision.

The main areas in which individual differences have been studied which are relevant to psychiatry are intelligence and personality. The practical value of these areas of study will be discussed below. However, their scientific value has been greatly reduced by their having developed over the last 80 years largely independently of the rest of scientific psychology. Thus, the items used in intelligence tests have little in common with the tasks used to investigate cognitive processes. Conversely, experimental psychology has tended to neglect individual differences in the processes which it has studied. Eysenck in particular has argued that the study of basic processes and of individual differences would both benefit from being integrated.

Statistical approach to assessment

The study of intelligence and personality are thus closely bound up with the assessment of individuals, often for practical purposes. Intelligence tests, and most measures of personality, are examples of standardised techniques. In these, the score of the person being assessed is compared against the scores of a normative group (norm-referenced measure) or against a criterion (criterion-referenced measure). The reliabilities and validities of the tests and measures have usually also been established. These and other relevant features of measurement are discussed in Chapter 9.

Intelligence

As noted above, cognitive processes can be studied with the aim of describing the features of the various stages of information processing and identifying the variables which affect them. However, they can also be studied from the standpoint of their adaptive function — what these processes, when interacting with and supporting one another, allow us to achieve. Looked at in this way, 'cognition' refers to a purposeful series of activities aimed at providing solutions to problems posed by our daily lives. People differ in the effectiveness with which they solve these problems; e.g. some are more likely than others to arrive at correct answers, to provide original and imaginative solutions, or to reach a solution quickly. These individual differences in the effectiveness of problem solving are the subject matter of the study of intelligence, and intelligence tests are intended to summarise and quantify these differences.

Intelligence or intelligences?

One major controversy is whether intelligence is a single, general ability (often referred to as 'g') or whether it comprises a number of different although related abilities; if the latter, the issues are how many of these abilities are there and how best they can be described. Most tests in current use in clinical, educational and occupational psychology assume that greatest practical benefit can be obtained by distinguishing between 'verbal' and 'non-verbal' intelligence or reasoning.

Tests of verbal reasoning assess the ability or abilities required to understand and use words and other verbal material; they do so by testing vocabulary, verbal fluency and the comprehension of written or spoken material.

Tests of non-verbal reasoning or performance intelligence typically assess the ability or abilities involved in understanding spatial relationships; they do so by using tasks which require diagrams and other spatial material to be understood or completed and objects to be assembled.

Numerical skills are included along with verbal items in some tests but with non-verbal items in others.

Verbal and non-verbal tests are usually found to be positively correlated (see Ch. 10), so to some extent they measure the same thing. However, the distinction is useful in educational and occupational settings, since verbal and non-verbal abilities are related to performance in different school subjects and types of work. Clinically, the distinction is important because of the long-held view that verbal abilities are relatively less affected than non-verbal abilities by dementia or other forms of brain damage.

Features of tests

Intelligence tests differ considerably from one another in several ways. These differences are not arbitrary, but reflect the varied uses of such tests. The main differences are: (1) in the abilities which the test is designed to assess, so that some tests assess only verbal abilities, some only non-verbal abilities and some both; (2) in the age of those with whom the test is used, e.g. younger and older children and adults; (3) in the level of ability of those with whom the test is used, i.e. those of average, below or above average ability; (4) in whether the test has, or has not, to be completed within a set time, i.e. timed or untimed tests; and (5) in whether it can be given by one tester to a group of people simultaneously or is intended for use by one tester with one person, i.e. group or individual tests.

Indices of intellectual level

The score of an individual on an intelligence test is reported in terms of a comparison of his performance with that of the standardisation sample and hence of the population from which the sample was drawn (see Ch. 9). Thus, tests answer questions such as 'On a measure of verbal intelligence, how does Jane compare with other children of her age?' or 'Is Ms Smith's general intellectual ability above average compared with the UK adult population?'

Intelligence can be described in three main ways, for the purpose of comparing the score of one person with that of others.

Centile ranking. The centile (or percentile) ranking indicates the percentage of the standardisation sample which scored lower than the person in question. Thus, a centile rank of 80 means that on that particular test his score was superior to the scores of 80% of the standardisation sample.

Deviation scores. Several indices are based on the mean score and standard deviation (see Ch. 10) of the standardisation sample; they express an individual score in terms of the number of standard deviations which it is above or below the mean.

IQ. In some of the original childrens' tests, the intelligence quotient (IQ) was calculated from the mental age (MA) of the child, i.e. the age at which the average child scores the same as he does; the IQ is the MA expressed as a percentage of the child's chronological age. Although this use of IQ has now largely been superseded, some currently used tests for children and adults — including the widely used Wechsler series — continue to express scores as IQs because they are familiar to clinicians and the general public alike. However, these are calculated in a quite different way, from deviation scores, i.e. the difference between a score and the mean score of the standardisation sample, expressed as a standard deviation (see Chs 9 and 10).

Intelligence tests

Many different intelligence tests are in use. The two most commonly used in Britain with adults are described below.

Wechsler Adult Intelligence Scale — Revised. The 'WAIS-R UK' comprises 11 subtests, six of which deal with words or numbers (e.g. general knowledge, arithmetic and vocabulary) and whose scores are combined to give a 'verbal IQ'; the other five involve spatial patterns (e.g. completing pictures and assembling jigsaw-type designs) and give a 'performance IQ'. The verbal and performance IQs are combined into a 'full scale IQ' (as noted above, these IQs are based on the deviation of the score of the person being tested from the mean score of the

standardisation sample). The test has norms obtained from US populations although the UK version has replaced items which were specifically American in content.

The Wechsler Intelligence Scale for Children ('WISC') is a version of the WAIS intended for children aged 7–16 years of age and exists in revised forms with both UK and specifically Scottish norms ('WISC-R UK' and 'WISC-R S', respectively). The Wechsler Preschool and Primary Scale of Intelligence ('WPPSI-R UK') is a version for children aged 3–7 years with UK norms.

Raven's Progressive Matrices and Vocabulary Scales. The Matrices is a diagram completion test which exists in three versions: Standard, for use with people of average ability; Coloured for children and those of lower ability; and Advanced for those of above average ability. The vocabulary test is in two parts, one involving the recall and the other the recognition of the meaning of words, with different versions available for people of different ability. Scores are presented as (per)centile ranks based on UK normative data (which are now somewhat out of date).

Some research findings

The availability of reliable and objective measures has enabled a great deal of research to be conducted on various aspects of intelligence. Studies of clinical relevance include those on the effects on intelligence of age and of various psychiatric disorders.

Age and intelligence. The accepted view of the effects of age on intelligence has undergone a change in recent years. Early research, which was based on cross-sectional comparisons, i.e. testing groups of people of different ages, suggested that quite substantial decline occurred in many aspects of intellectual ability, beginning in early adulthood — around 25 years — with the rate of deterioration gradually accelerating. Longitudinal studies, in which the same people are repeatedly tested over many years, give a more optimistic picture. These studies suggest that the decline in many important aspects of intellectual functioning starts later and occurs less rapidly than previously believed.

Psychiatric disorders. Although there is abundant evidence that intellectual functioning deteriorates in dementia, despite many studies it is not yet clear whether the pattern of change is similar — although more severe — to that in normal ageing or whether different changes occur. There is no evidence that most other disorders affect intelligence permanently, although test performance can be affected temporarily by inattention, poor motivation, etc. The main exception is schizophrenia, where there is evidence that some chronic patients do develop intellectual deterioration (see Ch. 18).

Clinical uses of intelligence tests

Purpose of intelligence testing. Intellectual assessment, involving the use of standardised intelligence tests, is used clinically in three main areas: (1) in the assessment and classification of people with learning difficulties; (2) to throw light on a person's educational and employment performance or potential; and (3) in the diagnosis and description of dementia, brain dysfunction and other organic conditions. In particular in the field of learning difficulties, the widespread introduction of intelligence testing in the 1950s led to a significantly decrease in the number of people who were incorrectly diagnosed as mentally handicapped on the basis of their poor educational attainment or of sensory or communication defects.

Limitations of testing. Standardised intelligence tests have four main limitations: (1) like any other measure they are subject to uncontrollable error, although the limits of this error can be specified statistically; (2) the norms may be inadequate or misleading, e.g. the standardisation sample might have been very different from the people with whom the test is currently being used; (3) any one intelligence test can assess only a small proportion of all mental abilities and some with important, practical implications, e.g. creativity, are under-represented among current tests; and (4) there are many factors which can cause an intelligence test score to give a misleading estimate of a person's true intellectual ability, e.g. low motivation, anxiety or a hostile attitude towards testing.

Statistically based judgement. The major advantage possessed by standardised assessments over other approaches, e.g. clinical judgement, is that it is possible to specify quite precisely in statistical terms the confidence which can be placed in a specific decision made on the basis of such an assessment. This is because the statistical properties of the test, e.g. its reliabilities and error of measurement, are known (see Ch. 9) and information will usually also be available about its validities. When a psychologist is carrying out an assessment for clinical or other professional purposes, his judgements and decisions will always be based upon these statistical and research data as well as upon his knowledge of the purpose of the assessment and the person being assessed (such as motivation and level of anxiety).

Personality

Definition

There are many competing definitions but most emphasise that personality is concerned with the relatively stable differences between people in those aspects of their emotional and interpersonal behaviour, motives and drives which determine their adjustment to social and other environmental situations.

Theories of personality

There have been several attempts to produce general theories to explain and describe all or most aspects of personality. Those with clinical relevance include the psychoanalytic theories of Freud and the post-Freudians, Rogers' self theory, Kelly's personal construct theory and that of Eysenck. The last decade has seen a decline in interest in comprehensive theories with a correspondingly greater use of 'narrow band' approaches (see below). Eysenck's theory, however, continues to influence British psychiatry and clinical psychology and will be described briefly.

Eysenck's theory of personality

From a statistical analysis (by factor analysis) of the performance of large numbers of people on many different types of measure, Eysenck concluded that many of the important differences between people can be summarised in terms of their differing along two, independent variables: neuroticism (N), which distinguishes people who are emotionally stable and calm (low N) from those who over-react to stress and are prone to worry (high N); and introversion–extraversion (E), which distinguishes between the quiet, retiring, controlled individual ('introvert' or low E) and the sociable, impulsive, excitement-craving person ('extravert' or high E). Later, a third dimension was added: psychoticism (P), which describes those long-standing features of personality which (Eysenck claims) distinguish psychotically ill patients (and some criminals) from normals.

Of these dimensions, E has been by far the most strongly supported by research and many studies have shown important differences in social, moral and emotional behaviour to be associated with differences in extraversion.

Eysenck postulates that the biological bases of neuroticism are variations in the reactivity of the autonomic nervous system; and those of introversion–extraversion are differences in the reticular activating system. The basis of psychoticism has not been described. These biological differences result in differences in conditionability. Compared to the extravert, the introvert is said to condition more readily and to develop responses which are stronger and more resistant to extinction. This, in turn, leads to introverts developing conditional anxiety more readily and hence becoming more socially controlled, rule-following and law-abiding than extraverts; for Eysenck, 'conscience' is no more than conditional anxiety.

People high on the N dimension are said to be more likely to develop neurotic symptoms under stress. People low on E but high on N are said to develop disorders characterised by excessive conditioned anxiety (phobias, generalised anxiety, obsessional states) whereas those high on E and N tend to develop disorders characterised by absence of control (hysterical and psychopathic conditions).

The theory has generated a great deal of research, the results of which defy summary; however, although this is a brilliant attempt to integrate a complex and diffuse field, its scientific status and clinical value remain in doubt. It is currently more widely accepted as a basis for the description of personality differences — in particular those associated with E — than as an account of their causes.

'Narrow band' accounts of personality

While Eysenck's theory aims to provide a comprehensive account of personality, there are many other theories or descriptions — often referred to as 'narrow band' theories — which do no more than identify and describe one aspect of personality. Those of clinical relevance include the following.

Type A personality. Friedman & Rosenman (1974) described the stress-prone individual, or type A personality, as being characterised by several behaviour patterns, such as taking on more than one task simultaneously, time urgency, inappropriate aggression and poorly defined goals. Although there have been difficulties in developing a reliable, valid and agreed measure of type A behaviour, there is strong evidence relating this aspect of personality to a variety of physical and psychiatric disorders, most notably ischaemic heart disease. There is also evidence that type A behaviour can be modified by psychological methods.

Locus of control. Rotter (1966) distinguished between people who view their lives as being under their personal control ('internal' locus of control) and those who regard themselves as powerless before authority and fate ('external'). This variable has been widely used in health research, distinguishing those who take, and who do not take, personal responsibility for their health and well-being.

Hostility and direction of hostility. Caine et al (1967) distinguished the various different ways in which individuals express hostility internally (guilt, self-criticism) and externally (criticism of others, projected hostility, acting out) and developed the Hostility and Direction of Hostility Questionnaire (HDHQ) to assess both this and the amount of hostility experienced. Scores on this measure have been associated with a variety of psychiatric symptoms and disorders.

Self-esteem. This is a very widely used personality concept, defined as: 'the sense of contentment and self-acceptance that stems from a person's appraisal of their own worth, significance, attractiveness, competence and ability to satisfy their aspirations' (Robson 1988). Low self-esteem is a symptom of several psychiatric disorders but, more interestingly, has been identified as a factor causing vulnerability to depression and also to several physical disorders. Various psychological methods have been described which are intended specifically to raise self-esteem and hence to reduce vulnerability.

Personality assessment

Of the many hundreds of different tests and techniques for assessing various aspects of personality, only a few have been developed from particular theories. Personality measures are of several types, and the three most widely used are described below.

Self-assessments. Most of the self-assessment measures of personality are in the form of questionnaires or inventories (see Ch. 9) which require the individual to indicate his typical attitudes or how he typically responds in various situations. Of these, one of the most widely used in the UK is the Eysenck Personality Inventory (EPI), which, in its various forms, assesses a person's scores on two or three of the personality dimensions (E, N and P) described above.

Projective methods. Although rejected by most psychologists because of their low reliability and often unknown validity, these methods continue to be used, in particular by clinicians with a psychodynamic orientation. They require the person being assessed to describe ambiguous stimuli, such as ink blots (e.g. the Rorschach test), and, in so doing, reveal aspects of his unconscious drives and motives.

Behavioural methods. These include direct observation of the individual in different settings, or laboratory procedures such as measures of psychophysiological variables.

Assessment of personality in clinical work

Although personality variables are increasingly invoked in theories of psychiatric and physical disorder measured in research, the formal assessment of personality by psychological methods currently plays little part in routine psychiatric practice. The main reason is that the great majority of those measures which satisfy the requirements of reliability and validity (see Ch. 9) — mainly self-report questionnaires — are useful only for distinguishing between groups of people. Because their items are couched in general terms which give little specific information, they reveal little of immediate clinical relevance about individuals.

CLINICAL PSYCHOLOGY

The profession of clinical psychology has the role of applying scientific psychology to health problems; clinical psychologists have expertise in the theories and findings of psychology, in the use of scientific methodology to investigate individuals and groups, and in the psychological assessment and treatment of clients and patients.

The role of the clinical psychologist has changed greatly over the past 20 years, with assessment occupying a diminishing part and many clinical psychologists now being almost wholly engaged in treatment. Unlike many of their colleagues in the USA and continental Europe, British clinical psychologists mostly have a 'cognitive–behavioural' orientation.

Clinical psychologists work alongside psychiatrists in areas such as geriatric psychiatry, learning difficulties, psychiatric rehabilitation, forensic psychiatry, child and family psychiatry and general, acute psychiatry. They are also increasingly working in other areas of the health services, e.g. general medicine, paediatrics, neurological rehabilitation and primary health care.

However, clinical psychology remains a comparatively small profession; in 1989, there were just over 2000 whole-time equivalent clinical psychologists employed in the National Health Service, with another 600 posts vacant — these vacancies being due mainly to the shortage of training places (MPAG 1990).

One recent development which will be important for the profession was the establishment by the British Psychological Society of a Register of Chartered Psychologists. This will be open to those with the necessary qualifications — an undergraduate degree plus at least 3 years of postgraduate training or experience — and who agree to abide by the codes of conduct of the Society. The Register is legally protected in that only those on the Register may refer to themselves as chartered psychologists, but it is as yet only voluntary and few employing authorities require psychologists to be registered.

REFERENCES

Argyle M 1978 The psychology of interpersonal behaviour. Penguin, Harmondsworth.

Ax A F 1953 The physiological differentiation between fear and anger in humans. Psychosomatic Medicine 15: 433–442

Bandura A 1977 Social learning theory. Prentice-Hall, Englewood Cliffs

Brewin C 1988 Cognitive foundations of clinical psychology. Lawrence Erlbaum, London

Caine T M, Foulds G A, Hope K 1967 Manual of the Hostility and Direction of Hostility Questionnaire (HDHQ). University of London Press, London

Cherry E C 1953 Some experiments on the recognition of speech with one and with two ears. Journal of the Acoustical Society of America 25: 975–979

Eysenck H J 1976 The learning theory model of neurosis: a new approach. Behaviour Research and Therapy 14: 251–267

Friedman M, Rosenman R M 1974 Type A behaviour and your heart. Knopf, New York

Gregory R L 1968 Visual illusions. Scientific American 217: 66–67

Heider F 1958 The psychology of interpersonal relations. Wiley, New York

James W 1890 The principles of psychology. Holt, New York

Kelly G A 1955 The psychology of personal constructs. Norton, New York

Lang P 1970 Stimulus control, response control and desensitization of fear. In: Levis D (ed) Learning approaches to therapeutic behaviour change. Aldine Press, Chicago

Lazarus R S 1966 Psychological stress and the coping process. McGraw-Hill, New York

Mandler G 1975 Mind and emotion. Wiley, New York

Miller G A 1956 The magic number seven plus or minus two: some limits on our capacity for information processing. Psychological Review 63: 81–97

Mowrer O H 1939 A stimulus-response analysis of anxiety and its role as a reinforcing agent. Psychological Review 46: 553–556

MPAG 1990 Clinical psychology project. Department of Health, London

Ost L-G 1985 Ways of acquiring phobias and outcome of individual treatments. Behaviour Research and Therapy 23: 683–693

Rachman S 1978 Fear and courage. Freeman, San Francisco

Ribot E 1882 Diseases of memory: an essay in the positive psychology. Kegan Paul, London

Robson P J 1988 Self-esteem: a psychiatrist's view. British Journal of Psychiatry 153: 6–15

Rotter J B 1966 Generalised expectancies for internal versus external control of reinforcement. Psychological Monographs 80 (No. 609)

Schachter S, Singer J E 1962 Cognitive, social and physiological determinants of emotional state. Psychological Review 69: 379–399

Seligman M P 1971 Phobias and preparedness. Behaviour Therapy 2: 307–320

Tyrer P 1976 The role of bodily feelings in anxiety. Maudsley Monograph 23. Oxford University Press, London

Weiskrantz L, Warrington E K 1970 A study of forgetting in amnesic patients. Neuropsychologica 8: 281–288

4. The biological determinants of personality

D. H. R. Blackwood

INTRODUCTION

Personality can be defined in various ways. One approach is to select particular traits which provide a description of how an individual thinks about himself and others and responds to his environment in different social and personal situations. Traits such as 'introversion' and 'extroversion' have an established place in our language and have some validity (Eysenck & Eysenck 1975), but attempts to define personality purely in terms of underlying relatively fixed traits has major limitations.

A trait theory of personality takes insufficient account of situation specific behaviours. Antisocial behaviour, for example, rather than being an enduring and pervasive personality attribute, may in many individuals be a response to quite specific environmental settings. Rutter (1980a) argues for an 'interactionist' view of personality, stressing the importance of person-specific traits and situation-specific behaviours, both of which may be the result of an interplay between genetic endowment and the effect of rearing and learning processes. A further important factor in development is an individual's ability not merely to react to his surroundings but actively to select a social environment by influencing the behaviour of others.

An adequate understanding of complex behaviours remains well beyond the scope of neurobiology. However, a knowledge of some specific neurobiological processes by which genetic endowment and environmental influences interact in the developing brain should increase our understanding of normal personality development.

For example, a neurobiological approach can now begin to unravel the complex cascade of genetic and endocrine events leading from the inheritance of the sex-determining gene on the Y chromosome in a male fetus to the expression of complex sex-related behaviours in childhood and adulthood. In another area, an understanding of the effect on the brain at different stages of its development of a severe environmental stress such as malnutrition may throw light on normal development and can also have an impact on the planning of effective intervention strategies.

HEREDITY

Genes are the molecular code which controls the synthesis of peptides, and hence the production of enzymes and structural proteins which give cells their differing characteristics. It is by the variations in the expression of genes — the mechanisms by which the production of enzymes and other proteins may be switched on and off in response to internal and external environmental cues — that the orderly development of the embryo can proceed in a largely predetermined manner unique to each species. It would be wrong to assume that this genetic control of development stops at birth. Throughout the entire lifespan, from childhood to old age, certain genetically determined physical characteristics and even complex patterns of behaviour are making their first appearance. The onset of puberty and hair loss in males leading to baldness are just two examples of changes, the timing of which is strongly influenced by genetic factors. The symptoms of Huntington's chorea, like many other hereditary illnesses, become manifest only in adulthood even though the person has been carrying the gene since conception. In these instances, environmental stress and learning may have little impact on modifying the expression of genetic endowment. However, in the development of characteristics such as IQ, personality traits and complex behaviour patterns such as sex role activity, the expression of a genetic predisposition may be radically influenced by the social environment in which the child grows up.

Behaviour genetics is concerned with the pathway from genes to behaviour and the lifelong interactions between the genotype and the environment. When considering the genetics of personality, it is perhaps more appropriate to consider 'how much' rather than 'whether' a given behaviour is determined by inheritance (Hay 1985). A rigid genetic determinism does not account for the many dissimilarities found between identical twins who have been brought up together in the same family, whereas a simple environmental approach fails to explain satisfactorily the many personality resemblances found between adopted children and their biological as opposed to their adoptive parents. Much of our present understanding of genetic and environmental interactions is derived from two research strategies, the study of twins and of adopted children.

Twin studies

Monozygotic (MZ) twins share exactly the same genes and are born into the same family and social environment. Dizygotic (DZ) twins have only approximately 50% of their genes in common and are rather similar to any pair of siblings within a family except that, by virtue of their similar age, their life experiences should be more similar than between siblings of different ages. In the rare instances when identical twins are separated at birth, adopted and reared in quite different families, the remarkable similarities in personality which are observed may be attributed entirely to the effect of their common inheritance (Holden 1980).

An early study of twins is that of Shields (1962). He traced 44 adult pairs of MZ twins brought up apart, 44 pairs of MZ twins brought up together (control) and 32 pairs of DZ twins brought up together. Over half of those who had been brought up apart had been separated from one another by the age of 3 months. Shields assessed the behaviour characteristics of the twins by personal interviews, by intelligence tests and by self–rating questionnaires of extraversion–introversion qualities.

As far as intelligence was concerned, the MZ twins, whether brought up together or apart, resembled one another more than the DZ twins. As a measure of the resemblance of one member of each twin pair to the other, Shields used intraclass correlation coefficients. For intelligence, the intraclass correlation coefficient was 0.76 for MZ twins brought up together, 0.77 for MZ twins brought up apart and 0.51 for DZ twins. Personality testing yielded some intriguing results. The measures of alikeness of the members of the twin pair to each other regarding extraversion–introversion and neuroticism were as shown in Table 4.1.

In terms of both extraversion–introversion and neuroticism, the MZ twins who were separated from

Table 4.1 Intraclass correlation coefficients for extraversion–introversion and neuroticism in MZ and DZ twins

	Extraversion–introversion	Neuroticism
MZ (control)	+0.42	+0.38
MZ (separated)	+0.61	+0.53
DZ	+0.17	+0.11

each other in early life were more alike in their adult personality than those twins who had been reared together! It seems that in order to establish their individuality, twins brought up together may tend to exaggerate their differences. Nevertheless, the control and separated MZ twins all resembled each other in personality much more than the DZ twins. In their little traits and habits, in their attitudes, and, especially, in their gestures and mannerisms, their sexual adjustment and their rapport with an interviewer, the MZ twins were strikingly alike.

The Louisville twin study (Wilson 1983), which began in 1957, followed the development of about 500 pairs of twins and their siblings from birth to adolescence. The twins were visited regularly at home by a social worker who carried out assessments of IQ and various cognitive abilities using several measures of mental development. The home environment was assessed, including play facilities, maternal temperament, maternal intellectual ability, and parental education. It is well recognised that normal mental development in the preschool years does not advance at an even rate for all types of physical and intellectual abilities but proceeds by a series of spurts and lags, the timing of which varies from child to child. A major finding of the Louisville study was that MZ twins show almost identical fluctuations in their rates of development during the first few years, and at 6 years of age their mental development scores were remarkably similar. In contrast, in DZ twins spurts and lags of development did not occur with the same synchrony, and these individuals often showed considerable differences in mental development by school age. As the children grew older, MZ twins continued to show strong similarities with one another whereas DZ twins tended to diverge in the same way as ordinary siblings. The study also made it clear, however, that features of the home environment were highly influential in the development of IQ. In particular, parental education and socioeconomic status were significantly related to the IQ scores achieved by these children. From this study it can be concluded that individual differences in intelligence progressively stabilise by the age of 6 years and in each child there is a distinct pattern of spurts and lags in mental development, the overall direction of which is under genetic control.

Heritable factors may play a part not only in determining the overall timetable of mental development but in the acquisition of quite subtle aspects of mental activity, as is suggested by an intriguing study reported by Rose & Ditto (1983) in which 2600 adolescents and adults, including more than 400 pairs of twins, were asked to complete a self-report questionnaire on commonly experienced fears. These included the fear of criticism and making mistakes; fear of small animals such as snakes, mice and spiders; the dislike of speaking in public and meeting strangers; the fear of dangerous places such as heights and crowds; the fear of death or the death of a loved one. Remarkably, MZ twins closely resembled one another in the intensity with which they experienced such fears, and the similarity between MZ twins but not DZ twins increased with age from adolescence to adulthood. This reinforces the view that genetic factors continue to make a major contribution to personality development throughout adult life.

Adoption studies

Several large studies initiated in recent years have examined adopted children from infancy to adolescence and compared their personality characteristics with those of their biological parents, their adoptive parents and siblings in their adopted families. From these adoption studies in Minnesota (Scarr & Weinberg 1983), Colorado (Plomin et al 1988) and Texas (Horn 1983), it is clear that children who have been adopted resemble their biological mothers more than they resemble their adopted parents in measures of IQ. The correlations are rather weak but nevertheless support the view that there is an important genetic component to the development of IQ. In the Texas adoption project, 300 families participated and both the biological and adopted mothers were assessed. The observed correlation for IQ between adopted child and its biological mother (shared genes) was 0.28, between adopted child and adoptive mother (shared environment) 0.15, and natural child and its mother (shared genes and environment) was 0.21. Although these correlations are small all three are statistically significant. Both the Texas and Minnesota studies also confirm that adoptees are responsive to the rearing environments of adoptive families, and in particular the ability of these families to provide adequate intellectual stimulus and exposure to skills.

The higher the intelligence of the child the more it is able to respond to an enriched environment. An interesting observation by Scarr & McCartney (1983) is that children, whether biologically related or adopted, grow less like their parents as they get older. To explain this they propose that a person's genotype may direct development by a number of indirect ways. A person's genetic make-up creates the environment he grows up in, as illustrated, for example, by the observation that smiling, 'easy' children are less likely to be the target of parental irritability (Rutter & Quinton 1984). Similarly, in adolescence, children will select friends, hobbies and academic pursuits in keeping with their genotype and, by identifying and selecting a niche, are likely to grow progressively dissimilar to their siblings.

A powerful opportunity for disentangling the influence of nature and nurture on personality development exploits the rare situation of twins being separated soon after birth and reared apart in separate families. The Minnesota study of twin pairs reared apart was started in 1979 and over 100 pairs have been fully assessed at an average age of 41 years (range: 19–68 years). These twins had been separated on average at 5 months after birth (range: birth to 4 years) and participation in the study involved approximately 50 hours of assessments which included measures of IQ, four personality inventories, and assessment of occupational and leisure interests. Over a range of tests, the findings showed that MZ twins had retained strong similarities despite being reared in different family settings. Seventy per cent of the variance in IQ measurement was associated with genetic variation but even more remarkable were similarities in temperament and interests. MZ twins reared apart were almost as similar as MZ twins reared together. The authors concluded that for almost every behavioural trait so far investigated, from reaction time to religiosity, an important fraction of the variation among people turns out to be associated with genetic variation (Bouchard et al 1990).

The authors stress that these findings should not, however, be interpreted to reinforce a deterministic view of behaviour: 'the remarkable similarity of MZ (reared apart) twins in social attitudes (for example traditionalism and religiosity) does not show that parents cannot influence those traits, but simply that this does not tend to happen in most families'.

Twin and adoption studies have provided impressive evidence in support of the notion that IQ and many behavioural and emotional measures are at least partly inherited. However, even in the case of MZ twins reared together, similarities of IQ and temperament are far from perfect and differences within families as much as differences between families require understanding if we are to explain the variability in personality development observed in children brought up together.

PRENATAL EFFECTS

Just as in childhood when the development of an individual's personality depends on the continuous interplay between genetically determined dispositions and social and cultural environmental factors, so in prenatal life fetal development may be modified at all stages by environmental happenings and fluctuations in the intrauterine chemical milieu.

Teratology is the field of research which is concerned with the causes of abnormal fetal development. Hereditary factors, including chromosomal aberrations and genetic mutations, are a major cause of fetal death or defect, and some environmental hazards such as exposure to radiation may be harmful to the fetus by a direct effect on the chromosomes. Interference with cell growth and differentiation in the early stages of development, such as that caused by infection with rubella virus, *Toxoplasma gondii* and cytomegalovirus during early pregnancy can lead to major abnormalities, including mental retardation, eye, ear and heart malformations. Fetal maldevelopment may also be due to maternal illnesses such as diabetes, phenylketonuria and obstetric complications which interfere with placental circulation. A variety of drugs have been implicated in fetal malformations and the effect may depend critically on the stage of fetal development during which exposure occurs. Thalidomide interferes with the development of fetal limbs. Retardation of fetal growth has been linked to the use of barbiturates, amphetamine and nicotine (Royal College of Psychiatrists 1987).

Drugs may also have more covert effects on the developing fetus, causing subtle changes in behaviour without being linked to physical deformities. This has given rise to the concept of behavioural teratology. It is postulated that departures from an optimal chemical environment in utero can affect the finer differentiation of the nervous system so as to cause enduring personality distortion in the offspring. Examples are methadone and heroin, neither of which causes gross physical abnormalities in the fetus, but children exposed to these drugs before birth show altered behaviour. In the neonatal period they may show an abstinence syndrome with unusually strong reflexes, irritability, sleep disturbance and failure to gain weight. At 4 years they are said to show short atten-

tion span and hyperactivity (Kolata 1978). There is now considerable evidence that persistently raised blood lead levels may cause cognitive impairment and increase the risk of behavioural difficulties in children (Rutter 1980b).

An understanding of teratogenic effects must take account of the gestational stage at the time of exposure, the health, nutrition and drug consumption of the mother and, finally, the genetic predisposition which may render some individuals more susceptible than others to specific insults. The prolonged period of development of the brain in utero renders this structure extremely susceptible to teratogenic effects. After about the third week of gestation the brain begins to differentiate from the anterior portion of the embryonic neural tube. By the fourth week, forebrain, midbrain and hindbrain vesicles have developed, and by the seventh week bulges appear which will later become the two hemispheres. Cerebellar growth starts during the second month, and in the latter half of pregnancy a period of rapid growth occurs during which the cerebral hemispheres become convoluted and there is active dendrite growth, synapse formation and axonal myelination. The vulnerability of the central nervous system may be greatest during periods of rapid brain growth, and these occur in the human during the first trimester and again from the third trimester to 18 months of postnatal life. Brain weight doubles during the first year of life and triples in 5 years, by which time it is 90% of its adult size. Early disruption of brain development by a teratogen during the stage of organogenesis is likely to lead to permanent, irreversible structural damage affecting the brain, limbs and other organs and be associated with severe mental retardation. Later in gestation, toxins may cause more selective impairments.

Animal studies of the effects of alcohol on the fetus illustrate the variety of ways in which a single teratogen may affect the nervous system. The cerebellum appears particularly vulnerable to alcohol exposure in rats during the period of rapid cerebellar growth during the later stages of gestation (Borges & Lewis 1982). When maternal rats are fed liquid diets containing ethanol their offspring show a number of fine histological changes, including abnormal distribution of nerve terminals in the hippocampus (West et al 1981), alterations in amine and peptide neurotransmitter systems (Schoemaker et al 1983), and impaired myelination (Druse & Hofteig 1977). The effect of alcohol on the fetus also illustrates the importance of genetic susceptibility. The expression of the enzyme alcohol dehydrogenase responsible for the metabolism of ethanol is under genetic control.

Embryos early in development do not possess this enzyme, and are thus rendered more susceptible to the direct toxic effect of alcohol on embryonic cellular proliferation. Chernoff (1977) showed that a strain of mouse with low alcohol dehydrogenase activity was more sensitive to the effect of ethanol on growth and morphology than a mouse strain with greater enzyme activity.

Teratogens may also affect the fetus indirectly, for example by causing hypoglycaemia or hypothermia or by interfering with placental transport of nutrients to the fetus. An advantage of animal studies is that effects of single teratogens can be studied in isolation. It becomes vastly more difficult in humans to isolate the effects on development of agents such as alcohol, where often quite subtle effects on development may be difficult to disentangle from associated social and medical factors affecting maternal health.

Alcohol and the human fetus

Alcohol is possibly the most widely studied of all teratogens, and recent interest in the effect of maternal drinking behaviour on fetal development has been comprehensively reviewed (Rosett & Weiner 1984, Plant 1985). During the 18th century in Britain, attempts were made by the London College of Physicians to draw public attention to the excessive consumption of gin by women as a cause of 'weak, feeble and distempered children'. In 1899 William Sullivan recorded a very high rate of infant mortality and severe malformations amongst children born to alcoholic mothers in a Liverpool prison. Several of these women later bore healthy children when prison confinement had forced them to abstain from alcohol.

Recent interest in the effects of alcohol on the fetus began with the study in France by Lemoine et al (1968). Of 127 children from families with chronic alcoholism, 25 children had physical malformations characterised by a common facial profile. They were below average IQ and had detectable behaviour problems, including hyperactivity and language and motor developmental delays. The term fetal alcohol syndrome (FAS) was later introduced to define a specific pattern of malformation which is found in some of the offspring of alcoholic mothers (Jones et al 1973). The diagnosis of FAS is based on the presence of the following signs (Rosett 1980):

1 Prenatal and/or postnatal growth retardation
2 Central nervous system involvement which often includes developmental delays and intellectual impairment, and

3 A characteristic facies which at its most severe includes microcephaly, thin upper lip, small palpebral fissures, flat maxillary area and poorly developed philtrum.

FAS is associated with severe mental retardation and behavioural disturbance but lesser degrees of abnormality are also reported in offspring of alcoholic mothers. These children are more prone to hyperactivity, disturbed language development, poor motor skills and sleep disturbance, effects which may be observed in the absence of facial dysmorphism. Many studies have confirmed the initial description of FAS, and it is likely that this reflects an extreme of a wide range of possible effects of maternal alcohol consumption on the fetus.

The effect on the fetus of moderate social drinking during pregnancy is less easy to quantify because failure to thrive is associated with a number of other risk factors, including age, parity, illness, malnutrition, cigarette smoking, drug use and abuse, and socioeconomic status (Miller & Merritt 1979). In a study by Plant (1985), more than 1000 women were interviewed when they attended antenatal clinics during the 12th week of pregnancy, and data were obtained on the pattern of alcohol consumption and other variables, including smoking habits, diet, drug abuse, medication, physical health and social status. Three groups of women were described: (1) abstainers, who had consumed no alcohol since conception (21.7%); (2) light drinkers who had consumed between 1 and 4 units on the maximum drinking day since conception (50.3%); and (3) heavy drinkers who had consumed 5 or more units (28%). Subjects were re-interviewed when 34 weeks pregnant, and pregnancy outcome was assessed by full paediatric assessment within 24 hours of birth and at 12 weeks after birth. The results showed that a number of birth abnormalities and perinatal difficulties were individually significantly associated with baseline alcohol consumption. Women whose maximum daily alcohol consumption during the first trimester had exceeded 10 units were significantly more likely than others to have produced babies with two or more abnormalities. These abnormalities included perinatal problems such as mild jaundice and lower birth weight. Further analysis was then conducted using stepwise multiple regression in an attempt to clarify the importance of alcohol as a cause of fetal harm. The results clearly showed that alcohol was not strongly predictive of fetal complications and the factors which accounted for the greatest variance in the multiple regressions were tobacco and illegal drugs. Although heavy drinkers were more at risk of producing damaged babies, factors such as smoking, maternal malnutrition and illicit drug abuse counted for as much of the variance as did alcohol consumption. In this group of women attending antenatal clinics, there was not one case of FAS.

However, the influence of moderate maternal drinking on fetal development remains controversial since some workers have obtained results suggesting that moderate alcohol consumption in pregnancy is a cause of fetal harm (Hanson et al 1978, Streissguth 1983). Landesman-Dwyer et al (1981) observed impaired attention and increased fidgetiness in 4-year-old children whose mothers had been moderate drinkers during pregnancy. However, factors such as maternal personality were not taken into account in this study.

In a detailed examination of the research literature on the effects of drinking during pregnancy, Knupfer (1991) found 'substantial evidence that very heavy drinking by pregnant women, such as that often consumed by alcoholics — a pint of whisky or 12 beers a day — does increase the risk of foetal damage', but no evidence that light drinking by pregnant women harms the fetus. Studies which claim to have found evidence of harmful effects on the fetus of moderate social drinking by mothers were criticised on the grounds that they inadequately classified the drinking practices of the mothers.

MALNUTRITION

The psychological, social and developmental implications of hunger have been studied in detail among several different groups, including deprived city dwellers in affluent countries, rural inhabitants of Third World countries, and following acute disasters such as the famine in Holland in 1944–1945 at the end of World War II. A description of the effects of maternal malnutrition on fetal development must take account of several factors:

1. The state of development when the child suffers undernourishment; are there critical periods for the fetus or neonate?
2. The severity of malnourishment and the effects of specific dietary deficiencies such as iodine
3. The mother/child relationship and cultural factor which in situations of poverty will interact with the effects of nutritional deprivation (Stein & Susser 1985, Martin et al 1990).

Effects of malnutrition on early fetal development

Specific nutritional deficits may profoundly affect early embryonic development. Iodine deficiency, which is endemic in many areas of the world, including the Himalayas, New Guinea and Indonesia, causes growth defects and later mental retardation. Connelly et al (1979) showed that deficits in psychometric testing attributable to iodine deficiency in the mother could be prevented by injecting women before conception with iodinised oil.

Both acute and chronic starvation during the first trimester of pregnancy increase the risk of neural tube defects in the fetus. This was shown in the Dutch famine in 1945. Women who experienced starvation during the early stages of their pregnancy subsequently showed an excess of stillbirths and low birth weight premature infants (Stein et al 1975). Amongst the surviving children followed up 19 years later there was an excess of cerebral palsy and neural tube defects (Stein & Susser 1976).

Maternal starvation during the second and third trimester of pregnancy also causes low birth weight and developmental delays. Winick (1976) has reviewed the relationship between malnutrition and human brain development. Studies from Africa, South America, India and the USA have shown that marasmic children who die have small brains, and studies in Africa indicated that children malnourished in early life continue in later life to have reduced head circumference (Hoorweg & Stanfield 1976, Stoch & Smythe 1976). An important question is how the low birth weight of these infants born to malnourished mothers affects subsequent mental performance.

Experiments in rats suggest that malnourishment of the mother when the embryo is at a critical period of rapid brain growth around the time of birth will cause loss of brain weight, reduction in total cell numbers, distortion of cellular composition and impaired development of neurotransmitter systems in the infant rat. However, nutritional rehabilitation after weaning can correct some of these aberrations in rats and can modify synaptogenesis (Balasz et al 1979). It appears that, in response to undernutrition, regulatory mechanisms cause a drop in cell numbers in the rat brain by slowing down the rate of DNA synthesis so that brain growth is delayed by a lengthening of the cell cycle time. The result is a slowing of growth, correctable by later nutritional rehabilitation, rather than a permanent alteration of structures. Humans, even more than animals, show a remarkable ability to restore mental functioning after a period of delayed development due to malnourishment.

Infants who had been exposed to the Dutch famine during the third trimester and who had showed evidence at birth of marked growth retardation were surveyed 19 years later when it was found that exposure to famine in infancy had produced virtually no permanent effects on mental or physical health (Stein et al 1976). In keeping with this observation is the absence of mental impairment in children whose malnourishment is caused by paediatric diseases, such as cystic fibrosis and pyloric stenosis, and who are brought up in a normal stimulating environment. However, this is not an argument for complacency about the effects of undernutrition, as it has been amply confirmed that poor nutrition is often associated with intellectual impairment.

In a major study in Jamaica, children who were admitted to hospital in the first 2 years of life on account of severe malnutrition were followed up to age 6–9 years. Their intellectual level was found to be significantly lower than that of controls consisting of the nearest sibling within the family exposed to a similar home environment (Hertzig et al 1972). Furthermore, these malnourished children had poor attention and were reported to have poorer social skills, especially in their ability to get on well with classmates (Waterlow 1974).

Social factors are important in determining the outcome of periods of undernutrition in children. Malnutrition may impair mental development by causing apathy, passivity and reduced exploratory behaviour in addition to any direct effects on the brain. Cravioto (1977) has carried out pioneering work among families in a Mexican village on the interaction between the effects of environmental stimulation and starvation in children's development. He described the low level of stimulation provided by a passive mother unaware of the needs of her child and responding to him poorly as the characteristic feature of a home environment which leads to severe malnutrition in children of poor families.

This view is supported by several large-scale studies. Winick et al (1975) studied 141 Korean orphans adopted before the age of 2 years by largely middle-class American parents. These children included a group who were severely malnourished before adoption, both height and weight being below the third percentile for the Korean average. The second group were described as moderately well nourished, being between the third and 24th percentile in height and weight, and the third group were well nourished, i.e.

above the 25th percentile. When examined a few years later during elementary schooling in the USA, all three groups were performing as well as expected from an average US population and the IQ of all three groups reached the mean for US children. Nevertheless, there were still significant differences in IQ and performance between the malnourished and the well-nourished group. It was concluded that the stigmata of malnutrition had not been entirely eliminated but that a prolonged programme of environmental enrichment and normal nutrition had resulted in IQ and achievement scores around the population mean.

More recently, Weber et al (1981) performed a study in Bogota, Colombia, to examine the effect of two types of intervention — nutritional supplements and maternal education — on the cognitive development of children who were undernourished. A door-to-door survey identified mothers during their first or second trimester of pregnancy. Families were selected if there was at least one child under the age of 5 years who showed signs of undernourishment. A total of 433 families were studied and allotted to a control group and five different treatment groups. One group were given food supplements for 3 years, starting when the mother was in her third trimester of pregnancy. A second group received no food supplement, but a trained home visitor carried out a programme to educate mothers in providing a stimulating environment to increase play and exploratory activity in the child. A third group received both types of intervention. Food supplements of 623 cal and 20 g of protein available to all family members were provided at special centres and infants were regularly tested for physical growth characteristics and mental development at intervals up to 3 years of age.

The principal finding of the study was that both food supplementation and the educational programme were beneficial and appeared to affect the children's behaviour independently. Food supplementation had a more marked effect on tests of motor skills, whereas the maternal education programme had a greater effect on improving language ability.

A further part of the study compared the effects of food supplementation given only until a child was 6 months old with that given to a child between 6 months and 3 years of age. The result showed that any food supplementation in the first 3 years of life was beneficial and there was no evidence that the first 6 months of life constituted a critical period. Children who received food supplements starting at 6 months of age did just as well as children in families receiving supplements from the time their mother was in the third trimester of pregnancy.

The response to nutritional and educational interventions following malnourishment attests to the remarkable plasticity of the developing nervous system, and also shows that under conditions of poverty and deprivation the quality of the child's immediate environment cannot be separated from purely physical considerations, such as protein and calorie intake.

Animals studies confirm the effects of an enriched environment on brain growth. If, during the time the brain is growing at its fastest, monkeys are reared in an interesting environment that calls forth exploratory behaviour, the brain grows larger and heavier than if the environment is a dull one and the detailed development of the neurones is altered, with more dendritic spines and branches (Floeter & Greenough 1979).

As part of a long-term study in the USA into the prevention of intellectual impairment in children of impoverished families, Martin et al (1990) have reported on the effectiveness of the early provision of stimulating day care to help the children achieve their potential in intelligence. Children who took part in the project were from low-income multi-problem families and their mothers were generally young with low IQs and low educational level.

One group of children who entered day care between 6 and 12 weeks of age and who continued with the provision of a stimulating and friendly environment for 5 days a week performed consistently better than a stay-at-home control group on tests of IQ and intellectual development. Some children have been followed up for over 4 years and the findings support the view that educational day care, maternal intelligence and home environment each contribute to the development of the children's intellectual abilities.

HYPOXIA AND LOW BIRTH WEIGHT

Numerous studies have shown how minor degrees of neural defect of early origin can be associated with subsequent subtle personality deviations. One example is provided by a study conducted in St Louis (Corah et al 1965). The children were all born in the same hospital in the same period, but 134 were normal full-term newborns and 101 were full-term newborns who, at the time, were recorded as showing signs of hypoxia. Corah et al successfully traced these 235 children when they were 7 years old. Neurological, psychological and psychiatric examinations were conducted throughout the whole of a day, without knowledge of their status at birth. Neurological examination failed to distinguish between those who had been hypoxic 7

years before and those who had not. However, psychological assessment showed that those who had been hypoxic at birth were, at the age of 7 years, more often 'explosive', 'obtuse' or 'lacking in social sensitivity'. They were more impulsive, more rigid and were liable to a greater degree of distractibility.

An even more striking illustration of relationships between personality maladjustment, multiple congenital handicaps, and family stress in early life is provided by the studies of low birth weight Edinburgh children by Drillien who followed them over a period of many years. The 600 children in her study were born between 1953 and 1955. One-third had a birth weight of under 2000 g. In the subsequent 5 years all children were seen at home by the same investigator on a minimum of seven occasions, and ratings of the parental relationship in the home, in terms of family stress, were made. The children were later assessed in their second year at school (Drillien 1963) and again when they were 11–12 years old (Drillien 1969).

Early in the study it became clear that children who had been of low birth weight frequently experienced intellectual difficulties at school, and also in their personality adjustment as rated by schoolteachers. When aged about 7 years, the children were more maladjusted if they had been of low birth weight and this was true irrespective of birth complications or family stress. However, if there was family stress a well-adjusted personality was less likely.

Where there had been complications of birth, the situation was also bad, and if there had been family stress and complications at birth, the liability to maladjustment was greater still. When family stress and complications of birth were combined with low birth weight, the mean score on the Social Adjustment Guide was 20 (the maximum), which indicates that the average child in these circumstances was severely maladjusted.

The children were reviewed again when aged 11–12 years. Those who had been of adequate birth weight scored more highly on group IQ tests than those who had been underweight. Boys were always worse affected by low birth weight than girls. At this later age the behavioural abnormalities, though causing less marked differences than at the age of 7 years, were still apparent in the case of boys from average working-class homes.

Neligan et al (1976) conducted studies on three groups of children aged around 7 years. They looked at babies who had been born too soon, the really premature who were born before day 255 of pregnancy; and they looked at another group who were born too small, being undergrown and underweight for their dates. There was also a group of random controls. Smoking more than five cigarettes per day by the mothers was associated with babies being born too soon and, even more so, too small.

On virtually every assessment the controls came out best, and children who had been underweight for their dates came out significantly the worst. Those who had been very underweight for their dates were of least intelligence, their linguistic skills the poorest and their ability to handle visual concepts and to read was worst. The controls came out best in tests of dexterity, and in psychiatrists' blind ratings covering such aspects as sociability, aggressiveness and anxiety. When the children were aged 7 years, schoolteachers made ratings of fidgeting, solitariness, fussiness, and being attention-seeking. Again, those children who were underweight for dates came out worst, and this also emerged when neurologists made assessments of needless gesturings.

While most studies suggest that low birth weight may lead to later intellectual impairment, the effect is greatly exacerbated when perinatal complications occur in children who are also socially disadvantaged. As is the case with malnutrition, alcohol exposure and other pre- and perinatal hazards, a 'good' postnatal environment can make up for these physical disadvantages except in instances of sever handicap. Women who are socially disadvantaged tend to be in poorer health, have less adequate nutrition and make less use of prenatal care than mothers who are better off. The evidence suggests that there is a causal connection between low birth weight and reduced IQ, but much of the effect is due to the relatively impoverished conditions in which the child is reared (Madge & Tizard 1980).

PHYSICAL ABNORMALITIES AND PERSONALITY

There is some evidence to suggest an association between multiple minor physical abnormalities at birth and subsequent behavioural disorder in children. Waldrop et al (1978) looked for physical abnormalities such as abnormal head circumference, malformed ears, low-set ears or a curved fifth finger in 30 newborn infants. Three years later ratings were made for such things as short attention span, aggression with fears and overactivity. These behavioural features were shown to be significantly correlated with the presence of minor physical abnormalities at birth.

There are a number of circumstances in which body build, physical attributes and the presence of minor physical anomalies may have an effect on an individual's development. Peripheral physical stigmata may be a consequence of early fetal maldevelopment which also affects the central nervous system. Dysmorphisms of hair, eyes, ears, fingers and toes appear to be selectively linked to central nervous system dysfunction and are frequently found in the mental handicap population, such as Down's syndrome and fragile X syndrome. Congenital influences may also indirectly lead to brain damage, as, for example, in children born with congenital heart disease who are at risk of ischaemic brain damage secondary to birth cyanosis. Physical appearance and body build may also influence personality development by the response of peers or parents to physical handicap. Unattractive preschool children are less popular than attractive children of the same age, and are therefore more likely to express aggressive or dependent behaviour (Rapoport 1980). However, in a study of boys treated for hyperactivity, the presence of minor abnormal physical signs was associated with birth complications and a father with a history of hyperactivity (Quinn & Rapoport 1974), which suggests that social, psychological and genetic mechanisms may each contribute to the weak associations observed between minor physical anomalies and behaviour disorder in children. Most studies suggest that children with cleft lip and palate are not significantly emotionally maladjusted, and the results of studies on disturbed children tend to the conclusion that the presence of minor physical anomalies indicates either genetic predisposition or environmental hazard early in development.

SEX DETERMINATION AND ENDOCRINE EFFECTS

Normal brain development can be affected when the internal milieu of the fetus is deranged by endocrine dysfunctions. Endocrine function in the fetus may also affect aspects of normal personality development rather specifically and this is illustrated by the way that oestrogens and androgens may influence adult sexual behaviour.

The presence of a Y chromosome in an embryo ensures that the embryonic gonad (the genital ridge) differentiates into testes about 6 weeks after conception. In a female the presence of two X chromosomes ensures that the gonad will differentiate into ovaries at around 12 weeks. The differentiation of testes rather than ovaries from the genital ridge in the embryo is the central event in sex determination and is due to the activity of a recently isolated testis-determining gene situated on the Y chromosome (Sinclair et al 1990).

Other differences between the sexes result from the action of hormones produced by the gonads. The developing testes synthesise androgens which promote the development of male genitalia and in the absence of these androgens, the embryo will develop female characteristics.

The testis-determining gene acting probably for a rather brief period during the first few weeks of embryonic development appears to be the critical switch for initiating sex differentiation and is likely to be part of a cascade of regulatory genes, each contributing to normal male and female development through the action of hormones.

Although sex-typed behaviours are to some extent influenced by the expectations of the culture, so that by the age of 2 or 3 years children are aware of the sex role which adults expect of them (Kuhn et al 1978), there is considerable evidence that a person's concept of himself or herself as male or female (gender identity), as well as sex-typed behaviour, are hormonally influenced.

Some clinical situations suggest that hormones may influence human sex related behaviour. In the adrenogenital syndrome there is an excessive prenatal production of androgens by the adrenal glands, which leads to virilisation in girls born with this condition. Ehrhardt & Baker (1974) observed that 17 girls with the fetal adrenogenital syndrome not only tended to behave as 'tomboys', but a third of them reported that they would prefer to be a boy or were undecided on their sex preference. These differences in sexual behaviour were significant when the group was compared with their unaffected sisters. Boys with the adrenogenital syndrome differ little from their brothers, apart from showing increased activity in outdoor play.

The importance of biological factors in psycho-sexual development is reinforced by the observations of Imperato-McGinley et al (1979) in their study of an unusual inherited form of male pseudohermaph-roditism identified from 23 interrelated families in three rural villages in the Dominican Republic. These subjects were born with female external genitalia due to a deficiency in dihydrotestosterone in utero. However, their plasma testosterone levels were normal. Eighteen subjects were raised as girls until puberty, at which time 16 of the 18 successfully adopted a male gender role. The authors concluded that the exposure of the brain to normal levels of testosterone during development ensured the formation of male gender identity and that this overrode the social and cultural effects of rearing as girls.

The effect of prenatal oestrogens on male development has been studied in boys born to diabetic mothers who had been given oestrogens during pregnancy (Yalom et al 1973). Aggression, assertiveness and athleticism were all reported to be reduced in this group of boys. In contrast, the administration of oestrogens to adult men with prostatic cancer, though responsible for the appearance of secondary sexual characteristics such as breast development, caused no alteration in either gender identity or sex-typed behaviours (Money & Ehrhardt 1972).

Animal studies have consistently shown that fetal exposure to gonadal steroids influences adult sex-related behaviour through an effect on the morphogenesis and survival of specific groups of neurones at critical periods of development (Arnold & Gorski 1984). The idea of structural sex differences in the central nervous system received support in 1973 when Raisman & Field found sex differences in rats in the fine dendritic structure of the preoptic area of the hypothalamus which could be reversed by manipulations of neonatal androgens. Since then, so-called sexually dimorphic areas of the brain have been identified in several species and in humans. The preoptic area of the rat hypothalamus is of interest because it has important regulatory functions in the control of masculine sexual behaviour and the cyclical release of gonadotrophins for ovulation. Within this preoptic area Gorski et al (1978) identified a distinct nucleus that was much larger in males than females and the development of this nucleus appeared to be almost totally determined by the hormonal environment during early development. Enlargement only occurred in the presence of androgens perinatally, and in the adult rat there was no further response to steroids (Arnold & Gorski 1984).

Sexual dimorphisms in the central nervous system are apparent not only in the structural morphology of specific brain regions but in the number of oestrogen and progestogen receptors in selected hypothalamic nuclei. Rainbow et al (1982) have suggested that these receptor changes could account for the sex-related neuroendocrine and behavioural responses to gonadal hormones.

Regions of the anterior hypothalamus have also been implicated in mating activities in monkeys. Stimulation of the preoptic area, lateral hypothalamus and dorsomedial nucleus of the hypothalamus induced sexual behavioural responses (Perachio et al 1979) whereas lesions to these structures reduced or completely eliminated sexual activity in male monkeys (Slimp et al 1978).

In the comparable region of the human hypothalamus, two small groups of neurones show sexual dimorphism and are found to be nearly twice as large in men as in women (Allen et al 1989). Further evidence that these hypothalamic regions are involved in the generation of human male sexual behaviour comes from a recent comparison of the volume of these nuclei in post mortem tissue obtained from three subject groups: women, heterosexual men and homosexual men. One of these small interstitial nuclei of the anterior hypothalamus was almost twice as large in heterosexual men as in women or in homosexual men (Le Vay 1991). Together with an earlier report (Swaab and Hofmann 1990), this finding suggests that sexual orientation at least in part has a biological substrate. To answer questions about what factors could influence the development of sexually dimorphic regions in the human hypothalamus, it may be useful to turn to animal studies. In rodents, a strong relationship has been established between male sexual activity, plasma testosterone level and the size of the sexually dimorphic nucleus in the hypothalamus (Anderson et al 1986). The growth of this nucleus is very sensitive to the presence of circulating androgens derived from the testis during critical periods of brain development before and immediately after birth.

The results of animal studies should still be interpreted cautiously and it is a large jump to apply findings in rodents and even primates to human development. Sexual differentiation of the brain involves systems concerned with social and aggressive, as well as specifically sexual, behaviours and there is as yet little substantial information about fetal hormonal influences on these aspects of human behaviour. Nevertheless, animal studies and recent human post mortem findings linking sexual behaviour to specific structures within the brain may lead the way to understanding the biological basis of other types of complex behaviour.

SPECIFICITY AND PLASTICITY IN THE NERVOUS SYSTEM

Although it is rarely possible to bridge the gap between brain structure and specific behaviours, it can reasonably be assumed that normal neurogenesis and maturation of the nervous system is a requirement for normal personality development. Experiments with rodents suggest that lesions to the visual system in young animals may lead to the formation of anomalous pathways and the development of quite abnormal visually related behaviours when the animals grow older (Sneider & Jhaveri 1974). The importance of anomalous neuronal connections resulting from early developmental events as a cause of behavioural and personality changes in humans remains specula-

tive, and ideas as to how genetic and environmental influences on personality operate at the physiological and neurochemical level are still in their infancy. However, two major topics in developmental neurobiology, the phenomena of specificity and of plasticity of neuronal connections, illustrate how genetic endowment and environmental inputs continuously interact during maturation and into adulthood.

The maturation of the nervous system is a highly ordered process beginning with the differentiation of cells into various subtypes of neurones and glia. A neurone differs from all other cells in the body in that its function is determined not only by what subclass of neurone it belongs to but also by its highly specific array of synaptic connections. Neurones in the human brain may make many synapses with other cells and, if information transfer between cells is to be discrete and reliable, connections between neurones must to a large degree be programmed genetically. However, total specificity of connections between neurones would not allow the nervous system to modify its responses according to experience. In other words, memory and learning require that some connections are continually being strengthened or weakened according to the pattern of activity within the neural network. The growth of a neurone in a particular spatial pattern which enables its dendrites to achieve highly selective synaptic connections with neighbouring groups of cells is termed neural specificity; the ability of neurones to adapt their synaptic connections according to use and disuse represents neural plasticity. Central neurones are generally not capable of division and are not replaced when they die, so it is by changes in the number of synapses between neurones and in the relative importance of one input as compared to another that neuronal populations adapt.

After the stage of proliferation of cells, which initially takes place in the germinal layer of the neural tube, neurones migrate to various locations in the central nervous system and begin to form what will later become specific brain structures. There is considerable redundancy of cells, and selective death of a proportion of neurones occurs. Differentiation continues by neurones adopting different types of neurotransmitter and developing axonal and dendritic projections, and it is at this stage, when synapses are forming, that specificity of connections is of great importance. For example, it is essential if the organism is to benefit from vision that the photoreceptors in the retina are precisely 'wired' through the visual pathways to the appropriate part of the visual cortex.

Over a century ago, Ramon y Cajal proposed his chemotropic theory of axon guidance and the work of Sperry (1963) on the optic system of amphibians developed the idea that specificity of synaptic connections is achieved through a process by which growing axons recognise specific chemical surface recognition sites on their target cell. In a classical experiment the optic nerve of a frog was severed and the eye rotated through 180°. In amphibia, unlike mammals, the retinal axons regenerate and grow back to the optic tectum so that vision is restored within a few weeks. Following eye rotation these animals recovered and behaved as if their visual world had been rotated, indicating a built-in specificity between the retina and the optic tectum which enabled the regenerating axon to be guided to and to recognise its postsynaptic target in a precise but rigid way.

Further studies have tended to confirm the importance of chemical recognition in guiding axons into making appropriate contacts. Recent work (Hankin and Lund 1991) has revealed that, during the development of the visual pathway in the embryo, axons growing out from the retina are guided to their correct target in the midbrain tectum by two processes. In the first stage, axons spread along the surface of the brain stem directed by surface chemical cues. The arrival of axons at their correct target in the tectum then triggers a second process by which target-derived homing agents are released which guide the growth of new axons and ensures the survival of those cells which successfully make the correct anatomic connection.

The neuronal response to injury is more readily studied in the periphery than in the central nervous system. By examining the pattern of re-innervation, which takes place in the superior cervical ganglion after preganglionic nerve injury, inferences can be drawn about synaptic specificity and plasticity which may be relevant to processes taking place in the central nervous system during development. Neurones in the superior cervical ganglion are innervated in a highly selective manner by axons arising in the spinal cord. In a remarkable process of regeneration, following injury to the preganglionic nerve fibres, preganglionic axons from the spinal cord seek out and connect with particular neurones in the sympathetic ganglion, which becomes re-innervated in such a way that specificity of function is fully restored.

The factors which bring about this selectivity in regeneration may include a 'chemoaffinity' process, but other mechanisms also operate. There is evidence that the release of trophic factors, the best charac-terised of which is nerve growth factor (NGF), helps to orchestrate the growth of axons and encourage re-innervation (Berg 1984). It has also been suggested that there are competitive interactions within the group of axons which reach a particular target, so that some connections are eliminated and others are stabilised. It now seems clear that it is the pattern of electrical activity in the axons themselves which enables some synapses to survive at the expense of others (Oppenheim & Chu-Wang 1983). The formation of neuronal circuits in the brain during development is a complex process which involves both a genetically predetermined growth of gross structures and a degree of 'fine tuning' of synaptic connections in response to use and disuse of pathways.

The work of Hubel (1982) and Wiesel (1982) provides an example of plasticity in response to visual experience in the development of binocular vision in the cat. In the visual cortex of adult animals stripes of cortex receive a visual input only from one or other eye. These so-called ocular dominance columns develop gradually after birth and form the basis of binocular vision. If activity in one eye is reduced by lid suture at birth, ocular dominance columns fail to develop for that eye when it is tested 6 weeks later. Visual experience and impulse activity in the visual pathway appear to be critical for the formation and stabilisation of these synapses. Further studies by Kasamatsu (1983) have suggested that, following depletion of neocortical noradrenaline in the visual cortex, ocular dominance failed to develop fully, implicating this neurotransmitter in neuronal plasticity of the visual system during a critical period of development.

Plasticity appears to be a property of the developing nervous system which is rapidly lost in many structures, including the visual cortex, after birth. However, in some regions of the brain, particularly the hippocampus and related limbic structures believed to be involved in the acquisition of learning and memory, there is evidence of continuing plasticity throughout life. In the perforant pathway of the hippocampus, brief trains of high-frequency electrical stimulation lasting for only a few seconds increase the amplitude of evoked potentials for several days, and sometimes weeks, indicating that the efficiency of these synapses can be dramatically altered by certain types of use (Bliss & Gardner-Medwin 1973). Much recent understanding of the cellular mechanisms of learning and memory is derived from this phenomenon known as long-term potentiation of synaptic transmission. It appears that trains of electrical stimulation or brief seizure episodes can set in motion, in some hippocampal pathways, a chain of synaptic events which includes alterations in gene expression, sprouting of fibres and the development of new synaptic contacts between neurones (Ben Ari & Represa 1990). This is only one example in neurobiology of a mechanism which can be studied at the cellular level and which can explain how genetic and environmental factors may react to determine behaviour.

REFERENCES

Allen L S, Hines M, Shryne J E, Gorski R A 1989 Two sexually dimorphic cell groups in the human brain. Journal of Neuroscience 9: 497

Anderson R H, Fleming D E, Rhees R W, Kinghorn E 1986 Relationships between sexual activity, plasma testosterone and the volume of the sexually dimorphic nucleus of the preoptic area in prenatally stressed and non stressed rats. Brain Research 370: 1

Arnold A P, Gorski R A 1984 Gonadal steroid induction of structural sex differences in the central nervous system. Annual Review of Neuroscience 7: 413

Balasaz R, Lewis P D, Patel A J 1979 Nutritional deficiencies and brain development. In: Falkner F, Tanner J N (eds) Human growth, vol 3. Plenum Press, New York

Ben Ari Y, Repressa A 1990 Brief seizure episodes induce long term potentiation and mossy fibre sprouting in the hippocampus. Trends Neurosci 13: 312–8

Berg D K 1984 New neuronal growth factors. Annual Review of Neuroscience 7: 149

Bliss T U P, Gardner-Medwin A R 1973 Long lasting potentiation of synaptic transmission in the dentate area of the unanaesthetised rabbit following stimulation of the perforant path. Journal of Physiology (London) 232: 357

Borges S, Lewis P D 1982 A study of alcohol effects on the brain during gestation and lactation. Teratology 25: 283

Bouchard T J, Lykken D T, McGue M, Segal N L, Tellegen A 1990 The sources of human psychological differences: the Minnesota study of twins reared apart. Science 250: 223

Chernoff G F 1977 The foetal alcohol syndrome in mice: an animal model. Teratology 15: 223

Connelly K J, Pharaoh P O, Hetzel B 1979 Fetal iodine deficiency and motor performance during childhood. Lancet ii: 149

Corah N L, Anthony E J, Painter P, Stern J A, Thurston D 1965 Effects of perinatal anoxia after seven years. Psychological Monographs 79: 3

Cravioto J 1977 Not by bread alone: effects of early malnutrition and stimuli deprivation on mental development. In: Ghai O P (ed) Perspectives in paediatrics. Indian Interprint, New Delhi

Drillien C M 1963 Obstetric hazard, mental retardation and behaviour disturbance in primary school. Developmental Medicine and Child Neurology 5: 3

Drillien C M 1969 School disposal and performance from children of different birth weight born 1953–1960. Archives of Diseases in Childhood 44: 562

Druse M J, Hofteig J H 1977 The effect of chronic maternal alcohol consumption on the development of central nervous myelin subfractions in rat offspring. Drug and Alcohol Dependence 2: 421

Ehrhardt A A, Baker S W 1974 Fetal androgens, human central nervous system differentiation, and behaviour sex differences. In: Friedman R C, Richart R M, Vande Wiele R L (eds) Sex differences in behavior. Wiley, New York

Eysenck H J, Eysenck S B G 1975 Manual of the Eysenck personality questionnaire. Hodder & Stoughton, London

Floeter M K, Greenough W T 1979 Cerebellar plasticity: modification of Purkinje cell structure by differential rearing in monkeys. Science 206: 227

Gorski R A, Gordon J H, Shryne J E, Southam A M 1978 Evidence for a morphological sex difference within the medical proptic area of the rat brain. Brain Research 148: 333

Hankin M, Lund R 1991 How do retinal axons find their targets in developing brain? Trends in Neurological Science 14: 224

Hanson J W, Streissguth A P, Smith D W 1978 The effects of moderate alcohol consumption during pregnancy on fetal growth and morphogenesis. Journal of Paediatrics 92: 457

Hay D A 1985 Essentials of behaviour genetics. Blackwell, Oxford

Hertzig M E, Birch H G, Richardson S A, Tizard J 1972 Intellectual levels of school children severely malnourished during the first two years of life. Paediatrics 49: 814

Holden C 1980 Identical twins reared apart. Science 207: 1323

Hoorweg J, Stanfield J P 1976 The effects of protein malnutrition in early childhood on intellectual and motor abilities in later childhood and adolescence. Developmental Medicine and Child Neurology 18: 330

Horn J M 1983 The Texas adoption project: adopted children and their intellectual resemblance to biological and adoptive parents. Child Development 54: 268

Hubel D H, 1982 Exploration of the primary visual cortex 1955-78. Nature 299: 515–524

Imperato-McGinley J, Peterson R E, Gautier T, Sturla E 1979 Androgens and the evolution of male gender identity among male Pseudohermaphrodites with 5 alpha-reductase deficiency. New England Journal of Medicine 300: 1233

Jones K L, Smith D W, Ulleland C N, Streissguth A P 1973 Pattern of malformation in offspring of chronic alcoholic women. Lancet i: 1267

Kasamatsu T 1983 Neuronal plasticity maintained by the central norepinephrine system in the cat visual cortex. In: Sprague J M, Epstein A N (eds) Progress in psychobiology and physiological psychology, vol 10. Academic Press, New York

Knupfer G 1991 Abstaining for foetal health: the fiction that even light drinking is dangerous. British Journal of Addiction 86: 1063–1073

Kolata G B 1978 Behavioral teratology: birth defects of the mind. Science 202: 732

Kuhn D, Nash S C, Brucken L 1978 Sex role concepts of two- and three-year-olds. Child Development 49: 445

Landesman-Dwyer S, Ragozin A S, Little R E 1981 Behavioural correlates of prenatal alcoholic exposure: a four year follow up study. Neurobehaviour, Toxicology and Teratology 3: 187

Le Vay S 1991 A difference in hypothalamic structure between homosexual and heterosexual men. Science 253: 1034–1037

Lemoine P, Harousseau H, Borteyru J P, Menuet J C 1968 Les enfants de parents alcooliques: anomalies observess. A propos de 127 cas. (Children of alcoholic parents: anomalies observed in 127 cases.) Ouest Medecine 21: 476

Madge N, Tizard J 1980 Intelligence. In: Rutter M (ed) Scientific foundations of developmental psychiatry. Heinemann, London

Martin S L, Craig T R, Ramey S 1990 The prevention of intellectual impairment in children of impoverished families: findings of a randomized trial of educational day care. American Journal of Public Health 80: 844–847.

Money J, Ehrhardt A A 1972 Man and woman; boy and girl: the differentiation and dimorphisms of gender identity from conception to maturity. Johns Hopkins University Press, Baltimore

Miller H C, Merritt T A 1979 Fetal growth in human. Yearbook Medical Publishers, Chicago

Neligan G A, Kolvin I, Scott D McI, Garside R F 1976 Born too soon or born too small. Heinemann, London

Oppenheim R, Chu-Wang I W 1983 Aspects of naturally-occurring motoneuron death in the chick spinal cord during embryonic development. In: Bernstock G (ed) Somatic and autonomic nerve muscle interactions. Elsevier, Amsterdam, pp 55–107

Perachio A A, Marr L D, Alexander M 1979 Sexual behaviour in male Rhesus monkeys elicited by electrical stimulation of preoptic and hypothalamic areas. Brain Research 142: 105

Plant M 1985 Women, drinking and pregnancy. Tavistock, London

Plummin R, De Fries J C 1983 The Colorado adoption project. Child Development 54: 276

Quinn P, Papoport J L 1974 Minor physical anomalies and neurological studies in hyperactive boys. Paediatrics 53: 742

Plomin R, De Fries J C, Fulker D W 1988 Nature and nurture during infancy and early childhood. Cambridge University Press, New York

Rainbow T C, Parsons B, McEwen B S 1982 Sex differences in rat brain oestrogen and progestin receptors. Nature 300: 648

Raisman G, Field P M 1973 Sexual dimorphism in the neuropil of the preoptic area of the rat and its dependence on neonatal androgen. Brain Research 54: 1

Rapoport J L 1980 Congenital anomalies, appearance and body build. In: Rutter M (ed) Scientific foundations of developmental psychiatry. Heinemann, London

Rose R J, Ditto W B 1983 A developmental-genetic analysis of common fears from early adolescence to early adulthood. Child Development 54: 361

Rosett H L 1980 A clinical perspective of the fetal alcohol syndrome. Alcoholism: Clinical Experimental Research 4: 119

Rosett H L, Weiner L 1984 Alcohol and the foetus: a clinical perspective. Oxford University Press, London

Royal College of Psychiatrists 1987 Drug scenes. Gaskell, London, pp 194–195

Rutter M 1980a In: Rutter M (ed) Scientific foundations of developmental psychiatry. Heinemann, London

Rutter M 1980b Raised lead levels and impaired cognitive/behavioral functioning: a review of the evidence. Developmental Medicine and Child Neurology (suppl 42). Heinemann, London

Rutter M, Quinton D 1984 Longterm follow up of women institutionalised in childhood: factors promoting good functioning in adult life. British Journal of Developmental Psychology 18: 225

Scarr S, McCartney K 1983 How people make their own environments: a theory of genotype environment effects. Child Development 54: 424

Scarr S, Weinberg R A 1983 The Minnesota adoption studies: genetic differences and maleability. Child Development 54: 262

Schoemaker W J, Baetge G, Azad R et al 1983 Effect of prenatal alcohol exposure on amine and peptide neurotransmitter systems. Monographs of Neural Science 9: 130

Shields J 1962 Monozygotic twins. Oxford University Press, London

Sinclair A H, Berta P, Palmer M S, Hawkins J R, Griffiths B L, Smith M J, Foster J W, Frischauf A M, Lovell-Badge R, Goodfellow P N 1990 A gene from the human sex-determining region encodes a protein with homology to a conserved DNA-binding motif. Nature 346: 240

Slimp J C, Hart B L, Goy R W 1978 Heterosexual, autosexual and social behaviour of adult male rhesus monkeys with medial preoptic-anterior hypothalamic lesions. Brain Research 142: 105

Sneider G E, Jhaveri S R 1974 Neuroanatomical correlates of spared or altered function after brain lesions in the newborn hamster. In: Stein D G, Rosen J L, Butters N (eds) Plasticity and recovery of function in the central nervous system. Academic Press, New York

Sperry R W 1963 Chemo affinity in the orderly growth of nerve fibre patterns and connections. Proceedings of the National Academy of Sciences of the USA 50: 703

Stein Z A, Susser M W 1976 Maternal starvation and birth defects. In: Hook E B (ed) Birth defects: risks and consequences. Academic Press, New York

Stein Z A, Susser M 1985 Effects of early nutrition on neurological and mental competence in human beings. Psychological Medicine 15: 717

Stein Z A, Susser M W, Saenger G, Marolla F A 1975 Famine and human development: the Dutch hunger winter of 1944–45. Oxford University Press, New York

Stoch M B, Smythe P M 1976 Fifteen year developmental study on the effects of severe under-nutrition during infancy and on subsequent physical growth and intellectual functioning. Archives of Diseases in Childhood 51: 237

Streissguth A P 1983 Alcohol and pregnancy: an overview and an update. Substance Alcohol Actions Misuse 4: 149

Swaab D F, Hofman M A 1990 An enlarged suprachiasmatic nucleus in homosexual men. Brain Research 370: 1

Waldrop M F, Bell R Q, McLaughlin B, Halverson C F 1978 Newborn minor physical anomalies predict a short attention span, peer aggression and impulsivity at age 3. Science 199: 563

Waterlow J C 1974 Some aspects of childhood malnutrition as a public health problem. British Medical Journal iii: 88

Weber D P, Vuori-Christiansen L et al 1981 Nutritional supplementation, maternal education and cognitive development in infants as risk of malnutrition. American Journal of Clinical Nutrition 34: 807

West J R, Hodges C A, Black A C 1981 Prenatal exposure to ethanol alters the organization of hippocampal mossy fibres in rats. Science 211: 957

Wiesel T N 1982 Postnatal development of the visual coreex and the influence of environment. Nature 299: 583–591

Wilson R S 1983 The Louisville twin study: development synchronies in behavior. Child Development 54: 298

Winick M 1976 Malnutrition and brain development. Oxford University Press, London

Winick M, Meyes K K, Harris R C 1975 Malnutrition and environmental enrichment by early adoption. Science 190: 1173

Yalom I D, Green R, Fisk N 1973 Prenatal exposure to female hormones: effect of psychosocial development in boys. Archives of General Psychiatry 28: 554

5. Personality development

Sula Wolff

DEFINITIONS

Definitions of personality are numerous but all have two features in common: first, personality refers to behaviour and to self-reports of subjective experience; second, it refers to relatively enduring and hence predictable human qualities. Some definitions exclude intelligence and aptitudes; some use the word only in relation to individual differences. These two restrictions are helpful in the practice of psychiatry when the focus is on personality disorders. When instead we are concerned with personality development in general, a broader view is needed. Intellectual and social–emotional development are intimately related, each crucially influencing the other. Moreover, for a useful perspective of individual variations, normal and deviant, we need to be clear that a great deal of behaviour is universal to the human race, much is common to all members of a particular culture or subculture, some characterises groups of individuals and only a portion is unique.

Personality development has been explored in a number of different ways (Wolff 1989). Developmental psychologists recorded the observable intellectual and social progress of children of different ages and set norms for the attainment of a variety of important skills. Psychoanalysts charted the internal historical connections made by patients (at first by adults; later by children) between their early life experiences and their present state as it could be observed and as the patients described it. Other child psychologists, Piaget and his followers, concerned themselves with how thinking and reasoning alter as children grow up. Ethologists defined and recorded items of social behaviour of infants and young children from a biological viewpoint. Learning theorists explored the changes in broader patterns of childhood behaviour brought about by rewards and punishments and by observations of the behaviour of others (modelling).

A difficulty often perceived as insuperable derives from the two different modes of explaining and understanding human behaviour and its development: the introspective, purposive and the scientific, causal. While much psychoanalytic activity is not in any conflict with the methods of scientific enquiry, psychoanalytic explanations as used in the course of psychotherapy are based on data quite different from the data of science and serve an altogether different purpose. A patient may be helped to understand how he has come to be as he is in terms of his past experiences. He feels better and his self-esteem rises as a result. But the next day he finds a different reason which also joins up his experiences in a meaningful way and adds to his inner comfort. Both explanations have a 'felt' truth about them and are valid as therapeutic tools. They may or may not tell us something about 'the causes' of the patient's present state and we cannot, from his varying inner connections, make calculated predictions for the future. Yet some of the patterns of these inner connections are shared by everyone and others appear repeatedly in individuals.

The two kinds of explanation used in the social sciences, reflecting the psychophysical dualism with which psychiatry is concerned, have been greatly clarified by Toulmin (1970). Reasons are subjective, retrospective justifications for conduct, and signals of intent. While a great deal of human behaviour, including subjective experience, especially when pathological, may be predetermined and obey the sort of laws Freud identified, much of our inner life springs from that part of the self which is free to make choices, unbound by deterministic, general laws. Subjective reasons are no basis for prediction. Causal explanations on the other hand derive from knowledge about more objectively observable relationships. They enable us to formulate general laws, within limits to make predictions for the future, and to take clinical decisions in the light of these predictions.

In psychiatry both types of explanation are necessary and our knowledge of personality development is based on objective and subjective data. The use we make of what we know will vary correspondingly. For decisions in child care, in education and in patient management we must rely as far as we can on science. But to understand and communicate with our patients we cannot do without a subjective view of human development.

THE COMPONENTS OF PERSONALITY

It is useful to think of three parts of personality: temperament, intelligence, and affect and motivation.

Temperament or style concerns the *how* of behaviour. It has been defined as '...a constitutionally based source of individual variation in personality functioning, emerging early in life' (Lamb et al 1991) and, unlike intelligence and motivation, it remains relatively stable with increasing age.

Intelligence defines levels of achievement and in childhood rates of development. It has to do with *how much* an individual is capable of (see Ch. 3).

Affect and *motivation* describe the component we identify as our self: the *contents* of our thoughts, our habitual choices, our intimate relationships, our moral standards, our public lives, our attitudes and opinions, our hopes and aspirations, our fears and our sorrows.

Both temperament and intelligence, although greatly influenced by events and opportunities, have firm biological roots. Our affective, motivational self is most open to change in the course of our lives and is patterned by our interactions with the family in which we are reared, the culture that surrounds us, the personalities of others who are close to us and by the life events that befall us. But there are biological determinants even in this field, especially in relation to human responses common to everyone, such as the child's attachment to his mother and the adolescent's search for a sexual partner. Moreover the child's cognitive development, tied in part to maturation of the nervous system, influences in a major way how at different ages he or she perceives and responds to the human and inanimate environment and to life events. The nature of perceptions and responses in childhood has long-term consequences for a child's future self.

SOME BASIC ASPECTS OF CHILD DEVELOPMENT

The empirical study of personality development is flourishing and what follows is a simplified outline, written from a clinical viewpoint, of a large and complex topic.

Human development is based on transactional processes

Human development, and indeed all human behaviour, is transactional. At any one moment, the individual as he is constituted is open to, seeks out and responds in a particular way to certain aspects of the environment, animate and inanimate. His particular constitution and behaviour in turn affect not only the material environment but also in part determine the responses of other people. We need to be clear also that the patients we see in clinical practice, for whom the processes of personality development have gone awry, may exemplify exceptional as well as common transactional patterns.

Heredity and environment

There is no question that both genetic and environmental factors contribute to human intelligence. But how much the variance of a population's intelligence depends on genetic or environmental influences changes with circumstances. Intelligence is environmentally impaired only under conditions of extreme adversity. More commonly, environmental influences affect educational attainments, competencies and motivation rather than intelligence itself. Rutter (1985) reminds us that heredity and environment tend to vary together because people with genotypic differences create different environments for themselves. The supposed psychosocial effects of parents on the intellectual development of their children may well in part be genetically determined.

Scarr & McCartney (1983) provide a helpful theory for the links between genotypic and phenotypic differences between people. The effect may be (1) a direct expression of genetic predispositions, or (2) indirect via three types of interactions with the environment: (a) *passive*, through the environment provided by biologically related parents (especially in infancy when self-selection of environmental input is limited); (b) *evoked*, through responses elicited from others by the individual's genetically determined attributes, such as appearance, intelligence and temperament; and (c) *active*, through the selection of different environments by different people. Theirs is an evolutionary theory based on the ideas that phenotypic variation is the raw material for selection, and that genetic differences prompt differences in the way in which environments are experienced and what effects they have.

Genes have a discontinuous action over time. When we consider not individual differences in intelligence but the processes of intellectual development during childhood (as well as the intellectual decline in later life), it is clear that only a common gene pool can account for the regularity of the sequence of unfolding of abilities despite individual differences. There are universal aspects as well as great individual variations both in our genetic endowment and in our environment, much of which we have created for ourselves.

The genetics of intelligence have been widely studied. More recently, temperament too has been shown to have a large genetic component, but we know little as yet about the genetic contribution to social and emotional development.

Sensitive periods in personality development

Both psychoanalytic theory of social–emotional development (not based on empirical observation before the work of Bowlby) and Piaget's theory of cognitive development (built from the start on direct observation of children) hold that the emotional and intellectual functioning of children differ qualitatively at different stages of development and that a regular sequence of such stages characterises the developmental process. At each stage children are open to certain selected aspects of their environment, and deal with these in characteristic ways. Psychoanalytic (and to a lesser extent cognitive) theory also holds that the child's particular experiences at each stage make long-lasting and specific contributions to his later personality. The notion of imprinting (Lorenz 1966) was based on the observation in geese and hens that chicks will permanently follow the first moving object they encounter (usually of course their mother) during a restricted period shortly after hatching. Perverse attachments to humans could be induced when goslings were exposed to a moving person rather than their mother during this 'critical period'. The concept of a critical period for learning certain specific patterns of social behaviour was later modified to a concept of 'sensitive periods'. It was found in rhesus monkeys that, although baby monkeys reared in isolation failed to develop normal social, sexual and maternal behaviour as adults, the period in which absence of maternal care or of peer relationships (which in monkeys can compensate) had such powerful effects was not so strictly confined, and later compensatory experiences could modify although not normalise social behaviour (Harlow & Zimmermann 1959, Rutter 1981).

The mediating processes between events and circumstances during sensitive periods and later personality are likely to be both transactional and experiential. For example, young children who lose their mothers normally react with anger to substitute care-givers. It needs exceptional understanding and self-control for such new parents not to withdraw or respond with counteraggression, and the chances of a poor relationship with the substitute care giver following the early loss are high. What part in such persisting difficulties is played by inner continuities, that is, by remembered childhood experiences, is only now being systematically explored (Radke-Yarrow et al 1988).

It seems reasonable, in the absence of sufficient empirical evidence, to adopt a view that is consonant with research findings, with clinical and personal experience and with biological principles. There is evidence for a biological programme within each person that determines physical, behavioural and subjective development in interaction with the environment. Children, and indeed adults too, learn different things at different stages of life and there is an extraordinary regularity and uniformity in this process which appears essential for procreation and survival within the human group. If what is learnt at any one stage did not have some permanence, we would be endlessly open to change in response to events and circumstances, with consequent decline of individual differences between people. It is the relative permanence of personality characteristics which fosters the maintenance of individual differences and these are thought to contribute to the preservation of the species within a changing physical and cultural environment. Of course the stages of the developmental process are not rigid. Flexibility increases the chances of survival in the face of accident or other adversity. For example, while the infant's attachment to his mother is largely mediated by vision, blind babies can use their healthy sensory modalities to develop early relationships although, as we shall see, this developmental process tends to be delayed. Likewise, later compensation for early environmental deficits can prevent personality impairments.

The great stage theorists, Freud and his followers and Piaget, were often proved wrong in detail by subsequent research, but the amazing fact is how accurately their often speculative ideas fit clinical experience. While research findings can refute and modify ideas, unproven but helpful theories cannot be abandoned for lack of empirical evidence. On the contrary, they act as a spur to further investigation.

TEMPERAMENT IN CHILDHOOD

Even healthy infants differ from each other from birth in mobility, irritability and vigour. Chess & Thomas

(1984) in the 1950s launched a systematic longitudinal study of New York children (the NYLS) to put these observations on a firmer footing. A homogeneous, middle-class group of parents was recruited both to minimise individual differences in life circumstances and to ensure continued participation in the study. Detailed descriptions of each child's behaviour in daily life were validated against systematic observations of the children. The temperamental qualities discovered were based on an initial content analysis yielding nine categories of responses which could be defined and reliably rated by independent raters: level of motor activity; intensity of response; sensitivity to stimuli (threshold); mood (whether mainly positive or negative); approach to or withdrawal from novelty; adaptability; rhythmicity (i.e. regularity of biological functions of sleeping, eating and elimination); persistence (in the face of frustration); and distractability. Approach/withdrawal, labelled by others as a disinhibition/shyness dimension, accounts for the greatest variance between children, and increased in stability from early to middle childhood (Kagan 1989). Activity level, intensity, threshold and, particularly, adaptability are all relatively stable over time (Plomin et al 1988, Thomas & Chess 1986). Even more stable are composite scores derived from temperamental profiles which, at the age of 3 years, had predicted good adjustment or behaviour disorders at the age of 7 years: 40% of children had at 3 years been 'easy' — regular, adaptable, approaching novelty, with positive mood and low intensity; 10% had a 'difficult child' syndrome — being irregular, withdrawing from novelty, non-adaptable, negative in mood and intense; 15%, with withdrawal and slow adaptation but mild intensity and regular biological functions, were called 'slow to warm up'.

The 133 children in the NYLS have all been followed into adult life (Chess & Thomas 1984). Those with a 'difficult child' syndrome at 3 years often had a poor adult adjustment, although early exposure to parental conflict predicted this even more strongly. The authors then, imaginatively, looked at the exceptions to these trends. Why did some children, at risk because of an early adverse temperament and parental conflict, nevertheless reach adult life unscathed? And why did others, not disadvantaged in this way, have a poor outcome?

Resilience in the face of high risk was attributed to the development of a gift in middle childhood or adolescence, commitment to a career, a good relationship with someone outside the family, and to a distancing from parents (sometimes geographical) of the young person. Poor outcome despite low risk factors was found in the few constitutionally impaired children of this cohort: those with brain damage, with depressive illnesses or with schizoid personality traits.

The authors view childhood maladjustment as the outcome of a 'poor fit' between the child's temperament and the demands made by parents and teachers. The counselling service offered to those parents whose offspring had developed behaviour disorders in childhood was more effective when the main risk factor was the child's difficult temperament rather than parental conflict.

A genetic basis for differences in temperament has been established by twin and adoption studies (Plomin et al 1988). Torgersen (1989) found activity level and approach/withdrawal to be among the most genetically influenced traits. This is congruent with the finding of Daniel & Plomin (1985) of high correlations for shyness between biological but not adoptive mothers and their children. Environmental effects are likely to contribute, since shy, socially anxious mothers tended to expose both themselves and their offspring less to novel situations. Aggression is one of the most stable, although largely acquired, personality characteristics, especially in boys, resembling IQ in its predictability over time (Olweus 1979). Its clinical importance is the high association with later antisocial conduct and criminality. Olweus (1980) found the determinants of aggression to be: high temperamental scores on activity level and intensity; mothers' early expectations and tolerance of aggressiveness in their sons; and parents' use of 'power-assertive' methods of child rearing. Moreover, aggression is transmitted from one generation to the next, with parental irritability as the major mediating factor (Patterson & Dishion 1988).

More rarely, neurological impairments, especially when associated with overactivity, poor attention and specific developmental delays, can contribute to the development of aggression and later antisocial conduct in children from vulnerable families (Taylor et al 1991). Cerebral damage at birth may be associated with subsequent irritability which may affect the later mother–infant relationship. Robson & Moss (1970) observed mothers' interactions with their babies and questioned them about their feelings. In the first months crying decreases. By the third month mothers of infants who were still inconsolable when held, and who maintained high levels of crying, experienced a decline in motherly feelings. If mothers ignore their children, crying increases. Which comes first in these mutually reinforcing interactions, the baby's irritability or the mother's inattentiveness is often not known. During training sessions, when irritable babies in a nursery were rewarded with smiles whenever they quietened or made social overtures, these now more friendly babies elicited more social responses from their nurses than they had during their preceding irritable state (Etzel & Gewirtz 1967).

SOCIAL RESPONSES AND RELATIONSHIPS IN INFANCY AND EARLY CHILDHOOD

The methods of animal ethologists have been applied with much success to the study of early childhood behaviour (Schaffer 1971, 1977). Soon after birth babies alert to the sound of a human voice, especially when female, and even show preferential head turning to the smell of their mother's milk. Their random but well-formed smiles are from the start endowed with meaning by their parents (Hinde 1976). Between 6 and 12 weeks babies show *indiscriminate attachment* behaviour, singling out human beings for special attention, smiling selectively at all human faces or pictures of these but only when seen in full front view. In the third quarter of the first year *specific social attachments* are formed, children now smiling selectively at familiar faces, those of their mothers and fathers, 'sobering' when confronted by strangers, and reacting from the age of 7 months onwards with a well-defined sequence of behaviour to the absence of their attachment figures. Fretting at temporary domestic separations has been used as an index of specific attachments, and this led to the discovery that, while the mother is usually the person with whom the baby forms its earliest and strongest bond, this is not always so. Fathers, grandparents or siblings may be chosen, depending on their sensitive responsiveness and their capacity to provide just the right amount of interest and contingent stimulation for the infant. As in rhesus monkeys, attachment is not primarily related to feeding.

A transient *fear of strangers* occurs after the appearance of specific attachments. The intensity of these reaches a peak at around 41–44 weeks, declines temporarily as the baby is diverted by the novelty of being able to crawl and walk, and then rises again.

The biological implications of the child's tie to the mother

Bruner (1972) held that the nature and duration of immaturity as well as patterns of interactions with others are as much subject to evolution and natural selection as any morphological variations. Because we live in a rapidly changing man-made environment, more and more knowledge and skills not stored in the gene pool have to be acquired in childhood, some by direct encounter, some by imitation, and even more from the culture transmitted through its artefacts. But the child's earliest learning, to recognise and follow its mother, is largely based on innately evolving responses.

Bowlby (1973, 1984) reviewed the studies of attachment behaviour in primates and man. Mothers and infants in these species behave in such a way that proximity between them is maintained. Bowlby regarded these mutual interactions as biologically adaptive to the ordinary, expectable environment (the 'environment of evolutionary adaptedness') and as fulfilling two main functions essential for survival and propagation: protection of the young against predators and other dangers, and promoting learning in the young of essential patterns of social behaviour in proximity to their mothers. In human babies one of the most important components of early learning is language, the basis for which is acquired by imitation of gesture and sound during the earliest social interactions between parent and child, at the stage of life when attachment behaviour is at its height (Howlin 1980). Bowlby viewed the behaviours of adult care givers and infants which mediate attachment as: mutually complementary; as instinctive, depending on universal, innate control systems which become effective at different stages of the life cycle; and as environmentally stable to a high degree in the sequence of their unfolding.

In human mother–child couples the mother at first takes responsibility for preserving proximity with her infant. After 18 months the baby takes a more active part and his proximity-seeking is at its height in the second and third years. It then decreases as the child becomes, and is encouraged to become, more independent and ventures forth into the world. The experiential (affective and cognitive) counterparts of proximity seeking, e.g. the child's sense of dependency on the mother and her protective affection for the baby, Bowlby regarded not as causes of the behaviours but as having a monitoring, appraising and signalling function.

Increasingly, the baby's role in initiating social interactions has become apparent, as has the variability in mothers' responses to the individual child according to his particular temperament and needs. Moreover, from a very early age mothers not only provide a 'secure base' from which babies explore the world, but they profoundly influence their children's reactions to the world. From about 7 months babies look to their mothers for cues about whether to be wary or respond with friendliness to strangers (Feinman & Lewis 1983).

Variability in the nature of early attachments

Although the sequence of social responses in infancy and early childhood, like the sequence of cognitive development to be examined later, is constant, depending on a common genetic heritage, actual life experiences influence the nature of early social behaviour. Intensity of attachment is greater when the number of care givers is low. The more people there are in a baby's life, the later the onset of the fear-of-stranger reaction. There is suggestive evidence too for a genetic component to individual differences in the timing and quality of early social responses: monozygotic twins are more alike than dizygotic twins (Freedman 1965).

Mary Ainsworth classified the attachment behaviour of 1-year-old infants in an experimental setting, in which they were exposed to brief separations from their mothers and encounters with a stranger, as 'secure', 'insecure ambivalent' and 'insecure avoidant'. 'Securely' attached infants were found to have had more sensitively responsive mothers as rated during home observations in the previous year than 'insecurely' attached babies. Moreover, at the age of 4 years, they were in a nursery setting less dependent on their teachers, more friendly to other children, more self-reliant and more resourceful. Of course, some of the constraints impeding secure attachment, such as a difficult temperament in the child, maternal depression and social stresses, may well have persisted in the children's lives (see Wolff 1989, Lamb 1991).

The separation reaction

An early focus of Bowlby's work and that of his colleagues was the separation reaction seen regularly in children aged 6 months to 3 years when removed from their parents and not visited, for example, in hospital. A period of *protest* with acute distress, crying and searching for the parent, during which no other person can provide effective comfort, is followed by a period of *despair* when searching for the mother ends and the child becomes withdrawn, inactive, weepy and lacking all interest in his surroundings. Finally, *detachment* follows, the parent(s) seem to have been forgotten, and the child once more becomes responsive to others. If the mother reappears in the first two stages, she may be greeted with anger or avoidance and has to woo back her child. If she reappears during the third stage, the child treats her like a stranger. The suddenness of separation and the quality of substitute care influence the child's reactions. In a setting of group care, in which attempts to form new bonds are con-

stantly frustrated, the above sequence is regularly seen. If instead the child is looked after by a familiar foster mother, separation reactions are mild and the return to the mother less troubled by anger (Robertson & Robertson 1971). All young children protest when their parents leave them (Bowlby 1973) and in a family setting this strengthens the bond and makes parents feel valued. But prolonged, traumatic separations arouse great anger in children, and their guilty parents or eager foster parents may then not know how to cope. Helplessness, guilt and, finally, irritation are common parental responses and the relationship with the child is endangered further. When children then perceive that their own anger threatens the security of their new-won home, they may repress their angry feelings and instead engage in destructive behaviour — soiling, wetting, stealing, fire-setting — over which they now have no control and which forms an even greater threat to their security.

The vicissitudes and long-term effects of the child's early social relationships

From the start, Bowlby developed the notion that when children's needs for secure early attachments are not met, there are likely to be serious later consequences for their own intimate relationships, including the care of their children. He also developed the idea of 'internal models' of human relationships, formed on the basis of early attachments, which determine a child's expectations of other people, his reactions to them and hence the relationships. Rutter (1981) has argued cogently that what had been loosely called 'maternal deprivation' is not all of a kind, and that specific deficits and distortions in a child's experience at specific times can have specific later consequences.

Personality development can be impaired when a child's readiness for activities and experiences is not matched by the environmental input necessary to activate these, especially during sensitive periods of development. Such interference can come from organic deficits, such as brain damage, blindness or deafness. Blind babies, for example, develop specific attachments more slowly than sighted children and elicit less social responsiveness from their care givers (Fraiberg 1968). They are often delayed in language and imaginative play as well, but catch up later (Howlin 1980).

During the *stage of indiscriminate social attachments*, between 3 and 6 months, what is essential is stimulation of the baby at an optimal individual level, and sensitive responsiveness on the part of the care giver. Understimulated infants (e.g. in the hospital wards of a former era) with few opportunities for social interactions and for watching interesting spectacles, declined in measures of infant intelligence, catching up only when returned to their parents. No such catch-up was seen in babies after brief spells in a children's home with much social stimulation (Schaffer 1966), and constitutionally very active babies suffered less of a set-back in the hospital setting, clearly being able to seek out and elicit more stimulation for themselves than others.

Serious personality impairments have been repeatedly described when, during the *stage of specific social attachments*, between 6 months and about 3 years, infants have no opportunities to form enduring relationships with a limited number of people but are instead cared for by multiple care givers and exposed to repeated disruptions of relationships. This is an unavoidable accompaniment of institutional care, and the consequences in terms of cognitive delays, especially of language, and of long-standing impairment of the capacity to form intimate affectional bonds with others, have been well documented (Bowlby 1984). The effects on child care services and hospital practices of this knowledge, while long delayed, have been dramatic. Children under 4 years are no longer admitted to homes or residential nurseries, but are fostered if family care breaks down, and all children's hospitals now encourage free visiting by parents and active play experiences for the children.

Rarely, under conditions of grossly pathological mothering, when mothers are mentally handicapped, psychotic or seriously personality disordered, young children's food intake may be impaired, leading to 'failure to thrive', that is, physical and sometimes intellectual stunting of development. The salient deficit is nutritional. Skuse and his colleagues (Matheson et al 1989) describe the usual origins of non-organic failure to thrive in young children as due to a negative cycle of maladaptive interactions between child and care giver, found particularly in socioeconomically deprived families. Minor neurological impairments of the infant which interfere with feeding, such as hypotonia of the lips, can also contribute.

Inadequate intellectual and linguistic stimulation can occur not only in institutions but also in socioeconomically deprived, large families where there may be affection, but where quiet conversational contacts between parents and children are few, and opportunities for learning from constructive play and books limited. Progressive educational retardation often follows when children from such a background arrive at school with poor conversational and other skills, and lacking in social competence and self-esteem. Later antisocial conduct is then common, especially in boys

and when there is also family disharmony or disruption. The evidence that good preschool education programmes can prevent such a development gives hope, but has not so far been widely acted upon in this country (Farrington 1985).

On the other hand, even children deprived of continuous mothering can be helped to make progress in language and cognitive development if brought up in an environment that fosters these accomplishments. Tizard et al (1973) some years ago showed that the language comprehension of young children in residential nurseries was improved when their care givers offered 'high-quality' conversations in the form of opinions, specific information, explanations and in play, as opposed to mere instructions, or global pleasantries uttered with a restricted vocabulary. 'High-quality' conversation in turn depended on how much autonomy the care givers had in the social and administrative organisation of their institution.

The effects of cultural understimulation are not limited to the early years. Children born into economically deprived families are not only more likely than others to experience family disruption and substitute care at some stage of their lives, they are likely to be brought up in an unstimulating environment with fewer opportunities to develop their skills, and then to get poorer schooling also.

Tizard's work has amply confirmed Rutter's thesis that childhood 'deprivation' is not a uniform hazard. In a comparative follow-up study of family-reared children and of children who spent their first 2 years in a residential nursery and were later adopted or restored to their own mothers, intellectual development and behaviour depended on the sort of family environment which followed the institutional experience. Children who returned to disorganised and disharmonious families did poorly; those who were adopted on the whole did well. But, while the family relationships in the adopted group were usually warm, unlike those in the 'restored' group, even at adolescence relationships with peers remained impaired in both; and, in contrast to children who had never been separated from their families, the adopted and 'restored' groups were judged by their teachers (although not by their adoptive parents) to be more disturbed than the never-separated group (Hodges & Tizard 1989).

The beginning of morality

Attachment is the behavioural system most intensively studied so far. Its origins lie in the first year of life, the psychoanalysts' 'oral' stage. But a start has now been made in elucidating the early development of self-appraisal and standards of right and wrong. Kagan (1981) identified a second stage in the biological maturation of children in which, for the first time, a built-in moral sense appears. Children exposed to experimental play settings at intervals during their second year (the psychoanalysts' 'anal' stage) suddenly became became aware of flaws in toys they had not noticed before, commented when things were not as they ought to be, and became aware also of what they themselves should be able to do, showing distress at the prospect of failure. At 14 months no child treated a damaged toy differently from others; at 19 months 57% expressed concern, saying 'broke', 'fix it', or taking the toy to their mother. The proportion increased with age. Because American and Fijian children reacted similarly, these changes in behaviour were clearly not culture bound. They immediately preceded the appearance of evaluative language, that is, the use of words such as 'bad', 'good', 'dirty' and 'nice'.

This developmental achievement coincides with changes in the capacity for empathy, thought to be a second essential component in the development of guilt and other aspects of morality (Hoffman 1987, see also Wolff 1991). Even newborns respond to the feelings of others: when one baby in a nursery cries, all the others do so too. This 'reflexive emotional resonance' occurs before the child can distinguish between his own feelings and those of others. In the second year true sympathy is seen, children attempting to comfort others in distress but with egocentric means, such as proffering their own comforters. In the third year, when children are capable of role taking, empathic responses become attuned to the needs of others, and in later childhood they extend to experiences beyond the here and now, such as the plight of famine victims in far-off lands. Although the research evidence in this area is still meagre, there is some evidence for Hoffman's notion that altruism, that is, empathic responsiveness and a cognitive awareness of the other person, constitutes a biological motive to help others in distress, independent of the prospects of reward or punishment.

Social relationships in the preschool years

A major contribution has been Dunn & Kendrick's study of siblings (Dunn & Kendrick 1982, Dunn 1988). Sibling rivalry is no myth. These authors quote a 4-year-old asking his mother after the arrival of the next child: 'Why have you ruined my life?' In this study many children were disturbed after the birth of the sibling, especially when the first born had a diffi-

cult temperament, when the mother was depressed and irritable, and when the older child's relationship with the mother had been especially close. Protective factors were a close relationship with the father, the birth of a sibling of the same sex, and when the mother treated her first born as a partner in interpreting and meeting the needs of the baby. Most striking was that the baby took his cues from the first born in their mutual interactions, and that the sibling relationship, whether positive or negative, was very stable over time.

Dunn & Munn (1985) studied the manifestations and resolutions of conflict between siblings and between mothers and young children. Physical aggression and teasing increased in the younger child's second year. Once this child was over 2 years, the older sibling assigned it responsibility in appeals to the mother. In the second year, but not before, children smiled teasingly at their mothers while doing forbidden things, now clearly aware of the rules, and mothers not only uttered 'dos' and 'don'ts' but referred increasingly to rules of social conduct.

Radke-Yarrow et al (1988), in an important prospective study of 108 pairs of siblings and their parents, complemented observations of videoed family interactions with interviews with parents and children as well as psychiatric assessments. Their sample included intact, middle-class families and very low-income, disrupted families; and mothers with and without a history of depressive illness.

When mothers had been depressed, their relationships with their children were more often negative; and when this was so, the relationships between the siblings were more often negative too. Clinically depressed mothers were less able to handle stressful situations involving their children and more likely to make negative attributions to their children who then, in turn, were less likely to be securely attached.

Family disorganisation and socioeconomic deprivation were associated with more expressed negative mood within the families and harsh maternal responses to children's non-compliance; while a high rate of children's compliance was related to the mother's more positive affects towards the children in stable families. In stable families, the child's affectionate relationship with the mother was the best predictor of social competence in later peer relationships. At 6 years, children who had had negative relationships with their mothers interpreted ambiguous pictures of mothers and children in a more punitive way, accurately reflecting the level of maternal hostility to which they had been exposed. Such children were also rated by psychiatrists as more disturbed.

The importance of experience

In this study, mothers' attributions to their children and children's views of their parents were seen as mediators in family relationships and social functioning. Perhaps the first attempt at an objective study of the effects of experience on mother–child interactions was Main & Kaplan's (1985) assessment of parents' reports about their own childhood memories. Using a semistructured 'adult attachment interview', they were able to relate parents' reactions to their own past experiences to the independent assessments of their child's attachment to them some 5 years earlier. Parents who reported happy early attachment memories or had come to terms with and realistically recounted poorer childhood experiences had had 'securely attached' infants. Babies of parents who defensively devalued their own childhood attachments or remained painfully preoccupied with these had been 'insecurely attached'.

COGNITIVE DEVELOPMENT

The child's intellectual level at each stage, that is, how he perceives and reasons about the world and himself in relation to people, things and ideas, is one of the major determinants of his social and emotional experiences. Knowledge about cognitive processes in childhood has been immeasurably advanced by Jean Piaget (Piaget 1932, 1951, 1960; Piaget & Inhelder 1969, Miller 1989). For this reason a full summary of his ideas follows.

Piaget described four factors contributing to the cognitive development of the child:

1. Maturation, that is, organic, neurological maturation determined by innate biological factors
2. Opportunities for the exercise of functions and for experiences of interactions with inanimate objects
3. Opportunities for social interactions and learning from being taught, and
4. Internal, psychological, mechanisms for constructing successive cognitive models (Piaget & Inhelder 1969).

These inner mechanisms, or 'schemata' as Piaget called them, depend on interactions between the first three factors. Piaget described a universally present sequence of qualitatively different cognitive models characterising the stages of personality development in childhood. Organic, maturational factors determine the maximum rate of development for the individual and his maximum adult level. Interactions with inanimate objects, with people and the child's culture, affect the specific contents of his thinking. Restriction of opportunities for such interaction can impede the rate of development and set limits to ultimate achievements. The sequence of transformation of cognitive models, however, depends on biologically determined and universally present potentialities.

Piaget's method was clinical. He was less concerned to establish norms of development than to find out why children think and behave as they do. He listened to the questions children of different ages tend to ask spontaneously and he modelled his own questions on these. He took as valid answers the types of responses commonly produced by children of a similar age, discarding totally idiosyncratic answers or random replies of the kind which children often give when at a loss. He observed his own three children in their first 2 years and groups of older Geneva nursery school and school children. He interviewed children and devised simple experiments for them to do. One of his salient discoveries was that children do not merely copy what they see or repeat what they hear, but from the start think up new ways of handling their environment and of talking about it. He saw the essential functions of intelligence as being understanding and inventing (Piaget 1972). To explain his findings Piaget postulated a very limited number of mental structures and mechanisms. *Schemata* govern the child's intelligent actions. Two processes mediate between these and the child's thoughts and actions. *Assimilation* is the incorporation of new objects, thoughts and activities into already existing schemata. The newborn, for instance, has a schema for turning his head towards an object that touches his cheek (the rooting reflex). He responds to every solid object — a nipple, his thumb, the corner of a pillow — with the routine he already knows and he attends only to those aspects of new objects that have their counterpart in the schema already in his mind, in this case, the touch of the object on his cheek. *Accommodation*, the second postulated process, is one whereby the schema is changed to fit in with novel experiences, provided these are not too different from what the child has already encountered and mastered. With experience of feeding, for example, the baby will search more effectively for the nipple (and in later months he sucks selectively at the nipple), his fingers, his own lips and small toys he can see, but no longer at everything that happens to touch his cheek. Whenever a schema has been changed, practice follows in the form of what Piaget has called the *circular reaction* until the novelty wears off.

1. The sensorimotor stage (birth to $1\frac{1}{2}$ or 2 years)

The behaviour of the newborn indicates that he cannot distinguish between himself and the outside world, and that he does not yet recognise objects as existing apart from his own activities, and as being permanent. He is born with a set of built-in reflexes, for example the sucking reflex. These become modified as a result of functional exercise so that after a few days the infant finds the nipple more easily and feeds with more assurance. Fortuitous, accidental behaviours, for example thumb sucking, are repeated for their own sake and develop into systematically pursued activities. At first the infant behaves as if the object he sees is not the same as the object he grasps or sucks. Then comes a time when he will reach out for an object he sees (vision and prehension become coordinated) but only if he can see both his hand and the object at the same time. If his hand is out of sight he behaves as if he had forgotten it and does not reach out even for a desirable toy. This is followed by a stage when he will invariably reach out for anything he sees, wherever his hand is. He discovers that he can make things happen. Accidentally his hand hits a row of rattles strung across his pram and he now deliberately repeats the activity (the 'circular reaction') to reproduce the interesting spectacle and noise.

Even when the child has detached himself and his actions from the object 'out there' (primary decentring), recognising it as the same object whether he looks at it, grasps it or sucks it (at around 4–5 months, coincidentally with his development of discriminatory smiling), he still behaves as if the universe consisted of 'shifting and unsubstantial "tableaux" which appear and are then totally reabsorbed' (Piaget & Inhelder 1969). When a child of 5–7 months is about to seize an object and this is covered with a cloth, he will withdraw his hand, and then in a moment his attention. For him the hidden object has disappeared, At 9–10 months he behaves quite differently, searching for the object and removing the interfering obstacle. His behaviour now indicates that for him the object does not cease to exist when it is covered over.

During the sensorimotor stage, in which the child becomes upright and mobile, he builds up inner representations of himself and of permanent outer objects, of practical relationships between objects in space and time, of simple causal relationships, and of his own effects on the objects and people around him.

2. The stage of animism and precausal logic (age $1\frac{1}{2}$–7 years)

Sensorimotor mechanisms are prerepresentational. Symbolic functions begin only during the second year of life. Now for the first time one can observe deferred imitation, that is, imitation starting after the disappearance of the model: symbolic play; verbal evocations of events not occurring at the time; and later, drawing. The child rapidly acquires an increasing vocabulary and changes from a creature of action to one of words and thoughts. His thinking and reasoning are, however, quite different from those of adults and, as a result, he misinterprets his environment. Just as the infant cannot distinguish between himself and the world around him so the animistic child cannot as yet detach words from the objects they symbolise, nor his own thoughts from the things thought about. At this stage a hostile intent is equivalent to a hostile deed.

There are four principal characteristics of this stage: egocentrism, animism, precausal logic and an authoritarian morality. Under the age of 7 years, children are *egocentric* and cannot imagine another person's point of view. They talk more in each other's company but there are few shared topics. Instead one observes what Piaget has called the 'collective monologue', each child talking about his own concerns. Children see themselves literally as the centre of the universe, believing that as they walk along the street the sun by day and the moon by night actually follow them. Explanations for events in the physical world are *animistic*. Everything is alive and has feeling and thoughts, resembling those of the child himself. Explanations are psychological in terms of motivation and everything that happens occurs by intent. There are no impartial, natural causes. The notion that some events happen 'by chance' cannot be grasped.

Reasoning is *precausal*, that is, non-scientific. It is based not on observations but on the child's internal model of the world. Children at this stage are insensible of contradictions and accept false explanations that others or they themselves may offer even if these are in conflict with their observations. This is the stage at which babies can be bought in shops and Father Christmas delivers presents the world over. When liquid is poured from a short, wide container into a long, narrow one it becomes 'more' because the level of water rises.

The child's *authoritarian morality* reveals itself both in his notions about the rules of games, which are believed to be sacrosanct even if they are incompletely understood, and in his ideas about crime and punishment. Under 7 years, children believe that bad events are punishments, that the punishment must fit the crime and that bad deeds are inevitably followed by retribution.

Piaget himself pointed out that this cognitive stage coincides on the social–emotional level with the genesis of duty, that is, with a unilateral sense of obligation, and later with the development of conscience and guilt. Perhaps it is not surprising that the fears and phobias of childhood are commonest in the animistic period and that the erotic longings of the oedipal stage can arouse such terrors.

3. The stage of concrete operational thought (age 8–12 years)

After the age of 7 years, when myelination of much of the central nervous system is complete (Combrinck-Graham 1991), children lose their egocentrism, their animism and their authoritarianism. In Piaget's terms a second 'decentring' of thoughts from objects, and from the subject himself, occurs. This enables the child to have multiple perspectives, to argue logically on the basis of observations (accurate deductions, for example, relating to number, to the conservation of weight and volume and to other physical relationships can now be made in an experimental situation with objects) and to engage in cooperative activities with others. Justice is now a more central concept than obedience.

4. The stage of abstract or propositional thought (age 12–15 years)

The child now succeeds in freeing himself from the concrete and is capable of logical operations using thought alone. In the preceding stage logic was tied to actual observations of objects, to their observed inter-relationships and to counting them. The final transformation of cognitive schemata consists of the differentiation of form from content so that the individual becomes capable of reasoning correctly in the realm of pure hypothesis. He can now draw conclusions from truths which are merely possible and this, Piaget thinks, constitutes the beginning of formal or hypotheticodeductive thought. To a large extent, however, abstract thinking at adolescence reflects the scientific knowledge available in the culture. Notions of chance and probability now taken for granted were not, for example, understood 300 years ago.

Piaget stressed the interaction at each stage of cognitive and emotional processes. Social and affective experiences foster exploration of the environment and constitute 'the energetics' or motives of cognitive behaviour. On the other hand, affectivity and the nature of social relationships are dependent on the child's cognitive level. The affective changes of adolescence, the preoccupations with ideologies, future lifestyles and social change, reflect the cognitive transformation achieved at this stage from concrete operational logic to abstract thought.

After Piaget

Piaget's work and writings have had two major effects: the transformation of primary school education from a system of rote learning to one which encourages practical experimentation; and the burgeoning of research into cognitive development in childhood. Piaget's main findings have, on the whole, been confirmed, though he has been proved wrong in many details and some basic principles (Donaldson 1978, Bower 1979, Miller 1989). He was not correct to suppose that sensorimotor experiments were essential for later logical thinking. Some of the apparent immaturities of children under 7 years of age are due to limitations of memory and to linguistic and social misunderstandings rather than to faulty logic. 'When a child interprets what we say to him his interpretation is influenced by at least three things...his knowledge of the language, his assessment of what we intend...and the manner in which he would represent the physical situation to himself if we were not there at all' (Donaldson 1978, p 69).

Some studies have failed to find Piaget's stage transformations in children's cognition. Such studies have often been cross-sectional, examining children of different ages, rather than longitudinal; and it is well known that cross-sectional studies mask growth spurts and qualitative changes with age, because of individual differences in the timing of their appearance. Only longitudinal studies can reveal such transformations. One such (Colby & Kohlberg 1987) confirmed Piaget's findings about the stages of moral judgement, matched by children's changing concepts of conscience (Stilwell et al 1991).

More recently, cognitive-developmental theory has moved towards studying children's representations of their social world, and has taken much more note than Piaget did of environmental and contextual influences on children's thinking (Case 1988). Real integration is now being achieved between children's cognitive and psychosocial development, and psychoanalytic ideas are no longer banished from scientific explorations of child development.

Language development

Piaget held that both language and logic arise from the coordination of actions and that general cognitive processes and language develop together. Bruner (1983) sees the basis of grammar in the preverbal social interchanges between mother and child that begin in early infancy. At first mothers imitate their babies' facial expressions, gestures and vocalisations. From the start there is a conversational type of to-and-fro in these interactions, with mothers pausing until their baby has made a response before 'replying' with a corresponding expression, gesture or utterance. In the last quarter of the first year of life babies begin to imitate their mothers in 'speech acts' and a language of gesture can be discerned. Mutual regard by mother and child of an object are equivalent to a sentence. Looking, pointing, giving and taking correspond to the earliest verbs. Noam Chomsky (1967) demonstrated that children do not copy the grammar of adults but process the language they hear and invent their own grammatical rules. A study of children's language errors revealed common features of immature grammar across different languages and suggests that, like cognition, language development is tied to a common neurological basis. In conversations between mothers and young children, language *structure* is never emphasised by the mother yet is always learnt by the child. Children become proficient in the *use* of language as a result of encouragement to speak rather than because of what they hear others say. Mothers can understand even unclear utterances from their own child and they also interpret and respond to their child's meaning accurately when what the child utters could convey a whole range of different meanings (Harris & Coltheart 1986).

In their responses mothers often repeat what the child had said in an expanded form. Young children in turn appear to learn language by first interpreting the meaning a speaker intends to convey and then working out the relationship between meaning and language. In her excellent review of language development, Howlin (1980) stresses its relation to cognitive and social development and its relative independence of any particular aspect of the mother's speech.

SOCIAL–EMOTIONAL DEVELOPMENT

Here some general comments will be made about the relationship between psychoanalytic and other theories of child development. An outline of Erikson's views about the development of the social self will follow.

Psychoanalysis and child development

Freud, like Piaget, viewed personality development in childhood as an invariant sequence of qualitatively different stages. Both were influenced by Darwin's biological and evolutionary ideas (Dixon & Lerner 1984). While Piaget was well informed about psychoanalytic theories and linked these to his own findings, Freud and his followers took little note of the work done by the Geneva school, although they often made similar observations.

From the start Freud (1953) stressed the importance of childhood experience, much of it forgotten, in the genesis of the psychoneuroses. Such forgotten or unconscious thoughts and memories obey different rules of logic (*primary process thinking*) from those of adult conscious thought (*secondary process thinking*). The characteristics of primary process thinking, as illustrated in dreams, in the material produced during psychoanalysis, or in emotionally motivated slips of the tongue and parapraxes, are quite similar to the characteristics of children's logic during the animistic stage. Moreover, the traumatic childhood experiences revealed by neurotic patients in the course of treatment generally occurred during the first three (oral, anal and genital) stages of emotional development, which coincide almost precisely with the years in which, as Piaget had discovered, prerational logic prevails. It must be stressed that, although children in a child-centred world can, as Piaget's followers have shown, operate with more advanced logic than he thought possible (Donaldson 1978), children spend much of their lives in an adult world and this fosters childish errors and misperceptions.

During the animistic stage children are more prone to anxiety than at any later time. They misperceive what they see, misunderstand what they are told and at the same time have great capacities for symbolic thinking and for storing their memories. It is not surprising that during this period even minor events can arouse major emotional experiences. It is also not surprising that when such experiences are repressed and the child misses out on reality testing, the manifestations of such repressed material in later life (neurotic symptoms and repeated acts of unintended behaviour) retain an animistic logic. Phenomena such as the Oedipus complex and castration anxiety make sense only in the light of the young child's inability to distinguish between thoughts and actions, between intentions and consequences on the one hand, and his authoritarian morality whereby the crime begets the punishment and the punishment must fit the crime, on the other.

The findings of both psychoanalysts and cognitive psychologists have helped clinicians to sharpen their emphatic understanding of children's perceptions of the world, and of how life-events are likely to impinge on them. This is especially important because young children cannot fully convey their feelings and thoughts, for example in a clinical interview. What is surprising is not that both Freud and Piaget were sometimes wrong in their postulates but that, so many years ago and in a different scientific era, they were so often right.

Bowlby (1980) views psychological defence mechanisms as one form of selective exclusion of information similar to the routine exclusion from further processing of much information overload and irrelevant distractions of attention. Under adverse circumstances in childhood, selective exclusion of some kinds of information is adaptive; but the persistent exclusion of the same sort of information during adolescence and adult life (the defensive process postulated by psychoanalysts) can be highly maladaptive, constricting the range of possible behaviour. He suggests that defensive exclusion differs from routine exclusion of information not in its mechanisms but in its content: information associated with suffering is most likely to be defensively excluded. Repression of traumatic experiences is one way in which childhood events can have long-lasting effects and lay the foundation for illness or personality disorder. But there is, as we saw earlier, another mechanism: the *transactional effect*, by which childhood experiences are perpetuated. Transactional effects between children and parents are not confined to individual stages of development. Their quality, however, does seem to depend on when they began. A 3-year-old, for example, whose mother enters hospital unexpectedly, may be angry and difficult with her when she returns. Depending on her own state of health and mood, the mother may misconstrue such signs of emotional immaturity and react in turn with disappointment and irritability. Her response now confirms the toddler's view that she does not love him and that if she had really loved him she would never have left. As his experience of rejection appears to be confirmed, he becomes more difficult and the stage is set for mutually reinforcing patterns of frustrating interactions between mother and child. The child's future intimate relationships are coloured by the memories of these interactions. They help to determine how he presents himself to others and how these others in turn respond to him.

An outline of Erikson's stages of social and emotional development

Psychoanalysts in focusing on internal mental mechanisms, had largely ignored the sociocultural environment in which children grow up. They had also paid quite insufficient regard to the actual catastrophes that commonly befall children and contribute to the course of their development and often, through the long-term personality distortions they induce, to the development of the next generation. Unlike Freud, Erikson (1968) does not set out to prove a scientific theory. Instead he uses a literary approach as a bridge between psychoanalysis on the one hand and the social sciences and history on the other. He too sees first experiences

as crucial for later personality, and he too views each stage of the 'life cycle', as he calls it, as opening up a particular new range of encounters for the future. His ideas can greatly help the clinician to understand and empathise with the patient's life experiences.

In the earliest stages the child's social interactions are associated with body functions and the experience of both is distorted by the child's immature modes of perception and reasoning. The events and circumstances in his life depend on his family setting and the behaviour and attitudes of his parents. These in turn spring from the parents' individuality but are influenced by the culture within which they live and by their personal standing within their community. Erikson suggests that the effects of child-rearing on personality ensure cultural continuity and the preservation of cultural differences from one generation to the next. He sees the individual as both absorbing and making history. Each stage of development poses specific conflicts whose solution depends in part on the degree of anxiety and the degree of satisfaction experienced at the time. First solutions become the prototype for the solutions of similar conflicts in later life.

The first year (the oral stage): trust versus mistrust

Ethologists have helped us to discard the 'secondary drive theory' of attachment between baby and mother, by demonstrating that attachment depends on her social attractiveness to the infant, not on her capacity to relieve hunger. Nevertheless, much early satisfaction comes from feeding, mouthing, sucking and biting. These activities remain important throughout the child's first year even when looking, smiling, reaching, grasping and holding have become additional sources of pleasure and interest.

In the early months of *adualism* the infant cannot distinguish between himself and the objects around him. It is assumed that he endows the world with his own good and bad feelings. Projection and introjection are postulated as the first mental mechanisms, linked symbolically with the incorporative activities of feeding, looking and grasping. The infant recognises objects and people as things in themselves only after about 6 months, when he engages in his first social relationship. This has three main qualities: it is a one-to-one relationship (when he engages with a second person, he forgets the first); he is totally dependent on the other for his very survival; and no demands are made of him. In the second half of the first year separation from the mother figure leads to anxiety and depression. Erikson holds that, depending on the infant's actual experiences in his first year, he develops basic attitudes of optimism and trust if all goes well; of distrust if for any reason his needs have not been met. Such attitudes are revived in later life when security is threatened or the individual finds himself dependent on others. If infancy has been gratifying but later stages are associated with high anxiety levels, regression to oral-dependent behaviour can occur. If the expressions of normal sibling rivalry, for example, are not handled sympathetically by parents, a previously independent child can revert to clinging babyish behaviour with demands to be bottle-fed. Of course the child continues to be dependent on parents far beyond his first year and parents are nurturing until their child is grown up. But their interactions in the child's first year set the stage for subsequent encounters of this type. Erikson relates attitudes of trust in the child to trustworthiness of the parents and to the parents' sense of security within their social environment. He also describes the more impersonal institutions of the culture as supporting each of the early modes of being. Faith and religion are the public counterparts of the trust that springs from infantile dependency. Erikson's ideas can explain the common clusters of personality attributes in adult life: for example the association of overeating or of addiction with depression and feelings of hopelessness, and with either unworthiness or suspicion.

The second and third years (the anal stage): autonomy versus shame and doubt

The child is now on his feet and can use his hands as he gets about. He can make his first choice: to hold on or to throw wilfully. He is acquiring control over his sphincters and can choose whether to tolerate discomfort for the sake of social conformity or give way to his impulses and get satisfactions from messing and smearing. His relationships are still mainly of a one-to-one type but he now follows his mother and can actively avoid separations. Her approach to him has also changed as she makes her first attempts to teach him the customs of the culture. Here she relies on his increasing capacity for self-control, self-appraisal and value judgements (Kagan 1981). The new experiences of this stage relate to learning the first rules, acquiring self-discipline and cooperating with a more powerful other in what has to be done. Pride can come from achievement; pleasure from praise, but also from the free exertion of one's own will; shame from failure. Because language is limited and memory not yet reliable, the child can contain his or her impulses only so long as others indicate what must or must not be done. Erikson suggests parents are now most helpful if

they are firm in their controls while protecting children from too great a sense of shame. The more permanent personality attributes laid down at this stage, depending on the individual child's experiences, relate to dirt, cleanliness and punctuality and to obsessional pre-occupations with rules; also to feelings of autonomy, if all goes well, or shame and doubt, if it does not, in subsequent cooperative relationships with others. Parents who themselves have a sense of controlling their destinies and who are in control of their own aggressive impulses are likely to cope well with this aspect of child-rearing. Parents with little autonomy in society and with poor impulse control often expect from their small children more control than they can manage. Such parents add to childish anxieties by not stepping in to provide safety and prevent destruction, merely warning the child before and punishing him after each calamity. The child's high anxiety level then leads to repeated testing out of the limits of safety and this, together with the impulsive and aggressive role models provided by the parents, engender personality attributes similar to theirs. In contrast, overcontrolled and overdisciplined children become inhibited, ashamed and full of doubt about their own capacities, over-compliant and unable to exert their will.

In later childhood the integrity and moral worth of parents reinforce the child's capacities for self-discipline, enabling him to incorporate parental standards and transform these into conscience. The more impersonal public counterparts of this stage are the judicial institutions. Like religion in relation to dependency, the legal framework acts as a safety net for those youngsters who in early life have acquired inadequate self-discipline.

From 3 to 6 years (the genital stage): initiative versus guilt

With the acquisition of language a remarkable transformation takes place in the child's person. He now has tools for imagining all sorts of things. His experience is no longer tied to the present and the actual: it encompasses the past and the future. This is the age of symbolic play, of listening to and telling stories, of finding out about history and envisaging the wider world as well as oneself grown up. Comparisons are possible, e.g. for size and sex. The child identifies himself as a person in imitation of his elders. Small girls become feminine and small boys adopt their father's demeanour. Children are now members of groups: the family and the play group. New conflicts and emotions arise: rivalry and jealousy and the need to postpone immediate satisfactions for the future.

This is the romantic age of childhood when erotic feelings arise. Family relationships are at first poorly grasped. A small boy will know he has a sister but cannot (because of his egocentricity) see himself as her brother. When he meets a married couple he is likely to think of the wife as the husband's 'mother'. Although children now ask endless questions, they often misunderstand the answers. They rarely comment on their feelings (introspection is rudimentary and in any case children believe grown-ups know what is in their minds) but, if asked, they reveal both their erotic longings for the parent of the opposite sex and their frequent misconceptions about sexuality, as about other aspects of life. Sexual enlightenment often does little to shift childish beliefs, for example that 'you have to have an operation' to get a baby; that a baby comes from eating a lot; or that all children were once the same and if the girl has no penis it must have been cut off, and if that could happen to her it can happen to him too. These discoveries and misunderstandings add to the anxieties aroused by the new conflicts of rivalry. At the same time a powerful new source of anxiety is born: the incorporation of parental edicts in the form of *conscience*. Because of the child's authoritarian morality his first conscience is a harsh one.

In this stage of primary identification the child builds up his first inner images of himself as he would like to be in future, that is his *ideal self*. Future attitudes towards sex and family life are laid down and also towards work and work status. But at this age, the future which the child envisages for himself and that which the parents envisage for him hold boundless opportunities.

Erikson believes that, according to the actual circumstances, life events and parental attitudes, the child emerges from this stage with his initiative unimpaired and a sense of himself as a future person. If anxieties at this stage are excessive, inhibition and guilt can stunt personality development and be a basis for later neurotic illnesses and personality difficulties. A society's kinship patterns form the public counterparts of this developmental stage.

From 6 to 12 years (latency): industry versus inferiority

The resolution of the Oedipus conflict through identification with the parent of the same sex is likely to be aided by the child's increasing rationality at around the age of 7 years, when he gives up the impossible for what is possible. Like Bruner (1972), Erikson observed the child's eagerness to learn from his elders and to copy what others do. He is now keen to engage in 'real' activities and these for the first time have real consequences. He is emerging from the stage of make-believe. His actual school work affects his future education. He now makes friends, some of whom may be lifelong. But this is also the most creative period of life when children become poets and painters. Artistic products often provide great sources of satisfaction and can compensate for work or social failure.

As he leaves his family for the larger world, the child becomes aware for the first time of his real place in society and of how others see him. This is the time of affiliative relationship with a group of peers. The ritualistic games of the playground can be viewed as the precursors of the laws and customs uniting the members of human societies. Latency is also the time when children become acutely aware of similarities and differences between themselves and others and *stigma* first appears. A child's appearance, his colour, his name, his family, his street and especially his competence are now under scrutiny. Social approval and work achievements become important sources of self-esteem and contribute to positive attitudes to work and to the community. Less well-endowed or socially handicapped children are stigmatised and now suffer a sudden constriction of their lives with profound loss of self-esteem. Unresolved conflicts from the past can also inhibit competence at this stage even in well-endowed children. Excessive dependency and separation anxiety can literally block the way to school; inadequate impulse control can disrupt the child's attention span and indeed the whole classroom; inhibition can lead to social isolation and work anxieties. Erikson sees the child as emerging from latency either confident in his capacities for work and peer group relationships or with a lasting sense of inferiority about his competence and social worth. The more impersonal counterparts to the experiences of this stage are the politics and the technology and work ethic of the culture.

Each of these four stages contributes in an important way to the tasks of adolescence and also to personality adjustment in later life.

Adolescence: identity versus identity confusion

The child, now capable of abstract thought, experiences a further transformation of perspective. He reviews his past and prepares himself for his future. The physical changes of adolescence not only affect his emotional state and open the path to adult sexuality; they also affect the expectations others have of him and contribute in an important way to his emancipation from his family and to his status in the community. He is no longer small enough to be controlled by others.

Instead he is endowed with responsibility for his own actions.

Erikson views much of adolescent activity as experimentation in order to achieve a sense of identity, that is, a more permanent inner image of one's self, one's nature, one's aims, beliefs, capacities and sources of pleasure.

Youngsters have to establish a work role for themselves, find a sexual partner, achieve independence from their families, and develop their personal ideology and belief systems.

Unresolved conflicts from earlier stages surface once more and call for new solutions. Successful adolescence ends with a number of life choices made and with a sense of inner continuity, of autonomy and purpose, with hope for the future and the capacity for intimate relationships with others. In contrast, if childhood stresses have been excessive or socialisation in childhood inadequate, or if the period of adolescence itself brought insuperable conflicts, the individual may emerge with a permanently unclear view of himself, with no commitments to other people, to a work role or an ideology, unsure of who he is and of his purpose.

Adolescent activity often oscillates between extremes, for example of compliance and opposition to parents, or in the choice of friends, jobs or social groups. Allegiances to movements and gangs may be very strong but temporary.

The dangers are that activities whose purpose is experimentation and identity development may have real consequences which then confirm a maladaptive part of the person that might otherwise have been transient. The birth of an illegitimate baby, parental intolerance of adolescent rebellion with a real disruption of bonds, a criminal conviction (sometimes reinforcing rather than preventing further misconduct) are examples.

Erikson sees the identity achieved at adolescence as the foundation for the main tasks, modes and conflicts of the subsequent life cycle. We saw earlier that there is much objective research evidence for the first two stages of his scheme. The features of later stages are still wide open for scientific exploration.

LEARNING AND CULTURE

No overview of personality development in childhood is complete without mentioning the work of learning theorists, also referred to in Chapter 3. Bandura (Bandura & Walters 1963, Bandura 1986) has extended ideas about operant learning (that is, that rewarded behaviour tends to be repeated while unrewarded or punished behaviour ceases) to include observation learning. This has made learning theory applicable and relevant to the study of human beings and indeed to animal species, like the higher apes, who learn by imitating others. Bandura's own experiments have shown, for example, that small children with dog phobias can overcome these by watching other children approach and pat dogs without coming to harm, and that children exposed to filmed displays of aggressive play will themselves play aggressively when put into a similar play setting.

While Piaget and the psychoanalysts focused on structural change with development, learning theorists concern themselves with the processes of change. They used to ignore developmental aspects of children's learning, focusing mainly on proximal causes of behaviour, but a more complex view has evolved (see Berger 1985, Miller 1989). Moreover, there is now much emphasis on cognitive processes, and on 'reciprocal determinism', that is, on transactional processes between the individual with his particular characteristics and the environment. Social learning theory holds that direct or vicarious reinforcement may not be necessary for learning, and that observation alone can be effective. Bandura's notion of 'abstract modelling' is that children can formulate rules by deduction, using important elements from a number of observations. This would account for aspects of language learning, e.g. that the past tense is denoted by the suffix '-ed', hence 'talked', 'walked', 'hitted', 'doed'. Bandura also discussed the importance of 'self-efficacy'. Children who attribute failure to lack of trying are likely to persevere and succeed; while those who attribute failure to inability are likely to give up and fail. The most efficacious self-assessment is a slight overestimation of oneself.

Modelling is an important concept for the understanding of cultural continuity between the generations, although genetic factors contribute to temperamental similarities between parents and children. There are cultural, subcultural and family differences in the personality of parents and these include their beliefs about how children should behave and also their child-rearing practices. There are corresponding differences in the behaviour of the children (Newson & Newson 1976). What is less well understood is the apparent effectiveness as a role model of a despised and often absent parent on the future behaviour of a child, and how it comes about that much of what is learnt in childhood, for example patterns of delinquency and aggression, is learnt involuntarily against the better judgement of both parents and child.

REFERENCES

Bandura A 1986 Social foundations of thought and action. Prentice-Hall, Englewood Cliffs

Bandura A, Walters R H 1963 Social learning and personality development. Holt, Rinehart & Winston, London

Berger M 1985 Learning theories, development and childhood disorders. In: Rutter M, Hersov L (eds) Child and adolescent psychiatry: modern approaches. Blackwell, Oxford

Bower T G R 1979 Human development. Freeman, San Francisco

Bowlby J 1973 Attachment and loss, vol II. Separation. Hogarth Press (Pelican Books 1975), London

Bowlby J 1980 Attachment and loss, vol III. Loss, sadness and depression. Hogarth Press and the Institute of Psychoanalysis, London

Bowlby J 1984 Attachment and loss, 2nd edn, vol I. Attachment. Penguin, Harmondsworth

Bruner J 1972 Nature and uses of immaturity. American Psychologist 27: 687–708

Bruner J 1983 Child's talk: learning to use language. Oxford University Press, Oxford

Buss A H, Plomin R 1984 Temperament: early developing personality traits. Lawrence Erlbaum, Hillsdale, N J

Case R 1988 The whole child: toward an integrated view of young children's cognitive, social, and emotional development. In: Pellegrini A D (ed) Psychological bases for early education. Wiley, Chichester, pp 153–184

Chess S, Thomas A 1984 Origins and evolution of behavior disorders. Raven Press, New York

Chomsky N 1967 The formal nature of language. In: Lenneberg E H (ed) Biological foundations of language. Wiley, New York

Colby A, Kohlberg L 1987 The measurement of moral judgement, vol I. Theoretical foundations and research validation. Cambridge University Press, Cambridge

Combrinck-Graham L 1991 Development of school-age children. In: Lewis M (ed) Child and adolescent psychiatry: a comprehensive textbook. Williams & Wilkins, Baltimore, pp 257–266

Daniels D, Plomin R 1985 Origins of individual differences in infant shyness. Developmental Psychology 21: 118–121

Dixon R A, Lerner R M 1984 A history of systems in developmental psychology. In: Bornstein M H, Lamb M E (eds) Developmental psychology: an advanced textbook. Lawrence Erlbaum, Hillsdale, NJ

Donaldson M 1978 Children's minds. Fontana/Collins, Glasgow

Dunn J 1988 Annotation: sibling influences on child development. Journal of Child Psychology and Psychiatry 29: 119–127

Dunn J, Kendrick C 1982 Siblings: love, envy and understanding. Grant McIntyre, London

Dunn J, Munn P 1985 Becoming a family member: family conflict and the development of social understanding in the second year. Child Development 56: 480–492

Erikson E H 1968 Identity, youth and crisis. Faber, London

Farrington D 1985 Delinquency prevention in the 1980s. Journal of Adolescence 8: 3–16

Feinman S, Lewis M 1983 Social referencing at ten months: a second-order effect on infants' responses to strangers. Child Development 54: 878–887

Fraiberg S 1968 Parallel and divergent patterns in blind and sighted infants. Psychoanalytic Study of the Child 23: 264–300

Freedman D G 1965 Hereditary control of early social behaviour. In: Foss B M (ed) Determinants of infant behaviour, vol III. Methuen, London

Freud S 1953 Three essays on the theory of sexuality (1905). In: The complete psychological works of Sigmund Freud VII. Hogarth Press and the Institute of Psychoanalysis, London, pp 125–245

Goodyer I M 1990 Life experiences, development and childhood psychopathology. Wiley, Chichester

Harlow H F, Zimmermann R R 1959 Affectional responses in the infant monkey. Science 130: 421–432

Harris M, Coltheart M 1986 Language processing in children and adults. Routledge & Kegan Paul, London

Hinde R A 1976 On describing relationships. Journal of Child Psychology and Psychiatry 17: 1–19

Hodges J, Tizard B 1989 Social and family relationships of ex-institutional adolescents. Journal of Child Psychology and Psychiatry 30: 77–98

Hoffman M 1987 The contribution of empathy to justice and moral judgement. In: Eisenberg N, Strayer J (eds) Empathy and its development. Cambridge University Press, New York, pp 47–80

Howlin P 1980 Language. In: Rutter M (ed) Scientific foundations of developmental psychiatry. Heinemann, London

Kagan J 1981 The second year: the emergence of self-awareness. Harvard University Press, Cambridge, MA

Kagan J, Reznick J S, Gibbons J 1989 Inhibited and uninhibited types of children. Child Development 60: 838–845

Lamb M E, Nash A, Teti D M, Bornstein M H 1991 Infancy. In: Lewis M (ed) Child and adolescent psychiatry: a comprehensive textbook. Williams & Wilkins, Baltimore, pp 222–256

Lorenz K 1966 Evolution and modification of behaviour. Methuen, London

Main M, Kaplan N 1985 Security in infancy, childhood, and adulthood: a move to the level of representation. In: Bretherton I, Waters E (eds) Growing points of attachment theory and research. Monographs of the Society for Research in Child Development 50: 66–104

Matheson B, Skuse D, Wolke D, Reilley S 1989 Oral–motor dysfunction and failure to thrive among inner-city infants. Developmental Medicine and Child Neurology 31: 293–302

Miller P H 1989 Theories of developmental psychology. Freeman, New York

Newson J, Newson E 1976 Seven year olds in the home environment. Allen & Unwin, London

Olweus D 1979 Stability of aggressive reaction patterns in males: a review. Psychological Bulletin 86: 852–875

Olweus D 1980 Familial and temperamental determinants of aggressive behaviour in adolescent boys: a causal analysis. Developmental Psychology 16: 644–660

Patterson G R, Dishion T J 1988 Multilevel family process models: traits, interactions and relationships. In: Hinde R A, Stevenson-Hinde J (eds) Relationships within families: mutual influences. Clarendon Press, Oxford, pp 283–310

Piaget J 1932 The moral judgement of the child. Routledge & Kegan Paul, London

Piaget J 1960 The language and thought of the child. Routledge & Kegan Paul, London

Piaget J 1972 The science of education and the psychology of the child. Longman, London

Piaget J, Inhelder B 1969 The psychology of the child. Routledge & Kegan Paul, London

Plomin R, De Fries J C, Fulker D W 1988 Nature and nurture during infancy and early childhood. Cambridge University Press, Cambridge

Radke-Yarrow M, Richters J, Wilson W E 1988 Child development in a network of relationships. In: Hinde R A, Stevenson-Hinde J (eds) Relationships within families: mutual influences. Clarendon Press, Oxford, pp 48–67

Robertson J, Robertson J 1971 Young children in brief separation: a fresh look. Psychoanalytic Study of the Child 26: 264–315

Robson K S, Moss H A 1970 Patterns and determinants of maternal attachment. Journal of Pediatrics 77: 976–985

Rutter M 1981 Maternal deprivation reassessed, 2nd edn. Penguin, Harmondsworth

Rutter M 1985 Family and school influences on cognitive development. Journal of Child Psychology and Psychiatry 26: 683–704

Scarr S, McCartney K 1983 How people make their own environments: a theory of genotype–environment effects. Child Development 54: 424–435

Schaffer H R 1966 Activity level as a constitutional determinant of infantile reaction to deprivation. Child Development 37: 595–602

Schaffer H R 1971 The growth of sociability. Penguin, Harmondsworth

Schaffer H R 1977 (ed) Studies in mother–infant interaction. Academic Press, London

Stilwell B M, Galvin M, Kopta S M 1991 Conceptualization of conscience in normal children and adolescents, ages 5 to 17. Journal of the American Academy for Child and Adolescent Psychiatry 30: 16–21

Taylor E, Sandberg S, Thorley G, Giles S 1991 The epidemiology of childhood hyperactivity. Maudsley monograph. Oxford University Press, Oxford

Tizard B 1977 Adoption: a second chance. Open Books, London

Tizard B, Joseph A 1973 Cognitive development of young children in residential care: a study of children aged 24 months. Journal of Child Psychology and Psychiatry 11: 177–186

Thomas A, Chess S 1986 The New York longitudinal study: from infancy to early adult life. In: Plomin R, Dunn J F (eds) The study of temperament: changes, continuities and challenges. Lawrence Erlbaum, Hillsdale, NJ, pp 39–52

Torgersen A M 1989 Genetic and environmental influences on temperament development: longitudinal study of twins from infancy to adolescence. In: Doxiadis S (ed) Early influences shaping the individual. Plenum Press, London

Toulmin S 1970 Reasons and causes. In: Borger R, Cioffi F (eds) Explanation in the behavioural sciences. Cambridge University Press, Cambridge

Wolff S 1989 Childhood and human nature: the development of personality. Routledge, London

Wolff S 1991 Moral development. In: Lewis M (ed) Child and adolescent psychiatry: a comprehensive textbook. Williams & Wilkins, Baltimore, pp 187–194

6. Functional neuroanatomy

E. Szabadi

INTRODUCTION

Neuroanatomy is the discipline dealing with the structure of the nervous system. There are two basic neuroanatomical approaches: a descriptive one, and a functional one. The *descriptive anatomy* of the brain is usually divided into macroscopic or gross anatomy, and into microscopic anatomy. Descriptive anatomy is based on the dissection of the brain, and deals with the brain on a regional basis (e.g. spinal cord, brain stem, cerebellum, etc.). This chapter will not deal with the descriptive anatomy of the nervous system, since there are excellent concise texts covering this field (e.g. Mitchell 1971, Smith 1971, Bowsher 1972, Gatz 1973). *Functional neuroanatomy* discusses the structure of the brain on a functional basis, and often encompasses topographically distant regions into functional entities (e.g. motor system, visual system, etc.). Functional neuroanatomy often uses 'wiring diagrams' in order to illustrate the interconnections between different parts of the brain.

The purpose of this chapter is to discuss some aspects of the functional anatomy of the brain, and thus to serve as a 'companion' to the reader during his journey through the disciplines of neuroanatomy and neurophysiology.

CELLULAR ELEMENTS OF THE NERVOUS SYSTEM

The cellular elements of the nervous system can be divided into three groups: (1) neurones (or nerve cells); (2) interstitial cells; (3) connective tissue cells (Noback 1967).

Neurones (nerve cells)

The neurones are cellular units of the nervous tissue which possess the two most characteristic features of the nervous tissue itself: excitability and conductivity.

Neurones are also a homogeneous population of cells from a developmental point of view: all the neurones of the body develop from a primordial cell type, the neuroblasts.

Neurones vary greatly in size and shape. A typical neurone (Fig. 6.1A) consists of a cell body and several processes.

The cell body (neurocyte, perikaryon) contains the nucleus and the neuroplasm. The nucleus is relatively large, and contains relatively little chromatin material. The chromatin material is composed of deoxyribonucleoprotein, the chemical substrate of the genes. The nucleus has a thick membrane, and contains the prominent nucleolus. Adjacent to the nucleus is situated a small DNA body, the paranuclear body or nuclear satellite. This body corresponds to the paired X (female) chromosomes, and thus it is present in the female, but absent in the male.

The neuroplasm contains different subcellular particles, of which the *Nissl substance* (chromophil substance) is the most characteristic of nerve cells. The Nissl substance appears as coarse granules under the light microscope; in electron micrographs each granule is the collection of flattened membranous sacs to which RNA-containing granules (ribosomes) are attached. The Nissl substance corresponds to the ergastoplasm of gland cells, and thus it is a protein synthesising cell organelle. Proteins synthesised in the cell body are transported by 'axoplasmic flow' down the axon to the synaptic terminals. When a neurone is injured, the Nissl substance seems to disappear, indicating that proteins are being synthesised at an increased rate for the reconstitution of the cell. *Neurofibrils* are also characteristic of neurones. These are filamentous structures whose function is uncertain. They are believed to play a role in the fast transport of materials within the cell body. *Mitochondria, Golgi apparatus,* and *lysosomes* are ubiquitous cell organelles, and thus not specific to neurones. An iron-containing melanin *pigment* is found in cell bodies of neurones in the substantia nigra and the locus coeruleus. It is of interest that these cells are the origins of the catecholamine-containing pathways of the brain: the dopamine-containing neurones are located in the pars compacta of the substantia nigra, whereas the noradrenaline-containing neurones are situated in the locus coeruleus (see below).

Neurones have two kinds of processes: dendrites and axons. The *dendrites* are extensions of the cell body, and thus they also contain Nissl substance. The pattern of arborisation of the dendrites is characteristic of particular types of nerve cells, and is thus the basis for the neurohistological identification of types of neurones. The dendrites greatly increase the surface area of neurones: it is estimated that on some neurones as much as 90% of the surface area is taken up by the dendrites. Dendrites often have small spine-like processes (dendritic spines) which form the subsynaptic part of axodendritic synapses (see below). Most

neurones have only one axon (axis cylinder, neurite) which is distinguishable from the dendrites on the basis of the absence of the Nissl substance. The axon originates from the axon hillock, an area of the cell body devoid of Nissl substance. The initial part of the axon (initial segment) is thin and never possesses a myelin sheath. The membrane of the initial segment is the point from which action potentials normally originate. The axon of a neurone can be as long as 1 m and it can have several thousand collaterals. Each collateral ends in a terminal arborisation (telodendrion) which contains the individual nerve endings (nerve terminals, axon terminals). The nerve terminals are usually enlarged endings (synaptic knobs, 'boutons terminaux'). They are the presynaptic elements of the synapse.

Synapses are sites of contact between one neurone and another, or between a neurone and a peripheral effector cell (muscle fibre, gland cell). The schematic

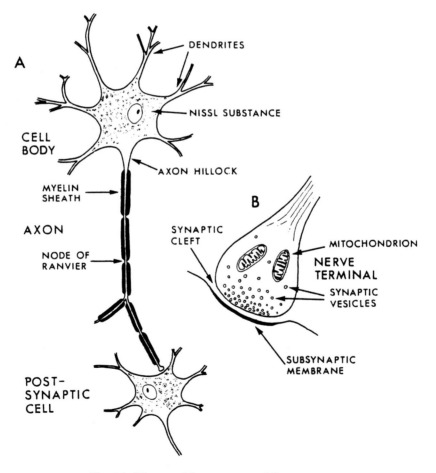

Fig. 6.1 Diagram of **A** a neurone, and **B** a synapse.

picture of a synapse is shown in Figure 6.1B. The synapse consists of the (pre)synaptic nerve terminals, the synaptic gap or cleft, and the subsynaptic membrane of the postsynaptic neurone. The presynaptic terminals contain (pre)synaptic vesicles which are believed to be the sites of the synthesis and storage of the chemical neurotransmitter agent. Synaptic terminals also contain mitochondria in large numbers which also play a role in the metabolism of the neurotransmitter. The number, size and appearance of synaptic vesicles varies between different synapses. It is believed that clear vesicles are indicative of the storage of acetylcholine, whereas the so-called dense-core vesicles are related to monoamines. The synaptic gap is about 200 Å wide. The subsynaptic membrane is usually somewhat thicker than non-synaptic areas of the postsynaptic membrane.

Interneuronal synapses usually connect an axon terminal of one cell and the cell body or dendrite of another. Axo-axonic synapses have also been described: in this case one nerve terminal synapses on to the terminal of another neurone. It is assumed that axo-axonic synapses are the anatomical substrates of presynaptic inhibition (see Guyton 1972).

The synapse is regarded by many neuroscientists as a specialised functional unit of the nervous system. A nerve impulse (action potential) arriving at the synaptic terminal depolarises the neuronal membrane, and this results in the release of the neurotransmitter from the vesicular stores. Transmitter release is probably achieved by exocytosis: the vesicles adhere to the membrane of the presynaptic terminal, then the fused membrane of the vesicle and the terminal breaks open, and the contents of the vesicle are 'poured' into the synaptic gap. The released transmitter diffuses across the gap to the subsynaptic membrane, where it interacts with specific receptors. The interaction between transmitter and receptors results in a change in the membrane potential: the membrane may become either depolarised (excitatory postsynaptic potential, EPSP), or hyperpolarised (inhibitory postsynaptic potential, IPSP). The EPSPs and IPSPs produced in response to different synaptic inputs to the same postsynaptic neurone are integrated by the cell, and if the net result is a sufficient degree of depolarisation, it will trigger off an action potential at the initial segment of the axon of the neurone. Action potentials are all-or-none events which are conducted in a non-decremental way along the axon and also along the membrane of the cell body. Action potentials reaching the nerve terminals can result in the release of the transmitter from the nerve endings. It is generally assumed that there is a direct relationship between the amount of excitatory

transmitter released and the degree of depolarisation achieved on the postsynaptic cell; a greater degree of depolarisation would result in a higher frequency of action potential production by the postsynaptic neurone. Thus the transmission of nerve impulses through synapses involves alternating translations of electrical signals into chemical messages, and of chemical messages into electrical signals.

It has been suggested (Grundfest 1959) that, on a functional basis, the membrane of the neurone can be divided into three parts: (1) a chemosensitive receptor area (corresponding to the membrane of dendrites and of the cell body); (2) a chemically largely insensitive conductile area (corresponding to the axonal membrane); (3) a neurosecretory effector area (corresponding to the nerve terminal). This functional differentiation of the neuronal membrane is of great significance. Firstly, it shows that the neurone itself possesses the differentiation which is characteristic of the entire nervous system: the spatial separation of the receptor part from the effector part. Secondly, since only a chemical released from the presynaptic terminal can transmit the nerve impulse from one neurone to another, the synapse acts as a one-way valve allowing the propagation of impulses in one direction only. Thirdly, as the postsynaptic membrane is chemosensitive, it is likely that many centrally acting drugs exert their effects on this membrane, either mimicking or blocking the effect of the natural transmitter.

Interstitial cells (neuroglia)

The interstitial cells (neuroglia) are of ectodermal origin and develop in close association with the neurone. These cells are interposed between neurones, between neurones and blood capillaries, and between neurones and the surface of the brain. Thus, each neurone is surrounded by a layer of interstitial cells. The bulk of the nervous tissue is made up by interstitial cells and their processes; there are about ten times as many interstitial cells as neurones in the brain. The interstitial cells completely fill the gaps between neurones, leaving only very thin (150–200 Å) clefts between the cellular elements of the nervous tissue. As a result of this, the extracellular space is much smaller in the brain than in other tissues of the body.

There are two kinds of neuroglia: astroglia and oligodendroglia (Fig. 6.2). The *astroglia* (astrocytes) are multipolar cells with several thick processes. The processes of these cells form a bridge between the capillaries and the nerve cell bodies, and it is believed that several nutrients and metabolites pass from the neurone to capillaries through astrocytes. The strate-

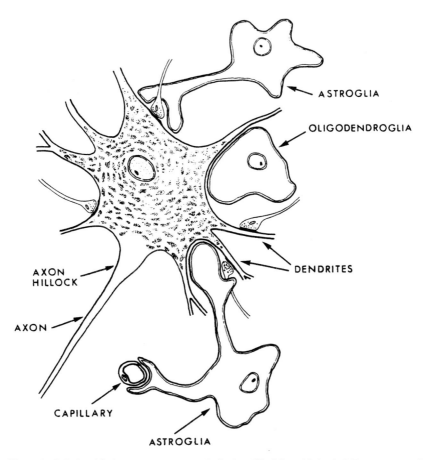

Fig. 6.2 Relationship between neurone and glia (modified from Noback & Demarest 1981).

gic position of the astrocytes and capillaries gives these cells a very important role in the metabolism of neurones. The glial processes reaching capillaries form the so-called perivascular feet which almost completely cover the outer surface of the capillaries (see Fig. 6.2). This 'gliovascular membrane' (composed of the processes of astrocytes) is regarded as one of the anatomical substrates of the blood–brain barrier. (The blood–brain barrier is not an anatomical, but a functional concept. One should not speak of the blood–brain barrier in general, but only with reference to a particular substance. The existence of a blood–brain barrier for a particular substance is indicated if after injection into the bloodstream, the substance fails to appear in the brain tissue while it is easily detectable in other tissues. Astrocytes may accumulate some substances, thus preventing them from reaching the neurones.)

The *oligodendroglia* (oligodendrocytes) are smaller spherical cells which have only a few processes. A certain number of these cells may participate together with the processes of the astrocytes in forming a glial protective layer around the neuronal cell body (see Fig. 6.2). These oligodendroglial cells are often referred to as perineuronal satellite cells, and are equivalent to the satellite cells encapsulating neuronal cell bodies in peripheral ganglia. However, most of the oligodendroglial cells in the central nervous system are arranged in long parallel rows alongside axons. These interfascicular oligodendroglia are equivalent to the neurilemma cells (lemmocytes or Schwann cells) of peripheral nerves. The Schwann cells in the periphery, and the interfascicular oligodendroglia in the central nervous system, form a protecting insulating cell layer around neuronal axons. In the periphery, a neuronal axon is usually embedded in the bodies of a row of Schwann cells, causing an invagination of the membrane of the individual Schwann cells (Fig. 6.3). This is the characteristic structure of unmyelinated nerve

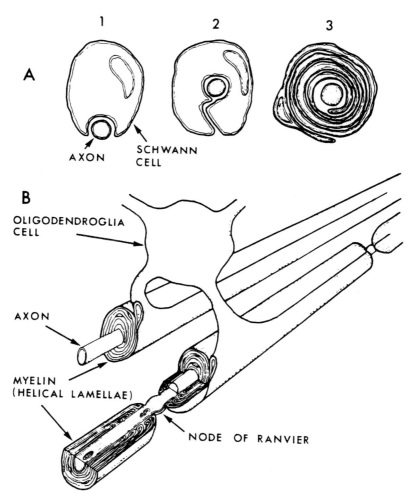

Fig. 6.3 Formation of the myelin sheath: **A** in peripheral nerves; **B** in the central nervous system.

fibres in the periphery. In the case of many peripheral nerve fibres the Schwann cells rotate around the axon, which results in the 'winding up' of the Schwann cell membrane around the axon. The layers of the Schwann cell membrane are the basis for the deposition of lipids, and thus the formation of the myelin sheath. In the central nervous system, the flattened processes of one oligodendroglia cell can wrap up several nearby nerve fibres (Fig. 6.3), thus forming myelin sheaths of more than one axon.

In myelinated nerves the myelin cover extends almost over the entire length of the axon. There are, however, three areas where even myelinated nerve fibres are devoid of a myelin sheath: (1) the initial segment of the axon; (2) the terminal arborisation of the axon, and (3) the nodes of Ranvier. The nodes of Ranvier are the

boundaries between segments of the myelin sheath formed by two neighbouring oligodendroglia or Schwann cells (see Fig. 6.3). The nodes of Ranvier are of great physiological significance. It is believed that the nerve impulses 'jump' from one node to the next one (so-called saltatory conduction of the nerve impulse), and this results in a much faster impulse propagation than is possible in non-myelinated fibres.

Connective tissue cells

Connective tissue elements in the brain are the microglia cells and the cellular elements of cerebral blood vessels. The *microglia* (or mesoglia) are of mesodermal origin, and thus they differ from the ectodermal neuroglia. The microglia cells are thin elongated cells with several thin processes. They are phagocytic cells and act as 'scavengers' within the nervous tissue. Being mobile, they can migrate for long distances. These cells often respond to pathological stimuli as a unified system, and are often regarded as the central nervous system equivalents of the reticuloendothelial cellular system of the body. In certain diseases (e.g. general paralysis of the insane, sleeping sickness) they may proliferate enormously, and may thus dominate the histological appearance of the brain tissue.

The cells of the *blood vessels* are similar to cells making up the vascular bed in other parts of the body. The capillaries have a continuous endothelial lining in contact with a continuous basement membrane. The endothelial cells of brain capillaries may possess metabolic features which distinguish them from endothelial cells elsewhere. Thus, for example, it has been shown that these cells have a high activity in γ-aminobutyric-acid transaminase (GABA-T), the enzyme responsible for the metabolic degradation of γ-aminobutyric acid (GABA), a putative neurotransmitter. This explains why intravenously injected GABA does not reach the brain tissue. Thus, in the case of GABA the blood–brain barrier is anatomically equivalent to the brain capillary endothelium (Katzman 1971).

DEVELOPMENTAL ORGANISATION OF THE BRAIN

The nervous system is highly specialised epithelium: it develops, together with the skin, from the ectoderm (outer germ layer) of the embryo (Fig. 6.4). The first stage of its development is the appearance of a shield-like thickening in the midline of the dorsal surface of the embryo (approximately 18 days old) called the *neural plate*. The neural plate gives rise to the development of three *placods* (optic, auditory and nasal) at its cephalic end, from which the sense organs develop, and to the formation of the *neural tube*. The neural tube arises from the closing of most of the neural plate into a tube that sinks beneath the surface skin and gets detached from it. A bilateral column of cells is separated from the neural ectoderm at its junction with the skin ectoderm to form the *neural crest*. The central nervous system (brain and spinal cord), including all neurones, oligodendroglia and astroglia, develops entirely from the neural tube, whereas the neural crest gives rise to all peripheral (sensory and autonomic) ganglia, the pia and the arachnoid, adrenal medulla and the receptor cells of the carotid body.

The primordial nervous system (neural tube) is recognizable in the anatomical organization of the adult brain. The cavity inside the neural tube is the

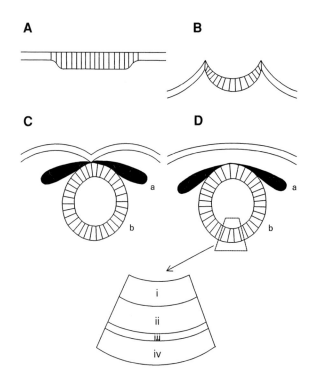

Fig. 6.4 Transverse sections through the human embryo showing early development of the nervous system. **A** Neural plate (18 days): hatched area, neural ectoderm; open area, skin ectoderm. **B** Neural plate with neural groove (19 days). **C, D** Neural tube (b) and neural crest (a) (21–25 days). At the bottom of the figure a segment of the neural tube is shown (i, ventricular zone; ii, subventricular zone; iii, intermediate zone; iv, marginal zone).

precursor of the central canal of the spinal cord and of the cerebral ventricles. Later in development three cerebral vesicles can be distinguished at the oral end of the tube corresponding to the head region of the embryo. These three vesicles are called: (1) the prosencephalon (forebrain); (2) the mesencephalon (midbrain); (3) the rhombencephalon (hindbrain). The hindbrain continues into the spinal cord (Fig. 6.5). The *midbrain* region changes very little, and it maintains its position anchored to the centre of the cranial cavity. The prosencephalon and rhombencephalon differentiate further. Two secondary vesicles (telencephalon) grow out from the prosencephalon; they are the precursors of the cerebral hemispheres. The cerebral hemispheres include the olfactory bulbs and olfactory lobes (rhinencephalon), the pallium (cerebral cortex), and the basal ganglia (corpus striatum). A part of the prosencephalon (the diencephalon) remains undivided in the midline. The diencephalon comprises the thalamus, hypothalamus and epithalamus. The

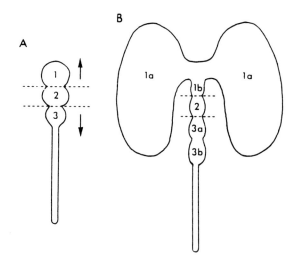

Fig. 6.5 Development of the cerebral vesicles **A** at an early and **B** at a later stage: 1, prosencephalon; 1a, telencephalon; 1b, diencephalon; 2, mesencephalon; 3, rhombencephalon; 3a, metencephalon; 3b, myelencephalon.

rhombencephalon divides into two secondary vesicles: the metencephalon and the myelencephalon. The metencephalon comprises the pons, the oral part of the medulla oblongata, and the cerebellum. The myelencephalon corresponds to the caudal part of the medulla.

The histogenesis of the central nervous system is a very complex process. The starting point is the neural tube, the wall of which has four cellular layers: (1) ventricular zone, adjacent to the lumen of the tube; (2) subventricular zone; (3) intermediate zone; (4) marginal zone (see Fig. 6.4). All cellular divisions take place in the ventricular and subventricular zones; the intermediate zone is populated mainly by neuronal migration, whereas the marginal zone gives rise to the future white matter of the brain. Four processes have been implicated in the histogenesis of the brain: (1) cell proliferation; (2) cell migration; (3) differentiation and connectivity; (4) cell death (for a review, see Jones & Murray 1991). Phylogenetically older parts of the brain (e.g. hippocampus, spinal cord) develop mainly by cell proliferation from a small number of progenitor cells situated near the ventricular surface, whereas newer structures (e.g. neocortex) develop mainly by cellular migration. Differentiation and connectivity involve axonal growth, the establishment of neuronal connections, and myelination of axons. Cell death is an important, but rather poorly understood, process of cerebral histogenesis by which redundant neurones and transient connections are eliminated. It is customary to differentiate between early and late develop-

ment, the former taking place in early prenatal life and consisting of proliferation and differentiation, and the latter taking place in late prenatal and early postnatal life, and consisting of growth. It is generally believed that neuronal proliferation does not take place after birth, and postnatal brain development is due mainly to growth (increase in size of neurones and glia, and myelination). Recent brain imaging and histopathological studies have revealed that some schizophrenic patients may show evidence of abnormal brain development, relating mainly to the temporal lobes and the hippocampus. All four processes of histological differentiation may be involved, indicating an early prenatal lesion. The aetiology remains to be determined; however, a genetic defect remains a likely candidate (Jones & Murray 1991).

FUNCTIONAL ORGANISATION OF THE BRAIN

We have seen above that the neurone itself shows a remarkable degree of functional polarisation: the receptor part of the neurone is spatially separated from the effector part (Fig. 6.6). This polarisation further develops with the appearance of the *reflex arc*. The reflex arc is a chain of at least two, but often of many, neurones. A simple two neuronal reflex arc is shown in Figure 6.6B. Each reflex arc consists of five parts: (1) a receptor; (2) an afferent branch; (3) an integrating centre (one synapse or a more complex neuronal network); (4) an efferent branch; (5) an effector. In the simple reflex arc the two neurones are functionally different: one neurone is capable of receiving stimuli from the environment (sensory neurone), whereas the other neurone is capable of causing a response in an effector tissue (motor neurone, effector neurone). Both the sensory neurone and the motor neurone are in contact with 'higher' structures of the brain (Fig. 6.7). The sensory neurone can pass on the 'sensory information' to another neurone located in the central nervous system (e.g. in the spinal cord), and this second neurone can pass on the information to a third neurone located in a 'higher' centre of the brain (e.g. in the thalamus). The route followed by nerve impulses evoked by a sensory stimulus is referred to as a sensory system. Similarly, the peripheral motor neurone is influenced by a series of higher structures (cerebral cortex, basal ganglia, brain stem). The assembly of the neurones which directly influence the activity of the peripheral motor neurone is known as a motor system. The sensory and motor systems of the brain are interconnected at different levels: in the spinal cord, in the brain stem, at the level of the basal

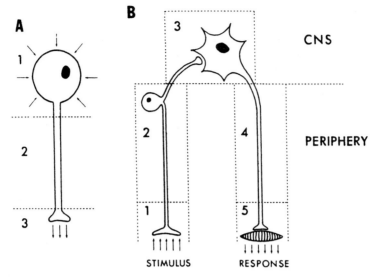

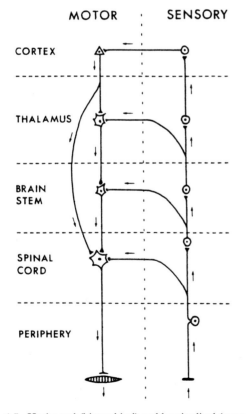

Fig. 6.6 Functional differentiation in the nervous system. **A** In the neurone: 1, receptor area; 2, conductile area; 3, effector area. **B** In the reflex arc: 1, receptor; 2, afferent branch; 3, integrating centre; 4, efferent branch; 5, effector.

Fig. 6.7 Horizontal (hierarchical) and longitudinal (sensory motor) organisation of the nervous system.

ganglia and at the level of the cerebral cortex (see Fig. 6.7). These connections between the two systems are the anatomical substrates of spinal, brain stem, sub-cortical and cortical reflexes.

On the basis of the organisation patterns described above, it is possible to distinguish between two basic principles: (1) the principle of functional polarisation into sensory and motor systems; (2) the principle of hierarchical organisation. Thus the simple reflex arc can be regarded as the basic unit of brain function: higher 'centres' of the brain influence this basic unit. However, the majority of neurones cannot be classified as either sensory or motor; these neurones form the integrative neuronal circuits which receive inputs from sensory neurones and may send outputs to motor neurones.

The sensory and motor divisions of the brain are separated anatomically. In the spinal cord and in the brain stem the motor parts take up a ventral position, whereas the sensory parts take up a dorsal position. Thus, in the spinal cord the ventral horns are motor and the dorsal horns are sensory and, in the brain stem, motor nuclei of the cranial nerves are in a ventral and more medial position compared to the dorsally and laterally located sensory nuclei. In the cerebral cortex motor areas are in a frontal position, whereas sensory areas are in a more occipital position; the two areas are divided by the deep central sulcus.

In the following sections of this chapter we shall follow the pattern of structural organisation described above. First we shall discuss the organisation of sensory systems, then we shall deal with the organisation of the motor system. Although the organisation of the autonomic nervous system follows similar principles, it will be discussed separately due to its unique role in the control of the internal environment of the organism. The hypothalamic and endocrine control of the internal environment will be discussed in conjunction with the autonomic nervous system. Areas of the brain with mainly integrative functions will be discussed under separate headings (limbic system, reticular formation, cerebral cortex). Finally, a brief description of the anatomy of the monoamine-containing neuronal systems will be given. This special treatment of this unique group of neurones is warranted by their postulated role in the genesis of functional psychoses (affective disorders and schizophrenia).

ORGANISATION OF SENSORY SYSTEMS

General principles

Sensory systems are parts of the nervous system which are concerned with (1) translation of stimuli into nerve signals; (2) conduction of signals into the brain and (3) processing of sensory information. On this basis, all sensory systems consist of three basic elements: (1) transducers (receptors); (2) conductors; (3) integrators.

Sensory transducers (receptors)

Receptors are sensory nerve endings which are capable of responding with depolarisation (generator potential) to environmental stimuli. The stimulus is a change in the level of a specific kind of energy in the environment, and the response is the generator potential in the sensory neurone which can trigger off action potentials at the nearest node of Ranvier in the sensory nerve fibre. Although every receptor can respond to every kind of energy, there are great differences between receptors in their sensitivities to different kinds of energy. The specificity of a receptor simply means that the receptor has a lower threshold for a particular kind of environmental energy (e.g. the rods and cones of the retina have a lower threshold for light than for mechanical or chemical stimulation). There is a close quantitative relationship between the size of the stimulus and the size of the evoked response: an increase in the size of the stimulus causes an increase in the size of the generator potential, which in turn causes an increase in the number of

action potentials generated in the peripheral neurone.

A stimulus can evoke the generator potential directly in the sensory nerve ending (simple receptors), or in a specialised sensory cell which is in synaptic contact with the sensory nerve ending of the peripheral sensory neurone (complex receptors). The sensory cells (or receptor cells) of complex receptors are specialised epithelial cells which are capable of responding with depolarisation to the environmental stimulus (e.g. hair cells of the cochlea). The depolarisation in the receptor cell (receptor potential) can spread to the adjacent sensory nerve ending and result in a generator potential.

Receptors can be classified using different criteria. On the basis of the *stimulus* one can distinguish four classes: (1) mechanoreceptors (cutaneous, deep tissue, auditory, vestibular and baroreceptors); (2) thermoreceptors (cold and warmth receptors); (3) photoreceptors; (4) chemoreceptors (taste, olfactory, pain and receptors sensitive to arterial oxygen and carbon dioxide tension). (The pain receptors listed under chemoreceptors are free nerve endings which are sensitive to chemicals (histamine, bradykinin) released by damaged tissues). A practical *anatomical* classification generally adopted in medicine considers whether the receptors are distributed diffusely throughout the body or localised in specialised sense organs. On this basis it is usual to distinguish between receptors subserving (1) somatic senses (mechanoreceptive, thermoceptive, nociceptive), and (2) special senses (visual, auditory, olfactory, gustatory and equilibrium). We shall follow this classificatory scheme in our further discussion.

Sensory conductors

Sensory conductors are a chain of neurones which constitute the sensory pathways between the receptors and the cerebral cortex. A sensory pathway consists of at least three neurones connected in series: (1) peripheral sensory neurone (primary sensory neurone); (2) secondary sensory neurone; (3) tertiary sensory neurone.

The *peripheral sensory neurones* are pseudo-unipolar or bipolar neurones with two axon-like processes. (Pseudo-unipolar cells are bipolar cells in which the two processes are fused together at their point of origin from the cell body, but separate again a few millimetres from the cell body; see Fig. 6.6.) The cell bodies of peripheral sensory neurones are situated in the intervertebral (spinal) ganglia and in the ganglia of the sensory cranial nerves. The two processes of the sensory ganglion cells carry nerve impulses from peripheral receptors to the central nervous system. The peripheral processes run out to the periphery, constitute sensory nerves, and terminate in sensory nerve endings. A peripheral sensory neurone can be connected to several receptors via its collaterals. A peripheral neurone and the receptors belonging to it is called a sensory unit. The area of the periphery belonging to one sensory unit is called its receptive field. Although the peripheral processes of sensory neurones have an axon-like structure, impulses are conducted along them in a cellulopetal direction (i.e. behave like dendrites). The central processes connect the ganglia to the central nervous system: they constitute the dorsal roots of the spinal cord, and the central branches of cranial sensory ganglia. Central processes of some primary sensory neurones can be very long (e.g. nearly 1 m in the case of the dorsal column pathway). The central processes terminate in sensory nuclei of the spinal cord or brain stem where they synapse with the *secondary sensory neurones*. There are four groups of sensory nuclei: (1) the dorsal horn of the spinal cord; (2) the dorsal column nuclei of the medulla (gracile and cuneate nuclei); (3) the sensory nuclei of cranial nerves V, VII, IX and X; (4) the vestibular and auditory nuclei. The secondary neurones send their axons to the thalamus. The *tertiary sensory neurones* originate in the thalamus, and send their axons to the cerebral cortex.

Sensory integrators

The sensory integrators are neuronal pools which receive collaterals from the sensory pathways, and thus participate in the processing of sensory information. Integration and information processing take place at every stage in the sensory pathway, i.e. in (1) the sensory nuclei of the spinal cord and brain stem, (2) the thalamus and (3) the sensory cortex. Apart from these 'primary' centres of sensory integration, there are four other structures of the brain which receive collaterals from every sensory pathway: (1) the reticular formation (maintenance of level of arousal); (2) the hypothalamus (organisation of autonomic responses); (3) the limbic system (organisation of emotional reactions); (4) the cerebellum (organisation of motor responses).

Somatosensory systems

The somatosensory systems carry information to the somatosensory cortex from three kinds of receptor: (1) mechanoreceptors, (2) thermoreceptors and (3) pain receptors. These receptors are located in the skin, subcutaneous tissues, tendons, ligaments and in the connective tissue of internal organs. There are two separate somatosensory systems: (1) the spinothalamic system and (2) the dorsal column system.

The *spinothalamic system* carries sensory information from all three types of receptor listed above — (1) mechanoreceptors (crude touch sensation, pressure sensation, tickle and itch sensation, sexual sensation), (2) thermoreceptors (warm and cold sensation) and (3) pain receptors. The peripheral sensory neurone sends its peripheral process to the appropriate receptors, and its central process to the spinal cord, where it synapses with the secondary neurone in the dorsal horn. The secondary neurone crosses over to the other side in front of the central canal, and ascends in the lateral or ventral tract of the spinal cord and terminates in the ventrobasal nuclear complex of the thalamus (spinothalamic tract). The secondary neurone is often damaged at the point of the crossover in syringomyelia; this damage results in the selective loss of pain and heat sensations in the dermatomal segments affected. The tertiary neurone ascends through the internal capsule to the somatosensory area of the cortex (Fig. 6.8).

The *dorsal column system* carries information only from mechanoreceptors. Four mechanical sensory qualities are related to this system: (1) fine, precisely localised touch; (2) vibration; (3) kinaesthetic sensation; (4) fine pressure sensation. This system contains thick myelinated fibres, and is capable of very fast transmission. The central processes of the primary sensory neurones enter the spinal cord via the dorsal roots, and ascend in the ipsilateral dorsal column to the dorsal column nuclei of the medulla. Any damage to the dorsal roots can separate dorsal column fibres from their cell bodies located in the spinal ganglia, and thus result in degeneration of the dorsal column (e.g. in tabes dorsalis). The secondary neurones originate in one of the dorsal column nuclei (cuneate or gracile nucleus). The secondary neurones decussate to the other side and ascend to the thalamus. This pathway is called the medial lemniscus. The tertiary neurones originate in the ventrobasal nuclear complex of the thalamus, and reach the somatosensory cortex through the internal capsule (Fig. 6.8).

The somatosensory cortex (somaesthetic cortex) corresponds to the postcentral gyrus (Brodmann areas 3, 1, 2). There is a distinct somatotopic localisation in this cortical area: sensory information from one part of the body is 'projected' to a distinct area of the cortex. The 'sensory homunculus' shows how the stimulation of peripheral receptors in certain regions of the body evokes neuronal firing consistently in well-defined cortical areas. The sensory homunculus is similar to the motor homunculus.

SPECIAL SENSORY SYSTEMS

The olfactory, visual and auditory systems developed in closed relationship to the three primordial cerebral vesicles (see above). The olfactory system is associated with the prosencephalon (rhinencephalon); the visual system is closely related to the mesencephalon (optic tectum); whereas the auditory system is connected to the rhombencephalon (auditory sensory nuclei). Later, with the development of the neopallium, both the visual and auditory systems obtain cortical representations. The lower and more ancient brain stem centres relay sensory information to these cortical projection areas for further analysis.

The olfactory system and the visual system differ significantly from other sensory systems in their anatomical organisation. The olfactory receptors are bipolar olfactory cells located in the olfactory membrane which lines the top of the nasal cavity. The peripheral process of each of these cells forms a knob with several olfactory hairs on it. The olfactory hairs are the chemo-

sensitive areas of the receptor cell which can respond with depolarisation to odours. The central processes of the bipolar sensory cells pass through the perforations of the lamina cribrosa and enter the olfactory bulb. The olfactory bulb is in fact a lobe of the forebrain. The olfactory cells synapse with the dendrites of large mitral cells in the olfactory bulb. The mitral cells (second olfactory neurones) send their axons via the olfactory tract to one of the olfactory areas of the cortex: (1) to the medial olfactory area (septum pellucidum, gyrus subcallosus, paraolfactory area) or (2) to the lateral olfactory area (pre-pyriform area, uncus, amygdaloid nucleus; Fig. 6.8). The two primary olfactory cortical areas are connected via secondary olfactory tracts to the thalamus, hypothalamus, hippocampus and brain stem nuclei. Through these connections the olfactory system is closely associated with the limbic system (see below).

The receptor area of the *visual system* is the retina. The retina is a sheet of modified cerebral cortex. There are three visual neurones linked in series in the

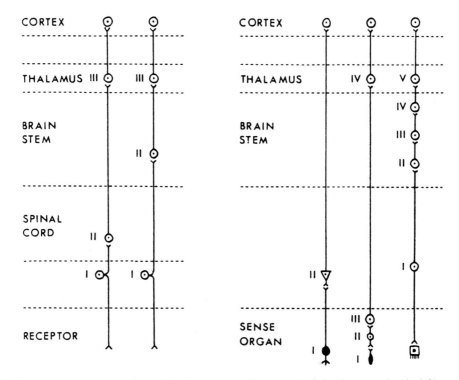

Fig. 6.8 Sensory neuronal chains. **A** Somatosensory systems: spinothalamic system (on the left) and dorsal column system (on the right). **B** Special sensory systems: olfactory system (on the left), visual system (in the middle) and auditory system (on the right).

retina: (1) receptor cells (rods and cones); (2) bipolar cells; (3) ganglion cells. There is a great degree of convergence in the retina: one ganglion cell receives inputs from many bipolar cells, and one bipolar cell receives inputs from many receptor cells. The axons of the third visual neurone constitute the optic nerve and the optic tract. From a structural point of view, the optic nerve is not a peripheral nerve, but a central neuronal pathway: the myelin sheaths of the fibres are produced by central oligodendroglia cells, and not by Schwann cells. The optic nerves partially decussate at the optic chiasma, and continue as optic tracts. For practical reasons, it is useful to distinguish between the two sections of the third optic neurone, the sections situated anterior and posterior to the chiasma; this distinction, however, does not correspond to any kind of structural or histological change in the pathway: the axons pass through the chiasma without interruption. The optic chiasma does not constitute a complete decussation; it is a hemidecussation: optic fibres orginating from the nasal halves of the retinae decussate, whereas fibres deriving from the temporal halves proceed on the same side. The third optic neurone (optic nerve–optic tract) terminates in the lateral geniculate body, which forms part of the thalamic nuclear complex. The fourth visual neurone originates in the lateral geniculate body, and its axons make up the optic radiation. The fourth visual neurone synapses on neurones in the visual cortex (Fig. 6.8). The visual cortex is located on the occipital pole of the cerebral hemisphere (Brodmann areas 17, 18, 19).

The *auditory pathway* originates in the hair cells (auditory receptor cells) of the cochlea. These cells are mechanoreceptors: the mechanical deformation caused in them by the dislocation of the basilar membrane of the cochlea results in the production of the sensory generator potential. The cell bodies of the primary sensory neurones are located in the spiral ganglion of Corti. The peripheral processes of these bipolar neurones are associated with the hair cells, whereas the central processes constitute the cochlear nerve (acoustic nerve), and terminate in the dorsal and ventral auditory nuclei of the brain stem. The secondary neurones originate from the auditory nuclei, and project to the superior olivary nuclei on both sides. The tertiary neurones originate from the superior olivary nuclei, and terminate in the inferior colliculus of the tectum of the midbrain. The axons of tertiary auditory neurones constitute the lateral lemniscus. The fourth auditory neurones originate in the inferior colliculus, and send their axons to the medial geniculate body of the thalamus. The fifth auditory neurones are located in the medial geniculate body. The axons of these neurones ascend through the posterior limb of the internal capsule (auditory radiation) and terminate in the auditory cortex (Fig. 6.8). The auditory cortex is located on the top of the superior temporal gyrus (Brodmann areas 41, 42). Each cochlea is represented in both hemispheres, due to the projections in the brain stem to the superior olivary nuclei of both sides. Thus, unilateral central lesions of the auditory pathway usually do not cause functional defects in hearing.

ORGANISATION OF THE MOTOR SYSTEM

The motor system is the part of the nervous system which is directly concerned with the control of the contraction of skeletal muscles. Because of the close anatomical and functional relationship between the skeletal muscles and the neurones controlling muscle contraction, it is appropriate to talk about a neuromuscular system. The role of the motor system is twofold: (1) to move the body or parts of it (locomotion); (2) to prevent the body from moving (i.e. to maintain the posture of the body by acting against the force of gravity). Both movement and posture are the results of muscle contraction elicited by the motor section of the nervous system.

The basic elements of the motor system are the motor neurones and the striated muscle fibres innervated by them. Higher structures of the brain ('higher motor centres') exert their influence by sending outputs to the peripheral motor neurones. Therefore, it is appropriate to discuss the two levels of organisation separately: (1) the basic machinery of motor function and (2) the motor centres.

Basic motor apparatus

Motor neurones are nerve cells which send their axons to muscle fibres in the periphery. There are two kinds of motor neurones: α motor neurones, and γ motor neurones.

The α *motor neurones* are large, multipolar cells which are located in the ventral horn of the spinal cord, and in the motor nuclei of cranial nerves. These neurones have thick myelinated axons (so-called Aα fibres) which can have several collaterals. Each collateral synapses with one individual muscle fibre. A motor neurone and the muscle fibres innervated by it is called a *motor unit* (Fig. 6.9). A motor unit functions on the basis of the 'all-or-none' principle: action potentials transmitted to the individual muscle fibres evoke maximal contraction. However, as each muscle of the body is innervated by several motor neurones, a graded muscle response is possible, the grade of contraction

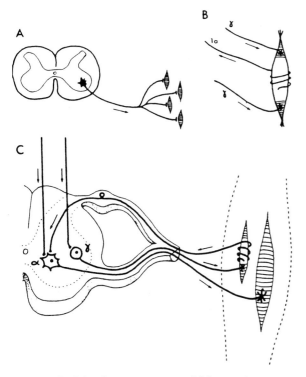

Fig. 6.9 Peripheral motor apparatus: **A** Motor unit; **B** intrafusal muscle fibre and its neuronal connections; **C** relationship between α and γ motor neurones (the γ loop).

depending on the number of motor units activated. In muscles in which very fine gradations of contraction are possible (e.g. external muscles of the eye), each motor neurone innervates only a small number of muscle fibres (innervation ratio 1:3). On the other hand, in muscles which are not capable of contractions of fine gradation (e.g. large muscles of the trunk), each motor neurone innervates several hundred muscle fibres (innervation ratio 1:500). The synaptic contact between the motor neurone and the striated muscle fibre is called the neuromuscular junction (myoneural junction). The presynaptic or prejunctional axon terminal of the motor neurone lies in a trough of the muscular membrane (this is the so-called endplate region of the membrane). The transmitter substance released from motor nerve endings is acetylcholine which causes depolarisation of the muscular membrane (endplate potential). The endplate potential can trigger off action potentials in the muscle fibre, which in turn result in the activation of the contractile machinery.

γ motor neurones are smaller cells located in the ventral horn of the spinal cord. These neurones have thin-ner myelinated axons (Aγ fibres) which reach the striated muscles. Within the muscle the γ motor neurones innervate only a special kind of muscle fibre: the intrafusal fibres of muscle spindles. These intrafusal fibres are specialised muscle cells: they have a central membranous region and two peripheral contractile regions at the end of the fibre (Fig 6.9B). The membranous region is connected to the peripheral process of a sensory neurone (so-called Ia afferent), the central process of which synapses with an α motor neurone innervating 'working' muscle fibres in the same muscle. The muscle spindles act as stretch receptors: stretching of the muscle initiates impulses in the sensory neurone, which in turn can activate the motor neurone, which results in muscle contraction. This is the anatomical basis of the stretch reflex (e.g. knee jerk). γ motor neurones innervate the muscular endparts of intrafusal muscle fibres, and thus, by contracting the endparts, can elicit the stretching of the central part; this in turn can activate the working muscle fibres via the stretch reflex (Fig 6.9C). Thus, neurones situated in higher structures of the brain can influence the contractile state of muscles in two ways: (1) directly, by acting on α motor neurones; (2) indirectly, via the so-called γ *loop* (γ motor neurones → muscle spindle → afferent neurone of the stretch reflex → α motor neurone).

Higher motor centres

There are two neuronal systems which can influence the activity of α and γ motor neurones: (1) the pyramidal system and (2) the extrapyramidal system.

The *pyramidal system* (corticospinal tract) is a group of cortical neurones which send their axons to the large α motor neurones of the spinal cord. The cell bodies are mainly situated in layer 5 of the precentral gyrus (motor cortex, Brodmann area 4); these are the huge Betz cells. The pyramidal tracts also contain fibres which originate in other neighbouring cortical areas such as the premotor cortex (areas 6, 8), parietal cortex (areas 3, 1, 2, 5) and temporal cortex (area 22). There is a distinct somatotopic localisation in the motor cortex: the electrical stimulation of a point in the cortex evokes muscle contractions in well-defined muscle groups (Fig. 6.10). The pyramidal tracts descend in the internal capsule, pass through the base of the midbrain and pons, and almost completely decussate in the pyramids of the medulla. (The fibres which do not decussate in the medulla decussate in the spinal cord before their termination.) The decussated fibres descend in the lateral, and the non-decussated fibres in the ventral tracts of the spinal cord. The pyramidal

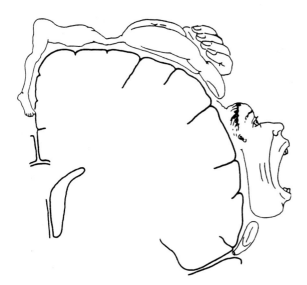

Fig. 6.10 The motor homunculus (after Penfield & Rasmussen 1954)

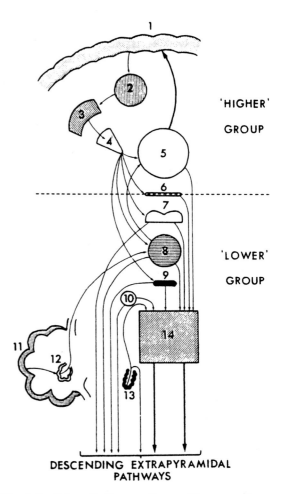

DESCENDING EXTRAPYRAMIDAL PATHWAYS

Fig. 6.11 Schematic diagram of some of the connections within the extrapyramidal system: 1, premotor cortex; 2, caudate nucleus; 3, putamen; 4, pallidum; 5, thalamus (ventrolateral nucleus); 6, subthalamic nucleus; 7, tectum; 8, red nucleus; 9, substantia nigra; 10, lateral vestibular nucleus of Deiters; 11, cerebellar cortex; 12, dentate nucleus; 13, inferior olive; 14, brain stem reticular formation.

fibres synapse either directly with alpha motor neurones, or with an interneurone, which in turn is connected to the motor neurone. The pyramidal pathway is thought to be responsible for the execution and control of skilled voluntary movements.

The *extrapyramidal system* comprises a number of neuronal groups which influence the motor neurones via pathways which reach the spinal cord outside the pyramids of the medulla. Figure 6.11 shows the schematic outline of the extrapyramidal system. The extrapyramidal nuclei can be divided into a higher and lower group. The *higher group* consists of the premotor frontal cortex (Brodmann areas 6, 8), the basal ganglia, and the thalamus. The basal ganglia are the striatum (caudate nucleus plus putamen of the lentiform nucleus) and the pallidum of the lentiform nucleus. An important neuronal circuit within the group is: cortex → striatum → pallidum → thalamus → cortex. The surgical interruption of this neuronal circuit is one of the treatment methods used in Parkinson's disease. It is a general organisational principle within the extrapyramidal system that higher structures send outputs to lower structures. The most important output from the higher nuclear group derives from the pallidum which is connected to the thalamus, subthalamic nucleus, red nucleus, substantia nigra, and reticular formation. The *lower group* consists of brain stem nuclei which are directly connected to the spinal cord. There are six nuclei in this group: (1) nuclei of the midbrain tectum; (2) the red nucleus; (3) the substantia nigra; (4) the lateral vestibular nucleus (Deiters' nucleus); (5) the

inferior olive; (6) the brain stem reticular formation. The pathways descending from these nuclei are located in different parts of the tegmentum in the brain stem, and descend in the lateral and ventral tracts of the spinal cord. Most of the fibres in these pathways terminate on γ motor neurones or on interneurones in the ventral horn of the spinal cord; the interneurones may be connected to α motor neurones. The brain stem reticular formation is the main collecting pool of outputs from subcortical motor nuclei: every cell group within the extrapyramidal system sends axon collaterals to the reticular formation. Thus the reticular formation of the brain stem can integrate all the extrapyramidal motor influences, and transmit the integrated 'message' to the spinal motor neurones. The most important outflow of extrapyramidal motor information comes from the brain stem reticular formation (the multi-neuronal reticulospinal pathway); the other connections from the brain stem to the spinal cord play a minor role in humans. The extrapyramidal system plays an important role in the distribution of muscle tone and in the maintenance of posture.

The *cerebellum* is interposed between the cerebral cortex and the spinal cord, and exerts an important controlling function on motor performance. It is possible to distinguish between three parts of the cerebellum on a developmental basis: (1) archicerebellum (nodulofloccular lobe); (2) paleocerebellum (anterior lobe); (3) neocerebellum (posterior lobe). The *archicerebellum* appears in fishes, and is closely related to the labyrinth, and thus to the maintenance of equilibrium. The *paleocerebellum* is highly developed in birds, and it receives an enormous projection from the spinal cord (spinocerebellar tracts). The *neocerebellum* achieves its greatest development in mammals, and it is connected to the neocortex (corticopontocerebellar pathway). The paleo- and neocerebellum probably function as a unit in higher mammals. It is believed that the cerebellum can 'compare' the cortical motor 'command' with the peripheral execution of the motor task: whenever a 'command' leaves the motor cortex through the corticospinal pathway, the cerebellum receives the information through the corticopontocerebellar pathway. The cerebellum also obtains the feedback about the execution of the motor task: this is achieved through joint and muscle receptors, their sensory connections, and the spinocerebellar pathways. It is believed that the cerebellum can compare the desired and actual motor responses, and can correct the motor performance, if necessary, in two ways: (1) by adjusting the function of the cortex (via the cerebello-dentatorubrothalamocortical pathway) (see Fig. 6.11) and/or (2) by altering the motor status in the periphery (via the reticular formation). It is thought that this 'error control' may be the most important function of the cerebellum. Although the cerebellum has a unique position in the nervous system, it functions as part of the extrapyramidal system.

ORGANISATION OF THE AUTONOMIC AND ENDOCRINE SYSTEMS

The *autonomic* (or *vegetative*) *nervous system* is the portion of the nervous system which is responsible for the maintenance of the constancy of the internal environment of the body. The autonomic nervous system accomplishes this in two ways: (1) through the control of visceral functions such as circulation, respiration, alimentary and excretory processes; (2) through the control of endocrine glands which can directly influence metabolism. The name 'autonomic' indicates that the functions controlled by this portion of the nervous system are usually not under voluntary control. The autonomic nervous system is often contrasted with the *somatic nervous system*, which is concerned with sensation and voluntary motor mechanisms (see above).

The visceral and endocrine portions of the autonomic nervous system work as one unified system. Similarly to the somatic nervous system the autonomic nervous system can be divided into a sensory and a motor division (Fig. 6.12). The *sensory division* of the autonomic nervous system consists of receptors and a chain of sensory neurones. The receptors can be either: (1) interoceptors located inside the body (e.g. in the walls of arteries, in the walls of the alimentary or respiratory canal); or (2) exteroceptors located on the surface of the body. The exteroceptors are identical to the receptors described under the heading 'Organisation of sensory systems'. Indeed, autonomic centres (e.g. hypothalamus) receive sensory information from every sensory modality. The primary sensory neurone is a pseudounipolar cell located in spinal ganglia or in the sensory ganglia of cranial nerves. The secondary and tertiary neurones are the same as those found in the somatic sensory system. Sensory neuronal chains give collaterals to the autonomic integrating neuronal pools of the spinal cord, brain stem and hypothalamus. Therefore it is hardly possible, on an anatomical basis, to separate the sensory division of the autonomic nervous system from the sensory division of the somatic nervous system.

The *motor division* of the autonomic nervous system consists of two sections: (1) the neuronal section and (2) the endocrine section (Fig. 6.12). The two sections are connected at the level of the hypothalamus. Both sections are organised on a hierarchical basis. First we shall discuss the organisation of the neuronal section, then the organisation of the endocrine section, and finally we shall deal with the connection between the two sections (the 'neuroendocrine interface').

Organisation of the neuronal section of the autonomic nervous system

Vegetative motor neurones

The peripheral effector cells ('vegetative motor neurones') are located in the intermediate horn of the spinal cord (i.e. between the ventral and dorsal horns)

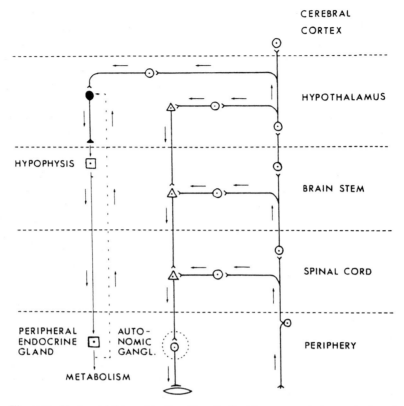

Fig. 6.12 Horizontal (hierarchical) and longitudinal (sensory motor) organisation of the autonomic and endocrine systems.

and in the autonomic nuclei of the cranial nerves (e.g the dorsal nucleus of the vagus). These neurones are smaller than the somatic motor neurones, and have fewer dendrites. The axon of a vegetative motor neurone never synapses directly with cells of the effector tissue: it synapses with another neurone which in turn is in synaptic contact with the effector cell (smooth muscle cell or gland cell; Fig. 6.12). Therefore, it is possible to distinguish between a first and a second vegetative motor neurone. The cell body of the second neurone can be located either (1) in a peripheral autonomic ganglion (e.g. a paravertebral ganglion, an autonomic ganglion of a cranial nerve) or (2) in the effector tissue itself. This two-neuronal effector chain is the uniform feature of the autonomic nervous system. The axon of the first neurone is usually called the preganglionic fibre (referring to its presynaptic position in relation to the autonomic ganglion); the axon of the second neurone is called the postganglionic fibre. The preganglionic fibres are always myelinated, whereas the postganglionic fibres either have no myelin sheath, or have only a very thin myelin covering. The axon of the second neurone usually terminates in

a diffuse arborisation (so-called vegetative ground plexus or terminal network). In a smooth muscle tissue only 1% of the muscle fibres has a synaptic contact with neuronal elements; other fibres, however, are also affected by the transmitter which diffuses slowly in the tissue. This anatomical arrangement explains why the stimulation of autonomic nerves evokes a slow and long-lasting peripheral response.

The motor division of the autonomic nervous system is usually divided into two parts: (1) the sympathetic system and (2) the parasympathetic system. This division is based on the observation that: (1) most organs receive autonomic innervation from two different sources; (2) the effects of the two nerve supplies are functionally antagonistic; (3) there are drugs which can selectively mimic or antagonise the functional effects of either of the nerve supplies.

The anatomical differences between the sympathetic and parasympathetic systems are as follows. *Sympathetic system*: the first neurones are located in the intermediate horn of the thoracolumbar region of the spinal cord; the second neurones are located in the paravertebral or prevertebral sympathetic ganglia.

Parasympathetic system: the first neurones are located either in autonomic nuclei of cranial nerves ('cranial autonomic outflow'), or in the intermediate horn of the sacral region of the spinal cord ('sacral outflow'); the second neurones are situated either in autonomic ganglia of cranial nerves, or in the effector tissue itself.

There are two neurotransmitters involved in the peripheral nervous system: acetylcholine and noradrenaline. *Cholinergic neurones* are: (1) the first neurones of both the sympathetic and parasympathetic divisions; (2) all the parasympathetic second neurones; (3) some of the sympathetic second neurones (those innervating sweat glands). *Adrenergic neurones* are: (1) most of the second sympathetic neurones; (2) the cells of the adrenal medullae. (These cells are modified neurones which secrete their 'transmitter' into the blood stream, and thus act as endocrine cells; Fig. 6.13.)

Autonomic 'centres'

Higher structures of the brain can send outputs to the first autonomic effector cells. These structures are located at different levels of the neuraxis, and a higher structure usually controls the function of a lower structure (Fig. 6.12). The following areas are important autonomic integrating centres: (1) the intermediate horn of the spinal cord; (2) autonomic nuclei in the brain stem reticular formation (e.g vasomotor centre, respiratory centre); (3) the hypothalamus; (4) the cerebral cortex (frontal lobe, cingulate gyrus).

The *hypothalamus* plays a key role in the integration of autonomic and endocrine functions. The hypothalamus comprises the walls and the floor of the third cerebral ventricle. It is possible to distinguish between three hypothalamic nuclear groups: (1) the anterior nuclei; (2) the central nuclei; (3) the posterior nuclei (Fig. 6.14). The *anterior nuclear group* consists of the preoptic nucleus and the supraoptic nucleus. The *central group* consists of three subgroups: (1) the medial hypothalamic nuclei (paraventricular, dorsomedial, and ventromedial nuclei); (2) the lateral hypothalamic nucleus; (3) the nucleus arcuatus (a small cellular group surrounding the infundibulum). The *posterior group* comprises the posterior nucleus and the mamillary nuclei. The hypothalamic nuclei receive inputs from: (1) every sensory pathway (see above); (2) the limbic system (from the hippocampus via the fornix, see below); (3) the cerebral cortex (frontal lobe). The following neuronal outputs are of great significance: (1) to autonomic areas of the brain stem (an ill-defined, multineuronal descending pathway); (2) to the cerebral cortex (via the anterior nucleus of the thalamus, see limbic system); (3) to the posterior lobe of the hypophysis (supraopticohypophysial tract).

The physiological anatomy of the hypothalamus is based mainly on results of experiments in which distinct areas of the hypothalamus were stimulated or destroyed. It is now well established that the hypothalamus plays an important role in the following regulatory functions: (1) cardiovascular regulation (the preoptic area decreases, whereas the posterior area increases the heart rate); (2) temperature regulation (cells in the anterior hypothalamus (preoptic area) are sensitive to blood temperature; a drop in temperature results in vasoconstriction, shivering, etc.); (3) regulation of body water (the supraoptic and ventromedial nuclei probably regulate drinking behaviour; neurones in the supraoptic and paraventricular nuclei act as osmoreceptors and secrete antidiuretic hormone (ADH) which is responsible for the reabsorption of water by the distal tubules of the kidneys); (4) regulation of feeding behaviour (the lateral hypothalamic area is regarded as the 'hunger centre', whereas the ventromedial nucleus is the postulated 'satiety centre').

Organisation of the endocrine section of the autonomic nervous system

The peripheral endocrine glands secrete their hormones into the bloodstream, and this can have a diffuse influence on metabolic processes in the body. The function of most of the peripheral glands is under pituitary control; the hypophysis secretes special 'stimulating' hormones (e.g. adrenocorticotrophic hormone (ACTH), thyroid-stimulating hormone (TSH)), which influence the activity of the peripheral glands. There is a hor-

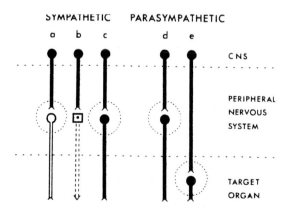

Fig. 6.13 Cholinergic and adrenergic neurones in the autonomic nervous system: black, cholinergic; white, adrenergic. a, sympathetic innervation of most peripheral organs; b, sympathetic innervation of the adrenal medulla; c, sympathetic innervation of sweat glands; d, parasympathetic outflow via cranial nerves; e, sacral parasympathetic outflow.

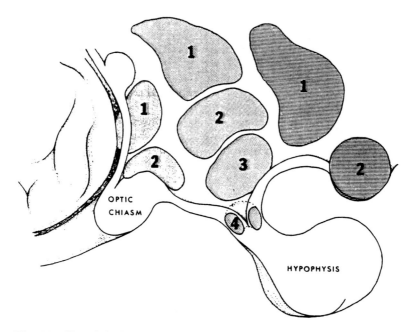

Fig. 6.14 Hypothalamic nuclei. Anterior group: 1, preoptic nucleus; 2, supraoptic nucleus. Central group: 1, paraventricular nucleus; 2, dorsomedial nucleus; 3, ventromedial nucleus; 4, nucleus arcuatus. Posterior group: 1, posterior nucleus; 2, mamillary nuclei. (Modified from Netter 1953.)

monal feedback from the peripheral gland to the hypophysis: the level of peripheral hormones can influence pituitary activity either directly, or indirectly through the hypothalamus (Fig. 6.12).

The neuroendocrine interface

The neuroendocrine interface is the connection between the neuronal and hormonal parts of the autonomic nervous system. This connection is based on the phenomenon of *neurosecretion.*

Each nerve cell is a specialised gland cell: it is capable of secreting a neurotransmitter. If the substance secreted by a nerve cell does not remain restricted to a synaptic region, but passes into the bloodstream, the nerve cell behaves like an endocrine cell. A nerve cell secreting a substance into the bloodstream is called a neurosecretory cell. The substance secreted by a neurosecretory cell can pass: (1) into the systemic circulation, or (2) into a local, so-called portal circulation. Examples for the first case are the secretion of adrenalin by the modified neurones of the adrenal medulla, and the secretion of ADH by the neurones of the supraoptic and paraventricular nuclei of the hypothalamus. Neurosecretion into a portal circulation is the basis for the neuroendocrine interface.

Some hypothalamic neurones situated in the infundibular region (i.e. near the floor of the third ventricle of the hypothalamus) secrete their hormone-like substance (so-called releasing factor) into a dense capillary network in the stalk of the hypophysis (Fig. 6.15). The venous blood collected from these capillaries mingles with the arterial blood supply of the anterior lobe of the hypophysis (so-called portal circulation of the hypophysis). In this way, the infundibular cells can influence the activity of pituitary gland cells. The infundibular neurones receive neuronal inputs from other parts of the hypothalamus. It is in this way that the endocrine system is connected to the neuronal part of the autonomic nervous system (Fig. 6.12).

ORGANISATION OF THE LIMBIC SYSTEM

The limbic system or ('visceral brain') is more a functional than an anatomical entity: the term limbic system is used to designate those parts of the brain whose activities are essential for the organisation of the emotional responses of the organism. From an anatomical point of view, 'limbic' means 'marginal': the limbic cortex is the ring-shaped band of the telencephalon which is situated on the borderline between telencephalon and diencephalon (see Fig. 6.16). Much of

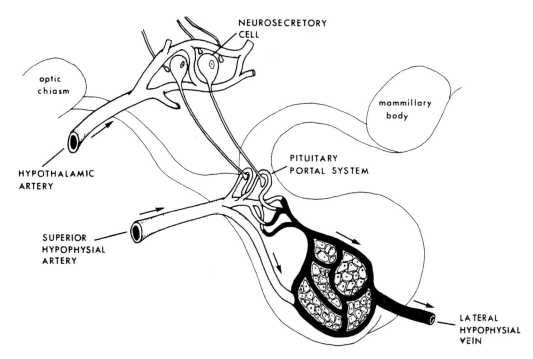

Fig. 6.15 Portal circulation of the anterior lobe of the hypophysis. (Venous blood is indicated with shading.)

the limbic cortex is identical to the 'rhinencephalon' of older descriptive anatomy textbooks.

Textbooks of neuroanatomy vary in their definitions of the limbic system: some use a very narrow, others a much wider, definition. Here it is convenient to distinguish between three parts within the limbic system: (1) the limbic cortex (or limbic lobe); (2) the subcortical limbic nuclei; (3) the associated nuclei.

The *limbic lobe* comprises cortical areas which are situated at the transition of the telencephalon into diencephalon; these areas surround the 'hilum' of the brain in the form of a ring on the medial surface of the brain (Figs 6.16, 6.17). The constituents of the limbic

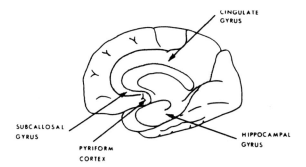

Fig. 6.16 The limbic lobe on the medial surface of the brain.

lobe are: (1) the primary olfactory cortex; (2) the septal cortex; (3) the hippocampal formation; (4) the cingulate (fornicate) gyrus. The *primary olfactory cortex* is the area in which the axons of the olfactory tracts terminate, i.e. the prepyriform cortex (rostral aspect of the uncus of the parahippocampal gyrus), the anterior perforated space (olfactory tubercle), and also the septal cortex. The *septal cortex* is the cortical area just below the knee of the corpus callosum (subcallosal gyrus). This cortical area is closely associated with the septum pellucidum and the septal nuclei. The septal cortex, septal nuclei and septum pellucidum are often referred to as the septal region. The *hippocampal formation* consists of: (1) the hippocampus; (2) the dentate gyrus; (3) the subiculum (the transitional cortical area situated between the hippocampus and parahippocampal gyrus); (4) the supracallosal gyrus (or longitudinal striae). The *cingulate gyrus* (Brodmann areas 24, 32) is the area of cortex overlying the corpus callosum. The histological structure of the limbic cortex (allocortex) differs from that of the neocortex (isocortex). The allocortex has fewer layers than the isocortex; the allocortex has only three layers, whereas the neocortex has six.

The *subcortical limbic nuclei* comprise the septal nuclei and the amygdala. The *septal nuclei* are a group of neurones underneath the septal cortex.

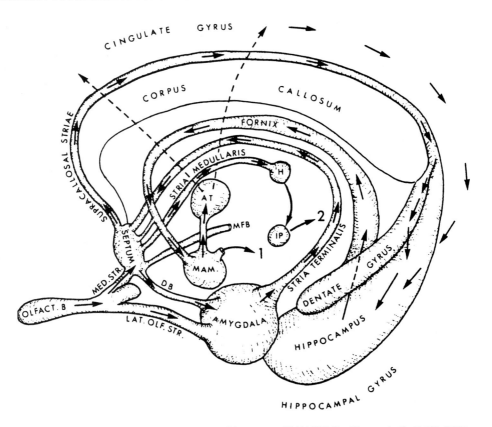

Fig. 6.17 Internal connections within the limbic system: OLFACT. B, olfactory bulb; LAT. OLF. STR., lateral olfactory stria; MED. STR., medial olfactory stria; AT, anterior nucleus of the thalamus; MFB, medial forebrain bundle; MAM, nucleus of the mamillary body (1, connection to midbrain reticular formation); DB, diagonal band of Broca; H, habenular nucleus; IP, interpeduncular nucleus (2, connection to midbrain reticular formation) (modified from MacLean 1949).

Three distinct nuclei can be distinguished within this group: the medial septal nucleus, the lateral septal nucleus, and the nucleus accumbens septi. The nucleus accumbens is interposed between the head of the caudate nucleus and the lateral septal nucleus. Although the nucleus accumbens is continuous with the head of the caudate nucleus, it can be distinguished from it by the presence of neurones which are larger than the characteristically small striatal nerve cells. The nucleus accumbens and the lateral septal nucleus receive a powerful dopaminergic innervation from the midbrain ('mesolimbic dopamine system', see below), and also an input from the hippocampus. The *amygdala* is located in the pole of the temporal lobe. It can be divided into two cell groups: (1) the corticomedial amygdaloid; (2) the basolateral amygdaloid. The former cell group receives its major input from the lateral olfactory

stria; the latter group is closely related to the neocortex of the temporal lobe.

The *associated limbic nuclei* receive inputs from the cortical and subcortical limbic areas, and thus they are often included in the limbic system. These nuclei are: (1) the anterior nucleus of the thalamus; (2) the nuclei of the mamillary body of the hypothalamus; (3) the habenular nucleus of the epithalamus; (4) the midbrain tegmentum (i.e. reticular formation); (5) the interpenduncular nucleus (Fig. 6.17).

The connections of the limbic system can be divided into three major parts: (1) connections within the system (intrinsic circuitry); (2) inputs to the system; (3) outputs from the system.

All parts of the limbic structures are interconnected with each other. Anatomically the most important connection is between the amygdala and the hippocampus (i.e. between the key structures within the system; Fig. 6.17). There is a two-way connection between these structures: (1) amygdala (stria terminalis) → septal region → supracallosal gyrus (longitudinal striae) → dentate gyrus → hippocampus; (2) hippocampus (fornix) → septal region (diagonal band of Broca) → amygdala.

The limbic system receives *inputs* from every sensory system. The olfactory system is closely connected to the amygdala and the uncus of the hippocampus and the parahippocampal gyrus. Most sensory collaterals reach the septal region through the medial forebrain bundle (Fig. 6.17). The medial forebrain bundle is a multineuronal pathway ascending from the midbrain through the lateral hypothalamus. There are also connections from the neocortex of the temporal lobe.

The *outputs* from the limbic system originate either from the hippocampus or the amygdala. The major output from the *hippocampus* is through the fornix to the nuclei of the mamillary body (Fig. 6.17). The fornix (hippocampo-mamillary tract) is composed of the axons of large pyramidal neurones in the hippocampus which synapse with cells in the mamillary body. Three important pathways originate from the neurones in the mamillary body: (1) the mamillothalamic tract (tract of Vicq d'Azyr) to the anterior nucleus of the thalamus; (2) the mamillotegmental tract to the reticular formation of the midbrain; (3) multineuronal connections to other hypothalamic nuclei.

The anterior nucleus of the thalamus is connected to the cingulate gyrus through the internal capsule. As the neurones in the cingulate gyrus are connected in a multineuronal chain in the allocortex to the hippocampus, a complete circuit results: hippocampus (fornix) → mamillary body → thalamus → cingulate gyrus → hippocampus. This is the famous 'reverberating circuit' which was suggested by Papez in 1937 as the basis for emotional behaviour. As the cingulate gyrus is connected to most neocortical areas through intercortical connections, the Papez circuit forms the link between the limbic system and the neocortex.

The most important *output from the amygdala* is through the stria medullaris to the habenular nucleus of the epithalamus (Fig. 6.17). The habenular nucleus is connected to the interpeduncular nucleus of the midbrain via the fasciculus retroflexus of Meynert. The interpeduncular nucleus itself sends its axons to the reticular formation. In summary, the limbic system sends outputs to the following structures of the brain: (1) the neocortex; (2) the hypothalamus (and from here to lower autonomic centres and to the hypophysis); (3) the brain stem reticular formation. Thus, sensory information filtered through the limbic system can influence conscious voluntary sensory motor activity, autonomic and endocrine functions, and the general level of arousal.

The functional significance of the limbic system has been established in experiments involving stimulation and lesioning of different parts of the system. *Electrical stimulation of the amygdala* usually evokes aggressive behaviour (anger, rage) in experimental animals. Another consequence of the stimulation of the amygdala is the appearance of so-called oral mechanisms (sniffing, licking, biting, swallowing). *Stimulation of the hippocampus* evokes respiratory and cardiovascular changes, generalised arousal, sexual responses (e.g. erection). *Stimulation of the septal* area can decrease aggressiveness in monkeys. Stimulation of certain limbic areas can be 'pleasurable' for the experimental animal; animals with implanted electrodes can quickly learn to press a lever when lever pressing is followed by electrical stimulation of the limbic system ('self-stimulation'; Olds 1971).

The bilateral *ablation* of the oral parts of the temporal lobes (i.e. the loss of the amygdala, uncus, parts of the hippocampal formation) results in the so-called Klüver–Bucy syndrome (Klüver & Bucy 1939). This syndrome is characterised by: (1) visual agnosia (i.e. inability to recognise objects by sight); (2) strong oral tendencies; (3) loss of fear and aggressiveness; (4) hypersexual behaviour.

In humans, lesions within the limbic system result in a characteristic disorder of memory: short-term memory is not consolidated into long-term memory. This type of memory defect is characteristic of Korsakoff's syndrome. The pathological basis of this condition is haemorrhages in the mamillary bodies and/or other parts of the limbic system. Post-mortem studies of the brains of schizophrenic patients have revealed an increase in the number of spiroperidol binding sites in a limbic area, the nucleus accumbens septi; this finding has been interpreted as an indication of the overactivity of the mesolimbic dopamine system in schizophrenic patients (Crow et al 1979; see also section on 'Monoamine-containing neuronal systems', below).

ORGANISATION OF THE RETICULAR FORMATION

The reticular formation consists of small aggregates of nerve cells and their diffusely organised fibre systems occupying the central core of the brain stem. The dendrites of these neurones are often arranged in small bundles creating a net-like ('reticular') pattern. The reticular formation extends from the substantia intermedia of the spinal cord through the tegmentum of the medulla oblongata, pons and midbrain into the diencephalon (intralaminar nuclei of thalamus). On both histological and functional grounds, it is possible to distinguish between three longitudinal nuclear columns; each nuclear column can be subdivided into a medullary, a pontine, and a mesencephalic section (Fig. 6.18). The three nuclear columns are: median (or midline) nuclear group; medial nuclear group; lateral nuclear group. The *median group* consists of the raphe nuclei (raphe = seam); the cells in this nuclear group contain 5-hydroxytryptamine (for details, see 'Monoamine-containing neuronal systems', below). The *medial group* consists of four subgroups: (1) the medullary nuclei (nucleus gigantocellularis); (2) the

pontine nuclei (nucleus reticularis pontis caudalis, nucleus reticularis pontis oralis, nucleus reticularis tegmenti pontis); (3) the mesencephalic nuclei (formatio reticularis mesencephali); (4) the diencephalic nuclei (subthalamic reticular formation including the zona incerta, thalamic reticular formation corresponding to the intralaminar nuclei and the centromedial nucleus of the thalamus). The medial nuclear group is also called the 'magnocellular reticular zone' since it contains relatively large neurones. The axons arising from these neurones usually bifurcate into long ascending and descending branches; some axons terminate within the confines of the reticular formation ('reticular relay cells'), others, however, ascend to the diencephalon or descend to the spinal cord. The *lateral group* can be divided into three subgroups: (1) the medullary nuclei (nucleus medullae oblongatae centralis); (2) the pontine nuclei (nucleus parabrachialis medialis, nucleus parabrachialis lateralis); (3) the mesencephalic nuclei (nucleus tegmenti pedunculopontinus). The lateral reticular formation consists of mainly small neurones ('parvicellular reticular zone'). Most of the medullary reticular formation belongs to this poorly differentiated parvicellular nuclear group.

The connections of the three nuclear columns will be considered separately. It should be noted, however, that this is a necessary simplification since the three nuclear columns are richly interconnected with each other. The connections of the *midline (raphe) group* are described in a later section of this chapter (see 'Monoamine-containing neuronal systems').

The *medial reticular zone* receives inputs from many parts of the brain. These inputs derive from four major sources: (1) the sensory relay nuclei of the spinal cord and the brain stem: (2) the motor nuclei of the so-called extra-pyramidal system (including the cerebellar nuclei and the premotor cortex); (3) the hypothalamus; (4) the limbic lobe. The outputs from the medial reticular formation can be divided into ascending and descending reticular pathways. The *ascending reticular* pathways consist of two pathways connected in series: the reticulothalamic pathway and the thalamocortical pathway. The reticulothalamic pathway ascends from the medullopontomesencephalic reticular formation to the intralaminar nuclei of the thalamus; this pathway also sends collaterals to the subthalamus (zona incerta) and to many parts of the hypothalamus. The reticular (or 'aspecific') thalamocortical pathway is a massive projection from the intralaminar nuclei of the thalamus to all parts of the neocortex. This pathway also gives collaterals to the following structures: the thalamus (ventrolateral nucleus, lateral posterior nucleus); the corpus striatum;

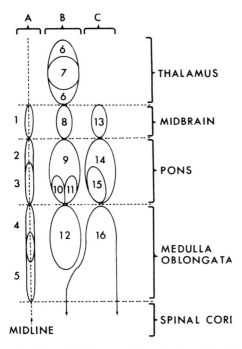

Fig. 6.18 Schematic diagram of the reticular nuclei. (A) *Median (or midline) group:* 1, nucleus raphes dorsalis (area B7 according to Dahlström and Fuxe 1964); 2, nucleus centralis superior (B6 and B8); 3, nucleus raphes pontis (B5); 4, nucleus raphes magnus (B3); 5, nucleus raphes obscurus (B2). Note that the nucleus raphes obscurus covers the nucleus raphes pallidus (B1) which is at the same level of the brain stem, but in a more ventral position. (B) *Medial (magnocellular) group:* 6, intralaminar nuclei of the thalamus; 7, centromedial nucleus of the thalamus; 8, mesencephalic reticular formation; 9, nucleus reticularis pontis oralis; 10, nucleus reticularis tegmenti pontis; 11, nucleus reticularis pontis caudalis; 12, nucleus gigantocellularis. (C) *Lateral (parvicellular) group:* 13, nucleus tegmenti pedunculopontinus; 14, nucleus parabrachialis lateralis; 15, nucleus parabrachialis medialis; 16, nucleus medullae oblongatae centralis. (Based on Nieuwenhuys et al 1979.)

the limbic lobe (septal region). It is possible to distinguish between two *descending reticular pathways:* the pontospinal tract and the bulbospinal tract. The pontospinal tract originates from the nucleus reticularis pontis caudalis and descends in the anterior funiculus; the bulbospinal tract originates from the nucleus gigantocellularis and descends in the lateral funiculus. Both reticulospinal pathways synapse, via interneurones, with α and γ motoneurons. The *lateral (parvicellular) reticular zone* receives inputs from cortical and subcortical motor areas. The output from this zone consists mainly of proprioreticular connections which form parts of bulbar reflex pathways.

Four different functions can be ascribed to the reticular formation:

1. 'Non-specific' alerting function ('ascending reticular activating system'): the ascending reticulo-thalamocortical pathway plays an essential role in maintaining the level of alertness (see Guyton 1972).
2. Sensory function: the spinoreticulothalamocortical pathway forms the so-called extralemniscal sensory system which is involved in pain sensation.
3. Motor function: the extrapyramidal motor system exerts its influence on spinal motoneurons via the powerful reticulospinal pathways (see 'Organisation of the motor system', above).
4. Vegetative function: the lateral reticular formation contains cellular groups which play an essential role in maintaining respiration and blood pressure ('respiratory and vasomotor centres').

ORGANISATION OF THE CEREBRAL CORTEX

The cerebral cortex (pallium) is a sheet of grey matter covering the surface of the telencephalon. In humans the total area of the cerebral cortex is about 0.75 m², its thickness varies between 1.5 and 4 mm, and it contains about 50% of all the neurones of the nervous system. From a developmental point of view, the cortex consists of three parts: (1) the paleocortex (primary olfactory area); (2) the archicortex (limbic formation); (3) the neocortex. The paleocortex and archicortex have the three-layered structure of the allocortex (see the limbic system). The neocortex becomes prominent in mammals, and it achieves its greatest development in primates. The neocortex constitutes about 90% of the cerebral cortex in humans.

The several million neurones located in the neocortex can be divided into five basic neuronal types: (1) pyramidal cells; (2) stellate cells (granule cells); (3) multiform (polyform) cells; (4) cells of

Martinotti; (5) horizontal cells of Cajal. The *pyramidal cells* have pyramid-shaped cell bodies (Fig. 6.19). There are two kinds of dendrites originating from the cell body: the single apical dendrite which ascends vertically in the cortex and divides into two side branches in the shape of a 'T', and the basilar dendrites. A single axon originates from the base of the pyramid, and it usually leaves the cerebral cortex. The axon almost invariably has a recurrent collateral which returns to the cortex. The *multiform cells* are modified pyramidal cells which are located in the deep layers of the cortex. The pyramidal cells and the multiform cells are 'corticofugal neurones': their axons leave the cortex, and thus form the outputs from cortical areas. The other three cell types are entirely intracortical: their axons arborise and terminate within the cortex. The most numerous of these are the *stellate cells* (or granule cells) which have small star-shaped cell bodies, short dendrites, and one short axon. The *Martinotti cells* are modified stellate cells. The stellate cells and the Martinotti cells form vertical connections within the cortex. The *horizontal cells* are located in the superficial layer of the cortex; their short processes form horizontal connections within the cortex.

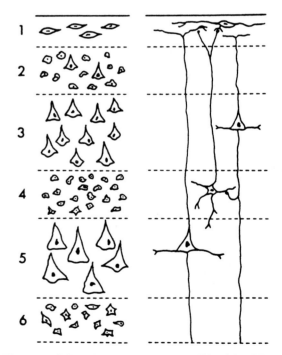

Fig. 6.19 Cellular layers in the neocortex. The right of the figure shows the connections between pyramidal and stellate cells.

On a morphological basis, it is possible to distinguish between six cellular layers within the neocortex. The six layers are: (1) the plexiform layer, or molecular layer (horizontal cells and dendrites of pyramidal cells); (2) the external granular layer (small pyramidal cells and a few granule cells); (3) the external pyramidal layer (pyramidal cells); (4) the internal granular layer (stellate cells, few small pyramidal cells); (5) the internal pyramidal layer (large pyramidal cells); (6) the multiform layer (mainly multiform cells (Fig. 6.19). In some areas of the cortex one layer may be more pronounced, whereas another layer may be present only in rudimentary form. Thus the primary motor cortex has only a scant number of granule cells ('agranular cortex'), whereas in the somatosensory cortex the granule cells predominate ('granular cortex' or 'coniocortex'). On the basis of the appearance of these layers, it is possible to create a cytoarchitectural map of the brain. There are several such maps in use, of which Brodmann's is the most generally accepted. Brodmann differentiated between 47 cortical areas (Fig. 6.20).

Apart from the horizontal organisation of the neurones in the cortex, there is also a *vertical organisation* which is regarded as the most important principle in cortical neuronal circuitry. Cortical neurones can be grouped into cortical columns or cylinders, each of which may function as a unit: excitation in one part of the column spreads to other neurones within the column via the stellate cells and the Martinotti cells, but it may not propagate to neighbouring columns. Indeed, the activation of a cortical column is often accompanied by inhibition in the neighbouring cortical columns, thus resulting in a greater contrast between the excited column and its neighbourhood.

Outputs from the cortex are usually divided into two groups: (1) outputs to other cortical areas, and (2) outputs to subcortical areas. The outputs to other cortical areas are either: (1) to other areas in the same hemisphere (association or intrahemispheric fibres), or (2) to homologous areas of the contralateral hemisphere (commissural or interhemispheric fibres). The commissural fibres form the cerebral commissures: (1) the corpus callosum; (2) the anterior commissure; (3) the hippocampal commissure; (4) the habenular commissure. Of these the corpus callosum is the most important interhemispheric connection in humans. Cortical outputs to subcortical structures are called projection fibres. The projection fibres terminate in the basal ganglia, diencephalon, brain stem and spinal cord.

From a functional point of view, it is possible to distinguish between three kinds of cortical areas: (1) primary sensory areas (i.e. cortical areas where sensory

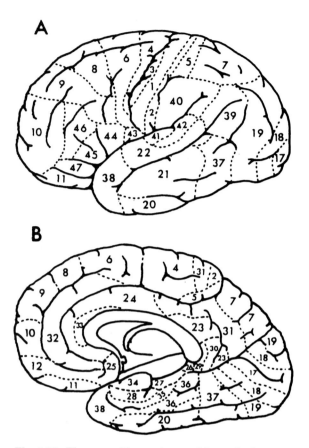

Fig. 6.20 The cytoarchitectural map of the cerebral cortex after Brodmann. **A** lateral surface; **B** medial surface.

pathways terminate); (2) primary motor areas (cortical areas from which long descending motor pathways originate); (3) association areas (cortical areas which cannot be classified as either sensory or motor; Fig. 6.18). The stimulation of primary motor areas results in movement in the appropriate muscle group, stimulation of the primary sensory areas simulates the experience produced by stimulation of the appropriate sensory receptors. The stimulation of association areas, however, does not result in either a motor or a sensory effect; for this reason the association areas used to be called 'mute'. The association areas achieved their greatest development in man, where they account for the bulk of the cortical surface. Animal experiments can thus give only partial information concerning the functions of these cortical areas. Most of our information has been supplied by clinical neurology. Descriptions of the syndromes arising from lesions of the frontal, parietal, or temporal lobes can be found in any textbook of neurology.

CHEMICAL NEUROANATOMY

Chemical neuroanatomy is a relatively new approach to the functional anatomy of the brain: different neuronal systems are identified on the basis of the neurotransmitter used by the neurones. The classification relies on the metabolic identity of neurones ('Dale's principle'): a neurone utilises the same neurotransmitter(s) at all its terminals (see Eccles 1964). The neurochemically identified systems can be classified according to the neurotransmitter: (1) acetylcholine; (2) monoamines (noradrenaline, dopamine, 5-hydroxytryptamine, adrenaline, histamine); (3) amino acids (GABA, glycine, glutamate, aspartate); (4) peptides (e.g. substance P, somatostatin, enkephalins; for details; see Nieuwenhuys 1985). The significance of this approach is that some diseases of the brain are associated with the selective loss of chemically identified neurones (e.g. the loss of dopamine neurones in Parkinson's disease, of acetylcholine and somatostatin neurones in Alzheimer's disease, of GABA neurones in Huntington's disease: see Legg 1978, Roth & Iversen 1986). Here we restrict ourselves to a brief description of the anatomy of the monoamine-containing neuronal systems of the brain; these systems have a special relevance to psychiatry (see below).

Monoamine-containing neuronal systems

The monoamines noradrenaline (NA), dopamine (DA), and 5-hydroxytryptamine (5-HT or serotonin) occur in well-defined neuronal groups in the brain (Dahlström & Fuxe 1964, Ungerstedt 1971), and it is generally assumed that each monoamine-containing neurone releases the stored monoamine as a neurotransmitter from its nerve endings. Although our detailed knowledge of the anatomy of the monoamine-containing neurones is based on studies conducted in animals, especially in rats, there is a growing body of information concerning the localisation and distribution of these neurones in the human brain (Nobin & Björklund 1973, Bogerts 1981).

The general feature of the anatomy of the 'monoamine neurones' is that the cell bodies are localised in a few circumscribed nuclei situated mainly in the lower brain stem, and the axons project to most parts of the brain and the spinal cord. The diffuse projection from the brain stem nuclei is the result of many axon collaterals arising from one neurone: in fact, any one neurone may send collaterals to several remote areas of the central nervous system (e.g. cerebral cortex, limbic areas, hypothalamus, cerebellum, spinal cord). The terminal branches of monoamine neurones arborise similarly to peripheral vegetative neurones, creating characteristic 'varicosities' (cf. sympathetic ground plexus or terminal network; Livett 1973.) The varicosities are enlargements along the terminal fibre which have the structure and function of presynaptic terminals or 'boutons'; they have been identified as sites of release. Although some of the 'monoamine boutons' form conventional synaptic contacts with adjoining neurones, many of them are located in interstitial gaps without any identifiable synaptic contact. The existence of non-synaptic boutons suggests that the monoamines, apart from acting as synaptic transmitters, may also have a more diffuse hormone-like action in the brain (Beaudet & Descarries 1978). As each monoamine neurone is characterised by the presence of one of the monoamines it is possible to distinguish between three distinct neuronal systems: (1) the NA neurones; (2) the DA neurones; (3) the 5-HT neurones (for a detailed review, see Nieuwenhuys et al 1979).

Anatomy of the NA neurones

The catecholamine (NA and DA)-containing nuclei have been designated as areas A1–A15 by Dahlström & Fuxe (1964): A1–A7 are the NA-containing cellular groups. All the NA-containing neurones are situated in the lower brain stem. It is customary to distinguish between three groups of nuclei: the caudal (or medullary) group, the central (or medullopontine group), and the rostral (or pontine) group. The rostral group is the largest and most important in man and consists of one nucleus: the locus coeruleus (area A6). The locus coeruleus is located in the dorsal pontine area: it appears as a dark patch on the floor of the fourth ventricle and contains almost 50% of all the NA-containing neurones in the brain.

The fibre projections arising from the NA nuclei can be divided into two major groups: fibres arising from the caudal and central nuclear groups, and fibres originating from the locus coeruleus. Neurones in the caudal and central nuclear groups (areas A1, A2, A5 and A7) give rise to both ascending and descending fibre systems. The ascending fibre system ('ventral NA bundle') innervates the following areas: (1) the midbrain reticular formation; (2) the entire hypothalamus; (3) parts of the limbic cortex. The descending fibres form two bulbospinal bundles terminating in the ventral and the intermediate nuclear columns of the spinal cord, respectively.

There are three major efferent pathways arising from the locus coeruleus. (1) The *ascending pathway* ('dorsal NA bundle') supplies the following areas of the brain: (a) the midbrain (periaqueductal grey substance, nucleus raphes dorsalis, superior and inferior colliculi); (b) the thalamus (anterior, ventral, lateral nuclear complexes, medial and lateral geniculate bodies); (c) the limbic system (amygdala, hippocampus, cingulate and parahippocampal gyri); (d) the neocortex (all areas of the neocortex receive a diffuse and uniform noradrenergic innervation). (2) The *cerebellar pathway* reaches the cerebellar nuclei and the cerebellar cortex via the superior cerebellar peduncle. (3) The *descending pathway* sends collaterals to some motor nuclei in the lower brain stem (dorsal nucleus of the vagus, inferior olivary complex), and then descends to the spinal cord ('coerulospinal pathway'). The massive coerulospinal pathway innervates the ventral horn and the basal part of the dorsal horn throughout the length of the cord.

Apart from innervating neuronal elements throughout the brain and the spinal cord, noradrenergic nerve terminals are also closely associated with cerebral arterioles and capillaries. This relationship suggests that the central noradrenergic system may play a role in the regulation of cerebral blood flow.

Anatomy of the DA neurones

The DA-containing neurones are located in the areas of the brain stem which have been designated as A8 to A15 by Dahlström & Fuxe (1964). It is possible to distinguish between three groups of DA nuclei: the mesencephalic nuclei, the diencephalic nuclei, and the telencephalic (olfactory) cellular group.

The *mesencephalic nuclei* comprise three cellular groups: A8, A9 and A10. Area A9 corresponds to the pars compacta of the substantia nigra. The *diencephalic nuclei* contain three nuclei in the hypothalamus, and one nucleus in the subthalamus; the two most important hypothalamic nuclei are the ventromedial nucleus and the arcuate (infundibular) nucleus. The *olfactory cellular group* is a set of DA-containing interneurones ('periglomerular cells') in the olfactory bulb.

The mesencephalic DA neurones give rise to two large ascending fibre system: (1) areas A8 and A9 send a massive innervation to the caudate nucleus and the putamen ('nigrostriatal DA system'); some fibres reach the amygdala; (2) fibres originating from nucleus A10 innervate both limbic ('mesolimbic DA system') and neocortical ('mesocortical DA system') areas. The following limbic areas receive a dopaminergic input: olfactory tubercle, septal nuclei (lateral septal nucleus and nucleus accumbens), interstitial cells of the stria terminalis, cingulate cortex, oral part of parahippocampal cortex (so-called entorhinal cortex). The dop-

aminergic innervation of the neocortex is restricted to the medial surface of the frontal lobe (Brodmann areas 10, 11, 12, 32; see Fig. 6.20).

The diencephalic DA neurones give rise mainly to short axons which remain within the confines of the diencephalic region. Neurones in the arcuate nucleus (A12) innervate the neighbouring infundibular area at the base of the third ventricle ('tuberoinfundibular DA system'), and neurones in the zona incerta give rise to short projections to the hypothalamus ('incertohypothalamic DA system').

Until recently, only ascending DA systems were known. There is, however, a growing body of evidence that there is also a descending DA system reaching the spinal cord.

Anatomy of the 5-HT neurones

All the 5-HT containing neurones are situated in the midline (or raphe) nuclei of the brain stem; these nuclei have been designated as areas B1 to B9 by Dahlström & Fuxe (1964). It is possible to distinguish between three nuclear groups: a medullary, a pontine and a mesencephalic group (Fig.6.20).

The *medullary raphe group* comprises three nuclei: nucleus raphes pallidus (B1), nucleus raphes magnus (B3) and nucleus raphes obscurus (B2). The *pontine raphe group* consists of two nuclei: nucleus centralis superior ('nucleus of Bechterew', corresponding to areas B6 and B8), and nucleus raphes pontis (B5). The *mesencephalic raphe nucleus* corresponds to the nucleus raphes dorsalis (B7). Areas B4 and B9 are insignificant in primates.

There are four major projections originating from the 5-HT-containing raphe nuclei:

1. The *descending bulbospinal 5-HT pathway* arises from the medullary raphe nuclei and innervates the ventral horn; a smaller contingent of fibres innervates the intermediate cellular column and the dorsal horn of the spinal cord.

2. The *pontocerebellar 5-HT pathway* arises from the pontine raphe nuclei and reaches the cerebellar nuclei and the cortex via the middle cerebellar peduncle.

3. The *propriobulbar 5-HT pathway* originates from the pontine and medullary raphe nuclei and sends fibres to many cellular groups in the reticular formation of the lower brain stem. Separate bundles from this pathway innervate the locus coeruleus and the inferior olivary complex.

4. The *ascending 5-HT pathway* is a massive system of fibres arising from the upper pontine and mesencephalic raphe nuclei.

This pathway supplies the following areas: (a) the mesencephalon (interpeduncular nucleus, substantia nigra); (b) the diencephalon (thalamus, lateral hypothalamus); (c) the telencephalon (striatum, neocortex via the internal capsule, limbic lobe). The following limbic areas receive a 5-HT innervation: olfactory bulb, olfactory tubercle, septal region (septal cortex and septal nuclei, including the nucleus accumbens), amygdala, hippocampus, cingulate and parahippocampal cortex.

The functional significance of the monoamine-containing neuronal systems is not fully understood. The nigrostriatal pathway of the DA system is part of the extrapyramidal motor system (see above). There is evidence that the mesolimbic and mesocortical DA pathways play an important role in the regulation of behaviour by positive reinforcers ('rewards') (see Liebman & Cooper 1989). 5-HT neurones have been implicated in sleep, temperature regulation, appetite and feeding behaviour, aggression, anxiety, and sexual activity (see Bevan et al 1989). There is evidence that NA neurones are involved in central autonomic regulation (see Bannister 1988), and it has been suggested that they may also play a role in selective attention and arousal, and contribute to positive reinforcement (see Liebman & Cooper 1988).

It is generally accepted that the selective degeneration of the nigrostriatal pathway is the pathological basis for Parkinson's disease. The 'dopamine hypothesis of schizophrenia' assumes that there is increased activity in the mesolimbic DA neurones in schizophrenia (see Murray et al 1988). The 'monoamine theory of affective disorders' assumes that alterations in the activity of the NA and/or 5-HT neurones are responsible for the symptoms of depression and mania (see van Praag 1978). In addition, both NA and 5-HT neuronal systems have been implicated in the pathogenesis of anxiety (Gray 1982), and disturbed function of 5-HT neurones has been associated with obsessive–compulsive disorder, aggressive and impulsive behaviour, suicidal behaviour and eating disorders (Eccleston and Doogan 1989).

ACKNOWLEDGEMENT

I am most grateful to Dr C. M. Bradshaw for drawing the figures.

REFERENCES

Bannister R 1988 Autonomic failure. Oxford University Press, Oxford

Beaudet A, Descarries L 1978 The monoamine innervation of rat cerebral cortex: synaptic and nonsynaptic axon terminals. Neuroscience 3: 851–860

Bevan P, Cools A R, Archer T 1989 Behavioural pharmacology of 5HT. Laurence Erlbaum, Hillsdale, NJ

Bogerts B 1981 A brainstem atlas of catecholaminergic neurons in man, using melanin as a natural marker. Journal of Comparative Neurology 197: 63–80

Bowsher D 1972 Introduction to neuroanatomy. Churchill Livingstone, Edinburgh

Crow T J, Johnstone E C, Owen F 1979 Research on schizophrenia. In: Granville-Grossman K (ed) Recent advances in clinical psychiatry, vol 3. Churchill Livingstone, Edinburgh

Dahlström A, Fuxe K 1964 Evidence for the existence of monoamine-containing neurons in the central nervous system. I. Demonstration of monoamines in the cell bodies of brain stem neurons. Acta Physiologica Scandinavica suppl 232: 1–55

Eccles J C 1964 The physiology of synapses. Springer-Verlag, Berlin

Eccleston D, Doogan D P 1989 Serotonin in behavioural disorders. British Journal of Psychiatry 155 (Suppl 8)

Gatz A J 1973 Manter's essentials of clinical neuroanatomy and neurophysiology. Davis, Philadelphia

Gray J A 1982 The neuropsychology of anxiety. Clarendon Press, Oxford

Grundfest H 1959 Synaptic and ephaptic transmission. In: Field J, Magoun H W (eds) Handbook of physiology. American Physiological Society, Washington, DC

Guyton A C 1972 Structure and function of the nervous system. W B Saunders, Philadelphia

Jones P, Murray R M 1991 The genetics of schizophrenia is the genetics of neurodevelopment. British Journal of Psychiatry 158: 615–623

Katzman R 1971 Blood-brain-CSF barriers. In: Albers R W, Siegel G J, Katzman R, Agranoff B W (eds) Basic neurochemistry. Little Brown, Boston

Kluver H, Bucy P C 1939 Preliminary analysis of functions of the temporal lobes in monkeys. Archives of Neurology and Psychiatry 42: 979–1000

Legg N J 1978 Neurotransmitter systems and their clinical disorders. Academic Press, London

Liebman J M, Cooper S J 1989 The neuropharmacological basis of reward. Oxford University Press, Oxford

Livett B C 1973 Histochemical visualization of adrenergic neurones. British Medical Bulletin 29: 93–99

MacLean P D 1949 Psychosomatic disease and the 'visceral brain'. Psychosomatic Medicine 11: 338–353

Mitchell G A G 1971 The essentials of neuroanatomy. Churchill Livingstone, Edinburgh

Murray R M, Kerwin R W, Nimgaonkar V L 1988 What have we learned about the biology of schizophrenia? In: Granville Grossman K (ed) Recent advances in clinical psychiatry, vol 6, Churchill Livingstone, Edinburgh

Netter F H 1953 The Ciba collection of medical illustrations, vol 1. Ciba, Summit, NJ

Nieuwenhuys R 1985 Chemoarchitecture of the brain. Springer-Verlag, Berlin

Nieuwenhuys R, Voogd, J, van Huijzen C 1979 The human central nervous system. Springer-Verlag, Berlin

Noback C R, Demarest R J 1981 The human nervous
system, 3rd edn, McGraw-Hill, New York
Nobin A, Björklund A 1973 Topography of the
monoamine neuron system in the human brain as revealed
in fetuses. Acta Physiologica Scandinavica suppl 338: 1–40
Olds J 1971 Emotional centres in the brain. In: Chalmers N,
Crawley R, Ross S P R (eds) Biological bases of behaviour.
Open University Press, London
Papez J W 1937 A proposed mechanism of emotion.
Archives of Neurology and Psychiatry 36: 725–743
Penfield W, Rasmussen T 1954 The cerebral cortex of man.
Macmillan, New York

Roth M, Iversen L L 1986 Alzheimer's disease and related
disorders. British Medical Bulletin 42: 1–114
Smith C G 1971 Basic neuroanatomy. University Press,
Toronto
Ungerstedt U 1971 Stereotaxic mapping of the monoamine
pathways in rat brain. Acta Physiologica Scandinavica
suppl 367: 1– 48
van Praag H M 1978 Amine hypotheses of affective
disorders. In: Iversen L L, Iversen S D, Snyder S H (eds)
Handbook of psychopharmacology, vol 13, Plenum Press,
New York.

FURTHER READING

Eccles J C 1973 The understanding of the brain. McGraw-
Hill, New York
McGeer P L, Eccles J C, McGreer E G 1978 Molecular neuro-
biology of the mammalian brain. Plenum Press, New York
Rohen J W 1971 Funktionelle Anatomie des Nervensystems.
Schattauer, Stuttgart

Schade J P, Ford D H 1971 Basic neurology. Elsevier,
Amsterdam
Williams P, Warwick R 1975 Functional neuroanatomy of
man. Churchill Livingstone, Edinburgh

7. Neuropharmacology and neuroendocrinology

L. J. Whalley

INTRODUCTION

Neuropharmacology is concerned with the effects of drugs on nervous tissue. The study of neuropharmacology forms the basis of psychopharmacology which concerns the effects of drugs on behaviour. The effects of a drug depend largely upon its concentration at its sites of action; its absorption, distribution, biotransformation and excretion determine these concentrations and a drug's passage through the body is referred to as its pharmacokinetics. A drug's pharmacodynamics comprises its biochemical and physiological effects. Clinical pharmacology is the study of drug effects in man and pharmacotherapeutics is the study of drug effects in the treatment and prevention of disease.

Neuropharmacological studies contribute extensively to the evaluation of drug treatments in psychiatry and may provide useful insights into the neurobiology of mental illnesses. The fact that mental illnesses cannot be fully understood from a pharmacological perspective is in part attributed to their complexity but is to some extent related to the present stage of development of neurobiology as a science. From a historical perspective, the current status of the neuropharmacology of psychiatric disorders resembles the position held by endocrinologists in the first decades of this century. At that time, diseases now known to be caused by defects in steroid and thyroid hormone function were clinically well described but basic physiological studies had yet to take place. An explosion of interest and knowledge made possible by technological advances in the physical sciences has led to the present position whereby the diverse effects of thyroid and adrenal cortical hormones are much more extensively described. Importantly, analysis of hormone receptors is now regarded as an essential prerequisite for a proper understanding of the genetics, abnormal metabolism, classification and treatment of thyroid and adrenal cortical diseases. Molecular mechanisms, especially those involving drug–receptor interaction and the control of genetic expression in the brain, form the focus of much current research in neuropharmacology.

PHARMACOKINETICS

The absorption, distribution, biotransformation and excretion of a drug depend upon its movement across cell membranes. This is determined by a drug's physical characteristics and the presence or absence of specific mechanisms to facilitate its passage across membranes. Passive movement of water-soluble substances of low molecular weight (less than 200 Da) is by filtration through aqueous channels. These are too narrow (less than 4 Å) for most drugs which must pass through the cell membrane to enter a cell. Many drugs are organic electrolytes and are weak acids or bases. Only the un-ionised fraction of a drug, not bound to plasma proteins, is free to cross the cell membrane. The pharmacokinetics of drug entry into the central nervous system (CNS) are summarised in Figure 7.1. The fraction labelled 'free' in this diagram is available to pass into the brain and its rate of movement is proportional to its concentration gradient from plasma to the extracellular fluid of the nervous system. The extent to which a drug is ionised is determined by the pH of its solution and the dissociation constant (K_d) of the drug. The un-ionised portion is usually 10 000 times more lipid-soluble than the ionised portion and consequently much more soluble in the lipid bilayer of the cell membrane.

Absorption and distribution

The passage of drugs into the brain is governed by the general principles of drug absorption and the specific properties of the blood–brain barrier. The important general principles are that drugs given in aqueous

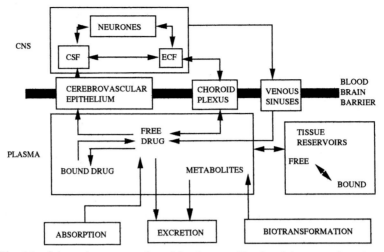

Fig. 7.1   Schematic representation of the pharmacokinetics of drug entry into the central nervous system. (CSF, cerebrospinal fluid; ECF, extracellular fluid).

solution are absorbed more quickly than those dissolved in oils or given as solids. Most drugs are given by mouth and the wide pH range encountered in the gastrointestinal tract influences absorption. Oral ingestion is the most convenient and economical method of administration and, because drugs are absorbed relatively slowly from the gut, is also relatively safe because adverse effects also develop slowly. Intravenous administration rapidly produces the desired plasma concentration of a drug, but, because the effects are immediate, so are adverse reactions. Table 7.1 summarises the properties of common routes of drug administration. After a drug is absorbed into the bloodstream, it is distributed between extracellular and intracellular fluids. At first, distribution is determined by the relative blood flow to the various regions of the body, so that highly perfused organs can reach peak concentrations within the first few minutes. Except in the brain, capillary endothelial membranes are highly permeable, allowing molecules as large as albumin (67 000 Da) to pass through their aqueous channels. As the plasma concentration of a drug falls, it may be released from body compartments which would allow its action to be sustained. The most immediate reservoir for drugs is formed by binding to plasma proteins, particularly albumin. Binding is relatively non-selective, so drugs compete for these binding sites. Drugs can also accumulate in other reservoirs such as muscle, fat or bone, and because many drugs are highly lipid-soluble they can be stored in body fat. In obese persons, this is an important drug reservoir.

Table 7.1   Properties of common routes of drug administration

Route	Absorption	Value	Limitations
Oral	Variable	Convenience Safety	Drugs of low solubility or high hepatic clearance have low oral availability
Subcutaneous	Quick in aqueous solution	Useful for some insoluble drugs and pellets	Pain, local necrosis Unsuitable for large volumes
Intramuscular	Quick in aqueous solution Slow from depot preparations	Useful for low to medium volumes and some irritating drugs	Contraindicated during anticoagulant therapy
Intravenous	May have immediate effects	Useful in emergency and suitable for large volumes	Can have immediate adverse reactions Unsuitable for oily or insoluble preparations

The blood–brain barrier

The brain and cerebrospinal fluid (CSF) are separated from the blood by the blood–brain barrier which regulates the movement of substances into and out of the nervous system. It is represented structurally by the capillary endothelium of the brain and subarachnoid space and the arachnoid membrane. The cells of these structures are so tightly bound together that diffusion between cells is negligible and the cells function as a single continuous sheet, behaving like a lipid membrane. Lipid-soluble substances pass readily through this membrane, whereas non-lipid-soluble substances and proteins enter the brain much more slowly.

The permeability of the blood–brain barrier to drugs (when there is no specific mechanism of entry) is determined by the general principles set out above. A ready guide to a drug's entry into the nervous system is provided by the 'pH partition hypothesis'. This states that the permeability of a cell membrane to a drug is proportional to that drug's partition parameter, which is the product of two fractional concentrations, one of the un-ionised drug in aqueous solution and the other the lipid solubility of the un-ionised drug. The latter is

usually measured as the optimal lipid/water partition coefficient. The pH of CSF can be regulated independently of plasma pH because un-ionised carbon dioxide passes across the blood–brain barrier much more readily than bicarbonate ions. CSF pH is usually 0.1 of a unit lower than plasma pH and, at equilibrium, concentrations of weak electrolytes may differ on either side of the blood–brain barrier, so that weak bases tend to accumulate in the CSF whereas weak acids tend to be excluded. The pH gradients between plasma and CSF can, therefore, produce concentration gradients at equilibrium for dissociated compounds. Figure 7.2 illustrates these principles by showing the relationship between the uptake by the brain of radiolabelled substances and their lipid/water partition coefficients. When a drug has a partition coefficient greater than 0.03, it is almost completely cleared from the blood after carotid artery injection during a single brain passage. A group of substances is encircled within a broken line in Figure 7.2 and these exceptions to the general rule show high clearance yet have very low partition coefficients.

Specific carrier transport systems related to lipid affinity are available for these substances. Large amino acids, essential for brain function, are not usually syn-

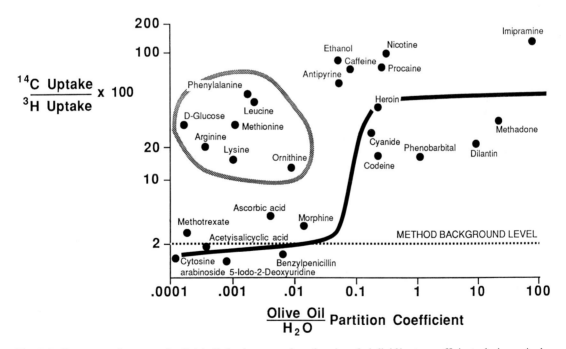

Fig. 7.2 Percentage clearance of radiolabelled substances plotted against their lipid/water coefficients during a single brain passage following carotid arterial injection. Drugs with a partition coefficient greater than about 0.03 show nearly complete clearance. The substances inside the broken line have very low lipid affinity but are effectively cleared brain metabolites which penetrate the blood–brain barrier by virtue of specific carrier transport systems. (After Oldendorf (1974) and Bradbury (1979).)

thesised in the brain and so need to be transported from the blood. For example, the rate of entry of tryptophan into the brain is directly proportional to the ratio of its plasma concentration to the sum of the concentrations of phenylalanine, leucine, valine and isoleucine. These other amino acids all compete with tryptophan for the same transport system. Amino acid transport mechanisms are stereospecific, preferring the laevo- to the dextro-isomer. Active transport can operate in both directions and against concentration gradients either from the brain to the blood or from the blood to the brain. Some nervous system metabolites do not have specific mechanisms to clear them from CSF, and so are removed when CSF passes back into the blood (the 'sink action' of CSF).

Endothelial capillaries vary in their permeability from area to area of the brain. In general, capillary endothelium is more permeable into grey than into white matter, and these high permeability areas may allow transfer of compounds such as peptides which cannot cross the blood–brain barrier elsewhere.

Biotransformation and excretion

Biotransformation of most drugs takes place in hepatic microsomal enzyme systems, though other systems — including plasma, gut, lung or kidney — may be involved. Lipid-soluble drugs are more readily metabolised by hepatic microsomes because of their ease of entry into the cell. Considerable individual variation in biotransformation can be related to genetic factors, the effects of age, hepatic disease or induction of microsomal enzymes by other drugs or environmental agents. The processes of biotransformation can lead to activation or inactivation of a drug and may involve numerous drug metabolites. Unchanged drugs or their metabolites are removed from the body by excretory organs such as the kidney or lung. Substances with high lipid solubility are not readily excreted until they have been metabolised to more polar compounds. The kidneys remove most drugs or their metabolites by renal excretion involving glomerular filtration, active tubular secretion and passive tubular reabsorption. Like all cell membranes, tubular cells are less permeable to the ionised portion of a drug, and more permeable to lipid-soluble compounds. Excretion of drugs in other body fluids is relatively unimportant with the exception of breast milk.

Clearance

In psychiatric practice, the usual aim is to maintain the concentration of a drug within its presumed therapeutic range. 'Steady state' concentrations are attained when the rate of drug elimination (clearance) equals the rate of drug administration. When complete bioavailability of a drug can be assumed, the rate of drug administration is, therefore, determined by its clearance. For most drugs used in psychiatry, clearance is typically constant within the range of concentrations seen in clinical practice. This arises because clearance mechanisms are not usually saturated and drug clearance is observed to be a linear function of the drug's blood concentration. A constant fraction of most drugs is cleared per unit of time, and when this happens the drug is said to follow *first-order kinetics*. When clearance systems for a drug are saturated, the pharmacokinetics of the drug become *zero order* and a constant amount of that drug is cleared per unit of time. Clearance is calculated as the total volume of blood (or other body fluid) from which a drug must be completely removed, not as the total amount of drug removed. Total clearance represents the sum of clearance by each organ of elimination (kidneys, liver, lung, etc).

In some circumstances, clearance of a drug by a specific organ becomes a matter of clinical concern, for example, the renal elimination of lithium. Clinical investigation of renal function of a patient on long-term lithium therapy might, therefore, use an alternative definition of clearance. Clearance can be defined by the blood flow to the organ under investigation (Q), arterial concentration (C_A) and venous concentration (C_V). The difference between the products of blood flow and blood concentration gives the clearance by an organ (CL_{organ}):

$$\text{Elimination} = QC_A - QC_V = Q(C_A - C_V)$$

$$CL_{organ} = \frac{Q(C_A - C_V)}{C_A}$$
$$= QE.$$

The expression $(C_A - C_V)/C_A$ defines the *extraction ratio* (*E*) for a drug by a specific sorgan.

Some drugs show dose-dependent clearance that varies with drug concentration in blood. Dosing schemes for these drugs can be difficult:

$$\text{total blood clearance} = V_M/(K_M + C_B)$$

where K_M is the blood concentration at which 50% of the maximum rate of elimination is reached (in units of mass/volume) and V_M is the maximum rate of elimination (in units of mass/time).

Drugs such as chlorpromazine and imipramine are mostly cleared by the liver. Hepatic clearance is largely determined by hepatic blood flow, i.e. the rate at which the drug can be transported to hepatic sites of biotransformation and/or excretion in bile. Although changes in drug binding to blood components and other tissues (Fig. 7.1) may influence hepatic or renal clearance, in present circumstances, when a drug's extraction ratio (E) is high, changes in protein binding due to disease or competitive processes should have little effect on drug clearance. However, when the extraction ratio is low, changes in protein binding and intrahepatic functions will substantially alter drug clearance, but changes in hepatic blood flow will have little effect. Because a drug bound to blood proteins is not filtered and thus not subject to active glomerular secretion and/or reabsorption, renal clearance is substantially influenced by protein binding and thus by those diseases that affect protein binding.

NEUROTRANSMISSION

Almost 40 years ago, intracellular recording techniques established beyond reasonable doubt the neurochemical nature of synaptic transmission in the CNS. Chemical neurotransmitters were shown to produce inhibition or excitation of neurones by briefly and rapidly increasing neuronal membrane permeability to specific ions. Table 7.2 shows the 'classical' criteria for the identification of neurotransmitters that were once widely accepted. Later, studies on single neurones identified noradrenaline, acetylcholine, serotonin, dopamine, γ-aminobutyric acid (GABA), glycine and glutamate as transmitters at synapses in the CNS. A major development in understanding the function of neurotransmitters in neural networks was provided by

Table 7.2 Criteria for identification of neurotransmitters

1. The transmitter must be shown to be present in the presynaptic terminals of the synapse and in the neurones from which those presynaptic terminals arise
2. The transmitter must be released from the presynaptic nerve concomitantly with presynaptic nerve activity
3. The effects of the putative neurotransmitter when applied experimentally to the target cells must be identical to those of the presynaptic pathway

Yamamoto & McIlwain (1966) who demonstrated the feasibility of recording from transverse hippocampal slices. This structure contains numerous neurotransmitters and their receptors and electrophysiological preparations preserve the precise laminar structure and much of the neuronal circuitry of the hippocampus. Although many accounts of neuropharmacology present information in terms of a single synapse (the functional unit of the nervous system) the data summarised in such accounts have often been obtained and characterised in model neuronal systems such as the hippocampal slice preparation (Bloom 1990).

Neutrotransmitters may open or close ion channels in the neuronal membrane and can do this directly or by activating adjacent proteins (Fig. 7.3). Initially, it was inferred that neurotransmitters caused a brief hyperpolarization or depolarization of the postsynaptic membrane. Now, it is known that neurotransmitters may have a much longer time-course of action produced by their altering the properties of voltage-sensitive (or 'voltage-gated') ion channels that are involved in the regulation of neuronal excitability. This is espe-

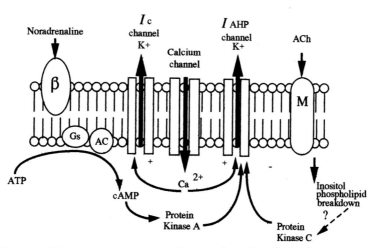

Fig. 7.3 The proposed mechanisms of action of noradrenaline and acetylcholine (ACh) in blocking the slow Ca^{2+}-activated K^+ conductance.

cially important in the case of K^+ and Ca^{2+} ion channels.

The release of neurotransmitters represents the 'final common pathway' of all neuronal functions. Table 7.3 summarises the properties of substances active at synapses. Neurotransmitters stored in presynaptic vesicles fuse with the presynaptic membrane at the nerve terminal. Synaptic vesicles are coated on their cytoplasmic face by synapsins, a particularly abundant group of extrinsic membrane proteins (Südhof et al 1989). The four synapsins appear to connect synaptic vesicles to each other and to the neuronal cytoskeleton and probably regulate vesicular position in the nerve terminal. None of the synapsins is the same but they share many common structural features and seem likely to comprise a single family of proteins with a common ancestor.

Calcium channels

Neurotransmitter release is Ca^{2+}-dependent and study of entry of Ca^{2+} across surface membranes is of intense interest to neuropharmacologists. In part this interest stems from technological developments and the availability of specific agents with which to study Ca^{2+} channels. The interest is also based on the ubiquitous nature of neuronal Ca^{2+} and its clinical relevance. Ca^{2+} channels open in response to membrane depolarisation and generate electrical and chemical responses. Ca^{2+} entry into the neurone carries a depolarising charge that contributes to paroxysmal phenomena such as epileptiform or pacemaker activity. It also causes the intracellular Ca^{2+} concentration to rise, and this in turn alters Ca^{2+}-dependent mechanisms involved in neurotransmitter release from synaptic vesicles, enzyme activation, Ca^{2+}-sensitive ion channels and many diverse aspects of neuronal metabolism.

Multiple types of Ca^{2+} channel exist in neurones and it is important to distinguish between them in order to understand neuronal function and its modification by drugs and neurotransmitters. Early electrophysiological studies demonstrated two classes of Ca^{2+} channel: 'low-voltage activated' (LVA) and 'high-voltage activated' (HVA) (Llinas & Yarom 1981). Subsequently, the HVA Ca^{2+} channel was found to comprise N and L subtypes (Nowycky et al 1985), yielding three subtypes designated T (or LVA), N and L. These acronyms should not be taken too literally but do have some mnemonic value: T for 'transient', L for 'long-lasting' and N for channels that are 'neither T nor L' (Tsien et al 1988). At present, none of the subtypes of Ca^{2+} channel is assigned an exclusive physiological role. However, T channels are important in pacemaker depolarization in heart cells and are the primary voltage-sensitive entry points for Ca^{2+} on contraction of certain smooth muscle cells. Ca^{2+} entry by L channels is associated with heart muscle contraction and substance P and noradrenaline release in the CNS. Only L channels are sensitive to blockade by Ca^{2+} channel-blocking drugs (the dihydropyridines, nicardipine and nimodipine and diltiazem, nifedipine and verapamil).

The complexity of the regulation of Ca^{2+} entry into neurones is not surprising in view of the central importance of intracellular Ca^{2+} in so many aspects of neuronal function. The fact that there are multiple types of voltage-sensitive Ca^{2+} channel and, as will be described later, multiple types of receptor-operated Ca^{2+} channel, indicates the adaptability available to the neurone in 'fine-tuning' intracellular Ca^{2+} concentrations (Miller 1987).

Pharmacological studies of the Ca^{2+} channel blockers have shown that each binds to a different

Table 7.3   Substances active at synapses

Substance	Properties	Example
Neurotransmitter	A substance found in neurone type A, secreted from it and acting on target neurone type B	Acetylcholine
Neurohormone	Peptide secretions of neurones directly into the blood that also act on other neurones as neurotransmitters	Corticotrophin-releasing factor (CRF)
Neuromodulator	A substance that influences neuronal activity and originates from non-synaptic sites	Steroid hormones
Neuromediator	Postsynaptic compounds that participate in generation of postsynaptic responses	Cyclic adenosine monophosphate (cAMP)

recognition site on a single protein–receptor complex. Although these drugs do not influence neurotransmitter release, their diverse chemical structures resemble many other clinically useful compounds (Snyder 1989). The neuroleptic drugs comprise several chemical classes: phenothiazines, butyrophenones and diphenylbutylpiperidines. This last class is as equipotent as a Ca^{2+} channel antagonist as the Ca^{2+}-blocking drugs listed above. Ca^{2+} channel blockade probably also accounts for some neuroleptic side-effects. Electrocardiogram (ECG) changes produced by thioridazine are similar to those produced by verapamil. Impaired vas deferens contraction and ejaculation observed in experiments using Ca^{2+}-blocking drugs probably explains a common side-effect of thioridazine that is rarely encountered with phenothiazines or butyrophenones. Cardiac and ejaculatory side-effects of thioridazine are probably caused by thioridazine-induced Ca^{2+} channel blockade.

Phosphatidylinositol (PI) metabolism

Protein kinase C (PKC) is a Ca^{2+}-dependent enzyme concentrated at presynaptic nerve terminals close to or in conjunction with synaptic vesicles. It is activated by diacylglycerol (DAG), a cleavage product of a group of membrane lipids called phosphatidylinositols. PKC activation in turn potentiates neurotransmitter release. These events are important components of the regulation of neurotransmission and are affected by lithium. Initially, in response to extracellular signals, lipases including phospholipase C (PLC) degrade phosphatidylinositols into precursors of two intracellular 'second messengers'. These are inositol phosphates (IPs) and DAG. Inositol 1,4,5–triphosphate (IP_3) synthesis is the major product of phosphatidylinositol degradation. The pathway is shown in Figure 7.4 (Majerus et al 1988). The PLC enzyme that initiates this cascade of events in fact comprises a group of at least five structurally dissimilar enzymes (Rhee et al 1989). This highly conserved diversity of enzyme structure is poorly understood but probably allows the two pathways (IP_3 and arachidonic acid) to respond selectively to specific extracellular signals and to be negatively influenced by products of these pathways. PKC activation by phorbol esters mimics the action of DAG and is blocked by lithium (Fig. 7.4). Since PKC activation also potentiates serotonin and noradrena-

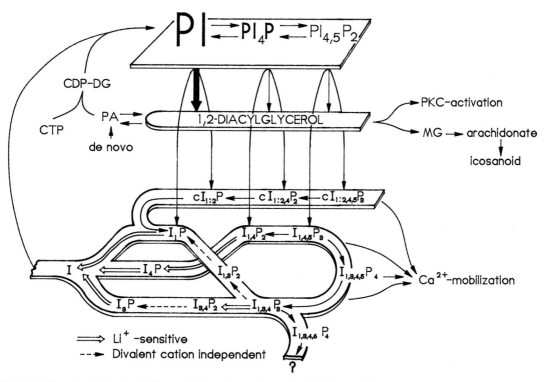

Fig. 7.4 Phosphatidylinositol (PI) metabolism shown schematically. Lithium effects are indicated. (After Majerus et al (1988).)

line release, this effect of lithium at therapeutically relevant concentrations may be relevant to understanding its mode of action in the treatment of mania and prophylaxis of manic depressive illness (Wang & Friedman 1989).

PHARMACODYNAMICS

Pharmacodynamics concerns the mechanism of action of drugs. Knowledge of drug pharmacodynamics in psychiatry is basic to their clinical use. Studies of drug action aim to identify chemical and physical interactions between drug and neurone. A proper understanding of the temporal order and scale of drug–neurone interactions provides the basis for understanding drug effects. It can be used to help design improved drugs and, potentially, may provide information of relevance to understanding neurobiological components of psychiatric disease.

Receptors

Early pharmacologists were impressed by the narrow physical requirements of novel drugs if these were to be effective. Although the term receptor was introduced to denote in a non-specific manner that part of the organism with which a drug interacted and so produced its effect, it soon became clear to early investigators that drug–receptor interactions took place at a molecular level. Receptors were conceptualised as large, functional molecules that played an established role in cellular function. This basic principle has two important implications. Firstly, drugs cannot produce novel cellular responses but can only modify established functions. Secondly, drugs can alter the rate at which cellular functions take place.

The physical and chemical features of receptor molecules may vary substantially. Some are protein constituents of the cellular membrane, others are proteins that are important in the maintenance of subcellular architecture and some are intracellular enzymes or proteins concerned with cellular transport. Likewise, interactions between drugs and receptors are of multiple types and include covalent, ionic, hydrophobic and van der Waals binding. Covalent binding tends to be of long duration whilst noncovalent high-affinity binding is usually irreversible. The physical configuration of the receptor largely determines the structural requirements of a drug designed to interact with that receptor. Several clinically important drugs in psychiatry have been developed from deliberate chemical changes to the structure of the endogenous ligand (*physiological*

agonist). Additionally, small changes of structure can alter the pharmacokinetic properties of drugs.

Most drugs produce their effects by interaction with receptive macromolecules and so start a sequence of biochemical and physiological events. Receptive macromolecules are termed 'drug receptors', of which cellular proteins that bind reversibly to endogenous ligands, such as neurotransmitters and hormones, are the most important. The term 'receptor' is also used in a wider sense to describe the mechanisms by which a neurotransmitter can change the functions of a cell. This wider definition includes recognition of the neurotransmitter (usually by a cell surface protein) and transduction of the message into alterations of cellular function, mechanisms that may involve changes in ion permeability and the formation of *second messengers.*

Drugs that bind to receptors and initiate a response in neuroeffector tissue are *agonists*. Drugs that produce a maximal response are *full agonists* and those producing less than maximal response are *partial agonists*. Drugs that have no intrinsic pharmacological activity but produce effects by preventing an agonist initiating a response are *antagonists*. Some antagonists can produce a partial pharmacological response ('partial agonist activity') at receptor binding sites where they compete with endogenous ligands. Some drugs combine both agonist and antagonist properties as *mixed agonist–antagonists*, and understanding these properties may have therapeutic potential. For example, a mixed opiate agonist–antagonist might have the advantage of providing relief of pain with much less risk of addiction than a full agonist such as morphine. Pharmacological antagonism is distinct from physiological antagonism produced by substances initiating an opposing response in neuroeffector tissue. For example, noradrenaline can act as a physiological antagonist of acetylcholine.

Classical receptor theory assumes that the effect of a drug is proportional to the number of receptors with which that drug interacts. The ease with which a drug attaches to a receptor is termed the *affinity* of the drug for that receptor. Receptors for neurotransmitters are components of the neural membrane. They are able to recognise specific neurotransmitters and produce physiological responses in neuroeffector tissues. Receptors can, therefore, be defined both in terms of their ability to recognise specific ligands and by the physiological responses they initiate.

Receptor sensitivity

Drug–receptor interactions may be modified by changes in receptor sensitivity. The sensitivity of receptors is influenced by complex regulatory and homeostatic factors. When receptor sensitivity changes, the same concentration of a drug will produce a greater or lesser physiological response. Changes in sensitivity occur, for example, after prolonged stimulation of cells by agonists and the cell becomes refractory to further stimulation. This is also termed 'desensitisation' or 'down-regulation'. Underlying mechanisms of desensitisation may involve receptor changes (e.g. phosphorylation) or the receptor may be concealed within the cell so that it is no longer exposed to the ligand. Long-term desensitisation may involve negative-feedback mechanisms that inhibit new receptor synthesis or cause a structurally modified receptor to be synthesised. Desensitisation involves at least two distinct 'closed' states of the nicotinic receptor. Both 'closed' states display a higher affinity for acetylcholine than does the resting (or 'active') conformation. Structural studies show that a specific segment of the lumen-facing part of the ion channel is crucial in the process of desensitisation in response to prolonged agonist exposure (Revah et al 1991). This segment of the ionic channel is highly conserved in other receptor types (e.g. $GABA_A$ and glycine receptors) where it may play a similar role. Supersensitivity ('up-regulation' or 'hypersensitivity') often follows prolonged receptor blockade. This may involve synthesis of new receptors so that an increased number of receptors is exposed on the cell surface to their physiological ligands.

Receptor families

Historically, there has been considerable debate about criteria for the characterisation of receptor subtypes. Practically, the identification of new receptor types has

Table 7.4   Criteria for identification of receptors

1. 'Possible': Radioligand binding sites
   a. Saturability and reversibility of radioligand binding
   b. Homogeneous population of sites
   c. Regional and species variation
   d. Pharmacological properties
2. 'Probable': Functional correlates
   a. Identification of special messenger links
   b. Delineation of physiological effects on membranes
   c. Behavioural or other models of action
3. 'Definite': Structural identification
   a. Unique amino acid sequence
   b. Cloned sequences mimic actions of natural receptor

After Peroutka (1988).

Table 7.5   Examples of 'superfamilies' of receptors

'Superfamily'	Neuroreceptor/ion channel
G protein–coupled receptors	Visual pigments Adrenergic Muscarinic, cholinergic Serotonergic
Ligand-gated ion channel receptors	Nicotinic cholinergic $GABA_A$ Glycine
Voltage-gated ion channel	Na^+ K^+

quickly followed the development of specific, potent agonists and/or antagonists that selectively bind to the new drug. Peroutka (1988) has used the example of receptor subtypes for serotonin to illustrate molecular, biochemical and physiological techniques of study. These are summarised in Table 7.4.

Molecular, biochemical and physiological techniques indicate the existence of several 'superfamilies' (probably less than ten) of receptor macromolecules (Table 7.5). Molecular biological techniques have provided the best classification of subtypes within receptor 'superfamilies'. Progress in this field has consistently led to revision of classification systems based on biochemical and physiological studies. Within each 'superfamily' of receptor types there can be considerable structural diversity of their endogenous ligands. Receptors within each receptor family, however, have many structural similarities with other members of the same family and share common mechanisms of signal propagation.

1. Steroid and thyroid hormone receptors. Receptors for steroid and thyroid hormones are members of a single family of receptor macromolecules. These are physiological regulatory proteins that each possess a region ('ligand-binding domain') to recognise steroid and thyroid hormones (ligands) and a structural part that couples the receptor to intracellular metabolic processes. Receptors for steroid and thyroid hormones, vitamin D and the retinoids are presently the best described prototypical 'receptor family' (Evans 1988). The part of these receptors that binds to the hormone is crucial to the receptor's function. Removal of this part of the receptor produces an active receptor fragment almost as effective in the regulation of genetic transcription as the natural hormone-bound receptor. Binding of the natural hormone to its receptor removes the inhibitory effect of the remainder of the receptor structure. The second of the three parts of the receptor binds to

Na$^+$ channel

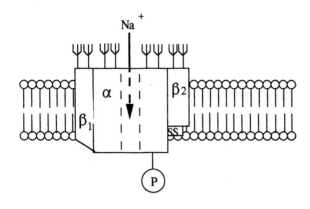

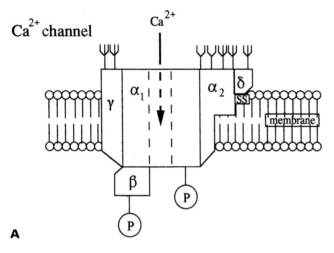

Ca^{2+} channel

A

Fig. 7.5 A Subunit structures of Na$^+$ and Ca^{2+} channels. The subunit structure and transmembrane organization of the rat brain Na$^+$ channel and the subunit structure of the rabbit skeletal muscle Ca^{2+} channel. Disulphide bonds (SS), glycosylation sites (f structures) and phosphorylation sites (P) are illustrated. (After Catterall (1988).) **B** Left: Ligand-gated channels (top) are made of distinct units, two for GABA$_A$ receptors or four for peripheral nicotinic-acetylcholine receptors (middle), each encoded by a separate gene. The units consist of four hydrophobic membrane-spanning domains (M1–M4) joined by a string of hydrophilic amino acid residues. Right: voltage-gated channels, such as the Na$^+$ and Ca^{2+} channels, are thought to be made of four structurally similar domains (motifs 1–4). These consist of six membrane-spanning domains (S1–S6) joined by a string of hydrophilic amino acid residues. K$^+$ channels have a single motif, with the same structure. (After Stevens (1987).)

B

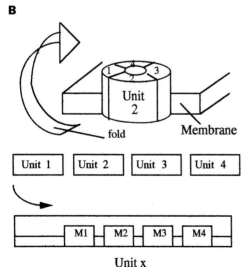

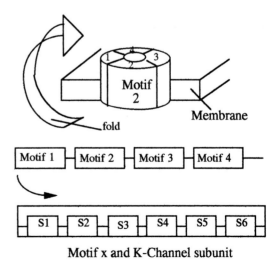

regulatory sites on nuclear DNA. These DNA-blinding receptors are soluble proteins that in their inactivated state inhibit transcription of the related gene. They are highly receptor-specific so that each type may mediate the effects of a specific endogenous ligand with the relevant ligand-responsive gene. The third component of the steroid/thyroid receptor is ill-understood but probably serves to promote the regulatory activity of the receptor macromolecule.

2. Voltage-sensitive ion channels. Voltage-sensitive ion channels have major roles in neurotransmission. Na^+, K^+ and Ca^{2+} channels consist of a principal transmembrane subunit which constitutes the core of the ion channel. Different cell types contain varying numbers of subunits for Na^+, K^+ and Ca^{2+} channels, and these are members of the same structural family whose ancestry shows many highly conserved structures, mostly around the core of the channel. These conserved regions are also found in second messenger-gated channels (Jan & Jan 1990). Figure 7.5 shows schematic models of Na^+ and Ca^{2+} ion channels (Catterall 1988, Stevens 1987). The primary structures of these ion channels are known and, especially in the case of the Na^+ channel, have led to proposals for advanced models of ion channel function. Figure 7.6 shows how depolarization leads to a sequence of conformational changes in individual α subunits. After each subunit changes, an open ion channel is formed by movement of the helical arrangement of amino acids that constitutes each subunit. The transmembrane subunits have a spiral ribbon of positive charge which, at resting potential, is paired with negative charges on adjacent transmembrane subunits. Forces maintaining the positive charges in this position are reduced by depolarisation. The helical subunit probably rotates in response to depolarisation and produces an unpaired negative charge on the inner surface of the membrane. The core size of the ion channel consistent with this model is 3×5 Å and would allow Na^+ to pass.

These voltage-sensitive ion channels require the movement of protein-bound positive charges from the intracellular to the extracellular surface of the membrane. Movement is said to be *voltage-sensitive* or *voltage-gated* and the current produced by movement of charges is detectable as 'gating current'. Voltage-sensitive ion channels are relevant to understanding the actions of many drugs in neuropharmacology.

3. G protein-coupled receptors. A family of cellular proteins called 'G proteins' (guanine triphosphate (GTP)-binding) link cell surface receptors to a variety of enzymes and ion channels. One class of receptor (summarized in Table 7.6) functions by stimulating a membrane-bound G protein. Members of this protein family are composed of three homologous subunits: α, β and γ. Figure 7.3 shows the likely organisation of receptors, G proteins and effectors (such as ion channels, adenylate cyclase and enzymes involved in phosphatidylinositol metabolism). Receptors coupled to G proteins have similar structures that include transmembrane helices (Fig. 7.7a). Sequence homology among the G protein-coupled receptors is found largely in the membrane-spanning regions. The cytoplasmic regions and loops between spans 5 and 6 show minimal sequence homology (Ross 1989). Neurotransmitter and hormonal ligands bind to G protein-coupled receptors in the pocket formed by the seven helices in Figure 7.7b. The G proteins are located on the intracellular surface of the plasma membrane and it is likely that that part of the receptor which regulates G proteins is also on the intracellular face. Binding of the ligand to the extracellular part of the receptor distorts the binding site to an extent sufficient to alter the cytoplasmic part of the receptor and to transform it from its passive to active state. The cytoplasmic loop between spans 5 and 6 is probably the G protein regulation site, as G protein regulation is sensitive to mutations in this region. The ligand-binding domain of the β adrenoceptor lies within the core of the receptor molecule. Structure–activity analyses of adrenoceptor ligands and the amino acid sequences in the receptor core have been greatly helped by the synthesis of 'mutant' receptors. These studies point the way toward the development of new drugs. They are also important in understanding molecular mechanisms of receptor desensitisation (Strader et al 1989).

Figure 7.8 shows the process of signal transduction by G proteins. A ligand binds at its receptor and produces a change in receptor–G protein interaction. This change allows GTP (in the presence of Mg^{2+}) to replace guanosine diphosphate (GDP) on the α subunit of the G protein. Now activated, the α-GTP

Table 7.6 Neurotransmitter ligands acting through G protein-coupled receptors

Neurotransmitter	Receptor subtypes	Effectors
Catecholamines	α_1, α_2, β_1, β_2, β_3	Adenylate cyclase
Cholinergic	M_1, M_2, M_3	PLC
Dopamine	D_1, D_2	Phospholipase A_2
Serotonin	$5\text{-HT}_{1A,B,C}$, 5-HT_2	Phosphodiesterases
Histamine	H_1, H_2, H_3	Ca^{2+} channels
GABA	$GABA_B$	K^+ channels
Glutamate	Angiotensin receptor	Guanylyl cyclase

A

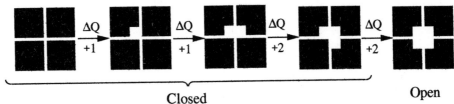

B

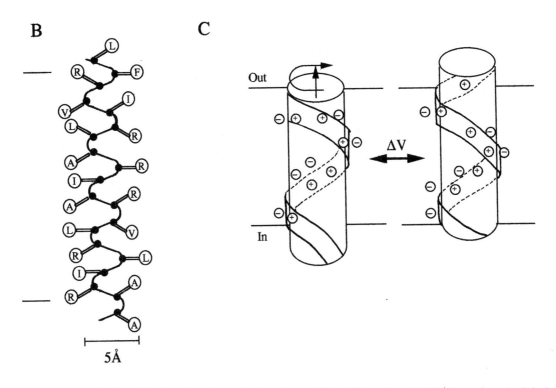

5Å

Fig. 7.6 **A** The sliding helix model of a voltage-dependent ion channel. Viewed from above, the Na$^+$ channel α subunit is shown as an array of four homologous domains around the central transmembrane pore. A sequence of voltage-driven conformational changes opens the ion channel. Each change is associated with an outward transfer across the membrane of a protein-bound positive gating charge (ΔQ). **B** A schematic representation of the S4 helix of the Na$^+$ channel. Solid circles represent the α carbon of each amino acid residue. Open circles represent the direction of projection of the side chain of each residue away from the core of the helix. **C** Movement of the S4 helix in response to membrane depolarization. The proposed transmembrane S4 helix is shown as a cylinder with a spiral ribbon of positive charge. At the resting potential (left) all positively charged residues are paired with fixed negative charges on other transmembrane segments of the channel and the transmembrane segment is held in that position by the negative internal membrane potential. Depolarization reduces the force holding the positive charges in their inward position. The S4 helix is then proposed to undergo a spiral motion through a rotation of approximately 60° and an outward displacement of approximately 5 Å. This movement leaves an unpaired negative charge on the inward surface of the membrane and reveals an unpaired positive charge on the outward surface to give a net charge transfer (ΔQ) of +1. Note that all intramembranous positive charges are paired in both conformations. In domains III and IV there are enough arginine residues to give a gating charge movement of +2. (After Catterall (1988).)

Extracellular

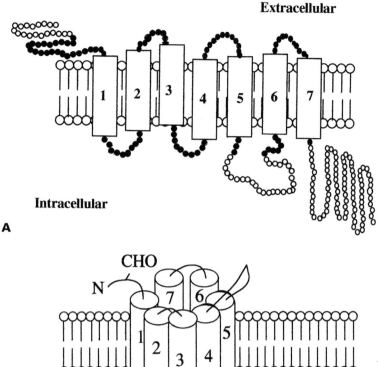

Intracellular

A

B   **Intracellular**

Fig. 7.7 **A** The peptide chains of the β-adrenergic and the G protein-coupled receptors are assumed to span the extracellular membrane as shown. **B** A three-dimensional array of the seven membrane-spanning helices shown in Figure 7.7A.

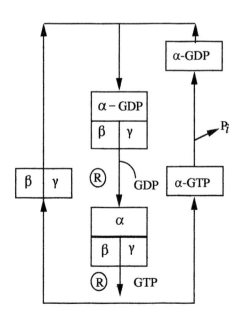

Fig. 7.8 The G protein cycle of activation in transmembrane signalling. (After Sternweis & Pang (1990).)

subunit dissociates from the βγ subunit allowing one or both subunits to interact with an effector (e.g. adenylate cyclase). The α subunit possesses intrinsic GTPase activity and hydrolyses GTP to GDP, releasing inorganic phosphate (P_i), and the cycle is terminated by α -GDP recombining with a βγ subunit. Throughout this cycle, the βγ subunit remains a single functional unit and all phases of the cycle take place in the cytoplasmic compartment. βγ subunits released in the cycle can interact with other effectors such as phospholipase A_2 (PLA_2) in some cell systems. The α subunit remains attached to the inner surface of the plasma membrane throughout this cycle (Neer & Clapham 1988).

G proteins can be subdivided by their susceptibilities to bacterial toxins. These subtypes are specific for: (1) cholera toxin only; (2) pertussis toxin only; (3) both toxins; (4) neither toxin. Cholera toxin-susceptible G proteins were initially thought to stimulate adenylate cyclase (G_s) and the pertussis toxin-susceptible G proteins to inhibit adenylate cyclase (G_i). These toxins modify different types of α subunit ($α_i$ and $α_s$) which then act upon a wide range of effectors. Structural analysis of the α and β subunits has revealed more subtypes than there are presently known functions. The $α_i$ subtype is divisible into $α_0$, $α_{i-1}$, $α_{i-2}$ and $α_{i-3}$. These are highly conserved and their individual genes probably derive from a common ancestor. The β and γ subtypes are also heterogeneous and the overall picture is of a loose spatial organisation of receptors, G proteins and their effectors. Receptors can interact with a single G protein and the same G protein can interact with several receptors or effectors. Probably up to 15 distinct kinds of receptor can stimulate adenylate cyclase through G_s. Interactions between G proteins and effectors, however, seem to be much more specific so that, for example, only G_s and not G_i or G_0 can stimulate adenylate cyclase. This capacity of G proteins to interact with multiple effectors underlies the advantages of G proteins as signal transducers. Multiple receptors, G proteins and effectors make up a complex signalling network. These networks sort extracellular signals and integrate incoming information (Birnbaumer 1990). The effector enzyme, adenylate cyclase, can be stimulated or inhibited by numerous hormones or transmitters either directly or along the G protein pathway. Structural studies have revealed multiple forms of adenylate cyclase that, surprisingly in view of its intracellular functions, contain numerous transmembrane spans (Krupinski et al 1989). The structure has many features shared with G protein-regulated Ca^{2+} channels and transporter molecules.

These similarities probably relate to hitherto unrecognised functions of adenylate cyclase.

AMINO ACID NEUROTRANSMISSION

Inhibitory amino acid neurotransmission (IAA)

GABA and the amino acid glycine are the major inhibitory neurotransmitters. GABA receptors are more abundant at inhibitory synapses in the brain whereas glycine receptors are more numerous in the brain stem and spinal cord.

Postsynaptic inhibition is mediated by the opening of ion channels in the postsynaptic membrane. These are selectively permeable to Cl^- and other small monovalent cations. Electrophysiological studies show that glycine and GABA receptors have similar properties.

1. Glycine receptors

Recent pharmacological and molecular biological studies of receptors for GABA and glycine have established that several receptor macromolecules are involved. The postsynaptic glycine receptor (GlyR) is a large membrane-spanning glycoprotein which on binding with glycine forms an anion-selective transmembrane (Fig. 7.9). GlyR is a member of the ligand-gated ion channel 'superfamily' of receptors (Betz 1987). Although these receptors are plentiful throughout the CNS and are of presumed biological importance, the neuropharmacology of glycine remains poorly understood. The amino acids taurine and β-alanine are effective agonists at GlyR but alanine, proline and serine are less effective. No non-amino acid agonists at GlyR have been detected and GABA has little effect at GlyR at physiological concentrations. GlyR antagonists include strychnine (a potent neurotoxic convulsant) which is believed to have its own specific binding site on GlyR close to the integral ion channel.

Betz and his colleagues at Heidelberg have shown GlyR to be like other ligand-gated ion channels (e.g. nicotinic acetylcholine receptor). It is composed of a core made up of four subunits, two of which are the same (Fig. 7.9). The role of GlyR in neurodegenerative disease is largely unexplored. In Parkinson's disease and motor neurone disease, GlyR–strychnine binding sites are reduced.

2. GABA receptors

GABA is the main cortical inhibitory neurotransmitter. Its inhibitory actions are Cl^-dependent and are

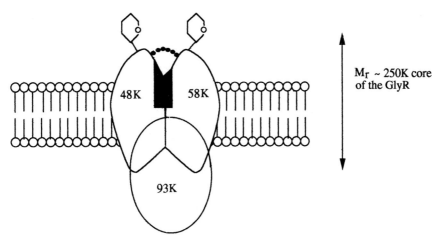

Fig. 7.9 Schematic representation of the postsynaptic glycine receptor (GlyR). The core of the receptor is likely to be made up of four subunits, but only one copy of each subunit is shown here. (After Betz (1987).)

blocked by the plant alkaloid bicuculline. Some effects of GABA are, however, insensitive to bicuculline, indicating the existence of two different types of GABA receptor. The classical GABA$_A$ receptor has an integral transmembrane Cl$^-$ channel that mediates GABAnergic transmission by opening and allowing Cl$^-$ entry. This type of channel is called a 'ligand-gated ion channel'. Less is known about GABA$_B$ receptors. They are linked to Ca^{2+} or K$^+$ channels and are coupled to G proteins (Fig. 7.10).

The GABA$_A$ receptor is the major inhibitory molecule in brain. It is present on most brain neurones, exists in several forms, and has at least four different sites at which ligands may bind (Fig. 7.10). These sites are for: (1) the GABA agonist/antagonist; (2) picrotoxin (where agents that block GABAergic transmission may bind); (3) benzodiazepine drugs and (4) CNS depressant drugs (these are multiple) where agents may bind and prolong GABAergic activation of the integral channel. Each of these sites may be occupied simultaneously by their respective ligands, implying that each is a physically distinct part of the same receptor molecule. A group of molecular biologists led by Eric Barnard achieved the first purification and then sequenced the GABA$_A$ receptor protein. The purified protein contains subunits of the types: α (about 53 000 Da) and β (about 57 000 Da). The receptor is composed of the combinations of four subunits which may be either α or β (i.e. it is a heterotetrameric protein). Electrophysiological studies show that occupation of both of the two binding sites for GABA is necessary to open the integral Cl$^-$ channel. These sites

are on the two β subunits and binding sites for benzodiazepine drugs are on the two α subunits. Receptor complementary DNA (cDNA) cloning and functional expression of full-length α and β subunits provide conclusive evidence that the α and β subunits constitute the receptor and its chloride channel. The genes for α$_1$, α$_2$, α$_3$, and β$_2$ subunits of the GABA$_A$ receptor have been cloned and expressed in cell lines to produce reconstituted ion channels. These have been made up of combinations of single GABA$_A$ receptor subunits and have characteristics (ion permeability and ligand binding) of the native receptor (Blair et al 1988) that suggest these characteristics are determined by substructures of the subunits that are shared by all subunits. The gene encoding the α$_3$ subunit of the GABA$_A$ receptor is on the X chromosome in a region previously linked to susceptibility to manic–depressive illness. The GABA$_A$-α$_3$ gene is a possible 'candidate' gene for this group of disorders (Bell et al 1989). The structure of the GABA$_A$ receptor is shown in Figure 7.10 and accounts for all its known pharmacological properties. The constituent amino acid segments of the receptor comprise parts that are sufficiently large to span the membrane and are also hydrophobic. Both α and β subunits contain four such parts (see Fig. 7.5) and have a cytoplasmic loop. The β subunit loop is longer and probably serves to modulate receptor function. The entire receptor thus contains 16 transmembrane subunits (α$_2$, β$_2$) and these crowd around the integral ion channel of 506 Å diameter. Only five α subunits are required to make up the necessary diameter but the likeliest solution is that one helix from

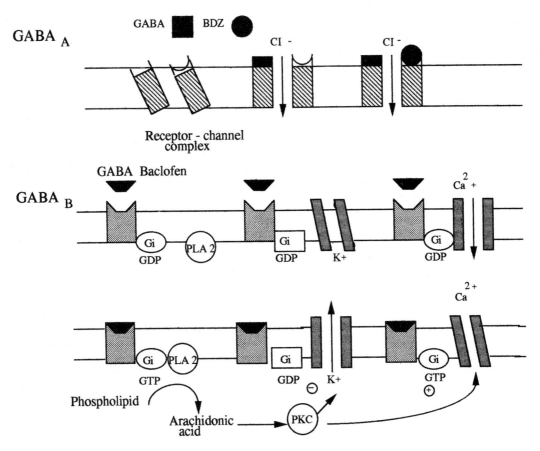

Fig. 7.10 Schematic models of GABA$_A$ and GABA$_B$ receptors. The GABA$_A$ receptor complex with its central Cl$^-$ ion channel is modulated by benzodiazepine binding (BDZ), which may increase Cl$^-$ currents (shown by an arrow). GABA$_B$ receptors are coupled to G proteins. + , positive effect; - , negative effect. (After Bormann (1988).)

each of the four subunits together form a single ion channel (Barnard et al 1987, Schofield et al 1987).

Benzodiazepine drugs are widely used as anxiolytics and anticonvulsants. They bind with high affinity to sites at the GABA$_A$ receptor and potentiate the actions of GABA. Pharmacological studies of benzodiazepine-binding sites show that the GABA$_A$ receptor may contain variants of α and β subunits. Expression of recombinant subunits produces functional receptors. When variants of the α subunit are coexpressed with standard β subunits the receptors produced are differentially distributed in the CNS (Lüddens et al 1990).

Inverse benzodiazepine receptor agonists of the β-carboline type decrease GABA$_A$ receptor-induced Cl$^-$ flow through the central channel. Epileptogenic agents like picrotoxin and t-butyl bicyclophosphorothionate (TBPS) block the Cl$^-$ channel by binding at a site close to the channel (Fig. 7.10). The convulsant actions of penicillin G and pentylenetetrazole involve blocking GABA$_A$ receptor function by an unknown mechanism. Barbiturates prolong GABA$_A$ receptor channel burst duration but do not affect conductance and directly activate Cl$^-$ channels. The synthetic steroid alphaxalone has similar actions to barbiturates and points to the possibility that endogenous steroids may modulate GABA$_A$ receptor function. The regulation of GABA$_A$ receptor function by intracellular mechanisms is little understood. GABA$_A$ receptor sensitivity is substantially reduced after a rapid increase in intracellular Ca^{2+} concentration and this suggests that Ca^{2+} may alter GABA$_A$ receptor function in vivo (Inoue et al 1987). The cytoplasmic loops of the α and β subunits contain phosphorylation sites for cyclic adenosine monophosphate (cAMP)-dependent protein kinase, and their presence indicates interactions between the GABA$_A$ receptor and protein phosphorylation of a second messenger system.

GABA$_B$ receptors are pharmacologically differentiated from GABA$_A$ receptors. They are unaffected by bicuculline and are not stimulated by GABAergic drugs such as isoguvacine. GABA binds at both GABA$_A$ and GABA$_B$ receptors, but only GABA$_B$ receptors are selectively stimulated by (−)-baclofen (β-p-chlorophenyl) GABA. There is, however, a paucity of specific antagonists at GABA$_B$ receptors with which to explore its pharmacology.

The GABA$_B$ receptor is not associated with an integral Cl$^-$ channel. Instead, it is coupled to adjacent Ca^{2+} channels by G proteins and its structure shows it to be a member of the seven helices membrane-spanning 'superfamily' of receptors. Binding between GABA or its agonist baclofen at the GABA$_B$ receptor selectively opens K$^+$ channels and closes Ca^{2+} channels (Deisz & Lux 1985). PLA$_2$ is stimulated via the GABA$_B$ receptor and, possibly, a membrane-bound G protein. There are thus two likely routes along which the GABA$_B$ receptor can modify K$^+$ and Ca^{2+}: one involves G protein and the other involves PLA$_2$. PLA$_2$ produces arachidonic acid by action on phospholipids. In turn, arachidonic acid may activate PKC which inhibits Ca^{2+} entry but increases K$^+$ flow.

GABA$_A$ and GABA$_B$ receptors share inhibitory functions in the CNS. They represent distinct receptor populations whose physiological functions are as yet poorly understood. The GABA$_B$ receptor may be more important in the regulation of Ca^{2+} entry and serves a major role in the modulation of Ca^{2+}-dependent neurotransmitter release. GABA$_A$ receptors are more widely distributed than GABA$_B$ receptors and may have important roles in the control of receptor sensitivity (Bormann 1988).

Excitatory amino acid neurotransmitters

Excitatory amino acid neurotransmitters (EAAs) are the focus of considerable current research. There is extensive evidence that EAAs provide the CNS with many useful functions that are essential in learning and memory and the structural and functional organisational changes (plasticity) that occur in neural development and in the neurodegeneration of ageing. The most abundant EAAs are glutamate and aspartate and, together with cysteic acid and homocysteic acid, are the most frequently encountered excitatory neurotransmitters in the brain.

EAA effects are mediated through at least five different receptor systems. The first four are ligand-gated ion channels and the fifth is coupled to G proteins and stimulates the IP–Ca^{2+} intracellular signalling pathway. The properties of these receptors are shown in Table 7.7. (Sladeczek et al 1988) and are pharmacologically defined as: (1) N-methyl-D-aspartate (NMDA); (2) quisqualate (Q); (3) kainate (K); (4) L-2-aminophosphorobutyric acid (AP4); and (5) the metabotropic glutamate receptor (mGluR). Non-NMDA receptors (Q or K) are widely distributed.

Table 7.7   Excitatory amino acid receptor subtypes

Receptor type	Agonists (most selective)	Competitive antagonists	Non–competitive antagonists	Allosteric agonist	Ions involved in ionotropic functions	Second messengers
NMDA	NMDA IBO	APV APH CPP	Ketamine MK–801, PCP SKF 10047 Mg^{2+}	Glycine	Ca^{2+} K$^+$ Na$^+$	Ca^{2+} (★★★) 1,4,5–IP$_3$/DAG (★★) cGMP? (★★)
K	K Domoate	γDGG, GDEE, GAMS, FG9065	JSTX		Na$^+$, K$^+$	Ca^{2+} (★) 1,4,5–IP$_3$/DAG (★)
Q	Q AMPA	γDGG, GDEE, GAMS, FG9065	JSTX		Na$^+$, K$^+$	1,4,5–IP$_3$/DAG (?) Ca2+ (?)
Qp IBOp	Q IBO	No antagonist APB, phosphoserine				1,4,5–IP$_3$/DAG (★★★) 1,4,5–IP$_3$/DAG (★★★)

After Sladeczek et al (1988).
APH, D-2-amino-4-phosphonobutyrate; PCP, phencyclidine; AMPA, α-amino-3-hydroxy-5-methylisoxazole-4-propionic acid; cGMP, cyclic guanosine monophosphate.
(★, ★★, ★★★), level of efficiency in producing second messengers.

They are highly concentrated in the cerebellum, and elsewhere in the brain their density is markedly different from NMDA receptors (Henley & Barnard 1990).

NMDA receptors are coupled through intracellular pathways to GlyR and also to a binding site for phencyclidine (PCP). Interactions between these receptor sites and the ion channels they regulate may prove as complex as the GABA–benzodiazepine ion channel. Although initially introduced as an anaesthetic, PCP is a potent psychotomimetic ('angel dust') and its drug-induced psychosis has been advanced as a useful model of schizophrenia. A similar psychosis can be induced by benzomorphan drugs, which are synthetic opiates (such as cyclazocine) that activate σ opiate receptors. PCP and σ opiate receptor activation antagonises the excitatory effects of NMDA activation but does not affect Q or K receptors (Sonders et al 1988).

Glutamate and its analogues are potent neurotoxins (Olney 1989). Exogenous NMDA agonist compounds are established neurotoxins. The legume *Lathyrus satirus* contains β-N-oxalylamino-L-alanine (BOAA) which, if ingested chronically, causes neuronal degeneration by excessive excitatory neuronal stimulation. This model of excitatory neurotoxicity by exogenous compounds (as in lathyrism) or endogenous compounds (as proposed for Huntington's disease (Beal 1986)) has been extended to include other neurodegenerative disorders, including Alzheimer's disease, head trauma, brain ischaemia and epilepsy (Olney 1989). Anti-excitotoxic agents are currently in development and some may soon enter clinical trials of their value in selected neuropsychiatric disorders (Honoré et al 1988).

Kainate receptors also mediate excitatory neurotransmission and are present on both neuronal and glial membranes, especially in the cerebellum. Their pharmacological and structural characteristics are those of the 'superfamily' of ligand-gated ion channels (Gregor et al 1989).

CHOLINERGIC NEUROTRANSMISSION

Acetylcholine is a widely distributed neurotransmitter present in the brain in the neostriatal interneurones and septal–hippocampal pathway. The effects of acetylcholine can be mimicked by muscarine and antagonised by atropine. These are termed 'muscarinic effects'. Other effects of acetylcholine are mimicked by nicotine, not antagonised by atropine but selectively blocked by tubocurarine. These are

Table 7.8   Cholinergic pharmacology

Presynaptic

Site of action	Effect	Drug	Use
Synthesis	Increases	Choline	Experimental
	Decreases	Hemicholinium	Experimental
Storage	—	—	—
Release	Increases	Black widow spider venom	Experimental

Postsynaptic

Receptor	Tissue	Agonist responses	Agonist	Antagonist	Molecular mechanisms
M_1	Cerebral cortex	?	Oxotremorine	Atropine	$\uparrow$PLC
	Sympathetic ganglia	Depolarization		Pirenzepine	$\uparrow$Ca^{2+}
M_2	Heart	Slowed depolarization		Atropine	$\uparrow$K$^+$ channels
	Sinoatrial node	Hyperpolarization			$\downarrow$Adenylate cyclase
	Atrium	Shortened action potential			
	Atrioventricular node	Decreased contractile force			
	Ventricle	Decreased conduction velocity			
M_3	Smooth muscle				$\uparrow$PLC
	Secretory glands				$\uparrow$Ca^{2+}

Degradation

Cholinesterase inhibitors (e.g. physostigmine)

'nicotinic effects'. The two types of cholinergic effect are mediated through two classes of cholinergic receptor: muscarinic and nicotinic. Cholinergic neuropharmacology is summarised in Table 7.8.

Nicotinic receptors are ligand-gated ion channels and, when activated by ligand binding, produce a rapid increase in cellular permeability to Na^+ and K^+. Muscarinic receptors are G protein coupled and are not necessarily linked to ion channels. The structures of nicotinic and muscarinic receptors show that they belong to two distinct 'superfamilies' of receptor types. The channel of the nicotinic cholinergic receptor is composed of five homologous subunits (Guy & Hucho 1987). The neuromuscular nicotinic receptor contains four distinct subunits (α, β, δ, γ) arranged as a pentamere (the γ subunit is replaced by an ϵ subunit in adult muscle). Nicotinic receptors in the CNS are also pentameres but comprise only two subunits (α and β). Brain nicotinic receptors are open to complex variation as there are multiple forms of both α and β subunits and it appears that different parts of the brain contain different combinations of α and β subtypes. The structure of the brain nicotinic receptor is shown in Figures 7.11 and 7.12. The four

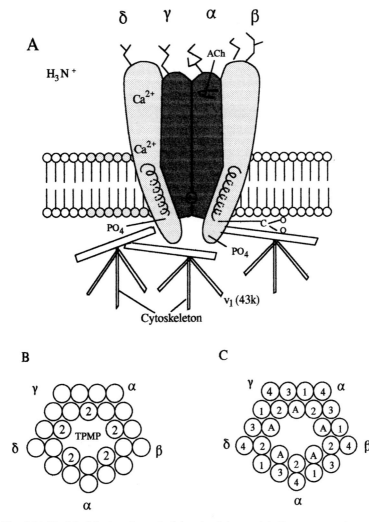

Fig. 7.11 Model of the ion channel of the nicotinic acetylcholine receptor. **A** Longitudinal section (ACh, acetylcholine) **B** Cross-section at the level of the site labelled by TPMP. **C** Alternative model in which TPMP can bind to segment M2 by fitting between MA segments. (After Guy & Hucho (1987).)

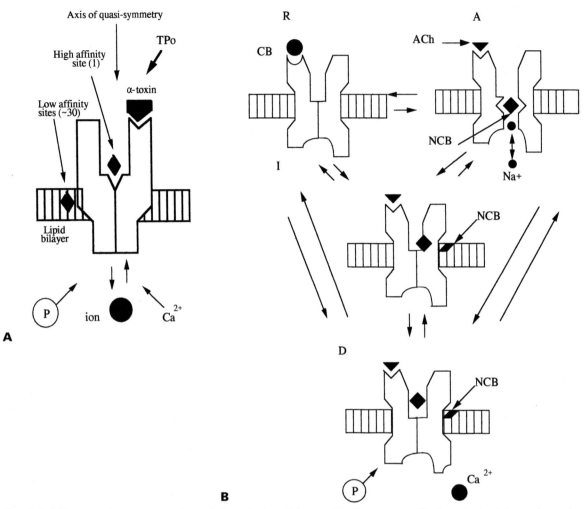

Fig. 7.12 A Transmembrane organisation and allosteric sites of the acetylcholine receptor. Cholinergic nicotinic agonists and antagonists compete with α-toxin at a site facing the synaptic cleft. Thymopoietin (TP$_o$) exerts its effect on the external face of the membrane while Ca^{2+} action and phosphorylation (P) take place on the internal face at the level of specific amino acids on the γ and δ subunits. The allosteric sites for the non-competitive blockers are subdivided into two main categories. In this model, the unique high-affinity site, sensitive to histrionicotoxin or phencyclidine, is tentatively located in the axis of quasi-symmetry of the molecule. The multiple low-affinity sites are distributed at the boundary of the protein with the lipid bilayer. (After Changeux & Revah (1987).) **B** Minimal four-state model for the allosteric transitions of the acetylcholine receptor. Binding of acetylcholine (ACh) to the receptor in its resting (R) state triggers the opening of the ion channel (active (A) state). Prolonged exposure of the receptor to acetylcholine provokes a two-step desensitisation process leading first to the I (intermediate desensitised) state followed by the D (desensitised) state. CB, competitive blocker; NCB, non-competitive blocker. (After Changeux & Revah (1987).)

genes encoding the α$_2$, α$_3$, α$_4$ and β$_2$ subunits of the nicotinic cholinergic receptor are differentially distributed in vertebrate brain (see Fig. 7.5b). All four mRNAs are present in the cerebellum, whereas only α$_2$ and β$_2$ mRNAs are found in lateral spiriform nuclei (Morris et al 1990). This indicates that neurones are capable of differential expression *in vivo* of nicotinic receptor subunits and points to nicotinic receptor heterogeneity in the CNS. The mRNAs for these subunits also show different temporal patterns of expression during brain development (Moss et al 1989).

Muscarinic cholinergic receptors also exist as various subtypes. Pharmacological studies had supported the subdivision of muscarinic receptors into M$_1$, M$_2$ and M$_3$. Structural studies have determined

Table 7.9   Properties of cloned muscarinic receptors

Property	m$_1$	m$_2$	m$_3$	m$_4$	m$_5$
Molecular weight	51387	51681	66085	53014	60120
Pirenzepine affinity	High	Low	◄———————intermediate———————►		
Phosphatidylinositol response	Stimulates	None	Stimulates	None	Stimulates
cAMP response	Stimulates	Inhibits	Stimulates	Inhibits	Stimulates
Arachidonic acid response	Stimulates	None	Stimulates	None	Stimulates
Ca^{2+}–dependent K$_A^+$ channel	Opens	No effect	Opens	No effect	?
mRNA distribution	Brain Glands	Brain Heart Smooth muscle	Brain Smooth muscle	Brain	?

After Bonner (1989).

three corresponding receptor subtypes termed m$_1$, m$_2$ and m$_3$. Two further molecules termed m$_4$ and m$_5$ have been detected, but little is known of their functions and distribution. Like all other G protein-coupled receptors, there are seven transmembrane domains, and the characteristics of muscarinic receptors are show in Table 7.9 (Bonner 1989).

Muscarinic receptors M$_1$ and M$_3$ activate a G protein that stimulates PLC activity. PLC stimulates hydrolysis of phosphatidylinositol phosphates to IP$_3$, which can release intracellular Ca^{2+}. DAG is also produced by PLC and this leads to PKC activation. Ligand binding to M$_2$ and M$_4$ receptors activates G$_i$ proteins which inhibit adenylate cyclase, and open K$^+$ and close Ca^{2+} channels.

Drugs affecting acetylcholine synthesis

Acetylcholine is synthesised in a single step from acetyl coenzyme A (produced in neuronal mitochondria) and choline (from the liver), which is catalysed by choline acetyltransferase. Synthesis of acetylcholine can be increased by choline administration because the synthetic enzyme is not fully saturated.

Drugs affecting acetylcholine release

Newly synthesised acetylcholine is preferentially released on stimulation from storage in presynaptic cholinergic terminals. Black widow spider venom produces a rapid release of acetylcholine and also causes morphological changes in the presynaptic storage vesicles.

Drugs affecting nicotinic receptors

Nicotinic receptors are excitatory and function by opening ionic channels. They are specifically blocked by α-bungarotoxin. Nicotinic receptors are present in the brain, particularly in the thalamus and cerebellar cortex. Outside the brain, the cholinergic input from the spinal cord synapses on to nicotinic receptors at the neurotransmitter junction. Most nicotinic receptor antagonists have profound effects at the neuromuscular junction. The best known agent is (+)-tubocurarine, which does not easily cross the blood–brain barrier, and that which does has little central effect because there are so few nicotinic receptors in the brain. Decamethonium and succinylcholine are also nicotinic receptor antagonists but, instead of competing with acetylcholine for the receptor site, they depolarise the receptor for a long period, making it insensitive to acetylcholine. Like (+)-tubocurarine, decamethonium and succinylcholine have almost no central effects. Agonists at nicotinic receptors include nicotine, dimethyl-phenylpiperazinium (DMPP) and phenyl-trimethylammonium (PTMA).

Nicotine is present in tobacco (*Nicotinia tabacum*) and most smokers identify 'stress reduction' as a major determinant of their habit, saying that smoking helps them to relax. Small, repeated injections of nicotine, similar to those received while smoking, produce increased cortical release of acetylcholine and electrocortical arousal. Adrenergic blockade has no effect on this action of nicotine but both muscarinic and nicotinic blockade prevent nicotine from activating the cortex. Lesion studies suggest that tobacco smoking increases electrocortical arousal by acting at sites in the cholinergic projections on to the cortex. Low doses of nicotine produce stimulation in the periphery while higher doses block nicotinic receptors and cause paralysis of neuromuscular junctions.

Drugs affecting muscarinic receptors

M_1 receptors are concentrated in the sympathetic ganglia, stomach and corpus striatum. They are selectively antagonised by pirenzipine and are closely associated with K^+ channels (ionophores). M_2 receptors are concentrated in the hind brain, cerebellum and heart. They are regulated by gallamine and GTP and inhibit adenylate cyclase. Muscarinic receptor antagonists, therefore, have both central and peripheral actions. Atropine and scopolamine are the best known and, in the periphery, they decrease secretion from the gut, nasopharynx and respiratory tract and increase the heart rate. Their central effects include confusion, lassitude and drowsiness, and higher doses can cause delirium ('atropine psychosis'). Agonists at muscarinic receptors include muscarine, pilocarpine, arecoline, methacholine and carbachol.

The tricyclic antidepressants commonly cause anticholinergic side-effects. These include dry mouth, excessive sweating, blurring of vision and urinary retention, which may be especially troublesome in the elderly. It is important, therefore, to know the relative potencies at muscarinic receptors of antidepressant drugs to guide prescribing, for example, in patients with glaucoma or prostatism. Amitriptyline has about 5% of the anticholinergic potency of atropine, but, as it is used in much greater doses (100–150 mg daily) than the well-known anticholinergics (0.6 mg), it can produce an extensive blockade of cholinergic receptors.

Parkinsonism

Until the introduction of L-dopa and decarboxylase inhibitors, anticholinergic drugs formed the mainstay of treatment for parkinsonism. These drugs remain useful for patients in the early stages of Parkinson's disease, patients unable to tolerate L-dopa and in addition to L-dopa in selected patients. They can be especially useful in drug-induced parkinsonism.

The anticholinergic drugs used to treat drug-induced parkinsonism are tertiary amines (benztropine, trihexyphenidyl and procyclidine). Their extra-CNS antimuscarinic effects are much weaker than atropine. Diphenhydramine is an antihistamine drug that has slight anticholinergic properties and is especially well tolerated by old people.

Anticholinesterases

Anticholinesterase drugs cause acetylcholine to accumulate at cholinergic synapses. These drugs inhibit the enzyme acetylcholinesterase, and the prototype drug is physostigmine. Others were developed as insecticides and investigated for use in chemical warfare. These latter types cause irreversible inhibition of acetylcholinesterase. The mechanism of action of anticholinesterases (including physostigmine) is based on their binding with the enzyme and, in the case of physostigmine and neostigmine, hydrolysing slowly. The terms 'reversible' and 'irreversible' as applied to anticholinesterases are only relative and refer to the speed at which the enzyme recovers function. In psychiatry, the main use of physostigmine is experimental in Alzheimer's disease where it may transiently produce a modest improvement in mental functions. Rarely, intravenous physostigmine may be used to reverse a brief psychosis induced by antimuscarinic drugs. Physostigmine does not reverse the anticholinergic cardiotoxic effects of tricyclic antidepressants.

NORADRENERGIC NEUROTRANSMISSION

An understanding of the classification and properties of the different types of adrenoceptor is essential to understanding the diverse effects of catecholamines and the neuropharmacology of this system. Physiological studies by Ahlquist (1948) supported the distinction between two types of adrenoceptor, termed α and β. This initial distinction was supported by observations on adrenergic antagonists at α adrenoceptors (e.g. phenoxybenzamine) and β adrenoceptors (e.g. propranolol). Subsequently, β receptors were subdivided into β_1 and β_2, and later structural studies identified a third type, termed β_3. The relative number of each of these subtypes varies with tissue type. α adrenoceptors are present in the iris where they stimulate contraction of the radial muscle, thus producing dilation. They are also present in the eyelid where their stimulation raises the lid. The heart contains β_1 receptors which mediate increases in both the rate and force of cardiac contractions. All β receptors are coupled through G proteins to the enzyme adenylate cyclase.

Table 7.10 summarises the sites of action, effects and uses of drugs that act on noradrenergic neurotransmission. Some drugs act specifically at noradrenergic synapses while others affect several monoamines. Tricyclic antidepressants are believed to have mood-elevating actions because of their inhibition of uptake of monoamines, particularly noradrenaline and

Table 7.10 Noradrenergic pharmacology

Presynaptic

Site of action	Effect	Drug	Use
Synthesis	False transmitter Decreased	α-Methyldopa α-Methyl-p-tyrosine	Hypotensive Experimental
Storage	Decreased (irreversible) Decreased(reversible) Increased	Reserpine Tetrabenazine Monoamine oxidase inhibitors (MAOIs)	Hypotensive Chorea Antidepressant
Release	Increased Increased Decreased	Amphetamine Tyramine Debrisoguine	Euphoriant Experimental Hypotensive
Re–uptake	Inhibits Inhibits Inhibits	Desipramine Amitriptyline Cocaine	Antidepressant Antidepressant Euphoriant

Postsynaptic

Receptor	Tissue	Agonist responses	Agonist	Antagonist	Molecular mechanisms
α_1	Vascular smooth muscle	Contracts	Isoprotenerol Phenylephrine	Prazosin	↑PLC ↑IP$_3$ ↑K$^+$channels ↑Intracellular Ca^{2+}
	Heart	Increased contractile force			
α_2	Neural	↓Noradrenaline release	Clonidine	Yohimbine	↓Adenylate cyclase ↑K$^+$ channels ↓Ca^{2+} channels
	Vascular smooth muscle	Contracts			
β_1	Heart	Increased contractile force			↑Adenylate cyclase ↑Ca^{2+} channels
β_2	Smooth muscle	Relaxation			↑Adenylate cyclase

Degradation

Monoamine oxidase (A and B) inhibition

serotonin, from the synaptic cleft. These actions of antidepressants have led to the 'monoamine hypothesis of affective disorders', which, simply stated, postulates that in depressive illness there is reduced efficiency of neurotransmission at noradrenergic and/or serotonergic synapses and that this may involve abnormalities in the affinity of monoaminergic receptors for their endogenous ligands (see Ch. 19).

Drugs inhibiting noradrenaline synthesis

Noradrenaline is synthesised from L-tyrosine by the following steps: L-tyrosine is hydroxylated to L-dopa (by tyrosine hydroxylase), L-dopa is decarboxylated to dopamine (by aromatic-L-amino-acid decarboxylase) and dopamine is then hydroxylated to noradrenaline (by dopamine β-hydroxylase). Tyrosine hydroxylase is

inhibited by α-methyl-p-tyrosine, and this drug is used experimentally to prevent the synthesis of dopamine, noradrenaline and adrenaline. Carbidopa inhibits aromatic-L-amino-acid decarboxylase at sites outside the CNS and can be given at the same time as L-dopa, when it will prevent enhancement of dopamine synthesis outside the CNS. Dopamine β-hydroxylase is inhibited by disulfiram and by FLA63. Synthesis of noradrenaline can also be disrupted by the structurally similar precursor α-methyldopa. This is synthesised to α-methylnoradrenaline, which then acts as a 'false neurotransmitter'.

Drugs affecting the storage of noradrenaline

Most noradrenaline is stored in a presynaptic complex of noradrenaline, adenosine triphosphate (ATP), metallic ions of magnesium, calcium, copper and proteins called chromogranins. Dopamine β–hydroxylase is present in noradrenergic storage vesicles, probably in association with the vesicular limiting membrane. Noradrenaline is taken up into storage by an active transport mechanism that is magnesium-dependent and requires ATP, although a little noradrenaline is available in the cytoplasm. The *Rauwolfia* alkaloids (e.g. reserpine) and tetrabenazine disrupt noradrenaline storage and inhibit noradrenaline uptake into storage vesicles; reserpine causes irreversible damage to granules whereas tetrabenazine has reversible effects. These processes can be relatively slow so that noradrenaline released from storage may be degraded by intracellular monoamine oxidase before it can bind with postsynaptic receptors. Reserpine can initially produce postsynaptic adrenoceptor stimulation by releasing noradrenaline.

Drugs affecting the release of noradrenaline

Noradrenaline is released from storage vesicles by a calcium-dependent process involving fusion of the vesicles with the presynaptic membrane and also involving prostaglandins (PGE_2 inhibiting and $PGE_{2\alpha}$ facilitating release). Release may be regulated by prostaglandins and other local hormones acting on noradrenergic nerve terminals. Presynaptic receptors (autoreceptors) are important in the regulation of impulse-induced noradrenaline release and such receptors may be sensitive not only to the local concentration of noradrenaline but also to acetylcholine, cAMP, prostaglandins and neuropeptides like thyrotrophin-releasing hormone.

Drugs that release noradrenaline quickly enough to bind with postsynaptic receptors are called 'indirectly acting sympathomimetic amines'. Examples are amphetamine, tyramine and ephedrine. Some drugs inhibit noradrenaline release from storage, for example, antihypertensive agents such as debrisoquine, bethanidine and guanethidine. These drugs do not readily cross the blood–brain barrier (their lipid solubility is low) and therefore have few psychotoxic effects.

Drugs acting on adrenergic receptors

There are two main types of receptor for noradrenaline, α and β adrenoceptors. The existence of these two types was deduced from studies on smooth muscle where catecholamines produce both excitatory and inhibitory effects. Later studies of drug-binding to adrenoceptors supported the original division into α and β receptor types. Phenoxybenzamine produces

selective blockade of α receptors and propranolol blocks β receptors. The development of more selective antagonist and agonists allowed these receptors to be further subdivided into β_1, β_2, α_1 and α_2 receptors. The relative number of the various subtypes of adrenoceptor varies with each tissue. Stimulation of α adrenoceptors in blood vessels causes vasoconstriction. Additionally, the pilomotor muscles and salivary glands are stimulated through their α adrenoceptors. The gastrointestinal tract has both α and β adrenoceptors and the smooth muscle in the tract relaxes in response to stimulation of either receptor type. Sphincter muscles, however, contract in response to excitation of α adrenoceptors.

The heart contains β_1 receptors which mediate increases in both rate and force of cardiac contraction. Stimulation of β_2 receptors in bronchial smooth muscle produces bronchodilation. They are also present in the gastrointestinal tract, uterus and bladder, where their stimulation produces smooth muscle relaxation. β receptors are also involved in the regulation of certain metabolic processes such as increasing lipolysis or gluconeogenesis and reducing insulin release. All β receptors are linked to the enzyme adenylate cyclase, so that stimulation of β receptors increases the synthesis of cAMP from ATP. Phosphodiesterases degrade cAMP to non-cyclic 5'-AMP. Drugs that inhibit phosphodiesterases (such as caffeine, aminophylline and theobromine) enhance the physiological responses to β adrenoceptor stimulation. α adrenoceptor agonists include noradrenaline and adrenaline. Noradrenaline acts mostly through α adrenoceptors and adrenaline largely through β adrenoceptors. Phenylephrine and clonidine are directly acting α adrenoceptor agonists with few β adrenoceptor effects, and their actions are therefore similar to noradrenaline. Isoprenaline is a synthetic catecholamine acting only on β receptors, where it is more potent than either adrenaline or noradrenaline. Salbutamol is a selective β_2 adrenoceptor agonist and has been used as an antidepressant. The rationale leading to this application is derived from the 'amine hypothesis of depression', where a postulated reduction in the functional efficiency of neurotransmission at synapses involving monoamines concerned with the regulation of mood is accompanied by increased postsynaptic sensitivity to those monoamines. Administration of a selective monoaminergic receptor antagonist such as salbutamol might, therefore, allow re-establishment of more efficient neurotransmission. α adrenoceptor antagonists are used mostly in experimental work, though phentolamine (a reversible α adrenoceptor antagonist) is useful in the emergency treatment of hypertension and the diagnosis of phaeochromocytomas. Some β adrenoceptor antagonists may have local anaesthetic-like activity on membrane fluidity as well as actions at adrenoceptors. These drugs are used mostly in the control of hypertension and the relief of angina. Their exact mode of action in the control of hypertension is unknown. Non-selective β adrenoceptor antagonists include propranolol and atenolol. Atenolol and metoprolol are selective β_1 adrenoceptor antagonists that in large doses affect all β receptors. These drugs act at both pre- and post-synaptic adrenoceptors. Presynaptic β_1 receptors facilitate noradrenaline release while presynaptic β_2 receptors are inhibitory. These receptors may be involved in the pathogenesis of affective symptoms and effective antidepressants could exert some or all of their effects at these sites.

Antidepressants and adrenergic receptors

There is a close relationship between the potencies of tricyclic antidepressants to occupy postsynaptic α_1 adrenoceptors and their sedative–hypotensive effects. The tertiary amines (e.g. amitriptyline) are more potent at these sites than secondary amines (e.g. nortriptyline) and are only slightly less potent than the better known α adrenoceptor antagonist phentolamine. Chronic administration of antidepressants, but not short-term treatment, reduces noradrenaline-coupled adenylate cyclase activity and also reduces the number of β receptors in brain tissue. These effects do not seem to be limited to one type of antidepressant treatment but are found with tricyclic drugs, mianserin, iprindole, monoamine oxidase inhibitors and also in an animal model of electroconvulsive therapy (ECT). Some antidepressants may act, therefore, by initially increasing the synaptic concentration of noradrenaline which in turn reduces the sensitivity and/or number of β adrenoceptors. The initial increase of noradrenaline may be caused by inhibition of noradrenaline uptake, blockade of presynaptic inhibitory autoreceptors, or actions at other sites.

Drugs affecting noradrenaline uptake

Antidepressants and euphoriants such as cocaine and amphetamine act rapidly on the presynaptic re-uptake of noradrenaline. The structure of the noradrenaline transporter is known and has much in common with the GABA transporter, so both may be members of a 'superfamily' of neurotransmitter transporters. The structure is shown schematically in Figure 7.13. Distribution of the transporter matches the localisation of noradrenaline cell bodies in the CNS (Pacholczyk et al, 1991). The transporter may be important in

neurodegenerative diseases. Potent neurotoxins (such as 1-methyl-4-phenylpyridinium (MPP^+) and 6-hydroxy-dopamine (6-OH-DA)) can be actively taken up by the noradrenaline transporter and, if allowed to accumulate in neurones, cause selective neuronal death. The transporter is an important site of action of mood-affecting drugs and its further study (e.g. binding to novel, potentially antidepressant compounds) may facilitate new drug development. It may also prove relevant to understanding the genetic contribution to affective disorders.

Uptake of noradrenaline from the synaptic cleft is an energy-consuming process that is sodium-dependent and involves ATP. Some drugs inhibit the uptake of monoamines from the synaptic cleft and this is thought to be the principal action of tricyclic antidepressants. These drugs affect both noradrenaline and serotonin uptake but have little effect on dopamine. The tertiary amines imipramine and amitriptyline mostly affect the uptake of serotonin. Secondary amines like desipramine and nortriptyline largely affect noradrenaline. Many tertiary amines are metabolised to secondary amines, so in reality, the tertiary amines often affect both noradrenaline and serotonin uptake. A number of drugs have been developed to act selectively on serotonin or noradrenaline uptake but there are no clear differences in antidepressant activity between the two. Inhibition of uptake is evident from pharmacological studies within 24 hours of administrative of the drug, but clinical effects are not typically seen for about 10–20 days. Because the tricyclic drugs and their related compounds were derived from the phenothiazines, they share several pharmacological properties with them. In particular, they have anticholinergic and antihistaminergic effects. The anticholinergic effects are evident within hours of first administering the drug and tolerance usually develops before the onset of the antidepressant effect. For these reasons, the anticholinergic effects of the tricyclics are probably not relevant to their antidepressant action. Further, the incidence of anticholinergic side-effects does not differ between patients who respond and those who do not respond to a tricyclic. The antihistaminergic effects of tricyclic drugs may prove relevant to their antidepressant actions. The commonly prescribed tricyclic drugs are amitriptyline, clomipramine, desipramine, dothiepin, doxepin, imipramine, iprindole, nortriptyline, protriptyline and trimipramine.

Drugs affecting degradation of noradrenaline

Noradrenaline that is not taken up by the presynaptic terminal from the synaptic cleft can be fused into the

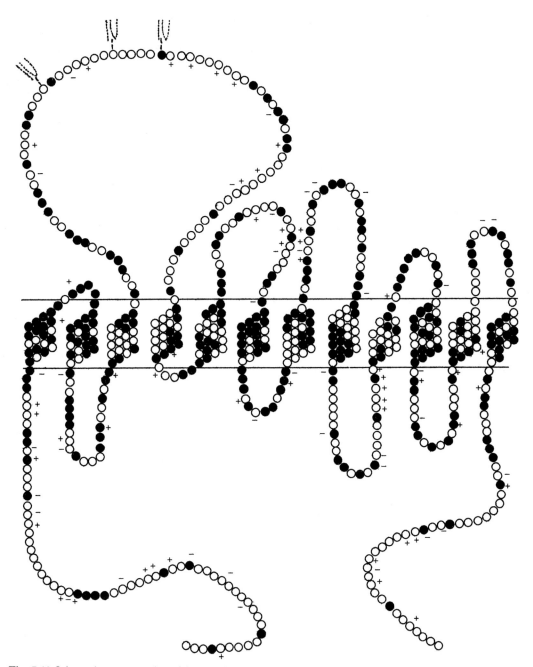

Fig. 7.13 Schematic representation of the noradrenaline transporter showing proposed orientation in the plasma membrane. Solid circles represent residues conserved with the GABA transporter. Glycosylation sites and charged residues are also indicated. (After Pacholczyk et al (1991) and Snyder (1991).)

postsynaptic membrane, where it is degraded by the enzymes monoamine oxidase and catechol-O-methyl-transferase (COMT). Monoamine oxidases are a group of enzymes that are present in a wide variety of tissues in which their substrate specificity and physical properties may differ. There are two types, known as A and B. Type A is more effective in the degradation of noradrenaline and serotonin whereas type B is more effective with dopamine. Tyramine (a naturally occurring amino acid present in many foods) is a substrate for both forms and the use of a monoamine oxidase inhibitor is associated with the hazard of toxic reactions to excessive amounts of tyramine. The antidepressant actions of monoamine oxidase inhibitors such as tranylcypromine, pargyline, phenelzine and clorgyline (a selective type A inhibitor) are produced largely by their inhibition of monoamine oxidase. They also affect aromatic-L-amino-acid decarboxylase and various other oxidases and in'.ibit uptake of noradrenaline and serotonin, but the clinical relevance of these effects is not known. The metabolism of concomitantly administered drugs may also be affected by monoamine oxidase inhibitors so that the action of barbiturates may be prolonged and the effect of amphetamine exaggerated.

Monoamine oxidase inhibitors also reduce the 'first-pass' presystemic degradation of tyramine after its intestinal absorption. Tyramine is selectively taken up into adrenergic neurones (by a high-affinity system), where it releases stored noradrenaline. Monoamine oxidase inhibitors thus potentiate the effects of tyramine and other indirectly acting sympathomimetic agents. New monoamine oxidase inhibitors have been developed that are selective for monoamine oxidase A and there are claims that these do not potentiate the tyramine response and are also effective antidepressants. Moclobemide is a novel reversible inhibitor of monoamine oxidase A. Since it spares the monoamine oxidase A present in the gut as a defence against ingested amines, it is potentially a useful antidepressant (Callingham & Ovens, 1988).

Table 7.11   Dopaminergic pharmacology
Presynaptic

Site of action	Effect	Drug	Use
Synthesis	Inhibits Increases	α-Methyltyrosine L-Dopa	Occasionally in phaeochromocytoma Parkinson's disease
Storage	Inhibits	Tetrabenazine α-Methyltyrosine Reserpine	Chorea As above Experimental Occasionally in treatment of refractory psychoses
Release	Increases Inhibits	Amphetamine γ-Hydroxybutyrate	Experimental Experimental
Uptake	Inhibits	Benztropine Nomifensine Cocaine Amitriptyline	Parkinson's disease Experimental Experimental Antidepressant

Postsynaptic

Receptor	Tissue	Agonist responses	Agonist	Antagonist	Molecular mechanisms
	Renal Mesenteric/coronary vessels Pituitary–hypothalamic axis	Vasodilation			↑cAMP
D_1	Cell bodies and presynaptic terminals of intrinsic striatal neurones		Pergolide SKF 38393	Lisuride SCH 23390	↑Adenylate cyclase
D_2	Neuronal cell bodies of striatum and presynaptic terminals of dopaminergic striatal neurones		Bromocriptine Pergolide Lisuride Apomorphine	Butyrophenones Sulpiride	↓Adenylate cyclase or no effect

Degradation

Monoamine oxidase (A and B) inhibition

DOPAMINERGIC NEUROTRANSMISSION

The modern era of pharmacotherapy in psychiatry began with the introduction of phenothiazine antipsychotics in 1952 and was quickly followed by the development of phenothiazine-derived tricyclic antidepressants. At first, the mode of action of these drugs was unknown, but during the past 25 years the effects of antipsychotic drugs on central dopaminergic transmission have been established as an important component of their antipsychotic actions. The neuropharmacology of dopaminergic neurotransmission is summarised in Table 7.11.

Dopamine synthesis

Dopamine is synthesised from the amino acid L-tyrosine by the following steps: L-tyrosine is hydroxylated to L-dopa (by tyrosine hydroxylase) and then decarboxylated (by aromatic-L-amino-acid decarboxylase) to form dopamine. Oral administration of L-dopa increases dopamine synthesis. In Parkinson's disease, dopaminergic neurones are damaged and have a much reduced capacity to synthesise dopamine. Adjacent glial cells retain dopamine synthetic capacity and, during L-dopa therapy, dopamine leaks out from these glial cells to stimulate surviving dopamine receptors.

Dopamine storage

Dopamine is stored in presynaptic complexes of dopamine, ATP, magnesium, calcium, copper and chromogranins. Drugs that disrupt the storage of noradrenaline, like *Rauwolfia* alkaloids and tetrabenazine, also disrupt dopamine storage complexes.

Dopamine release

Dopamine is released from central dopaminergic terminals by two discrete mechanisms that differ in their sensitivity to dopamine uptake inhibitors (Raiteri et al 1979). An energy-dependent transport mechanism for dopamine uptake is inhibited by nomifensine, benztropine and cocaine. A second carrierindependent mechanism for dopamine release is dependent upon extracellular Ca^{2+} concentrations and involves fusion of dopamine-containing vesicles with the presynaptic membrane. This type of release is facilitated by amphetamine at concentrations much lower than those required for amphetamine to stimulate postsynaptic catecholaminergic receptors. Amphetamines stimulate rapid release of dopamine, inhibit its uptake

from the synaptic cleft and also inhibit its degradative enzyme monoamine oxidase.

The dopamine hypothesis of schizophrenia

When the neuroleptic drugs were first introduced, their mode of antipsychotic action was unknown. At first, studies in the peripheral nervous system suggested that the antiadrenergic effects of chlorpromazine probably explained its antipsychotic action, perhaps by reducing arousal. However, the fact that potent antiadrenergic agents had no antipsychotic benefit clearly did not support this hypothesis. Carlsson & Lindqvist (1963) first suggested that dopamine receptor blockade was the basis of neuroleptic effects. The low activity of butyrophenone antipsychotics at dopamine receptor sites linked to adenylate cyclase stimulation was seen as evidence against this idea. It was supported, however, by the recognition of two types of dopamine receptor. One (called D_1) was linked to adenylate cyclase stimulation and another (called D_2) to adenylate cyclase inhibition and for which there was preferential binding of butyrophenones.

Neuropharmacological studies provide virtually all the evidence to support the 'dopamine hypothesis of schizophrenia'. Although some of the newer 'atypical' antipsychotic agents are weak dopamine receptor antagonists, all effective antipsychotics are believed to share the ability to impair dopaminergic neurotransmission. Post mortem studies of schizophrenic brains have demonstrated increased dopamine receptor (D_2) densities, but these densities are probably considerably influenced by ante mortem drug treatments. Positron emission tomography studies on D_2 receptor binding in neuroleptic-naive schizophrenic patients have provided conflicting results. Wong et al (1986) reported a two- to three-fold increase in D_2 receptor densities of drug-free patients when compared to controls, but a later more extensive study by Farde et al (1990) did not support the earlier finding (see Ch 18).

The CNS location of the site of antipsychotic action of neuroleptic drugs is unknown. Dopamine receptors are present in the basal ganglia, the mesolimbic system, the tuberoinfundibular region and, to a much lesser extent, in the cerebral cortex. Studies on the effects of dopaminergic transmission of pyschotomimetic agents such as amphetamine, PCP and benzmorphan point to a possible common mechanism of psychotic action. Carlsson (1988) has proposed that 'information overload' and 'hyperarousal' are integral features of many psychotic illnesses. He postulates that these features arise because of impairment of the protective effects on cortical function of the mesolimbic system. In health, Carlsson argues that mesolimbic glutaminergic neurones oppose mesolimbic dopaminergic pathways and maintain this protective function. Hypothetically, drug-induced psychoses are caused by blocking glutaminergic function (e.g. by PCP or benzmorphan) or by increasing dopaminergic activity (e.g. amphetamine).

The 'dopamine hypothesis of schizophrenia', simply stated, postulates that certain dopaminergic pathways are overactive in schizophrenia and so cause the symptoms of an acute schizophrenic episode. Clinical studies indicate that drugs like L-dopa or amphetamine which potentiate dopaminergic activity may induce or exacerbate schizophrenic symptoms.

Dopamine receptors

Pharmacological studies show that there are at least two types of dopamine receptor: D_1 and D_2. There is very good agreement between the affinity of an antipsychotic drug for D_2 receptors and the average daily dose of that drug used to treat schizophrenia. The structures of D_1 and D_2 receptors are now established and when expressed in cell lines are seen to possess the pharmacological properties predicted in earlier studies. Characteristics of dopamine receptor subtypes are summarised in Table 7.12.

Blockade of D_2 receptors is the likely cause of unwanted extrapyramidal system (EPS) effects and, therefore, if blockade of the D_2 receptor is also the site of antipsychotic action, all effective neuroleptics should be equipotent in the induction of EPS symptoms and in antipsychotic efficacy. Some newer drugs used to treat schizophrenia (sometimes termed 'atypical') have a lower tendency to produce EPS

effects than older neuroleptics such as chlorpromazine. ('Atypical' antipsychotic drugs include thioridazine, sulpiride and clozapine.) Pharmacological studies have not detected differences between D_2 receptors located in the striatum (where EPS effects arise) and in the mesolimbic system (where the antipsychotic action is presumed to be located). In large part, this issue has been resolved by recent molecular biological studies.

Structural analysis of dopamine receptor types has revealed a family of at least five similar G protein-coupled molecules (Sunahara et al 1990). The mRNA for D_1 is most abundant in the caudate, nucleus accumbens and olfactory tubercle with little in the substantia nigra (Dearry et al 1990). Structurally, D_1 receptors are most like the β adrenoceptor (Zhou et al 1990) and are functionally coupled to adenylate cyclase (Monsma et al 1990). Subsequently, similarities between the known structures of G protein-coupled receptors helped to isolate and characterise the D_2 receptor (Bunzow et al 1988). Structural studies also identified two D_2 receptor isoforms; one predicted by pharmacological studies but the other appearing to be novel (Giros et al 1989) and probably an alternative product of a single D_2 gene (Monsma et al 1989). The D_2 receptor isoforms are termed $D_{2(414)}$ and $D2_{(443)}$. Discovery of D_2 isoforms suggests a means by which different dopaminergic neuronal populations might adjust responses to stimuli (such as chronic exposure to neuroleptics) or be a source of genetically determined receptor variability of possible relevance to the aetiology of schizophrenia. However, no abnormalities of D_2 isoform structure in schizophrenia have been described, though linkage between the D_2 receptor gene (located in the q22–q23 region of human chromosome 11) has been reported in alcoholism (Blum et al 1990).

Table 7.12 Dopamine receptor subtypes (after Snyder 1990)

	D_1	$D2_{(short)}$	$D_{2 (long)}$	D_3
Amino acids	446	415	444	446
Highest brain densities	Neostriatum (caudate)	Neostriatum (caudate)	Neostriatum (caudate)	Olfactory tubercle
Adenylate cyclase	Stimulates	Inhibits	Inhibits	No effect
Affinity for dopamine	Micromolar	Nanomolar	Nanomolar	Nanomolar
Butyrophenone potency	Micromolar	Subnanomolar	Subnanomolar	Nanomolar
Phenothiazine potency	Nanomolar	Nanomolar	Nanomolar	Nanomolar

Further subtypes of dopamine receptor have been revealed by structural analysis. The D_3 receptor is located in the limbic system. It is present on both postsynaptic and presynaptic membranes and probably mediates the therapeutic effects of neuroleptic drugs (Sokoloff et al 1990). The neuropharmacology, CNS localisation and, possibly, connections with intracellular signalling systems of the D_3 receptor subtype all differ from D_1 and D_2. For example, butyrophenones are 10–20 times more potent at D_2 than at D_3 receptors but sulpiride, thioridazine and clozapine are only 2–3 times more potent at D_2 than D_3. These observations probably account for differences between antipsychotic drugs in their ability to induce EPS effects. The D_3 receptor forms the basis of current attempts to design new antipsychotic drugs with fewer EPS effects and to develop new drugs for Parkinson's disease (Snyder 1990).

The novel antipsychotic clozapine does not cause 'tardive dyskinesia'. Recently, a further subtype of dopamine receptor termed D_4 has been described and found to bind preferentially to clozapine (Van Tol et al 1991). It is structurally related to other members of the G protein-coupled receptor 'superfamily' and, as for D_3, understanding of its structure and functions may facilitate development of novel antipsychotic drugs. Sunahara et al (1991) have also described a further subtype of dopamine receptor (termed D_5) that is primarily located in the limbic system and may be involved in D_2 regulation.

Administration of dopamine receptor-blocking drugs can produce supersensitivity of dopamine receptors. The mechanism(s) underlying supersensitivity following chronic administration of neuroleptics are largely unknown. In some patients (postmenopausal women seem most susceptible) continuous administration of neuroleptics can cause a syndrome of involuntary movements to emerge. This 'tardive dyskinesia' characteristically affects buccolinguomasticatory musculature but may also involve choreic movements of limbs and dystonic contractions of the trunk. The syndrome is of major clinical importance (see Ch 36) and usually starts during therapy, but may worsen on cessation. Occasionally, the symptoms are relieved by reintroduction of neuroleptics, but no generally satisfactory drug treatment is available for this condition.

Dopamine uptake

Amphetamine and other drugs which release dopamine also inhibit its uptake and so potentiate the action of dopamine. Nomifensine and cocaine are also well-established dopamine uptake inhibitors. Benztropine and to a lesser extent benzhexol and orphenadrine inhibit the uptake of dopamine and also block cholinergic receptors, actions that contribute to the effects of these anticholinergic drugs in the treatment of parkinsonism.

Drugs affecting degradation of dopamine

Monamine oxidase inhibitors like tranylcypromine reduce the degradation of dopamine by monoamine oxidase. Tranylcypromine also reduces uptake of dopamine, but this is probably not relevant to its antidepressant action because drugs such as benztropine (a potent dopamine uptake inhibitor) are not effective antidepressants.

Parkinsonism

There is a substantial reduction of dopaminergic innervation of the basal ganglia in Parkinson's disease. The loss of dopamine leads to parkinsonian signs and symptoms and restoration of dopaminergic neurotransmission is the aim of all effective treatments. The neural connections of the basal ganglia are shown in Figure 7.14. The pathways that connect the caudate nucleus–putamen in the substantia nigra are of most importance in parkinsonism. Dopamine-containing cell bodies in the pars compacta of the substantia nigra degenerate in Parkinson's disease. The afferents of these cell bodies synapse on all types of cell in the caudate–putamen. The effect of dopaminergic inputs to the caudate–putamen is the modification of its output to other structures. Reserpine and phenothiazines can produce parkinsonism; the first by depletion of dopamine storage granules and the second by blocking dopamine receptors. In health, inhibitory dopaminergic and excitatory cholinergic activity in the caudate–putamen is balanced and because cholinergic cells are spared in Parkinson's disease, there is a relative excess of cholinergic activity. Blockade of cholinergic activity is thus a successful treatment of parkinsonism. Anticholinergic drugs are commonly used in psychiatry to relieve drug-induced parkinsonism. Currently they are regarded as less effective than L-dopa in idiopathic Parkinson's disease but can often be usefully combined with L-dopa in patients who have not fully responded. These drugs are muscarinic antagonists. Restoration of dopaminergic transmission by oral supplementation of L-dopa, a dopamine precursor, is also effective. Dopaminergic agonists that are useful in parkinsonism are mostly ergot derivatives: bromocriptine (often as

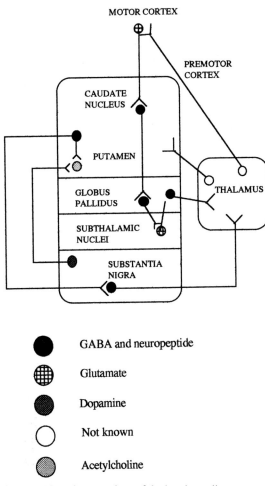

MOTOR CORTEX

PREMOTOR CORTEX

CAUDATE NUCLEUS

PUTAMEN

THALAMUS

GLOBUS PALLIDUS

SUBTHALAMIC NUCLEI

SUBSTANTIA NIGRA

● GABA and neuropeptide

⊕ Glutamate

● Dopamine

○ Not known

● Acetylcholine

Fig. 7.14 Neural connections of the basal ganglia.

an adjunct to L-dopa); lisuride; and pergolide mesylate. In experimental animals, deprenyl (a selective inhibitor of monoamine oxidase B) can prevent neurotoxin-induced parkinsonism by preventing the conversion of MPTP (1-methyl-4-phenyl-1,2,3,6-tetrahydropyridine) to its toxic metabolite MPP^+ by monoamine oxidase B.

SEROTONERGIC NEUROTRANSMISSION

Serotonin (5-hydroxytryptamine, 5-HT) is present in the enterochromaffin granules of the intestines and in blood platelets. Less than 2% of the total body serotonin is in the CNS. Early studies of serotonin indicated that disturbances of its physiology could produce abnormal behaviour, at times strongly suggestive of mental illness. Substances with marked

structural similarities to serotonin possess considerable pharmacological potency. Examples are N,N-dimethyl-tryptamine(DMT) and bufotenine (both present in the cahobe bean). Mexican hallucinogenic mushrooms also contain serotonin-related substances such as psilocybin. All three have a long history of abuse.

Serotonin is localised within specific neuronal pathways in the brain and their cell bodies are found in discrete brain nuclei, especially the midbrain and brain stem Raphé nuclei.

Serotonin synthesis

Serotonin is synthesised from L-tryptophan, being first hydroxylated to 5-HTP (by tryptophan hydroxylase) which is then decarboxylated to 5-HT (by aromatic-L-amino-acid decarboxylase). The capacity of the brain to synthesise serotonin is greatly in excess of requirements. Serotonin synthesis can be increased by oral tryptophan and takes place in neurones in both nuclei and nerve terminals.

Serotonin storage

Serotonin formed in the nucleus is transported to the terminals of dendrites and axons where it forms a readily releasable pool of serotonin. It is stored in presynaptic complexes comparable to those storing catecholamines. The *Rauwolfia* alkaloids and tetrabenazine reduce serotonin stores by disrupting these granules. When serotonin storage is disturbed, large quantities of serotonin are released and outside the CNS this causes side-effects such as diarrhoea and abdominal cramps.

Serotonin release

Serotonin release is a $Ca2^+$-dependent process and there is some evidence, as with dopamine, that release takes place by two separate mechanisms. The amphetamines and some tricyclic antidepressants release serotonin from storage granules. Amphetamine analogues containing halogen atoms (e.g. fenfluramine) are more effective in stimulating serotonin release than those without.

Serotonin receptors

Receptors for serotonin are found in the CNS as part of a diffuse serotonergic network. There are multiple 5-HT receptors (currently at least nine) and the neuropharmacological study of 5-HT receptor function in the CNS is a rapidly expanding field.

Subtypes of serotonergic receptors

Physiological responses to serotonin are mediated through multiple serotonin receptor subtypes. Individual serotonin receptor subtypes activate different intracellular signalling systems. $5-HT_{1A}$ and $5-HT_{1B}$ receptors regulate adenylate cyclase or couple to G proteins that directly activate ion channels. $5-HT_{1C}$ and $5-HT_2$ receptors activate PLC and stimulate phosphoinositol metabolism. 5-HT receptor classification is shown in Table 7.13. Continuing problems in receptor classification arise because of a lack of compounds with sufficient specificity to demonstrate differences between putative receptor subtypes. The

$5-HT_{1A}$ receptor is specifically activated by 8-hydroxy-2-(di-N-propylamino)tetralin (8-OH-DPAT). $5-HT_{1A}$ receptor density is highest in the CA1 region and dentate gyrus of the hippocampus and in the Raphé nuclei. Clinically useful drugs that are selective partial agonists at the $5-HT_{1A}$ receptor are buspirone and ipsapirone, both effective antianxiety agents. $5-HT_2$ receptors probably mediate excitatory effects; $5-HT_3$ receptors may act similarly but their exact functions are unknown. Little structural data are available about 5-HT receptors. The distinct ligand-binding properties of each subtype of serotonin receptor are based on important structural differences between them. Lübbert et al (1987) isolated a complementary DNA

Table 7.13 Serotonergic pharmacology
Presynaptic

Site of action	Effect	Drug	Use
Synthesis	Increases	Tryptophan	Antidepressant
	Blocks	p-Chlorophenylalanine	Experimental
	Blocks	5-Fluotryptophan	Experimental
Storage	Depletes	Reserpine	Experimental
	Depletes	Tetrabenazine	Chorea
Release	Increases	Amphetamine	Experimental
	Increases	Tricyclic antidepressants	Antidepressant
	Increases	Fenfluramine	Experimental
Uptake	Inhibits	Zimelidine	Experimental
		Clomipramine	Antidepressant
		Fluoxetine	Antidepressant
		Fluvoxamine	Antidepressant
		Paroxetine	Antidepressant
		Citalopram	Antidepressant

Postsynaptic

Receptor	Tissue (example)	Agonist responses	Agonist	Antagonist	Molecular mechanisms
$5-HT_{1A}$	Postsynaptic 5–HT neurones	Inhibits neuronal firing	LSD (partial) 8-OH-DPAT	Pindolol Metergoline Methysergide	↓Adenylate cyclase
$5-HT_{1B}$	5–HT presynaptic autoreceptor	Inhibits 5–HT release	RU 24969	Methysergide Metergoline	↓Adenylate cyclase
$5-HT_{1C}$	Choroid plexus and brain	Induction of specific behaviours (e.g. feeding)	TFMPP	Ritanserin ICI 169369	↑PI
$5-HT_2$	Postsynaptic 5–HT neurones	Induces slow wave sleep	LSD (partial)	Metergoline Ritanserin	↑PI
$5-HT_3$	Area postrema Limbic system	Emesis Modulation of dopamine and acetylcholine release	2–Methyl 5–HT	Ondansetron Granisetron Racopride Zacopride	Via ionic channels

Degradation

Monoamine oxidase (A and B) inhibition

(cDNA) clone that coded for a substantial portion of the 5-HT$_{1C}$ receptor and, subsequently, Julius et al (1988) cloned the entire 5-HT$_{1C}$ receptor. This receptor shares much in common with other members of the G protein-coupled 'superfamily' of receptors. There are seven membrane-spanning regions, the amino terminus is located on the extracellular side of the membrane and the carboxyl terminus is intracellular. Three intracellular loops link three extracellular loops to make up seven transmembrane domains (see Fig. 7.7).

The 5-HT$_2$ receptor has also been characterised by Julius et al (1990). It is homologous with the 5-HT$_{1C}$ receptor and is also a member of the G protein-coupled 'superfamily'. About 50% of the amino acid sequences are common to both 5-HT$_{1C}$ and 5-HT$_2$ receptors. These two receptors are further examples of the evolution of receptor subtypes within families that bind the same ligand (5-HT) and are coupled to the same signalling system (G proteins). However, the distinct structural differences between family members may provide the means for selective activation of intracellular pathways by different concentrations of the endogenous ligand or be relevant to a comprehensive understanding of the genetic regulation of neurotransmitter function. Because the many CNS effects of serotonergic drugs are mediated through subtypes of 5-HT receptors, these structural studies may eventually clarify individual differences in response to psychotomimetic drugs (e.g. LSD or other 5-HT agonists) and may in turn lead to a better understanding of some psychotic illnesses.

Chronic treatment with a wide range of antidepressant drugs (including the tricyclics, monoamine oxidase inhibitors and atypical antidepressants such as mianserin) is known to reduce the number of 5-HT$_1$ and 5-HT$_2$ receptors. Electroconvulsive shocks also decrease 5-HT$_{1A}$ receptors but increase 5-HT$_2$ receptor numbers. This difference may possibly explain why some depressive illnesses do not respond to a therapeutic course of oral antidepressant therapy but later respond to ECT.

Antidepressant drugs produce substantial decreases in 5-HT$_2$ receptor numbers after long-term treatment and these effects may be greater than their actions in catecholaminergic systems. For example, amitriptyline and imipramine reduce β adrenoceptor binding by about 20% but reduce 5-HT$_2$ binding even more, by about 40%. Monoamine oxidase inhibitors also reduce serotonin binding site numbers after chronic treatment, selective monoamine oxidase A inhibitors being most effective.

Abnormalities in serotonin receptor function have been put forward as part of the pathophysiology of depressive illness. Limited support for this hypothesis has been found in studies of ^{3}H serotonin binding to platelets and ^{3}H serotonin and ^{3}H spiroperidol binding to cortical tissue in suicide victims. The hypothesis has been extended to involve increased release of serotonin acting upon hypersensitive postsynaptic serotonin receptors and this has been suggested as a possible cause of depressive illness.

Cyproheptadine and methysergide are the most commonly used serotonergic antagonists. Structurally, cyproheptadine resembles the phenothiazines and also blocks histaminergic (H$_1$) and cholinergic (M$_1$) receptors. Methysergide is structurally similar to LSD, which can stimulate some serotonergic receptors and, especially in the periphery, be an antagonist at others. The physiological and biochemical actions of serotonergic receptors appear complex and study of their properties has been hindered by lack of specific antagonists or agonists. The recent development of such drugs is certain to add substantially to knowledge of the serotonergic system and will probably lead to better understanding of the mode of action of antidepressants as well.

Drugs affecting serotonin uptake

The re-uptake systems for serotonin resemble those for the catecholamines and are influenced by many antidepressant drugs. These may differ markedly in their relative affinities for serotonergic and catecholaminergic re-uptake mechanisms. The structure of the serotonergic transporter is known (Blakely et al 1991) and has much in common with the GABA and noradrenaline transporters. All three are members of a

Table 7.14 Relative potencies of antidepressants after oral administration to rats for inhibition of noradrenaline and serotonin uptake.

Drug	Inhibition of serotonin uptake	Inhibition of noradrenaline uptake
Paroxetine	0.4	—
Citalopram	2	>10
Fluoxetine	8	>100
Fluvoxamine	5	>30
Sertraline	—	—
Clomipramine	15	30
Imipramine	50	7
Amitriptyline	120	50
Desipramine	180	3

After Maitre et al (1982).

Table 7.15 Inhibition of radioligand binding in rat brain membranes in vitro by different types of antidepressant

Antidepressant	Receptor subtype/radioligand							
	α_1/prazosin	α_2/clonidine	β/DHA	D_2/spiperone	5–HT_1/5–HT	5–HT_1/ketanserin	Histamine H_1/mepyramine	Muscarinic/QNB
Paroxetine	>10 000	>10 000	>5 000	>7 700	>10 000	>1 000	>1 000	89
Citalopram	4 500	>10 000	>5 000	>10 000	>10 000	>1 000	>1 000	2 900
Fluvoxamine	>10 000	>10 000	>5 000	>10 000	>10 000	>1 000	>1 000	>10 000
Fluoxetine	>10 000	>10 000	>5 000	>10 000	>10 000	>1 000	>1 000	1 300
Amitriptyline	170	540	>5 000	1 200	1 000	8.3	3.3	5.1
Imipramine	440	1 000	>5 000	2 400	8 900	120	35	37
Clomipramine	150	3 300	>5 000	430	5 200	63	47	34
Desipramine	1 300	8 600	>5 000	3 800	2 500	160	370	68

After Thomas et al (1987).
QNB, quinuclidinylbenzilate; DHA, dihydroalprenolol.

'superfamily' of neurotransmitter transporters. The tricyclic antidepressant clomipramine was the first drug to inhibit serotonergic without also inhibiting noradrenergic re-uptake though its metabolite (desmethylclomipramine) is a strong inhibitor of noradrenergic re-uptake. The first truly specific serotonergic uptake inhibitor was zimelidine which, though an effective antidepressant, was withdrawn because of its hepatotoxic effects.

The currently available inhibitors of serotonin uptake comprise a class of antidepressants known as 'selective serotonin re-uptake inhibitors' (or SSRIs). Table 7.14 summarises potency and relative selectivity data. These show paroxetine to be the most potent inhibitor of serotonin re-uptake and citalopram to be the most selective. In vivo, the pharmacological profile of each of these drugs is changed by the formation of active metabolites, which may possess pharmacokinetic properties that differ markedly from their parent compound. For example, fluoxetine is metabolised to norfluoxetine with a half-life of 7–15 days. Since norfluoxetine is equipotent with fluoxetine and is equally selective, it probably contributes importantly to the antidepressant effects of fluoxetine. However, the metabolites of sertraline, fluvoxamine and paroxetine are considerably less active than their parent compounds and probably do not affect their clinical actions.

These drugs also interact with monoaminergic receptors (Table 7.15) but have considerably fewer effects on histaminergic, adrenergic and muscarinic cholinergic receptors than the tricyclic antidepressants.

Drugs affecting serotonin degradation

Most serotonin is oxidised by monoamine oxidase to 5-hydroxyindoleacetaldehyde and then to 5-hydroxyindoleacetic acid (5-HIAA) by aldehyde dehydrogenase. 5-Hydroxyindoleacetaldehyde is also reduced by alcohol dehydrogenase to 5-hydroxytryptophol. 5-HIAA is the major metabolite of 5-HT degradation. Monoamine oxidase inhibitors are the principal drugs to modify serotonin degradation.

PEPTIDERGIC NEUROTRANSMISSION

Neuroendocrinology is defined as the study of interaction between nervous and endocrine systems. Psychoneuroendocrinology is concerned with the same topics but with additional emphasis on the possible influence of psychological factors on the regulation and integration of neuroendocrine systems. Advances in neurobiology have demonstrated that the neural and endocrine systems are closely linked with many similarities. Previously, differences between the systems were apparent from a structural standpoint and seemed supported by the distinctive means of communication between the component parts of each system. Patterns of electrical activity in the nervous system were clearly not the same as the release of chemicals by endocrine tissue to act on distant target organs. The neural regulation of endocrine function is now seen to provide important insights into the working of the brain that are relevant to psychiatry. This view is based upon the following lines of evidence, many of which can be traced back to the writings of previous generations of psychiatrists who commented upon, and sought to explore, relationships between the signs and symptoms of mental disorder and abnormal functioning of the endocrine glands. In the modern era, the reasoning supporting neuroendocrine studies in psychiatry is much more cogent. First, there is extensive evidence showing that the neurotransmitter systems preferentially modified by effective psychotropic drugs (e.g. the dopaminergic and noradrenergic pathways) are also intimately involved in the limbic–hypothalamic integration and regulation of pituitary function. Putative abnormalities of these transmitter systems may extend from sites in the brain involved in the pathogenesis of mental illness to the hypothalamic–pituitary system and may therefore be detected in abnormal endocrine functioning. Secondly, the hypothalamus regulates the anterior pituitary by synthesising and secreting releasing factors into the pituitary portal vessel system to act upon anterior pituitary cells. These releasing factors are synthesised and released at sites elsewhere in the nervous system without any obvious endocrine function and there is experimental evidence that they may function as neurotransmitters or neuromodulators, and thereby play important roles in the neural regulation of certain behaviours. The abnormalities characteristic of severe mental illnesses may, therefore, be caused by pathological changes in the non-endocrine functions of the releasing factors. Thirdly, the hormones released by the pituitary regulate hormone production of target endocrine glands. These peripheral hormones can, in turn, act upon many aspects of neural function, for example by affecting neural development and classical neurotransmitters like noradrenaline. The actions on the brain of hormones such as testosterone, thyroxin and cortisol may be relevant to sex differences in the incidence of mental illnesses such as depression and the increased prevalence of psychological symptoms in endocrinopathies such as thyroid or adrenal cortical disease. Fourthly, releasing factors and 'classical neurotransmitters' can coexist in the same nerve terminal (e.g. serotonin and thyrotrophin-releasing factor, TRF). In this circumstance, the releasing factor may modify (or 'modulate') the actions of the neurotransmitter and this may be of relevance, for example, to the serotonergic hypothesis of the mode of action of some antidepressant treatments. Fifthly, stress responses to threatening or noxious stimuli include activation of the hypothalamic–pituitary system. These patterns of endocrine responses to stress are specific to the type of stressful stimulus. Since there is abundant evidence from clinical studies implicating stressful stimuli in the pathogenesis of mental illnesses, study of the neural regulation of endocrine responses to stress is likely to elucidate important individual differences relevant to variations in vulnerability to mental illnesses.

Molecular biology of peptidergic transmission

Most regulatory substances released by the nervous system are peptides, i.e. they consist of amino acids joined by peptide bonds. Unlike classical neurotransmitters, these compounds are synthesised as parts of larger molecules that are cleaved by proteolysis and carboxylation into active fragments of amino acid chains at the point of release. Local tissue-specific differences in the activity of processing enzymes can yield important topographical variations in the proportions of peptide fragments derived from a single precursor. However, with the exception of pro-opiomelanocortin, the specific degradative, cleavage and post-translational processing enzymes involved are usually unknown. Fundamental questions, relevant to proper understanding of the actions of drugs on the brain arise from this uncertainty. Neuropeptide fragments may be cleaved from widely available precursor molecules by enzymes specific to that cleavage site and/or general-purpose enzymes that are locally regulated.

The chromosomal localisation of neuropeptide genes are distributed widely throughout the human genome. Although some neuropeptides are close members of structurally related families, with the single exception of oxytocin and vasopressin, genes for these related family members are located on different chromosomes (Sherman et al 1989).

Neural regulation of neuropeptide synthesis and release

The hypothalamus controls the release of pituitary hormones in two ways, both of which involve neurones that synthesise and release neuropeptides. In the first, specialised neurones in the hypothalamus synthesise and secrete releasing factors. In the second, the magnocellular neurones of the hypothalamus synthesise precursor molecules (preprovasophysin and preproxyphysin) that are processed and transported to terminals in the posterior pituitary from which vasopressin, oxytocin and their related neurophysins are stoichiometrically released. The neuroendocrine neurones of the hypothalamus are influenced by many types of neurotransmitter. Releasing factor-producing neurones are richly supplied with noradrenergic, dopaminergic and serotonergic connections.

Cotransmission of neuropeptides

Neuropeptides are present in the central nervous system in concentrations between 10^{-12} and 10^{-15} mol/mg of protein. These are much lower than the concentrations of the 'classical neurotransmitters', which vary from 10^{-9} to 10^{-10} mol/mg of protein. The highest concentrations of neuropeptides in the brain are found in the hypothalamic–pituitary system but some neuropeptides (e.g. cholecystokinin and vasoactive intestinal peptide) have their highest concentrations in the cortex. Other neuropeptides (e.g. oxytocin and vasopressin) are present in cell bodies only in the hypothalamus and their presence in other brain or spinal cord areas is accounted for by the long projections of these cells into those areas. Some widely distributed neuropeptides (e.g. TRF and substance P) are found in cell bodies in numerous areas.

Hökfelt et al (1987) have demonstrated the coexistence of neuropeptides and 'classical neurotransmitters' within the same neurone at many sites in the nervous system. The physiological importance of coexistence is not yet known but a number of models have been put forward, some of which may prove to be of relevance to hypotheses concerning changes in receptor sensitivity in mental illness. In one model, a nerve terminal containing serotonin, substance P and TRF responds to low-frequency electrical stimulation by releasing serotonin. The released serotonin attaches to the postsynaptic receptors, where it generates a small postsynaptic potential. Some serotonin also attaches to the presynaptic serotonergic receptors (autoreceptors) which inhibit further serotonin release. As electrical stimulation is increased, TRF and substance P are also released. TRF and serotonin then act synergistically on the postsynaptic serotonin receptor to generate an increased postsynaptic potential, while substance P blocks the serotonergic autoreceptor preventing inhibition of serotonin release. The three substances thus combine to produce prolonged postsynaptic activation without inducing compensatory responses at a presynaptic level. These interactions between a monoamine neurotransmitter and neuropeptides may be relevant to long-term changes in homeostatic mechanisms, neural learning and long-term potentiation of synaptic activity. They have also been related to the mode of action of antidepressant treatments (including ECT) and pathological alterations in receptor sensitivity that may occur in affective disorders and schizophrenia.

Peptide regulatory factors

CNS peptide regulatory factors (PRFs) are not the same as neuropeptides. They act through a different class of receptor and are important in the normal development of the nervous system. PRFs are also important in neurodegenerative diseases, where they function in the restoration of neural circuits and the coordination of glial responses to damage.

Nerve growth factor (NGF) is the best known PRF. It is a neurotrophic factor and influences the synthesis of neurotransmitters, cytoskeletal proteins and neuropeptides (Hanley 1989). The survival and functional maintenance of neurones depends upon the presence of specific PRFs. Cholinergic neurones damaged in Alzheimer's disease contain high concentrations of mRNA for NGF and it is hypothesised that cholinergic loss in this condition may be reversed by NGF treatment (Perry 1990). Other PRFs include brain-derived neurotrophic factor (BDNF) (Maisonpierre et al 1990), which may be important in Parkinson's disease, neuroleucin, glial nexin, insulin-like growth factors, platelet-derived growth factor (Williams 1989) and epidermal growth factor. Since the cellular mechanisms that regulate PRF metabolism can be manipulated by noxious factors, study of psychological stress in humans has been extended to include effects on functions influenced by PRFs. Animal studies of electroconvulsive stimulation (ECS) of possible relevance to the mode of action of ECT have included direct measures of PRF metabolism. Repeated ECS probably alters the expression of many neural genes along a time-course that is relevant to the actions of ECT (Leviel et al 1990). Interleukins 1 and 2 are also PRFs and can be produced by the brain when stressed. Their functions may include integration of neural and immune responses to injury, studied in psychoneuroimmunology.

Peptidergic receptors

The receptors for most neuropeptides are unknown. As a group, neuropeptides appear to act on G protein-coupled receptors but the second messenger systems are largely unknown (Wollemann 1990). Opioid receptors appear linked to G_i and G_0 proteins (Wong et al 1989). Neuropeptides can function as (1) neurotransmitters released by one neurone at a presynaptic terminal to act on the adjacent postsynaptic membrane, (2) neuromodulators that act by modifying the turnover, release or action of classical neurotransmitters, or (3) as neurohormones released by one neurone to act at a site distant to the point of release. The most detailed understanding of a peptidergic receptor system currently available is provided by the pharmacology of opioid receptors. There is good evidence for the existence of three subtypes of opioid receptor.

Endorphins and enkephalins

The endorphins (literally 'endogenous morphine') are the endogenous ligands for the opioid receptors. Their study is a rapidly expanding field of research and has given rise to a confusing terminology. The term 'opiate' is used to describe drugs derived from the juice of the poppy *Papaver somniferum*. The word 'opioid' describes all substances with morphine-like actions. The word 'narcotic' is no longer used in pharmacology although originally it described drugs that induced sleep and was later applied to morphine-like analgesics. The sites of action of opioid drugs in the nervous system appear to be the receptors for a number of endogenous ligands which include the pentapeptides, leucine-enkephalin (leu-enkephalin) and methionine-enkephaline (met-enkephalin). The amino acid sequence of met-enkephalin is the same as the sequence contained in amino acid residues 61–65 in the pituitary hormone β-lipotrophin (β-LPH). Other opioid peptides are represented in fragments of the β-lipotrophin amino acid sequence. The carboxy terminus of amino acid residues 61–91 is called β-endorphin. Sequences of amino acid residues 61–76 are called α-endorphin and amino acid residues 61–77 are called γ–endorphin. The enkephalins and endorphins derived from β-lipotrophin probably belong to separate physiological systems. β-Endorphin is present in the hypothalamopituitary system, where it is derived from a larger precursor molecule, POMC, containing the amino acid sequences for both β-lipotrophin and adrenocorticotrophic hormone (ACTH). The enkephalins are not derived from POMC but are produced by cleavage of a separate precursor molecule.

The physiological role of endogenous ligands for opioid receptors is still unknown but they appear to be involved in the perception of pain and the neural control of certain aspects of endocrine function, the regulation of movement, mood and some aspects of behaviour. A large number of drugs are agonists at opioid receptor sites. Opioid agonist drugs appear to act largely at the μ receptor with a few actions mediated at the κ receptor. Opioid agonists include morphine, heroin (diacetylmorphine), dihydromorphine, codeine, pethidine, methadone, pentazocine, levorphanol and meperidine. Many of these agonists are structurally related to morphine but some, like meperidine and methadone, are chemically quite dissimilar. Naloxone, naltrexone and nalorphine are antagonists at opioid receptor sites. Pentazocine has both opioid agonist actions and weak antagonist activity. All the compounds listed above have clinical applications and their specific use has been determined by their pharmacokinetics, pharmacodynamics and liability to produce dependence. All opioid drugs, when regularly administered, appear able to induce tolerance and dependence. Tolerance may be innate or acquired. Innate tolerance is subject to wide individual variation, determined presumably by genetic factors and the age and reproductive status of the individual. Acquired tolerance is observed as the need to increase the dose of the opioid drug if the same effects are to be obtained with repeated administration. The mechanisms underlying the development of tolerance are ill-understood but may include the proliferation of new receptor sites or reduction in sensitivity of opioid receptors to their agonists. There is extensive cross-tolerance between opioid drugs. When they are administered regularly, tolerance frequently develops but this must not be taken to imply that withdrawal symptoms will always occur if the drug is removed. The manifestation of withdrawal symptoms (which may be either physical or psychological) demonstrates that an individual has become dependent (physically or psychologically) on the drug. Symptoms that can follow opioid withdrawal include insomnia, restlessness, anxiety, nausea and vomiting, abdominal cramps, myotonus, sweating, piloerection and rhinorrhoea. These symptoms may persist for several days and may be accompanied by a craving for the drug to be reintroduced. Tolerance may also develop to alcohol, barbiturates and hypnotic drugs. The withdrawal symptoms observed following prolonged administration of these substances are primarily rebound effects in the systems most affected by the drug. Depressant drugs tend to be followed by rebound hyperexcitability and mood-elevating drugs like the amphetamines by lethargy and depressed mood. Epileptic seizures may be seen in withdrawal from drugs that raise the seizure threshold.

Theories of drug dependence and withdrawal usually attempt to explain withdrawal symptoms in terms of some form of rebound phenomenon. Pharmacological explanations have included modification of receptor sensitivity, change in numbers of receptors, the utilisation of otherwise redundant neural pathways and the induction of enzymes involved in the synthesis of neurotransmitters.

REFERENCES

Ahlquist R P 1948 A study of the adrenotropic receptors. American Journal of Physiology 153: 586–600

Barnard E A, Darlison M G, Seeburg P 1987 Molecular biology of the $GABA_A$ receptor: the receptor/channel superfamily. Trends in Neurosciences 10(12): 502–509

Beal M F, Kowall N W, Ellison D W, Mazurek M F, Swartz K J, Martin J B 1986 Replication of the neurochemical characteristics of Huntington's disease by quinolinic acid. Nature 321: 168–171

Bell M V, Bloomfield J, McKinley M et al 1989 Physical linkage of the $GABA_A$ receptor subunit gene to the DX5374 locus in human Xq28. American Journal of Human Genetics 45: 882–888

Betz H 1987 Biology and structure of mammalian glycine receptor. Trends in Neurosciences 10(3): 113–117

Birnbaumer L 1990 G proteins in signal transduction. Annual Review of Pharmacology and Toxicology 30: 675–705

Blair L A, Levitan E S, Marshall J, Dionne V E, Barnard E A 1988 Single subunits of the $GABA_A$ receptor form ion channels with properties of the native receptor. Science 242: 577–579

Blakely R D, Berson H E, Fremeau Jr R T et al 1991 Cloning and expression of a functional serotonin transporter from rat brain. Nature 354: 66–70

Bloom F E 1990 Neurohumoral transmission and the central nervous system. In: Goodman A G, Rall T W, Nies A S and Taylor P (eds) The pharmacological basis of therapeutics. Pergamon Press, New York, pp 244–268

Blum K, Noble E P, Sheridan P J et al 1990 Allelic association of human dopamine D_2 receptor gene in alcoholism. Journal of the American Medical Association 263: 2055–2060

Bonner T I 1989 The molecular basis of muscarinic receptor diversity. Trends in Neurosciences 12(4): 148–151

Bormann J 1988 Electrophysiology of $GABA_A$ and $GABA_B$ receptor subtypes. Trends in Neurosciences 11(3): 112–116

Bradbury M 1979 The concept of the blood–brain barrier. Wiley, London

Bourne H R, Sanders D A, McCormick F 1990 The GTPase superfamily: a conserved switch for diverse cell functions. Nature 348: 125–132

Bunzow J R, Van Tol H H M, Grandy et al 1988 Cloning and expression of a rat D_2 dopamine receptor cDNA. Nature 336: 783–787

Callingham B A, Ovens R S 1988 Some in vitro effects of moclobemide and other MAO inhibitors on responses to sympathomimetic amines. In: Youdim M B H, Da Prada M, Amrein R (eds) The cheese effect and new reversible MAO-A inhibitors. Journal of Neurotransmission (Suppl) 26: 17–29

Carlsson A 1988 The current status of the dopamine hypothesis of schizophrenia. Neuropsychopharmacology 1: 179–186

Carlsson A, Lindqvist M 1963 Effect of chlorpromazine or haloperidol on formation of 3-methoxytyramine and normetanephrine in mouse brain. Acta Pharmacologica et Toxicologica 20: 140–144

Catterall W A 1988 Structure and function of voltage-sensitive ion channels. Science 242: 50–61

Changeux J-P, Revah F 1987 The acetylcholine receptor

molecule: allosteric sites and the ion channel. Trends in Neurosciences 10(6): 245–250

Dearry A, Gingrich J A, Falardeau P, Fremeau R T, Bates M D, Caron M G 1990 Molecular cloning and expression of the gene for human D_1 dopamine receptor. Nature 347: 72–76

Deisz R A, Lux H D 1985 Gamma-aminobutyric acid-induced depression of calcium currents of chick sensory neurons. Neuroscience Letters 56(2): 205–210

Evans R M 1988 The steroid and thyroid hormone receptor superfamily. Science 240: 889–895

Farde L, Wiesel F-A, Stone-Elander S et al 1990 D_2 dopamine receptors in neuroleptic-naive schizophrenic patients. Archives of General Psychiatry 47: 213–219

Giros B, Sokoloff P, Martres M-P, Riou J-F, Emorine L J, Schwartz J-C 1989 Alternative splicing directs the expression of two D_2 dopamine receptor isoforms. Nature 342: 923–926

Gregor P, Mano I, Maoz I, McKeown M, Teichberg V I 1989 Molecular structure of the chick cerebellar kainate-binding subunit of a putative glutamate receptor. Nature 342: 689–692

Guy H R, Hucho F 1987 The ion channel of the nicotine acetylcholine receptor. Trends in Neurosciences 10(8): 318–321

Hanley M R 1989 Peptide regulatory factors in the nervous system. Lancet i: 1373–1376

Henley J M Barnard E A 1990 Autoradiographic distribution of binding sites for the non-NMDA receptor antagonist CNQX in chick brain. Neuroscience Letters 116: 17–22

Hökfelt T, Millhorn D, Seroogy K et al 1987 Coexistence of peptides with classical neurotransmitters. Experientia 43: 768–780

Honoré T, Davies S N, Drejer J et al 1988 Quinoxalinediones: potent competitive non-NMDA glutamate receptor antagonists. Science 241: 701–703

Inoue M, Sadoshima J, Akaike N 1986 Different actions of intracellular free calcium on resting and GABA-gated chloride conductances. Brain Research 404: 301–303

Jan L Y, Jan Y N 1990 A superfamily of ion channels. Nature 345: 672

Julius D, McDermott A B, Axel R, Jessell T M 1988 Molecular characterization of a functional cDNA encoding the serotonin 1c receptor. Science 241: 558–564

Julius D, Huang K N, Livelli T J, Axel R, Jessell T M 1990 The 5HT2 receptor defines a family of structually distinct but functionally conserved serotonin receptors. Proceedings of the National Academy of Sciences of the USA 87: 928–932

Krupinski J, Coussen F, Bakalyar H A et al 1989 Adenylyl cyclase amino acid sequence: possible channel- or transporter-like structure. Science 244: 1558–1564

Leviel V, Fayada C, Guibert F et al 1990 Short- and long-term alterations of gene expression in limbic structures by repeated electroconvulsive-induced seizures. Journal of Neurochemistry 54: 899–904

Llinas R, Yarom Y 1981 Properties and distribution of ionic conductances generating electroresponsiveness of mammalian inferior olivary neurones in vitro. Journal of Physiology (Cambridge) 315: 569–584

Lübbert H, Hoffmann B J, Snutch T P et al 1987 cDNA cloning of a serotonin $5-HT_{1C}$ receptor by electrophysiological assays of mRNA-injected *Xenopus* oocytes. Proceedings of the Royal Academy of Sciences 84: 4332–4336

Lüddens H, Pritchett D B, Köhler M et al 1990 Cerebellar GABA$_A$ receptor selective for a behavioural alcohol antagonist. Nature 346: 648–651

Maisonpierre P C, Belluscio L, Squinto S et al 1990 Neurotrophin-3: a neurotrophic factor related to NGF and BDNF. Science 247: 1446–1451

Maitre L, Baumann P A, Jaekel J 1982 5-HT uptake inhibitors: psychopharmacological and neurochemical criteria of selectivity. In: Ho B T (ed) Serotonin in biological psychiatry. Raven Press, New York, pp 229–246

Majerus P W, Connolly T M, Bansal V S, Inhorn R C, Ross T S, Lips D L 1988 Inositol phosphates: synthesis and degradation. Journal of Biological Chemistry 263: 3051–3054

Miller R J 1987 Multiple Ca channels and neuronal function. Science 235: 46–52

Monsma Jr F J, McVittie L D, Gerfen C R, Mahan L C, Sibley D R 1989 Multiple D$_2$ dopamine receptors produced by alternative RNA splicing. Nature 342: 926–929

Monsma Jr F J, Mahan L C, McVittie L D, Gerfen C R, Sibley D R 1990 Molecular cloning and expression of a D$_1$ dopamine receptor linked to adenylyl cyclase activation. Proceedings of the National Academy of Sciences of the USA 87: 6723–6727

Morris B J, Hicks A A, Wisden W, Darlison M B, Hunts S P, Barnard E A 1990 Distinct regional expression of nicotinic acetylcholine receptor genes in chick brain. Brain Research. Molecular Brain Research 7: 305–315

Moss S J, Darlison M G, Beeson D M, Barnard E A 1989 Development expression of the genes encoding the four subunits of the chicken muscle acetylcholine receptor. Journal of Biological Chemistry 264: 20199–20205

Neer E J, Clapham D E 1988 Roles of G protein subunits in transmembrane signalling. Nature 333: 129–134

Nicoll R A 1988 The coupling of neurotransmitter receptors to ion channels in the brain. Science 241: 545–551

Nowycky M C, Fox A P, Tsien R W 1985 Three types of neuronal calcium channel with different calcium agonist sensitivity. Nature 316: 440–443

Ogata N, Narahashi T 1990 Potent blocking action of chlorpromazine on two types of calcium channels in cultured neuroblastoma cells. Journal of Pharmacology and Experimental Therapeutics 252: 1142–1149

Oldendorf W H 1974 Lipid solubility and drug penetration of the blood–brain barrier. Proceedings of the Society of Experimental Biological Medicine 147: 813

Olney J W 1989 Excitatory amino acids and neuropsychiatric disorders. Biological Psychiatry 26: 505–525

Pacholczyk T, Blakely R D, Amara S G 1991 Expression cloning of a cocaine- and antidepressant-sensitive human noradrenaline transporter. Nature 350: 350–354

Peroutka S J 1988 5-Hydroxytryptamine receptor subtypes: molecular, biochemical and physiological characterization. Trends in Neurosciences 11: 496–500

Perry E K 1990 Hypothesis linking plasticity, vulnerability and nerve growth factor to basal forebrain cholinergic neurons. International Journal of Geriatric Psychiatry 5: 223–231

Raiteri M, Cerrito F, Cervon A M, Levi G 1979 Dopamine can be released by two mechanisms differentially affected by the dopamine transport inhibitor nomifensine. Journal

of Pharmacology and Experimental Therapeutics 208: 195–202

Revah F, Bertrand D, Galzi J-L et al 1991 Mutations in the channel domain alter desensitization of a neuronal nicotinic receptor. Nature 353: 846–849

Rhee S G, Suh P-G, Ryu S-H, Lee S Y 1989 Studies of inositol phospholipid-specific phospholipase C. Science 244: 546–550

Ross E M 1989 Signal sorting and amplification through G protein-coupled receptors. Neuron 3: 141–152

Schofield P R, Darlison M G, Fujita N et al 1987 Sequence and functional expression of the GABA$_A$ receptor shows a ligand-gated receptor super-family. Nature 328: 221–227

Sherman T G, Akil H, Watson S J 1989 The molecular biology of neuropeptides: neuropeptide genetics. In: Magistretti P J (ed) Discussions in neuroscience, vol VI, No 1. Elsevier, Amsterdam

Sladeczek F, Récasens M, Bockaert J 1988 A new mechanism for glutamate receptor action: phosphoinositide hydrolysis. Trends in Neurosciences 11(12): 545–549

Snyder S H 1989 Drug and neurotransmitter receptors: new perspectives with clinical relevance. Journal of the American Medical Association 261: 3126–3129

Snyder S H 1990 The dopamine connection. Nature 347:121–122

Snyder S H 1991 Vehicles of inactivation. Nature 354:187

Sokoloff P, Giros B, Martres M-P, Bouthenet M-L, Schwartz J-C 1990 Molecular cloning and characterization of a novel dopamine receptor (D$_3$) as a target for neuroleptics. Nature 347: 146–151

Sonders M S, Keana J F W, Weber E 1988 Phencyclidine and psychotomimetic sigma opiates: recent insights into their biochemical and physiological sites of action. Trends in Neurosciences 11: 37–40

Sternweis P C, Pang I-H 1990 The G protein-channel connection. Trends in Neurosciences 13(4): 122–126

Stevens C F 1987 Channel families in the brain. Nature 328: 198–199

Strader C D, Sigal I S, Dixon R F 1989 Structural basis of β-adrenergic receptor function. FASEB Journal 3: 1825–1832

Sunahara R K, Niznik H B, Weiner D M et al 1990 Human dopamine D$_1$ receptor encoded by an intronless gene on chromosome 5. Nature 347: 80–83

Sunahara R K, Guan H-C, O'Dowd B F et al 1991 Cloning of the gene for a human dopamine D$_5$ recptor with higher affinity for dopamine than D$_1$. Nature 350: 614–619

Südhof T C, Czernik A J, Kao H-T et al 1989 Synapsins: mosaics of shared and individual domains in a family of synaptic vesicle phosphoproteins.Science 245: 1474–1480

Thomas D R, Nelson D R, Johnson A M 1987 Biochemical effects of the antidepressant paroxetinea specific 5-HT uptake inhibitor. Psychopharmacology 93: 193–200

Tsien R W, Lipscombe D, Madison D V, Bley K R, Fox A P 1988 Multiple types of neuronal calcium channels and their selective modulation. Trends in Neurosciences 11(10): 431–438

Van Tol H H M, Bunzow J R, Guan H-C et al 1991 Cloning of the gene for a human dopamine D$_4$ receptor with high affinity for the antipsychotic clozapine. Nature 350: 610–614

Wang H-Y, Friedman E 1989 Lithium inhibition of protein

kinase C activation-induced serotonin release. Psychopharmacology 99: 213–218

Williams L T 1989 Signal transduction by the platelet-derived growth factor receptor. Science 243: 1564–1570

Wollemann M 1990 Recent developments in the research of opioid receptor subtype molecular characterization. Journal of Neurochemistry 54: 1095–1101

Wong D F, Wagner H N, Tune L E et al 1986 Positron emission tomography reveals elevated D2 dopamine receptors in drug-naive schizophrenics. Science 234: 1558–1563

Wong Y H, Bemoliou-Mason C D, Barnard E A 1989 Opioid receptors in magnesium–digitonin-solubilized rat brain membrane are tightly coupled to a pertussis toxin-sensitive guanine nucleotide-binding protein. Journal of Neurochemistry 52: 999–1009

Yamamoto C, McIlwain H 1966 Electrical activities in thin sections from the mammalian brain maintained in chemically-defined media in vitro. Journal of Neurochemistry 13(12): 1333–1343

Zhou Q-Y, Grandy D K, Thambi L et al 1990 Cloning and expression of human and rat D_1 dopamine receptors. Nature 347: 76–80

8. Neurochemistry and neurotoxicology

A. J. Dewar

INTRODUCTION

The first attempts to apply chemical methods to the study of brain function were made several hundred years ago and information concerning the inorganic constituents of the brain was obtained as early as 1719. With the development of suitable chemical fractionation techniques in the 19th century, detailed investigations of the organic constituents of neural tissue became feasible. The term neurochemistry was first used by Julius Schlossberger in his *General and Comparative Animal Chemistry* — a book which devoted 135 of its 616 pages to the chemistry of neural tissues. This work stimulated a number of more extensive studies of the nervous system by the methods of organic chemistry, culminating in the most comprehensive of 19th century studies of brain composition: Thudichum's *Treatise on the Chemical Constitution of the Brain*, published in 1884 (see McIlwain 1990). As early as 1833 attempts were being made to relate mental disorders to alterations in the chemical composition of the brain.

The emphasis on studies of brain constituents in the early phase of the development of neurochemistry was due in part to the widely held, but erroneous, view that brain metabolism was a very slow process. Subsequently, with the advent of isotopic tracer techniques, it became apparent that the brain had one of the highest metabolic rates of any tissue and that most cerebral constituents are in a dynamic state undergoing rapid changes in association with changes in cerebral functioning. Knowledge of the chemical composition of the brain does not, therefore, in itself, afford much understanding of cerebral function. Indeed, it has been remarked that mere chemical analysis of the brain contributes no more to an understanding of brain function than the analysis of pigments to the appreciation of a painting (Hucho 1986). Although the composition of the brain is

altered significantly in a number of conditions (such as some of the inborn errors of lipid and amino acid metabolism) and analysis of brain tissue taken at autopsy has provided some valuable insights into the basis of schizophrenia (Reynolds 1988), most present-day research on the neurochemistry of mental disorders concentrates on dynamic processes such as synthesis, turnover, release, uptake and transport. The problems confronting the neurochemist in his quest to understand brain function in chemical terms should not be underestimated. Formidable practical obstacles exist, including the structural and functional complexity of the brain, its cellular heterogeneity and the enormous range of timescales over which reactions can occur.

There are, for example, two major cell types in the brain, neurones and glia (described in detail in Ch. 6), and the difference in their functional roles is reflected in their very different chemical composition and metabolic properties. However, even small samples of brain tissue will contain several types of neurone and glia, usually in close juxtaposition, and it is extremely difficult to separate the contributions of each cell type to the metabolism of the tissue as a whole. The problem is exacerbated if the tissue is homogenised (as it often is in neurochemical studies) because the cells are broken and all their constituents will be intermixed in an unphysiological manner. A further complication is that the intracellular concentrations of many chemicals within brain cells are not uniform. Each cell is composed of many types of organelle, each having a different chemical composition and different metabolic properties. The existence of different metabolic 'pools' within cells is known as compartmentation and is particularly pronounced in the brain. Many brain constituents, e.g. amino acids such as glutamate, are found in several intracellular pools which can differ in size and turnover rate.

For these reasons classical biochemical methods for studying metabolism (e.g. the use of tissue slices and homogenates in vitro) can, when applied to the brain, yield data that are extremely difficult to interpret. Although some of the problems can be overcome by use of such techniques as histochemistry (to assist in precise localisation of events) it has been necessary to develop fractionation and analytical techniques to enable the study of the metabolism of different cell types in isolation and the study of metabolism at the subcellular level. The successful development of such methods, particularly micromethods for single-cell analysis and fractionation methods that permit the study of isolated nerve endings ('synaptosomes'), has contributed greatly to progress in neurochemistry.

Since the 1970s the pace of advance in neurochemistry has accelerated markedly. In common with many other areas of chemistry, neurochemistry has benefited immensely from innovations in microelectronics which have led to the emergence of increasingly sophisticated analytical instrumentation and the widespread availability of hitherto undreamt levels of computing capability in the laboratory. The application of fundamental advances in molecular biology and immunology (notably recombinant DNA techniques and monoclonal antibodies) to the neurosciences has also contributed greatly to the speed of progress. Some insights into the diversity of techniques now available to neurochemists may be gained from Turner & Bachelard (1987) and Giacobini (1987).

The application of these modern methods is now leading to significant advances in our understanding of normal and abnormal brain function. However, it is important to recognise that, impressive though these advances are, our understanding remains limited in relation to the complexity of the functions studied. Although biochemical techniques have unravelled much of the complexity of the molecular workings of the neurone and the diverse mechanisms for transmitting information, the molecular approach will always remain limited in its ability to throw light on the *content* of this information. The neurochemist investigating the biochemistry of neurones can only explain the mechanism of the initiation and conduction of the signals. The specific content of the signal cannot be defined by his methods. Similarly, although the molecular events underlying the processing of the signals can be elucidated, the outcome of this processing (i.e. the 'information') cannot be accessed by neurochemical methods.

In spite of these limitations, the molecular approach has much to offer psychiatry. Knowledge of the biochemical aspects of the major psychiatric illnesses has advanced considerably and is now contributing significantly to methods of treatment. Furthermore, the advent of the new biotechnologies and advances in molecular genetics have yielded much of direct clinical relevance and importance (McGrath 1989).

Scope

Modern neurochemistry is the discipline that integrates the molecular and mechanistic aspects of neurosciences such as neurophysiology, neuropharmacology, neurotoxicology and neuroendocrinology. As a consequence the boundaries between neurochemistry and these other sciences have become increasingly blurred. For this reason important aspects of the subject such as the biochemistry of synaptic transmission and neurotransmitter metabolism are covered elsewhere (see Ch. 7).

This chapter is limited to a discussion of a small number of topics relevant to psychiatry which serve to illustrate the broad range of knowledge now available on the biochemistry of the brain. These include some examples of 'classical' biochemistry as they apply to nervous tissue (energy metabolism), an account of the biochemical aspects of brain development, and a brief survey of the manner in which biochemical techniques have been brought to bear on the challenging task of elucidating some of the underlying mechanisms of memory. The chapter concludes with an account of the rapidly growing field of neurotoxicology but focusing in particular on two problems of significance to psychiatry: the neurotoxicology of lead and ethanol.

ENERGY METABOLISM

The second law of thermodynamics states that 'systems in isolation spontaneously tend towards states of greater disorganisation'. This may be expressed mathematically as

$$\Delta F = \Delta H - T \Delta S$$

where ΔF is the change in free energy, ΔH is the change in heat content or enthalpy, T is the absolute temperature and S is the degree of disorganisation or entropy.

According to this equation, the existence of life appears to be thermodynamically improbable. However, the equation does imply that if free energy is supplied to a system the state of organisation of that system will increase. Living cells are effective transducers of chemical potential energy into other forms of energy which can be used to maintain their organised structure. From a chemical viewpoint, human cells are a collection of essentially unstable compounds dissolved in (or surrounded by) a salt solution of precisely controlled composition and maintained in general above the temperature of their surroundings. They also perform work at the expense of metabolic energy.

Although the tasks performed by the cells of the brain are less conspicuously energy-consuming than those of many other cells, since they do not involve mechanical work, osmotic work or significant external secretory activity, there are, nevertheless, many functions of brain cells that are energy intensive: the maintenance of membrane potentials, active transport and the synthesis and axoplasmic transport of cellular materials. It is not surprising, therefore, that, with its organisational complexity and wide range of endergonic activities, the brain has a high metabolic rate. Although it comprises a mere 2% of body weight it accounts for approximately 10% of the energy expenditure and 20% of the oxygen consumption of the body at rest. In children this percentage is even higher; the brain of a 5-year-old accounts for approximately 50% of the resting total body oxygen consumption. The oxygen consumption of a typical neurone is between ten and 100 times greater than that of a glial cell.

Energy metabolism is not responsible for all the oxygen consumption of the brain since the brain contains a variety of oxidases and hydroxylases that have a role in the synthesis and metabolism of a number of neurotransmitters. However, important though these are, they account for a negligible proportion of the total oxygen consumption of the brain.

As a consequence of its high energy requirement the brain is extremely sensitive to disturbances in the supply of its energy sources and many clinical conditions associated with disturbances of brain function can often be traced back to a deficiency in the production or utilisation of energy. Furthermore, in view of the poor regenerative abilities of nerve cells, an energy deficiency of any duration can have long-term implications for both functional and structural integrity.

Primary energy sources

The brain, like the rest of the body, obtains its chemical energy by the oxidation of foodstuffs. The energy derived from this oxidation is stored in a utilisable form as high-energy phosphate in molecules of adenosine triphosphate (ATP). The primary energy source of the central nervous system (CNS) is glucose, and in this the brain differs from other tissues which are able to utilise lipids and, to a lesser extent, protein. There is little storage of either lipid or glycogen. The glycogen content of brain is only 2–4 µmol/g and therefore the metabolism of the brain cannot be sustained by its carbohydrate reserves. Consequently, it is dependent on a constant blood-borne supply of glucose. Under normal conditions, the brain utilises approximately 16–20 µmol of glucose per gram of brain per hour and cessation of the blood supply of glucose and oxygen results in loss of consciousness within less than 10 seconds (the time taken to consume the oxygen within the brain and its blood) and irreversible brain damage within minutes.

In nutritional studies, a commonly used index for estimating the proportion of fat and carbohydrate being utilised is the respiratory quotient (RQ; calculated by dividing the volume of carbon dioxide produced by the volume of oxygen consumed). The RQ for fat oxidation is 0.71 and the RQ for carbohydrate oxidation is 1.00. The RQ calculated for the adult brain is 0.99. Under normal conditions, the amount of oxygen consumed in the brain is equivalent to that of the glucose removed from the blood (McIlwain & Bachelard 1985).

The normal arterial blood glucose concentration is approximately 80 mg/100 ml. When hypoglycaemia occurs, brain glucose consumption is reduced more than its oxygen utilisation and the total carbon dioxide produced by the brain can be increased to twice the basal level. Isotope experiments have shown that this increased carbon dioxide production is due to the oxidation of non-carbohydrate substrates, probably amino acids and lipids. As a result, hypoglycaemia may be associated with marked neurological manifestations, including convulsions. In insulin-induced hypoglycaemia the blood glucose concentration may fall to as low as 8 mg/100 ml and coma can result because, under these conditions, the reduced production of ATP is inadequate for normal brain function.

The pre-eminence of glucose as the substrate supporting the energy-requiring activities of the mammalian brain was first established over 50 years ago and remains unchallenged by more modern research. For recent reviews see Bradford (1986) and Sokoloff (1989).

Nervous tissue contains all the enzymes and metabolic intermediates of anaerobic and aerobic carbohydrate metabolism and is also able to utilise lipid and protein in vitro. The dependence of the brain on glucose as its primary energy source in vivo is due to the fact that the availability of other substrates is severely limited by the set of diverse homeostatic

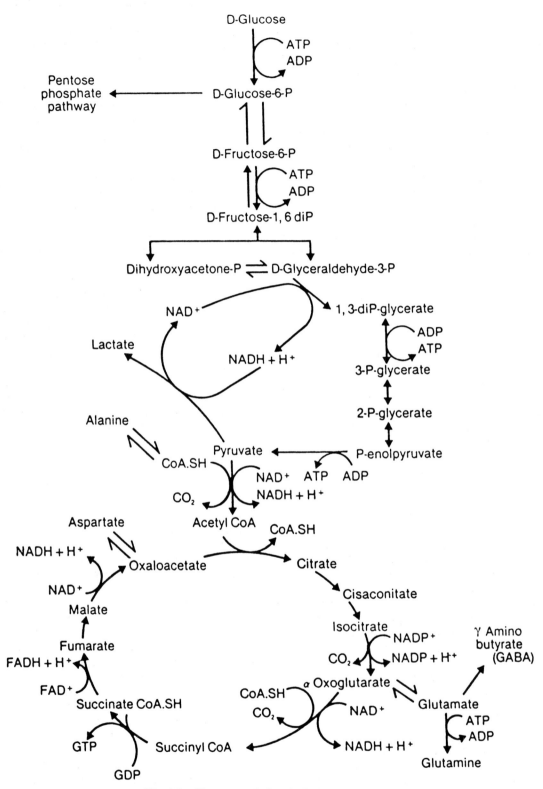

Fig. 8.1 Glucose metabolism in the brain.

mechanisms known as the blood–brain barrier. Whereas glucose has an unimpeded entry from the blood into the brain and rapidly reached tissue levels adequate for maintaining normal metabolism, the entry of fructose, lactate, pyruvate, succinate and glutamate is restricted and tissue levels comparable to those achieved by glucose are not reached.

The only modification to the view that the brain is essentially dependent on glucose is the realisation that certain other substrates may be used by the brain as energy sources if they are available in the blood at a sufficiently high concentration. For example, during the late 1960s it was discovered from observations on grossly obese persons subjected to total starvation for over 5 weeks that the brain is capable of maintaining its function by utilising certain ketone bodies such as hydroxybutyrate and acetoacetate. Under these conditions the RQ may fall as low as 0.63.

Glucose metabolism

The manner in which the potential chemical energy of glucose is captured and utilised for the synthesis of ATP in the brain is broadly similar to that in other tissues. It is achieved in three main stages. Firstly, glucose is converted to pyruvic acid by the glycolysis (Embden–Meyerhof) pathway in the cell cytoplasm. Although this glycolytic pathway is the main pathway of glucose utilisation, the pentose phosphate pathway is also functional and accounts for approximately 1% of the metabolic flux of glucose in human brain. Its primary role is to generate reduced coenzymes for use in biosynthetic pathways but the pentose phosphates it produces are also important for local nucleotide synthesis since, in the adult, there is a restricted entry of nucleotides from the blood to the brain. In the second stage of glucose breakdown, pyruvic acid is oxidised in the mitochondria to carbon dioxide via acetyl coenzyme A (acetyl-CoA) and the Krebs or tricarboxylic acid cycle. In the third stage, the electrons produced by the Krebs cycle enter the electron transport chain (flavoprotein–cytochrome system) where they are used in the reduction of oxygen. This process is coupled with the generation of ATP and is known as oxidative phosphorylation. A summary of glucose metabolism in brain is shown schematically in Figure 8.1.

ATP production

During glycolysis, direct transfer of high-energy phosphate from 1,3-diphosphoglyceric acid and phosphoenolpryuvate to adenosine diphosphate (ADP) results in the formation of two ATP molecules.

Under anaerobic conditions, therefore, there is a net synthesis of two ATP molecules since glucose breaks into two triose molecules, and two ATP molecules are used in the formation of glucose 6-phosphate and fructose 1,6-diphosphate. Under aerobic conditions, however, the reduced coenzyme nicotinamide–adenine dinucleotide (NAD) produced in the oxidation of glyceraldehyde phosphate is reoxidised through the flavoprotein cytochrome system, with the formation of three ATP molecules. Further oxidation of each pyruvate molecule to carbon dioxide and water via the tricarboxylic acid yields a further 15 molecules of ATP, i.e. a further 30 molecules per molecule of glucose. This ATP is produced by the reoxidation of reduced NAD, NAD phosphate (NADP) and flavin–adenine dinucleotide (FAD) by the electron transport chain, but ATP is also produced by reaction of ADP and guanosine triphosphate (GTP) formed in the conversion of succinyl CoA to succinate. Thus during the complete oxidative breakdown of glucose to carbon dioxide and water there is a net production of 38 molecules of ATP. This represents a theoretical efficiency of 42% in capturing the energy latent in the glucose. However, in practice, approximately 15% of brain glucose is converted from pyruvate to lactate and does not enter the Krebs cycle and therefore the net gain of ATP is nearer 33 molecules per molecule of glucose utilised (Clarke et al 1989).

Regulation: metabolism in relation to functional state

Anaerobic metabolism of glucose, yielding as it does a mere two molecules of ATP, cannot supply the energy requirements of normal cerebral function and, as a consequence, the brain is very dependent on the efficient working of the Krebs cycle. This dependence is reflected in the neurological dysfunctions which can ensue as a consequence of interference with its normal operation. Deficiency of thiamine, a cofactor in the conversion of pyruvate to acetyl-CoA, has profound effects on the CNS as does a deficiency of niacin (required for NAD synthesis). However, carbohydrate metabolism in brain is relatively insensitive to a number of factors that have pronounced effects on other organs. Thyroid hormones have been shown to have no effect on the cerebral respiration rate in the adult human although the development of the adult pattern of cerebral glucose metabolism is retarded after neonatal thyroidectomy. There is even doubt whether insulin affects glucose transport and utilisation in nervous tissue directly, although there have been reports that insulin does facilitate the entry of glucose in nervous tissues.

Cerebral carbohydrate metabolism exhibits considerable flexibility to supply energy according to functional need. For example, during anaesthesia glucose utilisation is of the order of 0.15 mmol/kg/min but during convulsions utilisation can increase to more than 10 mmol/kg/min. Such flexibility in the cerebral metabolic rate is possible because cerebral glucose metabolism is regulated at a number of different levels: by changes in cerebral circulation; by changes in glucose transport from the blood; and by changes in the rate of individual enzyme reactions brought about by environmental influences on the activity of key regulatory enzymes such as the glycolytic enzymes hexokinase and phosphofructokinase. Energy output and oxygen consumption in the brain are associated with high levels of enzyme activity in the Krebs cycle. The actual flux through the cycle depends on a number of factors: the rate of glycolysis and acetyl-CoA production which can 'push' the cycle, the activity of the pyruvate dehydrogenase complex which controls the rate of pyruvate entering the cycle, and the local ADP level, which is the prime activator of oxidative phosphorylation to which the cycle is linked. Another factor contributing to the flexibility in metabolic rate is the fact that the substrate levels found under normal physiological conditions are generally well below those required for maximum enzyme activities. For example, under normal conditions only half of the brain pyruvate dehydrogenase is active.

Although changes in cerebral metabolic rate occur during extremes of brain activity and a clear correlation between cerebral metabolic rate and level of consciousness has been demonstrated, it has proved more difficult to define metabolic correlates of more subtle changes in human brain activity. For example, attempts to demonstrate increased energy utilisation by the brain during periods of high mental effort (e.g. problem solving in mathematics) have failed, and no consistent changes in metabolic rate have been found in normal slow wave sleep or paradoxical (REM) sleep (Sokoloff 1989).

Cerebral energy metabolism and psychiatric disorders

Dementing illnesses like Alzheimer's disease, and other pathological states that lead to a progressive reduction in the level of consciousness, such as brain tumours, diabetic acidosis and coma, are associated with a measurable decline in the cerebral metabolic rate. However, most other psychiatric disorders (e.g. psychoses, neuroses and LSD-induced psychomimetic states) have only temporary or local effects on either cerebral blood flow or oxygen consumption. Similarly, anxiety or nervousness do not normally alter the cerebral metabolic rate although true panic attacks may be accompanied by an increase.

The γ-aminobutyrate (GABA) shunt

The metabolism of the adult brain is characterised by a high rate of incorporation of glucose carbon into free amino acids. In this respect the brain differs markedly from other organs such as the liver, kidney, lung, muscle and spleen. The explanation of this phenomenon is that the metabolism of certain glucose metabolites is closely related to that of the 'glutamate group' of amino acids. Members of this group (glutamate, aspartate and GABA) have a special role in the CNS and account for 75% of the free amino acids in the brain. They are found primarily in the grey matter and are associated with neuronal mitochondria. Glutamate, by its energy-dependent conversion to glutamine, plays an important role in the detoxification of ammonia in the brain and GABA functions physiologically as an inhibitory transmitter.

Aspartate and glutamate are glycogenic since they are readily and reversibly converted into oxaloacetate and α-oxoglutarate by transamination reactions. These reactions allow the extensive synthesis of non-essential amino acids from Krebs cycle intermediates and aid in regulating the concentration of metabolites entering this cycle. Another possible regulator of the Krebs cycle in the CNS is the metabolic sequence known as the 'GABA shunt' shown in Figure 8.2. This is a bypass around the cycle from α-oxoglutarate to succinate and accounts for approximately 10% of the total glucose turnover. Although this pathway is found at extremely low levels in some other tissues such as kidney, heart and liver it is, by far, most active in the brain. This is due to the relatively high levels in the CNS of the enzyme responsible for catalysing the decarboxylation of glutamate to GABA. This enzyme, glutamate decarboxylase, in common with the transaminase enzyme, requires vitamin B_6 phosphate (pyridoxal phosphate) as a cofactor. The importance of these interrelationships between the glutamate group of amino acids and glucose metabolism is illustrated by the deleterious effects of vitamin B_6 deficiency. Glutamate decarboxylase and transaminase inhibition caused by such a deficiency results in seizures. These seizures may be alleviated by the administration of GABA, suggesting that they are primarily due to the dysfunction of glutamate decarboxylase.

Earlier in this chapter it was noted that metabolic compartmentation is an important feature of brain metabolism. There is good evidence (Baxter 1976)

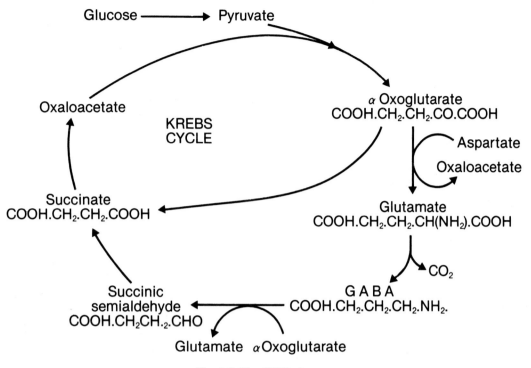

Fig. 8.2 The GABA shunt.

that this is true of the Krebs cycle and the GABA shunt. It is believed that there are at least two pools — one associated primarily with nerve endings and another associated primarily with glial cells.

THE BIOCHEMISTRY OF BRAIN DEVELOPMENT

Development of the nervous system proceeds in a series of interphased stages, commencing with embryological events and ending with maturity. These stages may be summarised as: organogenesis and neuronal multiplication; a maturation period (known as the 'growth spurt') during which there is axonal growth, dendritic arborisation, synaptogenesis, glial multiplication and myelination; and a period of generalised growth in size. The onset of these various events occurs at different times (in relation to birth) in different species.

In man the growth spurt (the time of the greatest rate of increase in the wet weight of the brain) commences before birth and extends for a period of up to 2 years after birth. Man is thus a perinatal brain developer. In contrast, the growth spurt of the rhesus monkey is predominantly prenatal, that of the guinea-

pig exclusively prenatal and that of the rat postnatal. The fact that rats are postnatal brain developers has proved to be convenient for the biochemical study of the growth spurt since during this most intensive period of development it can be easily subjected to various experimental procedures. Not surprisingly, a great deal of the early knowledge of the biochemistry of brain maturation (reviewed by Davison & Dobbing 1968) was obtained from studies using this animal.

Biochemical correlates of the principal stages of brain development

A variety of methods, including autoradiography, quantitative histology and the measurement of biochemical correlates of anatomical changes, have been used to elucidate the time-course of the main developmental stages. The advantage of using biochemical markers is that they permit a more quantitative assessment of the structural changes than is possible with most morphological techniques. Markers used have included DNA as an index of cell numbers, cholesterol and 2',3'-cAMP phospho-hydrolase as indicators of myelin, the 'protein/DNA ratio' as an indicator of cell size, acetylcholinesterase and gangliosides as indicators of nerve endings and synapses and the brain-specific protein S-100 as an indicator of glial cells.

Nucleic acid and lipids

DNA and cholesterol measurements have shown that in the rat, guinea-pig and pig the period of rapid deposition of lipid (i.e. myelination) is preceded by a peak rate of cellular multiplication (glial proliferation). Evidence from lipid biochemistry indicates that the period of neuronal multiplication and synaptogenesis also precedes myelination. Gangliosides are lipids primarily associated with neurones, plasma membranes and synaptic membranes and in the rat brain the rate of their biosynthesis is maximal approximately 12 days after birth. In contrast, the rate of biosynthesis of cerebrosides and sulphatides (major constituents of myelin) is maximal at approximately 22 days.

Application of similar techniques to human fetal and infant brain have indicated that the sequence of biochemical changes in man broadly resembles that in the rat brain, although the timing of the events in relation to the time of birth is different. However, in the rat brain there is a homogenous rate curve for DNA accumulation due to an overlap period of neuronal and glial multiplication, but the increase in DNA in the developing human brain is bimodal. The two peaks correspond to neuroblast proliferation between the tenth and 18th weeks of gestation and to glial multiplication between 3 and 18 months postnatally. Glial multiplication is followed by myelination, which proceeds rapidly for 4 years after birth but continues, albeit considerably more slowly, until 20 years of age.

Not all areas of the brain develop at the same rate. DNA measurements have shown that the cerebellum develops faster than other areas of the CNS, although some of its neurones divide at a later stage than in other brain areas.

Carbohydrate metabolism

In the fetal brain, glucose is metabolised exclusively by the glycolytic pathway. During the growth spurt of the developing brain the activities of the glycolytic enzymes remain relatively constant but the activities of the enzymes involved in the Krebs cycle increase markedly. In the rat their activity remains low until 10 days postpartum but thereafter increases steadily until maximum activity is attained at 40 days. During this period the mitochondrial content of succinic dehydrogenase and cytochrome oxidase increases four-fold. Changes of this type do not occur in the liver. The increased activity of the Krebs cycle during the brain growth spurt is necessary to fulfil the energy requirements of this period of heightened metabolic activity when anabolic processes such as RNA and protein synthesis are functioning maximally. For example, in the white matter of the brain the peaks in blood flow and metabolic rate coincide with the period of active myelination.

Studies in changes in cerebral circulation and metabolism in man have shown that a peak is reached at around 5–6 years of age when the oxygen consumption of the brain accounts for over 50% of total body oxygen consumption (see Sokoloff 1989).

Blood–brain barrier

In the adult, entry of many metabolites, including amino acids, is restricted by a blood–brain barrier (Pardridge 1977). There are indications, however, that the penetration of ions and metabolites from the blood into the brain is faster and less restricted in the neonate, and that the blood–brain barrier is either missing or considerably less effective in young animals. However attempts to demonstrate this by use of the dye trypan blue have failed; the idea that the blood–brain barrier is absent early in life and gradually develops is now discredited. The increased entry of metabolites such as amino acids is now held to be a reflection of metabolic activity and the activity of specific transport mechanisms.

Cell differentiation and synaptogenesis

The previous section summarised some of the biochemical changes that accompany the gross changes that occur during brain development. However, it did not address the key question — how does the elaborate network of specific connections between nerve cells develop? The adult human nervous system consists of a network of more than 10^{10} neurones and each neurone, typically, has of the order of 100 000 synaptic connections with other neurones.

The biochemical mechanisms underlying the development of the neuronal network are still far from being understood and their elucidation remains one of the most challenging tasks facing neurochemists. Most of our current knowledge in this area has come from the use of cell culture techniques. Although cell culture of vertebrate nervous tissues started as long ago as 1907, techniques have grown considerably in scope and sophistication during the last 30 years (Saneto & de Vellis 1987). This has been aided by parallel development of immunological methods (particularly monoclonal antibodies) which have met the need for molecular markers to enable the precise identification of cell types. Many cell cultures of developing nerve cells from vertebrate (and invertebrate) species are now available and, as a consequence, the neurochemical dissection of the development process has advanced considerably in recent years, revealing a growing range of regulatory molecules that participate in neural development.

Differentiation

The human genome contains approximately 10^6 genes but the number of synapses in the mature nervous system is approximately 10^{14} (10^{10} neurones each with 10^4 synapses). It follows, therefore, that it is not the genetic programme alone that determines the final structure of the neural network. The developing neurone migrates through numerous cell layers towards its target site where it becomes integrated as part of the mature organ. After reaching its final site each neurone begins to generate dendritic and axonal processes. This growth enables it to make and receive contacts from other cells. One theory, proposed by Sperry, is that each nerve cell acquires a particular genetically determined chemical identification and that specific macromolecules present on its surface, or released to its immediate environment, enable the cell to be recognised and either accepted or rejected. Although this hypothesis is by no means proven, there is, nevertheless, a growing body of evidence that both the migration and growth phases of neuronal development are mediated, at least in part, by chemical signals.

The existence of surface recognition molecules (termed cognins) has been demonstrated and a group of cell surface glycoproteins, known as cell adhesion molecules (CAMs), has been isolated. The best characterised of these is the neuronal adhesion molecule (N-CAM) discovered by Edelman. As its name implies, this molecule mediates cell-to-cell adhesion, thus fixing migrating cells in their correct place. N-CAM is a protein containing a substantial carbohydrate moiety, particularly polysialic acid. The polysialic acid content strongly influences the binding properties of the molecule but does not participate directly in the binding itself. N-CAM undergoes dynamic changes in amount, distribution and sialic content during development and various subclasses

appear at different stages of development. One such subclass is Ng-CAM, which appears on neuronal surfaces prior to glial differentiation and mediates the adhesion of neurones to glial cells. Although several dozen structurally related groups of CAMs are believed to exist, there is no evidence for the existence of the thousands of distinct CAMs that would be required by Sperry's chemospecificity theory to code for the unique neural addresses of developing neural processes.

The chemospecificity theory postulates that growth and differentiation of a nerve cell is stimulated by diffusible factors, known as trophic factors, which can be produced by its target organ, by one of its innervating neurones or by surrounding glial cells. In addition to their role in influencing the homing of the developing axons or dendrites on to their target, trophic factors also assist in the formation and stabilisation of specific synapses. Moreover, trophic factors are believed to influence cell survival and synapse formation in the mature as well as the developing nervous system.

The biochemistry of these trophic factors is not well defined and only a few have been isolated and chemically characterised. They can be proteins, ions (primarily Ca^{2+}, Na^+ and K^+), transmitters, metabolites or hormones. The best researched is the protein known as nerve growth factor (NGF), whose discovery by Levi-Montalcini and Hamburger in 1950 was a landmark in the history of developmental neurochemistry. This protein has been isolated from a variety of sources, notably from the submaxillary salivary gland of the male mouse and from snake venoms. Its structure varies depending on its source but, in essence, it is a zinc-containing complex with an active subunit of 118 amino acid residues. Unlike CAM it is a protein free of carbohydrate and lipid.

NGF is believed to regulate the differentiation, survival and target-oriented growth of nerve cells and its influences are thought to be initiated by the formation of complexes with specific NGF receptors in neuronal plasma membranes. Trophic effects on cell survival and development were demonstrated by experiments in which anti-NGF antibodies were added to cultures or injected into neonatal mice. In each case the NGF antibodies inhibited the formation of sympathetic ganglia. NGF has been shown to induce sympathetic neurones and basal forebrain cholinergic neurones to undergo biochemical and morphological differentiation, including neurite growth and changes in anabolic activity. There is also considerable evidence that NGF can guide neurite outgrowth; for example, neurites grow up an artificial

NGF concentration gradient. NGF also stimulates protein phosphorylation but no causal relationship between this effect and its physiological functions has been demonstrated. The mechanism of action of NGF within the cell remains unknown.

There is evidence to suggest that NGF is but one of a series of trophic factors that affect the development of neurones. Its action is primarily on adrenergic neurones, and other trophic factors are believed to exert similar influences on the growth of other neuronal cell types. The biochemical aspects of neuronal development are reviewed by Edelman (1985) and Arenander & de Vellis (1989).

Synaptogenesis

When growing axons reach their target cells, axonal elongation ceases and synapse formation commences. The mechanisms underlying synaptogenesis remain far from clear. It is known that it is not dependent on the electrical activity of the cells involved, nor is it conditional on the presence of transmitters, active receptors or Ca^{2+}. However, it is known that, at a specific time in embryonic development, 50–80% of neurones die. This observation led to the so-called 'cell death hypothesis' (Changeux & Danchin 1976), which postulates that all neurones which do not form permanent synaptic contacts die and that there is a trophic factor, transported retrogradely from the synapse, which is necessary for the stabilisation of the cell. This selective stabilisation of the 'correct' synapses may partly explain the specificity of synaptic connections. An alternative hypothesis is that specific macromolecules on the axonal surface provide recognition sites complementary to those on the postsynaptic membrane. The identity of these macromolecules is, at present, unknown but it is possible that they may be related to the cognins and N-CAM described earlier.

Factors influencing brain development

Malnutrition

The incidence of protein and calorie deficiency in human infants is widespread and it has been long established that this deficiency is associated with impaired intellectual function. Undernutrition is the commonest cause of mental retardation and worldwide over 100 million children are believed to be at risk (Davison 1977). As early as the beginning of this century it was discovered that the brain weight of rats was barely affected by undernutrition after weaning, but undernutrition during the period from birth to the time of weaning resulted in brain weights well below normal. Furthermore, the brain weights of rats underfed before weaning did not return to normal even if the rats were subsequently well nourished. In more recent times these observations have been confirmed in other species, including man, and extended by the use of neurochemical techniques. For example, the brains of human children who suffer from undernutrition during the early postnatal period have significantly less DNA than those who are adequately fed. Furthermore, undernutrition instituted during the period of active myelination permanently reduces the brain myelin content, whereas the myelin content of the adult brain is largely unaffected by starvation.

It is clear from such findings that the period of fastest developmental change (i.e. the 'growth spurt') is one of heightened vulnerability. In the human this 'vulnerable period' extends to 2 years after birth and field studies have confirmed that malnutrition during the first 2 postnatal years, but not later, can result in irreversible intellectual deficit and a smaller brain weight. In addition to affecting glial multiplication and myelination, malnutrition during the growth spurt reduces neuronal connectivity by interfering with dendritic arborisation and synaptogenesis. The brain areas that develop the most rapidly after birth are often especially vulnerable — particularly the cerebellum. The principal effects of malnutrition are believed to be disturbances in the balance of essential amino acids (thus interfering with protein synthesis) and an interference with the phasing of the cell generation time due to a reduction in the rate of DNA synthesis. These and other effects of malnutrition on the developing nervous system have been reviewed in detail by Dobbing (1981).

Toxic chemicals and disease

Malnutrition is but one of many factors that can produce irreversible changes during the vulnerable period of brain development. The developing brain is particularly susceptible to the effects of neurotoxic chemicals such as lead and certain CNS-active drugs such as the phenothiazines (Nelson 1985). Many inborn errors of metabolism produce their most deleterious effects during this period. Both phenylketonuria and leucinosis can produce severe mental retardation, but this can be avoided if during the early postnatal period the abnormally high concentrations of phenylalanine and leucine are reduced and low levels maintained by dietary restriction. High concentrations of phenylalanine have relatively little effect on the highest mental functions in adults.

Hormonal and environmental influences

Hormonal imbalances arising during the vulnerable period can result in permanent damage whereas, in the adult, mental changes produced by endocrine dysfunction are generally reversible. Exposure of rats or mice to steroid hormones during the first few days of life results in permanent effects on proliferation and differentiation of the CNS. For example, androgens exert a permanent masculinising influence on the developing brain (Balazs 1984). Of particular importance is the functioning of the thyroid gland. Thyroid deficiency during the vulnerable period leads to severe physiological, biochemical and behavioural effects. Neonatal hypothyroidism lowers the rate of cell proliferation, reduces average size and causes defective myelination. It also interferes with the development and organisation of neuronal processes, leading to a reduction in the number of interactions between neurones and a reduction in the electrical activity of the brain. The actions of thyroid hormones at the metabolic level have been extensively investigated and it is believed that they exert their primary influence by stimulating synthesis of specific proteins in almost all cell types (for a review see Nunez 1984).

The structural and functional organisation of the developing CNS is also very sensitive to environmental influences. Electrical activity begins in the brain well before the greater part of its substance has been synthesised and during its developmental period the brain is, therefore, receiving sensory input and other signals from the rest of the body. Reference has already been made to the fact that the genetic programme alone cannot account for the final structure of the neural network. For example, information theorists have calculated that to specify all the connections between individual retinal elements and individual cortical cells would require more information than could be represented in the neuronal DNA.

There is abundant evidence that environmental inputs during development increase synaptic complexity (see Bailey & Chen 1988, Greenough & Bailey 1988). There is also evidence that lack of environmental stimulation has the reverse effect. Thus, rats and mice reared in the dark have a reduced number of spines on the apical dendrites of their visual cortex pyramidal cells. The neurons of the outer layer of the visual cortex are also more closely packed and there is an alteration in their neurophysiological recognition properties. Similarly, the brains of rats kept in isolation in a severely restricted environment have a lower cortical weight, protein content and acetylcholinesterase activity compared with those of rats reared in conditions of environmental complexity and constant behavioural stimulation. Sudden changes in environment during the neonatal period, e.g. exposure to electric shocks or temperature extremes, can also exert profound effects on brain development and significantly influence subsequent behaviour.

THE BIOCHEMISTRY OF MEMORY

Memory is the capacity to receive, store and retrieve information. It is a general property of living things and exists in a number of forms, including genetic, epigenetic, immunological and neuronal. Neuronal memory is one of the fundamental brain functions and the mechanisms involved have intrigued neuroscientists for many years. In addition to the potent stimulus of man's desire to understand how his own mind works, the study of memory mechanisms has been motivated by important biomedical implications. With the ageing of the population, memory deficits and disorders are becoming increasingly significant as medical problems.

From studies of retrograde memory disruption experimental psychologists have inferred that there are two main stages in the process of memory storage. Between the registering of a new experience and its storage there is a period of variable duration known as short-term memory. During this period (which lasts for approximately 30 seconds to 1 minute) the record is very labile and easily abolished by anoxia, concussion, electroshock, epileptic fits, anaesthesia or indeed anything that tends to disrupt the electrical activity of the brain. At some stage, however, this labile record may be (but is not invariably) consolidated into a more durable form known as long-term memory, which is resistant to treatments that disrupt electrical activity. These observations suggested that short-term memory was primarily an electrical phenomenon, whereas long-term memory had a structural — and hence chemical — basis. This, however, is too simplistic. Advances in neurophysiology have now shown that long-lasting electrical changes can occur in the brain (e.g. heterosynaptic facilitation) and modern biochemical techniques have now made it possible to detect very rapid biochemical changes occurring within nanoseconds (e.g. phosphorylation of enzymes). There is also evidence that there is an intermediate stage between short- and long-term memory known as labile memory (Gibbs & Ng 1977). It is now believed that each stage is likely to have electrical and chemical consequences, although their precise nature is far from being understood. The search for a biochemical basis of memory has been pursued with considerable enthusiasm for more than 40 years and has passed through many phases and fashions influenced by the state of biochemistry at the time. In the 1940s and early 1950s came the dramatic advances in molecular biology that led to the understanding of how the genetic information of living cells is stored in the cell nucleus in the form of DNA, how it is transcribed into RNA and how it is translated into protein. The realisation that the genetic memory was stored in coded form in a macromolecule and that proteins stored immuno-logical memory in their amino acid sequence inspired the idea that neuronal memory could be stored in a similar way, i.e. as a stable informational macro-molecule. Since DNA is stable in non-dividing cells and the neurones of the brain do not divide, DNA was ruled out as the memory molecule. RNA and protein appeared to be more likely candidates since they can be synthesised according to the needs of the cell. Furthermore the brain (and particularly the neurones of the brain) possesses a rate of RNA and protein metabolism comparable to that which occurs in rapidly dividing cells and exocrine cells.

Since the 1950s there has been a considerable body of research relating to the role of RNA and proteins (and, latterly, peptides also) in memory formation. Most investigators have addressed the mechanism of behavioural memory, i.e. the enhanced performance of an experimental subject in a defined task as the result of past experience. The problems inherent in such studies should not be underestimated. A particular difficulty is the design of adequately controlled experiments since learning is only one aspect of the behavioural response to a particular situation. Others include sensory stimulation, arousal, locomotor activity and stress — all of which have metabolic correlates. The problem is to isolate the chemical events specifically associated with learning.

Past studies can be separated into two principal categories: the correlative and the interventive. In the former, animals are subjected to a learning task and biochemical changes resulting from the learning are sought — usually, but not invariably, using radio-isotopic precursors. Many different learning para-digms have been employed, including transfer of handedness (Hyden & Lange 1979), light and shock

avoidance (Glassman 1969) and imprinting in chicks (Rose 1980). In the interventive approach, agents known to affect specific biochemical actions are administered and the effects on learning examined. Interventive agents used have included various inhibitors of protein synthesis (e.g. cycloheximide, puromycin, acetoxycycloheximide and anisomycin), inhibitors of RNA synthesis (e.g. actinomycin), antibodies to specific brain proteins and neurotransmitter agonists and antagonists (Agranoff 1980). A particular problem of the interventive approach is that agents of this type can have adverse effects on the general health of the animal that can significantly affect the ability of the animal to learn. A third category of investigation which may be regarded as a form of positive intervention is so-called transfer experiments. In these, certain active principles are extracted from the brain of trained animals and injected into untrained animals with the aim of transferring the memory of the training. Putative active principles have included RNA and peptides. It was claimed, for example, that dark avoidance training in rats could be transferred in the form of a peptide called scotophobin (Ungar 1974).

There is a voluminous literature resulting from such studies. Unfortunately, particularly in the mid 1960s, the biochemistry of memory became a somewhat fashionable 'bandwagon' and a number of extravagant claims were made on the basis of experiments that were either incapable of replication or so poorly controlled as to be uninterpretable. There is now a far greater awareness of the potential pitfalls and the more recent literature on the subject is considerably more critical. For detailed surveys of this work and some insights into the controversy surrounding it see Dunn (1980) and Kometiani et al (1982) and the representative references cited above.

Intraneuronal versus interneuronal memory hypotheses

It is now generally agreed that there is convincing evidence that RNA and protein metabolism have an important role in learning and memory. However, in spite of past claims that certain types of learning result in the synthesis of specific RNAs, specific proteins (such as the S-100 protein) and specific peptides (such as scotophobin) there is still no convincing evidence to support the view that individual memories are embodied in individual coded macromolecules. Intraneuronal memory hypotheses that postulated the existence of such memory molecules have now been largely superseded by interneuronal hypotheses that propose that information storage in the brain is accomplished by alterations in connectivity in neuronal pathways. Changes in neuronal connectivity can be produced by the formation of new synapses, by the reconstitution of pre-existing synapses or by functional changes in synapses. According to these interneuronal hypotheses, the changes in RNA and protein metabolism that were shown to occur in many correlative and interventive studies were simply biochemical correlates of these connectivity changes. This type of hypothesis need not postulate the existence of a large number of 'memory proteins'.

A major stimulus for the shift in emphasis from the intraneuronal to the interneuronal type of memory hypothesis has been the progress in the understanding of the sequence of biochemical reactions underlying synaptic transmission that has occurred during the past 20 years and the growing appreciation of the role of neuropeptides and neurotransmitters and modulators of brain function and behaviour. As a consequence of these advances, studies of the biochemistry of memory broadened in scope and increased considerably in sophistication during the 1980s. Of particular note has been the series of elegant experiments on the gill withdrawal reflex of the mollusc *Aplysia* (Camardo et al 1984) and the investigations of light avoidance in another mollusc, *Hermissendas* (Farley & Alkon 1985). On the basis of these and other studies, it is now clear that many different biochemical processes are involved in learning and memory — both short-term and long-term. Transient changes during the learning experience itself include alterations in localised metabolic rates, precursor utilisation, ion fluxes, levels of internal cell messengers such as cyclic adenosine monophosphate (cAMP) and phosphoinositides and the activities of enzymes associated with RNA synthesis and neurotransmitter metabolism. More lasting biochemical changes include localised alteration in the absolute amounts and turnover rates of membrane proteins and enzymes believed to be associated with connectivity changes.

Short- and long-term memory have been described as information-containing states analogous to a latent image in a film and a finished photograph (Agranoff 1980). Much of the experimental evidence is compatible with the view that the 'latent image' is maintained by a transient enhancement in the responsiveness to neurotransmitters of postsynaptic receptor sites, and that fixation of this image is achieved by the production of increased amounts or different types of membrane constituents that modify both pre- and postsynaptic properties more perma-

nently. There is growing evidence from studies on simple learning paradigms in molluscs that an important element in the permanent modification of membrane properties is the phosphorylation of membrane proteins — this phosphorylation being mediated by the cAMP-dependent enzyme protein kinase.

Long-term potentiation

Much of the work in this field has used reductionist models for learning in non-mammalian species. This is because very little is known about the neuronal circuitry involved in learning in mammals and this makes the study of its biochemistry extremely difficult. However, there are reasons for believing that the hippocampus is important in at least some types of memory. In 1973 it was found that if electrodes are implanted in one of the pathways leading into the hippocampus and given short bursts of high-frequency stimulation, the connections between that pathway and the area it communicated with are strengthened for several weeks or more. This long-lasting increase in the efficacy of a specific set of synapses is called long-term potentiation (LTP). Initially, LTP was merely regarded as an interesting phenomenon, but during the last decade it has become apparent that LTP could be the substrate of associative learning.

This stemmed from the discovery that LTP depends critically on the activation of *N*-methyl-D-aspartate (NMDA) receptors, one of the three types of receptors in the hippocampus that respond to the excitatory neurotransmitter glutamate. If NMDA receptors are blocked by the selective antagonist aminophosphonovaleric acid (AP5), this not only prevents LTP but also inhibits learning. AP5 has no effects on normal synaptic transmission or normal behaviour. However, when it is infused into the lateral ventricle close to the hippocampus of rats being trained to escape from a tank of opaque water (by swimming to a hidden underwater platform), it prevents the rats from learning a skill that control rats learn with little difficulty (Morris 1989). It also impairs acquisition, but not retention, of olfactory memory.

LTP is associated with an increase in intracellular calcium ions, but how this elevated Ca^{2+} leads to LTP is not clear. One hypothesis is that it stimulates a Ca^{2+}-activated protease (calpain) which degrades certain cytoskeletal elements, thus altering receptor distribution. LTP is also known to be associated with long-lasting changes in the structure of specific proteins in the synapse and these are brought about by protein kinase-mediated protein phosphorylation (Feasey et al 1986). Protein kinase is known to be stimulated by Ca^{2+}. The involvement of protein kinase in memory formation is now being intensively investigated and has recently been reviewed by Bank et al (1989). In addition to its role in LTP, it has been shown to have a role in a number of experimental learning paradigms, including the molluscan system referred to earlier and imprinting in chicks (Burchuladze et al 1990).

Current status of research and its applications

In spite of considerable progress we are still a long way from explaining the molecular basis of memory. This will require the identification of all the biochemical processes involved in encoding, the identification of the location (both within the cell and within the brain) of the code and a demonstration of how the code is involved in the events of recall. One particularly important question is the identity of the protein(s) whose production renders memory-related synaptic changes permanent. It is hoped that the availability of advanced antibody techniques and the use of genetic probes will assist in tracing these. In addition, much work is needed to clarify the roles of ion fluxes and protein phosphorylation.

It may be concluded from the above that we are not yet in a position to design drugs, on a rational basis, for dealing with specific memory disorders, although there are a number of potential leads that are receiving attention from pharmaceutical companies. Currently, there are over 160 cognition enhancers in development worldwide.

The study of the biochemical basis of memory has, over the years, produced many suggestions for 'memory drugs'. Most of these, including the idea of using RNA or protein extracts to improve memory, have been long discredited. However, some may still prove of value. It is known, for example, that adrenocorticotrophic hormone (ACTH) and other pituitary hormones are involved in the learning process and that certain neuropeptides have the ability to block the extinction of a learned task and may contribute in some way to the fixation of long-term memory. There is some evidence that neuropeptides such as vasopressin can improve recall in elderly patients and that certain fragments of the ACTH molecule can enhance short-term memory (De Wied & Gispen 1977).

The main focus of attention at present is on cognitive enhancers that act via an effect on neurotransmitter systems. Many screening programmes have employed a test system in which a behavioural deficit produced by one agent is reversed by a candidate drug. In such a system it was demonstrated that cholinergic agonists such as physostigmine can relieve the amnesia induced by scopolamine. However, these test systems are highly artificial and their results must be treated with caution. Increasingly sophisticated strategies (e.g. biochemical; see Briley 1990) are now being employed in the search for cognitive enhancers and some successes, backed up by clinical trials on forgetful elderly people, are being claimed. A recent example is Glaxo's drug ondansetron, which is believed to block the action of serotonin and enhance the release of acetylcholine. Nevertheless, this field remains a very controversial one and many authorities remain unconvinced of the validity of the claims made.

NEUROTOXICITY

General introduction

The nervous system, as a consequence of its role as a supervising system, its unique metabolic properties and its low capacity for regeneration, is particularly susceptible to toxic insult. Many toxic substances have either primary or secondary effects on the nervous system and, in view of the immense diversity of potential targets for chemicals within the complex structure and functions of the nervous system, it is not surprising that there is an enormous variety of symptomatology associated with neurotoxicity. This ranges from gross neurological damage to subtle changes of a purely functional nature (Table 8.1).

Classification

Neurotoxic effects may be acute or chronic. Acute neurotoxicity is generally due to functional changes in the nervous system and usually does not involve structural damage and degeneration of the cellular elements. Acute effects are usually reversible, occur after a single exposure and are commonly due to pharmacological effects on nerve cell membranes or neurotransmitter metabolism. In contrast, most chronic neurotoxic effects involve structural changes and degeneration of the cellular elements. They are not readily reversible and require repeated exposure. Chronic effects are usually due to metabolic lesions in the neurones and their axons or supporting cells such as Schwann cells and glia, or due to interference with cerebral blood supply. However, there are some exceptions — one important example being the

Table 8.1 Range of symptoms associated with neurotoxicity in man

- Motor disorders (e.g. weakness and incoordination of limbs, paralysis, fatigue, slurred speech, rigidity, tremor, convulsions)
- Sensory disorders (e.g. paraesthesiae in limb extremities, spontaneous pain, auditory deficits, tinnitus, visual deficits)
- Disturbances of autonomic function (e.g. impaired sexual function, impotence, postural hypotension, lacrimation, excessive salivation, sweating, incontinence, altered heart rate, vomiting, gastrointestinal disorders)
- Increase in the state of excitability of the CNS (e.g. hyperactivity, nervousness, agitation, irritability, hallucinations, euphoria, mania, seizures)
- Decrease in the state of excitability of the CNS (e.g. narcosis, lethargy, apathy, depression, repetitive stereotyped behaviour, coma)
- Impairment of short- or long-term memory, disorientation, confusion
- Psychosis
- Addiction
- Sleep disorders
- Impaired temperature regulation — hypothermia or hyperthermia
- Alterations in appetite, weight gain or weight loss

tardive dyskinesia that can result from prolonged phenothiazine therapy. This is clearly a chronic neurotoxic effect, but it is probably due to a functional change (dopamine receptor supersensitivity) rather than to any degenerative or structural change in the CNS. Many compounds are capable of exerting both acute and chronic neurotoxicity, but at different dose levels and by different mechanisms. One well-known example is n-hexane, a substance that has been intensively investigated because of the problems associated with glue sniffing. Exposure to relatively high doses of n-hexane for short periods results in a reversible narcosis, but exposure to far lower doses for a period of weeks leads to degeneration of peripheral nerves.

Mechanisms

Potential mechanisms of neurotoxicity are legion. Toxins may selectively interfere with: basic metabolic processes such as energy metabolism, lipid metabolism, and protein and nucleic acid synthesis; biochemical pathways responsible for myelin sheath maintenance; axonal transport; nerve membrane permeability or synaptic transmission. As knowledge in the neurosciences has grown, so has awareness of the number of potential mechanisms that may be

encountered. However, although a great deal is known of these potential mechanisms, understanding of the modes of action of many (even common) neurotoxins remains relatively meagre — particularly in the case of toxins that produce structural damage.

The effect of age

Age has an important influence on neurotoxicity. As noted above, the immature and developing nervous system has particular vulnerabilities to toxic insult, particularly during the period of cellular proliferation, myelination and synaptogenesis, and many chemicals not overly toxic to the mature system (e.g. inhibitors of DNA or cholesterol synthesis) may have grave effects on the developing nervous system. Some, such as lead, may affect both the mature and immature systems but do so in different ways. The ageing nervous system is also especially sensitive to some toxins such as manganese.

Neurotoxicity, medicine and psychiatry

A growing number of compounds are known to be associated with neurotoxicity. These include abused substances (notably ethanol, hexacarbon solvents in glues and narcotics), therapeutic agents (e.g. nitroimidazoles, vincristines, aminoglycosides and phenothiazines), products of living organisms (e.g. biological toxins), pest control products (e.g. organophosphates, pyrethroids), industrial chemicals, metals, food additives, fragrance raw materials and many other types of chemical encountered in the environment.

Until relatively recently, public concern and legislative activity has focused predominantly on possible carcinogenic effects of environmental chemicals but there are now signs that the importance of possible neurotoxic effects of chemicals is being more widely recognised. For example, during 1991, the US Environmental Protection Agency issued, for the first time, comprehensive testing guidelines for evaluating potential neurotoxic effects of pesticides. The need for physicians to be aware of the effects of the potentially neurotoxic chemicals now deployed in the environment, work place and in pharmaceuticals is also acknowledged in the growing number of publications in the medical literature that deal with neurotoxic disease (e.g. see Schaumburg & Spencer 1987).

Neurotoxic disease falls into a number of broad categories. Firstly, there is iatrogenic disease resulting from side-effects of therapeutic substances. An example already mentioned is the tardive dyskinesia resulting from prolonged phenothiazine therapy. Secondly, there is disease resulting from the abuse of known neurotoxic chemicals such as ethanol or by accidental over exposure to neurotoxic industrial chemicals such as organophosphates or mercury. The third category, and one where unequivocal identification is considerably more problematic, is the adverse effects attributable to more subtle exposure to neurotoxic chemicals in the environment such as lead or food additives. It is often extremely difficult to determine whether a symptomatic individual with an unclear history of chemical exposure has a neurotoxic disease or merely a coincident naturally occurring condition. A good example of this difficulty is illustrated by the recent debate surrounding the possible role of environmental toxins in the aetiology of Parkinson's disease.

The discovery of the toxin MPTP (1-methyl-4-phenyl-1,2,3,6-tetrahydropyridine), which produces a syndrome that is both clinically and anatomically similar to Parkinson's disease, has stimulated a search for structurally related environmental toxins that could have the same effect. A recent review of the available evidence (Tanner & Langston 1990) concluded that it is indeed possible that environmental toxins contribute to the development of Parkinson's disease, although other factors such as genetic or constitutional predisposition and ageing are also of importance.

Evidence that exogenous chemical factors may trigger neuronal changes of the type found in a number of important neurodegenerative diseases including Alzheimer's disease has come from prolonged and intensive study of a remarkable disorder (known as ALS/P-D) that has been found in three genetically distinct populations in the Western Pacific. This displays various clinical combinations of motor neurone disease (amyotrophic lateral sclerosis, ALS), parkinsonism (P) and progressive dementia (D). The evidence (reviewed by Spencer 1987) strongly suggests that this condition is caused by 'slow toxins' in food — in particular consumption of the toxic cycad seed. Findings of this type have given further impetus to the search for possible environmental agents that could have a role in the aetiology of Alzheimer's disease (Spencer 1990).

Space does not permit a detailed survey of a wide range of neurotoxicological problems so the remainder of this chapter will be devoted to two of the more important: the neurotoxicity of lead and the neurotoxicity of ethanol. The reader interested in a wider range of neurotoxic conditions is referred to the neurotoxicology texts of Spencer & Schaumburg (1980) and Blum & Manzo (1985). For a greater understanding of the many problems associated with the identification of, and testing for, neurotoxic effects the reviews by Dewar (1983) and Walum et al (1990) should be consulted.

Lead neurotoxicity

Lead is one of the most widely dispersed of all pollutants. The scale of its use, dispersion and accumulation, coupled with its known and postulated effects on health, make it unique among environmental pollutants. Lead is geologically more abundant that most other toxic heavy metals, and its ease of extraction has resulted in widespread industrial exploitation over the past 5000 years. As a consequence of the cumulative mobilisation of lead from buried ore into the ecosphere, air, water, food and soil are now heavily contaminated. Global anthropogenic emissions have increased nine-fold since 1900 to approximately 4.3 million tonnes during the 1970s. Ambient air lead concentrations in cities are now 10 000–100 000 times the 'natural' (i.e. preindustrial) level and the body burden of lead in man is now 100–1000 times greater than that against which we evolved as a species.

The biological effects of lead are wholly adverse; there is no evidence that it has any beneficial effects even at low concentrations. This toxicity is believed to arise from two main properties. A strong affinity for sulphydryl groups enables it to alter the tertiary structure of proteins and for this reason enzyme inhibition is a major feature of lead toxicology. In addition, the lead ion Pb^{2+} has the ability to mimic the ions of several essential elements, notably Ca^{2+} but also Zn^{2+}, Mg^{2+} and Cu^{2+}. These two properties enable lead to disrupt many essential metabolic processes. In addition to its neurotoxicity, lead also has adverse effects on haematopoeisis and on renal, hepatic, endocrine and cardiovascular functions.

The neurotoxicity of lead illustrates in microcosm the complexity of interactions between toxic chemicals and the nervous system: the diversity of mechanisms and sites of attack, the range of symptomatology, and the differences in response and sensitivity depending on age (Krigman et al 1980).

Lead poisoning in adults

Adult lead poisoning is now primarily an occupational disease but ingestion of contaminated illicit whisky is an important non-occupational cause in some areas (notably the south-eastern USA). Neurotoxic effects include encephalopathy and peripheral neuropathy. Encephalopathy is now rarely seen as a result of occupational exposure but abusers of lead-contaminated whisky can present with multiple seizures, mania, delirium, blindness, aphasia and dementia. In adults, peripheral neuropathy is a more sensitive indicator of lead neurotoxicity. Lead produces a predominantly motor neuropathy, the pathological changes being suggestive of a wallerian-type axonal degeneration, although segmental demyelination has also been suspected. Undetected lead exposure has also been implicated as a cause of a variety of diseases, including motor neurone disease, presenile dementia and amyotrophic lateral sclerosis. However, a causal relationship between these conditions and lead remains to be established.

A recent review of the effects of occupational exposure to lead (Roeleveld et al 1990) failed to find any epidemiological evidence of a relationship between such exposure and defects of the CNS in children. However, the results of animal experiments suggest that, potentially, occupational exposure to lead could have adverse effects on the developing brain of offspring.

Lead and children

That lead is a neurotoxin has been recognised since Roman times and the main features of its neurotoxicity to adults, following high levels of exposure, have been understood for over a century. Similarly, the sequelae of acute high-dose lead poisoning in children are well known. Such high exposures result in overt neurotoxic phenomena such as peripheral neuropathy and, more commonly, encephalopathy. Severe mental retardation or psychosis may be followed by lethargy, seizures, brain oedema and, eventually, coma and death. However, since the 1940s, there has been a growing realisation that young children are especially sensitive to lead (Lin Fu 1973).

The work of Byers and Lovel revealed that childhood exposure to doses of lead insufficient to produce clinical encephalopathy were nevertheless associated with a variety of deficits in psychological function, including poor academic achievement, behavioural disturbances and sensorimotor deficits. In the 1960s it was discovered that children consistently show higher blood lead levels than adults in identical environmental settings and that the distinction is most pronounced in children under the age of 5 years. This is a reflection not only of their distinctive behaviour patterns and their ingestion of lead-contaminated dust

and paint, but also of the fact that their intestinal absorption of dietary lead is higher (50% as opposed to 10%).

Fortunately, with the steps taken to phase out many of the sources of potential acute exposure (e.g. lead paints) the incidence of overt lead poisoning in children has declined markedly. However, during the last two decades, concern has shifted to the possible long-term effects of prolonged exposure to lower doses and considerable research effort has been devoted to investigating the possibility that subclinical levels of lead (i.e. levels producing no overt signs of lead encephalopathy) cause more subtle effects on the nervous system of children.

During the 1970s, a number of studies were conducted in the USA on children with blood levels in excess of 40 μg/dl. Many of these early studies were relatively crude and inadequately controlled but, in spite of some conflicting result, a review of the data (Rutter & Jones 1983) concluded that there was some evidence of an association between elevated blood levels of lead and neuropsychological deficits in children. In asymptomatic children with blood lead levels above 40 μg/dl there was on average a reduction in IQ of between 1 and 5 points.

Although findings of this type were controversial, they did contribute to a reduction in accepted safety levels and stimulated changes in the law to restrict the use of lead in petrol and other products. As these levels fell, attention became focused on potential effects of lead at even lower doses. With the search for ever more subtle effects, the importance of experimental design and methodology increased — as did the intensity of debate surrounding the findings and their interpretation. Methodological problems that have contributed to the controversy include the selection of methods for assessing exposure or internal dose, the measurement of the neuropsychological outcome with techniques of adequate sensitivity, the measurement and control of 'confounding factors' (i.e. factors such as social class that could either exacerbate or negate the effects of lead), obtaining a sample size large enough to enable statistical detection of small effects and the avoidance of biases in sample selection.

Much of the work in this area stemmed from the paediatric studies of Needleman and his colleagues. In 1979 they reported a series of studies in which the lead content of the dentine of deciduous teeth was correlated with IQ and the incidence of behavioural deficits. Dentine is laid down during the first 2 years of life and is therefore a good indicator of lead exposure during the critical period of brain development. Needleman found that children with high dentine lead concentrations achieved a mean IQ score on the Wechsler Intelligence Scale for Children approximately 4 points below that of children with low concentrations. Analysis of variance indicated that this difference could not be explained by any of 39 covariates such as age, sex, race, socioeconomic status or past medical history. In addition to a lower IQ, children with higher dentine levels had a higher incidence of negative ratings by teachers relating to 11 classroom behaviours, including hyperactivity, distractability, lack of persistence and lack of organisation.

Although findings of this type were corroborated in a number of other centres, doubts were still expressed concerning the methodology and, in particular, the control of confounding factors. Smith (1985), in her review of the cross-sectional studies of normal children with blood levels of 35 μg/dl and below, pointed out that body lead acts to a certain extent as a market for other socially disadvantageous factors; she concluded that in studies in which this is adequately controlled the functional effects of lead are so small that they cannot be detected with any certainty and that 'they may not exist at all'. A well-controlled UK study conducted by Smith and her colleagues in 1983 failed to demonstrate a significant relationship between lead in dentine and intelligence.

In spite of doubts such as these, reports of the effects of low-level lead exposure continue to mount. Since 1985, studies using larger sample sizes and sophisticated multivariate analyses claim to have demonstrated effects on the IQ of children at blood levels as low as 10 μg/dl. In a recent review Needleman & Gatsonis (1990) subjected 24 major studies of children exposure to lead in relation to IQ to a 'meta-analysis' using statistical aggregation techniques and concluded that there was a strong link between low-dose lead exposure and intellectual deficit. Epidemiological studies by themselves cannot, however, establish causal relationships. Nor can cross-sectional studies disprove the alternative hypothesis that the neurobehavioural deficits are the *cause* rather than the *effect* of excess lead intake. There is, however, some further evidence that addresses these points. Briefly summarised, it is as follows:

- Recent prospective studies of lead exposure employing longitudinal designs and beginning at birth have shown that umbilical cord blood levels above 10 μg/dl are associated with decrements in IQ scores up to 2 years later (Bellinger et al 1991).
- In most modern studies the adequate control of confounding factors such as social class and

circumstances reduces the magnitude of the lead/IQ effect but does not eliminate it.

- The developmental effects of lead have been clearly demonstrated in animals and the lowest levels of exposure at which developmental neurobehavioural effects have been observed are broadly similar (10–15 μg/dl in children, <15 μg/dl in primates and <20 μg/dl in rodents) (Davis et al 1990).

The weight of evidence, therefore, suggests that there is some causal link between low-level lead exposure and intellectual deficit in children. In 1988 the Agency for Toxic Substances and Disease Registry in the USA concluded that children's risk of developmental problems is increased at blood levels of 10–15 μg/dl — well below the 'elevated' level defined in 1985 (25 μg/dl) and very considerably below the levels considered safe in 1978 (30 μg/dl) and 1970 (60 μg/dl). Nevertheless, the importance of social factors must be recognised. There is good evidence that children from less advantaged circumstances express deficit at lower blood levels than those from a higher social status and that they 'recover' less readily from deficits incurred as a result of prenatal exposure (Bellinger et al 1991).

In view of the controversy that has surrounded the more subtle neurotoxic effects of lead it is not surprising to find that no conclusive biochemical explanation for them has yet been established. There is, however, some evidence that GABAergic neurotransmission is very sensitive to lead exposure and that it is the GABAergic system that is involved in the earliest expression of lead neurotoxicity (Silbergeld 1985).

The neurotoxicity of ethanol and the biochemistry of alcoholism

Introduction

Abuse of ethanol (ethyl alcohol) has many consequences and is responsible for a considerable range of pathology both in the nervous system and elsewhere in the body. Neurotoxic disorders generally associated with alcoholism include direct toxic effects on the nervous system, effects related to withdrawal from alcohol, neurological syndromes associated with liver damage and indirect effects largely attributable to malnutrition and thiamine deficiency (such as cerebellar degeneration, peripheral neuropathy and Wernicke's encephalopathy). The active mechanism responsible for the absorption of water-soluble forms of thiamine in the intestine is inhibited by alcohol.

Large sums have been spent on research on the

biochemical mechanisms underlying these neurotoxic effects of alcohol with the aim of developing new and more rational approaches to treatment and prevention. However, a central problem has been the lack of relevant animal and in vitro models for study. Much of the work performed in the past has fallen into disrepute for its failure to employ appropriate models and to achieve and study pharmacologically relevant active concentrations. Although techniques of forced chronic alcohol administration that permit researchers to control the onset of tolerance and physical dependence in animals have now been developed, the problem remains that it is almost impossible to reproduce the human situation, i.e. self-administration of alcohol by choice. Nevertheless, despite the inherent methodological difficulties, basic research is now progressing rapidly and in the last few years there have been a number of significant developments, notably the discovery that doses of alcohol typical of those commonly consumed affect specific proteins in brain cell membranes. This is in contrast to much of the earlier work based on higher doses of alcohol that focused on effects on the membrane lipid bilayer. Research is now proceeding on a broad front and there are many conflicting hypotheses about the mechanisms underlying the various facets of alcohol neurotoxicity. There are also some grounds for cautious optimism that novel forms of therapeutic intervention may emerge from this research.

Mechanisms of acute intoxication

In some respects the acute intoxicating effects of ethanol resemble those of typical CNS depressants. As a class, CNS depressants are lipid-soluble and exert their action by entering neuronal membranes and interacting with their lipid and/or protein constituents. One long-standing hypothesis proposes that ethanol acts as a non-specific membrane perturbant, changing membrane fluidity.

This 'membrane hypothesis' goes some way to explaining why very high doses of ethanol act as a sedative or anaesthetic (and why ethanol is a less powerful depressant and anaesthetic than other more lipid-soluble alcohols and anaesthetics) but it does not account for the euphoria and anxiety reduction that it elicits at lower doses.

It has now been discovered that certain neuronal membrane-based proteins are particularly sensitive to low doses of alcohol. One such protein is a macromolecular complex comprising the GABA type A receptor (GABA$_A$R), the chloride ionophore protein and the benzodiazepine receptor (BZPR). GABA is the major inhibitory transmitter of the mammalian brain. Under normal physiological circumstances GABA activates the GABA$_A$R to cause an increased frequency of opening of the Cl$^-$ ionophore in the membrane, thus reducing the likelihood of nerve excitation by diminishing the ability of stimuli to induce membrane depolarisation. Benzodiazepine drugs further increase the frequency of opening of the Cl$^-$ ionophore when GABA is activating GABA$_A$R. Whilst screening for drugs which bind to the BZPR, the Swiss drug firm Hoffman La Roche discovered a compound, an imidazobenzodiazepine, RO15-4513, which selectively and potently reversed ethanol-induced sedation. It also prevented both the GABA-induced Cl$^-$ flux and the antianxiety and intoxicating effects of ethanol. This and other evidence strongly suggests that ethanol exerts its intoxicating effects via an action on Cl$^-$ fluxes associated with GABA$_A$R activation (Suzdak et al 1986).

The GABA neurotransmitter receptor complex is not the only system affected by ethanol, however. It is now clear from parallel investigations that, in addition to potentiating the inhibitory actions of GABA, ethanol inhibits the excitatory actions of glutamate by interacting with the N-methyl-D-aspartate (NMDA) receptor.

Mechanisms of tolerance and dependence

Tolerance is the diminished effect of a drug upon repeated administration. One contributory factor to the development of tolerance to ethanol is the adaptive metabolic responses in the liver. These include an increased rate of ethanol metabolism via the conventional NAD-dependent alcohol dehydrogenase route and activation of alternative pathways for oxidising ethanol, particularly the microsomal ethanol oxidising system (MEOS) (Jenkins & Peters 1978).

In addition to this metabolic tolerance in the liver, there is the development of tolerance within the CNS itself. This is a complex adaptive response involving neurones acting either individually ('cellular tolerance') or in an integrated manner ('learned tolerance'). Two theoretical types of cellular tolerance can be recognised: 'decremental tolerance' and 'oppositional tolerance'. In decremental tolerance the cell adapts in such a way as to lessen the effects of a drug but the changes do not produce any functional disturbance in its absence. In oppositional tolerance the response is achieved by active opposition to the effect of the drug (Littleton 1985). Most hypotheses seeking to explain physical dependence to ethanol assume that the signs and symptoms associated with withdrawal represent the consequence of oppositional tolerance in the absence of ethanol, i.e. an adaptation that may be appropriate in the presence of ethanol becomes a liability in its absence and a functional rebound in the opposite direction causes the withdrawal symptoms.

The nature of the neurochemical events underlying tolerance and dependence have been studied intensively and numerous parallel lines of investigation have emerged — each yielding its distinctive hypothesis and its body of supporting evidence. Some of these are reviewed briefly below.

Tetraisoquinolines (TIQs). One of the earlier hypotheses, dating from the 1970s, grew from the discovery that the primary metabolite of ethanol, acetaldehyde, undergoes condensation reactions with catecholamines to form TIQ derivatives. These have a structural similarity to morphine alkaloids and this led to the suggestion that TIQs formed following ethanol ingestion functioned as opiates and could contribute to the physical craving for ethanol in alcoholics. This line of thought has been pursued and there is evidence that TIQs act as agonists at the binding sites for the endogenous opiates enkephalins and endorphins. The possible role of TIQs and opioid peptides in alcoholism has been reviewed by Trachtenberg & Blum (1987).

The role of essential fatty acids (EFAs) and prostaglandins (PGs). Another significant line of investigation has been the possible role of EFAs and PGs in alcoholism. The major essential fatty acid in the diet is *cis*-linoleic acid. This is converted to γ–linolenic acid (GLA) by an enzyme known as Δ6–desaturase. GLA is then converted to dihomo-γ-linolenic acid (DGLA), which in turn may be stored in the form of membrane phospholipids or transformed into PGs. PGs have an important regulatory role in many systems and organs of the body and exist in two main series, one of which, the 1 series, is derived from DGLA as indicated below:

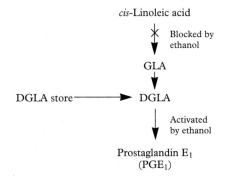

cis-Linoleic acid

Blocked by ethanol

GLA

DGLA store ⟶ DGLA

Activated by ethanol

Prostaglandin E₁ (PGE₁)

PGE_1 is of particular interest because it has profound effects on the nervous system and behaviour — effects that show marked similarity to those of alcohol.

Ethanol has been found to affect two steps in the metabolic sequence outlined above. Chronic alcohol consumption, both in alcoholics and experimental animals, inhibits Δ6–desaturase and hence the formation of GLA and DGLA from cis-linoleic acid. In contrast, studies using blood platelets have indicated that ethanol at clinically relevant concentration can enhance the formation of PGE_1 from DGLA by as much as 200%.

These and other findings have prompted a hypothesis to provide a biochemical explanation of alcohol tolerance and addiction (see Horrobin 1987). According to this hypothesis the acute effects of alcohol involve increased production of PGE_1. This increased production depends on a replete DGLA store. As DGLA stores become progressively depleted, ever increasing concentrations of alcohol will be required to achieve a given level of PGE_1. Alcohol tolerance could, therefore, be due in part to DGLA depletion. Similarly, a major cause of the acute withdrawal syndrome could be a precipitous fall in PGE_1 resulting from the depleted DGLA store being unable to maintain a normal PGE_1 production once alcohol stimulation has been removed. The finding that alcohol withdrawal symptoms in rats can be abolished by injection of PGE_1 is consistent with this idea. According to this EFA/PG hypothesis, alcoholics may drink to maintain a 'normal' PGE_1 level but this will require an increasing ethanol consumption as DGLA becomes depleted.

PGs often exert their effects by a common pathway by increasing the intracellular concentration of cyclic adenosine monophosphate (cAMP), a second messenger substance that affects many aspects of metabolism. An additional effect of ethanol that occurs at concentrations comparable to those found in heavy drinkers is a marked increase in the cAMP synthesis stimulated by PGE_1. This effect could stem from the ability of alcohol to increase the fluidity and disorganisation of cell membranes as PGE_1 binds to a specific receptor on the outside of the membrane. This activated complex then has to interact with the cAMP-synthesising enzyme adenyl cyclase which is positioned in the inside of the membrane. This interaction must occur through the membrane interior and could be facilitated if the fluidity of the membrane was increased by alcohol.

The role of the neuroadaptation. Since the mid-1980s, research into neurochemical mechanisms of ethanol tolerance and dependence has increasingly focused on effects on neuronal membranes and, in particular, on membrane proteins such as specific ion channels and receptors. To some extent this focus mirrors the explosive growth in this area of neurochemistry that has taken place over the same period. The resulting literature is, however, extremely complex with a bewilderingly wide range of effects being reported. Some insight into this complexity may be gained by reference to the reviews by Kuriyama & Ohkuma (1990) and Miller et al (1987) and to the comprehensive report on alcohol and health recently submitted to the US Congress (Secretary of Health and Human Services 1990).

Reference has already been made to the fluidising effects of ethanol on membranes and there is evidence that neuronal membranes become resistant to these fluidising effects after chronic exposure to ethanol. Increased membrane rigidity is an adaptive response and has been described as membrane tolerance. Recent work has indicated that a cellular trigger initiating this membrane adaption could be the activation of a membrane-bound enzyme, phospholipase C. This enzyme acts on specific components of membrane phospholipids, and this, in turn, could result in the structural modifications in the membrane lipid bilayer that account for membrane tolerance. More precise details of the stages in this cascade of molecular events are being sought; there are some indications that phosphatidylserine has an important role.

To date, several neurotransmitter/receptor systems, including the cholinergic system, the dopaminergic system, the serotoninergic system, the adrenergic system and the GABAergic system have been implicated in ethanol tolerance and dependence. There is also evidence that the neuropeptide arginine vasopressin (AVP) has a role both in the expression and maintenance of ethanol tolerance by interacting with one specific class of AVP receptors (VI receptors) in the brain. However, the recent insights into the mechanism of acute ethanol intoxication discussed earlier have led to a particular focus on the possible roles of the GABA system in tolerance and dependence. Since there is good evidence that the acute effects of ethanol are due at least in part to potentiation of the effect of GABA on Cl^- flux through the Cl^- ionophore, mechanisms are being sought which could produce the opposite effects (i.e. a reduction in the effects of GABA) to explain physical dependence. Possibilities would include a reduction in the number of $GABA_ARs$ or a reduction in the effects of GABA on Cl^- flux, but attempts to demonstrate

such effects have so far failed.

Consequently, attention has shifted to other forms of adaptation. Since the enhancement of the action of GABA on Cl^- flux reduces the ability of incoming stimuli to depolarize the neuronal membrane, one potential form of adaptation would be the restoration of neuronal excitability by an increase in the number of voltage-operated channels (VOCs) associated with excitability, i.e. either Na^+ or Ca^{2+} channels. Although there is no evidence that such changes occur in Na^+ channels as a consequence of chronic ethanol exposure, there is growing evidence that changes do occur in the voltage-operated Ca^{2+} channels (VOCCs).

There are three distinct groups of VOCCs in neuronal membranes. There are those that open at relatively low levels of depolarisation but open transiently (T channels) and those that require greater levels of depolarisation (N and L channels). The L channels open for a relatively long period (hence 'L') and therefore are attractive as a potential means of controlling the overall electrical excitability of neurones. An important piece of evidence for their involvement is the fact that calcium channel antagonists with a particular affinity for the L channel, such as the dihydropyridine (DHP) drug nifedipine, significantly delay the acquisition of tolerance in animals chronically exposed to ethanol (Wu et al 1987). Similarly, agents that block VOCCs reduce signs of alcohol withdrawal in both animals and humans, whereas agents that activate VOCCs induce a syndrome of seizures in animals similar to that produced by ethanol withdrawal.

Chronic ethanol exposure has been shown to produce an increase in VOCCs both in cell culture and in the brain. Furthermore, acute exposure of cultured cells to ethanol reduces the uptake of calcium, whereas prolonged exposure to ethanol increases it. This and other evidence strongly supports the view that the prolonged presence of ethanol in the immediate vicinity of neurones evokes, as an adaptive response, an increased sensitivity to agonists ('up-regulation') of the L VOCCs, and that this contributes significantly to the phenomenon of ethanol tolerance and dependence (Littleton 1989).

It will be recalled that ethanol also interacts with the NMDA receptor, thus inhibiting the excitatory actions of glutamate. There is now evidence that this receptor is also involved in tolerance and dependence. Chronic ethanol ingestion has been found to lead to up-regulation of the NMDA receptor — an action that would resist ethanol-induced inhibition. Chronic ethanol exposure might also affect the role of the

NMDA receptor system in memory through its effects on long-term potentiation. Long-term potentiation, as noted earlier, might be mediated via an NMDA receptor-activated Ca^{2+} flux. It is interesting to note that chronic ethanol exposure in rat model systems depresses long-term potentiation and that the effect is partially reversible following ethanol withdrawal. This may go some way to explaining a similar pattern of memory deficit and partial recovery in abstinent alcoholics.

Therapeutic implications

Until comparatively recently, treatments for alcohol abuse have been limited in scope. One approach has been the use of alcohol-sensitising agents such as disulfiram (Antabuse) and calcium carbimide to produce the unpleasant sensations associated with high blood acetaldehyde whenever ethanol is ingested. Disulfiram achieves this by reducing the activity of hepatic aldehyde dehydrogenase. Another approach has been to minimise the structural damage produced by chronic alcohol abuse by use of vitamin supplements, especially thiamine. As noted above, the active absorption of water-soluble forms of thiamine by the intestine is inhibited by alcohol. The use of passively absorbed fat-soluble forms of thiamine, such as thiamine propyldisulphide, is therefore a preferable option (see Madden 1985).

Useful though these treatments are, major advances are more likely to emerge from application of our increased understanding of the neurochemical mechanisms underlying ethanol-induced intoxication, tolerance and dependency. Although these mechanism are still not completely understood, some of the information already available is now being applied to devising novel forms of treatment.

One line of investigation is the search for an effective amethystic (sobering) agent. In the past, many of the agents suggested for this purpose were substances such as fructose that accelerated ethanol metabolism; unfortunately they have proved somewhat ineffective. With the discovery of the imidazobenzodiazepine RO15-4513 there is now the possibility of the rational design of drugs that interfere selectively with the molecular site of ethanol in the brain. There are, however, important ethical, legal and medical arguments against making an ethanol antagonist too readily available and the main purpose of such a drug would probably be in treating life-threatening overdoses (Littleton 1989).

The growth in knowledge of the factors involved in ethanol tolerance and dependency has also prompted attempts to develop new therapeutic approaches. For example, the EFA/PG hypothesis has led to a number of trials with agents such as γ-linoleic acid which modify EFA and PG metabolism and some success in ameliorating withdrawal symptons has been claimed (Horrobin 1987). Similarly, on the basis of the link between alcohol and opioid peptides, treatments designed to elevate levels of enkephalins and certain neurotransmitters have been used in alcohol detoxification programmes and beneficial effects have been reported (Blum et al 1988). However, one of the most exciting developments has been the recognition of the potential value of calcium channel antagonists in the treatment of alcoholism. In theory, calcium channel antagonists such as DHP could retard the development of ethanol tolerance and prevent the development of physical dependence (Whittington & Little 1988) although it is doubtful whether widespread prophylactic use of such drugs would be either feasible or desirable. It is in the suppression of the symptoms of withdrawal that the main opportunity lies, but this remains to be established in clinical trials.

REFERENCES

Agranoff B W 1980 Biochemical events mediating the formation of short and long term memory. In: Tsukada Y, Agranoff B W (eds) Neurobiological basis of learning and memory. Wiley, New York, pp 135–147

Arenander A T, de Vellis J 1989 Development of the nervous system. In: Siegel G J, Agranoff B W, Alberto R W, Molinoff P B (eds) Basic neurochemistry: molecules, cellular and medical aspects, 4th edn. Raven Press, New York, pp 479–506

Bailey G H, Chen M 1988 Long term memory in *Aplysia* modulates the total number of varicosities of single identified sensory neurones. Proceedings of the National Academy of Sciences of the USA 85; 2373–2377

Balazs R 1974 Influence of metabolic factors on brain development. British Medical Bulletin 30: 126–134

Bank B, LoTurco J J, Alkon D L 1989 Learning-induced activation of protein kinase C: a molecular memory trace. Molecular Neurobiology 3: 55–70

Baxter C F 1976 Some recent advances in studies of GABA metabolism and compartmentation. In: Roberts E, Chase T N, Tower D B (eds) GABA in nervous system function. Excerpta Medica, Amsterdam.

Bellinger D, Sloman J, Leviton A, Rabinowitz M, Needleman H L, Waternaux C, 1991 Low-level lead exposure and children's cognitive function in the preschool years. Pediatrics 87: 219–227

Blum K, Manzo L (eds) 1985 Neurotoxicity. Marcel Dekker, New York

Blum K, Trachtenberg M C, Ramsay J C 1988 Improvement of inpatient treatment of the alcoholic as a function of neurotransmitter restoration: A pilot study. International Journal of Addiction 23: 991–998

Bradford H F 1986 Brain glucose and energy metabolism: the linkage to function. In: Chemical neurobiology. Freeman, New York, pp 118–154

Briley M 1990 Biochemical strategies in the search for cognition enhancers. Pharmacopsychiatry 23: 75–80

Burchuladze R, Potter J, Rose S P 1990 Memory formation in the chick depends on membrane-bound protein kinase C. Brain Research 535: 131–138

Camardo J S, Siegelbaum A S, Kandel E R 1984 Cellular and molecular correlates of sensitisation in *Aplysia* and their implications for associative learning. In: Alkon D L, Farley J (eds) Primary neural substrates of learning and behavioural change. Cambridge University Press, Cambridge, pp 185–204

Changeux J P, Danchin A 1976 Selective stabilisation of developing synapses on a mechanism for the specification of neuronal networks. Nature 264: 705–712

Clarke D D, Lajtha A L, Maker H S 1989 Intermediary metabolism. In: Siegel G J, Alberto R W, Agranoff B W, Molinoff P B (eds) Basic neurochemistry: molecular, cellular and medical aspects, 4th edn. Raven Press, New York, pp 541–564

Davis J M, Otto D A, Weil D E, Grant L D 1990. The comparative developmental neurotoxicity of lead in humans and animals. Neurotoxicology and Teratology 12: 215–229

Davison A N 1977 The biochemistry of brain development and mental retardation. British Journal of Psychiatry 131: 5654–5674

Davison A N, Dobbing J 1968 The developing brain. In: Davison A N, Dobbing J (eds) Applied neurochemistry. Blackwell, Oxford, pp 253–286

Dewar A J 1983 Neurotoxicity. In: Balls M, Riddell, R J, Worden A N (eds) Animals and alternatives in toxicity testing. Academic Press, London, pp 229–283

De Wied D, Gispen W H 1977 Behavioural effects of peptides. In: Gainer H, Barker J L (eds) Peptides in neurobiology. Plenum Press, New York, pp 390–442

Dobbing J 1981 Nutritional growth restriction and the nervous system. In: Thomson R H S, Davidson A N (eds) Molecular basis of neuropathology. Edward Arnold, London, pp 565–577

Dunn A J 1980 Neurochemistry of learning and memory: an evaluation of recent data. Annual Reviews of Psychology 31: 343–390

Edelman G M 1985 Cell adhesion and the molecular processes of morphogenesis. Annual Reviews of Biochemistry 54: 135–169

Farley J, Alkon D L 1985 Cellular mechanisms of learning, memory and information storage. In: Rosenzweig M R, Porter L W (eds) Annual Review of Psychology 35: 419–494

Feasey K J, Lynch M A, Bliss T V P 1986 Long term potentiation associated with an increase in calcium dependent potassium-stimulated release of ^{14}C glutamate from hippocampal slices: an ex vivo study in the rat. Brain Research 364: 39–44

Giacobini E 1987 Neurochemical analysis of single neurons: a mini review dedicated to Oliver H Lowry. Journal of Neuroscience Research 18: 632–637

Gibbs M E, Ng K T 1977 Psychobiology of memory: towards a model of memory formation. Behavioural Reviews 1: 113–136

Glassman E 1969 The biochemistry of learning: an evaluation of the role of RNA and protein. Annual Reviews of Biochemistry 38: 605–615

Greenough W T, Bailey C H 1988 The anatomy of a memory: convergence of results over a diversity of tests. Trends in Neuroscience 11: 142–146

Horrobin D F 1987 Essential fatty acids, prostaglandins and alcoholism: an overview. Alcoholism: Clinical and Experimental Research 11: 2–9

Hucho F 1986 Neurochemistry: fundamentals and concepts. VCH, Verlaggesellschaft, FRG

Hyden H, Lange P 1979 Correlation of the S-100 brain protein with behaviour. Experimental Cell Research 62: 125–130

Jenkins W, Peters J J 1978 Mitochondrial enzyme activities in liver biopsies from patients with alcoholic liver disease. Gut 19: 341–344

Kometiani P A, Aleksidze N G, Klein E G 1982 The neurochemical correlates of memory. Progress in Neurobiology 18: 181–229

Krigman M R, Bouldin T W, Mushal P 1980 Lead. In: Spencer P S, Schaumburg H H (eds) Experimental and clinical neurotoxicology. Williams & Wilkins, Baltimore

Kuriyama K, Ohkuma S 1990 Alteration in the function of cerebral neurotransmitter receptors during the establishment of alcohol dependence: neurochemical aspects. Alcohol and Alcoholism 25: 239–249

Lin-Fu J S 1973 Vulnerability of children to lead exposure and toxicity. New England Journal of Medicine 289: 1229

Littleton J 1985 Biochemical pharmacology of ethanol tolerance and dependence. In: Edwards G, Littleton J (eds) Pharmacological treatment for alcoholism. Croom Helm, London, pp 119–144

Littleton J 1989 Alcohol intoxication and physical dependence: a molecular mystery tour. British Journal of Addiction 84: 267–276

McGrath J 1989 Psychiatry, molecular genetics and ethics: the new discoveries and the new issues. Australia and New Zealand Journal of Psychiatry 23: 67–72

McIlwain H 1990 Biochemistry and neurochemistry in the 1800s: their origins in comparative animal chemistry. Essays in Biochemistry 25: 197–224

McIlwain H, Bachelard H S 1985 Metabolism of the brain in situ. In: Biochemistry and the central nervous system, 5th edn. Churchill Livingstone, Edinburgh, pp 8–32

Madden J S 1985 What would a pharmacological treatment for alcohol dependence look like? In: Edward G, Littleton J (eds) Pharmacological treatments for alcoholism. Croom Helm, London, pp 197–218

Miller N S, Dackis C A, Gold M S 1987 The relationship of addiction, tolerance and dependence to alcohol and drugs: a neurochemical approach. Journal of Substance Abuse and Treatment 4: 197–207

Morris R G M 1989 Synaptic plasticity and learning: selective impairment of learning in rats and blockade of long term potentiation in vivo by the N-methyl-D-aspartate receptor antagonist AP5. Journal of Neuroscience 9: 3040–3057

Needleman H L 1990 Low level lead exposure: a continuing problem. Pediatric Annuals 19: 208–214

Needleman H L, Gatsonis C A 1990 Low level lead exposure and the IQ of children: a meta-analysis of modern studies. Journal of the American Medical Association 263: 673–678

Nelson B K 1985 Developmental neurotoxicology of environmental and industrial agents. In: Blum K, Manzo L (eds) Neurotoxicology. Marcel Dekker, New York, pp 163–201

Nunez J 1984 Effects of thyroid hormones during brain differentiation. Review of Molecular and Cellular Endocrinology 37: 125–132

Pardridge W M 1977 Regulation of amino acids availability to the brain. In: Wurtman R J, Wurtman J J (eds) Nutrition and the brain, vol 1. Raven Press, New York, pp 141–204

Reynolds G P 1988 Post-mortem neurochemistry of schizophrenia. Psychological Medicine 18: 793–797

Roeleveld N, Zielhuis G A, Gabreels F 1990 Occupational exposure and defects of the central nervous system in offspring: a review. British Journal of Industrial Medicine 47: 580–583

Rose S P R 1980 Neurochemical correlates of early learning in the chick. In: Tsukada Y, Agranoff B W (eds) Neurobiological basis of learning and memory. Wiley, New York, pp 179–191

Rutter M, Jones R R 1983 Lead versus health. Wiley, New York, pp 333–370

Saneto R P, de Vellis 1987 Neuronal and glial cells: cell culture of the central nervous system. In: Turner A J, Bachelard H S (eds). Neurochemistry — a practical approach. IRL Press, Washington, DC, pp 27–63

Schaumburg H H, Spencer P S 1987 Recognising neurotoxic disease. Neurology 37: 276–278

Secretary of Health and Human Services 1990 Seventh Special Report to the US Congress on Alcohol and Health. US Department of Health and Human Services, Rockville, MD

Silbergeld E K 1985 Neurotoxicology of lead. In: Blum K, Manzo L (eds) Neurotoxicology. Marcel Dekker, New York, pp 299–322

Smith M 1985 Intellectual and behavioural consequences of low level lead exposure: a review of recent studies. Clinics in Endocrinology and Metabolism 14: 657–680

Sokoloff L 1989 Circulation and energy metabolism of the brain. In: Siegel G J, Albers R W, Agranoff B W, Molinoff P B (eds) Basic neurochemistry: molecular, cellular and medical aspects, 4th edn. Raven Press, New York, pp 565–590

Spencer P S 1987 Guam ALS/parkinsonism–dementia: a long latency neurotoxic disorder caused by "slow toxins" in food. Journal Canadian des Sciences Neurologiques 14: 347–357

Spencer P S 1990 Etiology of Alzheimer's disease: a Western Pacific view. Advances in Neurology 51: 79–82

Spencer P S, Schaumburg H H (eds) 1980 Experimental and chemical neurotoxicology. Williams & Wilkins, Baltimore

Suzdak P D, Glowa J R, Crawley J N, Schwartz R D, Skolnick P, Paul S M 1986 A selective imidazodiazepine antagonist of ethanol in the rat. Science 234: 1243–1247

Tanner C M, Langston J W 1990 Do environmental toxins cause Parkinson's disease? A critical review. Neurology 40(suppl 3): 17–31

Trachtenberg M C, Blum K 1987 Alcohol and opioid peptides: neuropharmacological rationale for physical craving for alcohol. American Journal of Drug and Alcohol Abuse 13: 365–372

Turner A J, Bachelard H S (eds) 1987 Neurochemistry — a practical approach. IRL Press, Oxford

Ungar G 1974 Peptides and behaviour. International Review of Neurobiology 17: 37–60

Walum E, Hanson E, Harvey A L 1990 In vitro testing of neurotoxicity. ATLA 18: 153–180

Whittington M A, Little H J 1988 Nitrendipine prevents the ethanol withdrawal syndrome when administered chronically with ethanol prior to withdrawal. British Journal of Pharmacology 94: 385

Wu P H, Pham T, Naranjo C A 1987 Nifedipine delays the acquisition of tolerance to ethanol. European Journal of Pharmacology 139: 233–236.

9. Measurement in psychiatry

D. F. Peck

INTRODUCTION

At its current stage of development, psychiatry is seldom able to call on pathological services or on biochemical assays to provide quantified assessments of psychiatric conditions. However, some form of measurement is essential in any clinical discipline. Psychiatry, being predominantly concerned with a person's behaviour and subjective states, has largely relied on the methodology of psychological measurement.

Measurement in psychiatry has two main functions: to assist in making a diagnosis and to measure symptoms with a view to assessing change. This chapter will begin by examining some important basic concepts in measurement; it will then describe some standard measures of common disorders and give guidelines on how to devise new measures. It concludes by making some brief recommendations concerning measurement in psychiatric practice and research.

BASIC PSYCHOMETRIC CONCEPTS

Reliability

Reliability is concerned with how far errors of measurement have been excluded from an assessment. In particular, the question of reliability is often concerned with how far a test provides consistent results when apparently assessing the same characteristic under similar circumstances. Reliability can be measured in several different ways, of which the following are the most important in psychiatry.

Test–retest reliability. The same test is administered to the same people on two occasions, separated by a substantial time interval, usually of at least 3 or 4 weeks. The relationship between the two test results is expressed in terms of a correlation. This form of reliability is very commonly used, particularly when assessing stable characteristics. When assessing a characteristic which is expected to fluctuate (such as a psychiatric symptom), test–retest methods will provide an underestimate of reliability.

Alternative form reliability. Two alternative forms of a test are administered to a group and if they are measuring the same characteristic the correlation between them should be high.

Split-half reliability. Items in a test are divided into two halves (e.g. first half versus second half, or odd versus even-numbered items). If all the items are measuring the same characteristic a high correlation between the two halves can be expected. This is a measure of 'internal' reliability. Reliability is, however, partly a function of the number of items, and halving them this way may produce an underestimate. Use of the coefficient α helps to overcome this problem; it provides an estimate of the average correlation between all the items.

Inter-rater reliability. Two or more observers make judgements (e.g. about diagnosis, or children's interactions) based on the same material. Concordance between observers can be calculated in various ways, often in terms of percentage agreement, but also in the form of κ, a special type of correlation (Shrout et al, 1987) in which chance agreement is discounted.

Intra-rater reliability. This is similar to interobserver and to test–retest measures, except that observers base their judgements on the same material presented on two different occasions, normally using film or other audiovisual devices. Reliability is assessed by determining how far the two judgements by the same observer are in agreement.

The kind of reliability needed will be determined by the purpose of the measurement, but normally a measure of both temporal stability (e.g. test–retest) and of internal reliability (e.g. split-half) should be obtained. If a measure is to be used to make a judgement about an individual (for example in determining a diagnosis), reliability should normally be at least +0.70.

Validity

Validity is concerned with how far a test actually measures what it is supposed to be measuring, normally by reference to an independent external criterion. It is evaluated in several different ways in psychiatry, depending on the function of the test.

Face validity. This is the most basic but least satisfactory type, referring simply to whether a test looks as though it measures what it is supposed to measure; it is not reported statistically. For some purposes low face validity may be desirable, so that the patient is not so aware of what is being measured.

Sampling (or content) validity. When making a judgement, such as a diagnosis, on the basis of complex and wide-ranging information, care must be taken to ensure that the measure covers all aspects of the phenomenon being assessed.

Concurrent validity. A test is correlated with a concurrently available alternative measure of the characteristic being assessed. For example, a new anxiety scale may be compared with physiological measures of anxiety; or the scores of normals on a test may be compared with those of patients with a diagnosis of anxiety state, whose scores should be higher.

Predictive validity. This is one of the most critical forms of validity. Test scores are used to predict future behaviour (e.g. prognosis, or response to treatment). Correlations must be substantial (at least +0.70) to be useful in making decisions about individuals.

Incremental validity. This is closely related to the issue of utility and is concerned with whether the use of a test improves upon decisions that can be made from already existing information (e.g. base rates of a disorder) or from simpler techniques (e.g. patient self-rating).

The last two forms of validity are the 'acid test' or many measurements in psychiatry. However, they are often difficult and expensive to investigate, particularly predictive validity. Accordingly they are used less often than they should be.

To summarise, if a test (or any kind of measure) is to be used for categorising patients by comparing the individual patient's score with those of a reference group, one must ensure that the reference group sample is both large and representative. All measures should be investigated for reliability (external and interval) and for validity (at least concurrent, preferably predictive and incremental as well). Finally,

for decision-making about individual patients, the reliability and the concurrent or predictive validity should be at least +0.70.

It is not advisable to use any measure in clinical practice that does not meet these criteria, but research workers concerned with more theoretical issues may be content with lower levels. Whenever possible, the standardisation, reliability and validity data will be reported for the measures discussed in the following sections.

Advances in psychometric theory

Simple assessments of reliability based on correlation are useful, particularly in setting limits for validity, but they do oversimplify the situation; a measure may, for example, be reliable for males but not for females; or be reliable early in treatment but not later. It is more appropriate to ask under what circumstances and for what purposes a measure is reliable. Such considerations have led to *generalisability theory*, based on analysis of variance, in which the main sources or facets (and the interactions between them) which contribute to overall variability in a measure can be identified. For example, in recording the behaviour of mentally handicapped children, one could determine how much variability is accounted for by differences between the children themselves, the days of the week, the setting (e.g. ward versus playground), the occasions of observing and the observers, plus the interactions between these variables. Several forms of consistency are measured simultaneously and this represents a considerably more sophisticated approach to psychometrics. Unfortunately, the impact of generalisability theory on measurement of psychiatric problems has so far been slight, apart from its use in naturalistic observation (e.g. see Jones et al 1975). Latent trait theory is a further development which is increasingly being applied to psychiatric measures. Andrich & Van Schonbroeck (1989) used it to conduct a detailed analysis of the item structure of the GHQ (see later), which enabled them to highlight differences between the positive and negative items and to examine the detailed structure of the scale.

STANDARD MEASURES OF PSYCHIATRIC SYMPTOMS

Diagnostic instruments

Present State Examination (PSE) (Wing et al 1974)

The PSE is a semistructured interview with suggested probes for each symptom designed for use by experienced clinicians. It covers patients' symptomatology during the previous 4 weeks and abnormalities of speech and behaviour manifest during the interview itself. There are 140 items and each symptom is rated on a 3- or 4-point scale; there is a detailed manual giving definitions of the symptoms to be rated and indicating the levels of symptomatology required for each point on the scale. The interview takes at least 40 minutes, or longer if symptoms are acknowledged. Rigorous training in its use is recommended.

The PSE was originally designed for hospital patients but there is a short 40-item version for non-patient populations. The PSE does not collect the information necessary to diagnose alcoholism, personality disorder, mental retardation or organic states.

For the full version administered by psychiatrists, inter-rater reliability for symptoms is satisfactory with a mean κ of +0.77. Items covering depressive symptoms are generally reliable, whereas items covering anxiety are less so. Inter-rater reliability for items describing behaviour during the interview is not satisfactory, with a mean κ of +0.45. Reliability for most sections is about +0.70. Inter-rater reliability of the 40-item version using non-professionals as interviewers is lower, with a mean κ of +0.67 for symptoms (Cooper et al 1977). The mean value for test–retest is reported as +0.41 for symptoms and +0.37 for behavioural items.

The rules for making a diagnosis, using information from the PSE, have been incorporated into a computer program (Catego). In addition, a diagnosis from ICD-8 can be given.

In order to assess concurrent validity, Catego diagnoses were tested against clinicians' ICD diagnoses during the US/UK diagnostic project (Cooper et al 1972) and the International Pilot Study of Schizophrenia (IPSS; WHO 1973). In the IPSS project only 9% of diagnoses were discrepant (i.e. different clinical and Catego diagnosis).

Cooper & Mackenzie (1981) describe a ten-item version, which takes about 5 minutes, for use in community surveys. McGuffin et al (1986) describe the use of a past-history schedule (PHS) to be used prior to using the PSE. They also examine the reliability of the PSE in assessing past episodes as well as symptoms in the previous month. They report the inter-rater reliability for the Catego diagnosis of past episodes (κ = +0.87) and their dating (κ = +0.54 to +0.99) to be satisfactory.

Schedule for Affective Disorders and Schizophrenia (SADS) (Endicott & Spitzer 1978)

This is a structured interview which assesses symptoms on a 7-point scale. Generally speaking, a score of 3 or more on the scale for a symptom is regarded as clinically significant. Each symptom and the criteria for rating it are defined in the SADS interview schedule itself. The schedule also assesses any previous episodes. There are three versions: SADS, SADS-L (lifetime version) and SADS-C (change version). The SADS-L is most suitable for studies where there is no current episode of illness and the SADS-C where changes are being measured. The interview takes about 1–2 hours to complete, depending on the severity of illness. The SADS is mainly designed for use with hospital patients and covers most disorders, including personality disorders, drug and alcohol abuse and bipolar depression. The schedule is not useful for patients with organic states or anorexia nervosa. It is recommended that it should only be used by specially trained mental health workers. As regards inter-rater reliability, for 90% of the items this was +0.60 or better. For 82% of the items the test–retest reliability was at a similar level. On the whole, items with the lowest test–retest reliability were not key items.

The information obtained by using the SADS can be used to make a diagnosis on Research Diagnostic Criteria (RDC; Endicott & Spitzer 1979). The data for completing the Hamilton Rating Scale (Hamilton 1967), for making a Feighner diagnosis (Feighner et al 1972) or a Newcastle rating (Carney et al 1965) can also be extracted, permitting flexibility and facilitating comparison with other studies.

Clinical Interview Schedule (CIS) (Goldberg et al 1970)

This is a partially structured psychiatric interview which assesses ten reported symptoms during the previous week and 12 abnormalities manifest at interview, each on a 5-point scale. Psychotic symptoms are not formally assessed but are included amongst the 'manifest abnormalities'; this reduces the reliability of their assessment. A detailed manual gives definitions of all the terms and criteria for rating each item of the interview.

The interview was designed for community surveys rather than for use with psychiatric patients. It takes 10–20 minutes for normal individuals and about 30–60 minutes for those with psychological symptoms. It is not suitable for assessing patients with psychotic disorders, organic states, alcoholism or personality disorder, but is useful for people with minor psychiatric disorders or people who may not see themselves as psychiatrically disturbed. It is recommended for use only by psychiatrists after special training.

As regards inter-rater reliability, the weighted κ ranges from +0.66 to +0.93 (except for histrionic behaviour where it is lower). No diagnostic criteria are given and the psychiatrist is expected to use his own judgement, on the basis of the information ascertained, to make an ICD diagnosis. The reliability and validity of the ICD diagnoses thus derived are not reported.

National Institute of Mental Health Diagnostic Interview Schedule (DIS) (Robins et al 1981a)

The DIS is a highly structured interview which collects data sufficient for making a diagnosis by three systems: DSM-III, the Feighner criteria and the Research Diagnostic Criteria (RDC). It assesses symptoms which may have occurred at any time during the patient's life and in more detail over the time periods of 2 weeks, the last month, 6 months and a year. All questions and probes are strictly specified. It takes 45–75 minutes for most respondents. It is possible to use it for a wide range of disorders, including alcoholism, drug abuse and anorexia nervosa, but not for mental handicap or organic disorders. The instrument was designed for use by specially trained lay interviewers. The agreement between a lay interviewer and a psychiatrist for DSM-III diagnoses is quite good, with a mean κ of +0.69, a mean sensitivity of 75% and specificity of 94%. The agreement for RDC diagnoses was not as good (κ +0.62, sensitivity 57%, specificity 93%) (Robins et al 1981b).

Folstein et al (1985) compared diagnoses derived from DIS ratings by lay interviewers with diagnoses made by a clinician at the end of a 2 hour interview and a full PSE. They found that specificity is generally good (94–99%) for major depressive disorder, alcoholism and antisocial personality disorder, but lower for schizophrenia. Sensitivity is not so good; 52–59% for alcoholism and major depressive disorder and 21–26% for schizophrenia and antisocial personality disorder. In a similar study McLeod et al (1990) attribute such discrepancies to 'inconsistent episode reports' (i.e. forgetting) by patients. These results conflict with those of Robins and her colleagues and raise serious doubts about the validity of the DIS, at least when administered by lay interviewers.

Instruments designed to define and identify psychiatric 'cases'

The above diagnostic instruments can also be used for assessing 'caseness' in a sample according to their own diagnostic criteria, but there are also a number of other instruments which serve this function.

PSE Index of Definition (ID) (Wing et al 1978)

Wing and his colleagues have developed the concept of an Index of Definition (ID) based on PSE data, using either the full or 40-item version. A computer program can allocate each patient, depending on their PSE symptoms, to an ID with a range from 1 to 8. An ID of 5 or above indicates that the patient probably has a psychiatric illness, with sufficient symptoms to allow classification as a psychosis or a neurosis; such patients can also be classified by the Catego program and given an ICD diagnosis. The full or 40-item version of the PSE can thus be used in epidemiological surveys to identify people who according to the system would be regarded as a 'case'.

The ID has been compared with an independently made global rating by psychiatrists. There was 90% agreement on the identification of 'cases' by the two methods. The ID was also able to discriminate between in-patient, out-patient and community cases.

The General Health Questionnaire (GHQ) (Goldberg 1972)

This is a self-rated questionnaire of 60 items. There are also shorter versions of 30, 28 and 20 items. Each question has four possible responses; less than usual, no more than usual, rather more than usual, or much more than usual. The full version takes 6–8 minutes; the shorter 30-item version takes 3–4 minutes. A score of 11 on the full version discriminated most accurately between 'cases' and 'non-cases' but researchers are recommended to conduct a pilot study testing the GHQ against their own clinical judgement or particular diagnostic criteria. The questionnaire was designed for use in community settings, primary care or general medical out-patients. It was not intended for the detection of psychoses.

Selecting patients whose clinical status had not altered over some time, the test–retest reliability was reported as +0.95. Correlations with clinical assessment in numerous studies range from +0.71 to +0.88, with 91% sensitivity and 94% specificity. As regards validity, Goldberg et al (1976) showed that consecutive attenders at a general practitioner's surgery have higher GHQ scores than a random sample of patients on that doctor's list. The GHQ has been used to predict short-term response to various therapies; for instance, patients with high GHQ scores after a coronary thrombosis were more likely to be re-admitted (Prince & Miranda 1977).

Huppert et al (1989) reported a large-scale factor analysis of the GHQ30 with over 6000 subjects. In addition to the analysis on all the subjects, they also repeated it ten times, each with a different subsample of 600 subjects randomly selected from the total sample; and then a further 12 times in groups selected according to age and sex. An impressive degree of factor invariance was found, each analysis obtaining virtually the same factor structure. Five factors were found, corresponding to anxiety, feelings of incompetence, depression, difficulty in coping and social dysfunction. This study provides strong support for the robust structure of the GHQ.

There are many published validity studies of the GHQ carried out in different settings and countries and the instrument is available in many languages. There is also a scaled version which has 28 items and four subscales: somatic symptoms, anxiety and insomnia, social dysfunction and severe depression (Goldberg & Hillier 1979).

Recent developments in diagnostic schedules

Despite the increasing rigour with which diagnostic schedules are being developed, major discrepancies in case identification and in diagnostic assignment are still found between, for example, the PSE and DSM-III (van den Brink et al 1989). Several problems have emerged in using instruments such as the PSE and DIS to identify cases: scales which are useful with patient populations may be less reliable, and prevalence may be overestimated, when used with the general population; item scores can be contaminated by social class and ethnic effects; and much lower agreement between psychiatrists and lay interviewers has been found than in earlier studies.

A recent innovation, developed through multinational collaboration, may help to produce more consistency across measures and diagnostic systems. Wing et al (1990) have given a preliminary description of SCAN (Schedules for Clinical Assessment in Neuropsychiatry); these schedules, for use by experienced professionals, permit DSM-IIIR, Catego and ICD-10 diagnoses to be made. A complementary instrument, the Composite International Diagnostic Instrument (CIDI) has also been developed. It was derived from the DIS and the PSE but is different in design and was intended for administration by lay interviewers; previously Farmer et al (1987) reported that agreement between the PSE and the CIDI was low for many individual questions but better when broader categories (Catego) were used.

Instruments for measuring psychiatric symptoms

Some of the above diagnostic instruments measure symptoms and symptom severity and can therefore also be used to assess change. The SADS and CIS are particularly useful for this purpose. As well as these instruments there are others which were not designed to make a diagnosis, but specifically to measure symptoms and to monitor change.

Global symptom rating scales

Brief Psychiatric Rating Scale (BPRS) (Overall & Gorham 1962). The BPRS contains 11 items to be rated mainly via verbal report; and five items based mainly on observed behaviour. Each item is scored on a 7-point scale (not present, very mild, mild, moderate, moderate to severe, severe, extremely severe) at the end of the suggested 18 minute interview. Definitions are given for each item but no guidance is given about the rating of severity. The way the symptoms are elicited is not standardised and inevitably leads to lower reliability. The time period over which the symptoms should be assessed is not stated. It is recommended for use with psychiatric inpatients, particularly psychotic or long-stay inpatients. It is unsuitable for patients with minor psychiatric illnesses.

If two interviewers rate the same interview, the inter-rater reliability for the various items ranges from +0.56 to +0.87. Only 'tension' is below +0.6. It is recommended that when using the BPRS patients should be interviewed jointly by two observers and the ratings should be completed independently, and subsequently averaged. This improves the inter-rater reliability and correlations of +0.73 and +0.94 are reported. It is possible to make a diagnosis by computer using the symptom profile obtained from the BPRS.

The Symptom Rating Test (SRT) (Kellner & Sheffield 1973). The SRT was developed to measure distress, and in particular changes in neurotic symptoms in therapeutic trials. It comprises a semistructured interview based on a checklist of 38 symptoms: 15 somatic and 23 psychological. These symptoms are then self-rated for severity. Four subscales are included: anxiety, depression, inadequacy and somatic concern. Several forms are available according to the timescale over which symptoms are to be measured: a day form, week form, and an hour form, although the latter has received relatively little attention.

The SRT is recommended mainly for use in neurotic patients. It is a very reliable instrument with a test–retest reliability of over +0.9 (over 24 hours), and internal reliability of changes in SRT scores of

+0.89. Validity has been consistently demonstrated by its ability to discriminate well between neurotic patients and 'normals', and by its sensitivity to change in drug trials.

Symptom Questionnaire (Kellner 1987). This is a 92-item list of adjectives describing affective state; it assesses anxiety, depression, hostility and somatic concern. Its psychometric properties appear to be satisfactory, but few reports of its use have yet appeared.

Depression rating scales

Hamilton Rating Scale for Depression (HRSD) (Hamilton 1967). This is designed to be filled in at the end of an unstructured interview lasting about an hour; the value of the scale therefore depends on the skill of the interviewer. It is, however, possible to get the information necessary for the scale from a standard interview like the SADS or the Clinical Interview for Depression (Paykel 1985). The scale is rated on the basis of the patient's condition in the previous few days and takes into account information from all available sources, including nurses and relatives. It contains 17 variables, each rated on a 3- or 5-point scale. The items are not defined but detailed information is given about scoring. The scale is mainly concerned with behavioural and somatic features of depression rather than psychological and cognitive ones.

The scale, not being designed as a diagnostic instrument, should only be used on patients who have already been diagnosed as having a depressive illness. The maximum score is 52, but in practice few patients score over 35, with a score of 30 indicating severe depression.

The scale is intended for use by clinicians and it is suggested that if two raters rate a dozen patients together and discuss their ratings, this will produce close agreement. Hamilton suggests that in order to increase the reliability of ratings two interviewers should be present, one to conduct the interview and the other to ask supplementary questions. The two raters record scores independently which are then averaged. The inter-rater reliability for the total HRSD was reported as +0.90, using 70 patients.

Construct validity has been demonstrated by the scale's ability to discriminate between medical students and depressed patients and also between depressed inpatients, outpatients and depressed patients in general practice. Concurrent validity has been demonstrated by comparing a psychiatrist's global rating with the score on the HRSD (Zealley & Aitken

1969); this study produced a correlation of +0.90 in depressed patients on admission, of +0.76 midway through their stay and of +0.55 at discharge.

Rehm & O'Hara (1985) examined the reliability and validity of the individual items on the Hamilton scale. Some performed very badly. The reliability for most was improved by the use of a supplementary set of guidelines and anchor points, but four items (agitation, gastrointestinal symptoms, loss of weight and loss of insight) did badly on all their reliability and validity assessments. Potts et al (1990) have produced an interview guide for the HRSD; good agreement between laymen and psychiatrists was reported, and the guide is said to be particularly useful for administering the scale by telephone.

A short six-item version of the HRSD has been recommended by Bech et al (1975). The inter-observer agreement is as good as with the 17-item version and they find the shorter scale better at distinguishing between levels of depression, and therefore more useful for measuring change.

Beck Depression Inventory (BDI) (Beck et al 1961). This is generally used as a self-rated inventory, though it was designed to be administered by a trained psychologist or sociologist. It comprises 21 items, each describing a specific behavioural manifestation of depression. In each instance there are 4–6 self-evaluative statements. These are read aloud to the patient, who also has a copy of the inventory. He then selects the statement which fits him best at the time of interview. Completion of the inventory results in a total score (maximum 60) which is a measure of the depth of depression. The inventory has been mainly used on psychiatric in-patients and out-patients. It is not a diagnostic tool but may be used to measure depth of depression in patients with any diagnosis.

Internal consistency was demonstrated by obtaining a significant relationship between each item and the total score. The split-half reliability is +0.86. Concurrent validity was assessed by comparing the total BDI score with a 4-point clinical rating of the severity of depression (none, mild, moderate and severe). A significant difference in mean BDI scores between the four levels of depression was demonstrated. Metcalfe & Goldman (1965) have demonstrated the BDI's sensitivity to change in that they found significant differences on the mean BDI scores of depressed patients on admission and on discharge. Validity has also been assessed by comparing it with the HRSD, with most workers reporting an overall correlation of around +0.60 to +0.68.

Montgomery and Asberg Depression Rating Scale (MADRS) (Montgomery & Asberg 1979). This device was derived from the Comprehensive Psycho-pathological Rating Scale (Asberg et al 1978). It has ten items, each rated on a 4-point scale. A description of each item is provided and a definition is given for each point on the scale. Half-steps can be used, extending each scale to a 7-point scale as a way of increasing sensitivity to change.

The scale is concerned exclusively with the psychological symptoms of depression, unlike the Hamilton scale which also contains somatic symptoms. It is particularly useful, therefore, for assessing patients with concurrent physical illness or who are likely to experience marked side-effects from treatment. It is said to be reliable in the hands of trained mental health workers (psychiatrists, psycho-logists and nurses). The ratings should be based on a flexible clinical interview.

Inter-rater reliability is reported as being between +0.89 and +0.97. Validity was assessed by comparing performance on the scale with a clinician's global clinical judgement. Patients were divided into responders and non-responders on the basis of clinical judgement. There was a correlation of +0.70 between the change score on the MADRS and the clinician's response category. Another test of validity was that the scores on the MADRS correlated +0.73 with the HRSD score before treatment for depression and +0.94 with the HRSD score after 4 weeks of treatment. The scale seemed to be more sensitive to change than the HRSD; there was a correlation of +0.59 between the change scores on the HRSD and the clinician's response category. The authors suggest that the instrument should be used to measure changes over a short period of time, ideally weekly but daily or monthly if necessary.

Snaith et al (1986) suggest that the MADRS is as good at measuring severity as the HRSD; the suggested cut-offs for severity are 0–6 recovered, 7–19 mild depression, 20–34 moderate depression and 35–60 severe depression

The Inventory to Diagnose Depression (IDD)
(Zimmerman & Coryell 1988). This is a self-report 22-item measure, designed to cover the entire range of symptoms and to comply with other requirements for assessing major depression for DSM-III; one can determine caseness as well as assess degree of symptomatology. A 5-point scale is used. Agreement with the DIS was good ($\kappa=+0.80$) when the two instruments were used within 2 days of each other, but was reduced with longer intervals. The authors consider that it would be most useful for survey research, but may also be useful for monitoring changes with treatment.

The Hospital Anxiety and Depression Scale (HAD)
(Zigmond & Snaith 1983). This is a 14-item self-rating scale, seven concerned with anxiety and seven with depression. It was designed specifically for use in non-psychiatric hospital departments. The items on the scale are all concerned with the psychological symptoms of neurosis; this makes the scale suitable for use in patients with concurrent physical illness. The internal consistency of the scale is reported; correlations between each item and the total score ranged from +0.41 to +0.76 for anxiety items and +0.30 to +0.60 for depression items. The validity of the scales was tested against a clinical rating of caseness. A score of 11 or more on both scales was used to distinguish cases. With this cut-off, HAD depression had a specificity of 94% and sensitivity of 67%; HAD anxiety had a specificity of 76% and a sensitivity of 87%. The validity of the scales was assessed by examining the correlations of the subscale scores and a psychiatrist's global score. The cor-relations were +0.70 for depression and +0.74 for anxiety. The scales appear, therefore, to be a reasonably valid measure of anxiety and depression.

The factorial structure of the HAD was examined in a study of nearly 600 patients with a variety of cancers (Moorey et al 1991). Separate but related factors of anxiety and depression emerged, and internal relia-bility (α) was approximately +0.90 for both. They concluded that 'the HAD seems to be the best instrument available for simple and rapid evaluation of psychological interventions in patients with physical illness'.

Anxiety rating scales

The State–Trait Anxiety Inventory (STAI)
(Spielberger et al 1970). This comprises two separate self-rated scales, one measuring state anxiety and the other trait anxiety. Each consists of 20 statements, the trait scale being concerned with how subjects *generally* feel, the state scale with how they feel at that *particular moment in time*. It is said to be a sensitive indicator of changes in levels of anxiety. It takes 6–10 minutes for each scale to be completed. The state scale can be given repeatedly to measure change over time. Normative data for both scales, based on samples of students, are available in a manual.

It is recommended that the examiner and examinee read the instructions out loud together to allow time for questions and to ensure that the examinee understands the instructions. The test–retest correla-tions for the trait scale are reported as +0.73 to +0.86, and those of the state scale as +0.16 to +0.54. The lower reliability of the state scale is to be expected as it is designed to measure change. Concurrent validity was indicated by its correlation with the Taylor Manifest Anxiety Scale (+0.80). Scores on the state scale were demonstrated to increase with stress and decrease with relaxation.

Hamilton Anxiety Scale (HAS) (Hamilton 1959). The scale is designed to be used with patients already diagnosed as having anxiety states and not for assessing anxiety in patients with other disorders. It has 13 items and is rated on the basis of an unstructured interview. Each item has a brief description and is rated on a 5-point scale. Inter-rater reliability is good with a mean correlation between raters of +0.89.

The HAS has been adapted (Clinical Anxiety Scale, CAS; Snaith et al 1982), retaining six of the original 13 items, the somatic and depressive items being excluded. There are more detailed definitions of each point on the scale than in the original HAS. The authors of this scale believe it may prove useful in the assessment of anxiety in any patients and not just those with a diagnosis of anxiety neurosis. No inter-rater or test–retest reliability data have yet been published. Validity was assessed by comparing the total score on the CAS with a clinician's global severity rating in two groups of patients. The correlations were +0.67 and +0.85. The instrument is sensitive to change and the change score on the scale before and after treatment correlated +0.74 with the change score on the clinician's global severity rating before and after treatment.

The SADS-L (Anxiety) (Mannuzza et al 1989). This measure is based on the SADS, and assesses anxiety across a wide range of situations, including panic, generalised anxiety, social phobias, animal phobias and so on. Inter-observer agreement is satisfactory (κ ranges from +0.60 to +0.90, but is lower for simple phobias). Further development is required before this promising instrument can be used in routine practice.

Mania rating scales

Manic Rating Scale (MS) (Beigel et al 1971). This is a 26-item scale, each item being rated on two 6-point scales, one for frequency and one for severity. The product of the two ratings is taken as the overall score for each item. The scale is rated on the basis of observation over an 8 hour period, and was designed for use by nurses as a means of providing an objective measure of severity.

The inter-rater reliability for items is reported to be +0.86 to +0.99 based on 13 manic depressive patients.

The validity of the scale was assessed by comparing the total score on the scale with a psychiatrist's 15-point global rating of mania, giving a correlation of +0.7. No data are given about its sensitivity to change.

Modified Manic Rating Scale (MMS) (Blackburn et al 1977). This is a modification of the MS for use by psychiatrists and clinical psychologists. It is a 28-item scale and the ratings are made on the basis of severity only. Generally, it is recommended that the ratings are made during a structured interview, but six items are completed on the basis of information gleaned from nursing staff, for example items such as 'makes threats' and 'seeks out others'. There is a glossary which describes the items on the scale, the rating points and the items which can be based on nursing reports.

The inter-rater reliability between pairs of raters on the basis of 16 manic patients was between +0.79 and +0.85. All individual items of the MMS, except that relating to depression, were significantly correlated with the total score. The validity was assessed by correlating the total MMS score, averaged over three raters, with nurses' and medical staff's global ratings. A correlation of +0.65 was obtained between MMS scores and nurses' ratings and one of +0.8 between MMS scores and doctors' ratings. These correlations also reflect changes over time as MMS scores and global ratings were made at intervals during hospitalisation and all rating occasions were compared. An indication of sensitivity to change is that the MMS scores at discharge were significantly lower than at admission.

Obsessive–compulsive rating scales

The measurement of change in patients with obsessive–compulsive disorders is complex because of the multiplicity and wide range of symptoms and disabilities. Frequently research workers use a battery of tests, including semantic differentials and visual analogue scales (see below), which can be tailor-made to suit the individual patient's symptoms.

The Leyton Obsessional Inventory (Cooper 1970). This comprises 69 questions dealing with the subjective assessment of obsessional traits and symptoms. Factor analysis has revealed four main components (being clean and tidy, feeling of incompleteness, checking and ruminating.) A card-sorting procedure is used, the patient indicating his reply to each question by sorting cards into 'yes' and 'no' boxes. It produces four separate scores for symptoms, traits, interference and resistance. It was originally devised for differentiating houseproud housewives from normal housewives. It is unfortunately rather long and tedious to administer, with the patient requiring supervision throughout. Its test–retest reliability is reported as +0.87 for the symptom score and +0.91 for the trait score. The test is valid in that it can differentiate between obsessional patients and normal subjects (Murray et al 1979) and between houseproud housewives and normal women. However, it is less sensitive in assessing changes in clinical state in patients with an obsessional illness.

The Maudsley Obsessional–Compulsive Inventory (MOC) (Rachman & Hodgson 1980). This is a 30-item 'true–false' self-administered inventory, which provides a total score, and separate scores for four subscales (checking, washing, slowness–repetition, doubting–conscientious). The subscales were derived from a principal components analysis, on data from 100 adult obsessionals. Internal reliability (α coefficients) for the subscales was around +0.70 and test–retest reliability was +0.80. Validity was reported to be satisfactory as determined by comparing questionnaire responses with clinician ratings; the MOC was also reported to be sensitive to change.

There are several new measures of obsessive–compulsive problems which appear promising but with as yet limited reports of their use: The Yale–Brown Obsessive Compulsive Scale (Goodman et al 1989) set out to measure obsessive–compulsive features exclusively, and explicitly avoided incorporating items which may have measured trait-like characteristics or anxiety and depression. It has very high inter-rater and internal reliability and seems to be sensitive to change. The Padua Inventory (Sanavio 1988) is a 60-item inventory which appears to be well designed with good internal and test–retest reliability as well as high factorial and concurrent validity.

Rating of long-term patients

There are a number of rating scales designed to assess the treatment and rehabilitation of long-term, mainly schizophrenic, patients and which are mainly based on observed behaviour.

Standardised Psychiatric Assessment Scale (Krawiecka et al 1977). This brief scale was designed to assess chronic patients and to be sensitive to changes in their clinical state. It is intended to be used by psychiatrists and there is a training videotape which explains the method of scoring as well as a manual. The rater is not intended to perform the ratings blind to information about the patient; he is expected to be at the very least familiar with the patient's case notes. The scale has eight items; the first four are based on the patient's replies to questions about symptoms during the previous week and the final four on the interviewer's own observations. Each item is rated on a 5-point scale and there are detailed descriptions for each point on the scale. There are also six additional items which rate side-effects if the scale is being used in a drug trial.

Inter-rater reliability was +0.58 to +0.87 for the items. The lower concordance was for flattened and incongruous affect. Three psychiatrists who had trained themselves using the videotape and manual were included in the reliability study, demonstrating that psychiatrists trained in this way can achieve adequate reliability. No data are given for test–retest reliability. The instrument is said to be sensitive to change and it has been used in many studies of rehabilitation and drug treatment.

Rehab (Baker & Hall 1988). This instrument was devised to provide a multipurpose assessment of long-term patients, with a view to their return to the community. It has two sections, one measuring 'deviant behaviour' (nine questions on a 0–2 scale) and one 'general behaviour' (17 questions on a 0–9 scale). The factorial and concurrent validity are acceptable, and inter-rater reliability is over +0.8 for both sections. It has been used successfully to select patients for rehabilitation programmes and to monitor change.

Katz Adjustment Scale—Relatives' Form (Katz & Lyerly 1963). An hour may be required to complete this 205-item scale designed to assess psychotic symptoms and social behaviour. It is probably most suitable for severely disturbed patients; psychometric properties are acceptable and it has been widely used.

Life Skills Profile (Parker et al 1991). This is a 39-item scale designed to assess the skills necessary for the successful rehabilitation of long-term patients. It measures self-care, non-turbulence, socialisation, communication and responsibility. It is simple to complete and special training is not necessary. Test–retest reliability was between +0.78 and +0.90; inter-rater between +0.77 and +0.83. It correlated quite well (+0.65) with the much longer Katz Adjustment Scale.

Morningside Rehabilitation Status Schedule (Affleck & McGuire 1984). There are four dimensions measured by this schedule, which takes up to half an hour to administer. They are dependence, activity, social integration and effects of symptoms. Inter-rater reliability for the total score is +0.83 but less for the individual dimensions; moderate correlations with the Krawiecka Scale and the SAS have been reported; the level of association suggests that the various scales may be tapping different aspects of patients' functioning (McCreadie et al 1987).

The Modified Rogers Scale (Lund et al 1991). The Modified Rogers Scale was designed to measure mainly the catatonic symptoms of schizophrenia, but also volition, speech and overall behaviour. Inter-rater agreement (Kendall's *W*) was over 0.80 for virtually all items but test–retest was lower (+0.67). Concurrent validity was assessed by relating it to scores obtained on a variety of other scales measuring schizophrenic symptoms. The scale and guidelines for its use are given in McKenna et al (1991).

Measures of social adjustment

There is increasing interest in the measurement of social adjustment, partly because of the need to evaluate the quality of life of chronic patients who have been rehabilitated into the community from long-stay hospitals and partly because social factors have been demonstrated to be good predictors of outcome in neurotic disorders. There are many instruments which may measure entirely different aspects of a social dimension; some may measure material conditions, some interpersonal relationships and others satisfaction with life or 'quality of life'.

Social Maladjustment Schedule (SMS) (Clare & Cairns 1978). This interview schedule has 40 items rated on a 4-point scale. There are six subject areas: housing, occupation/social role, economic situation, leisure/social activities, family and domestic relationships and marriage. Each area is rated under three headings: material conditions, social management and satisfaction. The interview takes about 45 minutes and can be administered by any trained professional. Information from a collateral informant can be included.

An inter-rater reliability study on 48 patients found κ to be between +0.55 and +0.94, mostly in the higher range. The instrument was used in three different patient populations: a group with known social problems, a sample with premenstrual tension and a chronic neurotic sample. The three show differences in total social maladjustment scores and the pattern of scores on the various items, demonstrating reasonable concurrent validity.

Self-report Social Adjustment Scale (SAS-SR) (Weissman & Bothwell 1976). This is a self-rating scale comprising 42 items. It assesses functioning over the previous 2 weeks in six major areas: work

(including homemaker or student), social and leisure activities, relationship with extended family, marital role as a spouse, parental role, and membership of the family unit. Question in each area fall into four main categories: the patient's performance at expected tasks, the amount of friction with others, finer aspects of interpersonal relations and inner feelings and satisfactions. Each question is rated on a 5-point scale. The scale has high internal consistency (+0.74) and test–retest reliability (+0.80).

Concurrent validity was demonstrated by correlations between self-report and interview of +0.40 to +0.76. The correlation between the overall adjustment score obtained by the schedule and the interview was +0.72; that for overall adjustment between the patient and an informant was +0.65 to +0.74. The scale discriminates well between patient and non-patient populations and between different types of psychiatric patients (depressives, alcoholics, schizophrenics). It is also sensitive to change in that there were significant improvements in scores with treatment for depression both as reported by the patient and by a relative. The schedule has been used with most psychiatric patient groups and also with a British sample (McCreadie & Barron 1984).

The Social Functioning Scale (Birchwood et al 1990). This carefully constructed scale measures seven areas of social functioning, including social engagement, recreation and employment. It is intended for use in family intervention programmes with schizophrenic patients, and for determining their social impairments and needs. Reliability (four aspects) was high, as was factorial validity and concurrent validity; it also seems sensitive to change.

Social Network Schedule (SNS) (Dunn et al 1990). In an interesting paper Dunn et al describe the psychometric properties of the SNS, a structured interview designed to assess the social activity of long-stay patients; inter-rater reliability was high (+0.95) and its promise was well supported by validating it against unobtrusive observations of patients at a hospital social club.

CONSTRUCTING NEW SCALES

Rating scales

The previous section has examined some of the standard rating scales which have been developed and which are currently in use. There will be circumstances, however, where standard scales do not exist, and it will be necessary to devise a scale for a particular purpose. Many methods are available and this section will outline those often used in psychiatry.

Numerical scales

This is the most straightforward kind of rating where numerical values are attached to verbal descriptions, with reference to a preliminary statement. For example: 'How disturbed is patient A? Not at all disturbed (1); Slightly disturbed (2); Disturbed (3); Very disturbed (4)'. Theoretically, any number of categories could be used, but when the number exceeds six or seven, raters experience increasing difficulty in discriminating between categories.

Graphic scales

With graphic scales, sometimes called 'visual analogue scales' (VASs), the observer is not constrained by having to choose just one option from several, but can make his judgement anywhere along a continuum represented by a straight line; for example

Not at all disturbed
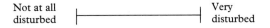
Very disturbed

The score is simply the distance from the left-hand end of the line to the point of endorsement. This type of scale is useful for measuring change in an individual, particularly when assessments need to be made at short time intervals. It also increases the potential variation in the ratings, is clear and easy to use and score, and fixes a continuum in the mind of the observer.

An excellent review of VASs, including the possible formats and correlations with external criterion measures of depression, anxiety, other mood, and pain, has been provided by McCormack et al (1988). With the exception of anxiety, concurrent validity is said to be high, as is inter-rater reliability. The authors also present a very useful discussion on such aspects as scoring methods, and appropriate statistics, when using VASs.

Attitude scales

Numerical and graphic scales can both be used to measure attitudes, although this is not their only function. Other scales have been developed specifically for this purpose.

Likert scales

These are the most widely used and most useful of a form of scaling called 'summated rating scales'. A series of statements are given, all of which are assumed to have approximately equal 'attitude values'; and the subject responds on a 5-point numerical scale from 'strongly agree' to 'strongly disagree'. The scores for each statement are then simply added together, with no differential weighting. The direction of scoring may have to be reversed in accordance with the wording of the statement.

For example, the following format might be used to assess attitudes to self-poisoning:

People who take drug overdoses are sick and need help.				
1	2	3	4	5
Strongly agree	Agree	Unsure	Disagree	Strongly disagree

Treatment of people who take overdoses is a misuse of hospital resources.				
1	2	3	4	5
Strongly agree	Agree	Unsure	Disagree	Strongly disagree

Thurstone scales

Thurstone scales are similar except that items are differentially 'weighted' in accordance with how extreme an attitude is portrayed. In order to determine the appropriate weights, a large number of judges are given many items reflecting a range of attitudes to a subject. The judges arrange the items into 11 categories with extreme attitudes at either end, and moderate views at the centre. Items where there is much disagreement between judges are omitted, and remaining items are assigned a number from 0 to 10. For example, the following might be extreme items from a scale used to measure attitudes towards the use of electroconvulsive therapy (ECT):

  0 ECT is the most effective and widely applicable treatment in modern psychiatry.
10 ECT is harmful, degrading and totally ineffective, and its use should be prohibited.

The full attitude scale would comprise a number of such items, and the subject's overall score would be the total of all the weights of items endorsed.

General comments on rating scales

Rating scales are generally easy for patients or observers to understand and use; they have a wide range of application and they are quick and easy to score. However, there are a number of serious problems. Rating scales are notoriously prone to 'response sets'; that is, for example, the tendency of some raters to avoid all extreme judgements and use only the middle of the scale. Observer-completed rating scales are particularly prone to the 'halo effect', or the tendency to rate an object or person in a consistent direction on a number of traits, in accordance with a general impression; for example, a person who is attractive may also be seen as warm, honest and intelligent. Such difficulties can be minimised if due regard is paid to the following guidelines:

1. The concepts used should be operationally and carefully defined.

2. Graphic or verbal scales are preferable to numerical scales.

3. If several people are to be rated on a number of traits, the results will be less subject to the 'halo effect' if all subjects being assessed are rated on one trait at a time rather than each individual being rated on all the traits successively.

4. Extreme wording (e.g. 'the worse possible') should be avoided, as extreme categories are seldom endorsed.

5. It is easier to complete and to score a rating if the 'positive' or 'desirable' end of the scale is consistently in the same direction. However, such an arrangement may encourage the appearance of response sets.

6. Where discrete ratings are to be used, six or seven is the ideal number. This permits sufficient variance to develop, but retains overall simplicity and ease of completion.

Leber (1990) pointed out some of the pitfalls in the use of rating scales to measure psychopathology; in particular, the importance of precise definition of phenomena for diagnostic purposes, obtaining external validation criteria, interpreting differences between global clinical assessments and rating scales, and valid statistical analysis and threats to this from data 'manipulation' and patient dropout.

INDIVIDUAL MEASURES OF SUBJECTIVE STATE

This section is concerned with measurement of the personal experience (i.e. feelings, emotions, attitudes, beliefs and symptoms) of individual subjects; that is, with experiential rather than observable phenomena. All the measurements discussed are subject completed although some are sufficiently flexible to be used in other ways. They are particularly useful to dynamic psychotherapists, but could also prove valuable in drug trials, behavioural therapies and other areas.

The Semantic Differential (SD)

The SD was developed by Osgood et al (1957) to measure the psychological meaning of concepts.

Although concepts have a common culturally accepted meaning, individuals also impose upon this meaning their own idiosyncratic interpretations, and the SD was originally developed to detect these variations. Clinically the SD is seldom used in this fashion, but rather to measure how patients see or evaluate particular concepts, and to assess changes in these evaluations. The format is similar to that of the visual analogue scale; it consists of a concept to be rated, and a number of scales on which to rate it. These scales are made up of bipolar adjectives, with a number of intervening points (usually, but not always, 7). For example, the following SD was developed in connection with a study on postoperative adjustment:

My reaction to pain

Controlled	Uncontrolled
Agitated	Relaxed
Well tolerated	Badly tolerated
Need drugs	Don't need drugs
Brave	Cowardly

This example illustrates that neither the concept to be rated, nor the scales, need consist of single words. The five items in the example form part of a 13-item scale used in the full study. There can be any number of adjective pairs per concept, and any number of concepts, each with the same adjectives, or with its own. The subject is required to insert a cross at whichever of the seven positions most accurately describes his view. If one feels quite neutral about the concept on a particular adjective pair, or that the pair is irrelevant to the concept judged, the cross is placed in the centre.

Adjective pairs can be selected to measure any domain of meaning, and should be chosen principally for their relevance to the concepts used. However, meanings are so complex that one can never be sure in advance whether an adjective pair will be seen as relevant or not.

Semantic differentials can be scored in a variety of ways. The simplest way, and the one most likely to be useful in clinical practice, is to assign a score of 7 to one extreme of the scale and 1 to the opposite extreme. If the scales are measuring approximately the same thing, scores can simply be summed.

In psychiatry, the SD has been used for a variety of purposes, including a measure of sexual interest. Its usefulness can be illustrated by reference to the work of Rutter (1979) who found that SD responses were more predictive of rehabilitation outcome in patients with chronic breathlessness than a number of other psychological and physiological measures. To conclude, the SD is flexible, sensitive, reliable and, above all, simple, and is particularly useful in the assessment of change.

The Personal Questionnaire (PQ)

Shapiro (1961) repeatedly advocated the intensive investigation of single cases as a clinical research technique, and he developed the PQ to this end. However, despite much agreement as to the value of this approach, few people have used it either for clinical practice or research, partly because of the complexity of the scoring system. However, Mulhall (1976) has described an ingenious version of the PQ which overcomes this problem.

PQs are intended to measure the intensity of symptoms and how they change over time, as seen by the patient. Patients themselves choose which symptoms (normally up to ten) are to be measured, and express them in their own words. Some guidance from the clinician may, of course, be required. Once the list of symptoms (or other variables) has been drawn up, the patient embarks on a series of paired comparisons whereby each symptom is assessed on a scale from 'maximum possible' to 'absolutely none'. In Mulhall's version, a booklet is provided in which all the relevant comparisons are systematically and simply presented. Two versions are available: the longer PQ14 has a range of scores from 0 to 13; the PQ10 ranges from 0 to 9. The former has a completion time of 15–20 minutes, the latter of 10–15 minutes. Scoring, by means of a template, takes a few seconds. A notable advantage of the PQ is that it incorporates a measure of internal reliability, enabling careless completion to be readily identified.

For the assessment of change in patients' perception of their symptoms, the PQ is one of the best available measures. It is individually tailored, simple and rapid and should have an important part to play in clinical practice and research.

Role Construct Repertory Test

The Role Construct Repertory Test, and the associated Repertory Grid Test, are closely linked to the personal construct theory of Kelly (1963). They are intended to reveal an individual's constructs or way of looking at the world. Kelly suggested that people use their construct system to attempt to anticipate events and make sense of, and gain some control over, their inner and outer worlds. Each individual has his own idiosyncratic system of personal constructs and the Grid Test was devised as a way of examining an individual's construct system.

A construct is represented by a bipolar adjective, such as good–bad, active–passive, tall–short or friendly–hostile. One way in which individuals' constructs can be discovered is by asking them to look at a series of cards, each naming a person with a significant role in their life; commonly listed people are 'father', 'a person I hated' and 'myself as I would like to be'. Such people are referred to as 'elements'. The individual is then asked to judge in what way two elements are similar, and how a third element is different from the other two. For example, the person may state that 'father' and 'a person I hated' are very authoritarian which is opposite to 'myself as I would like to be'. Thus, authoritarian/non-authoritarian would be one construct. Several others can be elicited in this way, by varying the three elements to be compared. Eventually a reasonably complete idea of the individual's construct system can be built up and, by ranking a number of elements on the constructs, correlations are generated which are assumed to reflect the psychological relationships within the construct system. Successive assessments may reveal changes in overall psychological functioning. A great deal of data is generated in the process, to a degree that it may lack immediate meaning and require extensive further analysis; special computer software is available for this purpose. Obviously the Repertory Grid is an idiographic test, since the constructs (and the elements) are supplied by the subject. Occasionally, and particularly when comparisons between subjects are to be made, constructs and elements are provided by the interviewer.

The Repertory Grid Test is generally used to plan treatment and assess change, usually within a psychotherapeutic framework. However, it can be used on any occasion when there is a need to assess the patient's 'inner world'. Unfortunately, the administration, scoring and interpretation of the Repertory Grid is very time-consuming and complex, and analysis by computer is essential. Clinicians may feel that its use is often unnecessary, since similar information may be available more simply via SDs. Adams-Weber (1979) has outlined the methodology and clinical applications of Repertory Grid Testing.

OBSERVATIONAL AND RELATED TECHNIQUES

The techniques of measurement discussed above have mostly attempted to assess characteristics at a distance; in other words, there has been a gap, temporal or spatial, between the occurrence of the phenomenon and the time and place of assessment. Inevitably, this introduces error since such assessment depends on unreliable phenomena such as memory. An alternative measurement technology has been developed, often called 'behavioural assessment' since it is based on overt behaviour and has been most extensively developed for use in behavioural therapy. However, these methods are equally useful in other treatments. There are three main types and each will be discussed separately. They are naturalistic observations, self-recording, and unobtrusive measures.

Naturalistic observation

The central characteristic of naturalistic observation is that it is concerned with the assessment of overt behaviour, at the time and in the place at which it occurs, hence the term 'naturalistic'. Little, if any, inference is needed to determine whether the behaviour has occurred. Studies using this technique frequently use trained observers.

It is, of course, impossible to record all events as they occur, especially in hospitals and homes; accordingly, some selection or sampling is required. Previous decisions must be made, often on the basis of a pilot study, as to which behaviours are to be recorded. The recording system should be designed so that it does not distract the observer from ongoing observations. A frequent solution to such problems is to use a coding system. For example, Jones et al (1975) have developed a coding system to record the behaviour of delinquent boys at home. Each person in the home is assigned a number, and 28 behaviours such as talking, crying, hitting and positive physical contact are assigned a code. All behaviours are carefully defined, and inter-observer reliabilities are generally over +0.90. As an example, the recording 3 CM-1 CO would mean that the father (3) told (CM) the boy (1) to do something, and the boy complied (CO). Similar coding systems have been developed for a number of behaviours, including marital interaction, social interaction of depressed patients, chronic psychotic behaviour, and nurse–patient interaction.

An important aspect of naturalistic observation is time-sampling. Since 24 hour observations are not practicable, the appropriate times for recording must be decided. Various methods of time-sampling have been used. In whole interval sampling, behaviour is recorded if it occurs throughout a whole interval; in partial interval sampling it is recorded if it occurs during any part of an interval; and in momentary time-sampling it is recorded if it is occurring at the end of an interval. The type of sampling used will depend upon the frequency and duration of the observed behaviour, and upon the resources available. For example, momentary sampling may be most appropriate for high-frequency behaviours, and partial interval for short-duration or low-frequency behaviours. The importance of careful time-sampling has been dramatically demonstrated by Russell & Bernal (1977), who found that the frequency of delinquent behaviours in 5–7-year-old boys varied greatly according to the time of day, the day of the week, and to the weather and outside temperature.

A major problem with naturalistic observation is that of reactivity; that is, how far a subject's behaviour is changed by the assessment procedure itself. There is no doubt that a subject who knows that his behaviour is being recorded may behave differently. Whether reactivity occurs depends on a number of factors, including the actual behaviour being observed, the degree of prior exposure to the recording method, and the characteristics of the subjects under study. Furthermore, when direct recording by a human observer is compared with video-recording, one-way mirrors or other devices, the evidence from a number of studies suggests that no major differences are produced by the recording method. Nevertheless, reactivity remains a potential hazard, and whenever possible naturalistic observations should be supplemented by unobtrusive measures (see below).

It is important to determine how far independent observers will agree on whether a behaviour has occurred, and it appears that reactivity can also influence measures of reliability of observation. It has been shown that inter-rater reliability is higher when the raters know that reliability is being assessed than when they do not. Accordingly, when reliability is being assessed, it should, on at least some occasions, be assessed unknown to the raters. A further hazard is that by a variety of subtle means (such as observer or experimenter expectations, knowledge of preliminary results and even knowledge of the findings of other observers) reported observations may be biased in a particular direction. Ideally, observers should be 'blind' to the nature of the study and should have minimal contact with all others involved. An excellent example of the usefulness of naturalistic observation is provided by Teplin & Lutz (1985). They devised an observation scale to assess alcohol intoxication, which correlated at +0.84 with blood alcohol levels.

Self-recording

The closer a clinical assessment is to the actual occurrence of a behaviour, the more accurate it should be. Often the people closest to the behaviour of interest are patients themselves and they may be the most accurate source of information. Much evidence now points towards the value of getting patients to record their own behaviour. Self-recording has been used to assess a wide range of psychological problems, including weight, obsessional thoughts, depressed mood, frequency of handwashing, hallucinations and frequency of headaches. It is particularly useful for behaviours where direct observation is impossible or impracticable; for example, for sexual or covert activity.

As with naturalistic observation, reactivity is a major methodological problem with self-recording. However, for clinical purposes, reactivity may not be a problem, since many studies report enduring changes in a clinically desirable direction during self-recording, before formal treatment has begun. This is the case particularly for mild self-injurious behaviour such as excessive scratching, lip chewing and fingernail biting. A change may occur when subjects do not know that a change is expected. Generally speaking, when subjects record behaviours which indicate failure or which have other negative connotations, desirable changes do not occur. However, when subjects record successes and other positive phenomena, desirable changes commonly occur. Thus, recording the number of cigarettes smoked may not lead to a reduction in cigarette consumption; but a reduction may occur if one records how often temptation to smoke has been resisted. Interestingly, recording weight as part of an obesity programme is not reactive, but recording calorie intake is. Weight does not respond immediately or closely to dieting, but a graph of changes in calorie intake is an immediate index of desirable changes in eating habits. When a patient is confronted with a graph indicating success this may add extra motivation to continue in treatment.

The validity of self-recording is an area of obvious concern. That is, do patients record their own behaviour accurately? A number of studies have compared self-recording with other measures of the same behaviour, such as biochemical measures of smoking and alcohol consumption, and generally the results support the validity of self-recording. More problematic is whether patients comply; several studies have found that, after a short while, patients simply stop self-recording. Some smoking cessation projects have floundered because clients found the required self-recording too onerous (Wurtele & Martin 1987). Frequent feedback and praise may go some way to overcoming this problem.

Unobtrusive measures

This term refers to methods of assessment in which the subject is not aware that his behaviour is being evaluated. Apart from this characteristic, unobtrusive measures have little in common and there are innumerable possibilities limited only by the ingenuity of the investigator. The main impetus for the development of unobtrusive measures derives from a desire to avoid the problem of reactivity, particularly to avoid the problems involved in asking people about themselves, and these measures do this very successfully. They often take advantage of remaining physical traces of the behaviour or of official records. As yet psychiatry has made little use of such measures, but their potential is great. Much of the work in the area has been described by Webb & Campbell (1981). A few examples will serve to give the flavour of methods that have been used.

Racial prejudice in different parts of a city has been measured by the researchers leaving a completed college application form (including a photograph so that ethnic background was obvious) in a telephone booth, with a note requesting 'Dad' to post it. Prejudice is revealed by a low rate of posting the form. The narrowness of perspective in various 'schools' of psychology was judged by the range of sources of references quoted in articles in specialised journals — the narrowest perspective being indicated by a tendency to quote references mainly from the journal in which the article itself appeared. A more clinical application has been the assessment of rehabilitation progress in quadriplegics: a pressure-sensitive recording device under the mattress, and a milometer attached to a wheelchair, were used to assess time out of bed and mobility. These measures correlated well with more complex and expensively obtained rehabilitation data. Uses in psychiatry have included the recording of the speed and intensity of speech to monitor changes in affective state; the recording of changes in soap usage in a ward self-care programme; and measuring hyperactivity via pressure-sensitive floor tiles.

General comments on observational and related techniques

There are a number of problems with these techniques, particularly in determining reliability and validity. It is important to note, however, that the problems associated with observational techniques are quite different in detail from those encountered with other techniques. All assessment methods leave some gaps through which errors may seep; however, the use of a wide range of methods, each with different gaps and different strengths, will facilitate the development of a reasonably watertight assessment battery.

Automated assessment

Many of the measures discussed in this chapter have been automated with much of the administration and scoring being done by computer. A wide range of measures have been automated, including the HRSD and the BDI. Burnett (1989) has reviewed developments in the use of computers in psychiatry, including assessment. The main advantages are savings in clinicians' time, more standard methods of administration and the potential for tailoring assessments for each patient using computer branching techniques. However, much work will need to be done to ensure that automated versions are comparable to standard versions; otherwise restandardisation may be necessary.

SUMMARY AND CONCLUSIONS

Some of the great variety of measurement devices available in psychiatry have been described, and the question arises as to the most appropriate choice in a given situation. Seldom can we unequivocally conclude that one is superior to another; some measures are more valid, others more reliable, and others easier and quicker to administer. Perhaps one or two examples will clarify things. If research workers want to investigate, say, a new antidepressant in hospital patients, they will need to select measures of depression which are sensitive to change. It would usually be advisable to choose an observer-rated and a self-rated scale, for example the HRSD and the BDI. If it was felt necessary to monitor the patient's mood

on a daily basis the patient could also be asked to complete a visual analogue scale. None of these instruments is diagnostic; so in order to select patients for the trial it would be advisable to use the SADS or PSE so that the selection criteria would be explicit.

If a research project requires the assessment of changes in subjective experience, for example the assessment of body image changes in the treatment of anorexia nervosa, the semantic differential would be a useful measure; PQs and Repertory Grid Tests might also be considered.

The most accurate assessment of overt behaviour can be obtained with naturalistic observation but this may be too expensive for routine use. However, in devising new rating scales an assessment of concurrent validity (i.e. comparison with an external criterion) will be necessary and this can be usefully accomplished by correlating the new rating scale with data from naturalistic observation. For example, a rating scale of obsessional behaviour could be correlated with direct observation of the frequency and duration of handwashing. If the validity of the new rating scale proves satisfactory, the use of observational procedures can be discontinued.

More than one measure should generally be used; for example, one patient-completed and one observer-completed rating. Measures not only differ in precisely what is measured, they may also detect different patterns of change over time; for example, observer-completed ratings often detect symptom change at an earlier stage than patient-completed ratings. The use of more than one instrument or technique greatly enhances the probability of detection of significant effects.

Finally, it should be remembered that, in many circumstances, patients will be the most accurate source of information about themselves. Accordingly, self-recording, for example by the use of daily diaries, or line ratings, should be used whenever possible as part of the assessment procedure. This may produce useful information with minimal use of staff resources.

REFERENCES

Adams-Weber J 1979 Personal construct theory: concepts and applications. Wiley, New York

Affleck J W, McGuire R J 1984 The measurement of psychiatric rehabilitation status: a review of the needs and a new scale. British Journal of Psychiatry 145: 517–525

Andrich D, Van Schonbroeck L 1989 The General Health Questionnaire: a psychometric analysis using latent trait theory. Psychological Medicine 19: 469–485

Asberg M, Montgomery S A, Perris C, Schalling D, Sedvall G 1978 A comprehensive psychopathological rating scale. Acta Psychiatrica Scandinavica suppl 271: 5–27

Baker R, Hall J N 1988 REHAB: a new assessment instrument for chronic psychiatric patients. Schizophrenia Bulletin 14: 97–111

Beck A T, Ward C H, Mendelson M, Mock J, Erbaugh J 1961 An inventory for measuring depression. Archives of General Psychiatry 4: 561–585

Beigel A, Murphy D L, Bunney W E 1971 The Manic-state Rating Scale: scale construction, reliability and validity. Archives of General Psychiatry 25: 256–262

Birchwood M, Smith J, Cochrane R, Wetton S, Copestake S 1990 The Social Functioning Scale. British Journal of Psychiatry 157: 853–859

Blackburn I M, Loudon J B, Ashworth C M 1977 A new scale for measuring mania. Psychological Medicine 7: 453–458

Burnett K F 1989 Computers for assessment and intervention in psychiatry and psychology. Current Opinion in Psychiatry 2: 780–786

Carney M W P, Roth M, Garside R F 1965 The diagnosis of depressive syndromes and the prediction of ECT response. British Journal of Psychiatry 111: 659–674

Clare A W, Cairns S V 1978 Design development and use of a standardised interview to assess social maladjustment and dysfunction in community studies. Psychological Medicine 8: 589–604

Cooper J E 1970 The Leyton Obsessional Inventory. Psychological Medicine 1: 48–64

Cooper J E, Mackenzie S 1981 The rapid prediction of low score on a standardised psychiatric interview (Present State examination). In: Wing J K, Bebbington P, Robins L N (eds) What is a case? Grant McIntyre, London

Cooper J E, Kendell R E, Gurland B J, Sharpe L, Copeland J R M, Simon R 1972 Psychiatric diagnosis in New York and London. Oxford University Press, London

Cooper J E, Copeland J R M, Brown G W, Harris T, Gourlay A J 1977 Further studies on interviewer training and inter-rater reliability of the Present State Examination (PSE). Psychological Medicine 7: 517–523

Dunn M, O'Driscoll C, Dayson D, Wills W, Leff J 1990 The TAPS Project 4: An observational study of the social life of long-stay patients. British Journal of Psychiatry 157: 842–848

Endicott J, Spitzer R L 1978 A diagnostic review: the Schedule for Affective Disorders and Schizophrenia. Archives of General Psychiatry 35: 837–844

Endicott J, Spitzer R L 1979 Use of the Research Diagnostic Criteria and the Schedule for Affective Disorders and Schizophrenia to study affective disorders. American Journal of Psychiatry 136: 52–56

Farmer A, Randy K, McGuffin P, Bebbington P 1987 A comparison between the Present State Examination and the Composite International Diagnostic Interview. Archives of General Psychiatry 44: 1064–1068

Feighner J P, Robins E, Guze S B et al 1972 Diagnostic criteria for use in psychiatric research. Archives of General Psychiatry 26: 57–63

Folstein M P, Romanoski A J, Nestadt G et al 1985 Brief report on the clinical reappraisal of the DIS carried out at the Johns Hopkins site of the epidemiological catchment area programme of the NIMH. Psychological Medicine 15: 809–814

Goldberg D P 1972 The detection of psychiatric illness by questionnaire. Maudsley monograph 21. Oxford University Press, London

Goldberg D, Hillier V P 1979 A scaled version of the General Health Questionnaire. Psychological Medicine 9: 139–145

Goldberg D, Cooper B, Eastwood M R, Kedward H B, Shepherd M 1970 A standardised psychiatric interview for use in community surveys. British Journal of Preventive and Social Medicine 24: 18–23

Goldberg D, Kay C, Thompson L 1976 Psychiatric morbidity in general practice and the community. Psychological Medicine 6: 565–569

Goodman W K, Price L H, Rasmussen S A et al 1989. The Yale–Brown Obsessive Compulsive Scale. Archives of General Psychiatry 46: 1006–1111

Hamilton M 1959 The assessment of anxiety states by rating. British Journal of Medical Psychology 32: 50–55

Hamilton M 1967 Development of a rating scale for primary depressive illness. British Journal of Social and Clinical Psychology 6: 278–296

Huppert F A, Walters D E, Day N E, Elliott B J 1989 The factor structure of the General Health Questionnaire (GHQ30): a reliability study on 6317 community residents. British Journal of Psychiatry 155: 178–185

Jones R R, Reid J B, Patterson G R 1975 Naturalistic observation in clinical assessment. In: McReynolds P (ed) Advances in psychological assessment, vol. 3. Jossey-Bass, San Francisco

Katz M M, Lyerly S B 1963 Methods of measuring adjustment and social behaviour in the community: 1. Rationale, description, discriminative validity and scale development. Psychological Reports 13: 505–535

Kellner R 1987 A symptom questionnaire. Journal of Clinical Psychiatry 48: 268–274

Kellner R, Sheffield B F 1973 A self-rating scale of distress. Psychological Medicine 3: 88–100

Kelly G A 1963 Theory of personality: the psychology of personal constructs. Norton, New York

Krawiecka M, Goldberg D, Vaughan M 1977 A standardised psychiatric assessment scale for rating chronic psychotic patients. Acta Psychiatrica Scandinavica 55: 299–308

Leber P 1990 Quantitative estimates of drug effects in psychopharmacology. Journal of Psychopharmacology 4: 53–62

Lund C E, Mortimer A M, Rogers D, McKenna P J 1991 Motor, volitional and behavioural disorders in schizophrenia 1: assessment using the Modified Rogers Scale. British Journal of Psychiatry 158: 323–327

McCormack H M, De L Horne D J, Sheather S 1988 Clinical applications of visual analogue scales: a critical review. Psychological Medicine 18: 1004–1019

McCreadie R G, Barron E T 1984 The Nithsdale schizophrenia survey IV. Social adjustment by self report. British Journal of Psychiatry 144: 547–550

McCreadie R G, Affleck J W, McKenzie Y, Robinson ADT 1987 A comparison of scales for assessing rehabilitation patients. British Journal of Psychiatry 151: 520–522

McGuffin P, Katz R, Aldrich J 1986 Past and present state examination: the assessment of 'life time ever' psychopathology. Psychological Medicine 16: 461–465

McKenna P J, Lund C E, Mortimer A M, Biggins C A 1991 Motor, volitional and behavioural disorders in schizophrenia 2: the 'conflict of paradigms' hypothesis. British Journal of Psychiatry 158: 328–336

McLeod J D, Turnbull J E, Kessler R C, Abelson J M 1990 Sources of discrepancy in the comparison of a lay-administrated diagnostic instrument with clinical diagnosis. Psychiatry Research 31: 145–159

Mannuzza S, Fyer A J, Martin L Y et al 1989 Reliability of anxiety measurement. Archives of General Psychiatry 46: 1093–1101

Metcalfe M, Goldman E 1965 Validation of an inventory for measuring depression. British Journal of Psychiatry 111: 240–242

Montgomery S A, Asberg M 1979 A new depression scale designed to be sensitive to change. British Journal of Psychiatry 134: 382–389

Moorey S, Greer S, Watson M et al 1991 The factor structure and factor stability of the Hospital Anxiety and Depression Scale in patients with cancer. British Journal of Psychiatry 158: 255–259

Mulhall D J 1976 Systematic self assessment by PQRST (personal questionnaire rapid scoring technique). Psychological Medicine 6: 591–597

Murray R M, Cooper J E, Smith A 1979 The Leyton Obsessional Inventory: an analysis of the responses of 73 obsessional patients. Psychological Medicine 9: 305–311

Osgood C E, Suci G J, Tannenbaum P H 1957 The measurement of meaning. University of Illinois Press, Urbana, IL

Overall J E, Gorham D R 1962 The Brief Psychiatric Rating Scale. Psychological Reports 10: 799–812

Parker G, Rosen A, Emdur N, Hadzi-Pavlovic D 1991 The Life Skills Profile: psychometric properties of a measure assessing function and disability in schizophrenia. Acta Psychiatrica Scandinavica 83: 145–152

Paykel E S 1985 The Clinical Interview for Depression: development, reliability and validity. Journal of Affective Disorders 9: 85–96

Potts M K, Daniels M, Burnham M A, Wells K B 1990 A structured interview version of the Hamilton Depression Rating Scale: evidence of reliability and versatility of administration. Journal of Psychiatric Research 24: 335–350

Prince R, Miranda L 1977 Monitoring life stress to prevent recurrence of coronary heart disease episodes. Canadian Psychiatric Association Journal 22: 161–169

Rachman S J, Hodgson R J 1980 Obsessions and Compulsions. Prentice Hall, Englewood Cliffs.

Rehm L P, O'Hara M W 1985 Item characteristics of the Hamilton Rating Scale for Depression. Journal of Psychiatric Research 19: 31–44

Robins L N, Helzer J E, Croughan J, Ratcliff K S 1981a National Institute of Mental Health Diagnostic Interview Schedule. Archives of General Psychiatry 38: 381–389

Robins L N, Helzer J E, Croughan J, Ratcliff K S 1981b The NIMH diagnostic interview schedule: its history, characteristics and validity. In: Wing J K, Bebbington P, Robins L N (eds) What is a case? The problem of definition in community surveys. Grant McIntyre, London

Russell M B, Bernal M A 1977 Temporal and climatic variables in naturalistic observation. Journal of Applied Behaviour Analysis 10: 399–405

Rutter B M 1979 The prognostic significance of psychological factors in the management of chronic bronchitis. Psychological Medicine 9: 63–70

Sanavio E 1988 Obsessions and compulsions: the Padua Inventory. Behaviour Research and Therapy 26: 169–177

Shapiro M B 1961 A method of measuring psychological changes specific to the individual psychiatric patient. British Journal of Medical Psychology 34: 151–155

Shrout P E, Spitzer R L, Fleiss J L 1987 Quantification of agreement in psychiatric diagnosis revisited. Archives of General Psychiatry 44: 172–177

Snaith R P, Baugh S J, Clayden A D, Husain A, Sipple M A 1982 The Clinical Anxiety Scale: an instrument derived from the Hamilton Anxiety Scale. British Journal of Psychiatry 141: 518–523

Snaith R P, Harrop F M, Newby D A, Teale C 1986 Grade scores of the Montgomery–Asberg Depression and the Clinical Anxiety Scales. British Journal of Psychiatry 148: 599–601

Spielberger C D, Gorsuch R L, Lushene R 1970 State–Trait Anxiety Inventory manual. Consulting Psychologists Press, Palo Alto, CA

Teplin L A, Lutz G W 1985 Measuring alcohol intoxication: the development of an observational instrument. Journal of Studies on Alcohol 46: 459–466

van den Brink W, Maarten W J, Koeter M A et al 1989 Psychiatric diagnosis in an outpatient population. Archives of General Psychiatry 46: 369–372

Webb E J, Campbell D T 1981 Non-reactive measures in the social sciences, 2nd edn. Houghton Mifflin, Boston

Weissman M M, Bothwell S 1976 Assessment of social adjustment by patient self-report. Archives of General Psychiatry 33: 1111–1115

World Health Organization WHO 1973 The international pilot study of schizophrenia (IPSS), vol. 1, Geneva

Wing J K, Babor T, Brugha T et al 1990 SCAN: Schedules for Clinical Assessment in Neuropsychiatry. Archives of General Psychiatry 47: 589–593

Wing J K, Cooper J E, Sartorius N 1974 The measurement and classification of psychiatric symptoms. Cambridge University Press, London

Wing J K, Mann S A, Leff J P, Nixon J M 1978 The concept of a 'case' in psychiatric population surveys. Psychological Medicine 8: 203–217

Wurtele S K, Martin J E 1987 Assessment of smoking. In: Nirenberg T D, Maisto S A (eds) Developments in the assessment and treatment of addictive behaviors. Ablex, Norwood

Zealley A K, Aitken R C V 1969 Measurement of mood. Proceedings of the Royal Society of Medicine 62: 993–996

Zigmond A S, Snaith R P 1983 The Hospital Anxiety and Depression Scale. Acta Psychiatrica Scandinavica 67: 361–370

Zimmerman M, Coryell W 1988 The validity of a self-report questionnaire for diagnosing major depressive disorder. Archives of General Psychiatry 45: 738–740

10. Statistics and research design

R. J. McGuire

INTRODUCTION

This chapter provides an introduction to the basic concepts of statistics by defining them and illustrating their use and calculation. The needs of the trainee psychiatrist or other professional preparing for a multiple-choice examination will not be neglected, nor will those of the working professional who has to understand the statistics used in research papers in order to keep abreast of the literature. But those who are likely to benefit most are those who have collected some data of their own and would like to get it into shape for a paper or a thesis. For this last group there are worked examples with suggestions for further exercises, because statistics does not stick very long unless you have actually worked something out for yourself. Not all the requirements of that group will be met nor all their questions answered, but they should acquire enough understanding to enable them to go to more advanced texts with some degree of confidence.

A major change that has taken place in the last few years is the increased availability not only of statistical packages on university computers, but also cheap microcomputers and electronic calculators with standard statistical programmes, so that only the most unfortunate researchers have the tedium of adding, subtracting, multiplying and dividing their own data. This development is particularly good news for the many who approach all mathematical techniques with what amounts to a phobia for numbers and an expectation of mystification and failure.

Research design is dealt with at the end of the chapter. The statistics section appears first because often the reason why one particular approach has been used in research is because the data can only be analysed competently and the correct conclusions drawn if that method is used.

Novice researchers sometimes believe that they can collect data in a way convenient for themselves and when it is all in take it along to a statistician who will, by some means beyond normal mortals, produce a set of neat conclusions. It is seldom wise to collect data in this way and hope to get answers. Only good questions get good answers.

STATISTICAL METHODS

Statistics has two main uses. The first is to simplify data either by illustrating them, as is done in graphs and diagrams, or by assigning a value, such as a mean which in one number represents all the scores of a group, or a correlation coefficient, which measures the relationship between two variables. This use of statistics is fairly common and most of us are already well acquainted with at least some of the forms described here. The second use is to provide a measure of our confidence in a given result. This is usually done by stating the probability that the result could have arisen by chance. The statement $p < 0.05$ printed beside a result means that it is likely to have arisen by chance in less than five out of 100 similar experiments. It follows that the smaller the fraction the more confidence we can have in the conclusions. Another way in which confidence can be expressed is to state the interval within which we are confident to a stated degree the true value of a measure lies. Statistics therefore gives us confidence by providing more accurate knowledge of our limitations.

DESCRIPTIVE STATISTICS

Most scientists in analysing data do not use illustrations frequently enough. Simple diagrams and graphs often display much more information in an understandable form than any number of tables or other numerical statistics and often reveal aspects of the data that would otherwise be missed.

Frequency distributions are diagrams in which the number of people, or occurrences, in each of several categories is represented by the height above a base level, preferably zero. The categories may be quite discreet, such as diagnostic categories, or may be formed from a continuous distribution such as age, in which case the categories will cover successive age intervals, e.g. 15–19 years, 20–24 years, etc. The range of each category, here 5 years, is called the *class interval* and the middle scores, here 17 years, 22 years, etc., represent the class interval. Figure 10.1 shows the frequency distribution of the ages of 25 patients involved in a drug trial. The data are drawn from column C4 in Table 10.1, which is given later in the chapter. A diagram such as this where the frequencies are represented by rectangles is called a *histogram*. Where frequencies are large and the class intervals are small, or where only the general shape of the distribution is to be indicated, the centres of the tops of the rectangles can be joined up to produce a *frequency curve*. It is important to remember that the area under the curve and not the height represents the frequency since the frequency depends on the class interval. In the histogram above, the frequency 9 is not the number who are aged 65 years but the number within the age group 65–69 years. In a frequency curve the total area under the curve represents the total frequency.

Cumulative frequency curves are curves where the height of the curve at any score represents the total number who have less than that score. Figure 10.2 is a cumulative curve formed from the same data as the previous figure. Cumulative curves can be useful in

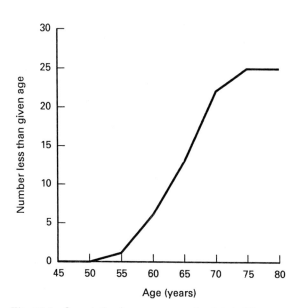

Fig. 10.2 Cumulative frequency curve for data in Figure 10.1.

smoothing out the irregularities in a frequency curve and for giving estimates of values in class intervals that are not supplied in the original data, e.g. the number who might be expected to be 57 years old or over. This can be estimated as 19.6; in fact it is 20.

Other types of diagrams, graphs and tables

There are other types of statistical diagrams such as pie charts and graphs which should not be neglected in simplifying data. Scattergrams and illustrative tables will be discussed later.

DISTRIBUTION AND PROBABILITIES

We have seen how the frequency distribution indicates the proportion of the sample, and therefore approximately of the population, who fall into a certain category or between two scores. This proportion measures the probability that a randomly chosen member of the population comes from that category or class interval. If we now look at some types of distributions we will see some practical applications.

Even distribution is when there are equal numbers in each of the categories. This is deliberately so for many games of chance, e.g. playing cards have four suits each of 13 cards, so the probability of drawing, say, a club from the pack is one in four. Similarly, the probability of drawing a face card (Jack, Queen or King) is three in 13. The probability of *not* drawing any of the

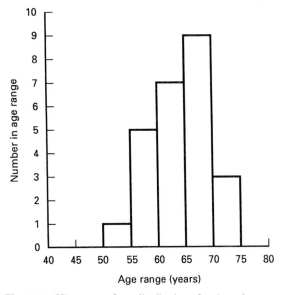

Fig. 10.1 Histogram of age distribution of patients from Table 10.1, column C4.

above is 1 minus the probability of doing so. If p is the probability of an event and q is the probability of the event not occurring then $p + q = 1$

A *binomial distribution* occurs when a trial can have two outcomes, a or b, with probabilities p and q, respectively, and a series of m trials is recorded. If we ignore the order of the results we have a number of possible outcomes, ranging from all m trials giving the outcome a to all giving outcome b. If we think of outcomes a and b being the birth of a boy or girl, respectively, then we are talking about the sex distribution with in a family of m children. For example, in a family of four children what is the probability that there are exactly two boys and two girls? *Pascal's triangle* gives us a means of answering this question (see Fig. 10.3). It is a triangular pattern of numbers where the numbers on the next line are given by adding the adjacent two numbers on the line above. Its use can be best illustrated by considering a situation where two events are equally likely, $p = q = \frac{1}{2}$. This is approximately true for the sex of a child. The sample size will refer to the number of children and the number of categories to the number of different combinations, ignoring birth order, or their sexes. If there are two children, there are three possibilities, two boys, one boy and one girl, and two girls. It will help to think of the left-hand side of the triangle as predominance of boys and the right hand side as a predominance of girls. Now, the numbers in the frequency distribution give the expected proportions of each. For a sample size of two there is one chance of there being two boys, two chances of one boy and one girl and one chance of two girls, making a total of four. The chance of one boy and one girl is therefore two out of four. (In case you are puzzled by the family size of zero there is only one possibility, i.e. no boys and no girl with a likelihood of one out of one, i.e. certainty.) Suppose a father of five children complained that he had only one son out of the five. How unlikely is this distribution? A sample size of 5 gives the probability of exactly that, namely one boy, as five out of 32, but we should also consider the mirror image of only one daughter which is also five out of

32 and also the more extreme cases of no sons and no daughters for which the probability is one in 32 each, so in families of five the chances of having an imbalance of the sexes as great or greater than one to four is 12 out of 32 or roughly one in three, which is probably more likely than would be guessed.

This example illustrates two features of the use of probability tables that may be overlooked by the beginner. The first is to remember to include the more unlikely probabilities in the consideration of the deviancy of a result and also to include the opposite result. This latter point is particularly relevant in statistics, and when it is applied gives the *two-tailed* probability. The *one-tailed* probability test, which assumes only one direction of improbability, should only be used if the opposite result is irrelevant or if it is so unthinkable that any consideration of it can be completely dismissed, for example the drug proving significantly less effective than the placebo — and even then wouldn't any respectable researcher have a closer look?

Pascal's triangle can also be used when the probabilities are unequal, i.e. $p \neq q$. Now the numbers refer to the coefficients of probabilities given p^m, $p^{m-1}q$, $p^{m-2}q^2$, ..., q^m. If $p = 0.9$ and $q = 0.1$ for a sample size of $m = 3$ these would be 1×0.9^3, $3 \times 0.9^2 \times 0.1$, $3 \times 0.9 \times 0.1^2$ and 1×0.1^3, which are 0.729, 0.243, 0.027 and 0.001, respectively, adding up to 1.000. These are the probabilities of cutting three times from a deck with no face cards and finding, respectively, no aces, one ace, two aces and three aces. This type of distribution is called a *binomial distribution*. It is clearly symmetrical if p and q are equal. In the last example it is *skewed*. A distribution is *negatively skewed* if the scores trail off to the left. For the example above, since the probabilities refer to zero, one, two and three occurrences, we would plot them as 0.729–0.001 for increasing scores and the distribution would be *positively skewed*.

The normal distribution

This is the most commonly occurring frequency distribution in nature. It arises, for example, if we plot the

Sample size	Number categories	Frequency distribution	Total frequency
0	1	1	1
1	2	1 1	2
2	3	1 2 1	4
3	4	1 3 3 1	8
4	5	1 4 6 4 1	16
5	6	1 5 10 10 5 1	32
6	7	1 6 15 20 15 6 1	64

Fig. 10.3 Pascal's triangle where the items in each successive row are derived by adding the two adjacent items in the row above.

frequency distribution of height, weight or IQ in boys of a given age from the same social background. The curve is bell shaped and is symmetrical about its mean (see Fig. 10.4).

The formula for the normal distribution is

$$f_x = [1/(\sigma\sqrt{(2\pi)}] \exp [-(x - \mu)^2/2\sigma^2]$$

where f_x is the frequency of occurrence of any given value, μ the arithmetic mean and σ the standard deviation.

Luckily you will never have to work out this formula. It is uniquely determined by its mean and standard deviation. The frequencies within certain intervals of the distribution are given in Figure 10.4 and are published in tables. They are the theoretical basis of many of the statistical tests of significance in standard use.

When $p = q = 0.5$ the binomial distribution resembles the normal distribution even for small sample sizes. With larger sample sizes, say $m = 50$, even for $p = 0.9$, $q = 0.1$, it is fairly close to the normal distribution. Since many natural characteristics are multi-

genetic where each gene is either switched on (p) or off (q) it is no wonder that such characteristics are normally distributed.

There is one more distribution that should be mentioned, namely the *Poisson distribution*, which is the distribution when there is some event that occurs rarely. Most trials will therefore have a score of 0, i.e. the event has not occurred, some have the score 1, but very many fewer will have the score 2 or higher.

In the early days of statistical theory, to simplify the task of working out the distributions of certain statistics it was usually assumed that the data were normally distributed. Only when this were so could one be confident that the probabilities quoted were accurate. It did not follow that if the data had not been normally distributed the tables were wrong. In fact, now that distributions can be generated by computers and various possibilities empirically determined it is clear that p values are seldom much altered by the non-normality of a distribution. This is usually expressed by saying that the statistic is *robust*. Most tests, e.g. the t test and the product moment correlation coefficient

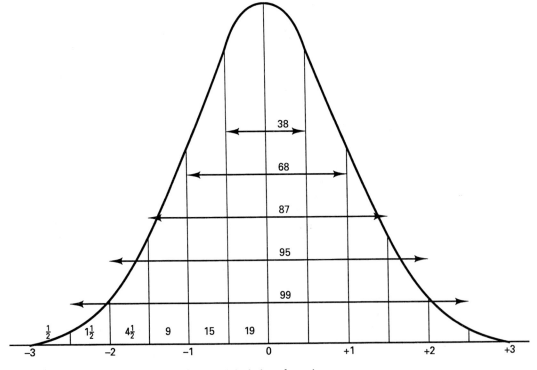

Standard deviations from the mean

Fig. 10.4 The normal distribution. Numbers on the left show what percentage of the total population lie in each half standard deviation interval. Numbers on the right show what percentage lie within the given number of standard deviations from the mean.

r, give valid results *except* when a distribution is significantly skewed. Some examiners and paper reviewers unfortunately seem to be ignorant of this and are more purist than most statisticians.

Measurements on frequency distributions

We have spoken so far about theoretical frequency distributions. In practice we collect data from a sample and by examining them we try to assess which theoretical distribution they most resemble; if the fit is reasonable we can use our knowledge of the theoretical distribution to make reliable estimates of the probability of the occurrence of events within the population. We usually look at our distributions by deciding on some measure of the central score of the sample and then looking at how the scores deviate from this actual score.

Non-parametric tests

Parameters have already been defined as measures, such as means and standard deviations, which refer to the population, and which can only be estimated from measures of the sample. When we are drawing conclusions about probability we are often making assumptions about the type of frequency distribution of the population, usually by assuming that it is normal. We then draw conclusions based on our estimates of the true population parameters as to the probability of our hypothesis being true or not. If our assumptions about our population are false, for instance because the distribution is not normal as we had assumed, then our conclusions may be false. However, there are occasions when we may prefer to play safe and use tests that do not assume a specific distribution. (They will incidentally not give wrong results if the population is actually normally distributed.)

There are also times when we cannot easily use parametric tests because our data are not in a suitable numerical form but are expressed in broad categories, such as mildly, moderately or severely depressed, or our data give us only an order of scores, such as the most disturbed to least disturbed patients, with no actual score for the degree of disturbance. These types of measure can usually fit into a form suitable for non-parametric statistics.

Non-parametric tests are also less dependent on sample size and can therefore be used when observations are too few to yield reliable results from parametric tests. Finally, many people are tempted to use non-parametric tests because they find the computations much simpler. Unfortunately, the tables used for assessing the significance of results are often more complex, so that the student who has worked out the statistics correctly enough may err when referring to the tables.

On the whole, non-parametric statistics are less *powerful* than their parametric equivalent, which means that for a given sample size they are less likely to detect a statistically significant result if one exists. For each problem I will try to mention both parametric and non-parametric procedures — indicated by 'par' and 'non-par'.

The null hypothesis

Although when we do research we are often trying to demonstrate differences, either already existing or produced by an experimental procedure, we have to start from the position that there is no difference until we have proved otherwise. That is what is meant by the *null hypothesis*. In t tests we assume that the true mean of x and the true mean of y are identical and that the difference found in the experiment had arisen by chance. We then calculate t and consult the appropriate tables to see how often this value of t would have arisen if the null hypothesis were correct. The t tables express this likelihood as a p value, for probability. If, for example, we had found $p = 0.001$ this would indicate that, if the true means of x and y were identical, a difference as large as we have found for our sample sizes would have occurred only once in 1000 similar experiments. This is very unlikely and we would therefore reject the null hypothesis with a high level of confidence and state that the two samples were not from the same population.

Levels of statistical significance

Before the advent of sophisticated calculators it was very difficult for experimenters to work out the exact probability of any result and they had therefore to refer to tables which gave the values of the significance statistic for certain values of p according to different degrees of freedom. Because of this the convention arose that p values were only quoted as being between the values given in the tables. A value of p greater than 0.05, i.e. the result could have arisen more often than one in 20, is, by this convention, regarded as *not statistically significant*. A value of p less than 0.05 but greater than 0.01 is regarded as *probably statistically significant* and the result is often labelled with the index * to show this level of significance. Similarly, p <0.01 is *statistically significant* and labelled ** and p <0.001 is *highly statistically significant* and labelled ***.

These levels are only conventional, and yet many researchers feel delighted when $p = 0.049$ and desolated when $p = 0.051$, as if there were some fundamental difference between the two. This artificiality does not arise when *intervals of confidence* are used, as will be discussed shortly.

Practical significance

Statistical significance should not be confused with practical significance and p values should not be confused with the clinical importance of the difference or the relationship. Statistical significance states the likelihood of a true difference or a true relationship, etc., but the actual size of such a difference may be quite small or even trivial from a clinical point of view. On the other hand, a difference may be important but fail to reach a level of statistical significance because of the small sample sizes used and *might* have done so with a larger sample size. Another factor which influences statistical significance is the variation within each sample. If samples can be made more homogeneous, for example by limiting the age range considered, a true difference might be more easily demonstrated.

DRUG TRIAL DATA

To give some cohesion to the statistical examples, some data are supplied in Table 10.1 and represent a simple drug trial. Let us assume that a new antidepressant drug is to be used and it is decided to compare it with an established antidepressant. One would measure the depression score of each patient before treatment, and column C5 is the rating of depression given by rater R1. He would also rate the patient for depression at the end of the treatment, and that result is recorded in column C7. With only these two scores one could in fact test the efficacy of the drug. However, it would be more convincing if we had shown that the rating method is reliable. For this purpose a second rater R2 also rates each patient for depression before the treatment begins, and this result is recorded in column C6. The patient's own rating of depression might also be used before and after treatment (columns C8 and C9). Besides being a useful measure in its own right, this rating can be used to validate the other depressive rating scale. If it had also been suggested in the literature that this new drug reduced anxiety, the patient's anxiety before and after the treatment would be recorded in columns C10 and C11. Other information about the patients is recorded in columns C1–C4: which treatment the patient is receiving (A or B) in column C2, sex in column C3, age in column C4 and

case number in column C1. The information in columns C1–C11 could be entered into a computer as it stands and all the later computations done using only these data.

Outcome will be evaluated by using change in scores. Recorded in columns C12–C14 are the change in rater R1's scoring, the change in the patients' own scoring of depression and the change in anxiety score. Finally, these three measures expressed as a percentage of their own original value are represented in columns C15–C17. Any computer could be used to calculate columns C12–C17 with simple instructions, but they are shown here for the benefit of those without computers. Also for the benefit of those without computers, the mean and standard deviation of each column is recorded at the bottom for the two treatment groups separately and combined. This table will be referred to in many of the worked examples that follow and students can attempt other examples of their own from the data and see what conclusions they can draw.

UNITS OF MEASUREMENT

Measures of central tendency

The most frequently used representative score is the *arithmetic mean* (par), which is what is commonly referred to as the 'average'. It is written $\bar{x}$, and is read as *x* bar, and is calculated by the formula

$$\bar{x} = (\Sigma x)/n$$

where Σx is the sum of the *x* values. For the age data in Table 10.1 the mean age is 1542/25, which is 61.68 years. The answer is often used for comparison with other means in statistical calculation and is therefore taken to a bit more accuracy than would be relevant for the individual. The mean of the sample is the best estimate of the mean of the population from which it was drawn, so we might predict that any group of similar patients would be aged about 62 years. The unit of the mean is obviously the same as the unit of the scores, whether this be years, milligrams or IQ. The mean is the most stable measure of central tendency, i.e. it will not change much if you enlarge your sample or take another sample from the same population.

The *median* (non-par) is also used. It is the score with half the sample score above and half the score below. In the example here there are 25 patients so the median will have 12 individuals older and 12 younger than the given age. One patient is 62 years old and 12 lie on either side of that age so 62 years is the *median*.

Table 10.1 Data from 25 subjects representing in columns C1–C4 experimental and personal variables, in C5–C11 mood variables and in C12–C17 calculated change scores. Means and standard deviations are given for the two treatment groups and for all the subjects. See text for explanation

Case	Tr. gp	Sex	Age (years)	Dep. bef. R1	Dep. bef. R2	Dep. aft. R1	Dep. bef. SR	Dep. aft. SR	Anx. bef. SR	Anx. aft. SR	Dep. chg. R1	Dep. chg. SR	Anx. chg. SR	Dep. pch. R1	Dep. pch. SR	Anx. pch. SR
C1	C2	C3	C4	C5	C6	C7	C8	C9	C10	C11	C12	C13	C14	C15	C16	C17
1	A	M	56	35	39	14	52	45	41	35	21	7	6	60	13	15
2	A	F	65	44	46	37	68	60	49	52	7	8	-3	16	12	-6
3	A	F	55	38	43	22	58	46	36	36	16	12	0	42	21	0
4	A	F	69	41	42	32	66	57	44	41	9	9	3	22	14	7
5	A	F	66	26	28	26	55	46	37	37	0	9	0	0	16	0
6	A	M	67	36	31	32	62	60	37	33	4	2	4	11	3	11
7	A	F	52	31	32	20	55	48	28	33	11	7	-5	35	13	-18
8	A	M	58	31	36	9	54	40	33	30	22	14	3	71	26	9
9	A	F	65	51	49	37	71	66	46	44	14	5	2	27	7	4
10	A	M	57	28	26	19	59	52	24	25	9	7	-1	32	12	-4
11	A	M	61	42	47	19	60	52	48	45	23	8	3	55	13	6
12	A	F	59	23	20	21	53	50	31	27	2	3	4	-6	6	13
13	A	F	68	35	31	37	63	60	44	39	-2	3	5	9	5	11
14	A	F	54	26	29	23	56	45	33	34	3	11	-1	12	20	-3
15	B	F	58	34	27	49	67	71	46	41	-15	-4	5	-44	-6	11
16	B	F	71	32	32	41	62	58	40	41	-9	4	-1	-28	6	-3
17	B	F	66	25	31	22	54	41	32	29	3	13	3	12	24	9
18	B	M	67	46	41	50	72	73	40	44	-4	-1	-4	-9	-1	-10
19	B	M	53	36	45	31	56	46	54	60	5	10	-6	14	18	-11
20	B	F	64	38	40	33	64	59	45	45	5	5	0	13	8	0
21	B	F	65	42	38	37	70	70	45	37	5	0	8	12	0	18
22	B	F	62	19	20	21	57	45	33	20	-2	12	13	-11	21	39
23	B	M	61	22	21	35	57	52	37	34	-13	5	3	-59	9	8
24	B	M	63	30	26	33	59	62	45	35	-3	-3	10	-10	-5	22
25	B	F	60	34	35	27	63	56	36	30	7	7	6	21	11	17
Group 1 Means (n=14)			60.9	34.8	35.6	24.9	59.4	51.9	37.9	36.5	9.9	7.5	1.4	25.6	12.9	3.2
SD			5.72	7.93	8.85	8.92	5.88	7.58	7.68	7.30	8.28	3.48	3.18	23.0	6.46	9.02
Group 2 Means (n=11)			62.7	32.6	32.4	34.5	61.9	57.6	41.2	37.8	-1.91	4.36	3.36	-8.09	7.73	9.09
SD			4.82	8.21	8.27	9.54	5.94	10.93	6.55	10.40	7.73	5.87	5.84	26.22	10.24	14.85
All Means (n=25)			61.7	33.8	34.2	29.1	60.5	54.4	39.4	37.1	4.7	6.1	2.3	11.9	10.6	5.8
SD			5.32	7.97	8.58	10.23	5.92	9.43	7.25	8.63	9.90	4.84	4.54	30.00	8.56	12.03

Rating (columns C5–C7: Dep. bef. R1, Dep. bef. R2, Dep. aft. R1)

The *mode* (non-par) is the score which occurs most frequently. Here it lies in the group who are aged 65–69 years. It is given as the mid-score of that group, in this case 67 years. In any distribution it is the score corresponding to the peak. In a small sample like this it is too unstable to be of much use as a representative measure but the definition is important in its use in describing some frequency distributions as *bimodal* because they have two distinct peaks. This happens when the sample, and hence the population, contains two different groups with different central points. In any unimodal distribution which is symmetrical, the mean, median and mode are likely to be very similar to each other. However, in a skewed distribution the mode will correspond to the peak and the median, and then the mean will occur in the direction of the long tail.

Measures of spread

Knowing only the mean of a distribution gives no indication of what proportion is different from that. We have to have some indication of the spread to know this. We will start with some simple but less useful measures of spread.

The *range* is the difference between the lowest and the highest score obtained. In the example, the age range is 19 years since the youngest patient is aged 52 years and the oldest 71 years, giving a difference of 19 years. The range is unstable for small samples since it depends only on the extreme scores. If one patient had happened to be 85 years old the range would have almost doubled (to 33 years) because of that one score.

The *standard deviation* (SD) is the most frequently used measure of spread of scores, because it is the most stable, using every score in its calculation. It is a very fundamental measure, as is its square, the variance of a sample or population. Its formula may look difficult and rather arbitrary, but many pocket calculators now do it automatically:

$$SD_x = \sqrt{[(\Sigma(x - \bar{x})^2)/(n - 1)]}.$$

Since it would be tedious and would introduce awkward figures to subtract the mean from each score before squaring it in the formula above, the formula is simplified, without any loss of accuracy, to the following:

$$SD_x = \sqrt{[(n\Sigma x^2 - (\Sigma x)^2)/(n(n-1))]}$$

For column C17, the percentage change in anxiety for all the patients, $n = 25$, $\Sigma x = 145$, $\Sigma x^2 = 4317$, so

$$SD_x = \sqrt{[(25 \times 4317 - 145 \times 145)/(25 \times 24)]}$$
$$= \sqrt{(144.83)}$$
$$= 12.03.$$

Standard (Z) scores

If a population is normally distributed it is often useful to express an individual's scores not in actual units but as the number of standard deviations above or below the mean. This is the standard score Z and the formula is

$$Z_{x1} = (x_1 - \bar{x})/SD_x.$$

One use is when scores in different units are being compared. For example, the first patient in the table was rated as having improved by 60% in depression (column C15) but rated himself as only having improved by 13%. Are these scores really as different as they look? This question can be answered by comparing him with the other patients in both measures and expressing his position on each in Z scores. This is the only simple method for comparing positions which are measured in different units. The means and standard deviations of the two measures are 11.88 and 30.00, respectively, for rating and 10.64 and 8.56 for self-rating. So

$$Z_{dep} = (60-11.88)/30.00 = +1.60$$
$$Z_{SR} = (13-10.64)/8.56 = +0.28.$$

Thus, he is well above the average for the rater while only slightly above average for his self-rating.

Standard errors

Not only scores have standard deviations. Any measure, such as a mean, can have a standard deviation. This is seen when we take several samples of the same population and therefore have several means which can be treated as scores. We can then calculate the mean of the means and the standard deviation of the means. The values of the means would form a normal distribution and the likelihood of any deviancy could be determined from it by referring to Figure 10.4. The standard deviation of the mean is known as the *standard error* of the mean (SE_{mean}) for reasons which arise from its use. If our number of samples was large enough, we would have the data to estimate how likely it is that a particular value for the mean could have arisen in the population. This would be done by expressing the particular mean as a standard score and by reference to tables of the normal distribution we could see how likely it was that the mean could, by chance, have that value in the given population of means.

Luckily, it is not necessary to take several samples to work out the standard error of the mean for a normally distributed population as it depends on the sample size and is calculated by the simple formula

$$SE_{mean} = SD_x/\sqrt{n}$$

where n is the number in the sample.

The mean anxiety score before treatment (column C10) for our 25 patients was 39.36 with $SD_x = 7.25$ and $n = 25$, so we find

$$SE_{mean} = 7.25/\sqrt{(25)} = 1.25.$$

This is a measure of the variability we can expect from this mean. Other uses of the standard error will be demonstrated shortly. Similar formulae are available to find the standard error of many descriptive statistics, including the standard deviation itself.

Type 1 and type 2 errors

When the results of an experiment are announced in statistical terms it is usually in the form 'treatment A was better than treatment B ($p < 0.05$)'. This means that in less than 5% of similar trials (i.e. same numbers, same standard deviations in each group) where a difference as large as that recorded in this experiment was found would there have been no *true* difference between the groups. One can therefore be 95% confident in saying that a difference exists in this case. The 5% refers to the chances of our having made an error of *type 1*.

Type 2 error represents the opposite danger, namely saying that no difference exists when in fact it does. Until recently this type of error has been almost ignored, largely because of the ambiguity as to what is meant by 'no difference'. In type 1 errors, unless the samples are very large, the differences have to be reasonably big to yield significant results. But to avoid type 2 errors one must start by defining just how big a difference one is prepared to ignore — which is a clinical question.

If one does not bear the type 2 error in mind one is in danger of assuming, fallaciously, that finding that a difference between two groups is not statistically significant ($p > 0.05$) is proof that no difference exists. To prevent falling into this trap two changes in the method of analysing and reporting results are available. The first is to work out the chances of a type 2 error in the experiment that is planned and if it is too great to increase the sample sizes until the risk is

at an acceptable level. This will be dealt with later. The second way is to report results in the form of *confidence intervals*.

CONFIDENCE INTERVALS

When the mean of a sample is measured it is assumed that it is close to the mean of the population — but how near? Luckily it is possible to answer that question with a certain level of confidence. One says, for example, that one would be correct 95% of the time in stating that the true mean of the population lay within a certain interval, called the 95% confidence interval of the mean and written CI_{95}. Corresponding intervals can be calculated for other parameters by using appropriate formulae. In every case we start off with the standard error of the measure.

Confidence interval for the mean

For a mean the standard error is found by dividing the standard deviation of the sample by the square root of the number in the sample. In Table 10.1, the depression score given by rater 1 (column C4) has a mean of 33.80, a standard deviation of 7.97 and there are 25 subjects in the sample. The SE_{mean} is therefore $7.97/5 = 1.6$. Now, in the normal distribution 95% of the items lie roughly between two standard deviations below and the same above the mean. So here 95% of the means lie between $2 \times 1.6 = 3.2$ above and below the measured mean, so the CI_{95} for this mean is 33.8 ± 3.2 or 30.6–37.0. For a more accurate answer one would not multiply by 2 but by $t_{0.05}$, which is the value of t found in statistical tables for $p < 0.05$ for degrees of freedom $(n-1)$. In this case there are 24 degrees of freedom, giving $t_{0.05} = 2.064$, which would have given an interval of 30.52–37.08. For further practice calculate the confidence interval for the percentage change in self-rating for depression (column C16): this gives a CI_{95} of 7.1–14.2% and suggests that it is unlikely (less than 5% risk) that there was no true change in this measure since a change of 0% is outside the confidence interval.

Confidence interval for the difference in means

For the difference in the means of two groups one has first to calculate the standard error of the difference of two means. If the two groups have roughly the same variances then first calculate the pooled variance estimate, which is done by multiplying each variance ($var_{A,B}$) by its degrees of freedom and dividing their sum by the sum of the degrees of freedom:

pooled variance estimate =
$[(n_A-1)\text{var}_A + (n_B-1)\text{var}_B]/(n_A + n_B-1)$.

This is then divided by each of the sample sizes in turn to yield the squares of their standard errors of the mean. The standard error of the difference of the means $SE_{diff} = \sqrt{(SE_{mean1}^2 + SE_{mean2}^2)}$. (If the variances of the two groups are different the calculation is simpler, since then the standard errors are just calculated in the usual way by dividing the standard deviation by the square root of the size of the sample.)

One now calculates the confidence interval for the difference as before by adding and subtracting two (or $t_{0.05}$) times the standard error of the difference from the measured difference. Worked examples are given later.

USING VARIOUS STATISTICAL PROCEDURES

COMPARING DIFFERENCES BETWEEN TWO GROUPS

Commonly we have two different groups, A and B, probably with different numbers in each, n_A and n_B, and with different mean scores x_A and x_B, and we wish to know if there is a real difference between the mean responses of the two groups. In our example, we can compare the different results from the 14 subjects of group A with the 11 subjects of group B. Let us consider this for the change in anxiety score (column C14). We wish to know if the mean change for group A (1.43) is significantly different from the mean change in group B (3.36). The appropriate procedures are t tests or one-way ANOVA (par) or the Mann–Whitney U test (non-par).

t test (par)

Group A with 14 patients has a mean anxiety change score of 1.43, SD = 3.18, while the 11 in group B have a mean of 3.36, SD = 5.84. The standard error for a mean is SD/√n, thus

$SE_A = 3.18/\sqrt{(14)} = 0.85$
$SE_B = 5.84/\sqrt{(11)} = 1.76$.

The formula for the standard error for the difference in the means is

$SE_{diff} = \sqrt{(SE_A^2 + SE_B^2)} = \sqrt{(6.72)} = 2.59$.

The observed difference of the means is

$(1.43 - 3.36) = -1.93$. The sign merely indicates which score was the greater and can be disregarded in the calculation:

$t = (\bar{x}_A - \bar{x}_B)/SE_{diff} = 1.93/2.59 = 0.75$
$$(DF = (n_A + n_B - 1) = 24).$$

If there was no real difference between the scores t would be zero. Here we are told that the observed difference is so many standard deviations away from zero. If it is too many (greater than 1.96) to be likely to have occurred by chance we will reject the hypothesis that the samples came from the same population.

Rather than use the normal distribution to work out the probability we usually refer to special 't tables'. This is because the normal distribution probability would only be accurate if our numbers were fairly large (say more than 100), but the t tables take account of the size of the samples by means of the *degrees of freedom* (DF).

You will come across degrees of freedom in other contexts and it is necessary to find the appropriate formula for degrees of freedom in each statistic. In tests of significance using normally distributed scores the degrees of freedom are usually one less than the number in a group. Here we have two groups in each of which the degrees of freedom is the number of the group minus 1. There is one degree of freedom represented by the two different means (again $n - 1$) and for the whole group we have therefore $n_A - 1 + n_B - 1 + 1 = n_A + n_B - 1$, which again obeys the rule of one less than the frequency. Degrees of freedom can be quite a difficult concept to understand, but fortunately it is not necessary to understand it to be able to apply it.

CI_{95} for the difference. $SE_{diff} = 2.59$ and the actual difference is 1.93, so

$CI_{95} = 1.93 - 2.06 \times 2.59$ to $1.93 + 2.06 \times 2.59$
$= -3.41 - 14.08$.

A value of zero (no true difference) obviously lies within this interval so one cannot with 95% confidence discard the null hypothesis. On the other it could be that the true difference is as great as 14.08, so one keeps an open mind — not proven rather than not true.

Mann–Whitney U test (non-par)

This tests for a difference in medians between two groups. The groups are combined and then the scores are ranked from the smallest to the largest (n_A to n_B), paying attention to sign if present. Remember that the largest negative number is the smallest number. Give the mean rank to tied scores. Now add the ranks of each group separately, giving T_A and T_B. (As a check $T_A + T_B$ should equal $(n_A + n_B)(n_A + n_B + 1)/2$.) For the smaller group, say A, find $U_A = n_A n_B + n_A(n_A + 1)/2 - T_A$ then calculate $U_B = n_A n_B - U_A$. Look up the smaller U in the appropriate tables.

For large samples ($n > 20$):

$$\text{mean}_U = n_A n_B / 2$$
$$\text{SD}_U = \sqrt{[n_A n_B (n_A + n_B + 1)/12]}$$
$$Z_U = (U - \text{mean}_U)/SD_U$$

which gives $p < 0.05$ for $Z > 1.96$.

Median test (non-par)

From the two groups combined find the median. Count the number above and the number below this median in each group. Do a χ^2 test on these data as shown below.

Matched pairs

We have considered the case where we are comparing results from two different groups. Sometimes there is only one group but each subject has two scores, e.g. before and after treatment. The appropriate techniques are the correlated t test (par) or the sign test (non-par) or Wilcoxon matched pairs test (non-par).

Correlated (paired) t test (par)

Where a subject has a before and an after score (columns C5 and C7 or C8 and C9 or C10 and C11), the differences should be tested using this technique. Computers can be used, with the data from, say, columns C8 and C9, and producing a value of t with degrees of freedom ($n-1$) where n is the number of pairs. The same t tables are used as for the unmatched t tests.

The procedure is better understood and more simply done if one forms a new variable, C13 = C8 – C9. If you are doing this using pencil and paper, do not forget the appropriate sign is negative when C9 is greater than C8. Column C13 now contains the change scores for each subject's self-rating in depression, '+' representing an improvement, '–' a deterioration, with '0' no change. The mean and standard deviation and standard error of the mean are then calculated in the usual way. Finally, we calculate

$t = \text{mean}/\text{SE}_\text{mean}.$

For column C13 for all 25 subjects

$t = 6.12/0.97 = 6.3$ (DF = 24).

From the tables, this is highly significant ($p < 0.001$). We can therefore conclude that there has been a change, presumably as a result of treatment.

CI_{95} for the mean. The mean is 6.12, SE_mean =0.97, DF = 24, $t_{0.05}$ = 2.06. The CI is therefore 6.12 ± 2.06 × 0.97 or 4.12 – 8.12.

Wilcoxon matched pair test (non-par)

Using the same data as above, we start off by finding the difference scores as before in column C13. Then, *ignoring the signs*, the scores are ranked, i.e. –9 and +9 are given the same rank. Start with the smallest and rank up to the highest, omitting zero changes. We are now going to compare the plus and minus scores. Take the smaller group, in this case the negative scores, and calculate $T = \Sigma(\text{ranks})$ for the smaller (negative) group = 1 + 4 + 6.5 = 11.5. Now refer to the tables in Siegel & Castellan (1988). For $n > 25$ tables are not available and so the calculation is

$$\text{mean}_T = n(n + 1)/4$$
$$= (24 \times 25)/4$$
$$= 150$$

$$\text{SD}_T = \sqrt{[n(n + 1)(2n + 1)/24]}$$
$$= \sqrt{[(24 \times 25 \times 49)/24]}$$
$$= 35$$

$$Z_T = (T - \text{mean}_T)/SD_T$$
$$= -138.5/35$$
$$= -3.96.$$

Reference to the proportion of the normal curve beyond this value of Z gives $p < 0.001$.

Sign test (non-par)

A very simple, but less powerful, test can be used even when all that has been decided is which is the higher of two scores, for example when each patient has expressed a preference for A rather than B or vice versa. Items where there is no difference are ignored. Still using column C13 data, we see that there are three subjects who have become more depressed and 21 who have got better. The smaller number, in this case 3, is referred to the appropriate table and again yields a significant result.

For $n > 25$ we can calculate the significance as follows:

$$\text{mean} = n/2$$
$$= 24/2$$
$$= 12$$

$$\text{SD} = \sqrt{(n)}/2$$
$$= 2.45$$

$$Z = (\text{sum} - \text{mean})/\text{SD}$$
$$= (3 - 12)/2.45$$
$$= 3.67$$

which again is highly significant, but note that, even though the data were the same, Z has reduced over the three different tests, because of the declining *powers* of the tests.

Chi squared ($\chi 2$) (non-par)

If we have some people or outcomes in each of several different categories it is possible to test whether the numbers (frequencies) in each category (cell) are distributed differently from what might be expected if chance alone were operating. This expectation might be based on theory, e.g. that those admitted to a hospital with a first attack of schizophrenia should show equal numbers of each sex, or the expectation might be based on results from some other group, e.g. that alcoholic patients treated as out-patients have similar rates of abstinence to those treated as in-patients. In the trial the groups differ in the numbers in each who have previously been treated for depression (scored as 1/0). For treatment A, four of the 14 have had previous treatment whereas for B this was true for seven out of 11. Is this difference statistically significant?

Usually such results are shown in a table, thus:

	Previous treatment				Previous treatment		
Observed data	Yes	No		Expected data	Yes	No	
Group A	4	10	14	Group A	6.16	7.84	14
Group B	7	4	11	Group B	4.84	6.16	11
	11	14	25		11	14	25

We have to calculate a similar table to show what might be expected by chance. The expected frequency in each cell is the row total for that cell multiplied by the column total divided by the grand total, e.g. $(14 \times 11)/25 = 6.16$.

The statistic χ^2 is calculated from the formula

$$\chi^2 = \Sigma[(f_0 - f_e)^2/f_e]$$

where f_0 is the number observed in each cell and f_e is the number expected in each cell.

In this example,

$$\chi^2 = \frac{(4-6.16)^2}{6.16} + \frac{(10-7.84)^2}{7.84} + \frac{(7-4.84)^2}{4.84} + \frac{(4-6.16)^2}{6.16}$$
$$= 0.76 + 0.60 + 0.96 + 0.76$$
$$= 3.07 \quad (DF = 1)$$

which is not statistically significant ($\chi^2 > 3.84$ for $p < 0.05$).

The formula above is sometimes modified by Yates' correction, which was claimed to make the result more accurate if small numbers were involved. For large numbers its effect is negligible. However, some doubt has been expressed as to the validity of the correction (Cammilli & Hopkins 1978), but some people may

insist on it, in which case the formula becomes

$$\chi^2 = \Sigma[(|f_0 - f_e| - \tfrac{1}{2})^2/f_e]$$

where $|...|$ indicates that the sign of the number inside should be ignored.

In the tables, notice that the totals in the margin are the same in the expected as in the observed tables. This must always be so if the expected frequencies have been calculated correctly.

The most commonly occurring table of results on which you might wish to apply χ^2 is the 2×2 table, e.g. males and females versus something happening or not, and for this so-called four-fold table χ^2 can be easily calculated by the simplified formula given below. This gives exactly the same results as the other formula and once mastered the method is very easily applied.

For the data already given:

	Previous treatment				Previous treatment		
Observed data	1	0			1	0	
Group A	4	10	14	Group A	a	b	e
Group B	7	4	11	Group B	c	d	f
	11	14	25		g	h	k

$$\chi^2 = [(ad - bc)^2 k]/efgh$$

For the data given,

$$\chi^2 = (16 - 70)^2 \, 25/(14 \times 11 \times 11 \times 14)$$
$$= 72\,900/23\,716$$
$$= 3.07$$

as before. With Yate's correction this formula becomes

$$\chi^2 = [(|\,ad - bc\,| - k/2)^2 k]/efgh.$$

Continuous variables such as duration of stay in hospital can be turned into categories by using cut-off points, so that category 1 could be less than 3 years, category 2 in the range 3–10 years and category 3 more than 10 years. Complex tables can be simplified by combining rows of figures with each other and also columns with each other. Statistical levels of significance are not reliable if the frequency in any expected cell is less than 5, but again see Cammilli & Hopkins (1978).

χ^2 is only valid if the items are uncorrelated. This will not be the case if the figures refer to, say, occurrences of a symptom and some individuals contribute several occurrences. For example, the number of epileptic fits reported in 1 year in a ward of 30 epileptics where half the patients are on anticonvulsant drug A and the other half on drug B is as recorded in Table

Table 10.2 Illustrating an example of a table where χ^2 is not the appropriate test although it may appear to be so

30 patients with epilepsy are treated with two different anticonvulsants. The observed frequencies of fits are given

| | Anticonvulsant | | |
	A	B	All
Patients	15	15	30
Fits			
Observed	112	63	175
Expected	87.5	87.5	175

10.2. The significance must not be tested using χ^2 since each fit was not completely independent of every other fit because some fits must have occurred in the same individual. Such data can be analysed by using the number of fits for each patient as his score and analysing the results by a *t* test. A useful tip in avoiding this error is to suspect any table where the total in the bottom right-hand corner is different from the number of individuals or units involved.

CI for a proportion. In the examples above we were comparing proportions, e.g. four out of 14 with seven out of 11. We can calculate the confidence intervals for these proportions as follows:

$$SE_A = \sqrt{(p_A q_A / n_A)}$$
$$CI_{95} = p \pm 1.96 \, SE_A \qquad \text{(for all } n\text{)}$$

and since we have $p = 0.29$, $q = 0.71$, $n = 14$ so $SE_A = 0.12$; therefore, $CI_A = 0.29 \pm 1.96 \times 0.12$ or 0.05–0.53. Similarly for B, $SE_B = \sqrt{(0.64 \times 0.36/11)} = 0.15$ and $CI_B = 0.36$–0.92, so that there is some overlap between the confidence intervals.

The confidence interval for the difference in proportions is calculated by finding the SE_{diff} by $\sqrt{(SE_A^2 + SE_B^2)}$ then applying the usual formula for the confidence interval. For the above, the difference in proportions is $(0.64 - 0.29)$ or 0.35 and $SE_{diff} = \sqrt{(0.12^2 + 0.15^2)} = 0.19$ so the CI is –0.02 to + 0.72 and therefore 'no true difference' is just within the 95% possibility and the null hypothesis cannot be rejected as we have already seen.

CORRELATION

Correlation refers to the relationship which may exist between variables such that any change in the value of one is associated with a change in the value of the other. For example, the two raters in Table 10.1 both tended to give high scores to some patients and low scores to others. If they had given identical scores there would have been a perfect correlation. How close were their scores to each other?

We can measure the relationship by a correlation coefficient (r), either the Pearson product moment correlation (par) or the Spearman rank order correlation (non-par).

Correlation coefficient (r) (Pearson product moment correlation)

The formula for the correlation coefficient is

$$r_{xy} = [n\Sigma xy - (\Sigma x)(\Sigma y)]/[n(n-1)SD_x SD_y]$$

where n is the number of pairs.

For the pairs of scores represented by columns C5 and C6, the correlation between the two raters is as follows ($n_{pairs} = 25$, $\Sigma xy = 30348$, $\Sigma x = 845$, $\Sigma y = 855$, $SD_x = 7.97$, $SD_y = 8.58$):

$$r_{xy} = (25 \times 30348 - 845 \times 855)/(25 \times 24 \times 7.97 \times 8.58)$$
$$= (36225 / 41030)$$
$$= 0.88.$$

Its standard error is

$$SE_r = \sqrt{[(1 - r^2)/(N - 2)]}.$$

For columns C5 and C6 this is

$$SE_r = \sqrt{[(1 - 0.78)/23]}$$
$$= \sqrt{(0.010)}$$
$$= 0.10$$
$$t = 0.88/0.1$$
$$= 8.8 \qquad \text{(DF = 23)}$$

As $t > 3.767$, $p < 0.001$.

The correlation coefficient r varies in value from –1 to +1. A value of 0 signifies that there is no linear relationship between the pairs of scores. In normal life we frequently come across pairs of variables which are so directly related to each other that they correlate exactly to the value of +1. For example, length in yards compared to length in metres gives a correlation of +1, and note that this is so even though the pairs of numbers are not the same but are arithmetically related. Correlations of any size are unaltered if we add, subtract, multiply, or divide either of the scores by a constant value. Negative correlations, i.e. $r < 0$, arise when one quantity appears to decrease when the other quantity is increasing, e.g. the scores of individuals on an intelligence test and the clinical estimate of their dementia. Figure 10.5 illustrates different degrees of linear relationship.

Occasionally relationships exist but they are curvilinear. Figure 10.6 illustrates this and might represent the raw scores on some cognitive test of people between the ages of 5 and 80 years. Up to the age of 16 years (part a) the older the child is the more likely he is to obtain a good score, therefore up to this point the cor-

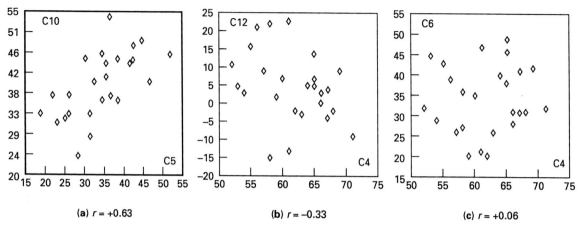

(a) $r = +0.63$ **(b)** $r = -0.33$ **(c)** $r = +0.06$

Fig. 10.5 Scattergrams illustrating different degrees of correlation between selected variables from Table 10.1.

relation coefficient measuring the relationship between age and raw score would be positive. Between 16 and 60 years (part b) there may be little change in score with age, and therefore r will be found to be close to zero, but after 60 years the older person may obtain lower scores so that r becomes negative. Over the whole range of ages from 5 to 80 years the correlation will depend on the number in each group, but with an even spread is likely to be close to zero. For this reason when one is interested in the relationship between two variables it is often worthwhile plotting the pair values on a graph to gain some idea of the form of relationship.

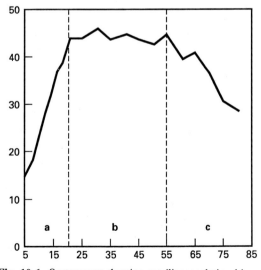

Fig. 10.6 Scattergram showing curvilinear relationship between variables.

Some relationships are curvilinear but do not reverse, e.g. length of hospitalisation and degree of social deterioration might be represented by a graph such as Figure 10.7a. In such cases the relationship might be strengthened by changing the method of measuring one of the variables, e.g. by plotting the log y rather than y itself, as in Figure 10.7b. This is known as a transformation procedure. At first thought it may seem slightly dishonest to change the values so as to produce a higher correlation, but if you are trying to find a relationship it is important to look for it in the form which is most relevant and it may give some suggestions about the nature of the relationship to make such transformations. It is no less honest than expressing the dose of a drug in terms of milligrams per kilogram bodyweight rather than by just the amount given, and the former is often a more meaningful way of measuring the dose.

Regression

Besides measuring the strength of the relationship, correlations are also used to improve the prediction of the value of one variable by another in a particular case. If we know the mean and standard deviation of each of the variables and the correlation between them and we know the value (x_1) of a new case but not the value of y for that case we can predict its most likely value by the formula

$$y_{1pred} = \bar{y} + r(\text{SD}_y/\text{SD}_x)(x_1 - \bar{x}).$$

If rater R1 gives a patient a score of 50, what will rater R2 give? Predicted DepR$_2$ = 34.20 + 0.88(8.58/7.97)(50 − 33.80)

= 34.20 + 15.35

= 49.55.

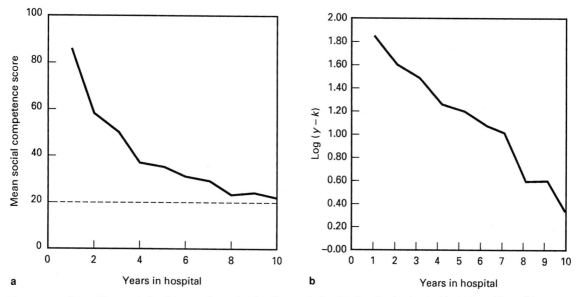

Fig. 10.7 **a** A curvilinear relationship transformed to **b** a linear relationship by plotting log (y–k), the logarithm of the y variable minus its asymptotic value k.

Note that if we know y and wish to predict x the formula is

$$x_{1\mathrm{pred}} = \bar{x} + r(\mathrm{SD}_x/\mathrm{SD}_y)(y_1 - \bar{y}).$$

These regression equations are equivalent but not identical.

Regression to the mean

'Regression to the mean' is a phrase used to describe a phenomenon where the most likely value of the unknown variable is always less deviant, i.e. nearer the mean, than the known variable was. For example, assume x_1 is 2 standard deviations from $\bar{x}$, then if the correlation is 0.5 the y_1 predicted will be only 1 standard deviation from $\bar{y}$, but if the correlation is –0.75 the y predicted will be 1.5 standard deviations from $\bar{y}$, and in the opposite direction. Only when the correlation is 1 is the predicted value as far from its mean as its predictor was. When the correlation is 0 the predicted value is its mean, no matter how deviant the predictor was because the predictor has no implications for the likely value of y.

Common variance

The correlation coefficient reflects the amount of information that the two correlated variables have in common. More specifically, r^2 is a measure of the common variance, so if $r = 0.5$ then $r^2 = 0.25$, which means that 25% of the variance of one variable is predicted from knowledge of the other and the remaining 75% is produced by other completely different factors — usually unknown. To explain half the variance r has to be 0.7 ($r^2 = 0.49$) and even $r = 0.9$ explains only 81% of the variance.

Causality and correlation

If there is a causal relationship between two variables they will correlate, but it does not follow that if two things are correlated one is the cause of the other. Quite frequently there is a third variable which is more directly related to each. The third variable is often time. For example, before 1939 the number of storks nesting in German towns in any year was found to correlate significantly with the birth rate in Germany for that year, presumably because both were being reduced by industrialisation.

Rank correlation (Spearman) (r_s) (non-par)

When it is only possible or advisable to arrange one or both variables in order of magnitude rather than give an absolute value it is still possible to measure the correlation by this technique. Arrange each of the variables in turn in order of magnitude and number each from 1 upwards to n. Now for each pair subtract the rank (position) score on one variable from the rank on the other; this gives d for each pair. Square these and sum them for Σd^2; n is the number of pairs of scores. Then,

$$r_s = 1 - (6\Sigma d^2/n(n^2 - 1)).$$

(Many purists who insist on using this formula if there is even the suspicion of non-normality in the data probably do not realise that the rank order correlation is itself derived by applying the Pearson formula to the ranks, which are certainly not normally distributed.)

For the correlation of rater R1 with the patient's self-rating of depression before treatment (columns C5 and C8), $\Sigma d^2 = 745$, and

$$r_s = 1 - [(6 \times 745)/(24 \times 25 \times 26)] = 0.71.$$

For the same data, $r = 0.76$.

As with r, r_s varies from -1 to $+1$, with 0 signifying no relationship. If data are normally distributed, r and r_s should be fairly similar. The standard error of r_s is calculated in the same way as for r, namely

$$SE r_s = \sqrt{[(1 - r_s^2)/(n - 2)]}$$

and as usual $t = r_s/SE r_s$ (DF $= n - 2$).

VARIANCE

When some variable, e.g. depressive score, is measured for each of n individuals, it is unlikely that all the scores will be the same. This variation between individuals is the basis of most statistical measures. The aim is often to explain the source of the variation. Does it arise from present or past circumstances? Has it been altered by treatments? Is it related to the age, personality or other characteristic of the subject? Statisticians find it convenient to measure this variation by a measure known as variance, where the variance of each individual is the square of his difference from the group mean. We can then have the total variance, which is the sum of the individual variances, and the mean variance, which is the total variance divided by $(n - 1)$. The square root of the mean variance is the standard deviation.

Statisticians like to work with variance because it can be simply dealt with, e.g. variances can be added and subtracted in a meaningful way, and the total variance of two groups combined is equal to the sum of each group's variance within itself plus the variance calculated from the difference between the means of the two groups. This is the basis of the powerful technique called 'analysis of variance'. Thinking in terms of variance gives insight into many other statistical procedures from regression to factor analysis.

Analysis of variance (ANOVA)

If we measure the mean of a variable for two or more groups it is highly unlikely that all the means will come out at exactly the same value even if there is no

real difference between the groups, so we need some way of telling whether the difference among the means is just due to this kind of sampling error or if some factors exists which is generating a difference in their means. Our null hypothesis is that there is no real difference among the means and that all the groups are random samples from just one population. If that is so, the variance we get within the samples gives us an estimate of the variance of the population, as we have already described. Moreover, the different means for our groups should also give us a method of estimating the variance of the population (see the discussion on the standard error of a mean). We can compare these two estimates and see if they are too different from each other to allow us to be confident that they are estimates of the true variance of the same population. This is the basis of the statistical technique known as *analysis of variance*.

For example, three groups of patients are given different kinds of treatment — 20 in group A are given a placebo, 40 in group B are given a new treatment and 40 in group C are given the standard treatment. The mean improvement scores are found to be 2, 4 and 5, respectively, which looks as if the new treatment is not as good as the old and both are better than the placebo. To test this we start off with the null hypothesis that there is no real difference and that the three means are just the results of random sampling differences. An analysis of variance is done and yields Table 10.3. The method of working out this table will not be given here but can be found in any of the textbooks on statistics mentioned later and in any case would probably be supplied by the computer, but it is still important that you should be able to understand the results as quoted.

Some of the variance is due to the fact that even within each group there are differences. The variance

Table 10.3 Illustrating one–way analysis of variance

100 patients treated in three separate groups are rated for degree of improvement. The differences between the mean scores are examined by one–way ANOVA

	Treatments: Placebo	New	Standard	All
N	20	40	40	100
Σx	40	160	200	400
Mean	2.0	4.0	5.0	4.0

Source of variation	Sum of squares	DF	Variance estimate	F	p
Treatments	120	2	60.0	6.00	<0.01
Residual	970	97	10.0	—	
Total	1090	99	—		

of each group was 10 and this is also the answer given in the estimate for variance within each treatment group. The degrees of freedom amount to 97 (19 + 39 + 39). The rest of the variance comes from the fact that even if in each group every subject had exactly the same score, namely its mean, there would still be differences for the whole group. There are three groups, and therefore two degrees of freedom. This gives a variance estimate of 60. There are two degrees of freedom in the greater estimate and 97 in the lesser estimate of variance. Consulting tables for F we find that for those degrees of freedom if $F > 3.1$ then $p < 0.05$ and if $F > 4.9$, then $p < 0.01$. Therefore, since our value of F is 6 we can reject with 100 to 1 confidence the idea that the differences among the three groups have just arisen by chance. It would be safe to accept that the placebo is not as good as the others. Unfortunately, we still do no know whether the new treatment is really poorer than the old and further analysis would be necessary to test this hypothesis using methods of comparing the means of groups such as that suggested by Tukey and which would probably be contained in the computer statistical package.

Two-way analysis of variance

In the above example, we considered only one way in which the three groups differed from each other, namely treatment. Sometimes we can see two or more ways in which they differ from each other and which might influence the scores. For example, if the subjects consisted of both in-patients and out-patients and we suspected on clinical grounds that that might alter their responses, we could use treatment setting as a second factor. In which case our results and analysis of variance tables might have been as shown in Table 10.4.

Table 10.4 is different from Table 10.3, and includes not only the new hospitalization effect but also an interaction effect which measures whether the main effects are consistent in their action. Overall, for example, out-patients fare slightly better than in-patients but, within treatment B, out-patients do very much better than in-patients whereas in A and C the opposite is true. The interaction effect in this example is not statistically significant although it is nearly so. (From the tables for F with degrees of freedom of 2 and 94 it is seen that F needs to be 3.1 for $p < 0.05$.) If an interaction effect is significant, it is not permissible to draw conclusions about the main effects. Here for example, if F had been greater, it would have been incorrect to state for all the groups that the treatment results differ from each other. We would have had to

do separate analyses by looking only at out-patients and then only at in-patients and drawing separate conclusions for each. This error is frequently made in analyses.

Analysis of covariance (ANCOVA) (par)

Sometimes we know that the differences in individual results arise from an effect that can be measured, e.g. age. If we know that older patients respond less well to treatment and can demonstrate this by showing that, within each group, age and improvement correlate, say, -0.5, we can correct for this age effect by regression and calculate the variance effects due to this regression. This would have the effect of reducing the unexplained variance in the residual, thus making the variance estimate less and so increasing the F ratio for the other effects, since we would be dividing by a smaller denominator.

Apart from an additional term measuring the regression variance the analysis would look exactly the same as those we have previously dealt with and would be interpreted in the same way. The method of doing an analysis of covariance will not be explained here. It is dealt with in standard textbooks on statistics and there will be a computer procedure for carrying out the analysis in most statistical packages.

Table 10.4 Illustrating two–way analysis of variance

100 patients are given one of three treatments, half as in–patients, half as out–patients. The differences between the mean improvement scores attributable to the two factors are examined by two–way ANOVA

		Treatments:			
		Placebo	New	Standard	All
OP	N	10	20	20	50
	Σx	14	100	96	210
	Mean	1.4	5.0	4.8	4.2
IP	N	10	20	20	50
	Σx	26	60	104	190
	Mean	2.6	3.0	5.2	3.8
Both	N	20	40	40	100
	Σx	40	160	200	400
	Mean	2.0	4.0	5.0	4.0

Source of variation	Sum of squares	DF	Variance estimate	F	p
Treatments	120	2	60.0	6.12	<0.01
OP vs IP	4	1	4.0	0.41	NSS
Interaction	44.8	2	22.4	2.29	NSS
Residual	921.2	94	9.8	—	
Total	1090	99	—		

OP, out–patients; IP, in–patients; NSS, not statistically significant.

RESEARCH DESIGN

Choice of a research topic

The best place for the novice researcher to find a topic for research is not in his imaginative speculations but in published research work. Every good research worker is usually well aware when he submits a paper for publication that it would have been a better paper if he had thought beforehand of measuring this or had had time to include that, and he is likely to have expressed these thoughts explicitly, knowing that it is better to disarm critics by himself drawing attention to deficiencies. Do not be afraid, therefore, to repeat respected research incorporating minor alterations that appear likely to clarify aspects of a problem. Progress in research comes more frequently by small steps than by giant leaps.

If you are tempted to carry out research on a topic that has come to you as 'I wonder if ...' or 'It appears to me that ...', the essential first step is to see what previous research has been done on the topic by consulting the literature or discussing it with more experienced colleagues. Medical or psychological abstracts and various bibliographic retrieval systems such as Medlars, Medline or the Science Citation Index can be helpful in tracing published work on a subject and thus suggest what useful work remains to be done. Computer-assisted retrieval systems, usually referred to as CD-ROM since they use compact disks to hold massive amounts of data, are now available in many university libraries.

Feasibility of a topic

Not every topic for research is feasible. There are frequently restrictions imposed by lack of subjects, time and/or facilities. There is a hoary joke among researchers that no matter how prevalent an illness is, as soon as you start to collect patients with that complaint, they become as rare as lepers. The reason is that for research we often wish to exclude patients who have other characteristics that may complicate the picture. Consequently, your chronic schizophrenics who fill several wards dwindle when it is decided that no subject in the study must have a measured IQ below 85 or have evidence of brain damage or have had a leucotomy or be older than 60 years. In such ways your 200 patients may very easily shrink to 25.

Do not unnecessarily restrict your patient choice. Remember that a wide age range of patients will produce more generally valid results and, provided you use appropriate statistical techniques, is almost as likely to yield significant results. For example, even if old and young patients respond differently, analysis of covariance not only allows measurement of the age effect but also compensates for it at a cost equivalent to one additional patient, because of the one degree of freedom used up by the regression sum of squares.

Lack of time is important. Research always takes longer than you think. Save time by doing research on patients you will be seeing anyway. Collect only relevant data rather than everything you can think of. Team up with a colleague. Two people can work twice as fast as one and you will find it helpful to have someone who is equally involved with whom to discuss progress. It can also be very encouraging to have someone to help you over periods of despair! If you have chosen a project that is relatively simple, you will have a better chance of finishing it before your time and enthusiasm have run out. You may then feel inspired to do more research.

If the facilities you require are not immediately available, think twice before trying to get them. It is very easy to convince yourself that some piece of apparatus, of which you have no experience, will make a big difference to your planned research, but you may find when you get it that it is a 'white elephant' that only complicates your life. It is a different matter if you know from personal experience that a piece of equipment will do what you want it to do. Then by all means try and get it. There is, even in hard times, a fair amount of research money available for equipment. Find an appropriate authority, drug firm or charity and write to them. Most of them are willing to sponsor research in a subject that is their responsibility. Salaries are rather harder to come by.

Design of the research

If the research topic can be put into the form of a question to be answered, this will often suggest the design and the statistics to be used in evaluating the results.

If you believe the results of your research will have an application, then be sure that the design yields usable results. For example, if you suspect that a certain type of depressed patient responds better to antidepressant A than B, devise if possible an operational definition of what that type is so that, if you are right, others will be able to choose the best patients to put on drug A.

Cross-over trials, in which patients are given treatments A and B successively (and vice versa), are beloved by clinicians but there are many practical and theoretical objections to them. The statistics are always complicated unless you can guarantee that neither treatment has any lasting effect, which is seldom the case. The argument for cross-over designs is that each patient acts as his own control and therefore individual differences are reduced, but order effects and carry over effects introduce differences which are much less easy to quantify. Only when subjects are rare can cross-over designs be justified. Individual differences can be greatly reduced if, for example, improvement is measured by a simple change in scores, or by the ratio of after to before scores for each patient.

Analysis of variance or covariance suggests excellent models for design of experiments which can take account of several factors and your attempt to draw up a two- or three-way analysis of variance table may suggest the necessary control groups to measure the main effects.

Measurement

To yield significant results, measures should be as reliable as possible. Standard procedures with standard scoring should be used where suitable. An advantage of using, say, the Hamilton Depression Rating Scale rather than your own method of assessing depression is that the former has a large background of published literature; you will be able to compare your results with other research data; its limitations are already known and people have learned to trust it. Thus, you will find it easier to convince people of the validity of your results, and remember that the function of research is to convince other people.

Ad hoc scales do have uses. For example, where there is no standard method of assessment available it is better to use your own direct measures rather than use a published scale which only approximates to what you are interested in.

Devising a scale

You will usually choose items that have *face validity*, i.e. that seem to be measuring what they claim to measure or which have generally accepted *clinical validity*. You can assess whether several items are measuring the same thing by finding the correlation of each item with the full scale (item analysis) or by a more elaborate factor analysis. You can also measure reliability by one of the ways already described. Some common pitfalls for people devising scales are: firstly, confusing two dimensions, e.g. an item measures both frequency of headache and its intensity instead of having one or more items for each; secondly, numerical values are given to possible answers which do not correspond to clinically equal intervals. If you are devising a scale of intensity which is going to be used to measure improvement, try and give numerical values so that clinical improvement from any point to any other point yields a numerical difference which, as far as can be arranged, corresponds to the amount of clinical improvement. It is, in fact, often easier to devise a scale so that the percentage reduction, i.e. the difference divided by the initial score, corresponds to the amount of clinical improvement.

A *visual analogue scale* is a 10 cm line, on which the patient places a cross to indicate his subjective position between two extreme positions, appropriately labelled, and the distance from one end measured in millimetres is a simple, but effective, means of recording the patient's rating of his state. It is particularly useful for measuring sequential changes over time.

The power of an experiment

In the past, most researchers, at least at the publication stage, were anxious to have positive results with type 1 errors clearly unlikely ($p < 0.05$). Results which were non-significant tended to be consigned to the wastepaper basket. Nowadays, more attempt is made to ensure that the results of an experiment are decisive in one direction or the other, which means that the sample has to be large enough to conclude that hypotheses being tested have been either proved or disproved, so that attention has to be paid to both type 1 and type 2 errors. Proposed research will often not be funded or results published if it is felt that the sizes of the samples involved may fail to produce significant results.

The probability of a type 1 error, i.e. incorrectly rejecting the null hypothesis, is usually represented by the Greek letter α. The possibility of a type 2 error, i.e. incorrectly accepting a null hypothesis, is represented by β. α is straightforward through having the long convention of 5, 1 and 0.1% levels being acceptable. β is less straightforward. It is suggested that β should be approximately 4α, therefore the corresponding β values would be 20, 4 and 0.4%. The power of a test is represented by $(1 - \beta)$. The size of the difference that one expects to detect d, *the size effect*, must also be stated, usually in terms of standard deviations. For example, at the planning stage one may decide that if two means differ by half of a standard deviation one ought to be able to detect it. For example, in an IQ test, where the standard deviation is 15, one is looking for a difference between two groups of children being tested as being about 7, and anything less than 7 would be regarded as being unimportant or not representing a practical difference between the two groups. Before an investigator starts an experiment, he has to know or estimate what the means and standard deviations of the groups are likely to be. This is done by reference to previous work in the area, or by a pilot study done before the main study is undertaken, or just by guesswork.

Let us consider a case where one is trying to compare the efficacy of two drugs. One may say that one would like to be 95% confident before accepting that there is a true difference between the drugs, and to be 80% confident before concluding that there was no real clinical difference, which you have defined as a difference in efficacy at least half of one standard deviation in magnitude. (On theoretical grounds one might like to detect an even smaller true difference, but this might require very large numbers, and be impracticable for this reason.)

With these figures one can calculate the sizes of the samples necessary to reach a decision. The method of calculating sample sizes will be illustrated for only the simplest, but most powerful, arrangement where the two samples are of equal size. For 95% confidence in rejecting the null hypothesis, $\alpha = 0.05$. It has to be two tailed since one is prepared to accept either treatment being better, so one looks up $\alpha = 0.025$ in one-tailed tables. For 80% confidence, β has to be 0.20, and this is one tailed since there is no sensible alternative. We have said d is to be 0.5. Then the approximate required sample size is given by

$$n_1 = n_2 = 2(Z_{1-\alpha} + Z_{1-\beta})^2/d^2$$

where the Zs are obtained from the normal distribution table. In this example

$$\begin{aligned}n_1 = n_2 &= 2(1.960+0.842)^2/0.5^2 \\ &= 2 \times (2.802)^2/0.25 \\ &= 62.8\end{aligned}$$

and thus it needs 63 in each group. If one were content to detect as the smallest difference one standard deviation between group means, the required sample size drops to 16 per group.

If this is a matched pairs design, d' is detected where $d' = d(1 - r)$ and r is the correlation between the pairs of scores, which shows why a matched pairs design is more powerful than unrelated groups. If r is not known it can be assumed to be 0.5.

To find the power of an experiment that has been presented, say, in a research proposal, $(1 - \beta)$ is found from

$$Z_{1-\beta} = d\sqrt{(2n_1)}/[2 + (1.21(Z_{1-\alpha} - 1.06))/(n_1 - 1)] - Z_{1-\alpha}.$$

To detect a d of 1 standard deviation with $\alpha = 0.05$ and a sample size of 20:

$$\begin{aligned}Z_{1-\beta} &= 1 \times \sqrt{(40)}/\{2 + [1.21(1.960 - 1.06)]/(19)\} \\ &\quad - 1.960 \\ &= 1.1124\end{aligned}$$

which gives $\beta = 0.16$ or $(1 - \beta) = 0.84$, so the power of the design is 84% (i.e. you would get a decisive result five out of six times).

Power calculations can be done for a large variety of research designs and statistical procedures (see Singer 1986).

Pilot studies

Before starting any piece of research it is usually worthwhile conducting a trial of your procedure on a few patients to see if there are any problems. You can estimate the power of your plan and you might reveal difficulties, such as patients being scarce, non-cooperativeness, procedures taking too long, difficulties in collecting some of the data, the data coming out in a form which you had not anticipated, etc. If you find these things out before you begin your experiment, they can be put right. Without a pilot study you might be tempted to carry on collecting the data despite such problems.

Time intervals

The question of how long to continue a treatment before assessing results is clearly a clinical question. If you have a good idea that a drug takes 4 weeks to work or that some other form of therapy takes several months, the trial must last at least that length of time. Also, if a patient has been on some relevant active drug you must wait until you are sure that its effects have ceased before the patient is entered for a new form of treatment.

Controlled trials

A controlled trial refers to the fact that at least one comparison (control) group is available which differs from the experimental group in only one way, so that it can be validly assumed that differences between the two groups are due to that factor alone. The factor could be diagnosis (schizophrenic versus normal), treatment (drug A versus drug B) or any other variable (e.g. hospitalised longer than or less than 1 year). Sometimes more than one control group is used so that several questions can be answered. One group may be given nothing at all to see if the new treatment is better than just ignoring the patient. A second group may be given an inert substance (placebo) to see if the experimental treatment has an active component. A third group may be given the most effective current treatment to see if the new treatment differs from it. The fourth group (the experimental group) would naturally be given the new treatment.

Matching groups

When one is forming groups for a treatment trial, it is crucial to avoid systematic bias in assigning subjects to groups. One must therefore decide if a patient is to enter the trial before deciding to which group he is to be assigned. Otherwise, if one knew that the patient was to be assigned to a non-treatment group, one might decide, because of the patient's needs, not to include him in the trial. (One would probably not make this decision if the assignment had been to the treatment group and thus only the less ill patients would be included in the no-treatment group with consequent distortion of the results.)

Sampling definitions and procedures

A *population* consists of *all* the individual members of any specified group. It can be narrow, namely, all males patients admitted to a particular ward in the last 3 months with a first attack of schizophrenia, or wide, namely all schizophrenics who have lived or will live in the whole world.

A *sample* is a group, from one to all, drawn from a population. Our group defined above as a narrow population could itself be regarded as a sample of the group defined as a wide population. Frequently, therefore, we sample a known population, e.g. a particular group of patients in a hospital who are themselves a sample of a more universal population, namely all patients in the world with that diagnosis and for whom we hope our conclusions, whatever they are, may be valid.

Observations are usually made on the sample with the intention of drawing conclusions, not only about the known population sampled, but about a wider population. Measurements that are calculated for the sample are called statistics and they are represented by Latin letters, e.g. M for the mean. The equivalent terms for the population are called parameters and are represented by Greek letters, e.g. μ for the population mean. These are seldom directly measured since every member of the population would have to be measured and this would usually be impossible or expensive, but they can be estimated from the sample statistics.

A good sample is one which represents the population fairly. A bad sample may fail to be representative for several reasons. For example, a male group of schizophrenics is not likely to give results which accurately represent all schizophrenics. A sample which is unrepresentative in an irrelevant characteristic may, however, be quite representative in all the relevant characteristics. It is important therefore to have a *clinical* knowledge of which characteristics are relevant and which are irrelevant in deciding how to choose one's sample. Several methods have been devised to avoid systematic bias and thus increase the likelihood of a representative sample being drawn.

A *random sample* from a population is obtained by ensuring that every member of the population has exactly the same probability of being included in the sample. Such a sample is fair, that is, not biased, but may not be truly representative. A table of random numbers can be used to select a random sample from a known population, e.g. to draw 30 patients for a drug trial from a patient population of 88, number all the patients 1–88, then go through the random numbers taking them two at a time and selecting each case that those numbers represent until 30 have been collected. Numbers 89–99 if they occur are ignored as are any repeats of numbers already selected.

A *stratified sample* provides a more representative sample. It consists of random samples drawn from subpopulations. The subsample size, in each group, should be proportional to the size of the subpopulation. The subpopulation might, for example, be defined according to age, sex, severity of illness, etc. One subpopulation might then be females, aged over 50 years and who have the illness only to a mild degree. The other subpopulations would be represented by all the permutations of the alternatives of each category. The numbers in each sample would then be a fixed proportion of the known numbers in the corresponding subpopulation. There are sometimes advantages in using a larger sample size than appropriate, but the results for this group must then be scaled down.

Occasionally, because of the difficulties in getting hold of a certain group their sample might have to be scaled up. If this is done, care has to be taken in deciding what the true degrees of freedom for the sample are. Only relevant factors have to be balanced when making up samples for control and experimental groups.

The term *double-blind* means that neither the subject nor the experimenter, particularly where he is assessing the subjects, is aware which group the subject belongs to. This is necessary because of the following sources of variation.

The *placebo effect* refers to the fact that any treatment will produce beneficial results if given or taken with enough faith and enthusiasm. It is important therefore, if one wishes to know if a drug is effective, to make sure that the active drug is compared to an inert substance which is identical in appearance and given with as much confidence and enthusiasm as the active drug. To ensure equal enthusiasm it is usually necessary that the therapist as well as the patient is ignorant of which treatment is active and which inert. This makes the trial double-blind. This is essential in the assessment of any treatment where the prejudice of the experimenter, whether for or against the treatment under test, is able to influence his assessment of its efficacy.

The *Hawthorne effect* refers to a better response from people who believe that an interest is being taken in them. Although it derives from an experiment in industrial psychology the effect can arise in any setting and is particularly liable to occur where patients or staff who have hitherto been ignored are suddenly involved in a research project.

Natural remission, while welcomed by the clinician and the patient, can be a nuisance to a researcher since it introduces unknown variation into the results. If natural remission is likely to occur to any great extent after *x* days, the trial must be completed before that time if the treatment results are not to be seriously influenced by the natural response.

The *practice effect* refers to the fact that as successive assessments are carried out the performance of the patient and the experimenter may alter as they become used to or more skilled in the procedure. In other tasks the subject may become bored, with consequent deterioration. It is well known that in the first assessment of most subjects, and in particular of institutionalised patients, there are many artifacts which obscure their basic state. In such situations it is worthwhile, if time allows, to assess the patient several times and only start the experimental procedure when it is clear that a steady state has been reached by each subject.

In some circumstances it is difficult to arrange a double-blind trial, for example in comparing electroconvulsive therapy (ECT) with antidepressant drugs, but allocation must still be random, and assessment of improvement should be made by a rater who is unaware of which treatment has been given to the subject being rated (i.e. the trial should still be single-blind).

The *reliability of a measure* refers to how consistent a result is obtained when two different raters use the measuring instrument on the same subject (inter-rater reliability), *or* when the same rater assesses the same subject after some interval of time (test–retest reliability), *or* when two distinct but similar measures are used at the same time (alternate form reliability), *or* when some items within the scale are compared with other items (split half or internal consistency reliability). All of these assume that the subject has not changed between the two assessments. Reliability is usually measured by the correlation between the pairs of scores obtained by any of the methods described above for a group of subjects. For our data in Table 10.1, the reliability of rating is measured by the correlation between the scores of rater R1 and rater R2 over all 25 subjects. This comes out as $r = 0.88$, which would be excellent for a trial of this sort. One often has to be satisfied with a reliability of 0.70 for such data.

The *validity of a measure* is how well a test measures what it claims to measure. Duration of hospitalisation of chronic schizophrenics may be a very reliable measure since it does not leave much room for disagreement or error, but it may not be a very valid measure of the degree of institutionalisation, since some very long-term patients may show little personality deterioration. Validity is not nearly so easy to assess as reliability since often no truly valid criterion exists against which the results can be gauged. It is usually assessed by comparing the measure in question with some different measure(s) of the same thing, e.g. a questionnaire versus doctor's ratings.

In Table 10.1 the estimate of validity we have is the correlation between the doctor's and the patient's rating of depression, i.e. columns C4 and C7. This gives $r = 0.76$, which would be acceptable for this sort of trial.

PUBLISHING YOUR RESULTS

Having chosen a research topic, planned the experiment, selected the subjects, assessed them, analysed the data and drawn valid conclusions, all that remains is to publish the findings. This is most easily done by reading a paper to colleagues at a local scientific meeting. The important rule is to be lucid. In the usual 20 minute paper you will have to introduce the topic to the audience and tell them as much about your research as they can absorb, which from your own experience you know is not very much. Written papers, on the other hand, give the reader the chance to go back to something they did not understand or even to refer to other papers, and can therefore be more detailed and more concise. Another difference is that an offer to read a paper is likely to be immediately accepted while a journal editor will reject, demand alterations and shortening and take a year to publish an accepted paper. Do not be discouraged. It is worth it in the end and research is a drug of addiction. It is hoped that this chapter may have helped you to get hooked on it.

BIBLIOGRAPHY

A list of references would be inappropriate for this chapter. The techniques discussed appear in most textbooks and the experiments quoted are either invented or have been altered to simplify the figures. References to confidence intervals and power calculations have been given since these are often neglected in textbooks. The books listed below are likely to be helpful to the beginner and they will supply references to more advanced texts where necessary.

Bulpitt C J 1987 Confidence intervals. Lancet i: 494–497

Camilli G, Hopkins K D 1978 Applicability of Chi-square to 2×2 contingency tables with small expected cell frequency. Psychological Bulletin 85: 163–167

Gardner M J, Altman D G 1986 Confidence intervals rather than p values: estimation rather than hypothesis testing. British Medical Journal i: 746–750

Geigy Scientific Tables (2) 1982 Introduction to statistics, statistical tables and mathematical formulae. Geigy Pharmaceutical Company, Manchester. (This is different from the other texts in that it is mainly statistical tables. A more comprehensive battery would be difficult to find, and it includes clear explanations of their uses)

Harper W M 1982 Statistics. Macdonald & Evans, Plymouth. (A very handy paper-back, brimming with worked examples on the main procedures)

Hill A B 1984 A short textbook of medical statistics. Hodder & Stoughton, London. (Covers the basics from a medical point of view, bringing in clinical, ethical and epidemiological concepts)

Robson C 1985 Experiment, design and statistics in psychology. Penguin, London. (Covers both parametric and non-parametric statistics with the emphasis on the latter. It uses the 'cook-book' approach with step-by-step details of procedures and will therefore particularly appeal to the beginner who wants to work out statistics on his own data)

Siegel S, Castellan N J 1988 Non-parametric statistics for the behavioural sciences. McGraw-Hill, New York. (This is a new edition of the standard text on this subject. Each test is discussed and the calculation described in detail with many worked examples. The serious student will find it well worth buying)

Singer B R 1986 Sample size and power. In: Lovie A D (ed) New developments in statistics for psychology and the social sciences, vol 1. Methuen, London

11. The principles of psychiatric epidemiology

N. Kreitman

INTRODUCTION

The aim of this chapter is to outline the epidemiological approach to psychiatric disorders. No attempt will be made to deal with the technical complexities of the subject, for which the reader is referred to any comprehensive textbook of general epidemiology (for example MacMahon & Pugh 1970) or the excellent short book by Susser (1973). Similarly, it will not be possible to review all the findings which have accumulated regarding specific psychiatric disorders; these data are to be found under their subject headings.

Epidemiology enjoys a plethora of definitions, such as 'the study of the mass aspects of disease' or 'the study of the distribution of illness in populations over time and space'. In a closely argued paper, Dunham (1966) refers to epidemiology as the numerate aspect of human ecology. Essentially, these definitions point to the study of disorder (treated or untreated) in relation to the population among which it occurs, and its variation among subgroups of that population and over time. The framework of study is thus drastically wider than is the case in clinical studies. The clinical features of a disorder may be the same in two different communities yet the frequency with which it is found may be markedly different. Conversely, two disorders may have very different prevalences within the same population. Observations of this kind must be incorporated into any general theory purporting to explain the origins, evolution, or outcome of illness, and in this sense the epidemiologist must be considered to be contributing to basic psychiatry. His first task is to provide an accurate enumeration of the frequency of disorders in different groups, but this is essentially a preliminary step on the way to causal explanations. For the latter he will need to draw freely on a host of related disciplines ranging from neurophysiology to sociology.

These strategic objectives in practice devolve into more limited tactical aims, an excellent account of which has been provided by Morris (1976). Some of these relate to the central issues of explaining differences in the origin, course, or outcome of disorders in different groups, while others represent more incidental uses of epidemiological techniques. They may be summarised as follows.

Perhaps the commonest objective pursued in epidemiological enquiries is to determine whether the prevalence of a condition differs between two or more populations which have been selected because they differ in some respect judged to be of practical or theoretical interest. The essential principle is that of comparison, and all the technical procedures of 'case' definition and ascertainment must be uniformly applied so that the two groups can sensibly be compared.

A variant on the above is the contrary situation in which the distributions of two disorders are examined in the same population. This approach is particularly apposite when there is genuine doubt as to whether two clinical syndromes should be viewed as basically similar or as distinct. If the two syndromes are found to have different profiles in terms of their prevalence in different subgroups of the population, then a 'differential diagnosis' has been established which would tend to support a separatist view.

Another objective is to test hypotheses concerning factors postulated to have an effect on the genesis or evolution of a disorder. The design of such enquiries approximates to that of an experiment. Usually the groups considered are those of individuals with and without the condition in question, who are then examined for the presence or absence of the factor being investigated. Alternatively, a group may be selected which is known to have been exposed to the factor, and the incidence of disease compared with that obtained in a non-exposed but otherwise comparable group. Similar strategies are of course used in many disciplines in psychiatry, and there is

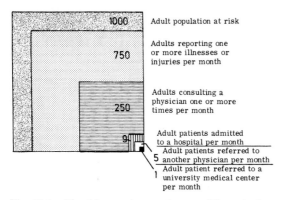

Fig. 11.1 Monthly prevalence estimates of illness in the community and the provision of general medical care (White et al 1961).

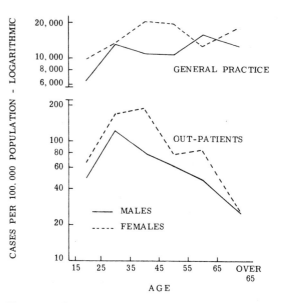

Fig. 11.2 One year period prevalence rates for neurosis in general practice and psychiatric out-patient departments (Kessel et al 1962).

surely no place for demarcation disputes. But in any comparative study of this kind where an investigator is using groups with a defined relationship to their parent population he is operating, knowingly or not, within an epidemiological framework.

A rather different purpose is to 'expand the clinical picture' by the study of individuals with the disorder of interest but without confining attention solely to those who have sought a particular type of care. It is well established that the patients who reach the clinician, especially the hospital-based doctor, have passed through a whole series of filters (Fig. 11.1). Selection begins among the general population in that even those who present to front-line agencies, such as the general practitioner, are self-selected since there are other individuals with similar symptoms who do not define themselves as potential patients and do not seek medical help (Ingham & Miller 1979). General practitioners in turn select patients, by criteria which are poorly understood, for referral to psychiatric services, where further screens operate in series until ultimately an in-patient group results. Studies of groups situated on either side of a particular filter can illuminate its 'permeability' (Gold-berg & Huxley 1980). Those individuals further along the referral pathway will be fewer in number but, what is equally important, may show quite different *qualitative* characteristics. Thus the view that neurosis is chiefly encountered among young adults is supported by hospital experience but is untrue for patients seen in general practice (Fig. 11.2). The important point is that the findings from a study can be generalised only to other patients at the same level of care.

Lastly there is the important use of epidemiological methods for determining the provision of services. It is not always possible to devise a detailed prescription for services derived solely from factual data since resources are always less than are ideally required, so that value judgements must then enter the planning process. Nevertheless, sound information is obviously essential for rational planning; it should include an estimate of the prevalence of the disorders to be treated and of the optimal provision of the facilities required for its treatment according to the best contemporary evidence. Models can be constructed illustrating how many patients, with what charac-teristics, requiring what pattern and cost of treatment can be successfully cured or rehabilitated with a given range of facilities; conversely, if one starts with a structure such as a hospital, a model can be derived of the flow of patients through it. Studies of how services and institutions function, sometimes termed operational research, lead on naturally to comparisons of the costs, benefits, and relative efficiency of alter-native patterns of care.

These general statements are necessarily somewhat abstract and require to be made more precise by consideration of some of the concepts and methods they entail.

BASIC CONCEPTS

One of the definitions of epidemiology cited above was 'the study of the mass aspects of disease'. A moment's reflection will suggest that this must be a complex exercise: a disease may be described not only in terms of its frequency but also its chronicity, its tendency to relapse, the likelihood of recovery or death, the therapeutic provision which may be required and so forth. Obviously not all these aspects can be captured by one descriptive term, and different measurements must be employed to measure these various features. The optimal selection among the various descriptive possibilities for any particular purpose will be considered later; first it is necessary to have some general grasp of what kinds of measures are commonly employed.

Perhaps the most basic concept in epidemiology is that of a *rate*. A rate describes the relationship between two numbers. One refers to the number of 'instances' of whatever it is that is being measured and is referred to as the numerator. The second is the devisor or denominator and represents the total reference group (usually a population of some kind) within which the instances may or may not occur and which defines the sole source from which they are derived.

Rates are of essentially two kinds. The first may be considered true rates; both the numerator and the denominator refer to the same units of observation over the same period of time. Thus, a rate which expresses the number of individuals who die in a given city in relation to the total number of inhabitants is a true rate. With such rates all the individuals counted in the numerator are also present in the denominator; in the mortality example those dying during the period will have been counted as part of the total living population at the beginning of the study period. A 'true' rate is thus simply a proportion.

The second type of rate is really a *ratio* or 'false' rate, in that the numerator and denominator refer to different units. A common example is the hospital 'admission rate' in which the number of admissions, which are essentially *events*, are divided by a local population estimate of *persons*. Expressions of this sort are logically equivalent to the familiar ratios of miles per hour, cost per metre, and the like. The distinction between rates and ratios should always be recognised to avoid illogical comparisons.

The instances or numerators of a rate may be of different kinds. One has already been mentioned and refers essentially to events such as episodes of illness, admissions to hospital and so forth, all of which may befall an individual on more than one occasion. As usually expressed, that is, as events/persons, such a rate cannot be interpreted in terms of individuals. For example, in a village of 100 people where there have been five episodes of illness in a given period, giving

an event/person rate of five per 100, it will not be possible to say if Mr A has been ill five times or if five different people have each succumbed once only.

The second type of numerator is of the kind used in computing person rates. This in essence is an unduplicated count of the individuals being studied during a unit time. If the denominator used in deriving such a rate is that of the total number of individuals at risks, then a patient rate is a true rate in the sense defined above. In the village example just cited, if only Mr A became ill then the patient rate is only one per 100.

There is a third type of numerator in which only individuals suffering an illness for the first time (or displaying some other characteristic on the first occasion) are counted.

Comparison of these three types of rate over time can be very useful in resolving such fundamental issues as whether a disorder is involving more members of a community, or changing in its tendency to relapse or chronicity, or both.

The types of denominator which may be used in the calculation of rates are similarly diverse. For most purposes the denominator is the population in which the researcher is interested, 'population' being considered in a mathematical sense as the total aggregate of actual and potential instances and not necessarily as any geographic or demographic entity. A population may be defined in a great variety of other ways. For example, one may speak of a population of mothers of schizophrenics, of wives of alcoholics, or of those exposed to a given intensity of aircraft noise. One of the creative components of epidemiology lies precisely in the designation of populations to be studied. How populations are counted or estimated is a technical matter outside the scope of this chapter, and it must suffice to say that data on demographic characteristics such as age, sex, social class, and population density are usually obtained from some form of census material, while the use of more elusive but possibly more fruitful parameters usually involves surveys, in which enumeration of the population is carried out as part of the project. Thus, the number of friends a person has and the quality of those friendships have been used to identify subpopulations among whom rates of disorder have been calculated (Miller & Ingham 1976).

The type of population so far considered has been that of persons, but this is not a necessary constraint. Events may also be used. An admission rate for a particular disorder is often better expressed as a proportion of all admissions per unit time than in relation to some population of persons, though of course everything depends upon the use that is intended to be made of the resulting estimate.

In all the preceding discussion there has been an implicit reference to the use of a time base when determining a rate. Figure 11.3 represents a population consisting of only five individuals spanning a period from t_0 to t_3, the horizontal bars constituting episodes of illness. At t_1 there are three affected individuals. Hence one can speak of a *point prevalence rate* at t_1 of three-fifths or 60%. For t_2 the corresponding point prevalence rate is two-fifths or 40%.

Alternatively, one may consider the number of individuals who are ill during a specified period of time, whether or not their illness persists throughout that period. Thus, in the interval between t_1 and t_2 there are four affected individuals, giving a *period prevalence rate* of four out of five or 80%. For many purposes it is convenient to take 1 year as the study period but alternatives are often used.

Lastly, one may consider the number of individuals who are healthy at the beginning of a period but then fall ill. Thus, for the interval between t_1 and t_2 there is only one such individual (D), while there are two individuals (D) and (E), who were well at t_1. For the t_1–t_2 interval there is thus an *inception rate* of one in two, or 50%. Note that it is only the status of individuals at the beginning of the period t_1 that matters; illnesses occurring prior to that time but from which the individual has recovered are not relevant to this type of inception rate (which is concerned with spells or episodes). If, however, attention is confined to those who had *never* previously suffered from the disorder one would refer to a 'first ever' rate. This is also 50% if it is assumed that neither (D) nor (E) had an illness prior to t_0.

In summary, the different types of rates may be formally defined as follows:

Point prevalence rate. The proportion of individuals in a population who have the disease at a given point in time.

Period prevalence rate. The proportion of individuals in a population who have the disease during a given interval of time.

Inception rate. The proportion of individuals in a population who are initially free of a disease but who acquire it within a given interval of time.

Note that of these the second, namely the period prevalence rate, is the sum of the other two; it is the rate referring to all individuals who are cases on the first day of the study period (the initial point prevalence rate) plus all those who subsequently become ill within the relevant time (the inception rate). Note too that the term *incidence* does not have a very clear meaning — though it is sometimes used synonymously with inception — and is probably better avoided.

Finally, the question may be posed as to how many individuals in a population may be expected to develop an illness (at least once) during the course of a specified period or during their lifetime. If, in Figure 11.3, t_0 represents birth and t_3 death, then it is evident that four out of five persons will be affected. In less obvious situations the lifetime expectations may be calculated by subtracting from unity the conjoint probability of remaining well over all the time intervals considered. The probability of remaining well during a discrete interval is 1 minus the probability of falling ill (the inception rate). Thus for Figure 11.3 the expression becomes

$$1 - (1 - 0.6)(1 - 0.5)(1 - 0.0) = 1 - 0.2 = 0.8.$$

However, where inception rates are low an acceptable approximation can be obtained by simply summing the inception rates for each consecutive period (e.g. see Hagnell 1966).

Some uses of rates

Different rates serve different purposes. The point prevalence rate can serve, for example, to indicate to someone planning a service how many individuals with a particular disorder he needs to be able to contain in treatment at any one time — assuming of course that all cases both need, and come forward for, care. If the prevalence rate remains stable then new cases will arise at the same frequency as established

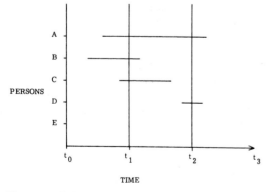

Fig. 11.3 Episodes of illness in a hypothetical population (see text).

cases recover or die, and the rate will indicate how many beds or other units of provision are required. But it may also be that it is the initial assessment of a patient that requires the most attention from staff, rather than the later phases of the disorder. In that situation the planner also needs to know the inception rate if he is to make appropriate provisions.

Different kinds of rates may also be used to characterise different types of disorder. The common cold, for example, is widespread in winter, but on any given day only 2 or 3% of the population (the point prevalence rate) may be afflicted. On the other hand, in the course of the winter months perhaps the majority of the population will have an attack, which is to say that the 6 month inception rate may approach 100%. Thus the (point) prevalence rate is much lower than the (period) inception rate. But for schizophrenia as traditionally defined, where the illness tends to be chronic, the prevalence rate will be high while the inception rate over a short period of time will be comparatively low. Thus the salient features of these two disorders are succinctly exemplified by comparing how their inception and prevalence rates relate to each other.

The schizophrenia example will also serve to show another feature which the reader may have already spotted. The relationship between the prevalence of a disease in a population (point prevalence) and the frequency with which new cases arise (inception rate) is a function of its chronicity, i.e. inception × chronicity = prevalence when all are measured by a common period of time such as a year. Hence, knowing any two of these values the third can be readily calculated. This strategy may be very useful in situations in which direct assessment of the average duration of a disorder may be very difficult to determine, as indeed will be true for any very chronic illness. Data on chronicity are important not only for service planning but also for more basic epidemiological purposes, for example to determine whether social factors conduce to a more chronic course of illness in some subgroups of the population, as appears to be the case with depressive disorders in different social classes and in different age groups.

Rates or frequency distributions

Rates were first employed in epidemiology in connection with mortality but their continuing use is based on much more than tradition. Rates have the great advantage that they can be expressed simply and compared with each other by elementary statistical procedures. This point is of some importance, since as a rule of thumb the more complex the statistical analysis the less certain the conclusion. Such a relationship is not due to failure of statistical technology but to the need for an increasing number of mathematical assumptions to be met if elaborate statistical procedures are to be employed properly, and it is often difficult to be certain that the data available do in fact meet the mathematician's requirements. In addition, a rate provides the service planner with estimates of the number of individuals or illness episodes he may expect to meet in a given period of time.

These advantages should not be lightly sacrificed (Wing et al 1978) but there are also certain problems involved in the use of rates. The principal difficulty of the concept is the implication that the members of the study population can be unequivocally differentiated into those who do and who do not have the characteristics in question. With mortality there is no problem. But with morbidity the matter is more complex. For certain disorders, status or behaviours, clear-cut distinctions are feasible, at least in principle: a woman is either pregnant or she is not. For the major psychoses or for specific forms of mental handicap the issue is a little less clear-cut in that there is argument as to precisely what criteria should be adopted to designate a patient as schizophrenic, manic and so on. Such debates have taken up much energy, but the majority opinion is still that a condition like schizophrenia should in principle be viewed as discontinuous from normality. The acceptance of standardised assessment procedures, and firm rules for classification following assessment, have done much to resolve difficulties of this kind (see below).

More formidable difficulties arise when at a conceptual level the phenomenon under examination is not obviously all-or-none. Examples include primary mental defect and the large and varied group of neurotic and personality disorders. In some instances a cut-off point on what is essentially a continuous distribution may be imposed if external reasons can be adduced to justify the particular level chosen. These may have to do with the requirements for special accommodation, as in the case of severely defective individuals, or that the individuals are suffering from disorders of an intensity which warrant psychiatric intervention, or that the symptoms are of an intensity and show a sufficiently clear-cut pattern (that is, a syndrome) which permits differential diagnosis. But all such cut-off points are arbitrary, and the epidemiologist is obliged to spend much care on the perennial problem of 'what is a case?'

(Bebbingston & Wing 1981), or to put the matter more accurately, on what convention should be adopted to designate a case. The important point is that rates can only be interpreted in conjunction with the definitions of a case which the investigator has used (as well as the intensity of his search). Minor shifts in threshold will make a substantial difference to the figures. It must also be realised that an inception rate will include a number of individuals who have crossed the threshold represented by the 'case' criteria but who formerly just failed to meet them. In clinical terms the difference may be minimal.

Accordingly, it has been proposed that for certain purposes frequency distributions presenting the different degrees of severity of a disorder should be used instead of rates (Ingham & Miller 1976, 1979). Comparisons between populations then become a matter of comparing distribution curves. The approach is perhaps most useful when studying single symptoms of differing degrees of intensity, or psychological characteristics such as intelligence. Note too that any study which reports classical inception or prevalence rates for a disorder but distinguishes different levels of severity is implicitly adopting a dimensional view and beginning to approximate to the notion of a frequency distribution.

In recent years there has been increased interest in using distribution curves to characterise populations. Evidence has accumulated to suggest that case *rates* may be related to population *means* for certain continuously distributed characteristics. For example, the number of hypertensives in different communities (the hypertension case rates) has been shown to be related to the average blood pressure found in those societies. Similarly, there is evidence that the rates for heavy alcohol consumption reflect average consumption, and the same relationship may hold for depressive disorders and depressed mood. Such findings are of great importance both for theories of aetiology and for strategies of prevention (Rose & Day 1990).

Ecological correlations

It has already been said that the epidemiological approach is essentially comparative, seeking to compare groups of individuals with respect to the frequency of some phenomenon of interest. For person rates this implies that each *individual* in the study is categorised both as regards the presence or absence of the phenomenon in question and his membership of one or other of the groups being compared. A different strategy is adopted in ecological studies. Here the unit of study becomes the population itself, and a comparison is carried out between the gross characteristics of each collective. Thus, towns may be compared with regard to the frequency of different kinds of illness, social circumstances, and demographic characteristics, but there is no information at the individual level. It may be reported that, say, cities with a high proportion of manual workers also have high rates of illness, but it will not be known whether it is the manual workers who are the more likely to be ill.

Such an approach was first used in psychiatry in the classical investigations of the 1920s associated with the Chicago school, most notably the work of Faris & Dunham (1939). They showed that the rate of schizophrenia was higher in the central than in the peripheral zones of a city, and that the inner areas were characterised by extensive social disorganisation. This concentric distribution of cases was not shown by other forms of psychosis. They therefore proposed that there was a special association between social disorganisation and schizophrenia and began the debate as to how that association was to be interpreted. The subsequent history makes fascinating reading, but the point at issue here is that the controversy led to the clearer recognition of what has come to be known as the 'ecological fallacy'. Simply stated, the error is to assume that phenomena which are correlated at a gross or population level are necessarily correlated within a population of individuals. Robinson (1950) cited data to show how illiteracy and the proportion of immigrants in a community could be positively associated ecologically, although there was a negative association between the two characteristics when studied at an individual level. Table 11.1 illustrates how this can be so in a hypothetical date set.

Subsequent studies using the ecological method have been much more clearly aware of what kinds of conclusions may legitimately be drawn. Thus, in a study of suicide in London, ecological correlations suggested a variety of characteristics of suicide. These correlations were then treated as hypotheses which were subsequently tested and largely confirmed at an individual level (Sainsbury 1955). Ecological matching of cities into pairs to provide groups with and without a Samaritan service has been used in studies looking at the effect of such provision on the suicide rate (Bagley 1968, Barraclough & Jennings 1977). But apart from such uses the method remains an interesting way of characterising populations even when there is no question of the phenomenon occurring within the same individuals. For example, in

Table 11.1 Association at the ecological and individual level

	Percentage voting for party X	Percentage middle class
Ecological level		
Town A	10	20
Town B	20	30
Town C	30	40

	Total voting for party X	
	Yes	No
Individual level		
Town A		
Social class		
Middle	0	200
Lower	100	700
Town B		
Social class		
Middle	0	300
Lower	200	500
Town C		
Social class		
Middle	0	400
Lower	300	300

There is a perfect ecological concordance between voting for party X and being middle-class, yet not a single middle-class person votes for that party in any of the three towns. Within each town the two variables are *negatively related*.

an analysis in Edinburgh it was shown that areas high in perinatal mortality were also high in rates of referral to child psychiatrists (Buglass et al 1980). In this example, of course, it is not possible for the same children to be responsible for the high values for both variables; the correlation presumably points to a common mediating factor such as maternal health. Ecological analysis can also serve to disprove a hypothesis that two behaviours or disorders are basically the same. Thus, Buglass & Duffy (1978) demonstrated that suicide and parasuicide have quite different ecological settings, a finding which adds further weight to the thesis that they are better considered as distinct rather than variants (see Ch. 32).

Recently, statisticians have begun to specify conditions under which correlations at an individual level can legitimately be inferred from ecological or aggregate data, but the practical usefulness of this work is uncertain. For the present it would be prudent to interpret ecological correlations as pertaining only to whole populations.

GENERAL EPIDEMIOLOGICAL STRATEGIES

Enumeration of *cases* may be based on data which have been collected for some other purpose, usually administrative, or alternatively the data may be specifically sought. These two classes of information differ in a number of important respects which will be briefly discussed. It is also evident that study *populations* can vary greatly, most importantly with regard to size. In theory there is no necessary correlation between the types of data on cases and on population size, but in practice the two are so closely connected it is necessary to consider both at the same time.

In certain obvious situations, a study will have to be based on a very large population. Rare disorders cannot be accumulated in sufficient numbers to yield a trustworthy rate without drawing on a large base, sometimes over several years. It is less obvious that *differences* between rates can only be sensitively detected if the difference is due to a reasonably large discrepancy in the numerators. Population A may show only half the rate of a disorder of population B, yet if the illness is rare the discrepancy may be within chance expectations, while a similar two-fold difference for a common disease may be statistically highly significant.

Generally speaking, logistic constraints dictate that the study of large population entails the use of prerecorded information, i.e. of data which are collected routinely and not as a research study. This is particularly true if it is hoped to monitor changes over many years, or to compare the experience of different countries.

The most important data available at the national level are those for mortality and hospital-treated morbidity. (A useful review of routine data-collecting systems in England and Wales has been provided by Fraser et al (1978).) Apart from being virtually the only recourse, such data have certain incidental advantages. They are, for example, relatively inexpensive, and may be available in a form, which, with due care for confidentiality, is suitable for purposes of secondary analysis.

Such data, however, pose some very substantial difficulties. The first is to ensure that the information has been collected with equal diligence across or between, for example, nations, and over time. The second problem is that of case definition. Among suicide researchers, for example, there has been extensive controversy as to how a suicide verdict is derived by coroners, and hence just what meaning should be attached to the official figures. Numerous studies have been needed to determine how far what the legal authority declares to be suicide coincides with how a psychiatrist might categorise unnatural deaths; of national practices in the ascertainment and recording of suicide; and of the epidemiological profile of officially recorded suicide compared with that of suicides plus open verdicts and selected causes of accidental death (Adelstein & Mardon 1975). The balance of evidence is somewhat reassuring in that it seems that official suicide statistics are sufficiently uniform for most practical purposes. But the general point is that much caution is required before accepting the validity of nationally collected data of any kind.

Even greater care than that required for mortality is needed in interpreting national or regional differences in hospital-treated morbidity: death is usually unequivocal, but disease may or may not be recognised or treated. The number of beds or out-patient departments available in different regions may vary very markedly, as may referral and admission practices, social service provisions, and so forth. Treated morbidity rates measure the supply of services and not the prevalence of disease (Matthew 1971), a disparity which is less marked for the psychoses and greatest for the minor neuroses and personality disorders.

But perhaps the most salient difficulty in interpreting statistics for treated morbidity is diagnostic uncertainty. The use of the International Classification of Diseases (ICD) is widespread but even though successive editions have sought to provide increasingly explicit criteria for particular diagnoses, the consistency with which it is used is uncertain. Under routine service conditions the reliability of ICD diagnoses is low (Foulds 1955, Kreitman 1961). More rigorous diagnostic schemes have been proposed and are widely used in research, but they do not as yet provide the basis for national reporting.

Finally, routine morbidity data often differentiate poorly, if at all, between events and persons (see introductory paragraphs). An attempt at clarification is provided by separate enumeration of first contacts, usually with reference to inpatient care, and, in the UK, hospital admission rates are usually presented both for first admissions and for all admissions. It is intended that the term 'first admission' should refer to any psychiatric facility, but often the coding functionary is aware only of previous admissions to the same institution. In consequence, official first admissions rates tend to be markedly inflated.

Case registers

With smaller units of population a new source of data may become available, namely the regional psychiatric case register. The principle of the case register is to ensure that all contacts with a psychiatric service by all the individuals living within a defined population are duly recorded and collated. In its most primitive form such a register can provide prevalence data for treated morbidity over any period of time, but the chief asset of case registers lies in their potential for record linkage. This means that it is possible to reconstruct the evolution of a cohort of patients (subject to loss by migration and the like from the area). Such studies add substantially to understanding of the natural history (including the effects of treatment) of psychiatric disorders. The principle of the case register may be applied to any size of population unit. Operation at a national level is shown most comprehensively in Sweden and Denmark, where the use by each member of the population of a unique identification number for a host of medical and social purposes enables the construction of interlinking registers capable of collating a remarkable variety of events or disorders. Several registers now exist in the USA and in the UK (DHSS 1974, Hall et al 1974) and a national system operates within Scotland (Heasman & Clark 1979). Registers are expensive to maintain and for that reason many have recently been discontinued. Their cost is most evidently justified where they can be used both for service planning and for scientific enquiry.

Case registers may operate with population units much smaller than that of a region or city. The principle may be applied not only to hospital services but also to a general practice, either for routine purposes (Gruer & Heasman 1970) or for a limited period to cover a specific study (Shepherd et al 1966). A register can also be extended to include paramedical services (Ebie 1971).

Special studies

Two main strategies can be used to overcome the limitations of routinely collected data. One is the focused study, in which investigators in different areas agree upon diagnostic criteria and prospectively categorise series of patients at each collaborating centre. To date, the outcome of the few studies which have used this design has been to show that putative difference evaporates once diagnostic uniformity is achieved (e.g. Cooper et al 1972) or the population more closely defined (e.g. Leff et al 1976). Enquiries of this kind, which have invariably been hospital based, do not entirely overcome the problem of possible differences in thresholds of referral or admission. However, comparisons of the severity of illness among the groups in care go some way to resolving the threshold problem, especially for psychotic disorders and in relatively affluent societies. For minor disorders the strategy is of less value since so many different kinds of filter are known to operate. For example, two populations may differ in their rates for hospital-treated neurotic illness even if uniform criteria are applied and only cases of comparable severity are accepted for treatment: the difference may be due to a greater tolerance by the families in one area, even though the prevalence of illness may be identical. By definition, treatment-based studies take no account of untreated illness.

It is in such a context, amongst others, that the population survey becomes especially valuable. It is indeed the only way in which information can be obtained about the frequency, variety and course of a disorder in the general population uncontaminated by treatment selection effects.

The population survey

Surveys are costly in time and money, and if clumsily carried out may be quite uninformative. Every survey should have a clear purpose, which will in turn influence the definitions used and the overall design.

It is useful to consider surveys and their attendant problems under the following three broad headings: (1) the definition of the individuals entering the numerator of a rate, that is, cases, or alternatively the definition of points on a frequency distribution curve; (2) the choice of a denominator or population; and (3) the problems that arise in the execution of the study itself.

The difficulties of case definition have already been touched on in connection with routine morbidity data but the issue becomes central in surveys. Whereas the giving and receiving of treatment provides an operational definition of illness when treated morbidity is studied, there is no such guide when total populations are considered. It therefore falls to the investigator to select appropriate criteria himself. Normally he seeks to find a way of identifying individuals in the population who in key respects are like those diagnosed in clinical practice. That is to say, he has to draw on traditional clinical knowledge, and would wish to proceed so that his criteria for a 'case' would be validated by clinical judgement. A direct application of this principle is to have an experienced psychiatrist personally interview every member of a population, or a sample thereof, using informal clinical judgement (Essen-Moller 1956, Hagnell 1966), or to apply such judgements to data collected

by assistants (Leighton et al 1963). The assumption is that other psychiatrists confronted with the same data would arrive at similar diagnoses even though the diagnostic criteria remain unspecified: alternatively, that although psychiatrists may differ somewhat in their concepts and threshold criteria the overall pattern of the results (e.g. differential associations with age or social class) would be the same. But contemporary investigators have become increasingly dissatisfied with an approach in which the basic definition of a case is so vague. Clinical judgements are rarely sufficiently explicit to be stated in operational terms, and are often particularly hazy about the threshold of severity which must be crossed before an individual may be given a diagnosis, to say nothing of the inconsistencies of the criteria for applying a particular diagnostic label. Comparisons between surveys become very difficult and independent replication almost impossible.

Another method is to attempt to bypass the diagnostic question altogether and to count single symptoms or to use 'degrees' of disturbance, without diagnostic specification (e.g. see Srole et al 1962). Much earlier work in the American tradition adopted such methods. Such a strategy was in keeping with an interest in psychopathology rather than diagnosis, but that emphasis has changed and it is now generally accepted that differentiation by diagnosis is important in the epidemiological as well as the clinical fields. The trend has been towards the use of more sophisticated instruments which permit diagnoses more or less analogous to those employed in clinical practice, are applicable to individuals identified in community surveys and are based on explicit criteria.

The assessment of individuals seen in surveys involves several distinct stages. There is first the eliciting of information concerning the presence or absence of symptoms. Standardised instruments are often rather weak in specifying exactly what psychological features are to be taken as representing a symptom, the implication being that a clinical training will suffice to educate the interviewer for this purpose. Once a symptom is identified as present, then formalised ratings can be made of its frequency and severity according to specific rules. When this is achieved, the third stage can be applied, which is the grouping of symptoms into syndromes or diagnostic categories. This last stage may be quite automatic and can be carried out by computer.

A minimum requirement of any interview procedure is that it should be of demonstrable reliability. It is clear that, given reasonable training of the users, the standardised instruments mentioned below have acceptable reliability. In the future attention will shift from the issue of reliability to that of validity (Brockington et al 1978).

One of the best known diagnostic interviews is the Present State Examination (PSE) by Wing et al (1974, 1977) which has been widely employed (e.g. WHO 1972). It has been through several editions and will be amended again in the near future. The PSE was derived from detailed study of patients in hospital care, and is therefore particulary useful for describing the more severely ill. The strength of the PSE is that it provides a reasonably clear operational definition of each symptom which is to be rated, and provides criteria for different levels of severity. Training is required if it is to be employed properly, and it was intended for use by those who already had some clinical experience, though recently it has been shown to be possible to train non-professionals in its use, at least for certain limited purposes. Assessment is based on the respondent's mental state at interview and over the preceding month. A computerised classification known as Catego can be applied to the ratings to produce a diagnosis according to the ICD as well as according to certain more specialised schemata. All these are based on a hierarchical principle whereby certain major disorders take precedence over lesser conditions when the criteria for both are met. A useful feature of Catego is that it can also generate an Index of Definition. This is a grading presenting, in effect, seven levels of severity of illness although 'syndromic clarity' or 'typicality' also influences the level.

In the USA a widely used interview schedule is the Schedule for Affective Disorders and Schizophrenia (SADS). It covers a wide range of symptoms and is intended to embrace such conditions as personality disorders and alcohol-related syndromes as well as the psychoses and neuroses. In this respect it is much more comprehensive than the PSE. Again, training is required in its use. The time base to which the ratings are applied is variable, and the instrument has often been used to characterise past illnesses at any point in the lifetime of the respondent as well as his or her present state. Diagnostic groupings are derived by applying the rules set out in the Research Diagnostic Criteria (RDC; Spitzer et al 1978). These involve consideration of non-symptomatic aspects of the disorder, such as impairment of function, which together with the symptom data permit the derivation of a diagnosis subject to hierarchical principles. Computer processing to generate these diagnoses is possible but not necessary. The number of alternative ways of classifying illnesses which it provides has

made the RDC particularly useful in clinical research as well as epidemiology, for example in defining subgroups of depressives for clinical trials.

More recently another interview schedule, the Diagnostic Interview Schedule (DIS; Robins et al 1981, 1982), is being widely employed in the USA. It is essentially intended for survey work and for use by lay interviewers with little training. For that reason the schedule is very precisely worded and the interviewer is not permitted to probe in the manner of a clinician. The time base is adjustable and in recent versions attention is directed to dating the duration of all current symptoms as well as noting those which were present in the past. Diagnoses corresponding to the RDC and other systems, including DSM-IIIR, can be derived, but a particular feature of the DIS system is the ease with which multiple diagnoses can be produced without regard to hierarchical rules. The DIS is simple to administer and cheap to use in population studies, but on the other hand there is current uncertainty about the validity of the diagnoses it generates when these are compared with those of experienced clinicians.

The interested reader will find these and other interview procedures extensively reviewed by Weissman et al (1986) but the field is one of rapid change. New systems will continue to be developed over the next decade, bringing together the advantages of the PSE and DIS, while others are being designed for specialised fields such as neuropsychiatry.

There is another important consideration. Reid (1960) has pointed out that the epidemiologist's 'diagnostic' label, like any other diagnostic term, is only useful if it serves some purpose. But the purpose may vary. Thus, in the case of tuberculosis, the public health physician may be centrally concerned with how many 'open' cases there are. The radiologist, on the other hand, may base his diagnosis on the extent of X-ray changes, while the general physician may be primarily concerned with whether the patient feels ill, is able to work, and so forth. Estimates based on any one set of criteria may coincide poorly with those based on any other. Exactly the same is true in psychiatry. Usually, case criteria consist of definitions applicable to the diagnosis of fairly ill patients in hospital. There are obvious historical reasons why this strategy should be adopted, even though such fully developed cases are likely to be rare in population samples. But the retention of such criteria may defeat the very object of the study if it is intended to 'complete the clinical picture' by describing prodromal syndromes, *formes frustes*, or defect states following illness. For these purposes hospital-derived criteria must be modified, and an important task for the near future is the derivation of an agreed nosology applicable to the large numbers of the psychologically disturbed who are inadequately covered by existing schemata. Further, the purpose of a survey may quite legitimately have little to do with diagnosis; surveys of disability are an example. A comprehensive service for the elderly should be planned according to how many old people cannot walk, or get lost when out of doors, rather than according to whether their disability is due to chronic arthritis or dementia (see Isaacs & Neville 1976). The development of measures of impairment, disability and handicap, and of the concepts involved, is receiving much attention at present (see WHO 1980).

In comparison with these intricacies concerning definition of numerators the definition of populations to be studied is relatively straightforward. The ideal procedure is to enumerate each member of the population and subsequently to draw a random sample: these individuals are then approached for their cooperation in the survey. The initial framework may be obtained in various ways, as by a private census or more commonly from the electoral roll. The latter has the disadvantage of omitting the homeless and vagrants — groups which might be particularly important to disorders such as schizophrenia and alcoholism — as well as children. The accuracy of electoral rolls even at the date of publication is uncertain; thereafter they lose individuals through migration or death at the rate of approximately 1% per month. An alternative procedure is to draw a sample, not of individuals but of addresses, weighted according to household size, and within each address to sample at random (Kish 1965, Blyth & Marchant 1973). Other methods involve stratification, whereby a group of census units is first sampled randomly, and then at a second stage further sampling is carried out within each selected unit. Yet another strategy is deliberately to oversample from certain subgroups of the population in order to obtain a large number of cases from that subpopulation (for any of a variety of reasons). Variations from straightforward probability sampling are generally more economical but raise statistical problems when standard errors are calculated. (The detailed implications of the different types of sampling strategy can be found in more special texts, e.g. Cochran (1977)).

In practice, whatever procedure is used a discrepancy will be found between the characteristics of the sample actually obtained and those of the base population. These discrepancies are of three main kinds. The first is simple sampling error, which is well covered by statistical theory. The second class of errors is the failure of the sample frame, such as the electoral roll or a general practice register, to reflect the real population accurately. Some of the listed individuals will have moved out of the area while others will have died or be missing because they are in hospital or prison, and it cannot be assumed that these differ in no important respects from those who remain. Thirdly, there is the special problem of non-cooperation. If those who agreed to participate in surveys differed in no important respect from those who refused there would be no difficulty that could not be dealt with by simple arithmetic. However, there is substantial evidence that refusals may be particularly common among those who are manifesting the disorder being investigated (see Cox et al 1977). The response rate of a survey is therefore of cardinal importance. No survey based on a probability sample has ever achieved 100% coverage, and the further the figure falls from this ideal the less confidence can one have in the rates derived by the study. Similarly, it is impossible to compare rates obtained by different surveys, even if they have used identical methods and criteria, if the response rates vary markedly.

Though non-response is a major source of bias, distortions in the data may also arise through unequal honesty of report among the survey respondents. Thus, those who are heavy drinkers or are clinically alcoholic may under-report their alcohol consumption to a greater extent than those in the moderate drinking range (Popham 1970, Schmidt 1972).

Cohort studies

A cohort is simply a group, and a cohort study is one in which a defined group of individuals, healthy or sick, is studied over a period of time, in order to ascertain the frequency with which selected characteristics change or develop. Such studies may be prospective or retrospective, or may use a combination of both methods according to the ease and completeness with which the relevant information can be obtained. The most satisfactory, if most expensive, procedure is to define and collect information from a sample at time 1 and then monitor the progress of the group until time 2. The alternative strategy of beginning with those individuals available at time 2 and working back to time 1 often leads to difficulties due to inadequate initial data recording. Moreover, if there have been many deaths or emigrations in the interim it may be impossible to reconstruct the original sample.

The larger and most ambitious studies have defined the starting cohort in demographic terms; thus, Douglas & Blomfield (1958) have reported on a sample of births occurring in England and Wales in 1 week in 1946 and followed for 40 years, while Helgasson (1964) constructed retrospectively an account of all Icelanders born in the period 1895–1897 and followed till 1957. Other long-term studies have started with clinically defined groups of children to determine the relationship of childhood and adult psychiatric disorder (e.g. see Robins 1966). But the principles of cohort studies can equally be applied to samples followed over relatively short periods. If the sample is composed of known patients such a study then becomes indistinguishable from the standard clinical follow-up investigation: the cohort study technique is not the prerogative of the epidemiologist, although certain statistical problems that arise in such contexts should be particularly familiar to him. The only distinction which may be drawn between epidemiological and other types of cohort study is whether the cohort itself is capable of definition in population terms.

Cohort designs, appropriately modified, can also be applied to total hospital populations (e.g. see Fryer 1974). Here the interest is in ascertaining what proportion of patients present in a service on a given date will have been discharged at varying intervals thereafter. The rate of decline in the numbers remaining in care is itself informative about the characteristics of the service, especially in relation to subgroups such as patients with schizophrenia or dementia. If supplemented by additional data on the numbers of patients newly recruited to the hospital, such information can also provide a guide to the likely future needs for hospital accommodation. Obviously, if in such investigations reliance is placed upon administrative criteria alone the results will merely be descriptive of what happens and not in any sense an evaluation of how well patients fare.

Certain points need to be borne in mind in interpreting the results of any cohort study. A cohort followed for an appreciable period will show three distinct effects. There are first those associated with the evolution of the disease, or if normal individuals are being studied, with the onset of new illnesses, or with mortality. These changes are usually of primary interest, and the study will usually have been undertaken precisely in order to investigate them. Secondly, it is evident that all the individuals in the cohort will age over the period of the investigation,

and such changes must be distinguished from those of disease process. For example, alcohol consumption tends to decrease with age, and the risk of suicide tends to increase. Appropriate control (or reference) data are required if the effects of ageing are to be separated from those of chronicity. Thirdly, the group being studied may also be affected by changes occurring at some particular time during the study follow-up period, but which may equally effect the population at large. Thus, a cohort of, say, depressed patients followed for a period which happens to include the outbreak of war or an economic slump may show a very different suicide rate from an identical cohort followed for a similar length of time in more tranquil circumstances. Such so-called period effects may be very elusive. For example, the diffusion of new ideas on the management of patients may be difficult to specify or to date accurately, yet may explain why the results for a particular cohort differ from similar studies carried out in the past. (Sequential cohort studies may be designed specifically to measure such effects, but are difficult to conduct prospectively.)

Another point to be kept in mind when interpreting cohort studies is how rapidly they become out of date. A sample which may be random with respect to some designated group at the beginning of the study and followed for a number of years will not be random with respect to the *contemporary* group at the point of follow-up. Not only will the cohort have aged, but the characteristics of the population it is designed to represent will often have changed substantially during the interim. Thus, a cohort of long-stay psychiatric in-patients drawn in 1970 and followed for 10 years will not be comparable, even at its starting point, to the long-stay population of 1980, since so many changes in hospital policy were introduced during the decade.

Finally, it is worth pointing out a simple fallacy sometimes made with cohort studies. Suppose a clinician follows a cohort of 100 patients for 5 years and finds that ten have died. There is thus a 10% mortality over the period, which might be reported as 2% mortality per annum. Another clinician might follow a similar group of 100 but over 10 years, and again find that ten had died, corresponding to a an average mortality rate of 1% per annum. Are these results different? The answer is clearly 'no' if in both studies all the deaths occurred in, say, the first year of follow-up and none thereafter. The example illustrates the danger of uncritically attempting to derive averages — in this example, annual values — for rates (as well as the importance of examining distributions before calculating means in any data set). Incidentally, the analysis of survival data is now a somewhat specialised branch of statistics, and expert advice is often necessary.

Matching and case controls

When examining a patient a clinician operates with a set of informal standards in mind which act as a yard-stick against which he evaluates his observations. For scientific purposes this comparative procedure requires to be formalised, and a number of steps can be distinguished in so doing. The first level requires only that the patient group be carefully described. This may appear a trivial point but in practice epidemiological studies are often hampered by the inadequacies of existing clinical descriptions and concepts. This first stage might be described as that of uncontrolled observation. Secondly, an additional group may be included for purposes of comparison and as an aid to interpretation but without specific reference to the patient sample. At his level one can speak of comparative observation, leaving unspecified the criteria used to select the comparison group. Though profoundly unsatisfactory, this situation does in fact pertain to many of the 'norms' available for psychometric tests and for biochemical evaluations, which are often based on ill-described 'samples of convenience'. Finally, there is the construction of a comparison group dictated by the characteristics of the study group in question and differing *only* with respect to some specified criteria, most commonly diagnosis. Such a group represents a matched control group.

Thus, a matched control group is constructed so that all the main features of the patient group, such as for example their age, sex or social class, are faithfully reproduced, but without reference to the one variable of primary interest. Any differences which then remain between the patient group and the comparison group cannot be due to the variables on which the matching has been carried out. The primary justification of the matched control procedure is to eliminate the effects of unwanted variables.

It follows that matching should be employed only if it is certain that the variables to be eliminated are indeed of no further interest. If a group of patients is matched with a control group in terms of age then it may no longer be possible to investigate the effects of age per se within the same study. Less obviously, the same consideration applies to other variables which, though not used directly in the matching procedure, are nevertheless closely associated with the

characteristics on which the selection has been effected. Thus, in the age example it would not be surprising to find that the patient and control groups were also very similar with respect to fertility, frequency of consultation with general practitioners, or marital status since each of these is known to be linked to age itself. It is of course possible that the original matching was carried out precisely to determine whether these variables can distinguish the groups once the age effect has been eliminated, but surprisingly often the selection of control variables is inappropriate in that it eliminates more from the investigation than the researcher had intended, including items he had hoped to examine (so-called 'overmatching'.)

Further it should be appreciated that a matching group constructed to reflect the salient characteristics of a study group will not be a random sample of the total population from which it is drawn. In a study of dementia a group of age-matched normal subjects will show a grossly skewed age distribution which is clearly atypical of the general population (though the sample should be random within the constraints of the specified age parameters).

Case–control procedures are by no means unique to epidemiology and are commonly used in clinical research. Indeed the only distinction between the two settings is that in the former the relationship of the study samples to their parent populations can be defined. Controls may be selected according to a number of different strategies, and these may entail different statistical procedures in the analysis of the results. The most powerful and economical strategy is to match each individual in the study group pairwise with a control subject; designs are also available in which more than one control individual is selected for each member of the study group (Pike & Morrow 1970). The main constraint on the use of *precision* matching of this kind is its practical difficulty. An alternative is the use of *group* controls, whereby a group is constructed in such a way that the means and standard deviations for the matching variables are the same for the two groups, but without the one-to-one correspondence of the members who make up the samples. The design of a control group in any specific context is in part dependent upon the level of precision required and in part upon what is possible.

Mistakes due to simple oversight can occur in constructing control groups for common conditions. A sample of hospital-referred schizophrenics might reasonably be contrasted with an appropriate sample of the general population since the latter will contain very few, if any, schizophrenics. But if neurosis is being investigated then an unscreened general population sample would not contribute to a powerful design, since some members of the general population sample will be neurotics. Judgement would then be required in interpreting the results of such a study, especially if they were negative.

It is also worth noting that an investigation in which control of more than three or four variables is attempted at the design stage is unlikely to be fully successful. The adequacy with which matching has in fact been achieved should always be checked and reported, and statistical corrections, as by covariance analysis, should be freely used even for minor failures.

REFERENCES

Adelstein A, Mardon C 1975 Suicides 1961–74. Population Trends 2: OPCS, pp 13–18

Bagley C 1968 The evaluation of a suicide prevention scheme by an ecological method. Social Science and Medicine 2: 1–14

Barraclough B, Jennings C 1977 Suicide prevention by the Samaritans. Lancet ii: 237–240

Bebbington P, Wing J 1981 What is a case? Proceedings of WPA 1980 Conference. Grant McIntyre, London

Blyth W, Marchant L 1973 A self-weighting random sampling technique. Journal of the Market Research Society 15: 157–162

Brockington J, Kendell R. Leff J 1978 Definitions of schizophrenia: concordance and prediction of outcome. Psychological Medicine 8: 387–398

Buglass D, Duffy J 1978 The ecological pattern of suicide and parasuicide in Edinburgh. Social Science and Medicine 12: 241–253

Buglass D, Duffy J, Kreitman N 1980 A register of social and medical indices by local government area in Edinburgh and the Lothians, part I. CRU papers, Scottish Office, Edinburgh

Cochran W G 1977 Sampling techniques. Wiley, London

Cooper J, Kendell R, Gurland E, Sharpe L, Copland J, Simon R 1972 Psychiatric diagnoses in New York and London. Maudsley monograph 20. Oxford University Press, London

Cox A, Rutter M, Yule B, Quinton D 1977 Bias resulting from missing information: some epidemiological findings. British Journal of Preventive and Social Medicine 31: 131–136

DHSS 1974 Proceedings of the conference on psychiatric case registers: Aberdeen 1973. Statistical and research reports series, No. 7. Department of Health and Social Security, London

Douglas J, Blomfield J 1958 Children under five. Allen & Unwin, London

Dunham H W 1966 Epidemiology of psychiatric disorders as a contribution to medical ecology. Archives of General Psychiatry 14: 1–19

Ebie J 1971 Identification of mother–children and sibling groups among social casework clients by a method of manual linkage. Applied Social Studies 3: 161–164

Essen-Möller E 1956 Individual traits and morbidity in a Swedish rural population. Acta Psychiatrica et Neurologica Scandinavica suppl 100

Faris R Dunham H 1939 Mental disorders in urban areas. Chicago University Press, Chicago

Foulds G 1955 Reliability of psychiatric and validity of psychological diagnoses. Journal of Mental Science 101: 851–862

Fraser P, Beral V, Choulders C 1978 Monitoring disease in England and Wales; methods applicable to routine data systems. Journal of Epidemiology and Community Health 32: 294–302

Fryer T 1974 Psychiatric inpatients in 1982: how many beds? Psychological Medicine 4: 196

Goldberg D, Huxley P 1980 Mental illness in the community: the pathway to psychiatric care. Tavistock, London

Gruer K, Heasman M 1970 Livingston new town—use of computing in general practice medical recording. British Medical Journal ii: 289–291

Hagnell O 1966 A prospective study of the incidence of mental disorder. Soenska Bokforlaget, Lund

Hall D, Robertson N, Eason R 1974 Proceedings of conference on psychiatric case registers Aberdeen 1973. Statistical and Research Reports 7. Her Majesty's Stationery Office, London

Heasman M, Clark J 1979 Medical record linkage in Scotland. Health Bulletin 37: 97–103

Helgasson T 1964 Epidemiology of mental disorders in Iceland. Acta Psychiatrica Scandinavica suppl 173

Ingham J, Miller P 1976 The concept of prevalence applied to psychiatric disorder and symptoms. Psychological Medicine 6: 217

Ingham J, Miller P 1979 Symptom prevalence and severity in a general practice population. Journal of Epidemiology and Community Health 33: 191–198

Isaacs B, Neville Y 1976 The needs of old people. British Journal of Preventive and Social Medicine 30: 79–85

Kessel W, Shepherd M 1962 Neurosis in hospital and general practice. Journal of Mental Science 108: 159–166

Kish L 1965 Survey sampling. Wiley, London

Kreitman N 1961 The reliability of psychiatric diagnosis. Journal of Mental Science 197: 876–886

Leff J, Fischer M, Bertelsen A 1976 A cross-national epidemiological study of mania. British Journal of Psychiatry 129: 428–437

Leighton D, Harding L, Maklin D, Macmillan A, Leighton A 1963 The character of danger. Basic Books, New York

MacMahon B, Pugh T F 1970 Epidemiology: principles and methods. Little, USA

Matthew G K 1971 Measuring need and evaluating services. In: Mahaghlan G (ed) Portfolio of health. Oxford University Press, London

Miller P McC, Ingham J C 1976 Friends, confidants and symptoms. Social Psychiatry 11: 51–58

Morris J N 1976 Uses of epidemiology, 3rd edn. Churchill Livingstone, London

Pike M, Morrow R 1970 Statistical analysis of patient—control studies in epidemiology. British Journal of Preventive and Social Medicine 24: 42

Popham R 1970 Indirect methods of alcoholism prevalence estimation; a critical evaluation. In: Popham R (ed) Alcohol and alcoholism. Toronto University Press. Toronto

Reid D D 1960 Epidemiological methods in the study of mental disorders. Public health paper 2: World Health Organization, Geneva

Robins L 1966 Deviant children grown up. Williams & Wilkins, Baltimore

Robins L N, Helzer J E 1981 National Institute of Mental Health Diagnostic Interview Schedule. Its history, characteristics and validity. Archives of General Psychiatry 38: 381–389

Robins L N, Helzer J E, Ratcliffe K S, Seyfried W 1982 Validity of the diagnostic interview schedule: version II:DSM-III diagnoses. Psychological Medicine 12: 855–870

Robinson W 1950 Ecological correlations and the behaviour of individuals. American Sociological Review 15: 351

Rose G, Day S 1990 The population mean predicts the number of deviant individuals. British Medical Journal 301: 1031–1034

Sainsbury P 1955 Suicide in London. Maudsley monograph 1. Chapman & Hall, London

Schmidt W 1972 Analysis of alcohol consumption data. The use of consumption data for research purposes. Report of conference on epidemiology of drug dependence. World Health Organization, Geneva

Shepherd M, Cooper B, Brown A, Kalton G 1966 Psychiatric illness in general practice. Oxford University Press, London

Spitzer R, Endicott J, Robins E 1978 Research diagnostic criteria. Archives of General Psychiatry 35: 773–782

Srole L, Langer T, Michael S, Oples M, Rennie T 1962 Mental health in the metropolis: the midtown Manhattan study. McGraw-Hill, New York

Susser M 1973 Causal thinking in the health sciences. Oxford University Press, London

Weissman M, Myers J K, Ross C E 1986 Community surveys of psychiatric disorders. Rutgers University Press, New Brunswick

White K, Williams T, Greenberg B 1961 The ecology of medical care. New England Journal of Medicine 265: 885–892

WHO 1972 Report of the international pilot study of schizophrenia. World Health Organization, Geneva

WHO 1980 International classification of impairments, disabilities and handicaps. World Health Organization, Geneva

Wing J, Cooper J, Sartorius N 1974 The measurement and clarification of psychiatric symptoms. Oxford University Press, London

Wing J, Nixon J, Mann S, Leff J 1978 Reliability of the PSE (ninth edition) used in a population survey. Psychological Medicine 7: 505–516

12. Genetic aspects of psychiatric disorders

R. M. Murray   P. McGuffin

INTRODUCTION

The observation that psychiatric disorder has a tendency to run in families is an ancient one. However, the history of psychiatric genetics has been a series of ups and downs. The founding fathers of modern psychiatry such as Kraepelin and Freud may have disagreed markedly over other issues but were of one mind that the major psychoses had a constitutional and probably hereditary basis. Against this background of general consensus, the study of psychiatric genetics began in earnest in the 1920s and 1930s with the Munich school taking a leading role. However, the image of psychiatric genetics became marred by the misdirected enthusiasms of the eugenics movement, culminating in the introduction of horrific sterilisation laws in Nazi Germany, and the whole subject of psychiatric genetics suffered a sort of guilt by association. This, together with the increasing optimism in the 1950s and 1960s concerning social, psychological or psychodynamic explanations of psychiatric disorders, conspired to make genetic studies unfashionable.

Despite this, research continued and by the early 1970s there was a substantial body of evidence accumulated from family, twin and adoption studies that genes make an important contribution to the aetiology of schizophrenia, major affective disorders and various other forms of psychiatric illness. Elsewhere at this time, dramatic advances were occurring in the understanding of molecular genetics and by the early 1980s it had become clear that various techniques collectively described as the 'new genetics' held enormous potential for the understanding for inherited diseases at a molecular level (Weatherall 1991). Success in the investigation of disorders with simple patterns of inheritance then resulted in the same sorts of approach being applied to more complex disorders, including psychiatric illness. As we shall discuss later in the chapter, this is (with certain provisos) appropriate and feasible, but we need to recognise that there is a danger of seeking to find simple solutions to complex problems.

In particular, we need to be aware that family members may resemble each other because of shared genes, shared environment or a combination of the two; characteristics which are wholly or mainly environmentally determined can simulate genetic patterns of transmission. Therefore, having established familiality (i.e. that a condition runs in families) is not sufficient evidence of genetic involvement. Twin and adoption studies provide the classic, and the still most efficient, methods of determining the extent to which complex characteristics are influenced by genes or family environment. Once it has been established that genes play a part in the aetiology of a condition it may then be justifiable to use newer methods to locate genes, to explore the ways in which they become expressed and to examine the ways in which genes and environment co-act and interact to produce their joint effect.

SOME BASIC PRINCIPLES IN GENETICS

As most readers should already have some grounding in basic genetics, it is our intention to provide only a brief review of those concepts which are necessary for a proper understanding of what follows in this chapter. Emery (1982) has provided a short but very readable introduction and texts by Vogel & Motulsky (1979) and Emery & Rimoin (1983) offer a more comprehensive coverage.

Chromosomes

Although concepts have been somewhat modified by recent advances in molecular genetics, it is still convenient to think of a gene coding for a defined characteristic, e.g. an enzyme, as the basic unit of inheritance. The genetic material which is contained

227

in the cell nuclei is arranged on chromosomes which can be thought of as long strings of genes. In the non-dividing cell, chromosomes are highly elongated structures and not distinguishable microscopically. In order to examine them, the process known as karyotyping is carried out. Leukocytes from peripheral blood are cultured and stimulated to undergo mitotic division, during which chromosomes contract in length, increase in breadth and become visible under the microscope. Mitosis is then arrested, and the chromosomes are spread out and fixed. Modern staining techniques reveal transverse bands, the pattern of which enables individual chromosomes to be identified and accurately distinguished.

All normal humans have a pair of sex chromosomes (XX in the female, XY in the male) and 22 pairs of autosomes. The normal male karyotype is often written as 46 XY and the normal female as 46 XX. Valuable information on sex chromosomes can be obtained without resorting to full karyotyping. In the normal (XX) female, a chromatin body (Barr body) can be seen in the nuclei of cells from buccal smear preparations or granulocytes. In 1961 Lyon hypothesised that in normal females only one X chromosome is functionally active and it is now believed that the Barr body represents inactivated X chromosome material. Individuals with Turner's syndrome who have a female-like appearance (phenotype), but an abnormal XO genetic constitution (genotype) do not show Barr bodies in their nuclei. Like normal males, they are said to be chromatin-negative. On the other hand, persons with predominantly male-like appearance who have the genotype XXY (Klinefelter's syndrome) are chromatin-positive. Preparations from individuals with the constitution XXX, so-called 'superfemales', show two Barr bodies. In general, therefore, the number of Barr bodies detectable is equal to the number of X chromosomes minus one.

In germ cells, double cell division — called meiosis — takes place, resulting in gametes which normally contain 22 autosomes plus one sex chromosome and therefore said to be haploid. The successful fertilisation of a normal ovum by a normal spermatozoon results in the diploid state. However, an anomalous meiotic division may result in gametes with more or less than the normal complement of chromosomes. Most products of such gametes prove to be non-viable, but a minority result in individuals who have an abnormal number of chromosomes (aneuploidy) and exhibit a variety of mental or physical stigmata depending on their particular karyotype.

An outline of molecular genetics

Molecular genetics is currently one of the most rapidly advancing branches of science and here we can provide only the briefest of reviews to enable the reader to grasp the broad principles and the possible applications in studies of psychiatric illnesses. Whatley & Owen (1991) provide a more detailed summary.

DNA and recombinant DNA

Each gene is endowed with its characteristic properties by its DNA structure. DNA has the biochemical role of directing the synthesis of enzymes and other proteins. A DNA molecule is composed of two long chains made up of nucleotide base groups, the pyrimidines thymine (T) and cytosine (C) and the purines adenine (A) and guanine (G). The two nucleotide chains are held together by hydrogen bonding between bases, always in the pairs A-T and G-C, forming the characteristic spiral staircase or double-helix structure. A vitally important property of DNA is its ability to replicate. This it does by unwinding and unzipping the chains, after which each resultant single strand picks up a complementary set of nucleotides so that a precise replica of the original double chain is produced. Certain base triplets (codons) code for particular amino acids. Since there are 64 possible three-letter codes, but only 20 amino acids, some amino acids are coded for by more than one triplet (e.g. UUU and UUC both code phenylalanine; U indicates the pyrimidine uracil). The sequence of base triplets determines the sequence of amino acids in polypeptide chains and three of the triplets are non-coding so that they can effectively act as 'full stops'. Information stored in the form of DNA is transported to the extranuclear part of the cell by messenger RNA (mRNA) and the code is translated into protein production.

Remarkable advances have taken place over the last 25 years in the area now called genetic engineering or recombinant DNA technology. This brand of 'new genetics' (Weatherall 1991) began with the discovery of two classes of bacterial enzymes. Restriction endonucleases recognise specific DNA sequences of 'restriction sites' at which they bring about cleavage of the molecule. Thus, it is possible to cut out a fragment containing a particular gene. Reverse transcriptases provide a means of tagging and identifying such genes. These enzymes enable the synthesis of DNA from mRNA (reversing the usual direction of information flow). Therefore, by isolating the cells in which certain genes are expressed and extracting specific mRNAs, it is possible to synthesise the complementary DNA. The DNA can be labelled with a radioactive marker (^{32}P) and the resultant probe is then used to find a section of DNA with the complementary base sequence, to which it will stick or *hybridise*.

Genetic markers and 'reverse genetics'

Probably the most important series of advances offered by new DNA technology has been the construction of a human genetic linkage map, which is now nearly complete and spread over the whole human *genome* (i.e. the 23 pairs of chromosomes). The map is constructed from a series of genetic markers which have been assigned to specific *loci* on particular chromosomes and hence provide a series of reference points for tracking disease genes. Until the beginning of the 1980s the only available genetic markers consisted of blood types, HLA antigens, variations in chromosome bands using special stains, and certain protein polymorphisms found in red cells or in plasma. However, there are now several ways of detecting variation in DNA sequences and mostly these depend on differences in the length of fragments which result when DNA is digested using restriction enzymes. Variations in fragment length can occur because of point mutations when a single base is inserted or deleted. Such changes will have no functional effect if they occur either in the long stretches of non-coding DNA which separate genes or within the non-coding sequences (*introns*) within genes. The function is only likely to be altered if the mutation takes place within coding sequences (*exons*). The fact that most of such changes are biologically 'neutral' and carry no disadvantage means that they will tend to be passed on from one generation to the next, creating variability in the population. Point mutations result in changes in DNA fragment length because restriction sites are lost or new ones are created. However, variations in fragment length may also occur because of repetitive sequences of DNA occurring in 'tandem', so-called variable number tandem repeats (VNTRs), or because of accumulated repeats of very short sequences, most commonly the dinucleotide A-C.

The standard way of detecting variation in DNA fragment length, so-called *restriction fragment length polymorphisms* (RFLPs), was devised by Southern (1975) in Edinburgh. DNA is digested into fragments with an endonuclease and the fragments are separated by electrophoresis. The double-stranded DNA is converted into single strands, and the DNA is transferred to a cellulose nitrate filter which is blotted

onto the gell (hence it is called the 'Southern blot' technique). The relative positions of fragments are unchanged and they are then hybridised with a radiolabelled DNA probe (which may consist of complementary DNA or genomic DNA) which will then cause the gene of interest to 'light up' when the filter is exposed to an X-ray film. More recently introduced methods make use of a technique called the *polymerase chain reaction* (PCR) to carry out gene amplification. The PCR may be used to produce many copies of a gene.

The availability of many DNA markers means that it is feasible to detect and localise disease genes, making use of the phenomenon of *genetic linkage*, by which genes close together on the same chromosome tend to be co-inherited within families. Subsequently, it became possible to search for more closely linked markers using such techniques as the graphically named chromosome walking and chromosome jumping, and eventually isolate the disease gene itself (Davies & Reid 1988). The DNA sequence can then be studied and the abnormal gene products discovered. This process is called *reverse genetics* because it provides a means of identifying a biochemical defect without prior knowledge of the disease process. This is in contrast with more traditional biochemical genetics where knowledge of the biochemical 'lesion' is used to infer the structure of the abnormal gene. The approach is obviously attractive in disorders where there is a known genetic basis but the pathogenesis is otherwise obscure. Furthermore, providing genes of major effect exist, this 'reverse' approach can be applied to complex diseases as well as disorders with simple patterns of inheritance. However, we will postpone further discussion of the methods of linkage and association studies using DNA markers until we have considered the laws governing patterns of inheritance.

Mendelian patterns of inheritance

Gregor Mendel knew nothing of chromosomes or of the biochemical basis of inheritance but his remarkable experiments published in 1864, and then ignored for 30 years, came to influence the whole of modern biology. Mendel chose to experiment with clear-cut all-or-none characteristics (e.g. dwarfness versus tallness and smooth versus wrinkled seeds in pea plants); his main findings are briefly summarised as follows.

Consider two alternative genes or alleles, *A* and *a*, at a certain locus on a chromosome. A mating between two individuals of the types *AA* and *aa* (homozygotes) can only produce offspring of the type *Aa* (the law of uniformity). But a mating between two individuals of the type *Aa* (heterozygotes) will result in offspring of the types *AA*, *Aa* and *aa* in the ratio 1:2:1 (the law of segregation).

If we now consider two loci with alleles *Aa* and *Bb*, a mating between a double heterozygote (*Aa/Bb*) and homozygote (*aa/bb*) will result in four types of offspring, *Aa Bb*, *aa Bb*, *Aa bb* and *aa bb*, which occur with the same frequency (the law of independent assortment).

A character or trait is said to be dominant when it is expressed in the heterozygous condition and recessive when it is expressed only in homozygotes.

The main principles of autosomal dominance are as follows:

1. All individuals who carry the abnormal gene exhibit the abnormal trait
2. On average, half of the offspring of an affected heterozygote exhibit the abnormal trait
3. In the (in practice unlikely) event of two affected heterozygotes marrying, we would expect to find three-quarters of their offspring affected
4. All offspring of an affected homozygote will be affected
5. The trait does not 'skip' generations.

In the case of recessive inheritance it is important to note the following:

1. The mating of two unaffected heterozygous 'carriers' results on average in one-quarter of their children being affected
2. On average, half of the offspring of an affected individual will be affected if his or her mate is a heterozygous carrier
3. However, the more usual case will be where an affected individual (if he or she mates at all) will do so with a normal homozygote; all offspring will then be unaffected carriers of the trait
4. Most commonly the parents of affected individuals will be unaffected carriers (heterozygotic) so that the disorder frequently 'skips' generations.

Huntington's chorea and acute intermittent porphyria are examples of dominant disorders which may be seen in psychiatric practice, while phenylketonuria (PKU) and Wilson's hepatolenticular degeneration are examples of recessive disorders. It is worth pointing out that dominance and recessivity are properties of the phenotype rather than of the genes themselves and that at the biochemical level the terms become less meaningful. Thus it is possible to detect heterozygous carriers of the PKU gene by testing for blood levels of phenylalanine and tyrosine after phenylalanine loading.

Sex-linked inheritance is said to be present when the gene coding for the trait or disorder is carried on the X chromosome (no known disorders are carried on the Y chromosome). For X-linked recessive inheritance we should note that:

1. Half of the sons of a female carrier will be affected and half of her daughters will be carriers
2. All of the daughters of an affected male will be carriers but none of the sons will be affected
3. Affected females will be rare.

If the X-linked trait is dominant, this does not materially alter the pattern of inheritance observed in males (who necessarily have only one X chromosome and are thus said to be 'hemizygous' for X-linked genes). However, in females the heterozygote will now exhibit the trait and the segregation ratios in females generally will follow the same rules as for autosomal dominant traits. We must also note that whether an X-linked trait is dominant or recessive, father–son transmission cannot occur.

Non-Mendelian patterns of inheritance

The majority of common familial disorders, including most psychiatric illnesses, do not follow the inheritance patterns which we have just described, and for these it is necessary to consider more complex models of genetic transmission. In addition, there are many characteristics such as height, weight, skin colour, blood pressure, IQ scores, etc., which are in part genetically determined but which are continuously distributed within the population and therefore cannot be considered as discrete (present or absent) Mendelian characters.

Single-locus inheritance

A continuous distribution of a genetic character can sometimes be due to just two alleles at one locus. Let us consider a hypothetical blood enzyme coded for by alleles *E*, *e* and suppose that neither is dominant, and that the effect of the combination of alleles is therefore always additive. If possession of *e* confers a mean blood enzyme level of x units per 100 ml and the possession of *E* gives $2x$ units per 100 ml and if the two alleles are equally frequent in the population, then we would expect to see three types of individuals, *ee*, *Ee* and *EE*, in the ration of 1:2:1. Their respective mean levels of enzyme will be $2x$, $3x$ and $4x$ units per 100 ml of blood. However, for non-genetic reasons

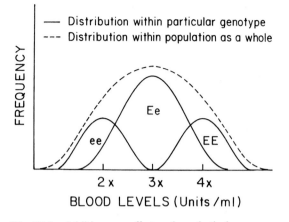

Distribution within particular genotype
Distribution within population as a whole

Fig. 12.1 Additive gene effects: a hypothetical enzyme whose blood levels are coded for by two alleles (*E, e*) at a single locus.

the actual values of enzyme may vary about the mean and there may be some overlap between genotypes, so if we were to sample the population as a whole, the ranges of value of the enzyme would appear to be continuously and normally distributed, as shown in Figure 12.1.

Discrete (present or absent) characters due to single-gene inheritance may show non-Mendelian ratios when penetrance is incomplete. For example, a dominant disease gene *D* with a normal alternative *d* might be expected to result in the disorder in all *Dd* individuals. However, prevailing environmental influences may mean that only a proportion of heterozygotes show signs of the disease. Acute intermittent porphyria is a dominantly inherited enzyme defect in which some of those affected never develop clinical symptoms. It has also been suggested that schizophrenia is due to a defect of this sort but, as we shall discuss later, recent analyses suggest that this is unlikely (O'Rourke et al 1982).

A further complication which is sometimes encountered is variable gene expressivity. Thus, a dominant disorder such as congenital myotonia leaves cataracts as the only stigmata in some individuals, but may be present as the full-blown muscle disorder in their relatives. Again there have been attempts to draw an analogy with some psychiatric disorders. For example, it has been suggested that non-psychotic relatives of schizophrenics who have personality disorder, neuroses, or who are even in some cases conspicuously successful and creative, might all be carriers of the same dominant gene which exhibits a wide range of expressivity (Heston 1970).

Unfortunately, these attractive speculations, as even their protagonists admit, have proved difficult to substantiate.

Polygenic inheritance

It is probable that the majority of inherited characteristics which are continuously distributed in the population are due to the combined effects of many genes at different loci acting additively. Assuming that each gene on its own has only a small effect, that there are no dominant effects and that there is no interaction between genes at different loci, a polygenic character tends to follow a symmetrical bell-shaped (normal) distribution in the population. A simplified hypothetical example would be if height in adult males were due to two loci each with two equally common alleles *Aa* and *Bb* respectively, where *A* or *B* on average confer 3 inches and *a* or *b* on average confer 1 inch over and above a basic minimum height of 5 feet. We should then see (Fig. 12.2) five types of genotypic values with the following means: 5 feet 4 inches, 5 feet 6 inches, 5 feet 8 inches, 5 feet 10 inches and 6 feet. These would occur in the ratio of 1:4:6:4:1. If in addition there is variation within each genotypic value due to environmental factors it becomes possible to envisage a normal distribution. Clearly, the approximation to normality will increase with increasing numbers of loci. The combination of polygenes and environmental effects is usually referred to as multifactorial inheritance.

Some common familial diseases are probably multifactorial in aetiology. This may at first seem implausible, for although it is possible to conceive of a continuous distribution of those who are affected (e.g. on a continuum of mild to severe) the distribution in

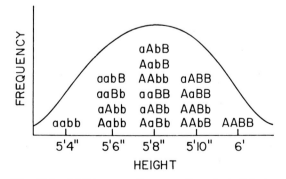

Fig. 12.2 Additive gene effects: two (hypothetical) loci, each with two alleles *A*, *a* and *B*, *b*, coding for height in adult males.

the population as a whole is clearly dichotomous (i.e. individuals are either affected or unaffected). However, we can postulate that the liability to the disease is continuously distributed, but that the disorder is only expressed when a certain threshold in liability is exceeded (Falconer 1965). This is illustrated in Figure 12.3. First-degree relatives (parents, offspring, siblings) of affected individuals are more commonly affected than members of the general population because their mean liability is increased (shifted to the right in Fig. 12.3) and, therefore, more are found beyond the threshold. The first application of a polygenic threshold model in psychiatry was the analysis of schizophrenia carried out by Gottesman & Shields (1967). Subsequently the introduction of more complex (but arguably more realistic) threshold models, including models with multiple thresholds (Reich et al 1972) has provided an important influence on recent thinking about the inheritance of mental disorders.

METHODS OF STUDY IN PSYCHIATRIC GENETICS

Family studies

An individual's first-degree relatives (parents, siblings and children) share on average 50% of his genes,

while his second-degree relatives (grandparents, grandchildren, aunts and uncles) share on average some 25%. Consequently, the sine qua non for a genetic disorder is that there should be, on average, greater similarity between an index case or proband and his close relatives than between persons drawn from the population at large. Since psychiatric disorders have variable ages of onset and may run remitting and relapsing courses, the most useful way to compare relatives is according to whether or not they have ever had an illness in their entire life. This is called the lifetime incidence, lifetime expectancy, or morbid risk of a disorder. In practice some relatives may be too young to be affected by a particular condition at the time they are studied while others may only have lived through part of the age of risk; therefore, the proportion of observed affected relatives in a study may need to be corrected for age, for example by the method of Weinberg (Slater & Cowie, 1971).

Although familial aggregation of a particular disorder is necessary for the condition to be considered genetic, it is by no means sufficient to prove the case. Shared environment can also be a powerful source of resemblance between relatives, particularly for behavioural traits. Traits such as going to medical school or contracting pulmonary tuberculosis have been observed to run in families, but it is unlikely that either is primarily genetic in origin. Fortunately, two types of investigations based upon 'natural experiments' can be used to distinguish between genetic and environmental influences. These are twin studies and adoption (or fostering) studies.

Twin studies

Monozygotic (MZ) twins are the product of the division of a single fertilised ovum and therefore genetically identical. Dizygotic (DZ) twins are, on the other hand, the result of near simultaneous fertilisation and implantation of two separate ova and, therefore, like full siblings, have on average 50% of their genes in common. The important assumption in twin studies is that the degree of environmental similarity is the same for MZ and DZ twins, so that any greater resemblance within MZ than within DZ pairs is likely to be due to genetic factors. This assumption is largely justified, at least when MZ twins are compared with same-sexed DZ twins, but it must be admitted that some of the intrapair similarities in MZ twins may be present because of a tendency to share activities and to identify psychologically with one another to a greater extent that DZ pairs (Kendler 1983).

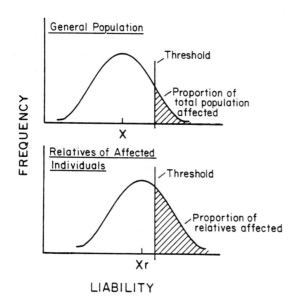

Fig. 12.3 The multifactorial/threshold model of inheritance of disease (*X*, mean liability in general population; *Xr*, mean liability in relatives of affected individuals).

Resemblance between twins for continuous variables such as IQ is expressed in terms of an intraclass correlation coefficient and for discrete traits is expressed in terms of concordance rates. Concordance may be expressed as a pairwise rate, which is simply the number of pairs in which both are affected divided by the total number of pairs, but recently and preferably (Smith 1974) the probandwise rate has been used. This is equal to the number of affected co-twins of an affected proband divided by the total number of co-twins. Pairwise and probandwise rates may be numerically different because in the latter some concordant pairs may be counted twice, since they may be ascertained (that is to say, included in the sample) through both members of the pair being in the initial sample of, for example, patients. It is important to remember that high MZ concordance rates do not necessarily reflect a genetic aetiology; after all the concordance rate for speaking Chinese among MZ twins living in Peking will be 100%, but so will that for DZ twins. It is the ratio of the MZ:DZ concordance rates that indicates the extent of the genetic contribution.

The method of ascertainment is of great importance in twin studies, but unfortunately has often been overlooked in the past. In the ideal situation all affected individuals within a certain population who were born a twin would be studied. This is feasible in some Scandinavian countries where a national twin register is available. Less complete forms of ascertainment are by a hospital twin register, such as the Maudsley Hospital twin register in London where all patients who are twins are consecutively listed, or by registers of all twins who have served in the armed forces. Hospital-based registers tend to be biased in the direction of greater morbidity, while registers based upon servicemen are biased towards health, but either form of ascertainment is greatly preferable to a non-systematic approach. Almost inevitably, haphazardly collected twin samples result in bias in the direction of concordance and an increase in the number of MZ pairs. A rough measure of the degree of bias is the extent to which the ratio of MZ:DZ pairs differs from that found in the general population. (In most white European populations the MZ:DZ ratio is about 1:2.)

Two further sources of bias in twin studies concern clinical diagnosis and determination of zygosity. For example, if, as has happened in some studies, a lone investigator makes a psychiatric diagnosis on both members of a pair and is also responsible for deciding zygosity on the basis of physical resemblance, the potential for error is considerable. Usually this will again overestimate the proportion of MZ concordant pairs, although the preconceptions of the investigator may bias results in either direction. These difficulties can to a large extent be overcome by using explicit psychiatric diagnostic criteria, by providing sufficiently detailed clinical accounts in published reports, or by obtaining a diagnosis on each subject from raters who are blind to the zygosity of the pair and to the diagnosis of the co-twin. While a dispassionate skilled observer can usually decide zygosity with a high degree of accuracy, greater objectivity results from a comparison of anthropometric measures, fingerprint patterns or, most satisfactory of all, by determination of genetic markers in the blood.

A special type of twin study is to examine MZ twins reared apart (MZA twins) where, theoretically, resemblance within pairs can be attributed entirely to genetic causes. In practice the rarity of MZA twins makes unbiased samples of sufficient size extremely difficult to obtain. Furthermore, the degree of separation and dissimilarity of environments of rearing is often questionable. Nevertheless, a concordance rate in MZA pairs which does not differ substantially from that in MZ twins reared together is highly suggestive of a genetic influence.

A number of studies have focused on discordant MZ twin pairs, particularly in the study of psychosis. Any difference within MZ pairs is almost certainly non-genetic, so that studies of discordant patients can provide evidence of environmental aetiological factors. Although the interpretation of isolated case reports needs to be circumspect, a single pair of discordant MZ twins who have lived through the period of risk for a disorder does provide compelling evidence that a condition is not entirely genetic.

Adoption studies

Individuals who have been separated early in life from their biological parents and raised by unrelated individuals provide a potential means of obtaining a 'clean' separation of environmental and genetic influences for particular traits. Rosenthal (1970) has outlined a number of different study designs, of which three have been important. These are adoptee studies, adoptee family studies and cross-fostering studies, The principles of each are summarised in Table 12.1. Adoption studies are only feasible in countries or regions where adoption/fostering registers are available. This apart, one of the main flaws in the experiment is that the placement of adoptees is almost never a random procedure, for the agencies managing adoption generally try to 'match' adoptees and

Table 12.1 Adoption studies in psychiatric disorders

Type of study	Who is studied	Comparisons made
Adoptee study	Adopted-away offspring of patients	Rate of illness versus rate in control adoptees
Adoptee's family study	Biological and adoptive relatives of probands who were adopted in early life	Rate of illness in biological versus adoptive relatives
Cross-fostering study	Individuals with an ill biological parent but raised by healthy adoptive parents; individuals with healthy biological parents but raised by an ill adoptive parent	Rate of illness in two types of adoptees

adopting parents so that the usual assumption of no correlation between the environments of biological and adopting families is not completely assured. In addition, parents who put their children up for adoption tend to be more deviant than ordinary parents and have been shown to be more likely to appear on criminal and alcohol abuse registers (Bohman 1978).

GENETIC EPIDEMIOLOGY AND NEWER METHODOLOGIES

Genetic epidemiology has recently become established (Morton 1982) as the branch of human genetics concerned with the familial distribution of common diseases. These include, for example, coronary heart disease, diabetes and some forms of cancer as well as psychiatric disorders. In the main, genetic epidemiology therefore deals with complex phenotypes where both genes and environment contribute and where simple, single-gene models are inadequate. While 'traditional' methods of investigation exemplified by family, twin and adoption studies provide empirical evidence for a genetic contribution to a complex disorder, it is necessary to go beyond this and attempt to discover modes of transmission, gene locations, and mechanisms of gene expression and of the interplay between genes and environment.

Biometric approaches

Where conditions are obviously not due to simple single-gene mechanisms, it may be useful to quantify how much genes or environment contribute to the phenotype. Assuming a liability/threshold model of transmission (see above) and knowing the frequency of a disorder in the population and the frequency in a particular class of relatives, it is possible to calculate the *correlation in liability* (Falconer 1965, Reich et al 1972). This in itself may be a useful measure of the strength of the familial effect but if information is also available on multiple categories of relatives (e.g. twins, siblings, parents, offspring, etc.) it is possible to look more closely at the possible contributors to familial aggregation. The basic notion is that a phenotype is due to a (mainly additive) combination of genetic and environmental effects. Environmental effects in turn can be divided into *common environment*, which is shared with siblings or other family members, and *non-shared environment*, which is special to the individual and includes any events which do not also impinge on his relatives. As already noted, a trait may be familial either because of genetic effects or because of common environmental effects or a combination of the two. Biometric analyses aim to estimate such quantities as the proportion of variance in liability due to additive gene affects or heritability (often written as h^2) and the proportion of liability due to common family environment (often written as c^2).

Where the aim is to elucidate the mode of transmission of a trait rather than simply estimate its variance components, a segregation analysis is carried out. The methods for simple mendelian characters have long been established (Elandt-Johnson 1971). However, the availability of high-speed computers now makes it feasible to perform segregation analysis for inherited traits in which environmental factors complicate the picture and patterns of transmission are irregular. The most widely used approach is to assess whether the inheritance of a disorder is most likely to be explained by a *mixed model* consisting of a major gene against a multifactorial background, by a multifactorial model, or by a single major locus alone (Morton 1982).

Linkage and association

We have already introduced the terms *genetic marker* and *linkage* in the section on molecular genetics. It is now necessary to define these terms more precisely. Genetic markers are reliably detected traits which have simple modes of inheritance and are polymorphic (i.e. there are two or more alleles with a gene frequency of at least 1%). As also mentioned earlier, there are two main groups, classical markers such as blood types, HLA, etc., and DNA markers. In linkage studies, the co-segregation of a marker and a disease is investigated within families. Linkage is inferred if there is a departure from Mendel's law of independent assortment (see above), so that a marker allele and the disorder are co-inherited within pedigrees at a higher frequency than would be expected by chance. This occurs when the two loci are close together on the same chromosome. For example, earlier in describing independent assortment we considered a mating between one parent who was a double heterozygote of the type *Aa/Bb* and another who was homozygous at both loci, *aa/bb*. Suppose that the two loci are close together and that in the double heterozygous parent *A* and *B* are on the same chromosome. Then, on average, offspring of the same type as the parents, *Aa Bb* and *aa bb* (non-recombinants) will outnumber those of the types *aa Bb* and *Aa bb* (recombinants). The number of recombinants divided by the total number of offspring is called the *recombination fraction*, and within certain limits is proportional to the physical distance between the two loci. This is because a pair of genes very close together on the same chromosome are rarely separated by crossing over during meiosis in gametes, whereas genes lying far apart on the same chromosome or on different chromosomes stand a 50:50 chance of either remaining together or of recombining.

The possible range of values for the recombination fraction is therefore from nearly zero, indicating tight linkage, up to 0.5, indicating independent assortment. The conventional statistical method of detecting linkage and estimating the recombination fraction is to compute *lod scores* over a range of values from 0 to 0.5 (Morton 1982). A lod score is the common logarithm of the odds that the recombination fraction has some postulated value as against a value of 0.5. Where the lod score curve reaches its peak is the *maximum likelihood* estimate of the recombination fraction. Conventionally a lod score of 3 (representing odds on linkage of 1000:1) is accepted as reasonable proof of linkage. Conversely, a lod score of − 2 (odds against of 100:1) is the accepted exclusion criterion.

However, the lod score method was originally devised for linkage studies with regular Mendelian traits. In carrying out linkage analysis with an irregular trait such as schizophrenia it is necessary to invoke the concept of *incomplete penetrance*, where penetrance is the probability of manifesting the disorder given a certain genotype. Although the mathematics become more complicated it is possible to calculate lod scores in the presence of incomplete penetrance and methods for doing this have been implemented in various computer programs (Ott 1985). The main problem is that with psychiatric disorders the true values of the penetrances are unknown, and in practice the investigator has to make a 'best guess' at their values based upon the distribution of the disorder in the population and in various classes of relatives. Indeed, in practice it is usual to take several different sets of guesses at the values of penetrance and the frequency of the putative disease gene. In addition the investigator may want to explore the effects of different diagnostic classifications, so that in one analysis individuals with mild or borderline disorder are classified as 'affected', while in another analysis they are classified as 'unaffected'. The combined effects of applying a range of single-gene models and a range of diagnostic classifications means that multiple tests are carried out and the investigator faces a problem, quite familiar to statisticians, of needing to apply some correction factor to take multiple testing into account. This is particularly pertinent for linkage studies in psychiatric disorders where, as we shall see, there has been much recent confusion and debate regarding failure of replication.

Association studies are in most respects less complicated. They compare the frequency of a particular marker phenotype in patients with a certain disorder and in healthy controls. Among the best known associations in medicine are those between blood group O and duodenal ulcer and between various HLA types and diseases such as juvenile diabetes mellitus, ankylosing spondylitis and multiple sclerosis. Association can arise either because of *pleitropy*, the phenomenon whereby the same gene affects two or more (apparently) different phenotypes, or because of *linkage disequilibrium*, when a disease and marker locus are so close together that the recombination fraction is very low (less than 0.01), so that combinations of alleles remain undisturbed over many generations. Association strategies are attractive in the study of polygenic disorders since they may enable the detection of genes accounting for a very small proportion of variance in liability.

SCHIZOPHRENIA

Family studies

The lifetime expectancies of schizophrenia in the relatives of schizophrenics are summarised in Table 12.2, where the figures represent the weighted average

Table 12.2 Lifetime expectancy of schizophrenia in the relatives of schizophrenics

Relationships	Percentage schizophrenic
Parent	5.6
Sibling	10.1
Sibling (when one parent also affected)	16.7
Children	12.8
Children (both parents affected)	46.3
Uncles/aunts/nephews/nieces	2.8
Grandchildren	3.7
Unrelated	0.86

From data compiled by Gottesman & Shields (1982).

of many studies. There is clearly no evidence of simple mendelian segregation, but the overall risks are compatible with the genetic hypothesis because the frequency of illness increases with the degree of genetic proximity to an affected individual. An apparent anomaly is the low rate of illness in the parents of schizophrenics. The probable explanation lies in the fact that schizophrenia is a disorder which greatly impairs the individual's ability to marry and produce offspring, so that it is likely that the parents of schizophrenics who transmit a liability to the disorder are unaffected 'carriers' of the disorder, or are drawn from that portion of affected individuals who produce offspring before developing the disorder. It has frequently been noted that affected parents are more often mothers than fathers. The probable explanation is that women who develop schizophrenia are more likely to reproduce than men. This is because women tend to marry and produce offspring earlier than men, while the onset of schizophrenia is usually later (Slater 1968).

The risk of schizophrenia increases when more than one relative is affected and thus the siblings of a proband are more likely to be affected when one parent is also ill. The rate is highest of all in offspring of two affected parents. Such data are in keeping with a liability/threshold model of transmission in which individuals with the greatest proportion of relatives affected tend to occupy a position towards the more severe end of the continuum of liability. It has also been noted that secondary cases among relatives are more common where the proband has a 'typical', severe or early onset form of schizophrenia. For example, in studies such as that of Kallman (1938), the risk of schizophrenia was over 20% in the children and siblings of probands classed as 'nuclear' cases, compared with 11% in the relatives of 'peripheral' cases. Formal model fitting has shown that such data

are compatible with a two-threshold model where nuclear schizophrenia represents the severe, high-liability form and peripheral schizophrenia is the less severe, low-liability type (McGuffin et al 1987a). Similarly, a study based on multivariate statistical classification of schizophrenics found that family members were more likely to be affected if the patient had an early onset subtype of schizophrenia characterised by poor premorbid adjustment and symptoms such as affective flattening than a disorder presenting with later onset, preserved affect and well-organised delusions (Farmer et al 1983, 1984). In particular, schizophrenia presenting in late life seems to be associated with lower risks to relatives (Castle & Murray, 1992). Once again a threshold model where the more severe cases occupy a more extreme position on the liability continuum offers a possible explanation.

Adoption studies

Heston (1966) followed up the grown children of women with a well-established diagnosis of schizophrenia who gave birth while they were patients in Oregon State psychiatric hospitals. The 47 offspring who, because of the state laws of the time, had been separated from their mothers within the first 3 days of life, were age and sex matched with a control group of fostered children and blind diagnoses were made on each group. The findings were striking. The offspring of the schizophrenic mothers had a generally higher psychiatric morbidity, but more specifically the incidence of schizophrenia (five out of 47) was very much in keeping with that expected in the children of schizophrenics from intact families, while the rate in controls (none out of 50) was consistent with the general population expectancy.

A more extensive set of studies was begun at about the same time, as a collaborative project between American and Danish psychiatrists, and led to the publication of an influential series of papers. The studies followed the three designs outlined in Table 12.1. Rosenthal et al (1975), like Heston, compared 69 adopted-away children of schizophrenics raised by normal parents with 79 control adoptees. As in the Heston study, a variety of psychopathologies other than schizophrenia were found in the adoptees. The researchers considered that some of these, in particular borderline schizophrenia and schizoid or paranoid traits, might be biologically allied to schizophrenia, and included such diagnoses under the rubric 'schizophrenia spectrum disorder'. Of those with schizophrenic biological parents, 18.8% were within the schizophrenia spectrum compared with 10.1% of controls, a statistically significant difference. The study was able to answer a criticism levelled against Heston's findings concerning possible early postnatal factors. In the Danish study most of the index adoptees were born before the parent's first psychiatric admission. Thus, arguments that the findings were simply a reflection of early mother–child cultural transmission are weakened.

The study of Kety and his colleagues (1976, 1983) was of the adoptees' family type. This took as its starting point probands who had been adopted away from natural parents early in life and who had subsequently become schizophrenic. The principal findings were that 20.3% of 118 biological relatives of adopted-away schizophrenics had chronic schizophrenia (including 'latent' or uncertain cases) compared with 5.8% of 224 adoptive relatives of schizophrenics and the relatives of control adoptees. A study of half-siblings (Kety et al 1976) was able to address the criticism that similarities between schizophrenics and their biological relatives could simply be a product of environmental influences occurring in utero. It was found that eight (13%) of the paternal half-siblings of schizophrenics were diagnosed as schizophrenic compared with one (1.6%) of 64 half-siblings of controls. Since paternal half-siblings separated early in life share neither intrauterine nor early maternal influences, the case in favour of genetic transmission is therefore compelling. The Kety adoption study material was subsequently reassessed using DSM-III criteria by Kendler et al (1981). On applying diagnoses blindly, it was found that 13.5% of the biological relatives of schizophrenics had schizophrenia or schizotypal personality compared with 1.5% of adoptive relatives and relatives of controls.

The third type of study, cross-fostering design, was employed by Wender et al (1973). The frequency of shizophrenia spectrum disorder was 10.7% in 28 children of normal biological parents raised by adopting parents who later became schizophrenic. A significantly higher rate (18.8%) of schizophrenia spectrum disorder was found in the biological children of schizophrenics raised by normal adopting parents.

Although the American and Danish adoption studies published in the 1960s and 1970s were enormously influential in persuading all but the most sceptical that schizophrenia is genetically influenced, they did have certain methodological shortcomings. These included a lack of explicit diagnostic criteria and a fairly scant investigation of family environment. A large study by Tienari attempting to remedy these problems is currently in progress in Finland. Preliminary results follow earlier studies in finding that 13 out of 138 adopted away offspring of schizophrenics are schizophrenic compared with two out of 171 control adoptees.

Twin studies

Early twin studies were subject to many of the methodological problems which have been discussed earlier and consequently have been criticised for overemphasising the role of genetic factors. More recent studies have taken care to avoid such biases and the results of five studies in which there was systematic ascertainment via twin registers are summarised in Table 12.3. With the exception of Fischer's (1973) study the probandwise concordance in DZ twins is comparable with the expectation of schizophrenia in ordinary siblings, but here, as in all of the other studies, the concordance rate in MZ twins is markedly higher. Taking a weighted average from all of the studies gives a probandwise concordance in MZ twins of 46%, compared with 14% in DZ twins.

These consistent results argue strongly for a genetic role in schizophrenia and any alternative explanation would have to explain why concordance is greater in MZ twins than in DZ twins by showing that MZ twins have obviously more shared environment of an aetiologically relevant type. One ingenious explanation based on psychoanalytic theory is that growing up as a member of an identical twin pair might result in confusion and weakness of 'ego identity' and thus produce an overall higher rate of psychosis in MZ twins (Jackson 1960). However, this effect can be ruled out by an examination of 12 pairs of MZ twins reported in the literature who were separated early in life (Gottesman 1991). Seven of these (58%) were concordant for schizophrenia, strongly supporting a genetic interpretation of the twin data.

Table 12.3 Probandwise concordance in schizophrenia twin studies (after Gottesman & Shields 1976)

	MZ pairs		DZ pairs	
	n	Concordance (%)	n	Concordance (%)
Kringlen (1967)	55	45	90	15
Pollin et al (1969)	95	43	125	9
Tienari (1968)	16	35	21	13
Fischer (1973)	21	56	41	26
Gottesman & Shields (1972)	22	58	33	12

Another recent criticism of past twin studies stems from the current preoccupation with operational diagnostic criteria which have now become mandatory in psychiatric research. Although the carefully studied series of Gottesman & Shields (1972) was scrutinised by a blindfold panel of raters and resulted in markedly higher MZ and DZ concordance, the criteria applied were based on clinician judgement and were not explicit. To rectify this, detailed abstracts from the same series were re-examined and modern operational criteria were applied, resulting in MZ concordance of 46–53% and DZ concordance of 9–11% using the criteria of Feighner et al (1972) and the Research Diagnostic Criteria of Spitzer et al (1978), and closely similar findings when DSM-III criteria were applied (McGuffin et al 1984, Farmer et al 1987).

Discordant twins and environmental factors

Discordant MZ twins provide a powerful means of identifying environmental factors. It has sometimes been suggested that in such pairs the schizophrenic member represents an entirely environmentally caused 'phenocopy' of schizophrenia. This proposition was first tested by Luxenburger, who showed that the risk of schizophrenia among the relatives of discordant MZ pairs was no less than that among the relatives of concordant pairs. Subsequent similar studies have agreed (Kringlen 1968). Even more strikingly, Fischer (1971) demonstrated that the offspring of discordant MZ twin pairs showed high rates of schizophrenia whether their parent was the schizophrenic or the unaffected co-twin of a schizophrenic. This result was extended by Gottesman & Bertelsen (1989), who confirmed Fischer's original finding as well as studying discordant DZ twins. Here the risk was high in the offspring of schizophrenics but lower, at around the rate usually found for second-degree relatives (about 3%) in the offspring of the non-schizophrenic co-twins.

Nevertheless, the fact that the MZ co-twin of a schizophrenic has a better than evens chance of avoiding the disease, indicates an important role for environmental factors. But what factors? Focusing particularly on birth history, Pollin and Stabenau (1968) found that a schizophrenic twin was more likely to be of low birth weight, have a history of perinatal trauma, and to be more submissive and dependent premorbidly than his unaffected co-twin. Other studies have agreed on the question of premorbid personality and perinatal complications (McNeill and Kaij 1978). In addition, a number of studies have reported that obstetric complications

increase the risk for schizophrenia (Murray et al 1988) and that schizophrenics who have had obstetric complications are especially likely to show increased ventricular size (Lewis et al 1989).

However, Lewis et al (1987) demonstrated that the intrapair difference in birth weight is much greater in MZ pairs discordant for psychosis than in normal MZ twin pairs. This implies the operation of environmental factors before birth and recent interest has centred on influenza and other maternal viral infections (see Ch. 18).

Mode of inheritance

The longstanding evidence of genetic predisposition, and the more recent environmental data, has resulted in much research addressing the mode of transmission, and possible gene–environment interactions. Although it is clear that schizophrenia as conventionally defined is not a simple single-gene condition, it has sometimes been suggested that this is just a problem of diagnostic boundaries. For example, Heston's (1970) solution was to redefine the phenotype to include not just schizophrenia but also 'schizoid disease' and to propose a fully penetrant dominant gene. An immediate objection to this interesting proposal is that it would require all non-schizophrenic MZ co-twins of schizophrenics to be 'schizoid' and this appears not to be the case (Gottesman & Shields 1982). Other workers (e.g. Elston & Campbell 1970 , Slater & Cowie 1971) have fitted single-gene models to family data and proposed solutions where all homozygotes carrying a double dose of the aberrant gene are affected, where there are no sporadic cases, and where there is a penetrance of under 20% in heterozygotes. However, O'Rourke et al (1982) have shown that many of the twin and family studies in the literature are mathematically incompatible with single-locus inheritance.

A polygenic or multifactorial liability/threshold model was first suggested for schizophrenia by Gottesman & Shields (1967). They adopted the model of Falconer (1965), who proposed that a variable termed 'liability to develop the disorder' (see above) is continuously distributed within the population such that only individuals whose liability at some time exceeds a certain threshold manifest the disorder. In the multifactorial model, liability is composed of the mainly additive effects of many genes at different loci together with environmental effects. This has appeal in explaining the transmission of schizophrenia for several reasons. First, if severity of the illness can be equated with severity on a liability scale this would explain why concordance in twins or first-degree relatives of schizophrenics increases with the severity of illness of the proband. Second, the risk of schizophrenia for an individual increases with the number of affected relatives, which again would be explained by invoking the notion of a continuum of liability. Third, the persistence of schizophrenia in the population despite its selective disadvantage (i.e. the reduced chance of producing offspring) is more easily explained in terms of multifactorial than a single-locus model. Recent applications of multifactorial models claim heritabilities of liability of between 60 and 80%, depending on whether a broad clinical definition or stricter operational criteria are used (McGue et al 1985, Farmer et al 1987).

McGue and colleagues (1985) point out that although it is possible to exclude a 'pure' single-locus model, the familial aggregation of schizophrenia could be explained either by a polygenic/multifactorial model or by a major gene operating against a multifactorial background, a so-called 'mixed model' of inheritance. Theoretically the difference between these two could be resolved by segregation analysis with information from entire pedigrees rather than simply risk figures for various categories of relative. Unfortunately, so far the results of segregation analysis have been equivocal (Risch & Baron 1984).

Heterogeneity: are there several forms?

Most attempts at explaining the transmission of schizophrenia begin by assuming that it is a unitary condition. An alternative view is that the syndrome comprises a number of distinct entities. Most studies have found that classic subtypes of schizophrenia such as hebephrenic and paranoid tend to breed true (show *homotypia*) to a limited extent. A similar picture of incomplete homotypia is also seen in studies of more novel subtypes such as those derived from cluster analysis (Farmer et al 1983) or Crow's (1980) types I and II (McGuffin et al 1987a). It seems possible that these clinical typologies divide schizophrenia on a quantitative rather than a qualitative basis, where illness with greater impairment, and perhaps such features as early onset and 'negative' symptoms, occupy a more extreme position on a liability continuum than do disorders where there is greater preservation of affect, a later onset and more 'positive symptoms'. Such a view is compatible with the idea we discussed earlier that schizophrenia consists of 'nuclear' and 'peripheral' forms lying at different points on a continuum of liability.

An older and more radical view has recently been reintroduced (Murray et al 1985, 1988) that schizophrenia can usefully be separated into genetic and non-genetic varieties. The existence of organic phenocopies is well documented, but it has usually been assumed that these are comparatively uncommon in clinical practice. However, it is now clear that many patients with severe schizophrenia have brain abnormalities which are developmental in origin (Murray & Lewis, 1987). The 'neuro-developmental hypothesis' implies that these structural abnormalities must arise either from some aberration in the genetic control of early brain development (Jones & Murray 1991) or alternatively from some environmental impairment of this process.

At present, there is considerable controversy over whether distinct 'familial' and 'sporadic' forms of schizophrenia exist, or whether early environmental hazards such as maternal influenza or perinatal complications merely compound a pre-existing genetic predisposition. There are important gender differences in risk factors which have a bearing on this argument. Several recent studies (e.g. Goldstein et al 1990) have shown that the relatives of female schizophrenics have a higher risk of similar illness than the relatives of male probands. On the other hand, male schizophrenics are more likely than their female counterparts to exhibit childhood deficits, early onset, poorer outcome and structural brain abnormalities. Castle & Murray (1991) point out that these characteristics may be due to the fact that male schizophrenics have more frequently been subject to neurodevelopmental insult, and suggest that both these data and the differences in morbid risk in the relatives of male and female probands are compatible with the notion that early environmental factors play a greater aetiological role in male than female schizophrenia.

Genetic marker studies

If major genes are operating in schizophrenia, under either a single major locus or heterogeneity model, it should be possible to identify them. Genetic linkage studies with classical markers have proved disappointingly negative, though several studies suggested a weak association between HLA antigens and certain subtypes, particularly HLA-A9 and paranoid schizophrenia (McGuffin & Sturt 1986). More recently, the availability of a nearly complete map of DNA markers has resulted in widespread enthusiasm for performing genetic linkage studies in order to detect genes of major effect for schizophrenia

(Gill et al 1989). Of particular interest was the suggestion of a gene on the long (q) arm of chromosome 5. This possibility was first highlighted because of the interesting observation that an uncle–nephew pair were concordant for a schizophrenia-type illness and both had a translocation defect resulting in partial trisomy of chromosome 5 (Bassett et al 1988). A subsequent linkage study using RFLP markers in other families proved highly suggestive of a dominant-like gene on 5q (Sherrington et al 1988). Unfortunately, these provocative results could not be replicated elsewhere and now the original authors have re- examined their original pedigrees using other chromosome 5 markers, with negative results. Large-scale collaborative studies are currently underway which aim to carry out a systematic search of the whole human genome. So if major genes (not just polygenes of small effect) exist for at least some forms of schizophrenia, they are likely to be detected within the next few years.

AFFECTIVE DISORDERS

There is universal agreement among investigators that affective illness aggregates in families. However, the figures for different studies vary considerably so that it is difficult to give an overall estimate of the lifetime expectancy of the disorder in the various classes of relatives. Part of the difficulty is probably due to differences in diagnostic practice, but there may also be real differences in the prevalence of affective illness in different populations. McGuffin & Katz (1986) have reviewed the data from 15 different studies published over the past 20 years, and find rates of affective disorder in first-degree relatives of ill probands ranging from 6 to 40%. The risk varies according to the clinical features of the proband's illness but may also be affected by the proband's age of onset. For example, Gershon et al (1976) found that the morbidity risk for relatives of probands with an early onset (before 40 years of age) was 19.4%, compared with 10% in the relatives of probands with a later onset. An age of onset effect was subsequently supported in another study (Weissman et al 1986), but is not a universal finding (McGuffin et al 1986). Studies on affectively ill twins, like the family studies, are somewhat blurred by the use of different diagnostic criteria, but Gershon et al (1976) combined the results of six methodologically sound studies where relatively narrow diagnostic criteria were employed. Out of a total of 91 MZ pairs, 63 (69.2%) were concordant, whereas among 226 DZ pairs only 30 (13.3%) were concordant. A recent British study found that a variety of different diagnostic criteria all resulted in significantly higher MZ than DZ concordance rates (McGuffin et al 1992). Such findings are highly suggestive of genetic transmission and are supported by Price's (1968) survey of 12 reported MZ twin pairs reared apart, of whom eight were concordant for affective illness.

Unipolar and bipolar disorder

So far we have discussed affective illness taking a broadly Kraepelinian perspective and assumed that manic depressive illness is a unitary condition. This was the rule in genetic studies until Angst (1966) and Perris (1966) both produced evidence from family studies supporting the view of Leonhard (1959) that there were two types of disorder, unipolar (UP) illness characterised by episodes of depression and bipolar (BP) illness characterised by episodes of both mania and depression. Perris found a high risk of BP illness and no increase in UP illness in the first-degree relatives of BP patients, while there was a high risk of UP illness and no increase in BP illness in the relatives of UP probands. Angst's findings were less clear-cut in that the relatives of BP patients had a high risk of both UP and BP illness while the relatives of UP probands had a high risk only of UP disorder. Although the exact risk figures differ considerably from one study to another, the overall pattern in subsequent investigations has been in close agreement with Angst's findings. The pooled results of a large number of studies based on a combined sample of several thousand first-degree relatives are shown in Table 12.4. The figures here need to be compared with the morbid risks in the general population, which are in the region of 3% for severe UP disorder and less

Table 12.4 Affective illness in the first-degree relatives of BP and UP probands

	Relatives		
	No. at risk (BZ)	Morbid risk (%)	
		BP	UP
BP	3710	7.8	
	3648		11.4
UP	2349	0.6	9.1

Pooled data from studies reviewed by McGuffin & Katz (1986).
BZ, Bezugsiffer (age-corrected denominator).

than 1% for BP disorder. It is noteworthy that not only do the relatives of BP probands have high rates of both BP and UP illness but that overall they have a higher rate of affective illness (weighted average 19.2%) than the relatives of UP probands (weighted average 9.7%).

A re-analysis of previous twin studies in terms of the UP/BP dichotomy also suggests that BP disorder is 'more genetic'. Where twin probands had BP illness the MZ concordance was found to be 72% and the DZ concordance 14%, whereas for the UP illness the MZ concordance was 40% and the DZ 11% (Allen 1976). There was a tendency for twin pairs to have the same subtype of affective illness but some overlap was also noted. More direct evidence comes from a Danish study based on the National Twin Register (Bertelsen et al 1977) from which 110 same-sexed pairs were identified of whom at least one twin had been hospitalised with affective disorder. The probandwise concordances are summarised in Table 12.5. This study, in which zygosity was based on blood testing and psychiatric diagnosis based on personal interview and explicit diagnostic criteria, suggests four conclusions:

1. There is a strong genetic contribution to affective illness
2. The MZ/DZ concordance ratio is higher (almost 4:1) where the proband has BP disorder than where the proband has UP disorder (ratio just over 2:1)
3. The tendency for concordance to occur with regard to BP and UP subtypes is confirmed
4. However, there is incomplete homotypia in that even MZ twins sharing 100% of their genes are discordant for UP/BP subtype in ten cases out of 46.

Table 12.5 Probandwise concordances for UP and BP affective illness in twins

Proband	Co-twins			
	UP	BP	Unaffected	Concordance (%)[a]
MZ				
UP	15	4	16	54
BP	6	21	7	79
DZ				
UP	3	1	13	24
BP	4	3	30	19

After Bertelsen et al (1977).
[a] Counting either UP or BP illness in co-twins as affected.

Table 12.6 Affective illness in the adopting and biological parents of adoptees with bipolar illness

	Affected parents (%)	
	Biological	Adoptive
BP adoptees (n = 29)	28	12
BP non-adoptees (n = 31)	26	—
Normal adoptees	5	9

Data from Mendelwicz & Rainer (1977).

In contrast with schizophrenia there is a disappointing lack of adoption data on affective illness. However, most of the available evidence supports a genetic aetiology. Mendelwicz & Rainer (1977) studied the families of adoptees, and their main findings are summarised in Table 12.6. In showing a high rate of affective illness in the biological parents but not the adopting parents of adoptees with BP disorder, the study strongly suggests genetic influences. However, it is noteworthy that the most common form of illness in the biological parents of BP adoptees was (in 12 out of the 16 affected) UP disorder. Cadoret & Gath (1978) carried out a smaller study dealing mainly with UP illness and found a significantly higher rate of affective disorder in the adopted-away offspring of biological parents with affective disorder than in adoptees whose natural parents had some other psychiatric conditions or who were psychiatrically well.

Despite the continuing debate over the finer points of classification, there is general agreement that typical affective illness approximating to Kraepelin's notion of manic–depressive insanity receives a substantial genetic contribution. However, we must ask whether this contribution extends to non-psychotic or non-endogenous forms of depression.

The family data here are at first sight confusing. Earlier Swedish studies (e.g. Stenstedt 1966) demonstrated high risks of depression in the relatives of typical endogenous probands but a risk of only 5.4% in the relatives of neurotically depressed probands, which was barely above the assumed population risk of about 3%. By contrast, a more recent multicentre collaborative study in the USA found no difference in the frequency of depressive illness between the relatives of neurotically and endogenously depressed patients (Andreasen et al 1986). It seems likely that these apparent differences reflect methodological and diagnostic disparities. A recent British study demonstrated that the pattern of

Table 12.7 Frequency (%) of depression in the first-degree relatives of probands with neurotic or endogenous depression

	Proband type		General population
	Neurotic	Endogenous	
Prevalence of current 'cases'	23.5	12.7	11.1
Morbid risk of moderate plus severe depression	23.7	25.7	8.9
Morbid risk of severe depression	7.9	14.7	2.6

From McGuffin et al (1987b).

results is to a considerable extent dependent on the breadth of diagnostic criteria (McGuffin et al 1987b). Some of the findings are summarised in Table 12.7.

Regarding lifetime risk there was no difference in the rate of moderate plus severe depression between first degree relatives of neurotically and endogenously depressed probands. However, when consideration was restricted to severe depression the rate in the first-degree relatives of endogenous probands was, at 14.7%, nearly twice that in the relatives of neurotic probands. In summary, the results are heavily influenced by the way in which the phenotype is defined.

The same effect almost certainly applies in twin studies of non-endogenous depression. An early study by Slater & Shields (1969) found no difference in the concordance for MZ and DZ twins, and these results were echoed by the more recent study of Torgersen (1986). By contrast, Shapiro (1970) found a broad concordance of 55% in MZ compared with 14% in DZ twins. However, it seems probable from their description that Shapiro's probands were more severely ill than in the two studies showing no genetic effect. A recent and larger British study has attempted to clarify the issue by paying closer attention to diagnostic criteria. The preliminary results confirm that there is a significant and substantial genetic contribution to major depression, with a concordance rate in MZ twins of 53% compared with 28% in DZ twins, and this is little influenced by an endogenous/non-endogenous breakdown of the data (McGuffin et al 1992).

Taken together therefore, twin studies of unipolar depression are suggestive of both environmental and genetic influences. Would a classification according to presence or absence of environmental factors help clarify the role of genes? There have been frequent

suggestions that depression which is clearly associated with stress should show a less prominent genetic component than depression arising 'out of the blue'. Pollitt (1972) found a high morbid risk of depression at around 21% in the relatives of probands in whom precipitants for depressive illness were absent or doubtful. The risk fell to between 6 and 12% when the proband's illness followed severe physical stress, infection or psychological trauma. However, a study using a more sophisticated means of assessing 'stress' based on the work of Brown & Harris (1978) provided no support for these findings. (McGuffin et al 1987b). Depression was no more common among the relatives of probands whose illness was unassociated with life events or chronic difficulties than among the relatives of probands whose depression followed adversity. Furthermore, the frequency of reported life events showed a highly significant increase among the relatives of depressives compared with a sample from the general population. Surprisingly, within families, exposure to life events showed only a weak and non-significant association with depression. These findings perhaps suggest that event-associated depression is something which occurs in hazard-prone rather than just stress susceptible individuals. The authors also suggested that the association between life events and depression, which has consistently been found in previous population-based studies, may at least in part be due to the fact that both show familial aggregation (McGuffin et al 1987b).

Mode of transmission and genetic marker studies

Liability/threshold models probably provide the best conceptual framework for understanding the transmission of affective disorders. However, it has proved difficult to distinguish between a major locus with incomplete penetrance, polygenic inheritance or a mixture of major gene plus polygenes. Segregation analysis of families ascertained through BP probands has provided some support for the presence of a major locus (O'Rourke et al 1982) and this encourages optimism in the application of genetic linkage strategies. In particular, a study of Amish communities in the USA suggestive of a gene for BP disorder on the short (p) arm of chromosome 11 provoked considerable interest (Egeland et al 1987). However subsequent investigations failed to confirm the finding and negative results were reported from an extension of the study on the original pedigree (Kelsoe et al 1989).

There has also been renewed interest in the possibility of X linkage in some forms of affective illness. X-linked pedigrees were first described over two decades ago (Reich et al 1972). However, X linkage can at best account for only a minority of inherited forms of affective illness. Father–son transmission has frequently been observed, effectively excluding X linkage in pedigrees where this occurs, and various groups have failed to find evidence of linkage with X chromosome markers. Two recent studies (Baron et al 1987, Mendelwicz et al 1987) at first sight appear mutually supportive in providing strong evidence for an affective disorder gene in the same region of Xq. However, a subsequent attempt at replication was unsuccessful and it has since become apparent that the different markers studied in the two positive studies are actually widely separated, making it unlikely that the same disease gene is linked to both.

The detection of a major gene or genes has provoked less interest in unipolar depression where more attention has been focused on devising models to explain the combined effect of genes and environment. The data on life events and depression in families referred to earlier suggest that the interplay is complex. Adopting a formal model-fitting approach to twin data where DSM-III criteria were applied provided evidence both of substantial heritability and of significant family environmental effects (McGuffin et al 1992).

CHILDHOOD PSYCHOSIS

There is general acceptance that infantile autism (Kanner's syndrome) is clinically and genetically distinct from the late-onset schizophrenic type psychosis of childhood. Compared with most other psychiatric disorders infantile autism is rare. Only a minority of autistic children grow up to lead independent lives and they marry rarely, so there are still no reported instances of parent-to-child transmission of autism. The siblings of autistic children have an increased risk of the disorder. Although at first sight this appears to be small at little over 2% (Rutter 1991), the frequency of the disorder in the general population is only 2–4 per 10 000. Thus, the risk in siblings is increased 50–100-fold. Simple Mendelian segregation ratios are not seen but some workers have selected families with two or more affected children and have claimed that the pattern of inheritance is compatible with autosomal recessive transmission. Basing such a conclusion on a non-systematically ascertained sample is very dubious. However, there does also seem to be a high frequency of cognitive and speech abnormalities in the non-autistic relatives of patients with autism (Rutter 1991) and it could be argued that these represent a different expression of the same major gene.

Support for a genetic rather than an environmental explanation of familial aggregation autism was first provided by a twin study in which four of 11 MZ pairs were concordant, compared with none of 18 DZ pairs (Folstein & Rutter 1977). This series has now been extended and the original findings confirmed (Rutter 1991). A criticism of twin studies in autism is that, since the condition is associated with mental handicap, high concordance in MZ pairs may be misleading because twin birth is itself associated with high rates of perinatal trauma and with a slight lowering in the average IQ (Hanson & Gottesman 1982). However, against such arguments is the absence of convincing evidence that twins in general and MZ twins in particular have an increased risk of autism. McGuffin & Gottesman (1984) have noted that if the estimates of 35% concordance in MZ twins and 2% concordance in siblings are accepted and a multifactorial/threshold model applied, then both figures are compatible with polygenic inheritance and a heritability of about 80%.

Although schizophrenia does occur in the relatives of autistic children the rate appears to be no greater than in the general population, so the transmission of autism and schizophrenia is almost certainly independent. By contrast, childhood psychosis occurring after the age of 7 years resembles adult schizophrenia in its symptomatology. It is much rarer than the adult disorder but there does appear to be a similar incidence of schizophrenia in the first-degree relatives of both adult and childhood forms, so these syndromes are likely to be genetically part of the same group of disorders (Kolvin et al 1971).

PSYCHOSES IN LATE LIFE

'Functional' psychoses

The available evidence suggests that psychoses in late life tend to have a less pronounced familial component than earlier-onset cases. Relatively few studies have specifically addressed familial aggregation in late onset schizophrenia but overall it seems that risks of schizophrenia in siblings are intermediate between those for siblings of early onset probands and the general population (Castle & Murray 1992). One suggestion is that genetic vulnerability, itself insufficient to cause schizophrenia in earlier life, acts in consort with environmental factors (social isolation, sensory impairment, age-related brain damage) to precipitate psychosis. In contrast to early onset schizophrenia, there is a large excess of females among late onset cases.

BP affective disorder occurring de novo in late life is uncommon, and when it does occur it is sometimes drug-induced or secondary to organic brain damage. UP depression occurring for the first time is common, and again the expectation in first-degree relatives is lower than in early onset cases.

Dementia

Alzheimer's disease

This shows a significant familial aggregation, occurring in first-degree relatives of index cases four times more frequently than in the general population (Larsson et al 1963). The risk to the relatives of early onset cases is much greater than that to the relatives of late-onset cases. This pattern suggests that early onset can be equated with increased severity and a greater genetic liability, while late-onset cases appear to merge into the elderly population; multifactorial inheritance would explain these findings (Wright 1991). Certainly the fact that MZ twins can remain discordant for Alzheimer's disease for many years implies that the disease is not wholly genetic. Nevertheless, there are many published reports of families showing segregation of autopsy-proven Alzheimer's disease in a manner consistent with autosomal dominant inheritance (Wright & Whalley 1984).

There the position rested until recently. The transmission of Alzheimer's disease seemed to be best explained by multifactorial inheritance but it remained possible that a rarer autosomal dominant form also occurred. It was Down's syndrome that provided the clue enabling progress to be made. Nearly all Down's syndrome individuals who survive past 35 years of age develop the characteristic senile plaques and neurofibrillary change of Alzheimer's disease; a proportion also show further intellectual decline (Oliver & Holland 1986). Researchers argued that if trisomy 21 is invariably associated with early development of Alzheimer's disease, perhaps a mutation in a gene on the 'obligate' Down's region of the long arm of chromosome 21 could be responsible for early onset familial cases. This seemed even more promising when it was shown that the gene for amyloid processor protein (APP) maps to the region. Such reasoning led St George-Hyslop et al (1987) to search for and to find evidence for genetic linkage between this form of the disease and RFLP markers

on the proximal long arm (q) of chromosome 21. These investigators studied four families, in which 54 members were affected in eight generations in one and 48 affected in eight generations in another; the mean age of onset in the four families ranged from 39.9 to 52.0 years. This report was subsequently confirmed in some but not all studies (Hardy 1991), and further research indicated that in a proportion of cases of early onset familial Alzheimer's disease, there is a point mutation in the APP gene. It is probable that only a small proportion of Alzheimer's disease is due to this mutation. Nevertheless, the identification of a pathogenic mutation in a gene coding for amyloid, which is known to be found in excess in the brains of patients with Alzheimer's disease, is an important pointer for research into the aetiology of the much more common sporadic cases.

The other common form of dementia, multi-infarct dementia, is, of course, most commonly a consequence of atheroma and/or hypertension, but may also be associated with other partly inherited disorders such as diabetes. The role of genes relates more to these conditions than to the dementia per se. Pick's disease, a less common cause of presenile dementia, appears to be due in some cases to an autosomal dominant gene (SjØgren et al 1952, Schenk 1959). The genetics of both multi-infarct dementia and Pick's disease have been much less studied than that of Alzheimer's disease. Recent research has, however, produced intriguing results in a rare group of dementias which appear to be both genetic and infectious! These are the spongiform encephalopathies which include Jakob–Creutzfeldt disease and the Gerstmann–Straussler syndrome. Both conditions can be autosomally transmitted in dominant fashion and involve mutation in the prion protein gene. Surprisingly, spongiform-type degenerative changes in the brains of experimental animals can be produced by infecting them with material from the brains of humans who have died of the inherited form of the disorder (Collinge et al 1991).

Huntington's chorea

This is an autosomal dominant condition with virtually complete penetrance. The age of onset is variable but most commonly between 30 and 40 years. Dementia and choreic movements are the principal features but considerable variation in gene expressivity has been noted (Harper 1986), and some cases only show chorea and no apparent mental change. Abnormalities in γ-aminobutyric acid (i.e. GABAergic) and dopaminergic systems in the basal ganglia have been demonstrated, but the precise mechanisms of gene expression are unknown.

Relatives of patients with Huntington's chorea often ask about their chances of developing the disease. Each child of an affected parent, whether male or female, is born with a 50% chance of inheriting the defective gene. Fortunately, one of the early successes of molecular genetics was the approximate localisation of the gene for Huntington's chorea. Gusella et al (1983) who studied two large Venezualan families with the disease using a DNA probe (G8) were able to detect close linkage with a polymorphism on the short arm of chromosome 4. Subsequent studies replicated this work, and showed no evidence of genetic heterogeneity. Soon newer and closer markers were also discovered.

These powerful new markers have allowed predictive testing to be available for the first time in this disease (Morris & Harper 1991). The two kinds of testing are (1) presymptomatic testing to determine whether an individual will develop the disease long before the first manifestation of symptoms, and (2) prenatal testing. These predictive tests are potentially of great importance for public health. For example, if individuals who have an adverse presymptomatic test result decide not to have children, the number of Huntington's genes transmitted onwards in the population will be reduced. In prenatal testing, the object is not to predict the risk in the individual at risk but rather to give that individual the possibility of having children with very low risk of the disease, irrespective of whether he or she subsequently develops it. There must be sufficient older, living relatives to establish which allele at the marker locus is linked to the Huntington's gene in the particular family and, at present, this is only so in about 40% of cases at risk (Crauford 1989).

The advent of presymptomatic testing has given rise to a number of difficult ethical dilemmas, and so far programmes offering such testing have proceeded with great caution (Crauford 1989, Morris & Harper 1991).

In deciding whether to offer the test to individuals, it is important to remember that none of the offspring of a choreic emerges totally unscathed. They may escape the disease itself, but they cannot escape its impact through family disruption and personal foreboding; a high proportion of unaffected siblings from Huntington's families develop psychological problems of one sort or another. In 1967 the widow of that famous sufferer Woody Guthrie founded a society to combat Huntington's disease in the USA, and this and similar societies in other countries can provide invaluable support for affected families.

One of the initial findings of programmes offering testing has been that a surprisingly high proportion of those at risk decline predictive testing. The obvious, and wholly understandable explanation, is that at present nothing can be done to prevent an individual who carries the Huntington's gene from developing the disease. For this reason, research continues with the aim of precisely identifying and characterising the aberrant gene. Unfortunately, this is proving more difficult than was originally estimated because of the gene's awkward position near to the tip of the short arm of chromosome 4. Nevertheless, that it will be identified and sequenced is certain and knowledge of the gene and its protein product will eventually allow some intervention which will prevent or ameliorate the symptoms of the clinical disease even in those carrying the gene.

Wilson's Disease

This is a rare autosomal recessive condition. It is of interest to the psychiatrist because it sometimes produces schizophrenia-like psychosis, and because it represents a potentially treatable form of presenile dementia. Homozygotes have abnormally low blood caeruloplasmin levels, and hence defective copper transport, resulting in hepatic cirrhosis and damage to the basal ganglia. Heterozygotes can be detected by their increased incorporation of a radioactive copper load into the serum and caeruloplasmin. Diagnosis in affected individuals can be confirmed by blood caeruloplasmin estimation and demonstration of excess urinary excretion of copper. The condition responds to treatment with the copper-chelating agent penicillamine.

NARCOLEPSY

Narcolepsy causes sudden episodes of unwanted sleep and drowsiness during daytime. Catalepsy or sudden loss of muscle tone also occurs in over half the cases (see Ch. 24). It has been known for many years that there is a tendency towards other family members being affected. It now transpires that narcolepsy is specifically associated with the DR15 split of the HLA-DR2 antigen. This is the closest disease association with an HLA type reported, though why HLA type should influence the risk of narcolepsy is unknown. Perhaps possession of this particular antigenic type makes an individual more likely to have an abnormal immunological reaction to some environmental agent (Parkes et al 1986).

PERSONALITY AND NEUROSIS

Personality and its roots are discussed in detail in Chapters 4 and 5, so here we will consider the origins of personality only so far as it is relevant to neurotic disorders. The supposition that neuroses and personality disorders are found most commonly in individuals who are towards the extreme ends of continuously distributed personality traits has been very influential in psychiatric genetics. An early proponent of this view was Eliot Slater who studied psychiatric breakdown among British soldiers in World War II. He showed not only that the relationship between type of personality and type of symptom was closer for some symptoms (e.g. obsessions) than others (e.g. hypochondriasis), but also that the degree of stress was directly related to the stability of the premorbid personality, i.e. the more stable the personality the greater the military stress required to produce neurotic symptoms. Slater & Cowie (1971) therefore put forward a model which is both polygenic and pluridimensional; in this, multiple genes and environmental factors combine to produce relatively enduring personality traits, and also a greater or lesser predisposition to neurotic breakdown under stress.

The majority of investigations of the influence of heredity on normal personality and behaviour have involved self-reports from MZ and DZ twins using personality questionnaires. Vandenberg (1967) reviewed all the available published studies, which involved a total of 785 MZ and 908 DZ pairs, and found that MZ twins were more alike in all but eight of the 101 variables investigated. Eaves et al (1989) carried out a similar review, this time concentrating on introversion–extraversion (E) and neuroticism (N); once again the correlations were significantly higher for MZ than for DZ twins.

Such studies confirm the importance of genetic effects on both E and N, and, surprisingly, show that intrafamilial environmental effects appear to be much less significant in forming personality than environmental effects specific to each twin. Such findings seem counter-intuitive to many psychologists and psychiatrists who believe that early infantile experience within the family has a crucial role in determining personality, and consequently considerable debate continues about this (Goodman 1991).

An obvious way to exclude the possible effects of shared family experience is to examine MZ twins reared apart (MZA twins). Several such studies have been carried out, the most elaborate being the Minnesota study of Bouchard & McGue (1990). These show a *higher* correlation for neuroticism among MZ twins reared apart than together, perhaps because MZ twins reared together try to develop traits to differentiate themselves from their cotwin.

Anxiety neurosis

Interest in a possible genetic contribution to pathological anxiety goes back over 100 years to Beard who wrote 'hereditary descent terribly predisposes to neurasthenia'. Nervousness and cardiac symptoms were also reported to be more common than expected in the families of those who had what was termed 'Da Costa's syndrome' in World War I and 'cardiac neurosis' in World War II.

McInnes (1936) and Brown (1942) collected information on the parents and siblings of anxiety neurotics while Cohen et al (1951) reported on the relatives of patients with what they termed 'neurocirculatory asthenia'. All three studies reported rates of about 15% among the combined relatives; comparative rates in the general population would be of the order of 3% in men and 6% in women.

Noyes et al (1978) used a structured history schedule to interview anxiety neurotics and surgical controls about their relatives. This more systematic approach gave results in close agreement with the earlier studies in that 15% of the parents and siblings were diagnosed as anxiety neurotics compared with 2.7% of controls. The risk for female relatives was twice that for male relatives, a ratio similar to that in most patient populations studied. The risk to first-degree relatives also increased as a function of familial 'loading'. When neither parent was affected only 9% of siblings also had anxiety neurosis. Where one parent was affected the rate rose to 24%, and, with both parents affected, 44% of siblings also had the disorder.

All of the above studies relied mainly on secondhand information about the relatives. Crowe et al (1980) carried out 'blind' structured interviews with the 99 first-degree relatives of 19 patients with strictly defined anxiety neurosis. Once again, higher morbidity risks for anxiety neurosis were found; and in a similar study, Cloninger et al (1981a) reported an 8% prevalence of anxiety neurosis among the relatives of anxiety neurotics compared with 3% among control relatives. Thus, there is no doubt that anxiety neurosis is familial.

There have been only two twin studies of anxiety neurosis which stand up to critical examination. Slater & Shields (1969) studied consecutive neurotic twins

Table 12.8 Twin studies of anxiety neurosis

	Probandwise concordance rates (%)	
	MZ	DZ
Slater & Shields (1969)	41	4
Torgersen (1983a)	34	17

seen at the Maudsley hospital and identified 17 MZ and 28 DZ probands with an anxiety state. Some form of psychiatric disorder was found in 47% of the MZ co-twins and 18% of the DZ co-twins. When the same diagnosis was taken as the criterion of concordance, the MZ rate decreased only slightly to 41%, but the DZ rate fell to 4% (Table 12.8). Slater & Shields (1969) then re-examined their series in terms of marked anxiety rather than a primary diagnosis of anxiety state. The concordance rate for MZ twins rose to 65% and that for DZ twins to 13%. Clearly these findings argue in favour of not only a general neurotic predisposition but also some genetic specificity for anxious personality. Torgersen (1983a) has reported a similar study from Norway. Probandwise concordance rates were 34% for MZ twins and 17% for DZ twins when all anxiety disorder probands were taken together.

The reader will know that there has been a recent trend, particularly in the USA, to subdivide anxiety states into distinct categories. Various researchers have attempted to justify this view through family and twin studies. The Iowa group claim that panic disorder is familial while generalised anxiety disorder is not (Crowe et al 1980, Noyes et al 1978). Some support for this claim has come from Torgersen's (1983a) twin data. As noted earlier, 34% of MZ and 17% of DZ pairs were concordant for anxiety neurosis; when generalised anxiety disorder was excluded, concordance rates increased in MZ but not DZ pairs (45 versus 15%). However, in both Torgersen's study and an Australian study (Andrews et al 1990) of a large number of volunteer twins, MZ pairs, even when concordant for an anxiety disorder, rarely had exactly the same DSM-III subtype. Thus, whether the various categories differ in kind as well as severity remains unclear. The data could be explained by supposing that panic disorder and generalised anxiety disorder occupy more extreme and less extreme positions on the same continuum of liability. This may seem an academic issue, but it has

important implications for the type of research that is carried out. For example, some of those who believe that panic disorder breeds true assume that this results from a major gene effect, and have started carrying out linkage studies, so far without success. On the other hand, those who believe in a continuum of liability running from normal anxiety through generalised anxiety disorder to panic disorder and agoraphobia at the severe extreme believe that twin studies of anxiety in the normal population may help us to understand the genetics of anxiety disorders. Less direct evidence for the continuum position comes from well-controlled selective breeding experiments with rats and dogs which show that emotional reactivity depends in part on polygenic factors. Twin studies in man have also shown that variation in autonomic function, which may constitute the psychophysiological substrate on which emotional responses are based, is to a large extent polygenic.

In summary, there is consistent evidence that anxiety neurosis tends to run in families, while twin studies suggest a genetic contribution to anxiety states which is greater than that for neurosis in general. However, whether there exist single major genes which have specific effects on some anxiety subtypes and not others is very controversial.

Obsessional and phobic neurosis

Estimates of the frequency of obsessional traits or symptoms in parents of obsessional neurotics have ranged from 3 to 37% (Macdonald et al 1991). Despite this discrepancy, which reflects the differing breadth of the investigators' diagnostic concepts, almost all studies agree that obsessionality is more prevalent in first-degree relatives of obsessive compulsive patients than in the population at large. The only exception is the study of McKeon & Murray (1987) who did, however, find an increased risk for neurosis in general among relatives.

The presence of obsessions among relatives could, of course, be due to transmission via a particular type of upbringing, or parental expectation. In favour of this hypothesis is the tendency for male obsessional neurotics to be first-born or only children, and the evidence that the children of obsessional mothers tend to have a rather solitary, restricted childhood with few easy-going, unstructured, and peer-oriented days. Obsessional neurotics are, in fact, less likely to marry than the general population, and within marriage their fertility is low. Hare et al (1972) noted that 'the proportion of childless marriages in obsessional neurosis is greater than in all the neuroses or in affective psychosis, and for females the proportion exceeds that in schizophrenia'.

Reports of twins have generally suggested a genetic contribution to obsessive–compulsive neurosis, showing frequent concordance in MZ pairs (about 70% over all published cases) and virtually none in DZ pairs. However, twins with this disorder are rare and most reports in the literature have consisted of one or two pairs, or of small non-systematic series. Inevitably, therefore, there has been bias in the direction of monozygosity and concordance. There have, though, been two more comprehensive investigations, one on abnormal and one on normal twins. The first, a study of a consecutive series of twin probands with obsessional neurosis presenting to the Maudsley Hospital, was initiated by Carey & Gottesman (1981) and has been expanded by MacDonald et al (1991). Preliminary findings from this ongoing study report probandwise concordance rates of hospital-treated obsessive compulsive disorder of 45.5% in MZ pairs versus 10.5% in DZ pairs.

The study of obsessional traits and symptoms allows the examination of much larger samples and the use of more sophisticated analyses than those which are available for categorical data, like diagnoses. Clifford et al (1984) administered the Leyton Obsessional Inventory (LOI) to 419 pairs of normal twins. The responses showed heritability estimates for the trait and symptom scales of the LOI that were very similar (47 and 44% respectively). Further examination of the relationship between the twins' scores on the LOI and the Eysenck Personality Questionnaire suggested two genetic factors, one influencing the development of obsessional personality characteristics, and the second transmitting a general neurotic tendency predisposing to the manifestation of obsessional symptoms. These results therefore support Slater's model (see above) for the polygenic contribution to neurosis.

Quite a different view has come from studies reporting an increased risk of obsessive–compulsive neurosis in the relatives of probands with Gilles de la Tourette syndrome. Pauls et al (1991), for example, suggest that obsessive–compulsive disorder may be a partial expression of putative 'Tourette's gene' in such families. Whether or not this proves to be the case, it seems unlikely to explain the majority of cases of obsessive–compulsive disorder.

There is a tendency for the relatives of phobics to have more phobic disorder, but not more psychiatric disorder overall, than the general population (Buglass et al 1977). A recent study showed that 31% of relatives of probands with simple phobias, compared with 11% of control relatives, were phobic themselves (Fyer et al 1990). Both Torgersen (1979) and Rose et al (1981), who gave fear questionnaires to normal twins, found that MZ pairs tended to be more alike in respect of common phobias than DZ pairs. Reports on more severely phobic twins are rare in the literature. Carey & Gottesman (1981) reported concordance for treated phobic neurosis in the co-twin of only one of eight MZ phobic probands, and in one of the co-twins of 13 DZ probands with phobic neurosis, clearly not a significant difference. On the other hand, seven out of eight MZ pairs were concordant for phobic features (whether or not treated) while only five out of 13 DZ pairs were similarly concordant.

It is noteworthy that the range of phobic cues affecting modern man is limited and not readily reconcilable with rational dangers in a predominantly urban society. Thus, fears of snakes and spiders are more common than fears of glass and reckless drivers. Charles Darwin was probably the first to suggest that phobias are inherited atavistic traits which may have had a survival value for our ancestors.

Hysteria

In 1931 Kraulis reported the results of a family study involving probands who had been diagnosed as having hysteria in Kraepelin's clinic. Of these probands, 9% of the parents and 6% of the siblings had also been hospitalised with 'hysterical reaction'. Subsequently, Brown (1942) classified 11% of the parents and siblings of patients with hysteria as also having hysteria. Ljungberg (1957) carried out a careful investigation into the first-degree relatives of 381 Swedish probands who had been treated for hysterical conversion symptoms such as disturbances of gait and fits. The risk of hysteria, at 2% for male relatives and 6% for female relatives, was well above the prevalence in the general population.

Slater (1961) set out to confirm what he originally thought was the hereditary nature of hysteria by studying 12 MZ and 12 DZ twins in whom the proband had been diagnosed as having hysteria. To his surprise, he did not find any co-twins or close relatives with hysteria. As a result of this and a follow-up study which revealed no consistent outcome in cases diagnosed as hysteria, Slater & Glithero (1965) became convinced not only that hysteria had no genetic basis but also that it was merely a label that doctors attached to patients they neither liked nor understood. Their views were very influential and for a time it seemed that, in the UK at least, the term hysteria would be superseded.

However, hysteria 'tends to outlive its obituarists'. The year after Slater published his negative twin study, the St Louis school (Arkonac & Guze 1963) began to develop a radically different notion of hysteria, which they originally called Briquet's syndrome and is now termed 'somatization disorder' in DSM-IIIR. This mainly affects women, and is characterised by the early onset of multiple, dramatically presented somatic complaints without a demonstrable organic cause, generally leading to frequent hospitalisation and surgery. They noted an increased rate of psychopathy in the male relatives of such patients and postulated that hysteria and psychopathy are sex-modified manifestations of the same underlying disorder. They assumed (Cloninger et al 1975) that liability to the disorder has a normal distribution in the general population. Meals (some 3%) whose liability is beyond a certain threshold exhibit psychopathy. For females there are two postulated thresholds. Beyond the first, the disorder manifests as hysteria, while beyond the second and more extreme threshold are found female psychopaths (approximately 2 and 1%, respectively, of the female population).

Thus, the picture remains very confused, with research seeming both to demolish and to validate the concept of hysteria as a genetic entity. As Shields (1982) says, 'considering the diversity of opinion about what hysteria is, it is hardly surprising that there should still be different views about genetics'. His parsimonious explanation was that mechanisms such as conversion and dissociation are within the repertoire of us all, but that heredity contributes more to the development of the hysterical personality. This view is compatible with Slater's finding of no role for heredity in dissociative and conversion states, and also with the more recent evidence of a familial, and possibly a genetic, effect on the tendency to somatise neurotic complaints.

ALCOHOLISM

No informed student of alcoholism would doubt that environmental factors are of major importance in determining the prevalence of alcohol-related problems in any society. But why is it that every study, irrespective of country, has shown higher rates of alcoholism among relatives of alcoholics than in the general population?

It was once widely assumed that this was all due to imitation and a shared environment rather than inheritance. However, Goodwin (1976) reported that the sons of alcoholics separated from their parents in early life and raised by foster parents, were nearly four times more likely to become alcoholic than adoptees without alcoholic biological parents (Table 12.9). They also compared adopted-away sons of alcoholics and their brothers raised by the alcoholic parent, and found similar rates of alcoholism in both. These findings have been supported by two other adoption studies. Cadoret & Gath (1978) investigated 84 American adoptees separated from their parents at birth and found alcoholism more frequently in those with heavy drinking biological relatives. Cloninger et al (1981b) used the Swedish criminal and alcoholic registers to examine the biological and adoptive parents of 2000 adoptees. Once again there was evidence for a genetic effect.

However, twin studies have not been so consistent. Kaij (1960) located twin pairs of whom at least

Table 12.9 Copenhagen adoptee study (Goodwin 1976) of sons

	Percentage ever alcoholic	Percentage ever depressed
Adoptees with no biological parent with alcoholism (*n* = 78)	5	20
Biological parent hospitalised for alcoholism		
Adopted (n = 55)	18	15
Not adopted (n = 30)	17	20
Adoptees with no biological parent with alcoholism (*n* = 47)	4	15
Biological parent hospitalised for alcoholism		
Adopted (n = 49)	2	14
Not adopted (n = 8)	3	27

one member had appeared on the Swedish register of alcohol abusers. When one twin was a heavy abuser so was the other in 70% of MZ but only 32% of DZ twins. A second study, from the USA, reported similar results; but when Gurling & Murray (1987) tried to replicate these findings among twins who presented to the Maudsley Hospital with alcoholism, they found no difference in concordance rates between MZ and DZ twins. These inconsistencies probably result from various methodological problems such as small sample sizes. Fortunately, a larger and more definitive study has now been reported by Pickens et al (1991) which showed higher, but not greatly higher, concordance rates in MZ than DZ twins. These results, approximately midway between the previous findings, were used to calculate the relative contribution of genetic and environmental factors; additive genetic factors accounted for 36% of the variance in male liability to alcoholism, 50% was accounted for by shared (i.e. intrafamilial) environmental factors, and only 14% by non-shared environmental factors.

The above studies were all concerned with pathological drinking. Partanen et al (1966) interviewed 902 'normal' Finnish male twins about their drinking habits. Although there was no difference between MZ and DZ twins with regard to consequences of drinking, the frequency of drinking and the amount drunk at a session showed moderate heritability. Clifford et al (1984) have reported results in 494 pairs of normal twins from the Institute of Psychiatry register. Thirty-seven per cent of the variance in alcohol consumption was accounted for by genetic effects, intrafamilial but non-genetic effects contributed some 42% of the variance, and environmental factors special to one twin and not shared by his co-twin contributed only 21%. These figures are rather similar to those calculated by Pickens et al (1991) for alcoholism. Thus, it seems that familial factors have a powerful effect in determining both alcohol consumption levels in the normal population and liability to alcoholism, but the familial effect comprises both a genetic component and intrafamilial cultural transmission. It's not so much nature versus nurture rather nature via nurture!

Now that we know that heredity contributes to the familial aggregation of alcoholism, the question is whether what is inherited is some predisposing personality or psychiatric trait, or alternatively some metabolic difference in reaction to alcohol. Cloninger (1987) used data from the Swedish adoption study to suggest the former. He proposed the existence of two forms of alcoholism. Type I, a mild form, occurred in both men and women, had a late onset, and was influenced by both genes and environment. Type II occurred exclusively in men and was transmitted genetically. It had an earlier onset — before 25 years — and was often associated with criminality in the father. Subsequent research has not altogether supported Cloninger's hypothesis, but it does seem that individuals with a positive family history of alcoholism exhibit many of the features encapsulated in the concept of 'Type II' alcoholism. Thus, familial alcoholics show an earlier age of onset and faster development of a more severe form of dependence than do those with no family history. Furthermore, familial alcoholics are more likely to have antisocial personalities than those without affected relatives. The simple division of alcoholics into familial and non-familial cases appears, therefore, to have as much to offer as Cloninger's more complex construction.

Cloninger's theory implies that what is inherited is primarily a predisposing personality type. An alternative view is that pre-alcoholics do not differ from the rest of the population in personality but rather in the way in which they metabolise alcohol. Martin and his colleagues (1985) gave challenge doses of alcohol to 200 pairs of twins and showed that the rate of alcohol elimination was under a substantial degree of genetic control.

What determines this? Most alcohol metabolism occurs in the liver via alcohol dehydrogenase (ADH), which converts alcohol to acetaldehyde, and acetaldehyde dehydrogenase (ALDH), which converts acetaldehyde to acetate. The $ALDH_2$ isoenzyme is responsible for most of the oxidation of acetaldehyde. Many orientals have a variant of $ALDH_2$ which is virtually inactive so, if they drink alcohol, acetaldehyde accumulates, producing tachycardia, nausea and flushing. Could this unpleasant reaction protect them against developing alcoholism? Harada et al (1985) examined the frequency of the 'flushing' variant among alcoholics and normals in Japan: 42% of normal individuals had the 'flushing' variant, but among alcoholics only 5% had the 'flushing' variant, implying that its presence confers some protective effect against alcoholism. Subsequently, Shibuya & Yoshida (1988) genotyped individuals with alcoholic liver disease in Japan. While 35% of their general population sample had the 'flushing' $ALDH_2$ allele, only 7% of those with alcoholic liver disease did; thus, Japanese with the 'flushing' $ALDH_2$ allele have a much lower risk of developing alcoholic liver disease, probably because they are less likely to drink heavily.

Might similar differences in gene frequencies among Europeans explain the increased predisposition of some to alcoholism? As yet, none have been found, but the search continues and is given added impetus by the existence of inbred strains of rats and mice with genetic differences in alcohol-metabolising enzymes, which show marked variation in alcohol preference (Hodgkinson et al 1991).

Another approach is to study genes which are known to have an important role in behaviour, such as the genes involved in catecholamine pathways. There was great excitement when Blum et al (1990) reported an association between alcoholism and the *A1* allele of the dopamine D_2 receptor gene located on the long arm of chromosome 11. They were credited with having found the 'gene for alcoholism'. However, their study was retrospective, based on a small sample, and attempts at replication have produced contradictory findings (Conneally, 1991).

It is extremely unlikely that a single gene will be found to account wholly for the transmission of such a complex disorder as alcoholism. It is much more likely that different genes will be shown to have effects on different aspects of the alcoholism syndrome. Thus, Murray & Gurling (1980) have proposed a polygenic model in which the pertinent genetic factors are conceptualised as operating at three related levels:

1. For pharmacokinetic reasons, some individuals experience an unusual excess of positive over negative effects of alcohol; such individuals are more likely to proceed to heavy drinking.
2. Liability to dependence on alcohol includes a genetic component which may be manifest only after exposure to chronic heavy drinking, but may be transmitted independently of heavy drinking.
3. Individuals differ in their genetic predisposition to alcohol-related disorders, but again this difference can only become manifest following chronic heavy drinking. For example, the possession of a particular HLA type may predispose the excessive drinker towards cirrhosis of the liver.

PSYCHOPATHY AND CRIMINALITY

As noted above, family studies by the St Louis group suggest that psychopathy in the male is the phenotypic equivalent of hysteria in females. There have also been adoptive studies of psychopathy. Crowe (1974) compared 52 adopted-away offspring of female offenders with a control group of adoptees. Six of the index offspring had antisocial personalities and 11 had committed a criminal offence. None of the controls had that diagnosis and only four had committed a crime. Unfortunately nothing was known of the fathers. Schulsinger (1972) used the Danish adoption register to identify the biological relatives of 57

Table 12.10   Crime in Danish male adoptees according to the criminal record of biological and adoptive fathers

	No. of adoptees	Percentage with criminal record
Neither father known to police	333	10.4
Adoptive father criminal, biological father not known to police	52	11.2
Biological father criminal, adoptive father not known to police	219	21.0
Adoptive and biological fathers both criminal	58	36.2

Data of Hutchings & Mednick (1974).

psychopathic adoptees and matched controls. He grouped together cases of psychopathy, doubtful psychopathy, criminality, alcoholism, and hysterical character disorder in the families as 'psychopathic spectrum disorder' and found the rate to be twice as high in the biological relatives of the psychopathic adoptees as in the adoptive relatives. Restricting the analysis to fathers the rate was 9.3% compared with 1.9%.

Criminality was one of the first behaviours to be studied genetically. Early studies found very high concordance rates in twins, but these were not wholly confirmed by later workers. Nevertheless, Christiansen (1974), who studied the records of all Danish twins born between 1870 and 1920, reported concordance rates for criminality of 52 and 22% for male MZ and DZ twins, respectively. Female concordance rates were lower but MZ:DZ difference and the contrast with the prevalence in the general population were even greater, suggesting that biological factors are more important in female than in male crime.

Adoption studies support the view that genetic factors contribute to criminality. Hutchings & Mednick (1974) checked 1145 males on the Copenhagen adoption register against the criminal register. They found (Table 12.10) that having a criminal adoptive father did not affect an adoptee's risk of being on the criminal register, whereas having a criminal biological father did. However, the highest risk for criminality in adoptees was found when both fathers were criminal, suggesting a gene–environment interaction. The same authors went on to make a more detailed study of 143 criminal adoptees. Of their biological fathers, 49% had criminal records compared with 28% of the biological fathers of non-criminal adoptees; the corresponding figures for adoptive fathers were 23 and 10%.

The above studies all point towards a genetic contribution, but the reader will not be surprised to learn that other studies are less positive. A Norwegian twin study, for example, gave little support for a genetic aetiology in criminality (Dalgard & Kringlen 1976). Much of the variation may be attributed to differences in the accepted definition of criminality in different cultures. However, on pooling the data from all available published twin studies, McGuffin & Gottesman (1984) concluded that the evidence for a genetic effect in adult criminality was consistently positive. Interestingly the same was not true for juvenile delinquency.

Initially, a Swedish study of adoptees born to biological parents registered for adult criminality failed to find evidence of a genetic effect (Bohman 1978). However, subsequent re-analysis (Bohman et al 1982) did show such an effect for petty criminality involving mainly non-violent property offences. Low social status by itself did not lead to criminality, but it did increase the risk in those genetically predisposed. An unstable period prior to adoption also contributed to later non-alcohol-related crime, as did prolonged institutional care, though only in women. Thus, the balance of the evidence is that genetic factors do contribute to a modest but significant extent towards liability to certain types of crime, particularly in combination with certain adverse environmental factors. Individuals are not, however, born destined to a life of crime, as was once suggested in the case of the XYY syndrome.

This suggestion arose when men with an XYY constitution were found with increased frequency in institutions for the criminally insane and the mentally retarded. Some 1.5/1000 live male births have such a constitution, but incidence rates as high as 2–3% have been reported in some special hospitals (Pitcher 1975). At one time it was thought that these tall men were predestined to become dangerous and aggressive criminals, and evidence that a defendant had this XYY syndrome was even accepted in a Court of Law as a mitigating factor for his crime. However, it has since been pointed out that the vast majority of XYY males lead blameless lives and go unnoticed in the community. Some suggest that the presence of the extra Y chromosome produces immaturity and lessened intellect (Hunter 1977). Others maintain that the excess of XYY males in special hospitals reflects the response of the judiciary to convicted felons who are tall and intellectually dull, rather than the result of an intrinsic predisposition to violent crime.

ANOREXIA NERVOSA

The aetiology of anorexia nervosa remains a matter of debate. Undoubtedly, social pressure towards dieting is important, but obesity, depression and alcoholism are all over-represented in the families of anorexics. Female relatives also have an increased risk of anorexia. Holland et al (1984) studied a series of pairs of twins in which the proband had anorexia nervosa. In the female pairs, 55% of the MZ and 7% of the DZ twin pairs were concordant for anorexia, supporting the operation of some genetic effect. An extension of this study confirmed the findings (Treasure & Holland 1991) but reported no genetic effect on bulimia. It may seem astonishing to some that anorexia nervosa is, in part, heritable but it is not so surprising when one realises that adoption studies and studies of normal MZ twins reared apart suggest that some 70% of variability in body mass is genetic (Stunkard et al 1990, Macdonald & Stunkard 1990). Furthermore, a recent study of normal female twins has shown that attitudes to eating and dieting are moderately heritable (Rutherford et al 1992) and this may also have some bearing on the aetiology of more extreme forms of self-imposed food restriction.

NON-PSYCHOTIC DISORDER IN SUMMARY

The global question of whether there is a genetic contribution to neurosis is not very meaningful. Torgersen (1983b) examined 229 same-sexed twins who presented to in-patient and out-patient units in Norway and found a modest and insignificantly greater concordance for neurosis among MZ than DZ twins. However the concordance ratios MZ:DZ increased from 1.2 in out-patient neurotics to 1.4 in those admitted to psychiatric units in general hospitals, and to 2.1 in those admitted to mental hospitals. This neatly demonstrates that heredity is more important among severe than mild neurotic disorders. He also found a greater genetic contribution to neurotic disorders in men than women, an observation compatible with the view that in contemporary society females are more exposed to adverse environmental pressures than men.

When one focuses on different conditions, further disparities emerge. There is now good evidence that heredity contributes to anxiety neurosis and to obsessional disorders. On balance alcoholism also appears subject to a modest but significant genetic contribution, and a case can perhaps be made for some contribution to psychopathy (at least as defined by criminal activity), to anorexia nervosa, and to fear of those phobic stimuli whose avoidance may have had survival value, e.g. snakes and spiders.

NORMAL INTELLIGENCE

Just as it was necessary to review the influence of heredity on normal personality before discussing neurosis, so mental retardation can only be fully understood in the context of a basic knowledge of the genetic contribution to normal intelligence. This is not the place to discuss the controversies concerning the measurement of intelligence; for the present purpose we shall assume that IQ tests provide reasonably accurate estimates of general intellectual ability.

While the IQs of unrelated persons are uncorrelated, it can be seen from Table 12.11 that the weighted average correlations between parents and their children have been estimated at 0.42 and those between siblings at 0.47. Bouchard & McGue (1981) reviewed all available studies of MZ and DZ twins reared together and reported intrapair correlations of 0.86 and 0.67, respectively. There have also been three reputable studies of IQ in MZ twins reared apart, giving intrapair correlations only slightly lower than those for MZ twins reared together. These various correlations suggest that at least half of the variance in IQ is due to genetic factors. Fulker & Eysenck (1979) point out that perhaps the most striking testimony to the importance of genetic factors to come from the investigation of reared-apart twins is simply that the largest intrapair IQ difference is 24 points. One would have expected a maximum difference of about 80 points among a similar number of unrelated individuals.

Studies of children adopted away from their natural parents show an adoptee–biological parent correlation of 0.32 (Table 12.11). This compares with a median correlation between adoptees and their adoptive parents of 0.19. Thus, there would appear to be not only a genetic contribution to IQ but also a comparatively important role for common family environment. This is supported by studies of unrelated children who happen to be raised together — their average IQ correlation is 0.29.

It is, of course, important to remember that there are more practical ways of assessing academic prowess than performance on IQ tests, and whether individuals reach their full academic potential is greatly influenced by environmental factors. Thus, a US study which examined the number of years of education that individuals achieved, concluded that genetic factors contributed 44% of the variance, common home environment 32% and specific environmental factors 24%. Thus, heritability is perhaps a little lower and the family environmental effect higher than for IQ.

Which environmental effects influence IQ? There is good evidence that first-born children on average show intellectual development superior to their younger siblings. Birth order 1 through 6 produces a total average drop in IQ of about 4 points. The reason for the difference is probably the quality of the attention available to the child when interacting with other members of the family. The first–born receives the undivided attention of two adults, but for subsequent children this advantageous parental effect is diluted by the presence of siblings.

Poor nutrition and physical illness appear to have little effect on IQ in modern industrial countries. However, IQ differences correlate substantially with differences in social and educational advantage. One study found that about 8% of IQ variation could be attributed to differences in social advantage. There has, of course, been an acrimonious dispute over whether the lower IQ scores of black US citizens are a consequence of their racial inheritance or social and educational deprivation (Eysenck & Kamin 1981). The effect of additional preschool education on such deprived children has been intensively studied in the USA following the massive government 'Head Start' programme initiated in the 1960s. The effects on later educational achievement and IQ appear to have been negligible, but this may have been because the programme was poorly structured.

More intensive and sharply focused preschool projects have raised infant IQ by as much as 15 points, though these gains tend to diminish after the

Table 12.11 Correlation coefficients for IQ scores in family, twin and adoptive studies

Unrelated individuals reared apart	−0.01
Unrelated individuals reared together	0.29
Biological parent–child	0.42
Biological parent–adopted-away child	0.32
Adoptive parent–child	0.19
Siblings	0.47
DZ twins	0.67
MZ twins reared apart	0.75
MZ twins reared together	0.86

controls have had a year or two of primary education. Perhaps the best evidence of the effects of an advantageous family upbringing comes from adoption studies. These show that being adopted by a high as opposed to a low socioeconomic status family can raise IQ by about 15 points in the long term (Fulker & Eysenck 1979).

The distribution of IQ in the general population approximates to the normal curve that one would expect if IQ were determined by polygenic factors co-acting with a variety of environmental effects. However, the curve is skewed to the left, i.e. persons of very low intelligence are much more frequent in the population than can be accounted for on this basis. This implies that severe mental retardation is not just the extreme lower end of the normal distribution, but that additional aetiological factors are present, and, of course, this is known to be the case. For example, the recent Minnesota study which examined 100 sets of reared-apart twins produced correlations in IQ of 0.88 for pairs reared together and 0.69 for MZ pairs reared apart (Bouchard et al 1990).

CHROMOSOMAL ABNORMALITIES

Most fetuses with chromosomal abnormalities do not survive. One-half of all fetuses that spontaneously abort before 12 weeks show major chromosomal abnormalities, and one in ten couples who are 'habitual aborters' show some minor chromosomal abnormality. Nevertheless, approximately six in 1000 live-born babies show a detectable chromosomal anomaly; two-thirds are autosomal and one-third are sex chromosome anomalies.

Autosomal abnormalities

Down's syndrome

This is not only the commonest autosomal defect, but also the disease entity most frequently detected in mentally retarded populations. It accounts for one-third of all those with an IQ less than 50, and 95% of cases have an extra chromosome 21 (trisomy 21). This arises when two homologous chromosomes fail to separate during meiosis (non-disjunction) and migrate to the same gamete. When such a gamete unites with a normal gamete the result is a zygote with trisomy 21 (Emery 1982).

The frequency of trisomy 21 increases with advancing maternal age, suggesting that the effect of ageing on the ovum increases non-disjunction. The risk of having a child with Down's syndrome is only one in 2300 for women of less than 20 years, but it rises, particularly after 35 years, until the risk for women over 40 years reaches one in 50.

Not all Down's children have trisomy 21. Some 4% are due to a translocation in which additional chromosome 21 material is fused onto another autosome (most frequently chromosome 14). Half of such translocations are spontaneous but in the remainder of the seemingly normal parents there may be found a balanced translocation, i.e. a translocation of a chromosome 21 without any extra material. These individuals are called 'translocation carriers'. The final 1% of Down's children are mosaics in whom some cells have a normal chromosome complement while others show trisomy 21. Such cases may show only limited stigmata of the disease, their intellectual retardation may be mild, and consequently the diagnosis may be missed (Baraitser 1980).

The fact that amniocentesis enables cytogeneticists to examine fetal chromosomes has profound implications for the prevention of Down's syndrome. If all mothers aged more than 40 years had amniocentesis and therapeutic abortion when indicated, the incidence of trisomy 21 could be reduced by 16%, and if all mothers over 35 years were screened the incidence could fall by 30%. Certainly all pregnant women over 40 years should be offered screening — 3% of their fetuses will have Down's syndrome and a further 2% some other chromosomal abnormality. These figures are higher than those for live births because some of the defective fetuses would later abort spontaneously. Since amniocentesis itself carries some risks there is some doubt about the optimum lower age limit for routine testing — most authorities would say around 35 years of age. In addition, amniocentesis should be offered to any mother who has had a translocation baby, since the risk of recurrence is significantly increased. Screening maternal blood for abnormal fetal cells is now being carried out on an experimental basis, and if successful may supplant amniocentesis, at least as an initial screening procedure for Down's syndrome.

Other autosomal anomalies

These include Edwards' syndrome (trisomy 18) and Patau's syndrome (trisomy 13). Both are more severe than and occur about one-tenth as frequently as Down's syndrome, but, similarly, both are associated with advanced maternal age. Partial deletion of chromosomes may also occur, that of the short arm of chromosome 5 producing the Cri-du-Chat syndrome.

The Prader–Willi syndrome is characterised by gross obesity from childhood, short stature, delay in secondary sexual development and varying degree of learning disability. Affected individuals fail to become satiated after even a huge meal, and therefore just keep on eating. Parents typically learn to lock away all food in the house as their affected child will simply eat their way through whatever is available (Holland 1991). Recent studies have shown that the syndrome results from an abnormality (usually a deletion) of the proximal long arm of chromosome 15 (15p11–13). Interestingly, this site is also associated with another quite different disorder, Angelman's syndrome. It appears that deletion of part of the maternal chromosome causes one syndrome and of the paternal chromosome, the other.

Sex chromosome abnormalities

It has been known for many years that among those with 'non–specific' mental retardation, males outnumber females by at least 25%. During the 1970s there were many reports of families in which mental retardation occurred in a pattern consistent with an X-linked mode of inheritance (Herbst 1980), and it was suggested that X linkage might account for the excess of retardation in males. This possibility was supported by the finding of an abnormality of X chromosome in many cases of familial retardation. For example, Primrose et al (1986) surveyed the population of a mental handicap hospital and found an overall male prevalence of 7% of what is now termed the 'Fragile X syndrome'. Among males with another retarded relative, the prevalence rose to 31%. A variety of other features has been reported as occurring sometimes, but the main one is large testes which are found in about half the cases (Turner 1982).

It is now evident that the Fragile X syndrome is second only to Down's syndrome as a cause of mental retardation in males. It is estimated to affect one in 1250 males and there is evidence that carrier females are at risk of some mental impairment. Indeed, 30% of carrier females are penetrant, while 20% of males carrying the fragile X chromosome are phenotypically normal but transmit the disorder and have fully penetrant grandsons. The abnormality is a tiny constriction or fragile site at the end of the X long arm (Xq27.3). Recent molecular studies have identified a gene (*FMR-1*) at the fragile site which is expressed in normal individuals but not in the majority of males with fragile X. Probably it is the lack of expression of this gene in the brain which causes the fragile X phenotype (Pierretti et al 1991). This 'Fragile X' can be demonstrated by culturing blood cells from affected males in a special medium deficient in folate, and it can also be detected in a proportion of female carriers. Diagnostic assay using molecular genetics will be available for fragile X in the near future.

This is a convenient point to discuss other sex chromosome abnormalities even though they are not invariably associated with mental retardation. About 1.7 per 1000 phenotypic males have an extra X chromosome and in consequence develop Klinefelter's syndrome. Affected individuals are sterile and have a eunuchoid body build, small testes, gynaecomastia and female distribution of body hair. They also tend to be withdrawn, timid and lacking in energy. Although many live apparently normal lives there is an increased incidence of mental retardation and about 40% present with psychiatric disturbance; neurosis, personality and sexual disorders are most common (Wakeling 1972), but the incidence of schizophrenia is also increased (Roy 1981).

The reason for the increased susceptibility to psychiatric disorder is unclear. While it could be a reaction to being sexually underdeveloped, other hypogonadal males are more stable (Nielsen et at 1980). However, there does appear to be a hormonal effect, as testosterone, which does little to enhance masculine appearance, does improve sexual and social adjustment. Psychiatric vulnerability may also be a direct effect of impaired brain development as there is a relationship between mental retardation and an extra X chromosomes in both phenotypic males and females. While only a minority of classic XXY Klinefelter's have noticeable mental subnormality, most of those with XXXY have profound mental retardation.

Similarly, most females with the XXX constitution (sometimes mistermed 'superfemales'), who occur with a frequency of about one in 1000 live births, have relatively mild retardation but the rarer XXXX or XXXXX females are almost invariably severely retarded. About one per 3000 phenotypic females has Turner's syndrome, which is characterised by: (1) short stature with underdeveloped secondary sexual characteristics, sterility and amenorrhoea; (2) outward displacement of the forearm on extension; (3) webbing of the neck; and (4) an increased frequency of various congenital abnormalities, including coarctation of the aorta. About half of these women have the sex karyotype XO, while the other half comprises a variety of chromosome aberrations — X deletions, translocations and mosaics.

The overall IQ distribution of females with Turner's syndrome appears to be near normal, although their mean scores on arithmetic and visuospatial tasks are lower than those of normal female controls. Unlike Klinefelter's males they are not predisposed to psychiatric disorder, and instead tend to be conscientious and conformist. They tend to have sexual intercourse and marry later than average, and some try to compensate for their shape by wearing very feminine clothes and jewellery (Nielsen et al 1977).

Autosomal dominant conditions

Tuberous sclerosis (epiloia) and neurofibromatosis (von Recklinghausen's disease) are both due to single dominant genes. Tuberous sclerosis may be associated with the so-called 'potato tumour' in the brain, epilepsy and various skin anomalies such as adenoma sebaceum; and about 40% of cases show mental retardation. Neurofibromatosis is characterised by 'cafe au lait' spots and tumours of the peripheral and central nervous systems; 10% of cases are mentally retarded, usually severely. The gene has been localised to a narrow region of chromosome 17.

One might suppose that it would always be easy to obtain a clear family history of these conditions. However, this is not so because, firstly, some affected relatives have such mild variants that they are not immediately detectable (e.g. neurofibromatosis may present merely with cafe au lait spots) and, secondly, in other cases the aberrant gene may arise from a fresh mutation in the germ cells of an unaffected parent. These factors explain why the gene for tuberous sclerosis persists in the population despite the fact that affected individuals have a reduced fertility. Any individual with even a mild variant of tuberous sclerosis should, of course, be told that there is a 50% chance of each child inheriting the gene, and that these children might be more severely affected.

Autosomal recessive disorders

A much larger number of autosomal recessive conditions are associated with severe mental retardation. Most of the 'inborn errors of metabolism' are due to autosomal recessive genes. Each step in a metabolic process is controlled by a particular enzyme and this in turn is the product of a particular gene — the 'one gene — one enzyme' concept. The activity of most enzymes can be reduced to a level under half the normal without serious harm. Consequently, the individual who is heterozygous for such a recessive gene and has around half the normal enzyme activity will show no outward manifestations of disease.

Nevertheless, this diminution in enzyme activity can often be used as a biochemical test for these unaffected heterozygous carriers.

When two heterozygous carriers of a recessive gene mate, the clinical disorder will be manifest on average in the one in four of their offspring who are homozygous. The chances of both parents being heterozygous for the same defective gene are, of course, greatly increased if the parents are themselves related. So, not surprisingly, the offspring of incestuous relationships (and cousin marriages) are most at risk of mental retardation due to recessive conditions (Editorial 1981).

Perhaps the best way of categorising autosomal recessive conditions is into those which affect (1) protein, (2) carbohydrate, and (3) fat metabolism.

Disorders of protein metabolism

Phenylketonuria is the most important of the autosomal recessive conditions; one in 50 of the population are heterozygous carriers and one in 10 000 live births are affected. Phenylketonurics are deficient in the enzyme phenylalanine hydroxylase, which converts phenylalanine to tyrosine. In consequence, phenylalanine tends to accumulate and some is diverted to form phenylpyruvic acid, which is then excreted in the urine. Screening tests for phenylketonuria depend on the detection of excess phenylalanine in the blood (Guthrie test) or phenylpyruvic acid in the urine. Heterozygotes are normal in intelligence and pigmentation but may sometimes be detected by the persistence of high serum phenylalanine levels and phenylpyruvic acid in the urine after a loading test.

Recent advances have now made available cloned DNA probes which are homologous for the gene for phenylalanine hydroxylase. This should enable not only prenatal diagnosis but also the identification of carriers in families with at least one affected child (Daiger et al 1986). Both the parents of a child with this recessive disorder must carry one defective and one normal copy of the phenylalanine gene. By examining DNA from the affected child and both parents, one can establish which restriction fragment is associated with the abnormal gene. Then, one can see whether the same fragment is also present in the unaffected child; if it is, the child must be a carrier.

The striking benefits of a low-phenylalanine diet are now well established, and many children homozygous for the defective gene now develop into intellectually normal adults. Some find as they get older that they can abandon their diets without ill effects. However, women who are contemplating becoming pregnant must return to strict avoidance of phenylalanine, since high circulating phenylalanine levels can have toxic effects on fetal development. Yu & O'Halloran (1980) have demonstrated that a high proportion of the children of such mothers are retarded, although only a small minority are homozygous for the defective gene. Apparently, heterozygous fetuses cannot withstand the effects of high circulating phenylalanine levels.

Disorders of carbohydrate metabolism

Galactosaemia is a recessive disorder in which the absence of galactose-1-phosphate uridyltransferase prevents the normal transformation of galactose to various glucose products. Many reports testify to the value of a milk (i.e. galactose)-free diet.

Disorders of fat metabolism

Tay–Sachs disease, which is largely untreatable and most common among Ashkenazim Jews, has produced one of the few successful attempts to prevent autosomal recessive conditions. Married non-pregnant couples in the Jewish population were chosen as the target group. An educational campaign among this cohesive and well-motivated population succeeded in identifying couples who were both heterozygous, and probably prevented a number of affected births (Kaback et al 1977). Tay–Sachs disease can also be detected by amniocentesis.

X-linked disorders

Lesch–Nyhan syndrome results from deficiency in an enzyme whose abbreviation is HGPRT, and which results in excessive purine synthesis and hyperuricaemia. Mental retardation is generally associated with aggression and self-mutilation. If a mother is a heterozygous carrier she will produce normal daughters (half of whom are carriers like herself), but half her sons will be affected. Fortunately, the female carrier state can be detected by cultivating skin fibroblasts and finding that they have the enzyme deficiency, and the presence of a defective fetus can be detected from enzyme levels in cells obtained at amniocentesis. DNA clones for HGPRT have now been developed and have shown that the enzyme deficiency can result from several different mutations at the HGPRT locus. Lesch–Nyhan syndrome can also now be diagnosed from samples of chorionic villi.

REFERENCES

Allen M G 1976 Twin studies of affective illness. Archives of General Psychiatry 33 : 1476–1478

Andreasen N C, Sheftner W, Reich T et al 1986 The validation of the concept of endogenous depression. Archives of General Psychiatry 43 : 246–251

Andrews G, Stewart G, Allen R et al 1990 The genetics of six neurotic disorders. Journal of Affective Disorders 19 : 23–29

Angst J 1966 Zur Atiologie und Nosologie endogener depressiver Psychosen. Monographien aus dem Gesamtgebiete der Neurologie und Psychiatrie 112. Springer-Verlag, Berlin

Arkonac O, Guze S B 1963 A family study of hysteria. New England Journal of Medicine 268 : 239–242

Baraitser M 1980 Down's syndrome. Hospital Update, October : 1021–1026

Baron M, Risch N, Hamburger R et al 1987 Genetic linkage between X-chromosome markers and bipolar affective illness. Nature 326 : 289–292

Bassett A S, McGillvray B C, Jones B et al 1988 Partial trisomy chromosome 5 co-segregating with schizophrenia. Lancet i: 799–902

Bertelsen A, Harvald B, Hauge M 1977 A Danish twin study of manic depressive disorders. British Journal of Psychiatry 130 : 330–351

Blum K, Noble E P, Sheridan P J et al 1990 Allelic association of human dopamine D2 receptor gene in alcoholism. Journal of the American Medical Association 263 : 2055–2060

Bohman M, 1978 Some genetic aspects of alcoholism and criminality. Archives of General Psychiatry 35 : 269–276

Bohman M, Cloninger C R, Sigvardsson S, von Knorring A L 1982 Predisposition to petty criminality in Swedish adoptees. Archives of General Psychiatry 39 : 1233–1241

Botstein D, White R L, Skolnick M, Davis R W 1980 Construction of a genetic linkage map in man using restriction fragment length polymorphisms. American Journal of Human Genetics 32 : 312–331

Bouchard T J, McGue M 1981 Familial studies of intelligence: a review. Science 212 : 1055–1060

Bouchard T J, McGue M 1990 Genetic and rearing environmental influences on personality. Journal of Personality Special Issue. Biological Foundations of Personality

Bouchard T J, Lykken D T, McGue M et al 1990 The Minnesota study of twins reared apart. Science 250 : 223–228

Editorial 1981 Children born as a result of incest. British Medical Journal i: 250–251

Brown F W 1942 Heredity in the psychoneuroses. Proceedings of the Royal Society of Medicine 35 : 785–790

Brown G, Harris T 1978 The social origins of depression. Tavistock, London

Buglass D, Clarke J, Henderson A S, Kreitman N, Presley A S 1977 A study of agoraphobic housewives. Psychological Medicine 7 : 73–86

Cadoret R J, Gath A 1978 Inheritance of alcoholism in adoptees. British Journal of Psychiatry 132 : 252–258

Carey G, Gottesman II 1981 Twin and family studies of anxiety, phobic and obsessive disorders. In: Klein D F, Rabkin J (eds) Anxiety: new research and changing concepts. Raven Press, New York

Castle D, Murray R M 1991 The neurodevelopmental basis of sex differences in schizophrenia. Psychological Medicine 21 : 565–575

Castle D, Murray R M 1992 Schizophrenia: aetiology and genetics. In: Copeland J R M, Abou-Saleh M T, Blazer D G (eds) The psychiatry of old age. Wiley, Chichester

Christiansen K O 1974 The genetics of aggresive criminality. In: de Wit J, Hartup W W (eds) Determinants of origins of aggressive behaviour. Mouton, The Hague, pp. 233–253

Clifford C A, Fulker D W, Gurling H M D, Murray R M 1981 Preliminary findings from a twin study of alcohol use. In: Gedda L, Parisi P, Nance W E (eds) Twin research 3. Alan R Liss, New York

Clifford C A, Murray R M, Fulker D W 1984 Genetic and environmental influences on obsessional traits and symptoms. Psychological Medicine 14: 791–800

Cloninger C R 1987 Neurogenetic adaptive mechanisms in alcoholism. Science 236 : 410–416

Cloninger C R, Reich R, Guze S B 1975 The multifactorial model of disease transmission: III The familial relationship between sociopathy and hysteria (Briquet's syndrome). British Journal of Psychiatry 127 : 23–32

Cloninger C R, Martin R L, Clayton P et al. 1981a A blind follow up and family study of anxiety neurosis. In: Klein D F, Rabkin J (eds) Anxiety: new research and changing concepts. Raven Press, New York

Cloninger C R, Bohman M, Sigvardsson S 1981b Inheritance of alcohol abuse. Archives of General Psychiatry 38: 861–868

Cohen M E, Badal D W, Kilpatrick J, Reed E W, White P D 1951 The high familial prevalence of neurocirculatory asthenia. American Journal of Human Genetics 3: 126–158

Collinge J, Palmer M S, Dryden A J 1991 Genetic predisposition to iatrogenic Creutzfeldt–Jacob disease. Lancet 337: 1441–1443

Conneally P M 1991 Association between the D2 dopamine receptor gene and alcoholism; continuing controversy. Archives of General Psychiatry 48: 664–668

Craufurd D 1989 Progress and problems in Huntington's disease. International Review of Psychiatry 1: 249–258

Crowe R R 1974 An adoption study of antisocial personality. Archives of General Psychiatry 31: 785–791

Crowe R R, Pauls D A, Slymen D J, Noyes R 1980 A family study of anxiety neurosis. Archives of General Psychiatry 37: 77–79

Daiger S P, Lidsky A S, Chakraborty R et al. 1986 Polymorphic DNA haplotypes at the phenylalanine hydroxylase locus in prenatal diagnosis of phenylketonuria. Lancet i: 230–232

Dalgard O S, Kringlen E 1976 A Norwegian study of criminality. British Journal of Criminology 16: 213–232

Davies K E 1988 Genome analysis. IRL Press, Oxford

Eaves L J, Eysenck H J, Martin N G 1989 Genes, culture and personality. Academic Press, New York

Egeland J A, Gerhard D S, Pauls D L et al 1987 Bipolar affective disorders linked to DNA markers on chromosome 11. Nature 325: 783–787

Elandt-Johnson R C 1971 Probability models and statistical methods in genetics. Wiley, New York

Elston R C, Campbell M A 1970 Schizophrenia: evidence for the major gene hypothesis. Behaviour Genetics 1: 3–10

Emery A E H 1982 Elements of medical genetics, 6th edn. Churchill Livingstone, Edinburgh

Emery A E H 1984 An introduction to recombinant DNA.Wiley,Chichester

Emery A E H,Rimoin D 1983 Principles and practice of medical genetics. Churchill Livingstone, Edingburgh

Eysenck H J, Kamin L 1981 Intelligence: the battle for the mind.Pan, London

Falconer D S 1965 The inheritance of liability to certain diseases, estimated from the incidence among relatives. Annals of Human Genetics 29: 51–76

Farmer A E, McGuffin P, Spitznagel E 1983 Heterogeneity in schizophrenia: a cluster analytic approach. Psychiatry Research 8: 1–12

Farmer A E, McGuffin P, Gottesman II 1987 Twin concordance for DSM III schizophrenia. Archives of General Psychiatry 44: 634–641

Feighner J P, Robins E, Guze S B, Woodruffe R A, Winokur G, Munoz R 1972 Diagnostic criteria for use in psychiatric research. Archives of General Psychiatry 26: 57–62

Fischer M 1971 Psychoses in the offspring of schizophrenic monozygotic twins and their normal cotwins. British Journal of Psychiatry 118: 43–52

Fischer M 1973 Genetic and environmental factors in schizophrenia. Acta Psychiatrica Scandinavica suppl 238

Folstein S, Rutter M 1977 Infantile autism: a genetic study of 21 twin pairs. Journal of Child Psychology and Psychiatry 18: 297–321

Fulker D W, Eysenck H J 1979 Nature and nurture: heredity. In: Eysenck H J (ed.) The structure and measurement of intelligence. Springer-Verlag, Berlin

Fyer A J, Mannuza S, Gallops M S et al. 1990 Familial transmission of simple phobias and fears. Archives of General Psychiatry 47: 252–256

Gershon E S, Bunney W E, Leckman, J F, Van Eerdewegh M, De Bauche B A 1976 The inheritance of affective disorders: a review of data and of hypotheses. Behaviour Genetics 6: 227–261

Gill M, Taylor C, Murray R M 1989 Schizophrenia research; attempting to integrate genetics, neurodevelopment and nosology. International Review of Psychiatry 1: 227–286

Goldstein J, Farone S, Weij et al.1990 Sex differences in the familial transmission of schizophrenia. British Journal of Psychiatry 156: 819–825

Goodman R 1991 Growing together and growing apart. In: McGuffin P, Murray R M (eds) The New Genetics of Mental Illness. Butterworth-Heinemann, Oxford

Goodwin D 1976 Is alcoholism hereditary? Oxford University Press, New York

Gottesman II 1991 Schizophrenia Genesis: the origins of madness. Freeman, New York

Gottesman II, Bertelsen A 1989 Confirming unexpressed phenotypes in schizophrenia. Archives of General Psychiatry 46: 867–872

Gottesman II, Schields J 1967 A polygenic theory of schizophrenia. Proceedings of the National Academy of Sciences of the USA 58: 199–205

Gottesman II, Shields J 1972 Schizophrenia and genetics: a twin study vantage point. Academic Press, London

Gottesman II, Shields J 1982 Schizophrenia, the epigenetic puzzle. Cambridge University Press, Cambridge

Gurling H M D, Murray R M 1987 Genetic influence, brain morphology and cognitive deficits in alcoholic twins. In:

Goedde H W, Agarwal D P (eds) Genetics and Alcoholism. Alan R Liss, New York

Gusella J F, Wexler N S, Conneally R M et al. 1983 A polymorphic DNA marker genetically linked to Huntington's disease. Nature 306: 234–238

Hanson D R Gottesman II 1982 The genetics of childhood psychosis. In: Wing J (ed.) Handbook of psychiatry, vol. III. Psychoses of uncertain aetiology. Cambridge University Press, London

Harada S, Agarwal D P, Goedde H W 1985 Aldehyde dehydrogenase polymorphism and alcohol metabolism in alcoholics. Alcohol 2: 391–392

Hardy, J 1991 The molecular basis of Alzheimer's type dementia. In: McGuffin P, Murray R M (eds) The new genetics of mental illness. Butterworth-Heinemann, Oxford

Hare E H, Price J S, Slater E T O 1972 Fertility in obsessional neurosis. British Journal of Psychiatry 121: 197–205

Harper P S 1986 The prevention of Huntington's chorea. Journal of the Royal College of Physicians 20: 7–14

Henderson N D 1982 Human behaviour genetics. Annual Review of Psychology 33: 403–416

Herbst D S 1980 Non-specific X-linked mental retardation. American Journal of Medical Genetics 7: 443–460

Heston L L 1966 Psychiatric disorders in foster home reared children of schizophrenic mothers. British Journal of Psychiatry 112: 819–825

Heston L L 1970 The genetics of schizophrenia and schizoid disease. Science 167: 249–256

Hodgkinson S, Mullan M, Murray R M 1991 The genetics of vulnerability to alcoholism. In: McGuffin P, Murray R M (eds) The new genetics of mental illness. Butterworth-Heinemann, Oxford

Holland A J 1991 Learning disability and psychiatric/behavioural disorders In: McGuffin P, Murray R M (eds) The new genetics of mental illness. Butterworth-Heinemann, Oxford

Holland A J, Hall A, Murray R M et al. 1984 Anorexia nervosa: a study of 34 pairs of twins and one set of triplets. British Journal of Psychiatry 145: 414–419

Hunter H, 1977 XYY males. British Journal of Psychiatry 131: 468–477

Hutchings B, Mednick S A 1974 Registered criminality in the adoptive and biological parents of registered male adoptees. In: Mednick S A et al. (eds) Genetics, environment and psychopathology. North Holland/American Elsevier, New York

Jackson D D 1960 A critique of the literature on the genetics of schizophrenia. In: Jackson D D (ed.) The Etiology of Schizophrenia. Basic Books, New York

Jones P B, Murray R M, 1991 Aberrant neurodevelopment as the expression of the schizophrenia genotype. In: McGuffin P, Murray R M (eds) The new genetics of mental illness. Butterworth-Heinemann, Oxford

Kaback M M, Shapiro L J, Hirsch P, Roy C 1977 Tay–Sachs disease heterozygote detection. Progress in Clinical Biological Research 18: 267–279

Kaij L 1960 Alcoholism in twins. Almqvist & Wiksell, Stockholm

Kallman F J 1938 The genetics of schizophrenia. J J Augustin, New York

Kelsoe J R, Ginns E I, Egeland J A et al 1989 Reevaluation of the linkage relationship between chromosome 11p loci and the gene for bipolar affective disorder in the old order Amish. Nature 342: 238–242

Kendler K S, 1983 Overview: a current perspective on twin studies of schizophrenia. American Journal of Psychiatry 140: 1413–1420

Kendler K S, Gruenberg A M, Strauss J S 1981 An independent analysis of the Copenhagen sample of the Danish adoption study of schizophrenia. II The relationship between schizotypal personality disorder and schizophrenia. Archives of General Psychiatry 38: 982–987

Kety S S 1983 Mental illness in the biological and adoptive relatives of schizophrenic adoptees: findings relevant to genetic and environmental factors in etiology. American Journal of Psychiatry 140: 720–726

Kety S S, Rosenthal D, Wender P H, Schulsinger F, Jacobsen B 1976 Mental illness in the biological and adoptive families of individuals who have become schizophrenic. Behaviour Genetics 6: 219–225

Kolvin I, Ounsted C, Richardson L M, Garside R F 1971 The family and social background in childhood psychoses. British Journal of Psychiatry 118: 396–402

Kringlen E 1967 Heredity and environment in the functional psychoses. Heinemann Medical, London

Kringlen E 1968 An epidemiological–clinical twin study on schizophrenia. In: Rosenthal D, Kety S S (eds) The transmission of schizophrenia. Pergamon Press, Oxford

Larsson T, Sjogren T, Jacobson G 1963 Senile dementia: a clinical, sociomedical and genetic study. Acta Psychiatrica Scandinavica suppl 167

Leonard K 1959 Aufteilung der Endogen Psychosen. Akademic Verlag, Berlin

Lewis S W, Chitkara B, Reveley A M et al. 1987 Family history and birth weight in monozygotic twins concordant and discordant for schizophrenia. Acta Genetica Medica 36:267–272

Lewis S W, Owen M J, Murray R M 1989 Obstetric complications and schizophrenia. In: Schulz S C, Tamminga C A (eds) Schizophrenia; a scientific focus. Oxford University Press, New York

Ljunberg L 1957 Hysteria: a clinical, prognostic and genetic study. Acta Psychiatrica Scandinavica suppl 112

Macdonald A M, Stunkard A J 1990 The body-mass index in British separated twins. New England Journal of Medicine 322:1530

Macdonald A M, Clifford C W, Murray R M 1991 The contribution of heredity to obsessional disorder and personality. In: Kendler K S, Lyons M J, Tsuang M T (eds) Genetic issues in psychosocial epidemiology. Rutgers University Press, Princeton

McGue M, Gottesman I I, Rao D C 1985 Resolving genetic models for the transmission of schizophrenia. Genetic Epidemiology 2: 99–110

McGuffin P, Gottesman II 1984 Genetic influences on normal and abnormal development. In: Rutter M, Hersov L (eds) Child psychiatry: modern approaches. Blackwell, London

McGuffin P, Katz R 1986 Nature, nurture and affective disorder. In: Deakin J F W (ed.) Biology of depression. Gaskell, Royal College of Psychiatrists, London

McGuffin P, Sturt E 1986 Genetic markers in schizophrenia. Human Heredity 36:65–68

McGuffin P, Farmer A E, Gottesman II, Murray R M, Reveley A 1984 Twin concordance for operationally defined schizophrenia. Confirmation of familiality and heritability. Archives of General Psychiatry 41:541–545

McGuffin P, Farmer A E, Gottesman II 1987a Is there really

a split in schizophrenia? The genetic evidence. British Journal of Psychiatry 150:581–592

McGuffin P, Katz R, Aldrich J et al 1987b The Camberwell Collaborative Depression Study II. British Journal of Psychiatry 152:766–774

McGuffin P, Katz R, Rutherford J 1992 The Maudsley twin study of affective disorder. Submitted

McKeon P, Murray R M 1987 Familial aspects of obsessive compulsive neurosis. British Journal of Psychiatry 151: 528–534

McNeill T F, Kaij L 1978 Obstetric factors in the development of schizophrenia. In: Wynne L C et al (eds) The nature of schizophrenia. Wiley, New York

Martin N G, Perl J, Oakshott J G et al. 1985 A twin study of ethanol metabolism. Behavioural Genetics: 15: 93–109

Mendelwicz J, Rainer J D 1977 Adoption study supporting genetic transmission in manic depressive illness. Nature 268: 327–329

Mendelwicz J, Simon PA, Sevy S et al 1987 Polymorphic DNA marker on X chromosome and manic depression. Lancet ii: 1230–1232

Morris M J, Harper P S 1991 Prediction and prevention in Huntington's disease In: McGuffin P, Murray R M (eds) The new genetics of mental illness. Butterworth-Heinemnann, Oxford

Morton N E 1982 Outline of genetic epidemiology. Karger, Basel

Murray R M, Gurling H M D 1980 Genetic contributions to normal and abnormal drinking. In: Sandler M (ed.) The psychopharmacology of alcohol. Raven Press, New York

Murray R M, Lewis S W 1987 Is schizophrenia a neurodevelopmental disease? British Medical Journal 295: 681–682

Murray R M, Lewis S, Reveley A M 1985 towards an aetiological classification of schizophrenia. Lancet i: 1023–1026

Murray R M, Lewis S W, Owen M J, Foerster A 1988 The neurodevelopmental origins of dementia praecox. In: Bebbington P, McGuffin P (eds) Schizophrenia: the major issues. Heinemann, London

Nielsen J, Nyborg H, Dahl G 1977 Turner's syndrome. Acta Jutlandica 45, Aarhus

Nielsen J, Johnsen S G, Sorensen K 1980 Follow up 10 years later of 34 Klinefelter males. Psychological Medicine 10: 345–352

Noyes R, Clancy J, Crowe R, Hoenk P R, Slymen D J 1978 The familial prevalence of anxiety neurosis. Archives of General Psychiatry 35: 1057–1059

Noyes R, Crowe R R, Harris E L, Hamra B J, McChesney C M, Chaudhry D R 1986 Relationship between panic disorder and agoraphobia. Archives of General Psychiatry 43: 227–232

Oliver C, Holland A J 1986 Down's syndrome and Alzheimer's disease: a review. Psychological Medicine 16: 307–322

O'Rourke D H, Gottesman II, Suarez B K, Rice J, Reich T 1982 Refutation of the single locus model in the etiology of schizophrenia.American Journal of Human Genetics 33: 630–649

Ott J 1985 Analysis of human genetic linkage. Johns Hopkins University Press, Baltimore

Parkes J D, Langdon N, Lock C 1986 Narcolepsy and immunity. British Medical Journal 292: 359–360

Partanen J, Bruun K, Markkanen T 1966 Inheritance of drinking behaviour. Finnish Foundation for Alcohol Studies, Helsinki

Pauls D L, Alsobrook J, Almasy B S, Leckman J F Cohen D J (1991) Genetic and epidemiological analyses of the Yale Tourette Syndrome Family Study Data. Psychiatric Genetics 2: 28

Perris C 1966 A study of bipolar (manic depressive) and unipolar recurrent depressive psychoses. Acta Psychiatrica Scandinavica suppl 294

Pickens R W, Sivikis D S, McGee M et al 1991 Heterogeneity in the inheritance of alcoholism. Archives of General Psychiatry 48: 19–28

Pierretti M, Zhang F, Fu Y et al 1991 Absence of expression of the FMR-1 gene in fragile X Syndrome. Cell 66: 817–822

Pitcher D R 1975 The XYY syndrome. In: Silverstone T, Barrachlough B (eds) Contemporary psychiatry. British Journal of Psychiatry Special Publication No 9. Headley, Ashford

Pollin W, Stabenau J R 1968 Biological, psychological and historical differences in a series of monozygotic twins discordant for schizophrenia. In: Rosenthal D, Key S S (eds) The transmission of schizophrenia. Pegamon Press, Oxford

Pollin W, Allen M G, Hoffer A, Stanbenau J R, Hrubec Z 1969 Psychopathology in 15 909 pairs of veteran twins: evidence for a genetic factor in the pathogenesis of schizophrenia and its relative absence in psychoneurosis. American Journal of Psychiatry 126: 597

Pollitt J 1972 The relationship between genetic and precipitating factors in depressive illness. British Journal of Psychiatry 121: 67 – 70

Price J 1968 The genetics of depressive disorder. In Coppen A J (ed.) Recent developments in affective disorders. Headley, Ashford

Primrose B A, El-Matmati R, Boyd E, Godson C, Newton M 1986 Prevalence of the Fragile X syndrome in an institution for the mentally handicapped. British Journal of Psychiatry 148: 655–657

Reich T, James J W, Morris C A 1972 the use of multiple thresholds in determining the mode of transmission of semi-continuous traits. Annals of Human Genetics 36: 163–184

Risch N, Baron M 1984 Segregation analysis of schizophrenia and related disorders. American Journal of Human Genetics 36: 1039–1051

Rose R J, Miller J Z, Pogue–Geile M F 1981 Twin family studies of common fears and phobias. In: Gedda L, Parisi P, Nance W E (eds) Twin research, vol. 3. Alan R Liss, New York

Rosenthal D 1970 Genetic theory and abnormal behaviour. McGraw-Hill, New York

Rosenthal D, Wender P H, Kety S S, Schulsinger F, Welner J, Reider R 1975 Parent–child relationships and psychopathological disorder in the child. Archives of General Psychiatry 32: 466–476

Roy A 1981 Schizophrenia and Klinefelter's syndrome. Canadian Journal of Psychiatry 26: 262–264

Rutherford J, Katz R, McGuffin P et al 1992 A twin study of attitudes to eating. Submitted

Rutter M 1991 Autism as a genetic disorder. In: McGuffin P, Murray R M (eds) The new genetics of mental illness. Butterworth-Heinemann, Oxford

St. George-Hyslop P H, Tanzi R E, Polinsky R J 1987 The

genetic defect causing familial Alzheimer's disease maps on chromosome 21. Science 235: 885–889

Schenk V W D 1959 Re-examination of a family with Pick's disease. Annals of Human Genetics 23: 325–333

Schulsinger F 1972 Psychopathy: heredity and environment. International Journal of Mental Health 1: 190–206

Shapiro R W 1970 A twin study of non-endogenous depression. Acta Jutlandica 42: 2

Sherrington R, Brynjolfsson J, Petursson H et al. 1988 Localisation of a susceptibility locus for schizophrenia on chromosome 5. Nature 336: 164–167

Shibuya A, Yoshida A 1988 Genotypes of alcohol-metabolising enzymes in Japanese with alcohol liver diseases. American Journal of Human Genetics 43: 744–748

Shields J 1982 Genetics studies of hysterical disorders. In: Roy A (ed.) Hysteria. Wiley, Chichester

Sjøgren T, Sjøgren H, Lindergren A G H 1952 Morbus Alzheimer and morbus Pick. A genetic, clinical and patho-anatomical study. Acta Psychiatrica et Neurologica Scandinavica suppl 82

Slater E 1961 Hysteria 311. Journal of Mental Science 107: 359–13

Slater E 1968 A review of earlier evidence of genetic factors schizophrenia. In: Rosenthal D, Kety S D (eds) The transmission of schizophrenia. Pergamon Press, Oxford

Slater E, Cowie V 1971 The genetics of mental disorders. Oxford University Press, London

Slater E, Glithero E 1965 A follow up of patients diagnosed as suffering from 'hysteria'. Journal of Psychosomatic Research 9: 9–13

Slater E, Shields J 1969 Genetical aspects of anxiety. In: Lader M H (ed.) Studies of anxiety. British Journal of Psychiatry Special Publication 3. Headley, Ashford

Smith C 1974 Concordance in twins: methods and interpretation. American Journal of Human Genetics 26: 454–466

Southern E M 1975 Detection of specific sequences among DNA fragments separated by gel electrophoresis. Journal of Molecular Biology 98: 503

Spitzer R L, Endicott J, Robins E 1978 Research Diagnostic Criteria. New York State Psychiatric Institute, New York

Stenstedt A 1966 Genetics of neurotic depression. Acta Psychiatrica Scandinavica 42: 392–409

Stunkard A J, Harris J, Pedersen N L et al 1990 The body mass index of twins who have been reared apart. New England Journal of Medicine 322: 1483–1488

Tienari P 1968 Schizophrenia in monozygotic male twins. In: Rosenthal D, Kety S S (eds) The transmission of schizophrenia. Pergamon Press, Oxford

Torgersen S 1979 The nature and origin of common phobic fears. British Journal of Psychiatry 134: 343–351

Torgersen S 1983a Genetic factors in anxiety disorders. Archives of General Psychiatry 40: 1085–1089

Torgersen S 1983b The genetics of neurosis: the effects of sampling variation upon the twin concordance ratio. British Journal of Psychiatry 142: 126

Torgersen S 1986 Genetic factors in moderately severe and mild affective disorders. Archives of General Psychiatry 43: 222–226

Treasure J L T, Holland A J 1991 Genes and the aetiology of eating disorders. In: McGuffin P, Murray R M (eds) The new genetics of mental illness. Butterworth-Heinemann, Oxford

Vanderberg S G 1967 Hereditary factors in normal personality traits. In: Wortis J (ed) Recent advances in biological psychiatry 9. Plenum Press, New York

Vogel F, Motulsky A G 1979 Human genetics: problems and approaches. Springer-Verlag, Berlin

Wakeling A 1972 Comparative study of psychiatric patients with Klinefelter's syndrome and hypogonadism. Psychological Medicine 2: 139–154

Weatherall D J 1991 The new genetics and clinical practice, 3rd ed. Oxford University Press, Oxford

Weissman M A, Merikangas K E, Wickramanthe P et al 1986 Understanding the clinical heterogeneity of major depression using family data. Archives of General Psychiatry 43: 430–434

Wender P H, Rosenthal D, Kety S, Schulsinger F, Welner J 1973 Social class and psychopathology in adoptees: a natural experimental method for separating the roles of genetic and experimental factors. Archives of General Psychiatry 28: 318–325

Whatley S A, Owen M J 1991 The cell, molecular biology and the new genetics. In: McGuffin P, Murray R M (eds) The New Genetics of Mental Illness. Butterworth-Heinemann, Oxford

Wright A 1991 The genetics of common forms of dementia. In: McGuffin P, Murray R M (eds) The New Genetics of Mental Illness. Butterworth-Heinemann, Oxford

Wright A F, Whalley L J 1984 Genetics, ageing and dementia. British Journal of Psychiatry 145: 20–38

Yu J S, O'Halloran M T 1980 Children of mothers with phenylketonuria. Lancet i: 210–212

Zerbin Rudin E 1967 Endogene Psychosen. In: Becker P E (ed) Humangenetik: ein kurzes Handbuch, vol. 2. Georg Thieme, Stuttgart

13. The psychiatric interview
G. P. Maguire

PURPOSE OF THE PSYCHIATRIC INTERVIEW

The key tasks include the obtaining of an accurate history of the patient's problems, assessing his personality, and making a formulation. The formulation seeks to characterise the key features of the patient's illness, list the most probable diagnoses and explain why the patient has become ill at this point in time. This explanation considers genetic predisposition, experiences and relationships in early and adult life and the occurrence of life events or chronic difficulties. The formulation then indicates the physical, social and psychological investigations that will be required to confirm the diagnosis and outlines a provisional treatment plan.

The psychiatrist needs, therefore, to know the areas that must be covered if a good formulation is to be made and the interviewing skills which will promote trust and disclosure. The psychiatrist also needs to know how to use the time available to maximum effect.

A HISTORY-TAKING SCHEME

Areas to be covered

History of the presenting complaints

Nature. The interviewer's first task is to help the patient communicate the nature of his current problems since this is why the patient has sought help. He should ensure that each problem is properly clarified before pursuing any other material. He should allow for the possibility that patients may initially volunteer a problem that masks the difficulties they really wish to communicate. Once the interviewer has elicited the patient's main problems he should summarise them by saying, for example: 'So far, as I understand it, you have been suffering from tiredness, low spirits and panic attacks — I'll go into each of these in a moment — but has there been anything else that you have not yet mentioned?'

For each problem elicited the interviewer should seek the following information.

The time of onset. The interviewer should take particular care to establish exactly when the problem began. Patients can often date what has happened accurately provided they are encouraged to do so. The use of anchor dates like birthdays, anniversaries or other events can help them do this. Otherwise they may give vague answers.

Development over time. The interviewer should next find out how each problem developed over the period between onset and the time of interview. He should be especially alert to any major changes in the intensity and frequency of the problem. Such 'change points' may provide important clues to the aetiology of these difficulties.

Precipitating or relieving factors. The interviewer should enquire whether the patient considers that the onset or major changes in his particular problems were related to any particular events or factors. He should be aware that many patients tend to search for a meaning. Thus, when people experience unpleasant events they often respond by striving to find an explanation in terms of why now or why me? This is particularly likely when they develop a psychiatric illness. It is still associated with much stigma and the early signs and symptoms are often interpreted by close relatives and friends as merely due to 'temporary weakness' or 'bloody-mindedness'. So, it might be more acceptable if a clear and understandable cause can be identified.

These pressures can result in patients and relatives unwittingly but falsely attributing the onset of problems to certain events. For example, a 46-year-old woman gave a history of a depressive illness. She said it had begun 2 months ago, a few days after she learned that her husband was likely to be made redundant. This seemed plausible since they already had financial problems. It later became clear that the depressive illness had developed 'out of the blue' some 6 weeks earlier.

False attribution may also occur when the event which triggered the psychiatric illness was very upsetting and still evokes painful memories which the patient prefers to avoid. Thus, a 34-year-old single woman attributed her problems to an acute onset of rheumatoid arthritis. She had been extremely fit and active and was fond of playing squash and riding and found her arthritis intolerable. However, a friend informed the doctor that the patient had become unwell within a few weeks of the death of her mother from a heart attack. When the patient was asked about this it became evident that she still found it very difficult to accept her mother's death and did not like to talk about it. It is important that the interviewer dates the onset of key symptoms and possible precipitants independently and cross-checks the dates if there is still any doubt.

The help given to date. Many patients who are referred have already been given some treatment. So, the interviewer must try to establish the exact nature, dose and duration of each treatment given. The interviewer should ask if the patient has noticed any changes since treatment was started and be on the look-out for both wanted and unwanted effects, especially adverse side-effects.

Impact of the problem. Many problems, particularly established physical and psychiatric illness, have an adverse effect on the day-to-day functioning of the patient, family and close friends. These effects may be serious and disrupt family life but often remain undisclosed. The interviewer should ask if the patient's problems have had any adverse effects on each of the following areas: his mood, his ability to do his job and level of job satisfaction; his ability to cope with his day-to-day chores; his ability to pursue and enjoy his usual hobbies, leisure and social activities; the quality of his relationship with his wife, immediate family and other close relatives.

Thus, the interviewer may begin this section by saying: 'I'd like now to find out how your problems have been affecting you and your family. Can I begin with your work ... has that been affected in any way since you became ill?' These data should help him assess the extent to which the patient's problems have burdened his family. He must allow for the tendency of patients who suffer from depressive illnesses to see themselves as a much greater burden than they are.

Availability of support. The amount of practical and emotional support available to a patient may determine how he copes with his problems and whether or not hospital admission is required. He

should, therefore, be asked if he has confided in anyone about his problems and the responses of such confidants established.

Some families react by being 'too understanding'. They take over from the patient and allow him to relinquish more of his roles than is justified by his illness. Alternatively, they may fuss over the patient and become too involved in his problems. Other families find it difficult to accept that one of them has become psychiatrically ill. They become irritated, impatient and frustrated and frequently tell the patient to 'pull yourself together'.

It is important to identify such reactions at the outset since they can hinder recovery or render relapse more likely. Thus, a patient whose family reacted to her agoraphobia by doing all her shopping for her is only likely to recover fully if her family begins to encourage her to do more for herself. A young schizophrenic whose parents have become very involved in his illness and spent much time with him runs a high risk of relapse if this level of emotional involvement continues. Similarly, a total absence of a confidant or support will create problems in management.

By now the interviewer should have obtained a vivid and reliable picture of what life has been like for the patient and his family since the onset of the main problems. To complete this phase of the psychiatric history the interviewer should establish the patient's view of his problems.

The patient's view of his problems. The patient should be asked what he thinks is wrong with him and whether he feels he needs help. He should also be asked if he believes that he can be helped. Unless the interviewer is fully aware of how the patient perceives the situation and why, he will be unable to provide effective reassurance and will remain unaware of factors that could hinder recovery or compliance with advice and treatment.

For example, a 50-year-old woman presented with a serious depressive illness. She said that she felt life was hopeless and that she had no future. She had been diagnosed as having cancer of the breast 4 months previously and had had a mastectomy. The cancer was at an early stage and there was no evidence of spread or involvement of the axillary lymph notes. The surgeon had told her that the prognosis was good and he was puzzled that she had become so depressed, especially as she had accepted the loss of a breast. When asked: 'How do you feel about your breast trouble?' it emerged that she did not believe the surgeon and had been ruminating endlessly about death from cancer. Her father had developed a swelling on the side of his jaw 6 years before. After investigation he was told that it was a small tumour but it had been removed successfully. The family, including his daughter, were told he had disseminated disease and had a year to live at most. She had no reason to believe that the doctors were being any more honest with her.

When another patient presented with a less severe depressive illness, the referral letter from his general practitioner said that he had failed to respond to amitryptiline 50 mg three times a day. When asked what he felt was wrong the patient said it was 'a lack of will power'. He found it shameful and intolerable that he had been referred to a psychiatrist. He had not taken the antidepressants because he hated not to be 'in control'. He was also afraid of becoming dependent on them since he thought they were tranquillisers like diazepam.

Past history of similar psychiatric problems

In order to put the patient's problems and attitudes into perspective it is helpful if the interviewer next finds out whether the patient has experienced similar difficulties before. If he has done so, the interviewer should clarify for each previous episode whether there was any particular trigger, its exact nature, how it affected him, how long it lasted and what treatments he responded to, if any. This will enable the interviewer to decide whether the patient is vulnerable to a particular type of mental illness and to particular stresses. For example, each episode of illness may have been precipitated by a loss event. It will also allow the interviewer to determine if the episodes are clinically different and to predict what treatments are likely to be most effective. He will usually leave asking about other past illnesses and problems until the personal history.

The interviewer should check how well the patient was actually functioning before the onset of the present problems. Otherwise he may set unrealistic goals for treatment and fail to realise that any impairment in functioning was due to factors other than the present illness. For example, a 44-year-old man presented with a history of agoraphobia and abuse of alcohol. His drinking appeared to be an attempt to forstall the panic attacks which he experienced as he was about to leave his house. It transpired that he had experienced an episode of 'hearing voices' 2 years previously. This responded well to trifluoperazine and he had been given this ever since. Enquiry about his functioning before the onset of panic attacks revealed that he often failed to go to work because he 'couldn't be bothered'. On such days he would usually stay in bed until midday. Even when he managed to get to work he would often sit around doing little. Similarly, he spent much of the time at home sitting in a chair. This was in marked contrast to his functioning before the episode of 'hearing voices'. Consequently, it was clear that even if his panic attacks responded to behavioural treatments he would still be seriously impaired by a loss of volition secondary to schizophrenia.

Screening questions

However well the interviewer has tried to establish the patient's main complaints it is possible that the patient will still not have communicated a key problem. It is likely that many psychiatric patients perceive the psychiatrist as principally concerned with their mental health. They may then not disclose an important physical complaint, as in the following example.

A 67-year-old married woman was referred by a physician to the psychiatric out-patient department. She had complained repeatedly of vomiting, and feeling tired and weak. Investigations had failed to reveal any physical causes for these symptoms. When seen initially no detailed enquiry about her physical health was made. It was assumed that the physician had excluded any serious illness. Instead, attention was focused on her mental state and it emerged that she had been experiencing symptoms of an anxiety state. It was arranged for her to be taught relaxation and to be reviewed in a month's time. When followed up, she seemed preoccupied and tearful. She was asked why she seemed so upset and replied that she had been very worried that something physical had been missed. Between seeing the physician and the psychiatrist she had begun to pass blood per rectum. She had been worried about this but had not felt able to mention it to the psychiatrist when she first saw him because 'I didn't realise you were interested in this kind of thing.'

Routine enquiry about 'How has your physical health been?' will encourage most patients to believe that the psychiatrist is genuinely concerned with any physical problems and to feel that it is legitimate to disclose such difficulties.

When the interview has been dominated by physical problems it is important that the interviewer should screen for any changes in psychological health along the following lines: 'So far, we have been discussing your heart trouble because you feel that is your main problem, but how have you been feeling in yourself, for example in your spirits?'

When these screening questions do not reveal further problems it is important to check that the patient has been mentally and physically well in all respects other than those concerned in the presenting problems.

Personal history

The next task of the interviewer is to find out about the patient's early life, subsequent development and experiences. This should enable him to throw light on the patient's personality and on the influences that moulded it. It may also allow him to detect particular areas of vulnerability and identify the factors which led to the patient's problems. He should be especially on the lookout for clear patterns of behaviour and experiences, e.g. repeated loss events.

Patients who have not seen a psychiatrist before may be puzzled by the change from talking about their current problems to asking about their early lives. It helps if this is explained in the following way: 'So far, we have been talking about your present problems. I'd like now to ask you some general questions about your self. Is that all right?' If the patient is uncertain, the interviewer can explain why the information might be important.

Family history. The interviewer should first establish whether both parents are still alive and their ages. If a parent has died, the date and circumstances should be established whenever possible. The patient should be asked how he reacted and whether or not he has got over it. The interviewer should be alert to evidence of continued feelings of anger, guilt or distress, especially on important anniversaries.

The patient should be asked how he got on with each parent from early childhood onwards. Were they loving and supportive towards him? Were there any major rows or disagreements? Did they encourage him to become independent or try to delay this? Has he been able to confide important worries to them? How have they responded? How well did the parents get on together? Has each parent achieved all he or she wanted in life? Has either of them experienced any major physical or psychiatric illness? If so, what was its exact nature? What treatment was given? How did the parent respond?

If his parents separated, the patient should be asked how he responded to this. Did it cause any particular problems? If he was brought up by others how did he react?

Similar general enquiries should be made about any siblings, and the patient should be asked if he felt his parents showed a preference for him or a sibling.

Finally, the interviewer should establish how often the patient sees any of his family and how he feels about this contact.

Early life and development. The interviewer should establish when and where the patient was born and enquire if there were any problems surrounding his birth. He should then be asked about his development. Did he pass the usual milestones on time? Were there any difficulties? What does he remember about his early childhood? Was it happy and secure or otherwise?

Schooling. Questions about schooling should initially cover when the patient first went to school and how he felt about this first separation from his mother. How did he get on with his peers? How did he progress at school academically and socially? How did he perceive his teachers? How did he compare himself with the other children? Were there any problems with discipline? Was there any school refusal? Did he experience any learning difficulties or problems in making friends?

Enquiry about his secondary education should include his reactions to the rules and constraints, teachers and peers. Did he progress scholastically as expected? Did he excel at anything? Did he have any particular problems? How well did he perform in public examinations? When did he leave school and why? How did his family and friends view his achievements?

If he moved schools the reasons for any move and his reactions should be explored. Such moves can lead to vulnerability, as the following example illustrates. A 22-year-old university student became very depressed after her boyfriend announced he had won a scholarship to go to America for a year. As a child she changed schools frequently because her father was in the army. As soon as she made new friends she seemed to lose them. Her boyfriend's news reactivated all her old fears and led her to feel depressed and hopeless.

If he went on to further education similar questions should be asked. The interviewer should look out for any evidence of a discrepancy between his potential and his achievements and explore possible reasons, for example the insidious onset of schizophrenia.

Behaviour problems. If the patient has not already disclosed such problems, direct questions should be asked, as follows: 'Was there any time in your childhood when you had problems with bedwetting? ... with nightmares?' Problems which should also be covered include temper tantrums, clinging behaviour, food fads, unexplained somatic symptoms, social or other phobias, hyperactivity, aggressiveness, truancy and delinquency or drug abuse.

Occupation. The jobs held by the patient should be established in chronological order and the reasons for any job change explored. Such enquiry may indicate a clear pattern, like a low boredom threshold or avoidance of responsibility.

He should then be asked how he feels about his present job, gets on with others at work, copes with any stresses and what his future prospects and ambitions are.

If unemployed, his response to this should be explored.

Personal relationships. The interviewer should first establish if the patient is married or has a girlfriend. If he has, he should be asked when and how they met, how they get on together, if they share any responsibilities and interests, and what their future plans are. The interviewer should check if the patient is able to confide his true worries in his wife or girlfriend. If he cannot do this does he turn to anyone else? Similar enquiries should be made about any important previous relationship and cover the reasons for it terminating and the patient's responses. If the relationship ended through bereavement the question already suggested about the death of a parent should be used. When relationships have gone wrong has the patient learned from his experience? When the patient has no current close relationship the reasons for this should also be explored.

Sexual history. Patients who are single, separated, widowed, young or elderly may be upset by questions about their sexuality. So it is worth following up questions about relationships by asking: 'Do you mind if I ask you if there has been a physical aspect to your relationship?' If the patient objects, his wishes should be respected. Otherwise, the interviewer may proceed as follows: 'Have you made love? How has it worked out? Have there been any difficulties? Could you tell me about them?'

The patient may then be asked about his early sexual history. How did he learn the facts of life? Did he have any early sexual experiences? How did he react? Does he masturbate and, if so, how often? What does he think about when he does so? Has he ever been attracted to his own sex? Did this lead to a homosexual relationship? Did this cause a problem?

A female patient should also be asked when her periods began, how she reacted and how regular her periods have been.

Children. The ages and names of any children should be noted and the following points covered: When was he born? Was he planned? Were there any difficulties with the pregnancy and birth? How has he progressed since? Have there been any difficulties?

How has his health been? How do you get on together? Do you plan to have more children? If not, what contraceptive precautions do you take?

Female patients should also be asked if and how well they bonded with each child and possible reasons for any bonding failure explored. Their reaction to any abortions or miscarriages should be determined. If the patient has lost or is separated from a child, he should be asked the effect of this.

Past medical history. Details of any previous major physical illnesses should be obtained and should include the exact nature of each illness, the duration, treatments given, the patient's responses and the short- and longer-term physical and psychological effects on the patient and family.

Previous psychiatric history. This should have been covered in the section on past history of similar psychiatric problems. However, it is always worth checking by asking: 'Have there been any other times when you have had trouble with your nerves?' and using similar probes if there have been.

Premorbid personality. The patient's account of his premorbid personality may be distorted by his illness or a general lack of insight. Thus, a depressed patient may describe himself in a misleadingly unfavourable way because of low self-esteem. A patient subject to recurrent illness may find it difficult to recall how he functioned before his first ever episode. While it is important to get an independent account from a close relative, it is still worth asking the patient what kind of a person he was before he first became ill. As he responds he should be asked to give examples of the behaviours he mentions.

Certain dimensions are worth covering routinely unless already volunteered. Is he usually a worrier? What is his mood like? How changeable is it? How concerned is he about high standards, order, tidiness and punctuality? How easy does he find it to form and sustain close relationships? Can he express feelings of love, anger, frustration and sadness? Does he ever lose control of his feelings? Has he ever been violent? Can he stand on his own two feet? Can he plan ahead? What are his hopes and ambitions? How assertive is he? Does he value himself? Does he have any special hobbies or interests? How does he react to stress? How much does he normally drink? Does he smoke? Has he ever used other drugs? (A detailed drinking history is particularly important in view of the contribution of alcohol to a wide range of psychiatric disorders.) Can he tolerate frustration? Does he appear to learn from experience?

When such enquiry generates hypotheses about the patient's personality these should be tested against the relatives' accounts and observations of the patient's subsequent behaviour within the out-patient clinic, day hospital or ward round.

Examination of the mental state

When the patient is able to give a history, the mental state is usually examined after the history has been completed. When the patient is very disturbed or is suffering from organic brain disease, this may not be possible. The examination of the mental state is then crucial. A scheme for the examination of patients with suspected organic brain disease is well described elsewhere (Institute of Psychiatry 1978).

Appearance and behaviour. As the interviewer examines the mental state his first task is to make systematic notes about the patient's general appearance and behaviour.

Does the patient appear appropriately dressed, clean and tidy? If female, is she wearing any make-up or jewellery? Does it seem excessive? Is it possible to establish and maintain a reasonable rapport? Can the patient make and tolerate eye contact or does he seek to avoid it?

Does the patient appear to be in reasonable touch with his surroundings and responsive to external stimuli? Is he able to maintain his attention or does he appear to be too easily diverted or distracted? If he is distractable is there any obvious reason for this and any pattern to it? Could he be experiencing hallucinations?

Can the patient sit still or does he have to keep getting up? If he sits still does he appear to find it difficult and seem restless or agitated? Is he generally responsive or unresponsive? If he is responsive, are his responses appropriate? Does he appear slowed down or speeded up? Does he make any particular gestures, exhibit any facial grimacing, perform any purposeful behaviours in an odd, stilted way (mannerisms), or carry out purposeless behaviours in a uniform way (stereotypies)?

What is his facial expression like? Is it devoid of feeling and movement? Does he appear agitated, perplexed, elated or sad?

How consistent is his behaviour? Does it change suddenly and unpredictably? Is there any reason for these changes?

Mood. Observation of the patient together with how he makes the interviewer feel should already have provided useful clues about the patient's mood. For example, when talking to a patient the interviewer may have found himself feeling sad. However, it is important that he checks how the patient is feeling by asking: 'How are you feeling in your spirits at the moment?'

The interviewer should also consider whether the patient's professed mood fits with what he has been saying, that is, is it appropriate or inappropriate? For example, a patient may report that he has felt 'terribly miserable' but appear cheerful when he says this. He may appear cheerful and even laugh as he says he has heard a voice telling him to murder his parents (inappropriate or incongruent affect).

Instead of appearing too high or low, tense and on edge, the patient's mood may appear flat. Indeed, he may complain that he can no longer exprience happiness and sadness as he did in the past (blunting of affect). Alternatively, his mood may be labile and change suddenly and frequently during the interview (lability of mood).

When enquiry about mood indicates depression, it is mandatory that the interviewer should determine if there are any other features of the mental state which suggest a high suicidal risk.

How low has he been feeling? Has he felt so low and miserable that he sees no point in going on? Has he contemplated taking his own life (suicidal ideas)? Has he made any plans (suicidal plans) and written a suicide note? Does he feel that the future is hopeless? How does he see himself as a person? Does he feel that he is of no use to anyone anymore (worthless) or that others would be better off if he were dead because he considers he has caused problems for them (feeling a burden)? Has he felt guilty in some way, even to the point of believing that he has committed a crime (feelings or delusions of guilt)? Is he worried about his physical health? Does he have fears or false beliefs that he is suffering from a fatal disease (hypochondriacal ideas or delusions)? Is he worried about his physical health? Does he have fears or false beliefs that he is suffering from a fatal disease (hypochondriacal ideas or delusions)? Has he ever felt that the world is such a terrible place that he and others close to him would be better off dead?

Has he got so low because of a recent bereavement? Is he still preoccupied with thoughts of the dead person? Is his intention to kill himself linked to a belief that this will enable him to join the deceased? Are his suicidal feelings related to the anniversary of the death or of another important date? Overall, how depressed does the patient appear (depth of depression)?

Replies to the initial probe about mood may reveal that the patient is feeling worried, anxious, tense or agitated. He should be asked to describe these feelings in detail and consider if anything triggers them. When the patient's mood appears flat he should be asked whether he has noticed any change in his ability to feel different emotions like sadness or happiness.

The interviewer should also consider whether the patient could be masking his true feelings.

Patient's speech

Stream. It is important that the interviewer notes how the patient talks. Does he speak in a uniform and regular way? Are there sudden and unexpected pauses? Is his speech slowed down or speeded up? Is there any pressure of thought? Is his speech clear? Is it slurred? Does he stammer or speak with a lisp?

Form. Does the patient say a lot or a little? Is his speech spontaneous? Does what he says seem a reasonable and logical response to the interviewer? Are his responses quick or slow? When he talks can he keep to the point or does it seem difficult for him to do so? Is it difficult to follow him? Is this because his speech is incoherent? Is it because there is little if any connection between consecutive thoughts? Such a lack of connection will become obvious if, as he should, the interviewer writes down verbatim examples of the patient's speech. He will then be able to decide if such 'thought disorder' is present. Does the patient seem to flit rapidly from one idea to the next (flight of ideas)? Does his speech contain any wholly new words (neologisms), rhymes or puns? Does he perseverate with particular ideas or phrases? Are his sentences grammatically constructed or not? Are there occasions when one thought sequence stops suddenly and a new unconnected sequence begins? Does his speech contain abstract ideas or is it concrete and dictated solely by obvious stimuli around him?

Content. The history taking and examination may have indicated already that the patient has particular worries and is suffering from free-floating anxiety, fears of specific objects, people or situations, obsessional ruminations and rituals, or suicidal ideas. If not, the interviewer may begin by asking: 'Have you any particular worries?' If the patient admits any such problems their nature should be clarified. He should also establish whether the patient can distract himself from these worries and whether they impair his day-to-day functioning. He will also find it useful to ask: 'Are there any situations you try to avoid — like going out alone, shopping, travelling on buses or meeting people?' If this reveals phobias their exact nature should be clarified and details obtained about the extent to which the patient takes steps to avoid these situations.

Probes like: 'Do you have any thoughts which keep coming into your mind? Do you try to resist them?' should elicit any ruminations. It is also worth asking: 'Do you ever find you have to do anything repeatedly — like checking that the light switches or taps are off — or cleaning something? How do you feel about it? How much does it interfere with your daily life?'

While the interview has been proceeding the interviewer will have been alert to any evidence of abnormal beliefs and experiences. Thus, is there any evidence that the patient holds a false belief (delusion) with conviction and against argument? Does it seem to arise out of his mood (secondary delusion) or did it arrive suddenly in a well-developed form (primary delusion)? How well developed are his delusions? How much is his behaviour influenced by them? Does he appear to be certain that something sinister is happening which will be harmful to him but does not know what exactly is happening (delusional mood)?

Has he attributed an abnormal significance to a normal percept (delusional perception)? Does he profess any overvalued ideas, that is, ideas such as a belief in witchcraft which are acquired from and shared by others? Does he believe that conversations between others and programmes on television or radio are referring especially to him (ideas of reference)? Does he believe that he is under the control of other forces or some external agency (ideas of influence)?

If such abnormal beliefs are not apparent, some general probes should be made as follows: 'How well have you been getting on with people? Do you ever feel that they are out to harm you in some way? Do you ever feel that your life has some special meaning or significance?'

Possession. The patient may complain that others are putting alien thoughts into his mind (thought insertion) or taking them out (thought withdrawal). He may believe that others know what he is thinking, even when he tries to keep his thoughts private (thought broadcasting). If such phenomena are not volunteered it is worth asking the patient: 'Do you ever feel that people are putting thoughts into your mind? Do they ever take them away? Can you keep your private thoughts secret from others?'

Abnormal perceptions. The patient's behaviour during the interview may suggest that he is experiencing auditory hallucinations. For example, he may keep turning his head towards a particular area of the room as though he has heard something. Enquiry about why he keeps turning his head may reveal that he is hearing voices which the interviewer is unable to hear (auditory hallucinations). When such hallucinations seem likely, their nature and content should be explored. Are they like real voices? Do they come from inside or outside the patient's head? Are they talking to him or each other? Are they pleasant, neutral or abusive? Do they comment on the patient's actions, carry on a conversation about him, or echo his thoughts aloud? Do they urge him to harm himself or others?

True hallucinations should be distinguished from hallucinations which the patient immediately or soon realises are the product of his own imagination (pseudohallucinations). Such pseudohallucinations often occur when the patient is falling asleep (hypnogogic) or waking up (hypnopompic). When hallucinations are not obvious, the patient should be asked: 'Have you had any odd, unusual or strange experiences lately? Have you heard anything unusual? Have you seen anything? Has there been any change in your sense of taste... or smell? What about touch? Have you noticed any strange sensations in your body?' If the patient has been hallucinating what exactly was the experience like? What is the patient's attitude to the hallucinations? Are they exciting or distressing? Can he account for them? Are they so distressing he finds them intolerable?

The patient may also complain that he feels unreal (depersonalisation) or finds everything around him unreal and dream-like (derealisation). He may state that he has recently been in a new situation but had a strong, albeit transient, feeling that he had been there before (*déjà vu*). Conversely, he may have been in a very familiar situation but had a strong feeling that he had never been there before (*jamais vu*). It may also be useful to enquire if objects have seemed any bigger (macropsia) or smaller (micropsia) than normal.

The interview may have revealed that the patient tends to misinterpret things. What matters here is whether the patient recognises this or attaches a delusional significance to it. For example, a woman suffering from a confusional state may perceive a doctor who approaches her with a syringe as a man with a knife who is about to murder her. Does she soon realise she is mistaken or believe she is about to be murdered?

Cognition. The cognitive state should be assessed in each patient. When organic brain disease is suspected, a more thorough examination should be conducted (Institute of Psychiatry 1978). The history may have suggested already that the patient has impaired memory. Otherwise he should be asked if he has noticed any problems with his memory and the nature of these clarified. He should then be asked if he minds if his memory is tested.

The interviewer should check if the patient is fully oriented in time, date and place; and record his answers. The patient should then be given a name and address to learn and asked to recall them at 3 and 5 minutes to test his short-term memory. If this suggests impairment this aspect of memory may be tested further by asking him to learn and recall pairs of words, like scissors and a pen, which have no logical connection. His immediate memory is tested by asking him to repeat an increasing number of digits first forwards then backwards to see how many he can remember. His memory and comprehension may be assessed by asking him to learn the Cowboy or Donkey story.

To test recent memory he should be asked when he was admitted to hospital and what has happened since then. His ability to attend and concentrate is judged both on his behaviour during the interview and his performance when asked to repeat the days of the week or months of the year backwards, and do the 'serial 7s' test. This requires the patient to subtract 7 from 100 and then continue to subtract 7 from the resulting number. Simple calculations may also be used to assess attention and concentration.

His general knowledge is judged by asking him to name the Queen, the Prime Minister and his predecessor, capitals of foreign countries, cities within Britain, and say what is currently in the news. His intelligence can then be judged by comparing his responses to what has been established about his scholastic and occupational achievements.

His attitude to his illness or problems should have been fully elicited in the first section of the history. If not, it should be explored here in the way recommended earlier.

Recording data

It is most important that the patient's mental state should be recorded carefully. Any abnormalities of behaviour which are observed should be noted in detail. Whenever the form or content of speech appears abnormal, verbatim examples should be recorded in the notes. Responses to the tests of cognition should also be noted.

Key interviewing skills

It is helpful to divide the psychiatric interview into six parts: the beginning; orienting the patient; obtaining the history; examining the mental state (and conducting a physical examination); the exposition; and termination.

Before the interviewer begins he should ensure that the setting is right. Talking to a patient across a desk or from a higher chair emphasises social distance and makes it harder for him to relax and confide. Chairs should, therefore, be of equal height and so placed that the interviewer and patient can sit comfortably and converse easily. They should neither be too close nor too far away. The interviewer should also try to ensure that he is not interrupted by others, by phone calls or his bleeper. When possible he should arrange for someone to take messages and interrupt only if it is urgent.

Beginning the interview

The interviewer should stand up as the patient enters the consulting room, establish eye contact, move towards the patient, greet him verbally with a clear 'Hello' or 'Good morning', using the patient's correct name and title, and shake hands.

Once the greeting is completed the interviewer should indicate clearly by words and a gesture of the hand where the patient should sit. He should then sit down himself, adopting a posture that conveys interest and friendliness. Thus he should lean slightly forward, look at the patient and smile. He should avoid extremes of posture such as lounging back in a casual manner or leaning so far forward that he infringes the patient's personal space.

Once they are both comfortable, the interviewer should introduce himself by name and explain his status. For example, he might say: 'I am Dr. Brown, Dr. Johnson's registrar'.

Orienting the patient

Patients who are seeing a psychiatrist for the first time are often apprehensive. They may be uncertain about the reasons for referral and resent being sent to a psychiatrist. They may fear that if they disclose what is troubling them the psychiatrist will judge them 'mad' and want to lock them up. They may feel ashamed that they have not been able to cope without seeking help and worry about the stigma of psychiatric illness. They may also find it hard to decide whether to disclose personal matters lest they be revealed to others. They will have little idea of what the psychiatrist wants to cover or how long he has at his disposal. They may fear that they will be overheard or interrupted.

The interviewer should, therefore, begin by explaining the exact purpose of his interview. For example, 'I would like to find out as much as possible about your present problems in the time we have available'. This emphasis on current problems is made in the hope that it will encourage the patient to talk about them rather than previous difficulties or episodes. The interviewer should next indicate how long he has got, since this helps the patient make sure he mentions his problems within the time: 'We have about 45 minutes if we need it.' He should explain that

he wishes to take notes to help him remember what was discussed, but add that these will be confidential.

He should then ask if the patient finds what he proposes acceptable. He should do this in a way that indicates he is genuinely interested in the patient's viewpoint: 'Are you happy with what I propose to do?' He must give the patient time to reply.

The patient may indicate that the time proposed is too short. The interviewer can respond by saying: 'Well, you could be right. If we do not have enough time today we can meet again next week. Is that all right?'. The patient may object to the interviewer's taking notes and the reasons for this can be explored. Any worries or resentments about referral may also be voiced at this time and can be discussed and usually defused.

Finally, the interviewer should ensure that the patient is as much at ease as possible before he pursues the history. He should be alert to any signs that the patient is uneasy. If the patient still appears worried the interviewer might comment: 'You seem worried.' The patient might then reply by saying he is afraid of being interrupted or overheard, or perhaps that he believes there is a plot to harm him and is afraid the interviewer may be part of it.

Obtaining the history

The interviewer should begin this part of the interview by asking an open-ended question which will encourage the patient to mention his main problems. Thus, the interviewer may ask: 'Can you begin by telling me what problems brought you to hospital?' He should be aware of the tendency of many patients to begin by explaining the likely causes of their problems rather than their nature. For example, a woman referred for advice about further treatment of her depressive illness responded to this initial question by launching into a detailed account of how she became divorced. The interviewer then had to interrupt and say: 'What you say is very helpful but I am still not clear what changes have occurred in you that led to your being here.' The patient immediately responded by saying: 'I've been so miserable. I've got no interest in anything. I just can't seem to get going.' Without such an interruption and redirection much time would have been wasted.

Verbal clues

Usually, the patient responds by giving a series of helpful verbal clues about his main problems, as in the following sequence:

Interviewer: What has brought you to see me?
Patient: I've not been right since I had the baby. I've been ever so down. I've felt on pins all the time. The slightest thing and I blow my top. I've been crying for no reason. It's just not like me. I'm frightened I'm going mad. I'm not sure I can trust myself any more.

The interviewer's problem is to take advantage of all these clues and yet still encourage the patient to tell her story in her own words. What he must do is try to note each clue down on his pad and wait until the utterance is completed. He should then acknowledge that he has heard each clue by saying: 'As I understand it, you feel you have not been well since you had your baby. You've felt down, been liable to blow your top and been weepy. You have worried that you are going mad and are not sure you can trust yourself. Is that right?'

The interviewer should then cover the possibility that the patient has other complaints by saying: 'I'll come back to these in a moment but can I ask whether you've noticed anything else wrong? Are you sure?' Such screening questions are vital if all the patient's problems are to be identified correctly.

Once the main problems have been identified in this way and the interviewer has checked whether there have been any other problems he has to decide which problems to ask the patient about first. He can best do this by recapping the problems and asking: 'Which of these has been troubling you the most?' He can begin with this problem and then work through the others systematically.

Initial clarification

The next step is for him to encourage the patient to tell him what she meant by each clue to a problem area. For example, 'You say you have been especially troubled by your blowing your top. What exactly do you mean by "blowing your top"?' He can then encourage the patient to continue talking by saying such things as 'Go on; tell me more about it, what exactly happened?' This is called verbal facilitation.

He can also use non-verbal methods of facilitation. These include nodding his head, looking attentive and smiling. The interviewer may feel that it is difficult to do this and take notes. The secret is to make sure that he looks at the patient at the end of each utterance. He can then indicate whether or not he wishes the patient to continue talking.

A major difficulty facing the interviewer is how to ensure that he clarifies and follows up each of the problems he has been cued to. An occasional glance at his notes should indicate which ones still have to be followed up. The aim of clarification is to encourage the patient to paint, in words, as vivid a picture of his experiences as possible. The interviewer should be wary of jargon words like 'nerves', 'nervous breakdown' and 'depression', for he must not assume that he knows what they mean until he has asked the patient. Instead he should check in the following way: 'You say you have had a depression. What exactly do you mean by depression? Can you tell me more of what it felt like?'

Further clarification

As the interviewer begins to sense what the patient has been experiencing he can try to further his understanding by sharing what he is thinking. Such educated guesses (understanding hypotheses) should be offered in a tentative (negotiating) style. Their use shows the patient that the interviewer is keen to understand him but is open to elaboration, correction or refutation.

Interviewer: It sounds as though you find these voices very unpleasant.
Patient: I don't think I can take much more.
Interviewer: How do you mean?
Patient: I feel my head's exploding and there only seems one way out.
Interviewer: What way?
Patient: To kill myself.
Interviewer: As we are talking I get the feeling you are miserable.
Patient: It's not so much miserable as angry and frustrated.

Empathic statements also promote further disclosure of experiences and feelings:

Interviewer: From what you say, losing a breast was an awful experience.
Patient: It was devastating, absolutely devastating.

The interviewer is now into territory which is emotionally distressing. How should he proceed? He should express a clear wish to explore her responses further but also signal that he will only continue if the patient agrees (negotiation).

Interviewer: You say it was devastating. Can you bear to tell me in what way?
Patient: I know it will upset me. But if I don't tell someone, I'll go out of my mind?
Interviewer: So can you tell me?

If the patient is recounting an extremely painful experience (for example, a fatal accident or sexual abuse) it is important to advise the patient to signal that if it becomes too painful the interviewer will stop exploring that issue. However, the aim, whenever possible, is to help patients describe not only their experiences but talk about *and* express the associated feelings. This conveys a willingness to get alongside and understand the true nature and extent of their suffering.

If the patient permits exploration, the key question is how long it should continue for. The answer is until the interviewer feels he has fully understood what the patient has experienced. Then permission should be sought to move on:

Interviewer: As I understand it, your mastectomy has left you feeling ugly and repulsive and also terrified that the cancer may come back. Is there anything you would like to add?
Patient: No.
Interviewer: Is it okay then if we move on?
Patient: Yes.

Control

Interviewers usually have little difficulty in getting their patients to talk but often experience problems in exerting control. Control is optimal when the interviewer is giving the patient enough time to respond to any question but does not allow him to take too long or get off the point.

An interviewer can only control a patient in a constructive way if he knows how to do this. Interrupting too quickly or not at all are equally unhelpful. The interviewer should have begun by agreeing with the patient that his main task was to identify any current problems. It should then be clear to him when the patient in moving on to irrelevant matters. When this occurs the interviewer should interrupt gently but firmly, and first check that what is being said is likely to be relevant to an understanding of the patient's present problems. For example:

Interviewer: What you say is very interesting, but is it relevant to your present problems?
Patient: No, not really.
Interviewer: Well, it would be helpful if we could return to what you were saying earlier about feeling very fearful. Is that all right? We can come back to this later.
Patient: Yes, fine.

Interviewers often fear that such interruptions will alienate their patients. In reality they usually welcome such direction and are happy to oblige because it indicates the information that the interviewer needs. Sometimes, a patient with an obsessional personality may insist on telling his story in his own lengthy and pedantic way. It is still worthwhile attempting to see if he can be encouraged to stick to more relevant areas and give his history more quickly.

Precision

Encouraging patients to be precise about the dates and exact nature of key events and experiences is important. It reduces the risk of falsely attributing an illness to an unconnected event. It also makes it more likely that the patient will connect with the feelings associated with a key event.

Interviewer: You say you lost your mother last year? When exactly was it
Patient: August.
Interviewer: Could you tell me what day it was?
Patient: The 23rd.
Interviewer: Can you bear to tell me what happened on the 23rd?

Such precision will reveal how distressed the patient still is about her mother's death.

The interviewer should be particularly alert to any uncertainties or inconsistencies in the information given and be prepared to disentangle these as soon as they arise. Thus, he might say: 'I'm still a bit confused about when your problem started. Can I try and get this clear before we go any further?'

Precision is also more likely if the patient is asked to provide actual examples of the problems he is discussing, for example: 'You say you have been sleeping badly over the last week. Can you describe a typical night from the time you went to bed until you got up in the morning?'

Non-verbal clues

During an interview patients may give hints of important problems or feelings by changes in tone, facial expression or posture. The interviewer has to be alert to this possibility and pursue such clues by commenting on them. Thus, he might say: 'You seem angry' or 'You look upset'; 'You seemed weepy when I asked you about your father.' It is all too easy to miss such clues or let them pass without comment.

For example, when a woman complained of abdominal pain and was asked if anyone in her family had similar trouble, she mentioned that her father had died of cancer of the stomach 10 months ago. As she did so she became very distressed and tearful. The interviewer noted her distress but elected not to comment on it because he did not want to upset her further. He continued the interview in a way that indicated he was preoccupied with possible explanations of her pain. Yet had he said 'You seemed upset when you talked of your father', she would have disclosed that she had not been able to accept his death, and that the pains had begun after his death and were identical to those he had complained of. This would have prompted him to consider the correct diagnosis of atypical grief.

Question style

The interviewer should use open-ended questions in the early part of the interview to establish the patient's complaints. Once he has followed up and clarified these he should begin to use more specific probes.

He should avoid putting questions in a way that presupposes an answer or limits the information given. Thus, he should ask: 'How have you been sleeping?' rather then 'Have you been waking early?', and 'Have you noticed any change in your appetite?' instead of 'Have you stopped eating?'

He should avoid asking multiple-choice questions like 'Was the depression worse in the morning or the evening?' since it is possible that the depression showed no diurnal variation or peaked both in the morning and the evening. He should avoid putting several questions at once, such as 'When you say you have been very miserable, was that at any particular time of the day? How have your sleep and appetite been? What about your weight?' The patient will usually answer only one element of such a question and the interviewer may fail to realise that he has obtained no response to the other elements.

Recapitulation

Once the interviewer has completed his history and examined the mental (and physical) state he should summarise what he considers are the patient's main problems in the following way: 'I would just like to check that I've got things right. As I understand it, you are convinced that there is a plot to harm you. People in blue Ford Cortina cars are keeping a close eye on you and relaying messages to the KGB. You have become so worried you have thought of throwing bricks at these cars. Is that right?'

The interviewer should then ask a final screening question: 'Before I explain what I think is wrong, is there anything that you would like to add to what you have told me? Are you sure?' This minimises the chance that he will miss something important, either that he has forgotten to enquire about or that the patient has not yet had the courage to mention.

Exposition

The interviewer should next explain what he thinks is wrong and what he plans to do. He should explain in plain English. He should present information about the diagnosis first and check that the patient has understood him before he proceeds to discuss treatment. For example:

Interviewer: I am sure you are suffering from a depressive illness. This is why you have felt so low and not been able to eat or sleep. It is also why you got so tired and irritable. Do you want to ask any questions about it?
Patient: What has caused it?
Interviewer: Well, it's clear you became depressed after your father died. I think the shock of that in some way upset your body chemistry. That's what caused you to feel so low.

The interviewer should then separately outline each component of treatment and again encourage the patient to ask questions. For example:

Interviewer: We will need to do two things. First, I am going to prescribe some tablets, an anti-depressant. This should restore your body chemistry to normal and help you feel more cheerful again. Is that all right?

The tablets are called amitryptiline. I am going to give you a dose of 75 mg at night to begin with. It will not shift your depression immediately. That will take a week or so, so do persevere with the treatment. The tablets may cause some unwanted effects. For example, they may make your mouth dry or make you feel sleepy to begin with. If you drive or handle machinery you should be especially careful. If possible it would be better if you did not do so for the first few days. You should also be very careful with alcohol since it may affect you more than it usually does.

Could you just repeat back what I have told you so that I can check that you have got it right.

If you like I can write it down for you. Is there anything else you would like to know?

The second thing I'd like to do is talk with you again about your father to see if I can help you get over his death. I would like to do this in 2 weeks' time. Is that all right? I can then also check how well the tablets are working. If you have any worries in the meantime, please ring me.

Termination

The interviewer should finally make a clear concluding statement: 'Well, if you have no more questions, I think we should finish now. I'll see you again in 2 weeks' time.'

Validation

Importantly, all the skills advocated here promote psychological disclosure and trust. But there are behaviours to avoid because they block disclosure. These include: normalisation (explaining emotional distress away as normal and to be expected); premature reassurance (giving reassurance before the problem has been fully understood); false reassurance (implying a much better outcome than there will be in reality); switching (changing from a topic before it has been fully understood); and the use of leading or closed questions. All the above behaviours serve to keep the interview at a safe level. In the following examples a patient was interviewed separately by two trainee psychiatrists. One had no additional training in interviewing skills while the other had received training.

Untrained

Interviewer: You said you were scared of walking on pavements with lots of rubbish. Is that because you're frightened by being contaminated?
Patient: Yes.
Interviewer: Any other things that scare you?

Trained

Interviewer: So you avoid walking on payments with lots of rubbish. Do you mind telling me (negotiation) exactly why that is (clarification) ?
Patient: I am scared.
Interviewer: What exactly scares you (clarification)?
Patient: That I'll pick up something very harmful.
Interviewer: What kind of harmful thing (clarification)?
Patient: An amoeba-like creature — I'm worried it would get into one of my feet.
Interviewer: And how might it harm you?
Patient (very distressed): I'm terrified it would travel up my body and enter my brain and destroy me.

IMPROVING INTERVIEWING SKILLS

Like other clinicians, psychiatrists vary in their interviewing skills and tend to use a consistent but inflexible style (Cox et al 1981) which is relatively insensitive to their patients' needs. They often miss key clues and ask leading, lengthy or multiple questions. Psychiatrists in training experience difficulty in establishing a productive relationship, listening properly and handling emotionally loaded material (Janek et al 1979, Harrison et al 1991). These deficiencies should not be surprising since most psychiatrists were, until recently, trained by the apprenticeship method. Thus, their interviewing skills were judged on what they wrote in the case notes and reported on ward rounds. Yet, these are unreliable indicators of the actual skill level. So, the key question is how best to overcome these problems and improve interviewing skills.

Training methods

Training will be effective if it includes the following components.

An appropriate model

The interviewer should first be given a detailed handout which explains the areas to be covered, the questions which should be asked, and the skills which should be used. The scheme described here is a suggested model of how to conduct a psychiatric interview and mental state examination.

It then helps to watch an expert covering the key areas and using the required skills. He can do this by watching an expert conduct live interviews via closed-circuit television or by watching demonstration videotapes specially made for the purpose.

Practice under controlled conditions

Once he has a clear grasp of what is required the trainee should practise a specific and limited aspect of the psychiatric interview and examination. Thus, he might begin by obtaining a history of the key complaints and proceed on a subsequent occasion to practise obtaining the personal history. Alternatively, he might practise examining the mental state. For practice he should choose patients who are likely to be helpful rather than difficult. He should also set himself a time limit since this will reveal how well he handles time constraints and whether he uses his time efficiently while still maintaining good rapport. He should record some of these practice interviews on videotape or audiotape so that he has an accurate and objective record of how he performed to review later. Patients are usually perfectly willing to cooperate in such practice interviews if the reason is properly explained to them. For example, 'I would like to talk with you for 15 minutes to find out what's been troubling you. I would like to record it so that I can see later if I was talking to you in the right kind of way. Is that all right?' A simple cassette tape recorder is all that is necessary for such recording.

Feedback

Feedback by videotape replay has the advantage over audiotape in that it provides valuable information about non-verbal aspects of interviewing and examination. However, feedback by either videotape or audiotape have been found to be very effective in helping ensure that the essential skills are acquired and maintained (Maguire et al 1986).

To be effective the interviewer must have some systematic way of assessing his performance. He will find it helpful to use a rating scale. These commonly consist of sets of 5-point (0–4) scales which require the rater to indicate how well he did in terms of eliciting specific items of information and whether he used the required skills (Maguire et al 1978, Verby et al 1979). Rating scales for assessing examination of the mental state and the exposition have yet to be developed.

Supervision

The interviewer will gain considerably from learning the model, practising aspects of it and scrutinising his own performance. However, after initial progress he is unlikely to improve further unless a supervisor is present. Providing the supervisor understands the skills to be taught he can help the interviewer better to identify his strengths and weaknesses and make further progress. The presence of a supervisor also makes this training more enjoyable and less time is wasted through unnecessary repetition.

Nothing is lost by carrying out this supervision with small groups of trainees rather than individually. Trainees can help each other learn from recordings of their practice interviews, especially if a supervisor is present. Supervision may be enhanced by asking the patient to comment on particular points in the interview or examination. It is also useful to have the same patient interviewed by two or more interviewers. Patients usually accept this and it reveals how much the outcome of an interview is determined by the interviewer's rather than by the patient's behaviours.

CONCLUSION

Most psychiatrists, like other clinicians, are less proficient in their essential clinical skills than they realise. Yet, these skills are central to psychiatric practice and teaching, and feedback methods are available which will improve them both in the short and longer term (Maguire et al 1986). Moreover, psychiatrists who are so trained are better able to recognise psychiatric illness in their patients (Goldberg et al 1980, Maguire et al 1990). The growing interest in the application of these methods within postgraduate training is, therefore, to be welcomed. But if reliance is still placed on the apprenticeship method the trainee should audit his or her skills by the use of a tape recorder when interviewing a new patient.

REFERENCES

Cox A, Hopkins K, Rutter M 1981 Psychiatric interviewing techniques. II Naturalistic study: eliciting factual information. British Journal of Psychiatry 138: 283

Goldberg D P, Smith C, Steele J J, Spivey L 1980 Training family doctors to recognise psychiatric illness with increased accuracy. Lancet ii: 521

Harrison J A, Creed F H, Gask L, Goldberg D P, Maguire G P, Tantum D, O'Dowd T 1991 Improving the interview skills of psychiatry trainees: evaluation of a teaching programme. In press

Institute of Psychiatry 1978 Notes on eliciting and recording clinical information. Oxford University Press, Oxford

Janek W, Burra E, Leichner P 1979 Teaching interviewing skills by encountering patients. Journal of Medical Education 54: 402

Maguire P, Roe P, Goldberg D et al 1978 The value of feedback in teaching interviewing skills to medical students. Psychological Medicine 8: 695

Maguire P, Tait A, Brooke M, Thomas C, Sellwood R 1980 The effects of counselling on the psychiatric morbidity after mastectomy. British Medical Journal ii: 1454

Maguire P, Fairbairn S, Fletcher C 1986 Consultation skills of young doctors I. Benefits of feedback training in interviewing as students persist. British Medical Journal 292: 1573

Verby J E, Holden P, Davis R H 1979 Peer review of consultations in primary care: the use of audiovisual recordings. British Medical Journal i: 686

14. Diagnosis and classification

R. E. Kendell

INTRODUCTION

Attitudes to psychiatric classification have undergone a revolution in the last generation. In the 1950s and 1960s, psychiatric diagnoses were held in low esteem. Their reliability was known to be low, it was becoming apparent that key diagnostic terms like 'schizophrenia' had different meanings in different parts of the world, and influential American writers like Rogers and Menninger were arguing that psychiatry would be better off without any diagnostic categories at all. Although the current situation is very different and it is no longer necessary to defend the importance of diagnoses, it is, nonetheless, important to understand why classification is necessary, and to appreciate the ways in which it may be harmful as well as helpful to a patient to attach a diagnostic label to him.

THE INEVITABILITY OF CLASSIFICATION

Every patient possesses characteristics of three kinds:

1. Those he shares with all other patients
2. Those he shares with some other patients, but not all
3. Those which are unique to him.

Insofar as the first of these three categories is dominant, classification or subdivision is pointless and unnecessary. All patients have fundamentally similar problems and even if there are a few superficial differences between them they all require the same treatment. Insofar as the third category is dominant, classification is impossible. Learning from experience and useful communication with others are also impossible. For if every patient is different from every other we can learn nothing useful from textbooks, from colleagues, or the accumulated wisdom of our predecessors. Indeed, we cannot even learn from our own personal experience if there are no significant similarities between our last patient and the next. Our attention has, therefore, to be focused on the second category. What is more, as soon as one begins to recognise features that are common to some patients but not all, and to distinguish those which are important from those, like eye colour, which are not, one is classifying them, whether one recognises it or not. And if we have more than one treatment available, as we have, and wish to use these different treatments with maximum efficacy, we must distinguish between one type of patient and another. Otherwise we are reduced to allocating different patients to different treatments by whim or the throw of dice. (Those who argued that diagnostic categories should be abandoned did indeed believe that all patients required the same treatment — the 'moral regime' of the asylum for Neumann and Prichard in the 19th century and psychotherapy for Rogers and Menninger in the 20th.)

A distinction between different kinds of mental disorder is therefore inevitable. The only open issues are whether this classification is going to be public or private, stable or unstable, reliable or unreliable, valid or invalid. Classifications of mental disorders may well be less useful than classifications of, say, cardio-vascular disorders or gastrointestinal disorders, for they are still largely based on differences in symptomatology rather than on differences in aetiology, but the only viable option in this situation is to try to improve the classification we possess. It cannot simply be abandoned, and the idea that a diagnosis can, or should, be replaced by a formulation is based on a fundamental misunderstanding of the nature of both. A formulation which takes account of the unique features of the patient and his environment, and the interaction between them, is often essential for any real understanding of his predicament, and for planning effective treatment, but it is unusable in any situation in which populations or groups of patients need to be considered. The essential feature of any population is that its members share at least one important characteristic in common. The essence of a diagnosis is that it embodies as many as possible of those characteristics which are common to several different patients (i.e. category 2 above), just as it is the essence of a formulation to embody those which are unique to the individual (category 3 above). Formulation and diagnosis are equally necessary, but for quite different purposes.

The shortcomings and disadvantages of diagnoses

If some form of categorisation or subdivision of mental disorders is inescapable, as it is, it is essential that we appreciate the limitations and potential ill effects of allocating patients to diagnostic categories. In the first place, psychiatric diagnoses are often a very inadequate means of conveying what the clinician regards as the essence of his patient's predicament, and the better he knows the patient the stronger this feeling becomes. To say that a woman has a depressive illness does not explain why she became depressed or how she came to medical attention, nor does it establish whether she is on the brink of committing suicide or merely despondent and dejected. She may have been ill for anything from a few weeks to several years and may require electroconvulsive therapy (ECT) or antidepressant drugs or psychotherapy. Another important problem is that many patients do not conform to the tidy stereotyped descriptions found in textbooks. They possess some, but not all, of the characteristic features of two or three different diagnostic categories and so have to be allocated more or less arbitrarily to whichever syndrome they seem to resemble most closely. As a result, disagreements about diagnosis are commonplace and hybrid terms like schizoaffective and borderline state have to be coined and pressed into service.

Many psychiatric diagnoses also have pejorative connotations. Terms like hysteric, neurotic, schizophrenic and psychopath are sometimes used as thinly disguised expressions of contempt, and even when this is not so the aura surrounding such terms can very easily have harmful effects on the behaviour and attitudes of other people, and so on the patient's own attitude to himself. Attaching a name to a condition may also create a spurious impression of understanding. To say that a patient is suffering from schizophrenia actually says little more than that he has some puzzling but familiar symptoms which have often been encountered before in other patients. To some psychiatrists, however, the impressive neologism 'schizophrenia' implies that the patient has a disease which

was discovered by Kraepelin, or perhaps by Bleuler, which is fundamentally different from other diseases like manic–depressive illness and whose cause will eventually be elucidated by medical science. Historically, of course, it has been very convenient for doctors to be able to conceal their ignorance from their patients by clothing it in Greek neologisms, but all too often they also deceive themselves. They 'reify' the diagnostic concept and treat the 'disease' instead of trying to relieve their patients' symptoms, anxieties and disabilities.

Diagnoses as concepts

It is important never to lose sight of the fact that all diseases and diagnostic categories are simply concepts. Schizophrenia and manic depressive insanity were not discovered by either Kraepelin or Bleuler. It is closer to the truth to say that they were invented by them, and we continue to use the terms nearly a century later only because the concepts they represent make it easier to comprehend the variegated phenomena of psychotic illness that it would be otherwise. The same is true, of course, of tuberculosis and migraine. To assert, as Szasz does, that 'there is no such thing as schizophrenia' is as trite an assertion as it would be to point out that there is no such thing as tuberculosis or poverty. None of these are objects; none has mass, velocity or position in space. All three are concepts which may in time lose their usefulness and pass out of use, as earlier concepts like phthisis and monomania have already done. But if this happens it will be because they have been replaced by other more useful concepts, not because of any sudden realisation that they do not exist. And, of course, to tell a bewildered patient who has been told he is suffering from schizophrenia that there is no such thing does not remove his disabilities, or prevent hallucinatory voices from tormenting him, any more than a man whose lungs have been destroyed by the tubercle bacillus would be prevented from dying by being told there was no such thing as tuberculosis.

Classification on the basis of symptoms

It is widely agreed that classifications of diseases should, wherever possible, be based on aetiology. This is so simply because physicians have learnt by experience that aetiological classifications are almost invariably more useful than others. Classifications of infections based on the identity of the infecting organism are, for example, more useful than those based on purely clinical phenomena — the patient's fever, tachycardia, malaise and limb pains, the appearance of his tongue and the fetor on his breath — because they provide more information about treatment, prognosis and the risk to others. Unfortunately, apart from a few conditions like delirium tremens, general paralysis of the insane (GPI) and Wernicke's encephalopathy, the aetiology of most psychiatric disorders is still unknown, or all that is known for certain is that both genetic and environmental factors are involved. For this reason, most contemporary classifications of psychiatric disorders are largely based on clinical symptoms, a term which is usually assumed to include abnormalities of subjective experience elicited by questioning and abnormalities of behaviour observed by the examiner or described to him by others, in addition to the symptoms the patient actually complains of.

In all branches of medicine diseases usually start by being defined by their clinical symptoms, largely because these are the overt manifestations of illness. They are the reason for the patient seeking medical attention in the first place, or being identified as ill by other people. But in most other medical disciplines, apart perhaps from neurology, this is no longer so. As their aetiology has slowly been elucidated they have come to be defined instead by the presence of some more fundamental characteristic — a distinctive morbid anatomy perhaps, or an infective agent or a biochemical defect. Phthisis, for example, which was originally defined by its symptoms and clinical course, became pulmonary tuberculosis, defined by a characteristic histology and the presence of the mycobacterium tuberculi, when it became clear that this organism was ultimately responsible for the symptoms; and myxoedema, originally defined by the patient's complaints and appearance, became hypothyroidism, defined by an abnormally low level of circulating thyroxine, when it was established that the syndrome was a consequence of thyroid deficiency. A few conditions, like migraine, dystonia deformans and spasmodic torticollis, are still defined by their symptoms, but during the last 100 years these have dwindled to a small minority. We assume that the same transition will eventually take place for psychiatric disorders also, as their aetiology is slowly unravelled, but so far this has only occurred for a few conditions like Alzheimer's disease and GPI. The majority are still defined by their clinical features. In Scadding's terminology their defining characteristic is still their syndrome (Scadding 1963).

This state of affairs has a number of important consequences. Decisions about the presence or absence of symptoms are relatively unreliable; and, because few psychiatric illnesses have pathognomonic symptoms, most conditions have to be defined by the presence of some or most of a group of symptoms rather than by the presence of one key symptom. In the jargon of nosology they are *polythetic* rather than *monothetic*. This invites ambiguity and lowers reliability still further unless operational definitions are adopted (see below). Another important consequence is that most psychiatric diagnoses can never be confirmed or refuted, for there is no external criterion to appeal to. If two clinicians disagree about whether a patient is suffering from Pick's disease or Alzheimer's disease their disagreement can eventually be resolved by post mortem examination of the brain, for the defining characteristic of both conditions is its histology. But if two clinicians disagree about whether a patient is suffering from a schizophrenic or an affective illness no comparable criterion is available, for both schizophrenic and affective disorders are defined by their clinical syndromes. There is therefore no way of resolving the disagreement except by appeal to authority. One can only conclude either that the two clinicians have elicited different symptoms, or that they have different concepts (or are using different definitions) of schizophrenia and affective illness.

For these and other reasons it has often been suggested that symptoms should be ignored and a new classification developed on an entirely different basis. Psychoanalysts have frequently advocated a classification based on psychodynamic defence mechanisms and stages of libidinal development. In the 1950s, clinical psychologists extolled the advantages of a classification based on scores on batteries of cognitive and projective tests. More recently, learning theorists have argued that we should classify patients on the basis of a comprehensive analysis of their total behavioural repertoire. In principle all of these approaches are perfectly legitimate. In practice, however, none of them has ever progressed beyond the stage of advocacy. Although a series of different professional groups has, each in turn, proposed new classifications based on the mechanisms, scores or behaviours they themselves were most interested in, none has ever made a serious attempt to develop, test and use the new classification they were advocating. It is likely that a classification based on psychodynamic defence mechanisms would be hamstrung by the low reliability common to all inferential judgements, that one based on cognitive and projective test results would yield even fewer useful prognostic distinctions than one based on symptoms, and that any classification aspiring to be based on an analysis of the patient's total behavioural repertoire would simply prove to be impracticable, but one can only suspect these things because such classifications have never been developed.

Two other alternatives are sometimes proposed — classification on the basis of treatment response and classification on the basis of the course or outcome of the illness. Unfortunately, neither is feasible. The fatal weakness of the treatment response proposal is that there are few if any specific treatments in psychiatry. Depressive, schizophrenic and manic illnesses may all respond to ECT; schizophrenic and manic illnesses both respond to neuroleptics; depressions and anxiety states both respond to cognitive psychotherapy; and so on. Worse still, these therapies are not mutually exclusive. The patient who responds to ECT often responds equally well to a neuroleptic. In any case, the fact that two disorders respond to the same treatment does not imply that they share the same aetiology. Depression, panic attacks and nocturnal enuresis all respond to imipramine, and bruises, dysmenorrhoea, rheumatoid arthritis and rheumatic fever all respond to aspirin. Classification on the basis of outcome is equally impracticable, though for rather different reasons. One of the main functions of a diagnosis is to indicate the need for treatment, and the relative merits of different therapies. But if outcome was the defining characteristic one would, logically, have to wait until the outcome was known before making the diagnosis and therefore knowing which treatment to use. In any case most disorders, in psychiatry as in other branches of medicine, can have a wide range of outcomes. The fact that the patient recovered within a few weeks does not prove that he was suffering from chickenpox rather than smallpox, it merely makes it more likely. It is sometimes assumed that Kraepelin's classification, or at least his distinction between dementia praecox and manic depressive insanity, was based on long-term outcome, but this is a misunderstanding. Kraepelin certainly emphasised the difference in the lifetime course of his two great rubrics, and perhaps subdivided the functional psychoses in the way that he did in order to maximise the difference in outcome between dementia praecox and manic depressive insanity. But he used outcome as a validating criterion (i.e. as evidence that his two rubrics were fundamentally different disorders), not as a defining characteristic. Otherwise, when patients with dementia praecox recovered completely he would automatically have changed their diagnosis.

As things stand, therefore, we have no choice but to use a classification which is largely based on symptoms, despite its shortcomings and imperfections, because no practical alternative has yet been developed.

THE DIAGNOSTIC INTERVIEW

So far, we have discussed why psychiatric disorders have to be classified and why that classification is largely based on symptoms. We have also noted that all diagnoses are arbitrary concepts, liable to be altered or discarded as circumstances change; and that psychiatric diagnoses are particularly likely to be misunderstood and misused. We must now consider the important practical implications of these decisions: in particular, how to elicit the patient's symptoms as completely and as reliably as possible, and how to make the appropriate diagnosis when this has been done. As the general principles of psychiatric interviewing have been described in detail in the previous chapter, only matters bearing specifically on diagnostic interviews need be discussed here.

The conduct of the interview

Traditionally, psychiatrists, like other physicians, have usually detected symptoms by holding a free-ranging interview with the patient, and sometimes with his relatives also, and have assumed that the symptoms they elicited were present and that those they failed to elicit were absent. Unfortunately, these happy assumptions are unwarranted, as the many reliability studies carried out in the 1950s quickly revealed. A well-known study of the reliability of clinical ratings made under ordinary National Health Service working conditions illustrates the scale of the problem. A series of 90 patients referred to an English mental hospital were each re-interviewed by one of two research psychiatrists a few days after being seen as out-patients or on a domiciliary consultation by one of three consultants. All five of these interviewers recorded the presence or absence of 24 key symptoms in each patient. Despite having discussed their criteria for rating these items beforehand, the average 'positive percentage agreement' between the first and second interviewers was only 46% (Kreitman et al 1961). In other words, when one psychiatrist recorded a symptom as present there was less than a 50:50 chance of his colleague agreeing with him.

Many factors contribute to this low reliability. There are behavioural differences between one interviewer and another. They ask different questions, show interest and probe further in different places, establish different sorts of relationship with the patient, and so on. Their preconceptions are also important. If two interviewers are expecting to find different symptoms both may succeed in fulfilling their expectations by means of subtle differences in the wording of their questions, and in the way in which they interpret ambiguous replies. Finally, important conceptual differences are often involved. Common terms like 'anxiety', 'delusion' and 'thought disorder' may be used in rather different ways by different psychiatrists without their being aware of the fact, and even when there is no disagreement over the meaning of a term, there is often disagreement over the extent to which graded characteristics like worry or tension have to be present to justify a positive rating.

Because of these problems, unstructured interviewing methods are no longer used for research purposes. Instead a variety of 'structured' or 'standardised' interviews are employed. These specify not only, as rating scales do, the way in which symptoms are recorded, but also the manner in which they are elicited. Definitions, implicit or explicit, are provided for each item, and subject to varying degrees of flexibility, the questions the patient is asked, and their order, are predetermined and ratings made serially as the interview progresses rather than collectively at the end. Several of these diagnostic instruments, including the Present State Examination (Wing et al 1974) and the Diagnostic Interview Schedule (Robins et al 1981) are described in Chapter 9, and with such instruments trained raters achieve considerably higher reliability than is possible under ordinary clinical conditions.

Structured interviews of this kind are generally unsuitable for ordinary clinical purposes, mainly because they are not sufficiently flexible. The need to cover a wide range of symptomatology makes them either too long or too sketchy, and they do not permit that rapid focusing on the patient's main difficulties that is the essence of a good assessment interview. Even so, much of the discipline involved in structured interviewing can be incorporated into any information-gathering interview. Most of the principles involved are simple enough, even self-evident, though this does not stop them being flouted, even by experienced clinicians who ought to know better. The art of interviewing can only be learnt by practice, and by observing others and being observed by them. The part that textbooks can play is very limited, though the little booklet produced by the Institute of Psychiatry (1987) provides some helpful advice on content, and on the format of case notes. The following suggestions and observations may serve to illustrate some of the main principles governing the so-called 'diagnostic interview':

1. Start by giving the patient free rein to describe his problems as he sees them, even if you think he is rambling off the point, but be prepared to control the topic of conversation more and more as time goes on, and if need be to end up asking the string of questions to which you want answers and which he has not yet answered spontaneously.

2. Although it is useful for trainees to take exhaustive histories from a few patients early in their training, working steadily through a set sequence of topics, this approach is not feasible in ordinary clinical practice and is probably undesirable. After hearing the patient's initial complaints the interviewer has to concentrate on those parts of the mental state and history which are most likely to be relevant. Knowing which these are is probably the most important of the skills acquired by experience.

3. Symptoms which are complained of spontaneously are always more convincing than those elicited only by direct questioning. A surprising amount of accurate and relevant information can often be obtained by letting the patient tell his own story and merely interjecting an occasional 'Can you tell me more about that?' or 'Can you explain what you mean by ...?'

4. The initial questions on any topic should always be as wide and open-ended as possible. For example, if you want to know if a patient has early morning wakening always start by asking 'How have you been sleeping recently?' not 'Have you been waking up earlier than usual?' Often one is eventually forced to ask direct questions, like, for example, 'Have you ever had the feeling that someone was trying to hypnotise you?' but if so little significance can be attached to an affirmative answer *unless* the patient can also provide a clear description of the experience or situation in question.

5. Never ask questions in such a way that you make it clear which answer you are expecting. 'You haven't been losing weight, have you?' for example, or 'You get on perfectly well with your father, don't you?' You may think you know what the answer is going to be but, if you do, why ask the question at all? (This is one of the commonest of the many ways in which poor interviewers distort the patient's story to fit their own preconceptions.)

6. Record the patient's replies to key questions, and any striking or unusual remarks, verbatim. It is particularly important to do this for the 'presenting complaints' and it is useful to do the same for other important topics — replies, for example, to questions about mood and thoughts of suicide in patients who are depressed. It is also important to distinguish clearly between evidence and the interpretation placed on it. Comments in case notes like 'obvious thought disorder' are of little value unless accompanied by verbatim examples of the abnormalities of speech on which the opinion is based.

Definitions for symptoms

Knowing how to conduct a diagnostic interview — when to give the patient free rein and when to interrupt him, which areas to concentrate on, and how to phrase one's questions so as to focus the patient's replies without putting words into his mouth — is an art which can only be learnt by experience, but which is not necessarily acquired with experience. Knowing how to interpret what the patient says and what information is necessary to establish the presence of particular symptoms is, or ought to be, a simpler matter. If the interviewer understands, and different interviewers agree, precisely what is meant by the technical terms like depersonalisation and delusion of control that are used to describe symptomatology, it will usually be clear to him what information he needs to establish the presence of the symptom in question. The problem is essentially one of definition. Unfortunately, adequate definitions are not provided in any systematic way in most textbooks, or even in psychiatric dictionaries or glossaries, and much of the low reliability of clinical ratings is attributable to this. Definitions of some of the terms which are most commonly misapplied are given below and a more comprehensive list can be found in the manual of the Present State Examination (Wing et al 1974).

Agitation. A state of restlessness and motor overactivity in which actions which are either purposeless or ineffectual because they are never completed are repeated over and over again, e.g. hand wringing or pacing up and down the room. Agitated subjects usually feel anxious or tense and this feeling is often transmitted to the observer, but agitation is a description of behaviour not of mood.

Alcoholic blackouts. A misleading term for episodes of amnesia occurring at times when the subject was intoxicated. Typically the subject cannot remember what he was doing the previous evening although he was sober enough to get himself home and to bed unaided.

Apathy A state of underactivity, with reduced responsiveness to stimuli, which the observer has good grounds for attributing to loss of interest or concern, rather than to any intrinsic difficulty in responding. (This is a difficult judgement to make unless one knows the patient well because it involves an inference about his motivation as well as observation of his behaviour.)

Blunting (flattening) of affect A state of reduced emotional responsiveness rather than a total loss of the ability to express emotion. It is a dangerous judgement to make on a single interview; the subject really needs to be seen in a variety of different situations before deciding. A superficially similar state may also be produced by depression, or by neuroleptics.

Confabulation. People with a severe impairment of recent memory (e.g. in a Korsakoff state) of which they are unaware sometimes 'confabulate' when questioned about recent events, i.e. they give replies which often sound plausible and which they themselves believe to be true, but which are actually false. Sometimes these confabulations have a grandiose, wishfulfilling quality but they are more commonly genuine memories displaced in time.

Confusion. A temporary state of fluctuating intellectual impairment characterised (and recognised) by some or all of the following features: disorientation in time, space or person, impaired concentration and attention span, inability to register new memories and imperfect comprehension of surrounding events.

Delusional mood. A state of perplexity sometimes seen at the onset of a psychotic illness. The subject is convinced, or at least strongly suspects, that something very unusual is going on around him, but he has not yet decided what this is. Mundane events suddenly acquire a new significance and delusions of reference are often widespread. Grandiose or persecutory ideas may be entertained and discarded in quick succession as the subject attempts to make sense of his experiences, but the prevailing mood remains one of perplexity and apprehension. It ends either in recovery or in the development of a relatively stable delusional system.

Delusional perception. A primary delusion (q.v.) which the subject attributes to his perception of an event or situation which is real but mundane and logically quite unconnected, e.g. he suddenly knew that he was on another planet because the other man in the carriage was sitting crosslegged.

Delusions of control **(passivity feelings).** The subject believes that his thoughts, his feelings, his actions or his will are in some way being influenced or controlled by an alien, external force. Vague ideas that God puts thoughts into people's minds, or that one is easily influenced by other people do *not* qualify. Nor do hallucinatory voices issuing commands. The sensation of being the passive recipient of some controlling or interfering force that is alien and external is crucial.

Delusions of reference. The subject is convinced that events — perhaps a programme on television or a conversation between two strangers in the street — that in reality are mundane and nothing to do with him have an important personal significance and were arranged deliberately.

Depersonalisation. A sensation of subjective change which the subject describes *as if* he had lost his feelings, is empty within or is watching himself from outside. The 'as if' quality is crucial. The subject is not deluded; he is simply trying to describe an unpleasant subjective state which involves a loss of normal emotional responsiveness.

Diurnal variation of mood. A variation in mood with a consistent 24 hour cycle. The commonest pattern is for deep depression first thing in the morning to life as the day progresses. It is important to make sure that the mood change is not simply a response to environmental events — like the departure of children to school, or the return of a spouse from work — and is the same at weekends as during the week.

Ecstasy. An elevation of mood which, unlike elation, is essentially private. The subject is no longer interested in the surrounding world. It is rare and the subject's thought content, when it can be discerned, is usually religious.

Elation. An elevation of mood which is pathological unless short lived and obviously warranted by circumstances. Unlike euphoria and ecstasy, the mood is infectious and the observer feels himself being invited and tempted to share it.

Euphoria. A state of unconcern and contentment which is not justified by circumstances and, unlike elation, is not in the least infectious. It is usually encountered in the presence of extensive brain damage and may be due either to inability to comprehend the true state of affairs or to loss of the ability to experience sadness or anxiety.

Ideas of reference. The subject feels that other people look at him or talk about him because they notice things about him of which he is embarrassed or ashamed. Insight is retained however. He realises, at least in retrospect, that these feelings originate within himself and that in reality he is probably no more conspicuous than anyone else.

Incongruity of affect. Emotional responses which are inappropriate to the situation or the topic of conversation, e.g. giggling while discussing serious matters.

Lability of affect. Rapidly changing emotional responses which are exaggerated but not necessarily incongruous, e.g. bursting into tears when talking of a long dead parent and laughing the next minute at a weak joke.

Obsessional symptoms. Repetitive thoughts or actions which the subject, although he recognises them as his own, feels compelled to resist, but fails to do so successfully. This unsuccessful resistance is crucial, though some subjects with long-standing obses-

sional rituals like checking or hand washing do sometimes stop trying to resist. Obsessional acts also — like Lady Macbeth's hand washing — have a symbolic significance which is more important than their overt behavioural content and which distinguishes them from unwanted habits like masturbation and smoking which may also be accompanied by unsuccessful resistance.

Overvalued ideas. Abnormal beliefs which are firmly held and often immune to rational argument, but differ from delusions in being comprehensible in the light of the subject's past experience and the belief systems of his family or subculture, e.g. insistence that the earth is flat or that a daily purgative is essential to health. Such ideas are evidence of eccentricity, not of psychiatric illness.

Panic attacks. Sudden episodes of anxiety which are so severe that behaviour ceases to be rational and controlled. At the height of the attack the subject is generally afraid either that he is dying or that he is going mad, and if the anxiety is phobic he usually flees the phobic situation.

Phobic (situational) anxiety. Anxiety which is experienced only in particular situations, like crowds or open spaces, which are not in reality dangerous or threatening. It may vary in severity from mild unease to uncontrolled panic and is accompanied by a tendency to avoid the situation in question.

Primary (autocthonous) delusion. A delusion which arises fully formed, without any identifiable precursors and apparently unrelated to the prevailing mood or recent events. The subject suddenly knows, for example, that he is God, or that the two halves of his brain have been transposed.

Retardation. The central feature of retardation is an observable slowing of motor responses, including speech, though the patient's subjective experience is usually one of increasing difficulty rather than slowing. Gestures and expressive facial movements may be lost completely and the slowing of speech is often only apparent, or much more severe, when emotionally charged topics are discussed. Retardation may be so mild that its presence is only recognisable in retrospect, or so severe that stupor supervenes.

Stereotypies Repetitive and apparently purposeless movements which differ from tics in being more complex and from ordinary mannerisms in being more gross and bizarre. They may also have symbolic meaning for the patient.

Stupor. A state in which the subject is conscious but makes no spontaneous movements and responds little or not at all to stimuli. Usually consciousness can be inferred from the presence of purposive eye movements but sometimes it can only be established in retrospect by the subject's ability to describe events during the period of stupor.

Information from relatives

It is a sound principle always to see a relative, or some other close acquaintance of the patient, if one is available before making even a provisional formulation of the problem. Often 10 minutes will suffice to establish that the relative's perception of the situation is essentially the same as the patient's, but it is commonplace for his account to be different in important ways. He may describe a more alarming situation than the patient has admitted to, or make it clear that the symptoms the patient complains of are not a new development but have been present to a greater or lesser extent for years. It is particularly important to get an independent history from someone else if there is any suspicion of alcoholism or drug abuse. The capacity of alcoholics to minimise or gloss over the ways in which their drinking has disrupted their lives is almost limitless and the diagnosis will often be missed if the patient's account is accepted without corroboration.

THE RELATIONSHIP BETWEEN SYMPTOMS AND DIAGNOSIS

For the reasons discussed previously, diagnoses are mainly based on symptoms — the patient's complaints and descriptions of abnormal subjective experiences and the behavioural abnormalities evident on examination or reported by others. Other factors, like the patient's age, sex and personality and the course of the illness in the past, are certainly taken into account, but the patient's symptoms, past and present, are the main determinants. Unfortunately, it is only comparatively recently that we have appreciated the need to specify the relationship between symptoms and diagnosis. Textbooks have always made it clear that the characteristic symptoms of schizophrenia were disorder, auditory hallucinations and delusions of control, that the characteristic symptoms of melancholia were severe depression, retardation and early morning wakening, that the characteristic features of obsessional illness were persistent and disabling compulsive acts or ruminations, and so on. They have not made it clear, however, which diagnosis should be given to someone with auditory hallucinations alone; or with obsessional ruminations in the presence of severe depression. As a result, psychiatrists frequently made different diagnoses when confronted with such situations and diagnostic reliability was low.

What was needed were *rules of application* or *operational definitions* specifying the appropriate diagnosis for every possible combination of symptoms. Instead of simply listing the typical features of diagnosis X as A, B, C and sometimes D, as they had generally done in the past, textbooks and glossaries needed to say something like this: before diagnosis X can be made A must be present, together with one or more of B, C and D, and E must be absent. As with symptoms themselves, the problem is primarily a matter of adequate definition. In the last 20 years, operational definitions of this kind have slowly come into everyday clinical use. In 1972 Eli Robins and his colleagues in St Louis published operational criteria for 15 major diagnostic categories (Feighner et al 1972) and since then many alternative operational definitions have been published for most of the main syndromes and their use has become the norm in clinical research. The most decisive change, however, was the American Psychiatric Association's decision to provide an operational definition for every diagnostic category in the third edition of its Diagnostic and Statistical Manual (DSM-III; APA 1980). As a result, American psychiatrists have since 1980 been committed to using operational definitions for all their diagnostic terms, not just in research but in routine clinical practice as well.

The difference between these two types of definition, the descriptive and the operational, is best illustrated by an example. In the previous (ninth) revision of the International Classification of Diseases (ICD-9), hysterical personality disorder was described thus:

Personality disorder characterised by shallow, labile affectivity, dependence on others, craving for appreciation and attention, suggestibility and theatricality. There is often sexual immaturity, e.g. frigidity and over-responsiveness to stimuli. Under stress hysterical symptoms (neurosis) may develop.

In contrast, the corresponding category, histrionic personality disorder, was defined in DSM-III as follows:

The following are characteristic of the individual's current and long-term functioning, are not limited to episodes of illness, and cause either significant impairment in social or occupational functioning or subjective distress.

A. Behavior that is overly dramatic, reactive, and intensely expressed, as indicated by at least three of the following:

   1. self-dramatisation, e.g. exaggerated expression of emotions
   2. incessant drawing of attention to oneself
   3. craving for activity and excitement
   4. overreaction to minor events
   5. irrational, angry outbursts or tantrums.

B. Characteristic disturbances in interpersonal relationships as indicated by at least two of the following:

1. perceived by others as shallow and lacking genuineness, even if superficially warm and charming
2. egocentric, self-indulgent, and inconsiderate of others
3. vain and demanding
4. dependent, helpless, constantly seeking reassurance
5. prone to manipulative suicidal threats, gestures or attempts.

Knowing that a patient was diagnosed as having a hysterical personality disorder using ICD-9 criteria was not much more informative than knowing that he was so diagnosed 'by an experienced psychiatrist' or 'in accordance with the description in so and so's textbook', whereas to know that the DSM-III criteria were used gives a fairly precise indication of the characteristics he must have displayed to qualify.

Diagnostic hierarchies

Insofar as there is a formal structure to the relationship between symptoms and diagnoses it is a hierarchical one. At the top of this hierarchy come the organic psychoses. If there is evidence of organicity — perhaps clinical or electroencephalographic evidence of epilepsy or definite cognitive impairment — this overrides all other considerations and whatever other symptoms the patient has, psychotic or neurotic, the diagnosis is organic. Schizophrenia has traditionally come next in the hierarchy. To many European psychiatrists certain symptoms are regarded as diagnostic of schizophrenia, regardless of which other symptoms are also present, provided only that there is no question of cerebral disease. The 'symptoms of the first rank' which Schneider (1959) regarded as pathognomonic of schizophrenia 'except in the presence of coarse brain disease' constitute an explicit statement of this convention, and other clinicians have attached a similar significance to symptoms like thought disorder and incongruity of affect. For Schneider and his successors, third place in the hierarchy is occupied by the affective disorders. Even if the characteristic features of mania or melancholia are unmistakably present, organic or schizophrenic symptoms take precedence. As a result, patients with both schizophrenic and affective symptoms are classified as schizophrenics, and were so classified in ICD-9. However, in ICD-10, schizophrenic and affective disorders are both at the same level. A diagnosis of schizophrenia cannot be made if the full depressive or manic syndrome is also present 'unless it is clear that schizophrenic symptoms antedated the affective disturbance'. Neurotic, stress related and somatoform disorders come at the bottom of the

hierarchy. As a result, patients with both neurotic and psychotic symptoms are regarded as having psychotic illnesses. Another consequence of the relative status of neurotic and psychotic symptoms in this hierarchy is that, for those who still employ the traditional distinction between psychotic and neurotic depression, the latter is characterised by the absence of the characteristic features of psychotic depression, rather than by the possession of typical symptoms of its own. In general, any given diagnosis *excludes* the presence of the symptoms of all higher members of the hierarchy and *embraces* the symptoms of all lower members.

It is no coincidence that the order in which diagnostic categories are arranged in the international and other classifications is the same as in this hierarchy, for both reflect the sequence of questions psychiatrists commonly ask themselves when making a diagnosis. Indeed, a very similar sequence is involved in the decision pathways of computer programs like Catego (Wing et al 1974). The psychologist Graham Foulds suggested that this structure was inherent in the nature of psychiatric illness but it is more likely that it is a man-made imposition. It is a firm principle in medicine that every effort should be made to account for the patient's symptoms in terms of a single diagnosis. In a situation in which most individual symptoms are liable to be encountered in the presence of a wide range of other symptoms this is not easy to achieve unless the defining characteristics of different illnesses are in a hierarchical relationship to one another, with the least common symptoms at the top and the most common at the bottom. There is also some empirical justification for this arrangement. For example, when schizophrenic and neurotic symptoms coexist, the patient's prognosis and response to treatment are determined more by the former than by the latter, so if only one diagnosis is allowable it is more appropriate to regard the patient as schizophrenic than as neurotic.

INTERNATIONAL DIFFERENCES IN DIAGNOSTIC CRITERIA

We have seen that until comparatively recently the relationship between symptoms and diagnoses was vague and ill defined and many technical terms — like thought disorder, dependency and immaturity — were also poorly defined. As a result, trainees were forced to learn how to make diagnoses by copying their teachers. In the absence of adequate rules the only way to learn which of their patients should be regarded as schizophrenics was to observe which patients their mentors gave this diagnosis to and do the same. As a result, diagnostic criteria were at the mercy of the personal views and idiosyncrasies of influential teachers, and also liable to be affected by therapeutic fashions and innovations, and changing assumptions about aetiology. This led to the development of substantial differences in the way in which several key diagnostic terms were used in different centres. The less contact there was between two centres — and of course national boundaries and language differences were substantial impediments to such contact — the more likely it was that progressive differences in diagnostic usage would develop.

The best documented of these differences in usage were those that developed between Britain and the USA in the 1940s and 1950s. The comparative studies carried out by the US/UK Diagnostic Project in the 1960s established that, in comparable series of patients, psychiatrists in New York diagnosed schizophrenia twice as frequently as their counterparts in London. Patients regarded in London as suffering from depressive illnesses or mania, or even neurotic illnesses or personality disorders, were all diagnosed as schizophrenics in New York (Cooper et al 1972). The International Pilot Study of Schizophrenia confirmed that American psychiatrists had an unusually broad concept of schizophrenia, and also showed that the same was true, for quite different reasons, of Russian psychiatrists (WHO 1973). Of the nine centres involved, seven (London, Prague, Aarhus in Denmark, Ibadan in Nigeria, Agra in India, Cali in Colombia and Taipei in Formosa) shared a very similar concept of schizophrenia, but Washington and Moscow both had a much broader concept. In Europe the situation was complicated by the fact that Scandinavian psychiatrists, particularly the Norwegians and the Danes, made frequent use of a diagnosis of reactive or psychogenic psychosis which embraced many patients who would have been regarded as having schizophrenic or affective psychoses in Britain or Germany. And French psychiatrists used a number of categories like *délire chronique* and *bouffée délirante* which had no counterpart in other nomenclatures. These differences are now disappearing, and for the younger generation of psychiatrists are already a thing of the past. The very broad American concept of schizophrenia was psychoanalytic in origin and the decline of psychoanalytic influence in the 1970s, together with a renewed interest in descriptive psychopathology and classification, led to a rapid change. Indeed, the contemporary American concept of schizophrenia embodied in the operational criteria of DSM-IIIR is

somewhat narrower that the current British concept. The widespread adoption of the operational definitions of DSM-III and DSM-IIIR by research workers in many different parts of the world has also played an important role in reducing international differences in usage.

It is important to realise that it is meaningless to ask who is right where any of these differences, past or present, are concerned. It two individual psychiatrists disagree about a diagnosis we are accustomed to assume that whichever of the two is more experienced, or whom we respect the more, is probably right. But if experienced psychiatrists in different centres disagree with one another when presented with identical information all one can say is that they have different concepts of that condition. The same is true of two psychiatrists using different operational definitions of the same syndrome. One can check that they are both using their respective definitions appropriately, but beyond that one can only concede that the two definitions embrace different populations of patients. However, although it is meaningless to ask who is *right* it is perfectly legitimate, and necessary, to ask which concept or definition is more *useful*. Essentially, the choice between alternative definitions is a matter of validity. If we knew more about the aetiology of psychiatric disorders we could easily decide which of the two alternative definitions of the syndrome correlated better with the underlying abnormality, just as we could easily decide which clinical definition of mitral stenosis was most reliably associated with narrowing of the mitral valve, or which clinical definition of Pick's disease was most reliably associated with the characteristic pathology of that condition. In the absence of this knowledge all we can do is ask which of the competing definitions most successfully meets some arbitrary criterion like homogeneity of outcome or treatment response. But as different criteria may be best satisfied by different definitions the problem is not resolved. For example, the definition of schizophrenia which most successfully identifies patients who subsequently develop a defect state and become chronic invalids is probably different from the definition which gives the highest monozygotic/dizygotic concordance ratio in twin populations. We must accept, therefore, that until we know more about the aetiology of the various syndromes we recognise and treat we cannot be sure how they should best be defined. As a result, we will probably have to accept the coexistence of a number of alternative operational definitions of syndromes like schizophrenia, and in some areas of alternative classifications, for some time to come.

CONTEMPORARY CLASSIFICATIONS

The international classification

International classifications of mental disorders have existed for over 100 years but until recently they had little influence and were almost universally ignored. Individual countries, and indeed individual organisations and hospitals, often had their own more or less private classifications, while others declined to be bound by any nomenclature, national or local. The crucial change occurred in the late 1960s. In response to strenuous efforts by the World Health Organization (WHO), most countries were persuaded to sacrifice their own traditions and aspirations in the interests of international communication and to use the nomenclature and definitions of the eighth revision of the *International Classification of Diseases, Injuries and Causes of Death* (ICD-8) which came into use in 1969.

This eighth revision was replaced by a ninth (ICD-9) a decade later. If one compares the successive revisions of the ICD from the sixth in 1948 to the ninth in 1979, each was undoubtedly an improvement on its predecessor. The mental disorders section of ICD-6 was primarily a classification of psychoses and mental deficiency. Its successors provided much more adequate coverage of neurotic and stress-related disorders, of childhood disorders and of the range of conditions attributable to alcohol and drug dependence and abuse. Many new terms were introduced, a few obsolete ones like involutional melancholia were dropped and every category was provided with a brief definition (and sometimes a list of synonyms and another list of incompatible alternative diagnoses as a further aid to consistent usage). Despite these improvements the inherent problems associated with an international classification became more apparent with each revision. The definitions provided in ICD-8 and ICD-9 were not operational definitions. They were simply thumb-nail sketches of the clinical concept in question. They described its essential features well enough but did not provide rules of application, as the ICD-9 definition of hysterical personality disorder described above illustrates. A more fundamental problem was that radical change of any kind was almost impossible to effect, because every country had to be willing to accept whatever innovations were introduced, and any attempt to force the pace risked damaging the fragile international consensus on which the whole enterprise was based. Another major problem was that, because national representatives were always prepared to argue more forcefully for the inclusion of their own favourite terms than they were to oppose the efforts of others to do likewise, there was a constant tendency for the classification to expand by incorporating alternative and sometimes incompatible concepts. ICD-9 contained no less than 13 categories for patients with depressive symptoms, because in effect two or three different ways of classifying depressions were included alongside one another.

The tenth revision (ICD-10)

Preparation of ICD-10 started as long ago as 1983 but it did not finally come into use in the UK and most other countries until 1993. It has a new title — the *International Statistical Classification of Diseases and Related Health Problems* — and a new alphanumeric format (WHO 1992). The main purpose of the latter is to provide more categories (there are 26 letters in the alphabet but only ten digits) and so leave space for future expansion without the whole classification having to be changed. Each section has either 100, 1000 or 10 000 categories, depending on how many digits are used. The general format of the section entitled 'mental, behavioural and developmental disorders' (F00–F99) is very similar to that of the American Psychiatric Association's recent classifications because it incorporates many of the radical innovations introduced in DSM-III (see below). The traditional distinction between psychoses and neuroses has been laid aside, though the terms themselves are retained, and all mood (affective) disorders are brought together in a single grouping (F3). All disorders due to the use of psychoactive substances, including alcohol, have also been brought together under a common format (F1). Most categories are provided with both 'diagnostic guidelines' for everyday clinical use and separate 'diagnostic criteria for research', providing unambiguous rules of application. There is also provision for multiple axes, as in DSM-III and its successors.

The section 'mental, behavioural and developmental disorders' is being published in a variety of different formats — the basic text, code numbers and titles; the clinical descriptions and diagnostic guidelines ('the blue book'); and the diagnostic criteria for research ('the green book'). It will probably remain in use for considerably longer that the 10 years for which ICD-6 to ICD-9 were each used. It is likely, therefore, to be the classification that today's young psychiatrists will use for most of their careers. Field trials of the 1986 draft text were held in 194 different centres in 55 different countries and the final text benefited greatly from the comments of users in these very varied settings, and the evidence they provided of the acceptability, coverage and inter-rater reliability of the provisional categories and definitions of that draft.

The American Psychiatric Association's classifications

The first edition of the American Psychiatric Association's *Diagnostic and Statistical Manual of Mental Disorders* (DSM-I) was published in 1952. Its format reflected the dominant Meyerian philosophy of the times and although its influence was limited it was the first official nomenclature to provide a glossary of descriptions of the diagnostic categories it listed. The second edition (DSM-II), published in 1968, was, like the corresponding English glossary (General Register Office 1968), a national glossary to the nomenclature of ICD-8, the American Psychiatric Association (APA) having been persuaded on this occasion to sacrifice its own diagnostic preferences in the interests of international conformity.

DSM-III

The third edition (DSM-III), published in 1980, was radically different from any previous classification (APA 1980). Its innovations were a response to the evidence that had accumulated over the previous 20 years that psychiatric diagnoses were generally unreliable, that there were systematic differences in the usage of key terms like 'schizophrenia' between the USA and other parts of the world, and that major changes were needed to the overall format of the international and other existing classifications. It was also evidence of a sea change in the orientation of American psychiatry; the end of the psychodynamic era and the dawn of a new biological or 'neo-Kraepelinian' era. For the first time in any classification of disease almost every diagnostic category was given an operational definition to make it as clear as possible which patients were and were not covered by that rubric. Although this made the manual five times the size of its predecessors — and involved much discussion, argument and persuasion as well as extensive field trials in order to secure the necessary agreement — the result, as the field trials demonstrated, was that the reliability of most of its 200 categories was far higher than in any previous classification.

DSM-III was also a multiaxial classification with separate axes allowing the systematic recording of five different information sets — the clinical syndrome (Axis I); lifelong disorders or handicaps like personality disorders and specific developmental disorders (Axis II); associated physical conditions (Axis III); the severity of psychosocial stressors (Axis IV); and the highest level of social and occupational functioning in the past year (Axis V). The clinical syndromes coded on Axis I were also arranged in a novel sequence; in particular, the traditional distinction between neuroses and psychoses was abandoned to allow all affective disorders to be brought together. A further important change was that most, although not all, diagnostic terms were either explicitly divested of their aetiological implications or replaced by new terms devoid of such implications. As a result, many of the hallowed terms of psychiatry, like hysteria and manic–depressive illness, and even psychosis and neurosis, were discarded and replaced by stark, utilitarian terms like somatoform disorder, factitious disorder and paraphilia.

Classifications always tend to be controversial, if only because they involve fundamental concepts and important philosophical assumptions. Initially, DSM-III and its principal architect, Robert Spitzer, were bitterly criticised by many senior American psychiatrists for introducing what they regarded as a crude 'Chinese menu' approach to diagnosis, and for discarding the concept of neurosis and with it most psychoanalytic assumptions about aetiology. Clinical researchers and the younger generation of American psychiatrists, on the other hand, welcomed the new classification with enthusiasm (Jampala et al 1986) and it was soon clear that DSM-III was going to have a major influence on the whole persona of American psychiatry, particularly on clinical and biological research. Indeed, within a few years of its publication it had become an all-time psychiatric best-seller and made huge profits for the APA. It had also been translated into 13 other languages and its definitions were being widely used throughout the world. DSM-III also led to important changes in American usage of several diagnostic terms (Loranger 1990). Fewer patients were labelled as schizophrenics and more were diagnosed as having unipolar or bipolar affective disorders. The creation of a separate axis for them also resulted in more extensive use of personality disorder diagnoses.

DSM-IIIR

DSM-III was replaced by an extensive revision, DSM-IIIR, in 1987 (APA 1987). No fundamental changes were involved but a substantial number of minor alterations were introduced. The classification of sleep disorders was expanded, mental retardation was moved from Axis I to Axis II, one or two categories were dropped (including homosexuality, even if egodystonic) and one or two new ones introduced. Three other more contentious concepts (late luteal phase dysphoric disorder and sadistic and self defeating personality disorders) were introduced in an appendix, candidates for future election as it were. Schizoaffective disorders were given an operational definition for the first time; the definition of paranoid disorders was enlarged to include patients with grandiose, somatic and erotomanic delusions as well as those with delusions of persecution and jealousy; the inappropriate stipulation that schizophrenia must start before the age of 45 years was dropped; and 'agoraphobia with panic attacks' was replaced by 'panic disorder with secondary agoraphobia' in deference to the emerging view that panic attacks were the primary phenomenon. Most important of all, the definition of the majority of disorders listed in the glossary was altered, usually in fairly minor ways.

Individually, most of these changes were improvements. They involved either the correction of mistakes or misjudgements, or rational responses to new evidence or a change in the climate of opinion. Even so, it is doubtful whether it was wise to introduce a new classification after only 7 years with all the disruption to newly established clinical concepts, to clinical research and to residency training programmes which new definitions inevitably involve.

DSM-IV

In 1987 the APA setup a new Task Force, chaired by Allan Frances, to produce yet another revision of its Diagnostic and Statistical Manual, DSM-IV, 'concurrently and congruently' with ICD-10. It was assumed that DSM-IV and ICD-10 would both be introduced in 1993. Unfortunately, the APA did not appreciate that by 1987 the major elements of the format of the mental disorders section of ICD-10 had already been decided. As a result, Dr Frances' Task Force has been forced to choose between accepting the in some cases rather unsatisfactory terminology and definitions of ICD-10 in order to harmonise the two classifications as much as possible; or alternatively to ignore ICD-10 and accept the recommendations of the 13 work groups it had set up to draft proposals for the format of each of the individual sections of DSM-IV (Kendell 1991). Each of these work groups has mounted a comprehensive review of the literature bearing on its group of disorders and consulted widely. Many have also mounted field

trials, explored the implications of potential definitional changes by reanalysing existing data sets, and used videotaped interviews to assess reliability and the sources of unreliability. The result of this impressive concentration of expertise is likely to be a classification and a comprehensive set of operational definitions more firmly based on empirical evidence that any previous classification of mental disorders. For the reasons referred to above, the differences between DSM-IV and ICD-10 are likely to be more extensive than they might have been if the DSM-IV Task Force had been set up 2 or 3 years earlier. Even so, these differences will be much less extensive and confusing than the differences between DSM-III and ICD-9, and are unlikely to prevent DSM-IV being widely used outside the USA, particularly for research purposes.

Future classifications of mental disorders

Until we know more about the aetiology of the major syndromes like schizophrenia, Alzheimer's disease and bipolar disorder it is unlikely that any future classification will be self evidently superior to the kind of classification DSM-IV is likely to be. Literature reviews, follow-up studies, family studies, therapeutic trials and laborious analyses of sets of ratings derived from structured interviews with representative populations of patients can only take us so far. Apart from one or two under-researched areas like the personality disorders we may already be approaching the limits of what can be achieved by traditional clinical and epidemiological means. We should not be in a hurry, therefore, to develop new versions of comprehensive, formal classifications like DSM-IV and ICD-10. It would be better to wait and see what novel concepts are introduced over the next decade by individual research groups, and what insights we gain from burgeoning developments in the neurosciences and human genetics. Other branches of medicine did not progress by a dogged pursuit of better and better classifications of their subject matter. They did so by acquiring new technologies, by developing radically new concepts and by elucidating fundamental mechanisms.

THE RELIABILITY AND VALIDITY OF PSYCHIATRIC DIAGNOSES

Reliability

The reliability of psychiatric diagnoses is usually measured in one of two ways. Either a diagnostic interview is watched by a passive observer who makes his own independent diagnosis at the end (*observer method*), or else a second diagnostician conducts an independent interview with the patient a few hours or days after the first (*re-interview method*). The former overestimates reliability because all variation in the conduct of the interview is eliminated; the latter may underestimate it because the subject's clinical state may change in the interval between the two interviews, and he may react differently to the second interview simply because it is a repetition of the first.

Many reliability studies were carried out in the 1950s and 1960s and most of them found reliability to be depressingly low. The studies of Beck in Philadelphia and Kreitman in Chichester are often quoted because they were well designed and the participants were all experienced psychiatrists. Both used the re-interview method. Beck obtained 54% agreement for the specific diagnosis, compared with the 15–19% agreement that could have arisen by chance alone. Kreitman, using a restricted range of 11 diagnostic categories, obtained 63% agreement. There are three main ways of reducing disagreement: using structured or standardised interviews to minimise variation in the conduct of the interview, and providing definitions for all the items of psychopathology covered by that interview, which together will help to minimise disagreements about which symptoms the subject exhibits; and using operational definitions to ensure that any given combination of symptoms always leads to the same diagnosis.

It has been shown repeatedly that research workers using standardised interviews can obtain considerably higher diagnostic reliability than is possible with unstructured interviews, and that further improvement can be obtained by adopting operational definitions for all diagnostic categories. For example, the field trials of DSM-III carried out in various parts of the USA in the late 1970s gave values for the reliability of the major diagnostic categories varying from 0.65 to 0.83, compared with values ranging from 0.41 to 0.77 in comparable reliability studies carried out between 1956 and 1972. (κ is a better statistic for measuring concordance than the percentage agreement used in the early reliability studies because it discounts chance agreement. It has a value of +1.0 if agreement is perfect, of zero if agreement is no better than chance, and a negative value if agreement is actually below chance expectation. (See Cohen 1960.)) Organic and psychotic disorders generally have higher reliability than neuroses and personality disorders and for this reason reliability studies based on in-patients tend to produce higher overall reliability than those based on out-patients. The comparatively low reliability of neu-roses and personality disorders is probably due to the frequency of neurotic symptoms and maladaptive personality traits in the general population, and the fact that quantitative as well as merely qualitative judgements are therefore involved.

In summary, although the studies conducted in the 1950s and 1960s demonstrated that the reliability of psychiatric diagnoses was often very low, the introduction of structured interviews and operational definitions has transformed the situation. In skilled hands, psychiatric diagnoses are now as reliable as the clinical judgements made in other branches of medicine, and sometimes more so. But reliability still does not, and probably never can, match the reliability of laboratory tests where the human eye is only required to judge the position of a needle on a scale or the timing of a colour change. Clinical judgements, whether they concern depersonalisation or bronchial breathing, are inevitably imprecise and imperfect, and the best we can do is to understand what the problems are and do our best to minimise them.

Validity

Reliability is a means to an end rather than an end in itself. Its importance lies in the fact that it establishes a ceiling for validity; the lower it is the lower validity necessarily becomes. (Suppose, for example, that in reality syndrome A always responds to lithium and other superficially similar syndromes never do. If diagnostic reliability is low and A is only correctly distinguished from B, C and D 50% of the time, this crucial difference will never be recognised. Instead, it will be believed that the chances of patients with syndrome A responding to lithium are about 50:50, and that B, C and D respond quite often as well.) The converse, however, is not true. Reliability can be high while validity remains trivial and, if so, high reliability is of little value. One could, for example, increase the reliability of the diagnosis of schizophrenia by agreeing to apply the term to all those, and only those, with clear-cut delusions of control. It would be silly to do this, though, because the response to treatment and long-term outcome of the population so defined would almost certainly be more variable and unpredictable than it is at present.

Textbooks of psychology usually describe four different types of validity — concurrent, predictive, construct and content. Predictive validity is the most important of these where psychiatric diagnoses are concerned. In the last resort all diagnostic concepts stand or fall by the strength of the prognostic and therapeutic implications they embody. The ability to predict the outcome of an illness, and to alter this course of events if need be, have always been the main functions of medicine. Diagnoses like pulmonary tuberculosis and bronchial carcinoma are useful and valid not because we understand what causes them — indeed, there is much about both that we do not understand — but because they enable us to predict fairly accurately what will happen to the patient, and which therapeutic measures will and will not improve that outcome.

Although numerous studies of reliability have been carried out in the last 30 years, few direct attempts have ever been made to assess validity, either predictive validity or validity of other kinds. Indeed, it is still an open issue whether there are genuine boundaries between the clinical syndromes recognised in contemporary classifications, or between these syndromes and normality (Kendell 1989). This is partly due to lack of agreement on how best to establish the validity of diagnostic concepts, and partly because much of the basic evidence for the validity of our diagnostic categories accumulated and became accepted before anyone began to ask questions about reliability and validity. Most psychiatrists, for example, accept that the distinction between schizophrenic and affective disorders is valid because they consider it to be well established that, generally speaking, the two respond differently to phenothiazines and lithium salts, and have different long-term outcomes, the former tending to run a progressive downhill course and the latter to relapse repeatedly but to recover fully each time. To demonstrate that this is really so it would be necessary to follow up a representative population of patients with schizophrenic and affective disorders for a decade or more and then show that the differences in outcome between the two were not simply, or mainly, due to other variables like age of onset, social class and treatment. Strictly speaking, this has never been done, though it has been shown many times that, although the overlap is considerable, there are substantial and consistent differences in outcome between schizophrenic and affective illnesses.

Family studies are a further source of evidence. The fact that the relatives of schizophrenics have a raised incidence of schizophrenia but not of affective disorders, and that the relatives of patients with unipolar or bipolar affective disorders have a raised incidence of affective disorders but not of schizophrenia even when the relatives' illnesses are diagnosed blindly (Tsuang et al 1980), is evidence for the validity of the two concepts, and of the distinction between them. There is also a good deal of evidence relevant to the issue of validity implicit in the results of the numerous therapeutic trials that have been conducted in the last 30 years. These clearly establish the existence of several effective treatments for psychiatric disorders — ECT, neuroleptics, tricyclic antidepressants, lithium salts, and some behavioural and cognitive techniques also. They also establish that each of these therapies has a limited sphere of action. ECT is highly effective with severe depressions, rather less effective with schizophrenic or manic illnesses and generally ineffective elsewhere. Neuroleptics are most effective with acute schizophrenic or manic illnesses, less effective with chronic schizophrenic or depressive illnesses, and largely ineffective in neurotic states. Lithium and the antidepressants show the same general pattern; one or two diagnostic categories where their effect is greatest, others where it is weaker but still demonstrable, and others where it is negligible. The fact that each of these treatments has a limited range of action, and that diagnostic categories are helpful in predicting treatment response, is indirect evidence that the categories concerned are useful and valid. On the other hand, the fact that none of these therapies is specific to a single diagnostic category, and none is effective in more than perhaps two-thirds of the members of even that category in which its action is most powerful, clearly puts limits on their validity.

Cluster analysis also provides evidence for the concurrent validity of some diagnostic categories. This is a generic term for a variety of statistical techniques designed to sort heterogeneous populations into subpopulations or 'clusters' of similar individuals, similar, that is, in respect of the ratings on which the analysis is based. If clinical ratings derived from large populations of patients are subjected to such procedures the resulting clusters usually correspond quite well with diagnostic categories such as mania, paranoid schizophrenia and melancholia, suggesting that these concepts do correspond to genuine groupings in nature (e.g. see Everitt et al 1971).

In summary, the existing evidence for the validity of most psychiatric diagnoses is rather meagre, but by no means non-existent. It is also considerably better for major syndromes like schizophrenia, mania and depression than it is for other less well-defined syndromes, or for subcategories of the major syndromes such as catatonic or paranoid schizophrenia. Eventually, of course, we assume that validity will be established by elucidating the underlying pathology, but despite many attempts to explore the biological basis of the major syndromes in the last 20 years, and many promising findings, this long-awaited objective is not yet within our grasp.

CATEGORIES OR DIMENSIONS

Traditionally, psychiatry has always used a categorical classification or typology. That is, it has divided its subject matter, psychiatric illness, into a number of separate and mutually exclusive categories like schizophrenia, mania and Alzheimer's disease. The reasons why it has done so are clear enough. Medicine is rooted in the biological sciences and physicians were deeply impressed by the advantages botany and zoology derived from the development of detailed classifications of their subject matter into species, genera and orders in the 18th and 19th centuries. More compelling still, the structure of our language is based on classification. Every common noun — like 'tree', 'star' or 'fairy' — denotes the existence of a category or class of objects. There is, however, an alternative way of expressing the relationship between the members of a heterogeneous population, namely to assign each to a position on one or more axes or dimensions.

There has been much debate about the relative merits of these two types of classification (see Table 14.1). In general, theoreticians like Eysenck have favoured a dimensional approach while most practising clinicians — though not Kretschmer or Jung — have preferred to use a typology. It is important to appreciate that, in principle, both options — dimensions and categories — are available; there is no statistical technique or other criterion capable of deciding which is 'right'. The choice between the two is essentially a matter of deciding which is more useful, and the answer may well vary with the purpose for which the classification is required. The main advantage of a dimensional classification is its flexibility. Consider, for example, the advantages of an IQ — a dimensional representation of intelligence — over a typology with two categories (clever and stupid) or three categories (clever, ordinary and stupid). Two individuals with IQs of 120 and 160 would both, presumably, be allocated to the 'clever' category, but this would involve losing sight of what in many situations would be an important difference between them. Conversely, two individuals with IQs of 98 and 102 are in reality almost identical, yet one would be classified as stupid and the other as clever. Moreover, a distribution of IQs can always be converted to any number of categories as occasion demands, and the boundaries of these moved up or down the scale at will. But if the members of a population are all assigned to one of the three categories (clever, ordinary and stupid) to begin with, this cannot subsequently be increased to four categories or reduced to two, except by splitting or combining some

Table 14.1   The relative merits of categories and dimensions

Advantages of categories
1. They are familiar
2. They are easy to understand, to remember, and to use
3. Categorisation is a ready prelude to action, e.g. the diagnosis is X and X is treated with drug D
4. They do not strain the resources of a conservative and largely innumerate profession

Advantages of dimensions
1. They convey more information because finer distinctions are possible
2. They are more flexible, because they can easily be converted into any desired number of categories, and back again
3. They do not imply the presence of unproven qualitative differences between members of different subpopulations
4. They do not impose boundaries where none may exist in reality, and do not distort the observer's perception of individuals lying near the boundary between adjacent categories

of the existing groups; nor is there any possibility of converting them to a dimension.

Another important advantage of dimensions is that they do not distract attention from the atypical in favour of the typical, or distort the observer's perception of individuals lying near the boundary between two adjacent categories. One of the most serious drawbacks of categorical classifications is the way in which they cause individuals who seem to lie halfway between two disorders, or between a disorder and a healthy state, to be overlooked or misrepresented. Patients exhibiting a combination of schizophrenic and affective symptoms illustrate this problem very clearly. Time and again in clinical research they have either been ignored and the study confined to patients with typical schizophrenic or affective illnesses, or if they were included one or other component of their symptomatology was glossed over or ignored. In other words, using a typology leads us to expect, and so to perceive, our patients as fitting neatly into one or other of its categories whether or not they do so in reality.

The great disadvantage of dimensions is that any system involving more than one dimension can only be handled geometrically or algebraically, and if there are more than three only the latter is possible. This is why the only dimensional systems used in everyday life are those like height, weight and intelligence which only involve a single axis.

The most important advantage of a typology, apart from its familiarity, is the ease of description and conceptualisation it provides. A description of a typical member of a category provides a simple and easily remembered means of defining, and subsequently of recognising, the essence of that clinical concept, and of the essential differences between it and other categories. It is also difficult to ignore the fact that categorisation is the norm in most other areas of study and is inherent in the structure of all language. If we had good evidence that psychiatric illnesses were distributed in discrete clusters *in rerum natura* and that interforms between one disorder and the next were relatively uncommon, the arguments in favour of categorical classification would be very strong. Unfortunately, we still lack such evidence. Attempts to demonstrate by discriminant function analysis that interforms between psychotic and neurotic depressions, or between schizophrenic and affective psychoses, are less common than typical members of these categories have mostly been unsuccessful (e.g. Kendell & Gourlay 1970a, b). The frequency with which psychiatrists are driven to employ such terms as schizo-affective, anxiety depression, borderline syndrome and the like, and the difficulty they have agreeing where to draw the boundary between one category and the next, is further evidence that in reality patterns of symptoms merge into one another and are not separated by convenient 'points of rarity'. It is said that the art of classification lies in carving nature at the joints, but where psychiatric illness is concerned we cannot be sure that we have found the joints, or even that there are many to be found.

Despite the considerable theoretical attractions it is unlikely that psychiatry will adopt a dimensional classification for ordinary clinical purposes in the foreseeable future. Old traditions die hard, and few psychiatrists are sufficiently numerate to handle algebraic relationships between multiple dimensions with any confidence. Nor is there any immediate prospect of the advocates of dimensional systems being able to agree how many dimensions are needed and what their identity should be. In the long run, though, it is difficult to believe that personality disorder, and perhaps neurotic illness also, will not be more conveniently and usefully portrayed by a set of dimensions than by the discrete types we attempt to delineate at present. There is already broad agreement that the protean variations of normal personality are better portrayed by dimensions, and the continuity between normal personality and the clinical categories of personality disorder and neurotic illness is increasingly difficult to ignore. Where psychotic illness is concerned, however, the balance of advantages and disadvantages is rather different and it may well be that here a typology will continue to be preferable even though the names of the disorders we recognise, and their defining characteristics, may change considerably as we come to understand their aetiology.

REFERENCES

APA 1980 Diagnostic and statistical manual of mental disorders, 3rd edn. American Psychiatric Association, Washington, DC

APA 1987 Diagnostic and statistical manual of mental disorders, 3rd edn, revised. American Psychiatric Association, Washington, DC

Cohen J 1960 A coefficient of agreement for nominal scales. Educational and Psychological Measurement 20: 37–46

Cooper J E, Kendell R E, Gurland B J, Sharpe L, Copeland J R M, Simon R 1972 Psychiatric diagnosis in New York and London. Maudsley monograph 20. Oxford University Press, London

Everitt B S, Gourlay A J, Kendell R E 1971 An attempt at validation of traditional psychiatric syndromes by cluster analysis. British Journal of Psychiatry 119: 399–412

Feighner J P, Robins E, Guze S B, Woodruff R A, Winokur G, Munoz R 1972 Diagnostic criteria for use in psychiatric research. Archives of General Psychiatry 26: 57–63

General Register Office 1968 A glossary of mental disorders. Studies on medical and population subjects, No 22. Her Majesty's Stationery Office, London

Institute of Psychiatry, Departments of Psychiatry and Child Psychiatry and Maudsley Hospital, London (1987) Psychiatric examination: notes on eliciting and recording clinical information in psychiatric patients. Oxford University Press, Oxford

Jampala V C, Sierles F S, Taylor M A 1986 Consumers' views of DSM-III: attitudes and practices of US psychiatrists and 1984 graduating psychiatric residents. American Journal of Psychiatry 143: 148–153

Kendell R E 1989 Clinical validity. Psychological Medicine 19: 45–55

Kendell R E 1991 Relationship between the DSM-IV and the ICD-10. Journal of Abnormal Psychology 100: 297–301

Kendell R E, Gourlay J 1970a The clinical distinction between psychotic and neurotic depression. British Journal of Psychiatry 117: 257–260

Kendell R E, Gourlay J 1970b The clinical distinction between the affective psychoses and schizophrenia. British Journal of Psychiatry 117: 261–266

Kreitman N, Sainsbury P, Morrissey J, Towers J, Scrivener J 1961 The reliability of psychiatric assessment: an analysis. Journal of Mental Science 107: 887–908

Loranger A W 1990 The impact of DSM-III on diagnostic practice in a university hospital. Archives of General Psychiatry 47: 672–675

Robins L N, Helzer J E, Croughan J, Ratliff K S 1981 National Institute of Mental Health Diagnostic Interview Schedule. Archives of General Psychiatry 38: 381–389

Scadding J G 1963 Meaning of diagnostic terms in broncho-pulmonary disease. British Medical Journal ii: 1425–1430

Schneider K 1959 Klinische Psychopathologie. Translation of the 5th edn by Hamilton M W. Grune & Stratton, New York

Tsuang M T, Winokur G, Crowe R R 1980 Morbidity risks of schizophrenia and affective disorders among first degree relatives of patients with schizophrenia, mania, depression and surgical conditions. British Journal of Psychiatry 137: 497–504

Wing J K, Cooper J E, Sartorius N 1974 Description and classification of psychiatric symptoms. Cambridge University Press, Cambridge

WHO 1973 Report of the international pilot study of schizophrenia, vol 1. World Health Organization, Geneva

WHO 1978 Mental disorders: glossary and guide to their classification in accordance with the ninth revision of the international classification of diseases. World Health Organization, Geneva

WHO 1992 International statistical classification of diseases and related health problems, 10th revision. Vol 1, pp 311–387 World Health Organization, Geneva

FURTHER READING

Kendell R E 1975 The role of diagnosis in psychiatry. Blackwell, Oxford

15. Organic disorders

M. R. Bond   Jean Reid

A number of psychological symptoms and symptom complexes indicate the presence of abnormal brain function. The physical conditions which give rise to them are classified as organic disorders, of which there are many. They include brain damage as a consequence of trauma to the head, cerebral degenerative diseases, viral infections and tumours. Diseases elsewhere in the body can effect the brain's function, as in the case of cerebral anoxia due to low blood pressure secondary to myocardial infarction, or the intoxication caused by hepatic failure. Disturbances of brain function also occur as a result of damage caused by external agents, such as infective organisms, by intoxication (e.g. with alcohol), and by deficiencies in the diet of the vitamins in the B group. Identification of the cause of an organic disorder is not difficult if: (1) the physical appearance of the patient is characteristic of the disorder as in myxoedema or Huntington's disease; (2) the history provides relevant information, for example a known addiction to alcohol, or a recent head injury; (3) focal neurological signs indicative of a certain cerebral lesion are elicited; or (4) systemic disease known to affect brain functions is present. In some cases, however, diagnosis is only achieved after prolonged observation of the patient, repeated mental and physical examinations, extensive laboratory tests and non-invasive investigations supplemented in some instances by exploratory surgical techniques.

Patients with suspected organic disorders frequently present at psychiatric clinics, or as referrals from wards in a general hospital. Their initial assessment will almost certainly be made by a psychiatrist. Support for the initial diagnosis may be sought from a clinical psychologist who conducts a battery of neuropsychological tests designed to identify specific areas of impairment of general cognitive and perceptuo-motor abilities. The psychologist's involvement is important because the results of his assessment may aid diagnosis or form a valuable quantitative baseline of mental functions and behaviour against which results of future examinations may be compared.

PRELIMINARY CLINICAL NEUROPSYCHIATRIC EXAMINATION

It is a cardinal rule that, when examining a patient suspected of having an organic disorder, the doctor should first establish the patient's level of consciousness. Impairment of consciousness is common in acute disorders of brain function irrespective of their origin (e.g. head injury, metabolic disorders, infections), but also occurs in a number of more slowly developing conditions (e.g. chronic subdural haematoma, cerebral tumour) and at a late stage in conditions such as the dementias, and where there are mass lesions in the brain. In contrast, patients with defects of cerebral function that remain after an acute event are usually fully conscious although recovery continues to occur (e.g. following strokes, head injury and post-infective states) for some time.

Assessing consciousness

Clinical assessment of consciousness is based upon the criteria of orientation, memory and behaviour, with supporting or background information about the duration of any abnormality from relatives or friends. Most patients in a state of altered consciousness will be acutely ill, in which case the history should be obtained from a third party. Such information is invaluable also where the condition has developed more gradually.

The patient should be assessed first regarding orientation for time (day, month, year, date and time of day) for orientation in terms of the place in which the examination is taking place because misidentification is common when patients have altered levels of consciousness. If orientation is noticeably impaired, memory will be affected but, if it is only slightly impaired, a false impression of normality may be gained. Short-term memory should be tested specifically by giving the patient a name and address, a colour, or the name of a flower to remember and asking him to repeat these after an interval of 5 minutes. Behaviour is a useful guide to the presence of altered consciousness. For example, errors and inconsistencies in the patient's statements, failure to remember significant dates, poor levels of attention and easy distractibility are all common and patients with such problems quickly become restless, fatigued and grow weary of testing. Often they show irritability and may even be hostile.

Assessing memory

Memory is usually the first intellectual function to be impaired in organic disorders of the brain where the pathological process is diffuse, for example in the dementias, or abnormalities where lesions are concentrated in both medial temporal areas, as in herpes simplex encephalitis. In most cases the primary deficit is one of a failure of, or difficulty in, retrieving information recently acquired. It is current practice to divide memory functions into: immediate or working memory, which is concerned with the moment-to-moment handling of information — both newly acquired and recalled; short-term memory, in which information is processed for storage but is vulnerable to disruption and 'forgetting' and long-term memory, which is concerned with consolidated information in store. Unless the intellectual deficits are severe, long-term memories are retrieved with relative ease. When testing short-term memory (recalled) it must be remembered that advancing years, apart from any pathological process, diminish the ease with which patients memorise facts. Failure to remember the names of people is often the first sign of memory difficulties. Where memory problems are very severe, for example in the Korsakoff state following herpes simplex encephalitis or in chronic alcoholism, the patient may unconsciously fill out the large gaps in his memory by the process of confabulation. In some cases the material is totally fictitious and easily prompted by suggestions from the examiner and, in others, memories for past events which appear relevant to the current situation are used to compensate for deficiencies. A fuller assessment of memory should be obtained by a clinical psychologist.

Assessing speech

Defects of speech must be detected early in the clinical examination because they are often linked to a disorder of understanding, and this combination of deficits interferes with other tests the clinician may wish to perform. The term aphasia is used in a specific manner to describe central disturbances of language involving all language modalities and components of the language system caused by localised brain damage. It is used only when other higher functions are left intact, although, in fact, certain functions which are dependent on the language may be disturbed, as in the case of arithmetical skills. The most common aphasic disorder is impaired word finding (nominal dysphasia), for example hesitations, groping for the appropriate word and circumlocution or periphrasis are terms applied to the patient's substitute definitions, often inadequate, for the forgotten word (e.g. 'you write it' for a pen). A simple test for nominal dysphasia requires the patient to (1) name a dozen objects from the commonplace to the, for him, unfamiliar, for example a stethoscope, whilst he handles each object in turn, and (2) to enumerate as many components of certain categories, for example flowers and animals, as he can remember.

EVIDENCE OF FOCAL LESIONS

During the first examination the clinician should perform simple tests to determine the possibility of a focal component in an organic disorder of brain function. Disorders of speech (non-fluent/expressive and fluent/receptive dysphasias), of praxis (ability to manipulate parts of the body correctly in space) and of gnosis (ability to recognise objects, faces, sounds or a part of the body) are all evidence of focal damage.

Frontal lobes

The frontal lobes have extensive connections with other areas of the brain, including all four sensory areas, the limbic system and the motor and pre-motor cortex. Also, there is evidence of focal activity within the lobes and of a degree of laterality of function. The range of connections with other brain areas gives the frontal lobes access to both the internal and external environments and, as a consequence, they are involved in the selection, organisation and verification of motor and behavioural activities. For example, three types of behavioural deficit have been identified, namely:

- Psychomotor disorders and planning disabilities
- Disorders of abstract thinking
- Disturbances of social and emotional behaviour.

Clinical examination for behavioural deficits reveals that psychomotor abnormalities include the appearance of primitive reflexes, for example the grasp reflex elicited when the palmar surface of the hand is lightly stroked, and the sucking reflex when the lips are touched. Perseveration of motor function may be demonstrated by asking the patient to copy a series of simple designs, and this abnormality is revealed by the Wisconsin Card Sorting Test. Planning is affected by the presence of impulsiveness, which may be demonstrated in the same test. Poor attention span leads to failure to match test results to the original request from the tester. An ability to work with abstract concepts is a further feature of frontal lobe damage and a need to work with concrete objects is an indication of its presence.

Damage to the frontal lobes by trauma, tumour, degenerative conditions (e.g. early Pick's disease), and infection, especially if bilateral, has a primary effect upon certain aspects of social and emotional behaviour which tend to overshadow the changes in intellect. A considerable amount of attention has been given to disorders of the frontal lobes since the first dramatic description of their manifestations by Dr J. M. Harlow to the Massachusett's Medical Society in 1868 in his patient, Phineas Gage. He was a railway worker who was injured when a long iron rod was driven through his skull as a result of an explosion. The rod entered through his cheek below the zygoma and emerged rostral to the right precentral motor area. Marked changes in personality followed survival from this remarkable injury and, whereas Gage had previously been a competent and reasonable man, he became unpredictable, impervious to advice or argument, and continually devised new plans which he failed to execute. He showed little concern for others and indulged in 'the greatest profanity'. In fact he was 'no longer Gage'. Later, in 1898, Phelps commented perceptively that 'there seems to be a law of a relationship between a very limited region of the brain and higher physical phenomena'. Thus, the typical features of a personality change following frontal lobe damage include disinhibition, facile euphoria, blunting of emotional responsiveness, egocentricity, interference with the behaviour of others, irresponsibility, lack of tact and concern, and childishness. Usually, patients exhibit purposeless drive and show loss of initiative and judgement; in a proportion, there is apathy and inertia and, in others, marked aggressiveness.

In mild cases of dysfunction, as might be seen in certain forms of early dementia, the changes are more subtle. They include reduced sensitivity to the feelings of others, less creative drive, less intellectual curiosity, less foresight together with some loosening of standards of ethical behaviour, a reduction in performance at work, and increased carelessness with regard to personal appearance. At this stage such changes may only be apparent to those who know the patient well.

This rather general account of the elements of changes in personality and behaviour does not reveal to what extent the symptoms bear a relationship to specific areas within the frontal lobes or to laterality, about which there is a growing body of information. Animal experiments have been used to demonstrate that the dorsolateral and orbital areas, which have quite different morphological structures, have different functions and different central connections. Clinical observations in man indicate that damage to the orbital–frontal regions leads to impulsiveness, distractibility and loss of social and emotional control. In contrast, damage to the dorsolateral surface produces deficits in word fluency, the verbal regulation of behaviour and perseveration (Stuss & Benson 1983). Luria (1973) proposed that psychomotor disorders occur most commonly with damage to the posterior part of the dorsolateral surface, whereas he was of the opinion that planning ability and defects in the regulation of speech are caused by damage that is more anterior.

The deficits caused by full prefrontal leucotomy, as described by Freeman & Watts (1942), were carefully assessed by Tow (1955). The operation effectively isolated the superolateral and orbitomedial prefrontal cortex from the thalamus, insula, amygdaloid and temporal areas, and Tow concluded that, following surgery:

There seems to be impairment in the powers of abstraction and synthesis, of perception of relations, and differences of the ability to deal with complex situations, planning and thinking out the next action and its consequences, together with appreciation of one's own mistakes. These are, of course, not several discrete functions, but they are several closely related aspects of intellectual activity which are impaired.

Williams (1979) commented further that prefrontal leucotomy and disorders causing bilateral frontal lesions impair patients' abilities to switch from one mental process or strategy to another, resulting in what is clinically called 'perseveration' in response to a request to perform serial tasks quickly. At a practical level this deficit is often specifically sought by neuropsychologists using the Wisconsin Card Sorting Test.

Commenting on the effects of war wounds, Jarvie (1954) and Lishman (1968) reported that features of frontal lobe dysfunction may occur after injury to only one lobe (Jarvie) but that the most severe effects are produced by bilateral injuries, especially those involving the orbito–frontal regions (Lishman). Jarvie pointed out that basic intellect may be spared in comparison with the severe changes that occur in affect and behaviour, and that patients may well retain insight into the fact that they are abnormal. The problem for the patient, therefore, is that he has minimal or no control over sudden shifts in mood, basic drives and behaviour, and such control as is retained is short lived. Jarvie also believed that the effects of frontal injury add nothing new to the personality, but rather reveal pretraumatic tendencies which were previously given very limited or no public expression — a point of view that would be contested nowadays. Lishman (1968) also commented upon the accentuation in the premorbid characteristics that may occur, although he also observed that severe frontal damage obliterates premorbid traits. It is of some practical interest that where there has been moderate-to-severe traumatic injury to the frontal lobes with impaired impulse control and the retention of insight, gradual though partial re-establishment of control occurs — the process being hastened by the use of operant behavioural techniques. Thus, insight is vital to the successful management of such patients. Clearly there are fundamental differences, however, between the traumatically brain injured individual in whom some degree of recovery may occur, and those with progressive disorders such as dementia.

At a neuropsychological level it has been shown that the frontal lobes do reflect, to some extent, the specialisation of the two hemispheres as a whole (Smith 1966). The left is more concerned with linguistic than with visuospatial functions and the right vice versa.

It has been shown that learning disabilities following frontal damage are largely due to greatly increased distractibility, perseveration, or a lack of attention by the patient to environmental cues, as described earlier.

Temporal lobes

The temporal lobes are rich sources of human experience and expression, and dysfunction due to injury and other causes presenting as a 'focal sign' is of major importance to the neurologist and psychiatrist. In addition, the temporal lobes are the site of abnormal activity giving rise to the epileptic phenomena peculiar to these regions of the brain.

Lesions of the dominant hemisphere, which is the left hemisphere in more than 90% of individuals, give rise to disorders of communication, including speech, reading and writing. In addition, involvement of the lower part of the optic radiation, or that part of it which loops down into the temporal lobe (Myer's loop) produces a contralateral, homonymous, upper-quadrantic defect of vision. Lesions of the non-dominant hemisphere are difficult to detect but may also give rise to a similar visual field defect as the only sign of abnormality. Bilateral medial temporal lesions are the cause of profound disorders of memory, or the dysmnesic syndrome.

The relation between dysphasia and handedness represents a complex subject. In summary, it is clear that language is more often mediated by the left than by the right hemisphere in both left- and right-handed subjects, but left-handed individuals appear to be less severely dysphasic than those who are right-handed after equivalent posterior temporal lobe lesions, and recover more quickly. These observations suggest that, in left-handed individuals, language function is bilaterally represented (Piercy 1964).

Abnormalities of communication

The main areas of the brain involved in speech are the posterior two-thirds of the inferior frontal gyrus (Broca's area) and the posterior third of the middle and central gyri, and the adjacent parietal lobe. Williams (1979) made the point that speech may be disturbed in both organic and psychiatric disorders. The chief differences between the two are that, in the person who has an organically produced defect, it is rare for all speech to disappear even though what remains is sparse and unintelligible. Dysphasic patients make strenuous attempts to communicate for the most part, whereas this may not be so in the case of schizophrenic patients, or the severely retarded depressed patient.

Classification of speech disorders is subject to variation and the method favoured by the authors is the separation of abnormalities into those in which speech is *non-fluent*, with a limited number of words or phrases being used, but not always correctly (Broca's aphasia, expressive dysphasia, motor dysphasia), and *fluent* dysphasia, in which there is normal or excess fluency, and the normal sequencing of words, but without sense (jargon aphasia). The latter condition is often termed receptive or sensory dysphasia.

Nominal dysphasia

Nominal dysphasia is a condition in which the patient has difficulty in finding words (lexical retrieval), usually names of objects or people. In the case of objects their function may be described quite correctly and, with time, or with prompting, the word may be remembered. In some cases it is only recognised when spoken by the examiner, although inappropriate words will be rejected. Interestingly, words which cannot be recalled on demand, as in the test situation (propositional speech), may be spoken quite spontaneously in other circumstances (spontaneous speech). Speech is grammatically correct but may be in a telegraphic style when word finding is very limited. Comprehension is usually intact, being impaired only in more severe cases.

Broca's dysphasia (non-fluent dysphasia, motor dysphasia, expressive dysphasia)

Pierre Paul Broca was a Parisian surgeon and anthropologist, who, on 2 April 1864, admitted a speechless, hemiplegic, handicapped man, named Leborgne, for treatment to his ward at the Bicêtre Hospital. He died from an infection several days later and at post mortem was found to have a superficial cortical lesion of the middle and inferior frontal gyri of the left hemisphere. A second, and clinically similar case, was seen some weeks later, and eventually Broca collected 22 cases of 'aphemia' or loss of speech associated with hemiplegia. As a result he was hailed as the discoverer of the 'centre for speech' in the brain (Critchley 1979). Complete loss of speech with such lesions is uncommon and the problem is chiefly one of disorganised motor control of the muscles of articulation, but word-finding difficulties always occur. Language comprehension difficulties are always present, although not prominently. As a consequence of the underlying vocal motor difficulties in frontal lesions, words are often mispronounced and so distorted or fragmented as to be unintelligible to the listener, although the speaker clearly knows what he wants to say. The frustrations so engendered may cause irritability, or even an aggressive outburst. The patient with a very localised lesion should be able to read and write without difficulty, but in most cases the extent of the pathological insult to the brain causes both dysphasia and a right-sided hemiparesis in which the involvement of the right arm and hand will be greater than that of the leg. Finally, under the influence of very strong emotion, for example fear or anger, the patient may utter words or short sentences which he cannot produce in normal circumstances (emotional speech).

Broca's aphasia is often termed an expressive or motor aphasia and, in contrast, involvement of comprehension to the extent that it is noticeably impaired, although word fluency is retained, results in a receptive or sensory aphasia. The latter condition is much less common than the former and was first described by Wernicke in 1881; it occurs in only 5–10% of all new aphasic admissions to neurological units. Patients with Wernicke's aphasia are unable to repeat words or phrases when asked and, when given objects to name, will use an incorrect though similar word if there is any response at all (paraphasia); alternatively, the patient may use a non-existent word (neologism). In addition to problems with single words, patients reveal grammatical abnormalities (paragrammatism). Speech is, however, fluent and rambling with many words (logorrhoea) and often delivered with bright manner, but the incoherence of speech renders it meaningless (jargon aphasia). Reading and writing are impaired to a significant extent also. The anatomical locus of the lesion causing this disturbance is in the white matter of the posterior temporo–parietal areas.

Parietal lobes

The parietal lobe is not a well-defined anatomical entity. It is demarcated by the drawing of somewhat arbitrary lines on the surface of the hemispheres, but this absence of natural boundaries only serves to emphasise its close functional relationship to the adjoining temporal and occipital lobes, for example in relation to dysphasia and dyslexia. Neurological signs indicating the presence of a parietal lobe lesion include cortical sensory loss, disturbances of the body image (agnosias), of visuospatial functions (apraxias), and, when the optic radiations are involved, visual loss.

Cortical sensory loss

Cortical sensory loss is a combination of a disturbance of simple sensation and discrimination. For example, patients with such deficits are unable to identify objects by palpation alone (astereognosis) or to recognise numbers or letters written on the palm of the hand when unseen (agraphaesthesia). The ability to discriminate the separation of two points (using a pair of dividers) on the finger pad is impaired or lost and, when the back of each hand is touched simultaneously, unseen contact with the hand to the opposite side of the brain lesion will not be reported — a phenomenon known as sensory extinction. In another form the same phenomenon may be discovered when it is found that the patient ignores half of the visual field on the side opposite to the lesion (visual inattention).

Disorders of body image

'Body image' refers to a person's awareness of his bodily self. A right-handed patient with a parietal lesion of the non-dominant hemisphere may 'neglect' the left side of the body, for example when asked to put out his hands he raises the right one only, although he will bring up the left hand in opposition to it when the omission is brought to his attention. Automatic acts, for example, are not affected, nor are actions requiring coordination of both hands. In acute conditions, such as strokes, or a later stage in a progressive lesion of the non-dominant hemisphere, the patient may neglect to wash the left side of the body, or to clothe the left limbs. In fact, if a patient has a left hemiparesis or hemiplegia he may ignore the disability (anosognosia), or deny that it exists when it is brought to his attention though, in the latter case, there is usually some clouding of consciousness. In the case of acute lesions the phenomenon usually fades quite quickly, but where it is persistent and there is 'denial' of the presence of a part of the body it may be treated as alien or be given a nickname. Why these phenomena are observed only in relation to left-sided neglect and lesions in the non-dominant hemisphere is not clear. It has been suggested that right-sided neglect does not occur because it is subordinate to the dysphasia and other major disorders which accompany lesions in the region of the parietal lobe in the dominant hemisphere. Finally, patients with lesions of the dominant parietal lobe may fail to recognise the faces of others — a condition known as prosopagnosia. Interestingly, a patient with this condition may fail to recognise his wife or children, but, nevertheless, be able to pick them out as soon as he hears their voices. Therefore, the deficit is specific to vision, although it may also be specific for speech.

Gerstman's syndrome. There is a particular form of body image disturbance traditionally regarded as a minor form of autotopagnosia in which there is hesitation and doubt about identification of one's own fingers. In 1924, Gerstman reported an association between this phenomenon and right/left disorientation, agraphia, acalculia, and colour agnosia. The condition may occur in the absence of any other form of body image disturbance. Critchley (1953) published summaries of 28 cases of this disorder, of which only five had abnormalities in the right hemisphere and, of the patients concerned, two were left-handed or ambidextrous. The predominance of left-sided lesions has also been reported by Gloning et al (1968). Although Gerstman himself was convinced that the lesion responsible for the syndrome lay 'in the region of the parieto-occipital convexity (of the dominant hemisphere), particularly in that part which is represented by the transitional region of the angular and middle occipital convolutions', Critchley (1953) came to the conclusion that it was not possible to say more than that the disorder relates to abnormalities in the parietal area. The existence of the syndrome, which is by no means always complete, can be elicited by asking the patient to name a finger touched by the examiner, to hold up the finger touched by the examiner, to point to a named finger on the examiner, or to carry out a complex command such as 'put the third finger of the right hand on the tip of the left second finger'. It may be found that the patient has greater difficulty in indicating fingers than in naming them (apraxia), or the reverse (finger aphasia).

Ideomotor and ideational apraxia. Ideomotor apraxia is an inability to imitate gestures and actions to command when the patient understands the request and does not suffer from paresis. The condition denotes a difficulty with the sequencing and spacial orientation of movements when attempting to execute complex actions, for example those requiring a sequence of willed acts. A characteristic finding is that similar actions may be performed automatically, or when the patient is suffering from emotional stress.

Dressing apraxia. Putting on garments in their proper order and manipulating buttons, buckles and straps is so much a part of personal routine that any deviation from it impresses the observer. The so-called 'dressing apraxia' is not an isolated disorder, however, but is a form of ideational apraxia. Alternatively, it may result from neglect of the left half of the body, described previously. Dressing will then be one sided with the patient ignoring the left arm and leg. In such cases the lesion is in the non-dominant hemisphere.

Constructional apraxia. This phenomenon is illustrated by an inability to copy two-dimensional designs using pencil and paper and/or matchsticks and to construct a three-dimensional model from bricks of different sizes and shapes. In everyday life it becomes evident when an individual makes mistakes in laying the table, or is no longer able to carry out normal constructional tasks in his work. It is said that constructional apraxia is twice as frequent in right- as in left-sided lesions, but it has also been reported in association with bilateral lesions and diffuse cerebral disease. In the latter it is often an early indication of the presence of organic disease.

Topographical orientation. Topographical orientation, namely the ability to find one's way about in familiar surroundings, may be disordered in disturbances of parietal lobe function, as may topographical memory, defined as the ability to summon up a clear mental picture of routes and landmarks, or the internal layout of familiar buildings, and to describe these features to others. Errors in route finding and/or topographical memory are often the first sign of a parietal tumour or generalised cerebral atrophy. These disabilities may follow either bilateral or unilateral cerebral diseases and available evidence indicates that most often the posterior right hemisphere is damaged.

Temporal defects

Defects in temporal awareness are also encountered in parietal disease, for example difficulty in estimating the approximate hour of the day, or judging the length of time occupied by a particular activity. Disorientation in time is more likely to denote clouding of consciousness.

Having made a general assessment of intellectual and cognitive function and carried out a search for evidence of focal elements in the patient's disorder, the clinician should proceed to a general clinical neurological examination prior to obtaining additional information from the patient's nearest relative or a friend, and possibly from the results of neuro-psychological tests.

NEUROLOGICAL ASSESSMENT (THE USE OF NEUROPSYCHOLOGICAL TESTS)

Neuropsychological tests are used in several ways in the assessment of the effects of, or recovery from, brain damage. First, they may be used to support a clinical diagnosis and, at times, help to distinguish between symptoms attributable to either brain damage or a functional mental disorder. Second, they are used to monitor changes in mental functions with time, as in the case of patients recovering from acute traumatic brain injuries. At times, tests are used to provide serial measures of the extent of mental deterioration in degenerative disorders. (In both cases the information yielded is often required for research purposes). In the recovering patient, neuropsychological tests may be used to assess the effects of various forms of rehabilitation.

Neuropsychological tests exist in two main forms. For example, batteries of tests have been designed for specific purposes, as in the case of assessment of dementia (e.g. the Cambridge Mental Disorders of the Elderly Examination, CAMDEX) or intelligence (e.g. the Wechsler Adult Intelligence Scale, WAIS). On the

other hand, individual tests may be extracted from such batteries, or be specifically designed to assess a single brain function (e.g. speech). It should be remembered that each test, whether part of a battery or not, measures a specific function. Groups of tests yield profiles which are often characteristic of a given disorder.

Certain difficulties may be encountered in the use of neuropsychological tests. For example, communication disorders interfere with a wide range of tests which, as in the case of tests of intelligence, depend upon adequate communication skills. Test results must always be evaluated in the light of clinical observations and, where appropriate, taking into consideration the results of other forms of investigation (e.g. imaging).

CLASSIFICATION OF ORGANIC DISORDERS

The classification of organically determined psychiatric states has been a source of confusion to clinicians for many years. In 1980, steps towards clarification of this problem were taken by the American Psychiatric Association in DSM-III. The method of classification adopted in DSM-III was an extension of, and an improvement upon, the method of classification of mental disorders adopted by the World Health Organization in ICD-9 (WHO 1978). ICD-10 will reflect these improvements. DSM-III has been revised (DSM-IIIR; APA 1987), but the method of categorisation of organically determined mental disorders has been retained.

In DSM-IIIR, two broad categories of disorder are described — the organic mental syndromes and the organic mental disorders. This distinction has been made because, not uncommonly, it is not possible to determine the cause of a particular group of symptoms of mental disturbance. However, if the origin of such symptoms becomes known, or is known from the outset, the condition is described as an organic mental disorder. For example, if a patient is delirious, but the cause is unknown, he suffers from an organic mental syndrome, whereas if it is known to be due to alcohol withdrawal, then an organic mental disorder (delirium tremens) is present. Causes of organic mental syndromes include (1) primary cerebral disorders, (2) cerebral disorders secondary to systemic diseases, (3) exogenous toxic agents affecting the brain and (4) withdrawal from abused substances such as alcohol or barbiturates (Lipowski 1984). Ten organic mental syndromes are described in DSM-IIIR but, for convenience, these may be grouped as follows: (1) the dementias, (2) the amnestic syndromes, (3) delirium,

(4) other mental disorders due to brain damage, dysfunction or disease, including organic delusional syndrome, organic hallucinosis, and organic affective syndrome, and, finally, (5) the organic personality and behaviour disorders due to brain damage, disease or dysfunction.

In groups 1 and 2, changes in cognitive function predominate, in group 3 there is a disturbance of consciousness and widespread but reversible mental changes, whereas in group 4 the chief characteristics are the presence of disorders of thinking (delusions), of perception (hallucinations), and of mood and emotion (depression, elation and anxiety) in normal consciousness. In group 5 the chief manifestation of the disorder is a change in personality. Clearly, symptom clusters may vary in composition and groups may overlap.

In this chapter a series of disorders are described which are directly related to the syndromes listed. For example, different types of dementia, delirium and its causes, and the amnestic syndromes are dealt with individually. In addition, conditions which form the basis for any or several syndromes may appear at some point during the natural history of several disorders, for example head injury, subarachnoid haemorrhage, general paralysis and multiple sclerosis are described as part of the symptomatology of such disorders. Clearly, in some cases, the syndrome may be the predominating feature, but more often it is part of a specific organic disorder which is easily recognised.

ACUTE AND SUBACUTE DISTURBANCES OF CONSCIOUSNESS

It is accepted that consciousness is a state of mental activity in which, to a variable extent, an individual is aware of both external and internal (mental) events. It is a state which reflects underlying patterns of activity in basic neurophysiological and psychological processes and ranges from full consciousness, in which these processes are optimally active, through states of altered consciousness, in which they are impaired, to coma, in which awareness of external or internal events is absent.

Very mild impairment of consciousness is often termed a confusional state and implies, primarily, a condition in which attention and thinking are impaired. A more severe disturbance of consciousness and cognitive function associated with disordered perception in the form of illusions and hallucinations, and of thinking in the form of delusions, indicates the presence of delirium. The state of stupor intervenes

between delirium and coma. It is a condition resembling deep sleep from which the individual can only be aroused by vigorous and even painful stimulation, on cessation of which he returns to the unresponsive state. This is of interest to psychiatrists because, although stupor may be due to diffuse cerebral dysfunction secondary to known organic factors, it may also be the result of a severe functional disorder — most often a severe depressive illness.

DELIRIUM

In 1967, Lipowski suggested that the term delirium should be defined by the following criteria:

1. The individual is awake and usually capable of responding verbally.
2. There is evidence of impairment of thinking, memory, perception and attention that fluctuates over time.
3. There is an impaired ability to comprehend the environment and the internal perceptions in accordance with the individual's past experience and knowledge.
4. There is usually concomitant change in the frequency of the EEG which varies pari passu with the level of cognition.

Delirium is an acute disturbance of consciousness which tends to develop rapidly and rarely lasts more than 4–7 days. At the bedside the delirious patient is recognised by the presence of a number of abnormalities of mental state and behaviour, including disorientation for time, place and person, disturbed attention span with distractibility, impaired memory, and decreased capacity for abstract thinking. Patients often exhibit a fearful or suspicious mood but, on occasions, may be withdrawn and apathetic. They reveal evidence of having delusions, of misidentifying those around them, of hallucinations which are usually of a visual nature, and of delusions which are almost always of the paranoid type. Restlessness, irritability, fatiguability and a reversed sleep pattern, which means that the patient is somnolent during the day, but restless and agitated at night, are also features of delirium. Symptoms fluctuate markedly over time, and lucid intervals, lasting minutes to hours, may appear. It has been observed that delirium is commonest at the two extremes of life and the disorder accompanies diffuse metabolic and multifocal cerebral illness. Its presence indicates generalised impairment of brain function or, at least, bilateral involvement of limbic structures.

Apart from bedside observations, the presence of the condition may be identified by abnormalities of the electroencephalogram (EEG). In general, the basic frequencies of the EEG are slowed, with the notable exception of delirium tremens associated with alcoholism, in which it is more common to see fast rather than slow activity.

Treatment of delirium and disordered consciousness

The first line of treatment of delirium is that of the primary cause, but certain measures are uniformly applicable. The patient should be nursed in a bright simple ward or room, preferably by the same group of nurses. No potentially dangerous objects should be within reach, and at night a light should be provided to prevent increasing disturbances of perception that would be brought about by darkness. It is important to allay restlessness, and the drugs most commonly used are thioridazine, chlorpromazine and chlormethiazole. When there is reason to believe that alcohol is the cause, or that vitamin B_1 deficiency attributable to other factors is present, then Parentrovite (which contains the whole vitamin B complex) should be given immediately and preferably intravenously by infusion.

AETIOLOGY OF ACUTE DISTURBANCES OF CONSCIOUSNESS

Acute disturbances of consciousness are caused by a variety of factors (see Table 15.1), some of which will be described in more detail. Despite the fact that a large number of disorders can give rise to acute disturbances of consciousness, the final common pathway is a disturbance of metabolism in those areas of the brain responsible for consciousness. At one time infectious diseases were the commonest cause of delirium, but nowadays intoxication by drugs heads the list, and alcohol withdrawal is the commonest cause of delirium developing soon after admission to hospital. Determining the cause of acute disturbances of consciousness, other than those where there is a proven history of head injury, or a stroke, may prove to be quite difficult. However, despite the possible lack of an accurate history or helpful neurological signs, careful clinical examination, including observation of the patient's respiratory pattern, analysis of blood pH, serum bicarbonate, determination of the blood sugar level, and a simple drug screen, should be helpful.

Table 15.1 Some causes of acute organic disorders

Hypoxia
Heart failure, myocardial infarction
Respiratory disorders

Infection
1. General — bronchopneumonia, urinary tract, tropical infections
2. Cerebral — meningitis, encephalitis

Metabolic disorder
Electrolyte disturbance
Uraemia
Hepatic encephalopathy
Porphyria
Hypoglycaemia

Vitamin deficiency
Thiamine (Wernicke's encephalopathy)
B_{12} deficiency

Endocrine disease
Myxoedema, thyrotoxicosis
Parathyroid disorder
Diabetes
Cushing's disease, Addison's disease
Hypopituitarism

Trauma
Head injury

Epilepsy
Psychomotor seizure
Postictal state

Space-occupying lesion
Tumours — primary, metastatic
Subdural haematoma
Cerebral abscess

Vascular disease
Transient ischaemic attacks
Multi-infarct dementia
Cerebral embolism
Hypertensive encephalopathy
Subarachnoid haemorrhage
Transient global amnesia

Toxic disorders
Drugs — alcohol, barbiturates, amphetamines, LSD, opiates, cannabis, cocaine, salicylates, phenacetin, tricyclic antidepressants, monoamine oxidase inhibitors, lithium, benzhexol, L-dopa, isoniazid, cycloserine, steroids, digoxin
Industrial metals — lead, mercury, manganese, etc.

METABOLIC DISTURBANCES GIVING RISE TO ALTERED CONSCIOUSNESS AND DELIRIUM

Cerebral ischaemia and hypoxia

Disturbances of cerebral oxygenation may be divided into anoxic anoxia, anaemic anoxia, hypoxia and ischaemia — a failure of adequate perfusion of the brain. In anoxic anoxia insufficient oxygen reaches the blood and, therefore, its oxygen content and oxygen tension are low. This may occur because there is insufficient oxygen in the environment. Anaemic anoxia develops when the level of haemoglobin in the blood is low for some reason, or because there is displacement of oxygen by another gas, such as carbon monoxide. Mild hypoxia, for example in respiratory diseases, is associated with increased cerebral blood flow, which can increase to a maximum of about twice the normal level. When this point has been reached and there is still insufficient oxygen to compensate for the hypoxic state, the cerebral metabolic rate for oxygen begins to fall and symptoms of hypoxia occur. The causes of ischaemic hypoxia include reduced cardiac output for whatever reason, stroke and cerebral vasospasm (e.g. migraine and subarachnoid haemorrhage).

Infections

Delirium can complicate many infections, the mental changes being caused by a number of factors, including toxins released by bacteria, pyrexia and specific problems such as anoxia in respiratory infections, and electrolyte disturbances in infections of the gastrointestinal and renal tracts. Respiratory and urinary tract infections account for many cases of delirium in the elderly. Tropical infections, such as malaria and trypanosomiasis, must be considered where a confused and febrile patient has recently been abroad. Finally, it is likely that with the increase in infection by the human immunodeficiency virus (HIV), physicians will encounter patients with neurological disorders caused by HIV or some form of opportunistic infection of the brain described later in this chapter.

Renal disease

Renal failure caused by renal disease or systemic diseases, such as malignant hypertension, bacteraemia, or vascular collagen disorders, gives rise to changes in a patient's mental state as uraemia develops. In addition, the treatment of uraemia by dialysis may lead to cerebral dysfunction in the form of the dialysis disequilibrium syndrome, or progressive dialysis encephalopathy. The precise cause of renal encephalopathy is uncertain. The blood urea nitrogen level itself varies widely in relation to changes in the mental state, and therefore urea itself is not thought to be the cause. Likewise, the electrolyte levels show very little correlation either. In fact, the cause is likely to be a neurotoxic compound normally excluded from the

brain, but which gains access to it by an increased concentration in red cells. The presence of such a substance in erythrocytes is facilitated by the uraemic state, which increases red cell permeability. In addition, raised levels of calcium, which also occur in uraemia and which are raised in the brain, may play a role in altering neurotransmitter release and, therefore, psychological function. Clinically, uraemia does not give rise to a specific set of mental symptoms. Patients usually exhibit fatigue, drowsiness, poor concentration and hyperpnoea. In addition, they may have a tremor, muscle twitching and peripheral neuropathy with epilepsy, but all are signs which occur only in the most severely ill. Usually, patients complain of excessive thirst. Uraemia may also produce a full delirious state with noisy agitation as described previously, but more often patients are dull, confused and apathetic prior to progressing to stupor and coma.

Although several metabolic disorders cause a severe acidosis with alterations in consciousness, as, for example, in uraemia, diabetes and lactic acidosis, only uraemia is likely to cause tetany, multifocal myoclonus and epilepsy. The others do not give rise to a raised urea in the early stages and, therefore, uraemia should be relatively easily detected even when the patient is in a delirium. Occasionally, patients develop Wernicke's encephalopathy with confusion when on a long-term dialysis regime if they are not given vitamin supplements.

The treatment of uraemia is by dialysis, which produces neurological symptoms in about half those treated, and a more severe disturbance of central nervous system function in only 5%. The latter includes delirium, stupor, coma, convulsions and myoclonus. These effects occur most often in those who have undergone haemodialysis rather than peritoneal dialysis, and in children rather than adults. The most likely cause of these changes is an alteration in osmotic equilibrium between the brain tissues and blood with the brain becoming hyperosmolar for a time.

Repeated dialysis over a period of 3 years or more may give rise to neurological abnormalities, beginning with stammering and hesitancy of speech, progressing to a delusional state and then dementia with accompanying seizures. It has been suggested that this condition is the result of aluminium intoxication, with the metal entering the body via the dialysate and local water supply.

Apart from the conditions described, the process of repeated dialysis often produces anxiety and depression, which may be a reaction to the stress of the procedure or a complication of the use of antihypertensive drugs.

Disorders of acid–base balance

The acid–base balance of the brain is not necessarily altered by disturbances of systemic acid–base balance because physiological mechanisms protect the former from the latter. Thus, of the four disorders of systemic acid–base balance (respiratory and metabolic acidosis and alkalosis), respiratory alkalosis may cause a minor disturbance of consciousness, and metabolic acidosis a delirium. There are specific poisons which may be ingested by chronic alcoholics which cause metabolic acidosis, of which methyl alcohol (methanol) and ethylene glycol are examples. Also, a drug overdose with preparations containing salicylate produces a tissue acidosis with a respiratory alkalosis.

Liver disease

Mental disturbances occur in liver disease because either blood in the portal system bypasses the liver and enters the systemic circulation, or liver function fails for some reason. Diagnosis is not usually difficult because of a history of chronic liver disease, perhaps with a past history of alcoholism, together with the familiar physical signs of jaundice, spider angiomata, an enlarged liver or spleen and fetor hepaticus. However, occasionally the onset of the condition might be mistaken for acute alcoholism, or even hypomania, because in a small proportion of cases (10–20%) the earliest symptoms of the encephalopathy resemble the latter condition. For the majority, however, hepatic encephalopathy begins as a state of dull or apathetic delirium which may progress to coma, or from which the patient may recover. A small number of patients who have had repeated episodes of acute encephalopathy progress to dementia associated with cerebellar and extrapyramidal signs. The cause of the encephalopathy is not known with precision, but most attention has been paid to ammonia intoxication caused by the products of digestion which have bypassed the normal urea-synthesising mechanisms in the liver. In the brain, ammonia interferes with the cellular chloride pump mechanism, possibly replacing intracellular potassium, thereby affecting sodium/potassium-dependent ATPase activity. Also, ammonia interferes with brain cell energy metabolism. Finally, hepatic encephalopathy may be caused, at least in part, by abnormalities of neurotransmitter mechanisms.

Porphyria

Of the three types of porphyria, intermittent acute porphyria, hereditary coproporphyria and variegate porphyria, the first is the most common in Britain.

Intermittent acute porphyria (IAP) is transmitted by a single autosomal dominant gene with variable penetrance. It occurs in a ratio of 3:2 in women to men and the onset is after puberty, though it is seldom seen after middle life. As a result of the primary genetic defect there is a generalised deficiency of the enzyme uroporphyrinogen-I synthetase, which is important in the synthesis of haem, predominantly in the liver. The effect is a depression of δ-aminolaevulinic-acid synthetase activity and an overproduction of δ-aminolaevulinic acid and porphobilinogen. Freshly voided urine turns a deep red colour on exposure to light as porphobilinogen is converted to uroporphyrin.

Attacks of porphyria may erupt spontaneously or be precipitated by (1) drugs, notably barbiturates, alcohol, sulphonamides, methyldopa and oral contraceptives, (2) infections, (3) pregnancy and (4) metabolic and nutritional factors (dieting and low carbohydrate intake).

The basic clinical defect is a neuropathy, which is manifested in several ways. The classical case presents with acute abdominal pain (with or without rigidity), vomiting and constipation, thus simulating an 'acute abdomen' perhaps leading in some instances to laparotomy. More clear-cut evidence of neuropathy may be apparent as weakness or paralysis of the limbs. Any one of the cranial nerves may be involved. Pain in affected muscles is a common symptom, but it is frequently experienced in other areas also, for example as headache. Hypertension and tachycardia may occur at the height of the attack and, less commonly, epileptiform convulsions develop. Attacks of IAP are self-limiting. Death, when it occurs, results most commonly from ventilatory failure. The formerly high mortality has decreased dramatically with the introduction of more effective methods of dealing with this complication.

Psychological disturbances are observed more often in IAP than any other form of porphyria. Florid delirium or a quieter confusional state, during which the patient may show mildly aggressive and disinhibited behaviour for which amnesia is subsequently claimed, are commonly reported and may be erroneously labelled as hysterical. Memory impairment has been observed during and after an attack, but usually clears. Both schizophrenia-like illnesses and affective disorders have been reported, and McAlpine & Hunter (1969) claimed that the mental illnesses of King George III were manifestations of porphyria.

Vitamin B$_{12}$ deficiency

Lack of vitamin B$_{12}$ gives rise to pernicious anaemia and may be accompanied by subacute combined degeneration of the spinal cord. There is also an association with mental symptoms, which may accompany the anaemia and cord degeneration, or precede them by many months.

In pernicious anaemia, mental symptoms may take the form of pronounced slowing of mental processes, confusion and memory defects associated with signs of neuropathy and spinal cord involvement. In some cases the mental symptoms appear before the anaemia or neurological signs. Mental symptoms tend to disappear or improve following parenteral administration of vitamin B_{12}. In pernicious anaemia, both functional and organic mental symptoms have been described and, of the former, depression, and sometimes paranoid delusions have been noted. Their relationship to the low serum vitamin B_{12} level is doubtful. More certain is the association of the low serum vitamin B_{12} level with organic symptoms, such as intellectual and memory impairment or confusional states. Schulman (1967) compared patients with pernicious anaemia with patients with other forms of anaemia, and showed that whilst psychiatric symptoms occurred in about a third of each group, only organic symptoms appeared to be related to low vitamin B_{12} levels. Studies of the brain in those who have died from the disorder show diffuse and focal degeneration of white matter in the brain as well as in the spinal cord.

The usual cause of low serum vitamin B_{12} levels is the absence of intrinsic factor in the stomach, preventing absorption of the vitamin, but it can also follow gastric surgery, or occur in the presence of carcinoma of the stomach. Poor nutrition, as a cause, is very rare.

Treatment of the condition with hydroxycobalamin, if started early, is usually satisfactory. Memory impairment improves, fatigue is lost, and there is a restoration of well-being.

Endocrine disorders

Hypothyroidism

Myxoedema is a disease of insidious onset and the mental symptoms that usually accompany it may easily be mistaken for primary psychiatric illness. Characteristic physical signs are often present, such as pale rather oedematous facial skin, dryness of the skin, hair loss, and lowering of the voice. Relatives may have noticed the physical changes which can easily be overlooked at a single interview. The common mental symptoms that occur with myxoedema are slowness of thinking, fatigue, apathy and poor concentration.

Memory difficulties are frequent and often noticed at an early stage in the illness. The patient may be thought to have depression or, if the memory and intellectual difficulties are more apparent, to have primary presenile dementia.

Sometimes the picture is more florid and can take the form of a paranoid psychosis with delusions and hallucinations. Some degree of mental confusion, however, is usually apparent. The cases described by Asher (1949) as 'myxoedematous madness' fall into this category. Several of his patients had paranoid ideas and hallucinations in addition to organic features. In terms of DSM-IIIR diagnostic criteria they presented with organic hallucinosis, the delusional syndrome, or a combination of both.

Neurological complications are also important. Jellinek (1962) drew attention to the quite frequent occurrence of epilepsy, fainting and transient ischaemic attacks in myxoedematous patients. Cerebellar ataxia has been noted and EEG changes are common, with slowing and flattening of the alpha rhythm. The risk of associated hypothermia and coma is very real and brain damage may be irreversible if treatment is delayed. Death from myxoedema is rare but may occur.

The exact cause of changes in neurological and psychological function are not fully understood. The two major hypotheses both relate to the effect of hypothyroidism upon brain oxygen consumption and nucleoprotein and protein synthesis in neurones and synapses. Thyroid hormone increases both oxygen consumption in most tissues and the metabolic rate of cerebral cortex. Hypothyroid patients certainly show decreased oxygen consumption and, perhaps, a decrease in cerebral blood flow, but these changes are almost certainly a reflection of more general circulatory changes rather than changes in brain metabolism.

Hyperthyroidism

Anxiety, overactivity and lability are common in thyrotoxicosis and the disorder may be mistaken for a primary anxiety state or an agitated depression. Clinical features that may help in establishing hypothyroidism are the presence of goitre, lid lag, a history of weight loss in the presence of good appetite, a warm, moist skin, and raised sleeping pulse. Confirmation is by appropriate estimations of thyroid hormone activity.

Both affective and schizophrenic psychoses have often been reported as occurring in thyrotoxicosis, but there is no good reason to suppose they are specific;

indeed, they are relatively infrequent considering the commonness of thyrotoxicosis. Patients with this disorder have been found to be vulnerable to mental illness and the thyrotoxicosis seems to act as a precipitant for psychosis, and agitation and excitement are often frequent features of a psychosis associated with this disease.

Parathyroid disorders

Hypoparathyroidism

This most commonly follows thyroidectomy when an abrupt fall in serum calcium precipitates psychiatric disturbance. The mental state is closely related to the serum calcium level. If this is borderline there may only be symptoms such as anxiety, depression and tension, but with lower levels acute confusion may result. The mental picture is quickly relieved by intravenous calcium gluconate. More chronic symptoms occur in long-standing hypoparathyroidism, such as poor concentration, emotional lability and impaired intelligence.

Hyperparathyroidism

The usual cause of hyperparathyroidism is a benign adenoma. The main symptoms are physical, but psychiatric features are also common, particularly depression and anergia. Memory and intellectual impairment occur with higher calcium levels and, in the extreme case of parathyroid crisis, there is acute confusion.

Hypopituitarism

Hypopituitarism may be attributable to any one of a number of factors, but those most frequently encountered are pituitary tumours and planned destruction of the gland by surgery or radiation. Clinical features include lack of energy and initiative, marked pallor of the skin — which is fine in texture and does not tan, loss of axillary and pubic hair, impotence in the male and amenhorrhoea in the female. Subsequently, intolerance of cold and somnolence develop and, not uncommonly, signs of secondary (pituitary) myxoedema. Apathy is a prominent symptom, which may be replaced periodically by acute emotional distress. A dysmnesic syndrome has been observed in cases which have gone untreated for years, and recurring confusional states are a warning of imminent coma, which was the usual cause of death before substitution therapy was

available. Weight loss is rare and, when it does occur, fails to reach the state of emaciation characteristic of anorexia nervosa. The symptoms described are a combination of adrenal and thyroid failure. They may appear in a variety of forms and may resemble a disorder of either gland. In this case, if treatment is given for failure of only one endocrine gland, signs of acute failure of the other are likely to develop. It should be remembered that patients with panhypopituitarism are sensitive to both narcotic analgesics and sedative drugs.

Cushing's disease

Excessive glucocorticoid production by the adrenal gland, which becomes hyperplastic in response to excessive production of adrenocorticotrophic hormone (ACTH) by the pituitary gland, frequently leads to changes in brain function, giving rise to an encephalopathy characterised by changes in mood and behaviour. Depression of mood is most common where the underlying cause is excessive production of ACTH by the pituitary gland. This contrasts with euphoria or elation, which is more common in patients who have been overtreated with glucocorticoids. These observations have led to the view that depression in Cushing's disease is due to ACTH rather than glucocorticoid production. In addition to the mental changes described, some patients develop paranoid delusions and hallucinations. On occasions, brief episodes of acute disturbance of behaviour occur which are characterised by excitement, anxiety or apathy. However, these disturbances do not in any sense resemble schizophrenia or true affective disorders.

In addition to the mental and behavioural changes described, patients with Cushing's disease have a characteristic appearance, with a red, moon-shaped face, hirsutism, obesity and a 'buffalo hump'. Also, diabetes, hypertension and associated neurological symptoms are often present.

At a time when treatment with steroid hormones is common it is as well to be aware that excessive consumption of these drugs over a period of time will produce Cushing's syndrome. For example, in an American study (Boston Collaborative Drug Surveillance Program 1972) of the side-effects of prednisolone in 676 patients, 21 developed acute psychiatric disorders with eight of these being euphoric and 13 frankly psychotic. The latter disorder was manifest as hallucinations, delusions and violent behaviour. In formal psychiatric terms two patients were depressed and six developed mania. All recovered when treatment with the drugs was withdrawn, although some required treatment with psychotropic drugs as well.

Addison's disease

Deficient production of adrenocorticosteroids by the adrenal gland alters brain function, which is corrected only by the administration of cortisone. Examination of patients' mental state reveals evidence of apathy, depression, lack of drive and initiative, resembling hypopituitarism. Mild disturbances of memory and attention are also quite common. Physically, patients show a dusky pigmentation of the skin and, biochemically, they have hyponatraemia, hyperkalaemia and hypocalcaemia in many cases. Hypotension is characteristic and may be sufficient to cause cerebral ischaemia.

Diabetes mellitus

Diabetes is an endocrine disorder which produces several different forms of metabolic dysfunction and directly, or indirectly, alterations in brain function leading to states ranging from mild confusion and irritability, through delirium and stupor, to coma. Thus, on the one hand there are those disturbances of metabolism which produce acute disturbances of cerebral functions (hypoglycaemia, ketoacidosis and lactic acidosis) and those which have a more chronic effect (renal insufficiency and cerebral arteriosclerosis). Ketoacidosis usually occurs in patients with relatively severe diabetes who fail to take insulin, or develop infections, and lactic acidosis occurs in patients on oral hypoglycaemic drugs. Interestingly, spontaneous hypoglycaemia can occur in individuals not known to have diabetes, but who are in an early stage of the disease, and also in some patients with renal insufficiency.

Spontaneous hypoglycaemia

Intermittent bizarre behaviour occurring before breakfast in the early morning, or after exercise in the late morning, when accompanied by symptoms of pallor, sweating, unsteadiness, anxiety and depersonalisation, is symptomatic of an insulin-secreting tumour of the pancreas (insulinoma). Frequently, the physical symptoms are the sole manifestations. The behavioural anomalies reflect altered consciousness, which, in some instances, may progress to coma. Focal neurological signs may be present but are gener-

ally transient. The symptoms described represent the classical picture, but this is not always present and, when incomplete, may lead to the patient's referral to a psychiatric clinic. Patients with this condition, who are submitted to psychiatric investigations, are not easily allotted to a psychiatric category, and the absence of specific psychiatric symptoms sometimes suggests the diagnosis. Recurring hypoglycaemic episodes may lead to brain damage. Low blood sugar levels during an acute episode are diagnostic, but these are not always witnessed. Patients suspected of having this disorder should be referred to a diabetic clinic for further investigation.

Visceral carcinoma

Prolonged and intermittent confusion is sometimes the first indication of a visceral carcinoma, notably bronchogenic carcinoma of the oat cell type. This tumour secretes an ACTH-like hormone which produces delirium. The appearance of altered mental function may antedate the appearance of the tumour by several months. As might be expected, examination of the brain at autopsy does not usually reveal evidence of cerebral metastases, given that the alteration in mental state has been caused by hormone secreted from the tumour. Patients of middle age who present with memory loss and signs of early dementia, who do not have a family history of dementia, head injury, or other conditions giving rise to signs of dementia, and who have normal brain scans, should be suspected of having an occult tumour.

AMNESTIC SYNDROME

For almost a century it has been known that dysfunction in certain medial temporal lobe structures, later identified as the hippocampus, amygdala and fornix, and in mid-line structures — in particular the mammillary bodies and dorso–medial nucleus of the thalamus — results in profound amnesia. Specific causes of the syndrome, discussed here, include Wernicke's encephalopathy, the Wernicke–Korsakoff syndrome and damage to the medial temporal area, which occurs commonly in severe head injuries and in herpes simplex encephalitis. There is a record of an unusual case of gross amnesia in a man injured in the region of his left dorso–medial thalamic nucleus by a mini fencing foil which entered his brain as a result of an accidental stab wound via his left nostril (Teuber, Milner & Vaughan 1968). Other causes of severe and permanent amnesia include infarction in the territory of the posterior cerebral arteries, and hypoxia.

Clinical features

The amnestic syndrome is defined as a state of profound amnesia, usually permanent, and manifest most obviously as a defect of short-term memory occurring in full consciousness. In addition to short-term memory difficulties there is also a defect of long-term memory. As a result, patients fail to memorise a current experience when fully conscious and when other intellectual functions are normal, or are much less impaired by comparison with the disturbance of memory. Thus, the individual is unable to remember other than momentarily what he or she currently sees, hears, thinks or feels and appears to live in a memoryless vacuum lacking the ability to add new information to that previously acquired even if now imperfectly remembered. However, experienced clinical psychologists are able to demonstrate that certain forms of memory capacity, for example those which do not require a verbal component (visuospatial and geographical memory), are retained. The patient is unaware of this ability but his behaviour may eventually prove the point in everyday life. At an early stage in the disorder, confabulation — the description of imaginary events to fill in gaps in memory — may be observed, but it tends to disappear with time. Also, though fully conscious, patients are disorientated for place and time, but usually not for person. Most of those with the disorder lack insight into their memory loss and, indeed, may deny it despite evidence to the contrary. Alternatively, the problem may be recognised but is treated as of little importance. Patients with severe amnesia, perhaps not unexpectedly, lack initiative and may appear apathetic. Usually they are friendly, but their mood is shallow.

Wernicke's encephalopathy

In 1881 Carl Wernicke described an acute neurological disorder with confusion in two male alcoholics and a woman poisoned by sulphuric acid. The symptoms included disturbances of eye movements (lateral nystagmus, external rectus paralysis, and paralysis of conjugate gaze), ataxia of gait, polyneuropathy in the limbs with mental changes including apathy, reduced attention span, disorientation for time and place, inability to recognise familiar faces, and inability to conduct a coherent conversation. All died, and post mortem examination revealed that they had small punctate haemorrhages in the grey matter around the third and fourth ventricles of the brain. The disorder was regarded as an acute inflammatory reaction of the oculomotor nuclei, and was fatal within 2 weeks.

Later work revealed that high doses of thiamine dramatically reduced high mortality rates in the acute phase and led to the resolution of neurological symptoms. Nowadays, with prompt and adequate treatment the ophthalmoplegias generally fade in a few days, but nystagmus, ataxia and neuropathy recover more slowly. Indeed, the latter two symptoms may be present in an attenuated form for many years after the original illness. Lateral nystagmus also commonly persists.

Wernicke–Korsakoff syndrome

In 1889 S. S. Korsakoff published the first of several reports of a disorder characterised by polyneuropathy, amnesia and confabulation — in many cases following long-term alcohol consumption, but also following conditions such as persistent vomiting, typhoid fever and puerperal sepsis. Almost a century later, Victor (1971) finally brought the discoveries of Wernicke and Korsakoff together under the name of the Wernicke–Korsakoff syndrome and it is now generally accepted that the two conditions are successive stages of a single disease.

The emergence of the Korsakoff defect coincides with the disappearance of a patient's confusion, which usually lasts about 2 weeks. The defect is not present in all patients, however, and Victor (1971) found that, of 245 patients, most of whom had been alcoholic, 186 survived and, of these, 84% developed Korsakoff's syndrome. Significantly, only about 25% of patients completely recovered their premorbid intellectual state.

Most patients who develop Wernicke's symptoms recover, but some do not and the post mortem examination of their brains reveals, in acute cases, petechial haemorrhages which are often visible to the naked eye in the mammillary bodies and less commonly in the walls of the third ventricle, periaqueductal grey matter, the floor of the fourth ventricle and inferior colliculi. Microscopic abnormalities may be present, and the characteristic lesions are seen in the mammillary bodies and commonly at one or more of the other sites previously mentioned from the optic chiasma to the vestibular nuclei.

Newer concepts include direct alcohol neurotoxicity causing dementia, and this diagnosis has been aided by computerised tomography (CT), confirming atrophy, and neuropathological evidence of cell loss involving both cortical and subcortical structures (Lishman 1990). There is some evidence to suggest that prolonged abstinence may, in the early stages, reverse these changes.

Family studies support the hypothesis that individual alcoholic patients differ in their susceptibility to cerebral damage as a result of genetically controlled biochemical factors. They may be unable to utilise thiamine normally (Pratt 1985), to form effective enzyme systems such as that of transketolase, which is involved in brain glucose metabolism and neurotransmitter formation, or they may have abnormalities of those enzymes involved in the metabolism and detoxification of alcohol itself.

Treatment

The possibility of the Wernicke–Korsakoff syndrome as a clinical diagnosis should be raised by a history of chronic alcoholism, which in fact accounts for the majority of cases. It should also be considered where patients have lesions of the stomach, duodenum or jejunum, causing malabsorption — for example in the postgastrectomy syndrome, where there is a carcinoma of the stomach, where there is extreme dietary deprivation such as occurs under famine conditions and, finally, where there is persistent vomiting from whatever cause. Immediately Wernicke's symptoms are recognised, 50 mg of thiamine is given intravenously supplemented by a similar amount intramuscularly. Intravenous thiamine is continued for several days, after which daily intramuscular injections are substituted until such a time as normal eating habits are re-established. It is then customary to give an oral preparation containing all the B vitamins together with a balanced diet. Instead of thiamine many clinicians prefer to give the whole vitamin B complex from the outset (e.g. Parentrovite), most frequently by the intramuscular route. If the Korsakoff component of the syndrome is present, daily intramuscular injections are continued for several weeks and, thereafter, if recovery has not taken place, once weekly for 6 months. This is in addition to oral vitamins and a suitable diet. Certain points require special mention:

1. Bed rest in the acute stage is obligatory because of the danger of sudden cardiovascular collapse
2. Large amounts of carbohydrates should *not* be given until the body is saturated with thiamine; a carbohydrate intake in the presence of thiamine deficiency exacerbates the latter and, indeed, has been known to precipitate Wernicke's encephalopathy in patients who have suffered prolonged thiamine deprivation.
3. If the basic deficiency is attributable to malabsorption, for example a gastric or intestinal lesion, daily parenteral administration of thiamine must be maintained.

Patients left with a memory defect require careful assessment. A patient with total amnesia requires constant supervision and this may have to be provided in hospital, or by round the clock nursing in the home. Moderate defects are not incompatible with some earning capacity, however, as such patients retain a topographical sense and can find their way around familiar surroundings.

With regard to outcome it is clear that little spontaneous recovery of cognitive function occurs in alcoholic Korsakoff patients (Victor et al 1971). However, the prognosis is thought to be less severe in patients who develop the Wernicke–Korsakoff syndrome in association with nutritional insufficiency, malabsorption or intractable vomiting, provided that in the last two instances the primary defect can be corrected.

The dysmnesic syndrome and the hippocampal formation

The first direct evidence for this association came from a series of bilateral and medial temporal lobe resections of varying extent carried out for the relief of the psychoses of epilepsy (Scoville 1954, Scoville & Milner 1957). Bilateral excisions limited to the uncus and amygdala were unattended by memory loss, but more extensive removals encroaching on the hippocampus and hippocampal gyrus were followed by memory deficits, the severity of which were more or less commensurate with the extent of the hippocampal resection. Total and permanent memory deficits were observed after bilateral removal of the anterior two-thirds of the hippocampus and hippocampal gyrus. Subsequently, it became known that a severe memory deficit could follow unilateral temporal lobectomy if there was extensive pathological change on the other side.

A further difficulty is that a memory deficit has been reported following ablation of either the left (dominant) or right (non-dominant) temporal lobe without EEG evidence of dysfunction of the opposite temporal lobe (Walker 1957, Dimsdale et al 1964). It is obvious, therefore, that Scoville's series of bilateral medial temporal lobe resections still provides the most convincing evidence that bilateral hippocampal damage is the necessary prerequisite for the development of a memory deficit. More recent confirmation has been obtained from patients suffering from encephalitis.

The dysmnesic syndrome in herpes simplex encephalitis

Herpes simplex virus (HSV) is the commonest cause of focal encephalitis in man. In acute necrotising encephalitis caused by HSV, the inflammatory reaction has a predilection for the structures within the limbic system, that is, the uncus, amygdaloid nucleus, hippocampus, hippocampal and cingulate gyri and the posterior orbital regions (Brierly 1966). HSV causes progressive cerebral oedema and necrosis. The damage is maximal in the medial portions of the temporal lobes.

Clinical features

The majority of patients present with a fulminating encephalitis. Pyrexia is marked with seizures irrespective of age. An acute confusional state can occur. On examination, focal neurological signs, as well as those of meningeal irritation, may be present.

Psychiatric sequelae are common, reflecting the primary damage to the temporal lobe and orbital structures. The patient may experience focal symptoms such as anosmia, olfactory or gustatory hallucinations. Memory is more severely affected than any other aspects of cognitive function. A pure dysmnesic syndrome has been described with preferential damage to the medial portions of both temporal lobes present at autopsy (Rose 1960). In a minority of patients the lesions are unilateral and the resulting symptoms are milder than those caused by a bilateral insult, particularly if only the right hemisphere is involved.

Diagnosis

The virus can only be cultured from the cerebrospinal fluid (CSF) in around 4% of cases. Tests for HSV antibodies and antigens in the CSF are rarely helpful in the early stages. However, HSV DNA in CSF can be amplified using the polymerase chain reaction, thus aiding early diagnosis and monitoring the response to treatment (Rowley 1990).

Treatment

Mortality is up to 70% in untreated cases and two-thirds of survivors will have neurological deficits.

The most effective treatment is acyclovir, especially if given in the early stages of the illness. Although the morbidity is reduced by prompt drug therapy, unfortunately long-term cognitive and memory impairments are not (Kennedy 1988, Gordon 1990).

Transient dysmnesic syndromes

Recovery is the rule in dysmnesic syndromes occurring after subarachnoid haemorrhage. Walton (1953) reported that six of a series of 312 cases of subarachnoid haemorrhage exhibited a Korsakoff syndrome which resolved within a few weeks. In one case the syndrome was observed a few hours after haemorrhage. Cerebral hypoxia, in particular carbon monoxide poisoning, can give rise to a similar transient dysmnesic syndrome, but there are recorded cases in which recovery does not take place (Robertson & Kennedy 1988).

Transient global amnesia

This name was given by Fisher & Adams (1965) to a dysmnesic syndrome, affecting either sex, which starts abruptly and which subsides within a matter of several hours. Typically, the patient will have an attack during which he is unable to retain impressions, other than momentarily, and repeats the same questions, seeming to be unaware of having asked them before. He is aware of his personal identity and conducts himself normally, though often appearing perplexed and anxious. This episode may be followed by sleep and, following recovery, the retrograde amnesia gradually shrinks, but the patient is left with a total and permanent amnesia for the period between the onset and the termination of the attack. Fisher & Adams observed this syndrome in middle-aged patients and attributed it to cerebrovascular disease. Croft and his colleagues (1973) reported that in nine of 24 patients studied, symptoms and signs consistent with brain stem ischaemia occurred during an attack and the authors concluded that transient global amnesia is probably attributable to bilateral temporal lobe ischaemia occurring as a consequence of vertebrobasilar disease. They described the EEG abnormalities, which provide further support for a vascular cause, but warn that, if the EEG is to be helpful, recordings should be made within a few days of an attack.

Single attacks predominate, perhaps many months apart, although recurrent attacks have been described. Since the attacks are of short duration and occur in middle-aged patients of stable personality, the possibility of hysterical amnesia seldom requires consideration.

CHRONIC ORGANIC DISORDERS

Long-term or permanent dysfunction occurs either as the result of sudden injury to the brain, which leaves residual deficits to which, in later life, the effects of ageing are added, or a progressive disorder leading to a gradual deterioration in function. Head injuries, strokes and subarachnoid haemorrhage are all potential acute causes of permanent deficits. By contrast, Alzheimer's disease, Huntington's disease, and Creutzfeld–Jakob disease cause progressive deterioration in brain function and, ultimately, the patient's death. There are conditions in which progressive deterioration may be reversed and they include certain benign cerebral tumours (meningiomas), chronic subdural haematomas when evacuated surgically, myxoedema, vitamin B_{12} deficiency and, though rare, syphilitic infection. Conditions which lead to severe changes in intellect, personality and behaviour (dementia) may occasionally prove to be reversible but, for the most part, are associated with severe mental and behavioural deficits and, ultimately, death. Most structural causes of gradual or sudden deterioration in mental function are associated with preferential destruction of certain areas of the brain although, at a late stage, a more generalised dysfunction occurs. Therefore, it is important to be able to recognise symptoms and signs of focal brain damage, described previously, because the pattern of involvement in any particular case is an important clue to the site of damage and, therefore, predictions about future developments and needs for management.

HEAD INJURY

Head injuries are very common though most do not lead to permanent changes in brain function. But there are, within the general population, about 150 markedly disabled head injury victims per 100 000 people, with a steady addition of approximately 1000 newly disabled individuals each year in Britain. Most head injuries in civilian life are caused by abrupt acceleration or deceleration of the head, chiefly as a result of motor vehicle accidents, but also as a result of falls, assaults and sports injuries (Field 1976).

The mechanism of brain injury was first described by Holbourn (1943), who concluded that, irrespective of the site of the blow to the head, the rotational movements induced deform the brain by causing a swirling movement. This, he argued, produces shearing, through stress, of the brain substance and, in particular, of small blood vessels and nerve fibres. The first proof of this in humans was produced in 1956 by Strich, who demonstrated white matter degeneration and hydrocephalus in the brains of five head injury victims who died some months after injury. In 1961 she produced a further paper describing 20 cases, including the five original ones, who had survived for a period ranging from a few weeks to 2 years. Despite the severity of head injury there was no significant cerebral laceration or haemorrhage, or raised intracranial pressure, and skull fracture was noted in only two cases. However, a prominent histological feature in those who survived for up to 5 weeks was the presence of axonal retraction balls, which denoted severed nerve fibres from which axoplasm had flowed, giving the appearance of blobs or balls. In other cases there were widespread changes in the cerebral white matter and long tracts of the brain stem typical of secondary or Wallerian degeneration, which follows disruption of nerve fibres from whatever cause. Strich considered that the cause of the degeneration was stretching and tearing of the nerve fibres which occurred at the moment of impact. As proof of this she cited one of the 20 patients whose accident was witnessed by a trained nurse, who observed that the patient took up a characteristic decerebrate posture with both legs and the right arm rigidly extended and the left arm flexed as soon as she hit the ground.

The primary injuries to the brain may be extended by secondary brain damage due to one or more of several factors which may be classified as intracranial or extracranial in the following manner:

1. Intracranial factors:
   a. Intracranial haematomas
   b. Brain swelling
   c. Infection
   d. Subarachnoid haemorrhage
   e. Hydrocephalus
2. Extracranial factors:
   a. Respiratory failure
   b. Hypotension

Whatever the primary factor, the ultimate mechanism responsible for secondary damage to the brain is usually hypoxia/ischaemia, leading to hemispheric swelling producing distortion and compression of the brain stem.

The precise nature of the mental consequences of injury depends upon the severity of the blow and the varying mixture of generalised and focal injuries it produces. In general, the severity of the injury is a reflection of the volume of brain injured, especially in the case of focal brain damage (Lishman 1968). The mental consequences of brain injury form broad categories: (1) mental disability consequent upon damage to the brain and (2) emotional reactions to the intellectual and physical changes brought about by the injury — reactions which are in themselves coloured by alterations in mood control and perhaps by increased irritability, aggressiveness and impulsivity. There is less evidence that brain injuries lead to the development of major mental illnesses, such as depression and mania. However, a relationship between injuries to the left hemisphere and schizophrenia has been established and psychotic symptoms do occur at times in certain stages during the process of recovery.

In general terms the psychological, behavioural and social consequences of severe closed-head injuries pose greater problems for patients and their families than do physical disabilities, the majority of which lessen with time, or even disappear. Most patients are young with an average age of 30 years. Many are on the threshold of adult life with regard to work and marriage and yet the rehabilitative facilities for such patients are almost non-existent in Britain. In most cases patients and their families do not wish for rehabilitation in psychiatric units, nor do they favour facilities provided for those with primary mental retardation. They are often too disruptive in their behaviour for units for the physically disabled and, as a consequence, impose an enormous emotional and social burden on their families in the home (McKinlay et al 1981, Thomsen 1984). In recent years, relatives of the brain injured have formed a national self-help group called 'Headway', which provides many centres throughout Britain giving practical help to the injured and their families.

Severity of injury

The severity of injury is an important guide to the short- and long-term outcome, although the prognosis must always be given with caution because the guidelines to be described are based on studies of groups of brain-injured patients and not on individuals who may show surprising variations in the extent to which they recover from any given injury.

Post-traumatic amnesia

Post-traumatic amnesia (PTA) is the period that elapses between the moment of injury and the restoration of memory for everyday events. Its duration was shown to be directly related to the severity of the injury by Russell in 1932, and in his original paper he produced the following scale:

PTA < 1 hour   — mild injury
PTA 1–24 hours   — moderate injury

PTA 1–7 days   — severe injury
PTA >7 days   — very severe injury.

In a modification of this scale Fortuny et al (1980) expanded the number of categories for milder injuries as follows:

PTA < 10 minutes   — very mild injury
PTA 10–60 minutes   — mild injury
PTA 1–24 hours   — moderate injury.

In a study of patients admitted to a hospital in Oxford, it was found that the proportion of patients in each category was 47, 17.3 and 20.8%, respectively. Only 6.6% of patients had a PTA exceeding 24 hours. In a study of 1000 patients with severe closed-head injuries, Teasdale et al (1981) showed that all had a PTA greater than 2 days, 94% of more than one week, 80% of more than 2 weeks and 60% for more than 4 weeks.

There are a number of limitations to the use of PTA as an indication of the severity of brain injury. For example, it is known that head injuries produce more severe effects in the elderly than in the young or middle aged. As a result the duration of PTA increases with age for any given injury. Also, PTA may not be of value where injury has occurred as a result of a penetrating wound caused by a sharp object or missile. Local brain damage may be severe but the effect is focal and the patient's conscious level is not impaired. Russell & Nathan (1946) found that 32% of a series of cases of gunshot wounds showed no amnesia, and 20% had amnesia for less than an hour.

Those involved in the management of the recently injured patient are interested in ways of assessing coma and linking it with the potential outcome. Much work has been done in this area and the Glasgow Coma Scale, devised by Teasdale & Jennett (1974), is used in many countries for this purpose.

In addition to assessment of the severity of injury by measurement of coma duration, or PTA retrospectively, methods have been developed for assessing overall outcome. In 1975 Jennett & Bond devised the Glasgow Outcome Scale in order to remove previously used value judgements like 'worthwhile' and 'tolerable' and to avoid assessment based solely on the difficult and shifting measurement of time to return to work. The scale, which is easy to use, has a high level of validity and reliability, and is shown in Table 15.2. In large-scale studies it has been revealed that the greater part of recovery, but by no means all of it, is achieved by 6 months after injury and that, of those who by 12 months have made a good recovery, or who are moderately disabled, almost two-thirds have already reached this level within 3 months of injury and 90%

Table 15.2   The Glasgow Outcome Scale in its original form and in extended and contracted forms

Extended scale	Original scale	Contracted scale			
Dead	Dead	Dead	Dead or vegetative	Dead or vegetative	Dead
Vegetative	Vegetative				
Degree of disability		⎫ Dependent	⎫ Severely disabled	⎫	⎫
5	Severely				
4	disabled ⎬		⎬	⎬ Conscious	⎬ Survivors
3	Moderately				
2	disabled	⎫ Independent	⎫ Independent		
1	Good				
0	recovery ⎬		⎬		
Total categories					
8	5	3		2	

have done so by 6 months. These figures apply to those functions directly attributable to basic brain mechanisms, for example neurological or cognitive functions; however, more complex activities, and especially behavioural and mood changes, improve over a much longer time-scale, in fact over several years. It is important to remember that these comments apply to most patients, because not all follow the pattern of recovery described. The value of both PTA and coma duration as predictors of outcome is greatest during the first 6 months after injury, but they are weak indicators of late behavioural and social functions.

For many years it has been usual to assess general intelligence, memory and language deficits, in addition to motor and perceptual deficits, as a basis for evaluating the severity of severe brain injury and comments upon such assessments follow. More recently, it has been appreciated that other fundamental defects are present and important both in terms of the distorting effects they may have upon conventional psychological tests and upon reasoning and conduct in everyday life. The key areas involved are outlined in Table 15.3.

Cognitive functions following closed brain injury

A range of test batteries (e.g. the Halstead–Reitan battery, and the WAIS) reveals that after severe head injuries there is general slowing of performance, memory impairment and poorer abilities on non-verbal or perceptual tests when compared with those based on language. However, in the past 15 years there has been a movement away from the use of standard test batteries to the use of selected tests of specific cognitive functions with increasing attempts to relate these to performance in everyday life.

Table 15.3   Major areas of psychosocial change following severe head injury

1. *Emotional change.* Characterised by apathy, silliness, lability of mood, irritability and an increased or (more often) reduced or absent libido
2. *Impaired social perceptiveness.* Characterised by selfishness in which feelings for others, self-criticism and an ability to reflect, are greatly diminished or absent
3. *Impaired self-control.* Characterised by impulsivity, aggressiveness, restlessness and impatience
4. *Increased dependency.* Characterised by lack of initiative despite talk of action, and by impaired judgement and planning ability
5. *Behavioural rigidity.* Characterised by inability to learn from experience even when the ability to learn new information is retained.

Intelligence

Of the tests available for the assessment of general intelligence, the WAIS has proved the most popular in practice and in experimental studies. It incorporates a series of subtests which give verbal and performance IQs. The Progressive Matrices Test, and the Mill Hill Scale, have been used for the specific assessment of non-verbal and verbal IQ, respectively. The results of testing reveal that performance deficits are greater than verbal deficits amongst the head injured. The work of Brooks & Aughton (1979) revealed that vocabulary-based intelligence appeared to be more resistant than non-verbal intelligence to the effects of trauma. Also, there is a slower rate of recovery on performance tests than on verbally based tests. Although the final level of function is often reached about 12 months after injury, many of the injured are not fully recovered by that time. The severity of injury does not seem to affect the rate at which an individual's intelligence recovers, but it does bear a direct relationship to the extent to which intelligence does recover ultimately. Studies of long-term outcome reveal very little change in levels of overall intelligence after the first year following injury, but this is of less significance than the changes that occur in emotional and behavioural functions, which have a significant effect upon daily life and adaptation to stresses and strains imposed by the effects of injury upon the person and his need to adapt to social difficulties of many kinds.

Memory

Loss of short-term memory is the classical cognitive deficit of the traumatically brain injured patient and is seen in tests involving recognition, recall and relearning of verbal and non-verbal material. The tests used to reveal such deficits are the reversed Digit Span Scale, the WAIS, and the use of simple stories where difficulty in immediate and delayed recall may be manifest and give evidence of impairment of logical memory. Paired associate learning, in other words the learning of new pairs of words, is a sensitive test of memory after brain injury and test results reveal that patients are less severely impaired on the immediate recall of simple information (e.g. digits forward as opposed to digits reversed). In general, there is a definite relationship between severity of injury judged on the basis of PTA and performance on tests of memory although, within groups of patients with similar injuries, there are variations in performance. The rate of recovery is less well understood, but it appears that the greater part of it takes place within 6–9 months of injury, but further recovery does occur at a much slower rate. It seems that simple learning recovers more rapidly and to a greater extent than verbal learning. In everyday life, memory deficits are manifest chiefly in a failure to remember names and recent events with relative preservation of information learned prior to the injury.

Language

Following head injury the most frequent deficits are 'expressive or non-fluent aphasia' and specific anomic defects. Thus, word fluency, that is, the number of words used, is reduced for periods of up to 12 months or longer. Najenson (1978) demonstrated that visual and auditory comprehension appears to recover before oral expression, reading and writing. Signs of recovery were seen within 3 weeks in those with milder injuries, being completed by 9 months, but with a delay of 5–7

months in the severely injured, who had persisting deficits 2 years later. It should be remembered that communication, a broader concept than language alone and one which incorporates general cognitive abilities, may be more impaired than simple language. In everyday life it is disorders of communication which cause patients their greatest difficulties.

Changes in personality and behaviour

Emotional and behavioural deficits cause significantly more problems for both the injured person and his family than physical deficits in at least 70% of cases of severe head injury. During the course of the first year after injury, deficits associated with emotion and behaviour increase and there is little improvement over this period in the absence of adequate rehabilitation. Most psychiatrists see very few severely brain injured patients, and those who do often find it difficult to make a diagnosis which leads to an appropriate course of management. One way of overcoming this problem is to use the criteria laid down in DSM-IIIR under the rubric of organic disorders, as suggested earlier. A general outline of the classification is shown in Table 15.4.

Organic personality syndrome. The definition of this syndrome is restricted in DSM-IIIR to:

> a persistent personality disturbance, either lifelong or representing a change or accentuation of a previously characteristic trait, that is due to a specific organic factor. Affective instability, recurrent outbursts of aggression or rage, markedly impaired social judgement, marked apathy and indifference or paranoid ideation are common.

The text indicates that the pattern of symptoms or behaviour depends chiefly upon the site of the physical pathological process or damage. All the components of the syndrome may occur following

Table 15.4 Emotional and behavioural characteristics of the severely brain injured

States that develop early in recovery (less than 6 months after injury)

Coma
Delirium (consciousness impaired)

Organic[a] personality syndrome	Organic[a] 1. Delusional syndrome 2. Hallucinosis	Organic[a] affective syndrome

[a] Consciousness unimpaired.

moderate to severe traumatic brain injuries, but for the purposes of management and prediction of outcome it is preferable to deal with them as different categories of organically determined mental syndromes. It should be remembered that, although the syndromes may represent an accentuation of pre-morbid personality traits, they may also arise for the first time after an injury. The syndrome characterised by loss of control of aggressive or sexual drive or, in contrast, by loss of all drive, is not specifically included in DSM-IIIR but is sufficiently distinctive to warrant separate identification. In contrast, both affective disturbances and states in which disorders of thought and perception occur are categorised as the organic mood syndrome, the organic delusional syndrome and organic hallucinosis.

Aggressive states marked by loss of control often interpreted as impulsivity, poor mood control or explosive anger, may be the result of three conditions. First, general irritability which is often manifest as periods of verbal aggression and occasionally physical violence. The behaviour shown in this situation is an exaggeration of pretraumatic tendencies to aggressive behaviour. Secondly, sudden and often unprovoked episodes of very aggressive behaviour occur which are regarded as equivalent to epileptic seizures, except that the level of consciousness does not appear to change. Nevertheless, the individual feels totally 'out of control'. Such disorders often respond to treatment with carbamazepine, preferably in combination with behaviour modification techniques. Lastly, aggressive behaviour may be the direct result of partial complex seizures. Again the treatment of the disorder is by means of carbamazepine and the extent to which control is gained is variable, but may be striking and complete.

Loss of control may present as sexual disinhibition. Management is difficult and although the behavioural problems tend to lessen over a period of months as self-control is regained, there may be continued need to provide contraception for a disinhibited female patient, and possibly suppression of male hormone in men using the anti-androgen cyproterone acetate. In all syndromes where disinhibition is marked, the presence of insight on the part of the patient is a good prognostic sign; but it is usually necessary to use behavioural techniques and, perhaps, pharmacological agents such as carbamazepine to obtain the best results in rehabilitation.

In general, phenothiazines are not particularly helpful for the long term treatment of the aggressive patient, but it has been noted that haloperidol in small doses may bring about substantial improvements.

Patients who lose their motivation and drive completely present a problem because they fail to respond to rehabilitation processes. For example, they do not show any interest in rewards for alterations in behaviour and, although in some cases interest in change is expressed, action does not follow. Over a period of many months drive may return, but in the severely injured this is minimal. At an early stage in recovery, that is, once full consciousness has been restored, the use of a drug such as amphetamine (a CNS stimulant), together with programmes of rehabilitation designed to maintain arousal and attention, may be of value, though evidence supporting a consistent effect is lacking.

Organic affective syndrome. Recovery from brain injury is often associated with mood changes. In part these appear to be the result of loosening in internal controls leading to rapid fluctuations of mood, especially in the early months after injury. There may be an accentuation or return of pretraumatic tendencies to dysphoria, or this condition may develop as a response to combined physical, emotional and social consequences of injury. Management involves counselling in most cases but, if mood change is severe or persistent, antidepressant drugs may be required. Of those available, trazodone and amitriptyline are useful, the latter especially so if the patient shows marked agitation. Hypomania occurs very occasionally after severe brain injury and usually at an early stage in recovery. Control of the mood state and hyperactivity may be gained with haloperidol. On occasion further episodes of hypomania or mania may develop and the use of lithium as a prophylactic treatment may be required.

The development of major depressive illness tends to be delayed until some months or years after injury and may be associated with suicidal thoughts or acts. The development of such states is probably best seen in terms of a reaction to the overall consequences of injury in psychological, physical and social terms and, to date, there is little evidence to support the view that brain damage as such is the cause of such disorders.

Organic delusional syndrome and hallucinosis. In the early stages of recovery, often within the period of delirium, patients may develop one or other of two prominent disorders of thought and perception. First, and by far the most common, is the development of a delusional state, usually of the paranoid type, considered to be the consequence of a long period of partial and disordered consciousness with grossly disturbed perception and orientation. However, on occasion, patients do develop paranoid delusions in clear consciousness during the early phase of recovery but, in some cases, the process may not extend beyond development of a delusional mood. It is felt that such developments are also the consequence of disturbed cognition and perception. Recovery tends to be spontaneous, but the agitated paranoid patient may require treatment with a phenothiazine, for example fluphenazine, which has less potential than other drugs for inducing seizure activity. Complex hallucinatory states, other than being part of the process of delirium, are very uncommon but do occur occasionally. Generally speaking they are self-limiting.

The amnestic syndrome. Injuries in which there is severe damage to both medial temporal regions of the brain lead to a disorder in which a profound disturbance of memory occurs. It is manifest as a total loss of recall, except of events preceding injury, and confabulation is a major consequence. The fact that patients often retain insight into their abnormality produces considerable unhappiness and depression amongst them. Over a period of several years, repetition of simple acts of daily life, for example recognition of friends seen frequently, and some inability to find rooms in the house, may develop. Management is chiefly by careful environmental cueing and constant repetition of very simple but necessary tasks, for example finding clothes, the toilet, etc.

Post-traumatic neuroses

Anxiety and depression

Marked anxiety and destruction of self-confidence occurs in many of the brain injured. Probably only where marked euphoria develops are such changes completely absent. The anxiety experienced by head-injured patients may amount to panic at times, especially if the person is left alone, or finds himself in an unfamiliar environment. In fact, some individuals become so dependent on their relatives that they will not be separated from them for more than a few minutes at a time. It is possible to reduce anxiety and increase self-confidence by intensive psychological treatment based on cognitive therapy, which aims to provide a very firm but simple structure for daily life which, once mastered, restores some feeling of self-control. Even those with lesser degrees of injury experience anxiety in relation to return to work and dealing with novel situations. As indicated previously, treatment should be by counselling and psychological techniques, and the use of benzodiazepines as anxiolytics is not indicated.

Dysphoria or depression in response to repeated failures is common as individuals with brain injury attempt to re-establish their lives. It is usually variable in intensity and occasionally requires treatment with antidepressant therapy, when drugs such as trazodone or amitriptyline may be used in normal doses.

Conversion disorder/hysterical states

In addition to disorders which may have their origins in early mental changes, two reactive conditions may appear late in recovery, namely hysterical neurosis and an obsessional state.

There appears to be an inverse relationship between the severity of brain injury and a tendency to develop conversion disorders. In other words, mild to moderate injuries are most often associated with this form of abnormality. The patient may exhibit neurological signs which do not have a physical basis, such as hemiparesis, sensory changes in the limbs, or pseudoseizures which, on occasion, are mixed with true organically determined seizures. Rare conditions in this category include the Ganser syndrome. This is characterised by a history of a mild to moderate injury, a period of good recovery, then depression of mood, and marked withdrawal into a monosyllabic state with all answers to questions being given in such a way as to indicate that the patient understands the question despite which his reply is never quite correct.

Obsessional states

True obsessional neurosis is seldom seen after severe brain injury, but there is a marked tendency for some patients to show what is known as 'organic orderliness'. This is a need to establish order and to structure all aspects of everyday life. It is manifest in terms of extreme tidiness, with anxiousness or anger if possessions are disturbed. The condition is seen as a response to the internal chaos brought about by cognitive and perceptual disturbances in head-injured victims.

Alcoholism

Excessive consumption of alcohol is a frequent contributor to head injury and heavy drinking is not uncommon amongst the injured before their accident. There is no doubt that brain injury grossly reduces tolerance for alcohol in most individuals and intoxication may occur after as little as one pint of beer. Nevertheless, the injured may drink heavily, relatively speaking, either because they fail to appreciate their limitations, or as a response to stress. Control of these problems is particularly difficult when insight has been lost and, indeed, the only solution may be to prevent access to alcohol.

Postconcussional syndrome

Traumatic damage to the brain ranges from the effects of trivial blows to the head to major insults. Until fairly recently it was thought that injuries causing PTA of less than 1–2 hours of duration produced little or no permanent injury, but evidence has accumulated to show that damage does occur and that, although it does not produce lasting neuropsychiatric abnormalities, it does cause short-term and subtle changes in psychological function. Neurophysiological studies show that there is a change in the blood–brain barrier, slowing of the cerebral circulation, impairment of brain stem function, and an increased sensitivity to light. Such deficits, which are almost certainly short lived, are not usually appreciated by an examining physician, but they may well form the basis of later disturbances in psychological function.

For many years arguments have raged over the origins of the physical and emotional symptoms following minor head injury, the most consistent of which are throbbing headache at the site of injury, dizziness, poor concentration, fatigue, irritability, sensitivity to sound and poor sleep — a collection of symptoms which form 'post-traumatic syndrome'. At one period the view was taken that symptoms were generated by psychological factors rather than having an organic basis. Certainly, as Trimble (1981) made clear in discussing this point, there is ample evidence from wartime and civilian studies that premorbid constitutional factors relate strongly to the development of postinjury neurosis and that in a proportion of patients 'gain' is an important factor in the maintenance of symptoms. For example, in a classical and often quoted study by Miller (1961a, b) he reported that, of a group of 200 individuals, men developed neurotic complications twice as often as women, that such symptoms occurred more often after accidents at work when compared with road traffic accidents, or sports injuries, and that those involved came from the lower end of the socioeconomic scale. He also described an inverse relationship between the duration of unconsciousness and severity of symptoms and between the intensity and duration of patients' symptoms and premorbid constitution. However, these observations must be interpreted with some caution because Miller's subjects came from a group of individuals involved in litigation.

Evidence is accumulating to support the view that minor head injuries do cause injury to the brain, probably by the mechanism of axonal shearing, but that it is mild and recovers rapidly. In fact, most patients have recovered within a month. However, in individuals predisposed by their premorbid personality, a history of psychiatric disturbance, or the circumstances of the injury, or some combination of these factors, subjective complaints may persist for months and be associated with a delay in returning to normal activities of daily life. In a few cases, for example where labyrinthine structures have been damaged, symptoms such as dizziness and diplopia have a genuine physical basis and persist for up to a year, by which time they should have disappeared. Obviously, prolonged physical symptoms of this type may also form a focus for the development of neurotic symptoms and prolonged abnormal illness behaviour.

Diagnosis

When patients suffering from postconcussional symptoms are referred for psychiatric assessment the condition has generally been present for at least several months. It is, therefore, advisable to bear in mind the late complications of head injury. For example, headache is also a feature of chronic subdural haematoma. In an ambulant patient the usual presentation of a subdural haematoma is headache, mild spastic weakness of a limb, and pyramidal signs or, alternatively, obvious intellectual impairment with few or no localising signs. It is common for symptoms to fluctuate with time. 'Blackouts' have to be distinguished from post-traumatic epilepsy and care must be taken in determining whether or not actual loss of consciousness has occurred. The overall risk of epilepsy, excluding seizures occurring within 7 days of injury, is in the region of 5%. Rather more than half the patients have their seizures within a year of injury and the development of epilepsy is more common in individuals who have had one or more seizures during the first week after injury (Jennett 1975). With penetrating wounds the incidence of epilepsy is higher and Lishman (1968) reported an incidence of 45% in a group of 670 patients who has missile wounds with penetration of the dura mater.

Intracranial haematoma

The most trivial, as well as the most severe head injuries may give rise to an intracranial haematoma and this lesion accounts for 75% of deaths amongst patients who have a period of clear or mildly clouded consciousness after injury and then lapse into coma.

They form what has come to be known as the 'talk and die' group. Intradural haematomas occur with greatest frequency in patients between 50 and 60 years of age. In contrast, 40% of extradural haematomas occur in patients under 20 years of age (Teasdale & Jennett 1981).

Intracranial haematoma due to trauma may be attributed incorrectly to a cerebrovascular accident or alcohol intoxication. For example, Galbraith et al (1976) reported that, of a series of 51 patients admitted to a teaching hospital with an intracranial haematoma, approximately 25% were undiagnosed until post mortem. In view of the number of mistakes in diagnosis that can occur, given the various possible causes of unconsciousness in patients who have evidence of injury to the head, Galbraith mentions such practical matters as the clues provided by a fracture of the skull and the importance of measuring the blood alcohol before attributing unconsciousness to the 'effects of alcohol'. He added that recognition of an intracranial haematoma is helped by the doctor's continued awareness of the possibility. The psychiatrist, of course, is not usually concerned with the problems of diagnosis, but more with the mental sequelae of brain injury and psychological reactions to the consequences of injury, together with the occasional need to detect the presence of a chronic subdural haematoma, which gives rise to alterations in the mental state over a period of weeks or months.

Intracranial haematomas develop after both focal and diffuse brain injuries, representing in the latter a focal component of more widespread damage. The neurological and psychological consequences of focal brain injury are dealt with elsewhere in this chapter, as are the psychological consequences of severe brain injury.

Chronic subdural haematoma

In contrast to the development of an acute subdural haematomata half the adults who develop a chronic subdural haematoma do not have a history of trauma (Teasdale & Jennett 1981). A number have a history of minor head injury, or merely a sudden jerk or jolt of the head. In a few, intracranial haemorrhage occurs secondary to a blood disorder or the use of anticoagulants. Chronic subdural haematomas usually occur in older individuals, with a peak incidence between 50 and 60 years of age.

Clinical manifestations make their appearance a few weeks or even months after the injury, but since the injury is so often trivial it is not always immediately recalled. Persistent headache is the most common presenting feature. Recurring fluctuations in the level of consciousness are quoted as the classical signs of a subdural haematoma but, surprisingly, this is not common, though when present serves as a valuable diagnostic indicator. In the latter situation the patient is drowsy and comatose one day and alert and wakeful the next. The transition is not always abrupt and frequently retardation, perplexity and memory defects mark the wakeful period.

Memory impairment is usually obvious in longstanding cases with a history of headache and neurological signs. It is more difficult to identify cases which present with moderately severe dementia without a history of trauma, no subjective complaints, and no neurological deficits.

Neurologically, a half to three-quarters of patients show evidence of spastic weakness, usually on the same side as the haematoma, together with hyperreflexia and an extensor plantar response. As with alterations in consciousness, so also the neurological symptoms may vary in severity. Dilatation of the homolateral pupil with ptosis is a further and more sinister neurological development, being due to compression of the oculomotor nerve by herniation of the temporal lobe through the tentorium. Epilepsy may occur, but it should be remembered that it might have been the cause rather than the result of the haematoma. Dysphasia has been reported where the haematoma overlies the dominant hemisphere.

Investigations and treatment. An abnormality on a radioactive brain scan will be present in more than 90% of cases and an added CT scan gives information about the shape and size of the haematoma and the extent to which midline structures of the brain are displaced. Little useful information can be gained from skull radiographs, or from the EEG which, though abnormal in 80% of patients, is non-specific. Treatment is by surgical drainage of the subdural fluid.

Subarachnoid haemorrhage

Subarachnoid haemorrhage accounts for approximately 8% of cerebrovascular accidents. The cause may be the rupture of a cerebral aneurysm, which occurs in more than half the cases, or primary haemorrhage from an intracerebral vessel, from an angioma or from an arteriovenous malformation. The initial mortality following the rupture of an aneurysm is high, with over 50% of patients dying before reaching hospital, or within a few weeks of haemorrhage. Of those who survive, 25% do so for more than 5 years but, of these, 30% are partly or totally disabled.

Cerebral aneurysms are most common at the junction of the division of the main trunk of the middle cerebral artery, the origin of the posterior communicating artery from the internal carotid artery, and at the junction of the anterior communicating and anterior cerebral arteries. Rupture of an aneurysm produces very sudden and very severe headache with patients describing a feeling of having been kicked on the back of the head. Temporary loss of consciousness or confusion is common and nausea, vomiting and photophobia, together with neck stiffness, are classical features. Blood-stained cerebrospinal fluid is found at lumbar puncture. There is evidence that subarachnoid haemorrhage may be precipitated by strong emotional events (Storey 1967, 1970), and perhaps, unexpectedly, this is most common in patients who do not have a demonstrable aneurysm on angiography.

Subarachnoid haemorrhage is associated with a high level of psychological and psychiatric morbidity. In addition to an early acute confusional state, patients may develop evidence of focal neurological damage (stroke), personality change and intellectual deterioration. There is an association between the level of the residual physical deficit and the mental changes. Storey (1967) reported that 41% of a group of patients he examined had personality change. However, this was severe in only 4% of them. The greatest risk of intellectual deficits and personality change follows rupture and treatment of middle cerebral artery aneurysms. The intellectual change is most evident as a disturbance of memory and not an overall decline in intelligence. Following anterior communicating artery haemorrhage there may be a quite marked personality change of the 'frontal type' with relative sparing of intellect. Alterations in personality include apathy with a tendency to tire easily, or a mildly disinhibited state which, in some cases, leads to a pleasing improvement in personality in terms of a more relaxed and contented style, much appreciated by relatives (Logue et al 1968).

The commonest changes in emotion following subarachnoid haemorrhage include irritability, anxiety — often with fear of a further haemorrhage — and moodiness with intermittent periods of mild depression. Difficulty in sustaining attention and concentration and a tendency to tire easily are also present in many cases. These symptoms are similar to those following traumatic head injury and, as in that case, the development of psychiatric disorders bears a relationship to the patient's premorbid personality, or to a history of previous psychiatric illness. Also, as in the case of traumatic brain injury, the recovery of the patient from the organically induced state takes place over a period of 3–6 months, with changes still evident in many cases a year or more later.

DEMENTIA

Dementia is defined as a state in which there is a decline in intellect, personality and behaviour, which is usually, though not always, irreversible. The frequency increases with age; 10% of those over 65 years and over 20% over 80 years of age are demented. Although more than 50 disorders can give rise to dementia (Haase 1977), Alzheimer's disease is the most frequent cause and accounts for more than 50% of cases (Roth et al 1985). Several recently described disorders, which meet the diagnostic criteria for Alzheimer's disease, appear to be clinically and pathologically distinct. These include multi-infarct dementia, Pick's disease, the prion group of disorders including Creutzfeld–Jakob disease, Huntington's disease and acquired immune deficiency syndrome (AIDS) dementia. Less common forms of dementia include dementia of the frontal lobe type, Lewy body disorders and progressive lobar atrophy. Reversible dementias include those due to metabolic conditions such as abnormalities in liver and renal function, alcohol abuse and other systemic or toxic disorders.

Differentiation of the various forms of dementia in life may be difficult and, therefore, a careful clinical examination is necessary and must be backed by questioning of relatives or close friends. Standardised psychometric tests, EEG studies, CT and tests of neurological function give supporting evidence, but are in themselves insufficient to make the diagnosis. Blood levels of vitamin B_{12} and folate, and liver, renal and thyroid function, should be assessed to detect conditions which may prove to be reversible, for example myxoedema has been shown to be so in up to 15% of cases. Failure to conduct a thorough examination leads to misdiagnosis. For example, there is often confusion between dementia and depressive illness since depression in the elderly may present with a confusional state. Frequently the cause of dementia can only be established conclusively at post mortem.

Alzheimer's disease

The disorder originally described by Alzheimer in 1907 was a dementia which developed before the age of 65 years, but the definition has been extended to include those beyond this age.

Presenile versus senile dementia

Differences exist clinically, genetically and pathologically between early and late-onset cases of Alzheimer's disease. Late-onset cases, that is, those over the age of 65 years, are described as type 1 (Roth et al 1985) and early onset cases as type 2. The former are more likely to present with abnormalities of speech, other focal neurological signs and abnormalities of gait, in addition to which progress of the disease is more rapid than in the type 2 form.

There is often a more obvious family history of dementia amongst type 2 patients (Heston 1981) and at autopsy there is greater neuronal loss and more marked neurotransmitter changes in the brain. However, despite these facts there remains doubt as to whether the differences quoted between types 1 and 2 are significant enough to warrant separate identities. More recently, studies have shown that the age of onset of Alzheimer's disease is variable even within families (Chui 1985), and there is often an absence of clinical or pathological difference between familial Alzheimer's disease and sporadic cases. Further, 'senile dementia', that is Alzheimer type 1, appears to have a genetic basis. Genetically determined subgroups of dementias may exist, such as those with a pattern of early onset or specific symptoms, but also an interaction may be occurring between genetic and environmental factors, such as aluminium, or infective agents, to give rise to the variations recorded.

Alzheimer type 1 (senile dementia) versus normal ageing

It has been argued that senile dementia is no more than accelerated normal ageing because post mortem examination of the brains of non-demented elderly patients contain both neurofibrillary tangles and senile plaques. However, there is a body of evidence that contradicts this view and supports the belief that senile dementia is Alzheimer's disease developing in individuals over the age of 70 years. In fact, Roth (1986) regards it as such and refers to it as type 1 Alzheimer's disease. For example, the pattern of neuropsychological test results, produced by normal ageing, differs from the results gained from patients with senile dementia. Thus, in normal ageing, which is benign by comparison with senile dementia, memory loss is usually compensated for by the preservation of other aspects of intellect and personality, particularly where interests and social stimuli are maintained. By contrast, senile dementia is a devastating process, destroying all semblance of previous mental activity within the space of a few years. The associated disruption in family and social life and the dependency it engenders is a major problem for relatives as well as for the health and social services.

Genetics

The results of several large studies suggest that in some families Alzheimer's disease is inherited as an autosomal dominant trait. Although the risk factor to first-degree relatives is said to be particularly high, around 50%, in early onset cases, Breitner (1988) has shown that a similarly high risk exists for relatives of elderly probands and suggests that death from other causes may, in the past, have given a lower apparent incidence of Alzheimer's disease in old age. Sporadic cases are also common as around 35% of patients do not have a family history of Alzheimer's disease (Chui 1985).

The few available twin studies show a concordance in monozygotic twins of less than 50%, implying that environmental factors are of major importance.

The association of Alzheimer's disease and Down's syndrome suggests that chromosome 21 might be implicated in the pathogenesis of the former condition and, in fact, in some families the locus for the Alzheimer's disease gene does lie on chromosome 21 (Tanzi 1987) but at a different site for the gene for the A4 protein, which is a major component of amyloid found in senile plaques. However, familial Alzheimer's disease may be genetically heterogeneous with more than one gene responsible for the phenotype (St George-Hyslop 1990).

Pathology

The major pathological changes in Alzheimer's disease include widespread cerebral atrophy, neuronal loss, neuritic plaques and neurofibrillary tangles.

Up to 50% of large neurones are lost in early onset cases in the midfrontal, superior temporal, inferior and parietal areas, and in the hippocampus. In late-onset Alzheimer's disease a smaller proportion of neurones is lost, approximately 25%, but the absolute number of surviving neurones is considerably less, due to normal ageing. A substantial loss of cells in the nucleus basalis of Meynert, which is the main site of choline acetyltransferase, may account for the decreased levels of acetylcholine found in the cerebral cortex of subjects with Alzheimer's disease.

Senile or neuritic plaques are extracellular argyrophilic bodies which occur in normal elderly individuals but in much larger numbers in Alzheimer's disease of both types. They are composed of a central amyloid core surrounded by a halo of abnormal neurites. Aluminium silicate is present in the cores of mature plaques and, as aluminium can interfere with neuronal metabolism, it may be involved in nerve cell degeneration. Alzheimer's disease plaques, though widely distributed, are particularly concentrated in the temporal cortex, hippocampus and amygdala, and are usually found in close association with blood vessels. The number of plaques correlates well with the degree of impairment of cognitive functioning.

Neurofibrillary tangles are intracellular structures with a core of paired helical filaments of uncertain nature. They are more numerous in type 2 Alzheimer's disease or in elderly patients with long histories. The tangle consists of 25% of a microtubule-stabilising protein, designated τ, and the rest is made up of cytoskeletal proteins which can be identified by immunocytochemistry. Neurofibrillary tangles are also found in individuals with the 'punch-drunk syndrome' and the parkinsonism dementia complex of Guam, where amyloid A4 protein is a major component of the tangles. Severe neuronal degenerative changes in the olfactory cortex and nasal epithelium cells in Alzheimer's disease have been suggested as evidence of nasal entry of an environmental pathogen (Talamo 1989) in some cases.

Other histological findings include amyloid deposits around small blood vessels (amyloid angiopathy), Hirano bodies (small eosinophilic neuronal inclusion bodies) and granulovacuolar degeneration of neurones which are found mainly in the hippocampus and are non-specific markers of cell damage.

Neurotransmitters in Alzheimer's disease

A wide range of neurotransmitter abnormalities occurs in Alzheimer's disease involving both catecholamines and neuropeptides, although the causes and the full significance of most of the changes to be described and their relation to mental deficits observed clinically is not known. The first major discovery in this field was of low cortical levels of acetylcholine with choline acetyltransferase activity between 35 and 75% of normal, particularly in the cortex of the temporal lobe (Davies & Maloney 1976). In the nucleus basalis of Meynert, the main cholinergic nerve cell nucleus, activity was found to be as little as 10% of normal. The loss in choline acetyltransferase closely reflects the fall in the number of cholinergic nerve cells in the nucleus basalis of Meynert. Finally, a close correlation has been found between cholinergic activity, the increased density of senile plaques and deterioration in cognitive function (Perry et al 1978).

Reductions have also been found in the levels of other neurotransmitters, including somatostatin, serotonin (5-HT), noradrenaline and corticotrophin-releasing factor (CRF). Alteration in the levels of noradrenaline and serotonin is apparent only in severely demented patients, compared with the cholinergic deficit which occurs in even moderate dementia.

In Alzheimer's disease there is shrinkage or atrophy of pyramidal neurones in the temporal and parietal cortices, which use excitatory amino acids such as glutamate and aspartate as their neurotransmitters. The number of receptors sensitive to them may be reduced, particularly the N-methyl-D-aspartate (NMDA) receptor, which is known to be involved in memory function. In the hippocampus the release of glutamate has been implicated in the death of cells bearing NMDA receptors.

The inhibitory neurotransmitter, γ-aminobutyric acid (GABA) may be greatly reduced in early onset cases of Alzheimer's disease.

A number of GABA-containing cells also express somatostatin and other neuropeptides such as cholecystokinin and neuropeptide Y. Somatostatin is consistently reduced in Alzheimer's disease in the cortex and hippocampus and has been found to be present in senile plaques at autopsy. Like somatostatin, cholecystokinin acts as both a neurotransmitter and neuromodulator, and similarly its levels are decreased in Alzheimer's disease. However, in contrast, CRF receptor density is increased, compared with the reduction seen in somatostatin receptor levels.

Clinical features

In broad terms, Alzheimer's disease has three stages.

The patient presents with marked deterioration of memory, impaired concentration and an increasing tendency to fatigue and anxiety. Often there is restlessness and fleeting depression of mood, together with exaggeration of pre-existing personality traits, for example obsessionality, anxiousness or hypochondriasis. Focal neurological deficits, on the other hand, are uncommon at this stage and such changes, or indeed nothing more than an obvious failure of memory, may be observed for a year or two because of the relatively slow progress of the disease. However, increasingly unusual incidents occur, giving rise for concern. For example, a cautious business man tells a convincing false story about a fraudulent transaction involving an associate, or a timid spinster quarrels with her neighbours. It should be remembered that the use of psychotropic drugs for any reason may cause confusion in the patient with early dementia. This is an important point because the first presenting signs of the disease may well be taken for the presence of depressive illness, or a paranoid disorder. Speech disorders in the early stages are usually limited to occasional difficulty in word finding, but the patient's letters may show altered handwriting, and perseveration of words and phrases.

In the second stage, further deterioration takes place with a decline in practical everyday skills. An individual's surroundings take on an air of squalor because he or she is no longer able to use domestic appliances such as the washing machine and vacuum cleaner. Similar deficits in work practices may lead to premature retirement. Neurological abnormalities appear; for example, 5–10% of patients develop epilepsy, and dyspraxias, such as dressing apraxia, and agnosias may develop. About half the patients at this stage become incontinent of urine. Disorientation in territorial space and time become apparent. Patients lose their way in familiar surroundings and are unable to tell the time, or name the day or date. Speech difficulties increase, leading to dysarthria, loss of vocabulary, and disintegration of the ability to use normal grammatical constructions. Patients appear to grope for words, to mispronounce words, to reiterate endlessly single syllables, or parts of words (logoclonia), or to repeat words and phrases spoken by the examiner (echolalia). Writing is similarly affected; words are misspelt and their component parts are duplicated. Reading ability wanes. The progressive impairment in the patient's speech is associated with simultaneous failure to understand the speech of others. There is a concurrent progressive memory loss which is non-specific and involves both recent and remote events. A curious misidentification phenomenon occurs at this stage. For example, the patient may completely misidentify his reflection in a mirror, the so-called 'mirror sign'. Such patients are to be seen looking in glass mirrors or polished surfaces and talking animatedly to their own image, which they may address by the name of a brother, sister, or friend of the same sex. Characteristically, they do not misidentify the image of another person looking into the glass with them. Pictorial representations of human figures in newspapers or on packages may be misidentified as actual people. Psychiatric symptoms are common in Alzheimer's disease. Between a quarter and one-third are depressed, 16% have delusions and around 15% develop hallucinations, particularly of a visual type. Behaviour disorders occur in approximately one-quarter of all patients.

It should be remembered that depression is often mistaken for dementia and that both conditions may coexist. Where depression is suspected, a history is crucial when making the diagnosis, because in depressive pseudodementia there is often a personal or family history of depression. Interestingly, patients with depression often complain of memory loss, although this is unusual in those who are demented, and the depressed patient is far better on memory tests than might be expected. In other respects also the nature of cognitive impairment is uneven. The similarities between the depressed and demented patient include apathy, loss of initiative and a general decline in performance.

Emotional liability is shown in rapid swings from tearfulness to laughter, or brief flashes of motiveless anger. The most striking affective component of the disease, however, is eagerness to maintain emotional rapport with others. The Alzheimer patient smiles happily when addressed and strives hard to accomplish all that is asked of him. For example, in the test situation a catastrophic reaction, consisting of extreme anxiety and tearfulness, follows failure to satisfy the examiner. Motor restlessness is prominent, but this may alternate with phases of inertia. Muscular rigidity is always present in the later stages and is sometimes associated with difficultly in walking, but the latter may equally denote apraxia of gait.

In the final stage of the illness all intellectual functions are grossly impaired, there is considerable neurological disability, sometimes with hemiparesis, increased muscle tone and a wide-based and unsteady gait. Double incontinence is common. The premorbid personality is completely replaced by fatuous and gross euphoria. All semblance of communication is lost and patients fail to recognise families, friends and themselves. Speech is replaced by jargon dysphasia and, towards the end of life, the patient loses all semblance of personality, becomes emaciated and may develop limb contractures.

The course of senile dementia is a relentless decline and Roth (1955) reported that 80% of patients with this diagnosis died within 2 years of admission to hospital; but this figure was less by 1976, perhaps because demented patients were being admitted to hospital sooner and because the care was better by that time (Roth 1986).

Investigation

The EEG shows typical changes with increasing age in normal individuals. There is a gradual slowing of the alpha rhythm frequency from the young adult, with a mean of about 10 Hz, to not less than 8 Hz by the age of 80 years. Low-voltage, fast beta activity (15–30 Hz) tends to increase between the ages of 20 and 60 years and persists into old age, diminishing only after 80 years. Slow diffuse theta activity (4–7 Hz) and delta activity (1–3 Hz) is rare under the age of 75 years, but focal delta activity is present in 30–40% of those over the age of 60 years in the anterior temporal region. Fenton (1986) indicated that the diffuse theta and delta activity with slowing of the alpha rhythm is common in dementia. Of those with histologically confirmed Alzheimer's disease less than 5% have a normal EEG, even in the early clinical course of the illness. Gordon & Sim (1967) stated that loss of alpha rhythm is in itself an indication of probable Alzheimer's disease.

Brain-imaging techniques have improved considerably in recent years, though the more advanced techniques are confined to use by research workers, or those in neurological centres. In addition to CT, the use of magnetic resonance imaging (MRI), positron emission tomography (PET) and single-photon emission CT (SPECT) are being investigated. The normal brain shows its greatest physical and biochemical changes between the ages of 60 and 80 years; the problem of establishing normal values for each age therefore produces difficulty in discriminating accurately between the normal and abnormal brain. However, CT is useful in the diagnosis of causes of dementia and, in particular, in identifying 'treatable' lesions such as normal pressure hydrocephalus, cerebral tumour and subdural haematoma. However, it is insensitive in early disease and there is poor differentiation between grey and white matter. The clinician is most likely to have access to CT scanning facilities, which may give support to a diagnosis of dementia if they reveal cortical shrinkage and ventricular dilatation. The scan also reveals any focal lesions within the brain, including infarcts and space-occupying lesions. It should be remembered, however, that dementia may be present without CT scan changes, and CT scan changes occur without dementia.

MRI, with superior resolution to CT, defines focal lesions more clearly and measures the volume of brain structures. This allows differentiation between the changes of normal ageing and those due to dementia or other pathologies. Demonstration of hippocampal atrophy may be a clue to early diagnosis.

In Alzheimer's disease, SPECT demonstrates reduced cerebral blood flow in the temporal and posterior parietal lobes; this has been shown to correlate with specific neuropsychological impairment (Beeson 1990). PET shows that brain utilisation of oxygen and glucose is reduced by up to 50% in Alzheimer's disease; mainly in the temporal and parietal lobes. In the later stages of dementia, hypometabolism also occurs in the frontal regions. The clinical features and the area of decreased metabolism correlate well.

Neuropsychological tests

Specific neuropsychological test results are useful augmentors of the information obtained from the mental state examination. Brief, easily administered tests include, for example, the Mini-Mental State Examination, the Abbreviated Mental Test and the Mental State Questionnaire (the MSQ). More complex tests include the Camdex and the Camcog (the computerised version of the Camdex). The WAIS has both a verbal and a performance component, and a discrepancy in favour of a relative preservation of verbal ability is suggestive of a diagnosis of dementia. Raven's Matrices (non-verbal intelligence), the Wisconsin Card Sorting Test (frontal lobe functions) and Verbal Fluency Tests can all be useful in aiding diagnosis, but their main importance perhaps is for measuring the decline in function over a period of time. Other dementia questionnaires and rating scales include the Geriatric Mental State Schedule, the GERRI (a relatives' observation rating scale), the Clifton Assessment Schedule, the Crichton Behaviour Rating Scale (a nurse rating scale), the Blessed Scale and the Global Assessment Schedule.

Treatment in Alzheimer's disease

A range of pharmacological treatments has been used based on the known neurotransmitter and cellular abnormalities in Alzheimer's disease. For example, the cholinergic hypothesis suggests that memory loss in Alzheimer's disease is the result of cholinergic deficit. As receptor levels appear to be unaltered, therapy has focused on transmitter replacement; but use of the dietary precursors of acetylcholine, such as choline and lecithin, have been unsuccessful as treatments. Cholinesterase inhibitors such as physostigmine and velnacrine produce only short-lasting benefits and severe side-effects. Tetrahydroaminoacridine (THA), an inhibitor of cholinesterase activity which also acts at NMDA receptor sites, influences monoamine oxidase inhibitor enzyme levels and modulates GABA transmission in animals, but has had to be withdrawn from use because of its hepatotoxicity, despite promising initial trials. Muscarinic or nicotinic receptor agonists, such as bethanechol or nicotine, provide only modest, brief memory improvement in some demented patients. Combinations of the various pharmacological agents mentioned, all of which act on the cholinergic system, have not yet resulted in successful treatment.

Using a different pharmacological approach to treatment, compounds which modulate NMDA receptor transmission and those which alter calcium ion movement are being assessed, but to date their effectiveness is not known.

In contrast to drug therapy, treatment using nerve growth factor, found in cholinergic neurones in the forebrain, and essential for their growth and viability, may have a role in Alzheimer's disease by preventing progressive neuronal degeneration and the restoration of function (Everall 1990).

Transplantation of embryonic cholinergic neurones into the septum or nucleus basalis is an approach which may produce improvements in Alzheimer's disease, using the technique of implantation already in use for patients with Parkinson's disease.

To conclude, it would appear that there are various clinical and pathological subgroups of cerebral atrophy, as well as mixed dementias such as Alzheimer's disease and vascular dementia. These factors, in addition to possible differences between early and late-onset Alzheimer's disease, make it unlikely that a single form of therapy will be successful in the treatment of the dementias.

Multi-infarct dementia (arteriovascular sclerotic dementia)

Multi-infarct dementia is a disease of the elderly, and probably accounts for around 10–15% of cases of dementia, although the incidence seems to be falling. The male preponderance previously seen is less marked in recent series. The onset of dementia is typically abrupt, with stepwise deterioration and a fluctuating course. There is often a history of hypertension, transient ischaemic attacks or peripheral vascular disease. Hachinski et al (1974) have included the clinical features of the disorder in a clinical rating scale which provides a summary in the form of an 'ischaemic score' that enables differentiation of multi-infarct dementia from Alzheimer's disease, or may suggest the combination of Alzheimer's disease with multi-infarct dementia, which accounts for around 10% of cases of dementia coming to autopsy.

Focal neurological signs often develop due to episodes of cerebral infarction. These include paresis, dysphagia, dysarthria, dysphasia, and slowness of movement. On examination, reflexes are brisk with extensor plantar responses. Headache, dizziness, and syncope often occur and epilepsy is present in about 20% of patients.

The progression of the disorder is intermittent; memory and intellectual failure become worse with each successive episode, but periods of partial recovery take place in between. The mental state fluctuates considerably and the onset of confusional episodes, particularly at night, is characteristic.

Personality is disproportionately well preserved and insight is often good, which may account for the high incidence of depression and anxiety which develops, often with marked somatic symptoms. To compensate for failing memory and difficulty in word finding, a patient may carefully write things down, or adopt an obsessional routine. Emotional control is often poor and behaviour may be disinhibited. Also, a catastrophic reaction may occur when the patient is faced with a task he cannot complete: recovery takes place very quickly and the person is easily diverted to another subject.

Investigations should include examination of the heart and peripheral circulation, a chest radiograph and ECG. Evidence of hypertension should be sought and, if under treatment, be monitored. The EEG is of less value in assessing multi-infarct dementia than Alzheimer's disease. Brain infarcts may not produce EEG abnormalities if they are small and remote from the cortical surface, but when lesions are large and close to the cortex persistent EEG asymmetries are seen.

CT and MRI demonstrate areas of low attenuation, mainly in white matter, corresponding to foci of infarction. While the degree of dementia correlates well with the volume of tissue lost (a minimum of 150–200 ml), it appears that the location of the lesions is also important. SPECT shows a patchy decrease in cerebral blood flow, mirrored by failure of oxygen utilisation on PET. In such cases there is lack of response on exposure to 100% oxygen, suggesting a failure of cerebral vasomotor regulation.

Treatment in dementias

Whilst relatively little can be done to halt or ameliorate the pathological processes in the dementias, sleep disturbance, agitation and depression are common and can be managed by the use of suitable drugs. Nocturnal restlessness is particularly wearing on the family members and sleep for the demented person may be aided by the use of hypnotics (chloral, chlormethiazole, or a combination of small doses of a chloral compound with a tranquillising drug such as promazine). However, improved sleep may be associated with increased incontinence of urine and relatives may need to use disposable absorbent pads, or use special laundry facilities if available. Barbiturates should be avoided for night sedation, or the control of agitation, because they tend to produce confusion in the demented patient. Phenothiazines, such as thioridazine, promazine or haloperidol, are helpful in relieving agitation, aggressive or repetitive behaviour, but care must be taken with the use of such drugs, as they have unwanted side-effects which must be minimised. When depression is marked it can be treated with tetracyclics, and the newer tricyclics, in order to avoid the cardiotoxic side-effects of the more traditional tricyclic group of drugs. Other drugs, useful in other aspects of treatment, include 5-HT re-uptake inhibitors, which may be useful in increasing serotonin availability and which have been used with effect in behaviour disorders associated with dementia. Selegiline, a monoamine oxidase B inhibitor reduces the breakdown of noradrenaline without causing peripheral side-effects and may also be useful in patients who suffer from a low mood.

The treatment of hypertension in multi-infarct dementia has to be approached with caution. High blood pressure is the principal risk factor in strokes, but it must be remembered that in those aged over 70 years a diastolic blood pressure up to 110 mmHg can be regarded as acceptable. In rapidly progressive dementias due to arterial disease associated with transient ischaemic attacks hypertension is best left untreated but, if there is evidence of embolic phenomena, 200 mg of aspirin once daily may be used prophylactically. Treatment with enteric coated aspirin preparations is recommended if there is a history of gastrointestinal bleeding.

The use of socially provided services for both patients and their relatives may be helpful and admission of patients to hospital over short periods reduces family stress, or allows family members to take reasonable holidays. Non-medical day centres, or clubs, and attendance at residential homes, may be of value for those with early dementia, and for relatives there are bodies such as the 'Alzheimer's Disease Society'. Assistance in the home may be gained from occupational therapists, physiotherapists, nurses and other professionals who are able to provide much needed help (Airey 1984).

Pick's disease

Originally described in 1892, Pick's disease is a dementia characterised by frontal lobe dysfunction, and presents typically with selective speech disorders.

Pathology

In contrast to Alzheimer's disease, Pick's disease is characterised by severe atrophy, usually limited to the frontal and temporal lobes; the gyri are so thinned as to warrant the description 'knifeblade atrophy'. Both white matter and subcortical grey structures are involved, particularly the caudate nucleus and putamen. Senile plaques and neurofibrillary tangles are not seen, but there is substantial neuronal loss and some neurones may show silver-staining inclusion bodies known as Pick bodies. Ballooned neurones may also be found.

Using immunocytochemistry and electron microscopy, Pick bodies can be differentiated from other intracellular inclusion bodies, e.g. Lewy bodies. Pick bodies are intensely argyrophilic and lack the central core and peripheral halo of Lewy bodies. They also display an intense reaction with antibodies to τ protein and to paired helical filaments, in contrast to Lewy bodies which either lack reactivity or react in a peripheral band. Electron microscopy reveals that Pick bodies are composed of smoothly contoured random filaments, which contrast with the fuzzy deposits radiating from the central core of the Lewy bodies.

Clinical features

The early symptoms are those of personality change consistent with the frontal lobe syndrome, with changes in social behaviour. There is emotional blunting and increasing egocentricity. The mood may be mildly euphoric with fleeting outbursts of anger. The reaction to formal psychological testing is unlike that generally seen in organic brain disease because those with Pick's disease never show a catastrophic reaction to failure.

In the middle stages of the disease, abnormalities of speech become evident, usually beginning with nominal aphasia, commonly progressing to echolalia, palilalia and perseveration, with mutism in the later stages. In contrast, other cognitive functions remain relatively intact.

Unlike Alzheimer's disease, the frequency of Pick's disease does not increase with age but peaks at about the age of 58–60 years and then declines. Inheritance is thought to be by an incompletely penetrant autosomal dominant gene.

It is striking that patients with Pick's disease, if restricted to the simple routines of everyday life, are not severely affected in their performance until relatively late. For example, patients are able to dress themselves without assistance, and they can cook, mend, embroider, and lay a table. However, their dexterity is impaired and also they show a certain stereotype, for example cooking the same dish for every meal. Therefore, there is a continuing awareness of spatial relationships and an ability to construct objects or designs from their component parts. Also, patients with Pick's disease are able to make long journeys unaccompanied, e.g. to shops, without losing their way, and in hospital quickly orient themselves to the ward. A sense of time is usually well preserved. Retention of one or other of these abilities suggests that the parietal lobe is not involved in the disease process and this helps to differentiate Pick's from Alzheimer's disease. Physical symptoms include mild obesity, episodic restlessness which is nevertheless always purposive, and minor anomalies of gait and posture which do not conform to any specific pattern. A curious generalised hyperalgesia, prominent in the middle stage, disappears as the disease advances (Robertson et al 1958). The final stage of Pick's disease is similar to that seen in the severe forms of other dementias, except that emaciation is not prominent.

Investigations

Neuropsychological tests which are specific for frontal lobe dysfunction, e.g. the Wisconsin Card Sorting Test, verbal fluency, motor programming and cognitive estimates may be difficult because patients find it hard to concentrate and they show a lack of cooperation.

At least half of patients with Pick's disease have a normal EEG. Even when diffuse theta and delta activities are present, alpha activity is better preserved than in Alzheimer's disease. CT and MRI show atrophy of the frontal lobe, and sometimes of the anterior temporal lobe, unlike the posterior changes in Alzheimer's disease, and changes may be seen early in the disease. However, this information cannot be used alone to make the diagnosis.

Prion dementias (subacute spongiform encephalopathy)

The human forms of spongiform encephalopathy,

Creutzfeld–Jakob disease, Gerstmann–Straussler syndrome and kuru, are characterised by the accumulation in the brain of an *abnormal form* of a normal host protease-resistant protein, PrP, hence the name 'prion'. The diseases present with rapidly progressive dementia. Spongiform encephalopathies have also been found in sheep and goats (scrapie), in deer, mink and, recently, in cats and cattle (bovine spongiform encephalopathy or BSE). BSE has almost certainly been transmitted to cows by scrapie-infected sheep carcasses in animal feed and may be transmissable to man via infected meat (Matthews 1990).

Iatrogenic horizontal transmission of Creutzfeld–Jakob disease has occurred, for example following corneal grafting, while kuru was transmitted by cannibalism. The nature of the infectious agent in these disorders is unclear as no nucleic acid has been identified.

The Gerstmann–Straussler syndrome is inherited as an autosomal dominant gene with complete penetrance, while Creutzfeld–Jakob disease is familial in 15% of cases (Collinge 1990). In affected or at risk individuals in families with Gerstmann–Straussler syndrome, or familial Creutzfeld–Jakob disease, three gene variants of the PrP gene on chromosome 20 (a 'candidate gene' for these disorders) have been identified.

Creutzfeld–Jakob disease

This condition takes its name from Jakob (1921), who described a series of five cases, and Creutzfeld (1920), who a year earlier had published details of a single case which Jakob considered similar to his own. The disorder is rare. In the few familial cases reported, the distribution of the disease is compatible with dominant inheritance.

Pathology. Cerebral atrophy is minimal or absent, but some degree of ventricular dilatation is commonly observed. Histologically, there is loss and degeneration of nerve cells with pronounced proliferation of astrocytes in the grey matter of the cortex, basal ganglia, thalamus, motor nuclei of the brain stem and anterior horn cells of the spinal cord. Also, an abnormal form of protease-resistant protein (PrP), accumulates, which has the characteristics of amyloid, and is deposited, forming plaques which can be distinguished from those of Alzheimer's disease by immunohistochemical staining with antibodies to PrP. There is little or no cerebral atrophy. The long descending tracts may also show degeneration. In the

Heidenhain form, neuronal loss and astrocytosis are most severe in the occipital lobes, but are also found in the striatum and sometimes in the thalamus. The brain stem nuclei, the anterior horn cells and the descending tracts of the spinal cord are always spared, despite their invariable involvement in the classical form of the disease. In the ataxic form the maximum impact is on the cerebellum, with cerebellar atrophy and severe loss of granular cells. Neuronal loss and astrocytosis occur in the cortex, striatum and thalamus.

'Status spongiosis' is a pathological feature occurring in all prion dementias and in the majority of patients with Creutzfeld–Jakob disease. It consists of numerous microcystic spaces scattered throughout the grey matter, so giving the brain a spongy appearance, but is not pathognomonic of Creutzfeld–Jakob disease since it has been observed in a number of cerebral degenerative disorders.

Clinical features. The onset of the disease is sudden and it has a rapid course, most patients dying within a year or two.

The clinical picture of Creutzfeld–Jakob disease differs from that of other presenile dementias in its lack of uniformity. To the disease originally described by Jakob — now known as the classical form of the illness — have been added several other syndromes which have pathological similarities, but each with its own distinctive features. The two most important, mentioned earlier, are those described by Heidenhain (1928) and by Brownell & Oppenheimer (1965), which are referred to as the Heidenhain form and the ataxic form of Creutzfeld–Jakob disease. These additions reveal that considerable variations exist in the clinical picture, which is a reflection of the varied ways in which the CNS may be involved in what is essentially a uniform pathological process.

In all forms of Creutzfeld–Jakob disease, intellectual deterioration terminates in dementia and there may be a prodromal phase of anxiety, depression or hallucinations, which is generally brief. The somatic features of the classical form comprise spasticity of the limbs or, alternatively, weakness and wasting associated with the fasciculation of the muscles. With spasticity there is tremor, rigidity and choreoathetoid movements (mycoclonus, dysarthria and dysphagia — the latter a terminal feature). Convulsive seizures can also occur. Visual defects, terminating in cortical blindness, are the most prominent somatic feature of the Heidenhain form. Extrapyramidal symptoms also occur, as does myoclonus. The ataxic form presents initially as a rapidly progressive cerebellar ataxia. This is followed by the appearance of involuntary movements, often in the form of myoclonic jerking. The final stage is one of muteness and generalised rigidity.

The EEG in Creutzfeld–Jakob disease in often abnormal, with increased slow wave activity and a diminution of alpha rhythm. As the disease progresses, bilateral, slow spike–wave discharges are typical and may be accompanied by myoclonic jerks.

Other forms of dementia

Dementia of frontal lobe type

Patients within this group have symptoms of the 'frontal lobe syndrome'. They present with a major change in personality and social behaviour followed by progressive impairment of speech, in contrast to a relative preservation of memory and visuospatial functioning (Neary et al 1988). The disorder occurs at an earlier age than Alzheimer's disease and there is a strong family history of dementia; approximately 50% have a parent with dementia (Gustafson 1987). The EEG is normal, but SPECT demonstrates hypoperfusion of the frontal areas, and at post mortem the frontal and temporal lobes are severely atrophic. There is loss of large cortical nerve cells, spongiform changes in the cortex, with cortical and subcortical gliosis. No plaques or tangles are present. The ratio of dementia of the frontal lobe type to Alzheimer's disease is thought to be between 1:4 in the UK and 1:10 in Sweden.

The important alternative diagnoses are Pick's disease and Creutzfeld–Jakob disease, but the nature of the dementia is often not known until post mortem examination of the brain has been carried out.

Lobar atrophy

This term refers to a group of conditions in which there is atrophy of all or part of a lobe, resulting in a focal neurological deficit.

Progressive aphasia is the commonest disorder due to focal atrophy as in the case described by Goulding et al (1989) in which clinically there was a slowly progressive aphasia leading to mutism with relative preservation of other neuropsychological functions. Neuro-imaging and autopsy localised the disorder to the left cerebral hemisphere. There remains debate as to whether this condition is a distinct disease entity or a focal manifestation of Alzheimer's disease or Pick's disease. Posterior cortical atrophy presents with selective apraxia, acalculia, agraphia, anomia, visual agnosia, disorientation, disorders of ocular fixation and sensory aphasia. CT and MRI show atrophy to be most marked in the posterior cortical regions. Pathological changes similar to those of Alzheimer's disease affect the parietal and occipital association cortex.

Lewy body disease

Lewy bodies are eosinophilic intracellular inclusions which are present in the basal ganglia and substantia nigra of patients with Parkinson's disease. Recently, similar, smaller, previously unrecognised bodies have been demonstrated in the subcortex and cortex of patients with dementia by immunocytochemistry, which identifies the protein ubiquitin (Lennox 1989).

In senile dementia of the Lewy body type, patients present with acute or subacute confusional states, depression with short-term memory loss and marked psychiatric symptoms, particularly visual hallucinations (Perry 1990). Extrapyramidal symptoms are less severe than in Parkinson's disease initially, and respond to L-dopa. There is mild nigrostriatal degeneration, a wide spread of cortical Lewy bodies and senile plaques, but no other pathological features typical of Alzheimer's disease. Perry (1990) demonstrated that senile dementia of Lewy body type accounted for 20% of cases of dementia in patients over the age of 70 years, many of whom had been diagnosed as suffering from multi-infarct dementia in life.

Lewy body disorders are now thought to represent a spectrum rather than one disease. The clinical presentation reflects the distribution of Lewy bodies in the cerebral cortex and brain stem.

Occasional Lewy bodies are sometimes found in other disorders, including Alzheimer's disease, progressive supranuclear palsy and ataxia–telangiectasia.

Huntington's disease

This hereditary disease, characterised by continuous involuntary movements and slowly progressive dementia, was described in 1872 by a Dr Huntington, the third in a direct line of a family of New England physicians who had witnessed this disease descend though successive generations of their patients. It has a worldwide distribution and affects men and women equally. The prevalence in Britain is five per 100 000 of the population. Its transmission is by a single dominant autosomal gene. This implies that 50% of the children of an affected parent will develop the disease and, while they in turn transmit it to their offspring in a similar ratio, the offspring of the unaffected children are not at

risk. Sporadic cases occur with no known family history and are presumably attributable to new mutations.

There is considerable variation in both the clinical features and age at onset of symptoms. At least three clinical subtypes appear to be related to the age of onset of the disease. In general, patients developing Huntington's disease in early adult life have inherited the condition from their father, while maternal transmission leads to a later presentation (Martin & Gusella 1986). It has been suggested that this occurs due to the action of 'genetic modifiers'; the effects of the Huntington's disease gene may depend on their interaction with the genes which control the rate of ageing. Therefore, if the patient has 'superior' ageing genes, the onset of the disease will be later than in those with 'inferior' ageing genes. Alternatively, a maternal protective factor may be present in the cytoplasm (possibly a mitochondrial gene) or a maternal genotype may delay the onset of the disease.

Pathology

There is generalised cortical atrophy, most marked over the frontal lobes, together with ventricular dilatation. However, the major microscopic changes occur in the corpus striatum, in which there is a marked loss of small nerve cells with relative preservation of larger motor cells. Atrophy of the head of the caudate nucleus and of the putamen is marked. Neuronal loss is also severe in the outer cortical laminae, notably in the frontal region. Striatal GABA neurones (which also contain either enkephalin or substance P) projecting from the striatum to the lateral part of the globus pallidus or substantia nigra are lost.

Neurochemistry

Studies on autopsy specimens from patients with Huntington's disease have shown a deficiency of GABA in the substantia nigra, putamen, globus palladus and caudate nucleus. GABA is the transmitter for inhibitory neurones which are widespread in the cortex and other parts of the brain and an imbalance between GABA and dopamine in the basal ganglia could lead to excess dopaminergic activity and, therefore, abnormal movements. In fact, because movements are diminished by dopamine-blocking drugs it was felt that, as with Parkinson's disease, the disorder must involve some abnormality of dopamine activity.

More recent studies suggest a role for excitatory amino acids which, in excess concentrations, can be selectively toxic to certain types of neurones. Glutamate, the most common of the amino acids, is an endogenous neurotransmitter in the nigrostriatal pathway and it activates at least three types of receptors: the kainate, quisqualate and NMDA receptors. Infusion of glutamate into the caudate nucleus destroys caudate neurones.

Neurones bearing NMDA receptors seem to mediate most glutamate-induced toxicity, and GABA-containing neurones seem to be more susceptible than the total neurone population to the NMDA-mediated insult. At autopsy, NMDA receptors are more significantly depleted than other receptors. They are selectively located on medium-sized spiny neurones which have a large glutaminergic cortical innervation and these neurones are lost extensively in Huntington's disease. Quinolinic acid, another excitatory amino acid, which is an endogenous metabolite of tryptophan, can produce pathological changes similar to those found in Huntington's disease when injected locally into the brain of primates. Moreover, there is an increase in the enzyme which synthesises quinolinic acid in the brains of patients with Huntington's disease (Di Figlia 1990).

In contrast, somatostatin, which is thought to increase striatal dopamine, is increased and this may exaggerate the motor disturbances (Martin & Gusella 1986). Choline acetyltransferase levels are also reduced but catecholamine levels in general are not.

Clinical features

The onset of the disease is insidious. The occasional grimace, shrug or body twist, or the intermittent tapping of fingers or feet, may impress the observer as no more than a general 'fidgetiness'. In the established case the abnormal movements are notable for their abruptness and variable form. Choreiform movements are usually first noticed in the face, head and arms. Head nodding, torticollis and facial twitching are common. Both voluntary and involuntary movements of the arms are typically choreiform in that they are ill-sustained and jerky. At a later stage, athetoid movements of the limbs become apparent. No part of the body is exempt, and speech, swallowing, respiration and locomotion are all affected. Speech is slurred and stumbling; spasmodic inspiration may render it at times explosive. The gait is distinctive and the patient walks on his heels with a wide base. Sudden lurching has been known to precipitate the sufferer through a shop window or down a staircase. Retention of insight in the early stages understandably results in extreme sensitivity to the reaction of other people to the disabling and ungainly movements and reactive depression may develop. Explosive outbursts, or irritability and rage, are not uncommon and may continue to recur after insight has been replaced by mild euphoria. Physical activity may be maintained until late in the disease, but some patients sink into a state of almost total inertia. Intellectual impairment is slowly progressive and, although some patients maintain a semblance of mental clarity to the end of their lives, others show profound dementia in its final stages. The average duration of the disease is 12–16 years.

Investigations

There is an absence of rhythmical activity of the EEG over all areas, a so-called 'flat' EEG, defined as activity below 25 μV in amplitude. However, this is not specific for Huntingdon's chorea as it is sometimes found in normal adults.

Imaging

CT scanning can be useful in demonstrating caudate atrophy, but may not be sufficiently sensitive to differentiate between Huntingdon's disease and other extrapyramidal disorders. The degree of atrophy correlates well with the functional disability. MRI gives better resolution but, like CT, demonstrates changes only in established diseases. In contrast, PET, by measuring glucose metabolism in the caudate nuclei, which is decreased in Huntington's disease, even in very early forms, allows the diagnosis to be made before the clinical onset of the disease. SPECT demonstrates decreased blood flow in the region of the caudate nuclei and putamen.

Prodromal emotional disturbance, personality disorder and psychiatric illness

Some degree of emotional disturbance may precede the physical manifestations of the disease. Depression, apathy and fleeting paranoid beliefs are among the commoner features described. Oliver (1970) found that 38 of 100 patients examined exhibited behaviour disorders and catalogued violence, cruelty to children, high divorce rate, sexual perversions, repeated petty crime, and refusal to work amongst the abnormalities detected. There is evidence that such behaviour disorders are predictive in that the abnormal member (or members) of the family at risk is more likely to carry the Huntington gene. However, many Huntington patients, particularly those who develop the disease relatively late, have been stable and diligent and had good employment records. Bolt (1970) found that only 10% of patients in her series were described by their families 'as always having been difficult'. In some two-thirds of cases, psychiatric disturbances developed after the onset of chorea. For example, in the largest UK series Bolt (1970) recorded that 17.1% of her patients were depressed and characteristic symptoms were of a psychotic type, including paranoid delusions and unipolar depressive mood swings. Huntington stated that suicide was 'one of the three marked peculiarities of the disease' and, interestingly, it not only occurs with a greater than expected frequency in individuals with Huntingdon's chorea, but also in their relatives; perhaps this is a response to anticipation of the development of the disease in certain instances.

Schizophrenia also occurs more often in Huntington's disease than would be expected in the normal population, but published figures for the incidence of this disorder vary. In a group examined by Dewhurst & Oliver (1970) at the time of admission to a mental hospital, 8% were schizophrenic. Brothers (1964) reported that schizophrenia was the most common mental disorder to occur prior to the onset of chorea and that hebephrenia occurred more often than paranoid schizophrenia. Bolt (1970) reported paranoid delusions in 33% of her patients and in one case observed that a psychotic illness preceded the onset of chorea by 19 years. Thus, the literature indicates that the onset of psychosis may precede the arrival of chorea by some years and that, although there is no evidence of an increased incidence of psychotic illness in unaffected relatives, the appearance of schizophrenia in a young person with a family history of Huntington's disease may presage the later onset of this disorder.

Between 50 and 70% of patients exhibit dementia shortly after chorea becomes evident, but it varies from patient to patient both in intensity and in its rate of development. However, there does seem to be a relationship between the severity of chorea and of dementia. The dementia of Huntington's disease appears to show some neuropsychological differences from other presenile dementias with extensive cortical destruction. For example, patients with Huntington's chorea do not develop aphasia, apraxia, agnosia, alexia or visual neglect, all of which are common in Alzheimer's disease. Memory loss occurs but is less severe than in Korsakoff's syndrome, being part of a general intellectual deterioration rather than a specific loss. At a later stage deficits in problem-solving and judgement occur, attention and concentration are impaired, and there is a general decline in intellectual ability. McHugh & Folstein (1975) noted that the development of apathy, progressing later to complete inertia — a state resembling akinetic mutism — tends to obscure intellectual functioning, giving the picture of a subcortical dementia. Caine et al (1978) examined 18 patients with Huntington's disease and, using tests of parietal lobe function from the WAIS and Projection Tests, discovered an inability to plan, organise, sequence and recall factual material, and suggested that patients lose detailed memory. Their patients also exhibited slowed information processing. Interestingly, although deficits in performance were noted on the parietal lobe battery, for example on block figure construction, other aspects of the battery were unimpaired. They suggested that the pattern of abnormality demonstrated was similar to that seen in patients with frontal lobe syndromes with loss of 'cortical executive function'.

Differential diagnosis

The condition has to be differentiated from senile chorea, where the symptoms are mild and there is no family history, and phenothiazine-induced tardive dyskinesia. If in addition to facial dyskinesia, abnormal movements are present in the trunk and limbs, Sydenham's chorea, Wilson's disease, and other choreiform disorders should be considered.

Treatment

There is no treatment that will halt the disease. Neuroleptics, which block dopamine, may help to control chorea and psychotic disturbances. Involuntary movements may be reduced by thiopropazate (20 mg three times daily) or tetrabenazine (25–200 mg daily). Treatments that influence GABA mechanisms, such as baclofen and sodium valproate, have not proved effective and other treatments which influence cholinergic activity, such as demethylaminoethanol (Deanol) and physostigmine, do not help. However, D_2 antagonists result in stimulation of neurones projecting from the striatum to the lateral globus pallidus, thereby partially overcoming the degeneration of this pathway. The use of antidepressants, minor tranquillisers and electroconvulsive therapy (ECT) are not contraindicated for the treatment of psychiatric disorders at an early stage in the disease.

Prevention

In 1983 Gusella et al identified a DNA sequence (G8) showing close genetic linkage to Huntington's chorea on chromosome 4. The detection of this marker opened up the exciting possibility of genetic predictions of the disease in affected families. However, a number of limitations prevent complete identification of subjects at risk at present, although the marker genotype is of value in about 75% of cases examined. Harper & Sarfarazi (1985) indicated that careful analysis of family structure allows a degree of prediction to be made for the unborn child in almost 90% of cases. They concluded that such analyses will remain crucial until the limitations of the Gusella probe technique have been overcome. Individuals at risk could bear children when the disease has been excluded in pregnancy, and those pregnancies with high risk of disease in the fetus (50%) could be terminated. Some doctors and some parents may not find this approach acceptable, in which case the couple may be advised, or decide, not to have children.

A national medical linkage system, together with registration of the pedigrees of the affected families, would aid effective control of the disease. Information can be made available to families through the 'Association to Combat Huntington's Disease'.

OTHER NEUROLOGICAL DISORDERS

General paralysis

This was formerly one of the commonest causes of an organic psychosis in mid-life but is now one of the rarest. Dewhurst (1969) found 91 cases admitted to several hospitals in one region in Britain between the years 1950–1965. He pointed out that the diagnosis had been missed in many cases, with the condition often being regarded as depression, mania or dementia. Several patients had been treated with penicillin for other reasons, and this modified the clinical picture.

The cause of general paralysis is infection with *Treponema pallidum* and the latent period between primary infection and the onset of general paralysis varies from 5 to 25 years. Examination of the brain reveals marked cerebral atrophy and meningeal thickening with neuronal loss and astrocyte proliferation at the cellular level. The spirochaete can be seen in the cortex of 50% of cases. The frontal lobes of the brain are particularly involved, and this leads to personality changes. Disinhibition and unconventional behaviour, which may be instrumental in bringing the patient to attention, are noticeable features and such behaviour can easily be mistaken for a hypomanic state, as uncontrolled excitement and overactivity may be present. Most patients, however, develop the disorder more slowly, with the gradual onset of memory and intellectual impairment, often with depression as a predominant feature. The classical presentation with grandiose delusions is seen rarely and only occurred in about 10% of Dewhurst's patients.

In over half the cases the pupils are small, unequal and irregular and fail to react to light but do so to accommodation (Argyll–Robertson pupils). Speech may be slurred and tremor of the lips and tongue may be present. Later in the disease a progressive weakness in the legs ensues, eventually leading to a spastic paralysis.

The Venereal Disease Research Laboratory (VDRL) test is positive in the blood in about 90% of untreated cases. The fluorescent treponemal antibody test (the FTA absorption test) is very reliable and almost always positive, both in CSF and blood in the modified forms of neurosyphilis found today. The automated *Treponema pallidum* haemagglutination (TPHA) test is also highly specific. If the diagnosis is in question, examination of the CSF is essential and the VDRL test is positive in almost every untreated case. There is also a lymphocytosis and a raised protein level with an increase in the globulin fraction. The colloidal gold (Lange) test gives a paretic curve.

Treatment is with high doses of penicillin, often used with steroids to prevent the Herxheimer reaction, which is an acute febrile state in which the patient's symptoms are intensified within 24 hours of penicillin therapy. Improvement can be expected and, although mental symptoms may diminish, the VDRL test in CSF and blood may not become negative for a number of years. Relapses in the patient's clinical state are normally preceded by changes in the CSF reaction.

Lyme disease

Borrelia burgdorferi is a tick-borne spirochaete first recognised in 1975 in Lyme, Connecticut, by Burgdorfer. It can infect almost any organ in the body and the skin, joints, heart and nervous system are commonly involved. In around 15% of cases a variety of neurological symptoms and signs occur as a result of direct infection of the nervous system, including meningoencephalitis, cranial nerve palsies and radiculopathy. Neuropsychiatric manifestations occur in some cases. Just under half of the patients develop profound tiredness and malaise accompanied by myalgia, which can last several years, and the diagnosis of Lyme disease should be considered in cases of chronic so-called 'postviral fatigue'.

Diagnosis is made on history and clinical grounds with raised antibody titres indicating a current or recent infection. Culture from specimens is slow and has a low yield (O'Neill 1988).

Early disease responds well to antibiotics, such as benzylpenicillin, erythromycin, tetracycline and some cephalosporins. In the later stages the disease is more difficult to treat, especially if the CNS is involved, and parenteral therapy may be required.

Multiple sclerosis

Multiple sclerosis is characterised by episodes of demyelination, which cause abnormalities of CNS function which are disseminated in space and time. These result in a combination of neurological symptoms and changes in mental state.

Aetiology

Genetic factors are important. Up to 18% of patients have a first-degree relative with multiple sclerosis and the concordance rate for monozygotic twins is about 50% and around 17% for dizygotic twins. An area on chromosome 6 has been identified as probably being responsible for the susceptibility to multiple sclerosis. An increased frequency of human leucocyte system A antigens (HLA-B7, -A3, -Dw2 and especially HLA-DR2) has also been shown to be present in patients with multiple sclerosis (Comston 1986). Whether there is a link between the specific changes in the immune system and the psychiatric symptoms has not yet been fully elucidated (but HLA-B7 may be a common factor).

Other evidence implicates environmental factors, for example the presence of a viral agent perhaps acquired in childhood (Skegg 1991). Abnormal fatty acid metabolism, viral infections and immunological reactivity to brain antigens have all been suggested as possible aetiological factors. However, as yet there is no definite answer.

Neurological changes in multiple sclerosis include blurring of vision, which is a common first sign, diplopia, vertigo, limb paraesthesia and weakness. Impotence and difficulty in micturition also occur. Psychiatric consequences include euphoria, mood lability, depression and intellectual impairment, particularly loss of short-term memory and conceptual thinking. Denial of disability is common. In a small number of cases the disease is rapidly progressive and may present as dementia. There is a high risk of suicide. Severe personality changes may be seen in patients with a very acute presentation, and frontal lobe symptoms can occur in more insidious cases. Depression may occur as early as 2 years before the onset of other symptoms, but more often accompanies clinically apparent multiple sclerosis, occurring in as many as 54% of cases. The depression may or may not be related to the severity of the physical symptoms. Emotional disturbance may be as high as 90% in those with progressive multiple sclerosis and 39% in those with stable multiple sclerosis. There may be a reactive element but it seems likely that neurobiological abnormalities are implicated in the depression, although the suicide risk is high in the rapidly progressive form of the disease. The presentation may be masked by other symptoms, particularly those of frontal lobe dysfunction.

The affective symptoms may vary; conventional treatment, for example antidepressants or ECT, is seldom successful. Lithium and carbamazepine can be useful.

Pathology

Multifocal abnormalities are found in the CNS. In the early stages there is infiltration of the perivascular spaces by lymphocytes, plasma cells and macrophages, and the blood–brain barrier breaks down. Patchy demyelination due to lipolytic and proteolytic enzymes is accompanied by white matter gliosis. Ultimately, glial scars with astrocyte proliferation are seen in many sites, particularly around the lateral ventricles and in the brain stem, and axonal loss can be seen within these plaques.

Investigations

MRI is particularly sensitive in those diseases causing changes in the white matter of the brain. Almost all cases of multiple sclerosis will show brain changes, such as 'bright areas', that is, areas of increased signalling on MRI. A significant number will also show changes in the optic nerves and spinal cord. Unfortunately, problems may be encountered in patients over 50 years of age who do not have multiple sclerosis but have similar changes on MRI, thought to be due to small areas of ischaemia. Steroids are still the only, if short-term, effective drug treatment.

Human immunodeficiency virus

The nature of HIV infection

HIV attacks the immune system, the brain and spinal cord. HIV-1, the most common cause of AIDS in America, Europe and Central Africa, is a cytopathic retrovirus of the lentivirus group. It consists of a central core containing two strands of RNA, the enzyme reverse transcriptase, structural proteins, and a lipid envelope bearing two glycoproteins, gp120 and gp41. HIV infects cells bearing the CD4 antigen, to which gp120 binds. Macrophages and microglia are the 'prime' targets for HIV infection of the CNS. Although HIV infection of neurones has been shown in vitro it has yet to be confirmed in vivo.

Pathology

Over three-quarters of patients dying of AIDS have neuropathological abnormalities at post mortem. The direct effects are HIV encephalopathy and a vacuolar myelopathy. The brain becomes atrophic with widened sulci and dilated ventricles, and the meninges are often thickened. Microscopic abnormalities are found mainly in white matter and in subcortical grey structures where collections of microglia and characteristic multinucleated cells are found. There may be focal demyelination and diffuse astrocytosis. In vacuolar myelopathy, there is spongy degeneration of the ascending and descending white matter tracts.

The mechanism of neurotoxicity of HIV remains unclear. Two main pathways of HIV-associated damage have been proposed (Budka 1991 – see Fig. 15.1). Firstly, there may be systemic plus local increase of the virus, leading to HIV encephalitis, which is confirmed by HIV production within these 'lesions'. Secondly neuronotoxicity may be produced by HIV proteins or factors secreted from infected cells. This is supported by histological changes and by 'selective' loss of frontocortical neurones.

The envelope glycoprotein gp 120 has been shown to inhibit neuroleukin selectively. This is a neurotrophic peptide which mediates sensory nerve growth. Also, it interferes with other neurotransmitters, for example vasoactive intestinal peptide. Recent studies have shown that quinolinic acid, a neurotoxic intermediate metabolite of tryptophan, is increased in the CSF. There is a significant correlation between the levels of these substances and the stage of dementia. The similarity of HIV to visna virus, which causes demyelination in sheep, suggests that loss of myelin may be immune mediated.

There may be evidence of secondary infection of the nervous system by other viruses (e.g. cytomegalovirus), fungi (e.g. cryptococcus), protozoa (e.g. toxoplasma) and bacteria (e.g. mycobacteria). Kennedy (1988), reviewing the neurological complications of HIV infection, stated that primary cerebral lymphoma occurs in around 5% of patients.

Clinical features

HIV dementia (AIDS–dementia complex) affects a third of patients with AIDS (Kennedy 1988), and is now the commonest form of dementia in young people. It is usually insidious in onset, and presents with impairment of memory and concentration, and with mental slowing. There are also changes in behaviour, including apathy and social withdrawal or, in contrast, disinhibited behaviour usually associated with frontal damage. Motor symptoms such as loss of balance and coordination and leg weakness also occur. In the early stages of the illness a routine mental state examination may be normal, although mild slowing in verbal and motor responses, and impairment of short-term memory, may be detected. Higher cortical functions are usually well preserved until late in the course of the disease. Neurological examination may reveal tremor, ataxia, hyperreflexia, frontal release signs and dysarthria. There may be hypersensitivity due to accompanying sensory neuropathy (Kennedy 1988).

Most patients rapidly develop severe global impairment and marked psychomotor retardation and finally become bedridden, mute and doubly incontinent. Death due to inanition, aspiration pneumonia or opportunistic infection occurs in 90% of cases within 2 years.

Investigations

Both total protein and immunoglobulin (IgC) levels are increased in the CSF; sometimes with an oligoclonal band. Reversal of the ratio of the T lymphocyte subsets (CD4:CD8) is reflected in the peripheral blood, and a mild mononuclear pleocytosis can occur. The virus, the HIV-1 antigen p24 and antibodies to HIV-1 can be detected. CT and MRI scans demonstrate widespread cerebral atrophy, with ventricular dilatation and widened sulci. Also, MRI shows a focal increase in the white matter signal which is at least partially reversible with azidodeoxythymidine (AZT, zidovudine) treatment. In the early stages, PET changes include increased glucose metabolism in subcortical structures such as the thalamus and basal ganglia, but later there is hypometabolism in the cortical and subcortical grey matter. The ratio of ATP to inorganic phosphate assessed by magnetic resonance spectroscopy is reduced in moderate to severe cases, indicating reduced brain energy metabolism.

The EEG is usually unchanged early in the disease but may show diffuse slowing in the late stage.

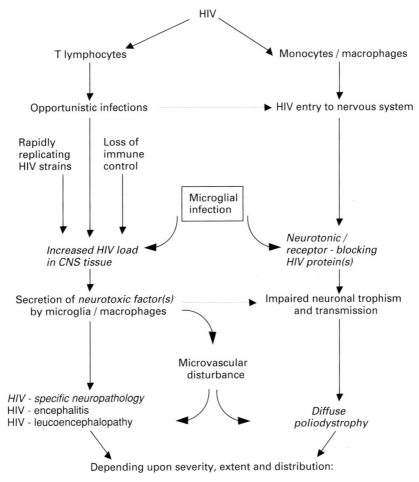

Fig. 15.1 Flow diagram of pathogenetic pathways for HIV-associated CNS damage as suggested from neuropathological and other data. Note the central role for infected microglia/macrophages and two major pathways: the first involves increased virus load in tissue leading to HIV-specific neuropathology (left part); and the second involves neuronotoxicity by HIV or macrophage products, leading to diffuse poliodystrophy (right part). (Budka 1991.)

Treatment

The aims of treatment are to halt the propagation of the virus, to restore immunocompetence and to prevent and treat opportunistic infections. Early diagnosis allows the introduction of antiviral therapy. AZT is the most effective of the drugs available and acts by inhibiting viral reverse transcriptase and thus prevents the transcription of viral RNA to DNA and its subsequent insertion into the host genome. In some cases AZT treatment results in an improvement in cerebral function and slows the course of the disease, but a major side-effect is bone marrow suppression. There is some evidence that calcium channel blockers are useful in preventing HIV coat protein-induced neurotoxicity. As yet, there is no safe effective vaccine against HIV infection.

Psychiatric sequelae of the diagnosis of HIV

Psychiatric problems occur at different stages of HIV infection (Maj 1990). Acute stress with anxiety and a brief period of depression may follow a positive antibody test and persistence of these symptoms is related to previous coping skills and perceived social support. Adjustment disorders similar to bereavement reactions may occur in otherwise asymptomatic HIV-positive individuals and in AIDS patients. Major affective disorders and acute psychoses are relatively common in AIDS, or the AIDS-related complex (ARC), and may be either functional or an early sign of organic brain disease. There is a high suicide risk, particularly soon after diagnosis.

Treatment includes counselling, and cognitive and behaviour therapies. Caution must be taken when prescribing tricyclic antidepressants, which may induce delirium, and phenothiazines, which are more likely to give extrapyramidal signs in patients with organic brain disease.

Psychiatric disorders also occur in subjects without HIV infection who develop the so-called 'worried well' syndrome, comprising hypochondriacal symptoms based on a persistent belief that HIV infection has occurred despite repeatedly negative tests. Affected patients often respond to cognitive therapy.

Primary prevention by appropriate counselling of high-risk groups and provision of a counselling service to those already HIV-positive, and their partners, may reduce high-risk behaviour and psychiatric morbidity. It should be remembered that General Medical Council guidelines insist that appropriate counselling is given before and after the antibody test.

Parkinson's disease

Primary Parkinson's disease is a disorder of movement consequent upon abnormalities of neurotransmission involving an imbalance between dopaminergic and cholinergic neurone systems and stemming from a deficit of dopaminergic activity in the striatum, resulting in akinesia, in the mesocortical systems, accounting for rigidity, and in the deep hypothalamic nuclei, causing tremor. Secondary parkinsonism occurs in patients with arteriosclerotic disease and, less often, amongst those who have had a head injury or encephalitis and, occasionally, in patients who have syphilis, manganese poisoning or carbon monoxide poisoning.

Pathology

As well as decreased dopamine levels, there is a fall in frontal choline acetyltransferase levels of 50% and neuropsychological changes in frontal lobe function. There are deficits in outflow from the caudate nucleus. Nucleus basalis cell loss is between 30 and 80% in patients with co-existing dementia, resulting in changes in the main ascending cholinergic pathways. The cholinergic deficit is probably sufficient to cause

the memory loss, but cortical pathology has to be present to result in dementia. The three main pathologies associated with the dementia are (coexisting) Alzheimer's disease, Lewy body neuronal degeneration in the nucleus basalis and cortical Lewy bodies.

Psychiatric symptoms

Psychiatric disturbances are common, with depression in 40–50% of patients; a figure similar to that obtained from others with chronic physical illness, for example rheumatoid arthritis. Obsessional symptoms, psychoses and changes in cognitive function occur. Mindham (1970) reported that 48% of patients with parkinsonism referred for psychiatric help, and 50% of those undergoing medical or surgical treatment for the disease, suffered from depression. Robins (1976) examined 45 patients with Parkinson's disease not on treatment with L-dopa and compared them with a group of 45 patients matched for age and who were physically ill. Depression scores on the Hamilton Rating Scale were significantly higher amongst patients with Parkinson's disease and examination of the items amongst the responses to the questionnaires showed that suicidal ideas, retardation, anxiety, somatic complaints and lack of insight were prominent. However, the results did not show a correlation between physical disability and mental state, as had been the case in Mindham's study. Clearly, depression may be part of the reaction to physical disability, but this does not appear to account totally for its presence. Depression can be relieved with antidepressant drugs in a high proportion of patients in whom further physical improvements are not possible.

Other psychoses are uncommon, but psychotic symptoms — hallucinations and delusions — do occur in association with treatment of the disease by anti-cholinergic drugs, L-dopa or bromocriptine.

The incidence of dementia (10–20%) is twice that in the general population and it occurs in all types of parkinsonism. As dementia is rare in younger patients, despite long survival, it is thought to be more a reflection of age than the disease process, occurring more often in older patients and those with cerebrovascular disease. However, Celesia and Wanamaker (1972) noted that the degree of dementia was related to the severity and duration of illness.

Intellectual impairment is frequently reported in Parkinson's disease and takes the form of subtle cognitive changes which are related to the duration and severity of the illness, occurring in between one-third and 40% of cases (Mindham 1970, Celesia & Wanamaker 1972).

Cognitive and perceptual function may be related more to the patient's akinesia than his level of rigidity (Ricklan et al 1959). Intellectual recovery occurred in half of a group of 40 patients who were examined 5–13 months after L-dopa therapy, which may have produced its effect by increasing arousal and levels of activation (Loranger et al 1972).

The differentiation between depression and dementia can be difficult. Patients may respond slowly to questions and have trouble mobilising thought processes quickly. Difficulties occur with word finding and verbal expression, but answers are usually correct if sufficient time is given. These problems are thought to be due to impaired subcortical afferent pathways from the brain stem and striatum to the cortex.

Depression and drug treatment both may simulate dementia and, if there is doubt, the Wisconsin Card Sorting Test and Verbal Fluency Test may be useful adjuncts to the mental state examination.

Patients with Alzheimer's disease are three times more likely to have a first-degree relative with Parkinson's disease than age-matched controls. Also, there is an increased prevalence of Alzheimer's disease in patients with Parkinson's disease, but those with this disorder can be demented without showing changes of Alzheimer's disease at autopsy (Gibb 1989).

Treatment

The basis of current treatment for Parkinson's disease is the substitution for dopamine within the brain by L-dopa or other means of altering neurotransmission within the dopamine system. L-Dopa is converted into dopamine by dopa decarboxylase. Because this process produces unacceptable peripheral side-effects, the action of dopa decarboxylase outside the central nervous system has to be blocked by a decarboxylase inhibitor, which is given with L-dopa. This does not cross the blood–brain barrier and thus does not impair the central effect of L-dopa. Compounds containing this combination include Sinemet and Madopar. This form of treatment is most effective in reducing rigidity and hypokinesia.

Interest in developing new forms of therapy led to the discovery of a monoamine oxidase B inhibitor, selegiline, which has been shown to slow the rate of progression of the disease in its early stages and to potentiate the effects of L-dopa in established cases. Also, L-dopa may be given in combination with lisuride, a dopamine agonist, at an early stage of the illness with a reduction in the fluctuations in symptoms and dyskinesia.

Amantadine (Symmetral), a drug with fewer side-effects than L-dopa and with a broader spectrum of action, is also used but resulting improvement is often only short lived. Patients unable to tolerate L-dopa may be given bromocriptine (Parlodel) as an alternative, or in association with it. This drug is a dopamine receptor agonist. Apomorphine, administered in bolus form, provides quick relief for unpleasant phenomena, for example dystonia. However, because of the side-effects its use is limited to those patients who are disabled by fluctuations in their symptoms despite other medication. Prior to the advent of drugs related to dopamine metabolism only anticholinergic agents, such as benzhexol (Artane), orphenadrine (Disipal), benztropine (Cogentin) and procyclidine (Kemedrin) were available for the treatment of Parkinson's disease and had their effects primarily upon rigidity.

Surgical treatment was used to control tremor and has re-emerged as a method of delivery for new techniques involving direct cell implants. Restorative treatment using cell implants from the patient's own adrenal medulla shows a time-limited benefit. A definite improvement occurs in the first 6–12 months after surgery, but it declines towards baseline levels at 18 months. Surgery is hazardous but there is evidence that it is more effective in younger, less severe cases. A more promising surgical technique is that of grafting the patient's own genetically modified cells which will produce L-dopa (Gage 1991). Fetal material from the ventral mesencephalon, or adrenal gland, has been grafted to the caudate nucleus with improvement in symptoms in older, more severe cases. Obviously, these techniques must be regarded as experimental at present and their long-term benefits and disadvantages have still to be established.

Over 90% of patients respond to initial treatment either with L-dopa or dopamine agonists. Initial failure is very uncommon and requires scrutiny as to the presence of other causes of symptomatic Parkinson's disease, or other akinetic-rigid syndromes. L-Dopa and dopamine agonists provide good symptom control for 5–10 years. All the drugs mentioned may produce changes in patients' mental states in addition to a range of physical symptoms. In particular, L-dopa therapy produces nausea and other gastrointestinal symptoms, abnormal movements, including choreoathetosis, tics, akathisia and restlessness, dystonias and dyskinesias. Depression is common, affecting 50% of patients after 6 months of treatment with L-dopa. Those with a previous affective illness are especially at risk. Elation of mood in schizophreniform states with delusions and hallucinations in a setting of

clear consciousness also occurs. Psychiatric disturbances are said to be even more frequent with
bromocriptine than with L-dopa, with a greater
likelihood of confusion, hallucinations and delusions.
Treatment of the side-effects of drugs is difficult,
requiring reduction of the antiparkinsonian drugs and
the administration of appropriate psychotropic agents.

Normal pressure hydrocephalus

This syndrome, described by Adams et al (1965), is
characterised by dilatation of the ventricular system
associated with normal CSF pressure on lumbar
puncture. In many cases there is obstruction to
normal circulation of CSF, sometimes by fibrous
adhesions (Editorial 1977) with failure of absorption
by the arachnoid villi. Clinically, there is a slow and
progressive deterioration of memory and intellect:
marked fluctuations of mental state over periods of a
day, or even longer, are characteristic. The patient's
gait becomes increasingly unsteady, broad based and,
eventually, spastic. Urinary incontinence develops in
the later stages of the disorder. The condition is
commoner in older individuals and may occur in
association with subarachnoid haemorrhage, cerebrovascular disease or meningoencephalitis, and may
follow intracranial surgery. In half of the cases
recorded, no underlying disease is found. It may be
difficult on clinical grounds to distinguish this condition from Alzheimer's disease or multi-infarct
dementia, but SPECT studies demonstrate a reduction in cerebral blood flow, particularly in the anterior
brain, in contrast to the pattern seen in Alzheimer's
disease (Graff-Radford 1987). Identification of
normal pressure hydrocephalus is helped by the use of
CT scans, which show symmetrically enlarged
ventricles without significant cortical atrophy. CSF
pressure on lumbar puncture is less than 200 mmHg,
but monitoring over several days reveals episodes of
increased pressure, particularly at night. Presumably
this explains the therapeutic value of ventriculoatrial
shunting, which results in clinical improvement in
30–50% of cases. Results of surgical treatment are
best in patients who show the full clinical syndrome,
who have a short history, and who have an obvious
cause for their condition. Postoperative infection or
malfunction of the shunt, a subdural haematoma, and
epilepsy, may occur in up to one-third of patients.

REFERENCES

Adams R D, Fisher C M, Hakim S, Ojemann R G, Sweet W
H 1965 Symptomatic occult hydrocephalus with "normal"
cerebrospinal fluid pressure. A treatable syndrome. New
England Journal of Medicine 273: 117–126

Airey T 1984 Dementia: implications for services. In:
Wertheimer J, Marois M (eds) Senile dementia: outlook
for the future. Alan R Liss, New York, pp 201–209

APA 1987 Diagnostic and statistical manual of mental
disorders, 3rd edn — revised. American Psychiatric
Association, Washington, DC

Asher R 1949 Myxoedematous madness. British Medical
Journal ii: 555–562

Besson J A O, Crawford J R, Parker D M et al 1990
Multimodal imaging in Alzheimer's disease: the
relationship between MRI, SPECT, cognitive and
pathological changes. British Journal of Psychiatry 157:
216–220

Bolt J M W 1970 Huntington's chorea in the West of
Scotland. British Journal of Psychiatry 116: 259–270

Boston Collaborative Drug Surveillance Program 1972 Acute
adverse reactions to prednisone in relation to dosage.
Clinical Pharmacol Therapeutics 13: 694–698

Breitner J C S, Silverman J M, Mohs R C 1988 Familial
aggregation in Alzheimer's disease; comparison of risk
among relatives of early and late onset cases and among
male and female relatives in successive generations.
Neurology 38: 207–212

Brierly J 1966 The neuropathology of amnesic states. In:
Whitty C W M, Zangwill O (eds) Amnesia. Butterworths,
London, ch 7

Brooks D N, Aughton M E 1979 Psychological consequences
of blunt head injury. International Rehabilitation Medicine
i: 160–165

Brothers C R D 1964 Huntington's chorea in Victoria and
Tasmania. Journal of Neurological Sciences 1: 405–420

Brownell B, Oppenheimer D R 1965 An ataxic form of
subacute pre-senile polioencephalopathy
(Creutzfeld–Jakob disease). Journal of Neurology
Neurosurgery and Psychiatry 28: 350–361

Budka H 1991 Neuropathology of human immunodeficiency
virus infection. Brain Pathology 1: 163–175

Caine E D, Hunt R D, Weingartner H, Ebert M H 1978
Huntington's dementia. Archives of General Psychiatry
35: 377–384.

Celesia G G, Wanamaker W M 1972 Psychiatric
disturbances in Parkinson's disease. Diseases of the
Nervous System 33: 577–583

Chui H C, Teng E L, Henderson V W 1985 Clinical
subtypes of dementia of Alzheimer type. Neurology 35:
1544–1550

Collinge J, Owen F, Poulter M, Leach M, Crow, T J, Rossor
M N, Hardie J, Mullen M J, Janota I, Lantos P L 1990
Prion dementia without characteristic pathology. Lancet
336: 7–9

Comston A 1986 Genetic factors in the aetiology of multiple
sclerosis. In: McDonald W I, Silberberg D H (eds)
Multiple sclerosis. Butterworth, London, pp 56–70

Creutzfeld H G 1920 Uber eine eigenartige Erkrankung des
Zentral-nerven Systems. Zeitschrift für die Gesamte
Neurologie und Psychiatrie 57: 1–18

Critchley M 1953 The parietal lobes. Edward Arnold,
London

Critchley M 1979 The divine banquet of the brain. Raven Press, New York, pp 72–74

Croft P R, Heathfield K W G, Swash M 1973 Differential diagnosis of transient amnesia. British Medical Journal 4: 593–596

Davies P, Maloney A J R 1976 Destruction of central cholinergic neurons in Alzheimer's disease. Lancet ii: 1403

Dewhurst K 1969 The neurosyphilitic psychoses of today. A survey of 91 cases. British Journal of Psychiatry 115: 31–38

Dewhurst K, Oliver J E, McKnight A L 1970 Sociopsychiatric consequences of Huntington's disease. British Journal of Psychiatry 116: 255–258

Di Figlia M, 1990 Excitotoxic injury to the neostriatum; a model for Huntington's disease. Trends in Neuroscience Research 13(7): 286–289

Dimsdale H, Logue V, Piercy M 1964 A case of persisting impairment of recent memory following right temporal lobectomy. Neuropsychologia 1: 287–298

Editorial 1977 Communicating hydrocephalus. Lancet (12 Nov): 1011–1012

Everall I P 1990 Editorial: The role of nerve growth factor in Alzheimer's disease. Psychological Medicine 20: 249–251

Fenton G W 1986 Electrophysiology of Alzheimer's disease. British Medical Bulletin 42: 29–33

Field J H L 1976 Epidemiology of head injuries in England and Wales. HMSO, London

Fisher C, Adams R D 1965 Transient global amnesia. Acta Neurologica Scandinavica 40(suppl 9)

Fortuny L A I, Briggs M, Newcombe F, Ratcliffe G, Thomas C 1980 Measuring the duration of post-traumatic amnesia. Journal of Neurology Neurosurgery and Psychiatry 43: 377–379

Freeman W, Watts J W 1942 Psychosurgery. Charles C Thomas, Springfield, IL

Gage F H, Kawaja M D, Fisher L J 1991 Genetically modified cells: applications for intracerebral grafting. Trends in Neuroscience Research 14(8): 328–333

Galbraith S, Murray W R, Patel A R 1976 The relationship between alcohol and head injury and its effect on conscious level. British Journal of Surgery 63: 138–140

Gibb W R G 1989 Dementia in Parkinson's disease. British Journal of Psychiatry 154: 596–614

Gloning I, Gloning K, Hoff H 1968 Neuropsychological symptoms and occipital lesions. Collection Neuropsychologia Monograph. Gautnier-Villars, Paris

Gordon B, Selnes O A, Hart J, Hanley O F, Whitley R J 1990 Long-term sequelae of acyclovir treatments in herpes simplex encephalitis. Archives of Neurology 47(6): 646–647

Gordon E B, Sim M 1967 The EEG in presenile dementia. Journal of Neurology Neurosurgery and Psychiatry 30: 285–291

Goulding P J, Northen B, Snowden J S 1989 Progressive aphasia with right sided extrapyramidal signs: another manifestation of localised cerebral atrophy. Journal of Neurology, Neurosurgery and Psychiatry 52: 128–130

Graff-Radford N R, Rezai K, Godersky J C, Eslinger P, Damasio H, Kirchner P T 1987 Regional cerebral blood flow in normal pressure hydrocephalus. Journal of Neurology, Neurosurgery and Psychiatry 50: 1589–1596

Gusella J F, Wexler N S, Conneally P M 1983 A polymorphic DNA marker genetically linked to Huntington's disease. Nature 306: 244–248

Gustafson L 1987 Frontal lobe dementia of the non-Alzheimer type. Clinical picture and differential diagnosis. Archives Gerontology Geriatrica 6: 209–223

Haase G R 1977 Diseases presenting as dementia. In: Wells C E (ed) Dementia, 2nd edn. Contemporary neurology, Series 15. F A Davis, Philadelphia, pp 27–67

Hachinski V C, Lassen N A, Marshall J 1974 Multi-infarct dementia: a cause of mental deterioration in the elderly. Lancet ii: 207–210

Harlow J M 1868 Recovery from the passage of an iron rod through the head. Massachusetts Medical Society Publication 2: 338–340

Harper P S, Sarfazi M 1985 Genetic prediction and family structure in Huntington's chorea. British Medical Journal 290: 1929–1931

Heidenhain A 1882 Klinische und anatonische Untersuchungen uber eine eigenartige Erkrankung des Zentral-nerven Systems in Praesenium. Zeitschrift für die Gesamte Neurologie und Psychiatrie 118: 49–114

Heston L L, Mastri A R, Anderson V E, White J 1981 Dementia of the Alzheimer type: clinical genetics. Natural history and associated conditions. Archives of General Psychiatry 38: 1085–1090

Holbourn A H S 1943 Mechanics of head injury. Lancet ii: 438–441

Jakob A 1921 Uber eigenartige Erkrankungen des Zentral nerve systems mit bernerkensverten anatomisches Befunde mit disseminierten degenerationsherdes. Zeitschrift für die Gesamte Neurologie und Psychiatrie 64: 147–228

Jarvie N F 1954 Frontal lobe wounds causing disinhibition. A study of six cases. Journal of Neurology, Neurosurgery and Psychiatry 17: 14–32

Jellinek E H 1962 Fits, faints, coma and dementia in myoedema. Lancet ii: 1010–1012

Jennett B 1975 Epilepsy after non-missile head injuries, 2nd edn. Heinemann, London

Jennett B, Bond M R 1975 Assessment of outcome after severe brain injury. A practical scale. Lancet i: 480–484

Kennedy P G E 1988 Neurological complications of human immunodeficiency virus infection. Postgraduate Medical Journal 64: 180–187

Kennedy P G E, Adams J H, Graham D J, Clements G B 1988 A clinico-pathological study of herpes simplex encephalitis. Neuropathology and Applied Neurobiology 14: 395–415

Korsakoff S S 1889 Etude medico-psychologique sur une forme de malades de memoire. Revue Philosophique 28: 501–530

Lennox G, Lowe J, Morrell K, Landon M, Mayer R J 1989 Diffuse Lewy body disease using correlative neuropathology anti-ubiquitin immunocytochemistry. Journal of Neurology, Neurosurgery and Psychiatry 52: 1236–1247

Lipowski Z J 1967 Delirium, clouding of consciousness and confusion. Journal of Nervous and Mental Disease 145: 227–255

Lipowski Z J 1984 Organic brain syndromes: new classification concepts and prospects. Canadian Journal of Psychiatry 29: 198–204

Lishman W A 1968 Brain damage in relation to psychiatric disability after head injury. British Journal of Psychiatry 114: 373–416

Lishman W A 1990 Alcohol and the brain. British Journal of Psychiatry 156: 635–644

Logue V, Durward M, Pratt R T C, Piercy M, Nixon W L B 1968 The quality of survival after rupture of an anterior cerebral aneurysm. British Journal of Psychiatry 114: 137–160

Loranger A W, Goodell H, McDowell F H, Lee J E, Sweet R D 1972 Intellectual impairment in Parkinson's disease. Brain 95: 405–412

Luria A R 1973 The working brain. Basic Books, New York

McAlpine I, Hunter R 1969 George the Third and the mad business. Lane, London

McHugh P R, Folstein M F 1975 Psychiatric syndromes of Huntington's chorea. In: Benson D F, Blumer D (eds) Psychiatric aspects of neurologic disease. Grune & Stratton, New York, pp 267–285

McKinlay W W, Brooks D N, Bond M R, Martinage D P, Marshall M M 1981 The short-term outcome of severe blunt head injury as reported by the relatives of the injured persons. Journal of Neurology, Neurosurgery and Psychiatry 44: 527–533

Maj M 1990 Psychiatric aspects of HIV-1 infection and AIDS. Psychological Medicine 20: 546–563

Martin J B, Gusella J F 1986 Huntington's disease: pathogenesis and management. New England Journal of Medicine 315: 1267–1276

Matthews W B 1990 Bovine spongiform encephalopathy. British Medical Journal 300: 412–413

Miller H 1961a Accident neurosis. British Medical Journal i: 919–925

Miller H 1961b Accident neurosis. British Medical Journal ii: 992–998

Mindham R H S 1970 Psychiatric symptoms in parkinsonism. Journal of Neurology, Neurosurgery and Psychiatry 33: 188–191

Najenson T 1978 Recovery of communicative functions after prolonged traumatic coma. Scandinavian Journal of Rehabilitation Medicine 10: 15–23

Neary D, Snowden J S, Northen B, Golding P 1988 Dementia of frontal lobe type. Journal of Neurology, Neurosurgery and Psychiatry 51: 353–361

Oliver J E 1970 Huntington's chorea in Northamptonshire. British Journal of Psychiatry 116: 241–253

O'Neill P M, Wright D J M 1988 Lyme disease. British Journal of Hospital Medicine 40: 284–289

Perry E K, Tomlinson B E, Blessed G, Bergmann K, Gibson P H, Perry R H 1978 Correlation of cholinergic abnormalities with senile plaques and mental test scores in senile dementia. British Medical Journal ii: 1457–1459

Perry R H, Irving D, Blessed G, Fairbairn A, Perry E K 1990 Senile dementia of the Lewy body type. Journal of Neurological Science 95: 119–139

Phelps C 1898 Traumatic injuries of the brain and its membranes. Kimpton, London

Pick A 1892 On the relation of senile atrophy and aphasia. Prager Medizinische Wachenschrift 17: 165–167

Piercy M 1964 The effects of cerebral lesions on intellectual function: a review of current research. British Journal of Psychiatry 110: 310–352

Pratt O E, Jeyasingham M, Shaw G K 1985 Transketolase variant enzymes and brain damage. Alcohol and Alcoholism 20: 223–232

Ricklan M, Weiner H, Diller L 1959 Somatopsychologic studies in Parkinson's disease. Journal of Nervous and Mental Disease 129: 263–272

Robertson E E, Kennedy R I 1988 In: Kendell R E, Zeally A K (eds) Companion to psychiatric studies, 4th edn. Churchill Livingstone, Edinburgh

Robertson E E, Le Roux A, Brown J H 1958 The classical differentiation of Pick's disease. Journal of Mental Science 104: 1000–1024

Robins A H 1976 Depression in patients with parkinsonism. British Journal of Psychiatry 128: 141–145

Rose F C, Symonds C P 1960 Persistent memory defect following encephalitis. Brain 83: 195–212

Roth M 1955 The natural history of mental disorder in old age. Journal of Mental Science 101: 281–301

Roth M 1986 The association of clinical and neurological findings and its bearing on the classification and aetiology of Alzheimer's disease. British Medical Bulletin 42: 42–50

Roth M, Wischik C M, Evans N, Mountjoy C Q 1985 Convergence and cohesion of recent neurobiological findings in relation to Alzheimer's disease and their bearing on its aetiological basis. In: Bergener M, Ermine M, Stahelim H B (eds) Thresholds in ageing. Academic Press, London, pp 117–146

Rowley A, Whitley R J, Lakeman F O, Wolinsky S M 1990 Rapid detection of herpes-simplex-virus DNA in cerebrospinal fluid of patients with herpes simplex encephalitis. Lancet 335: 440–441

Russell W R 1932 Discussion on the diagnosis and treatment of acute head injuries. Proceedings of the Royal Society of Medicine 25: 751–757

Russell W R, Nathan P W 1946 Traumatic amnesia. Brain 69: 280–300

Schulman R 1967 Psychiatric aspects of pernicious anaemia. A prospective controlled investigation. British Medical Journal iii: 267–269

Scoville W B 1954 The limbic lobe in man. Journal of Neurosurgery 11: 64–66

Scoville W B, Milner B 1957 Loss of recent memory after bilateral hippocampal lesions. Journal of Neurosurgery and Psychiatry 20: 11–21

Skegg D C G 1991 Multiple sclerosis, "nature or nurture". British Medical Journal 302: 247–248

Smith A 1966 Intellectual functions in patients with lateralised frontal tumours. Journal of Neurology Neurosurgery and Psychiatry 29: 52–58

St George-Hyslop P, Haines J, Farrer L 1990 Genetic linkage studies suggest that Alzheimer's disease is not a single homogeneous disorder. Nature 347: 194–197

Storey P B 1967 Psychiatric sequelae of subarachnoid haemorrhage. British Medical Journal iii: 261–266

Storey P B 1970 Brain damage and personality changes after subarachnoid haemorrhage. British Journal of Psychiatry 117: 129–142

Strich S J 1956 Diffuse degeneration of the cerebral white matter in severe dementia following head injury. Journal of Neurology Neurosurgery and Psychiatry 19: 163–185

Strich S J 1961 Shearing of nerve fibres as a cause of brain damage due to head injury. A pathological study of twenty cases. Lancet ii: 443–448

Stuss D T, Benson D E 1983 Emotional concomitants of psychosurgery. In: Heilman K M, Satz P (eds) Neuropsychology of human emotion. Guilford Press, New York, pp 111–140

Talamo B R, Rudel R A, Kosik K S 1989 Pathological

changes in olfactory neurons in patients with Alzheimer's disease. Nature 337: 736–739

Tanzi R E, Gusella J F, Watkins P 1987 Amyloid B protein gene, cDNA, mRNA distribution and genetic linkage near the Alzheimer locus. Science 235: 877–880

Teasdale G, Jennett B 1974 Assessment of coma and impaired consciousness. Lancet ii: 81–83

Teasdale G, Jennett B 1981 Management of head injuries. Contemporary neurology series. F A Davies, Philadelphia

Teuber H L, Milner B, Vaughan H G 1968 Persistent anterograde amnesia after stab wound of the basal brain. Neuropsychologia 6: 267–282

Thomsen I V 1984 Late outcome of very severe blunt head trauma. A 10–15 year second follow-up. Journal of Neurology Neurosurgery and Psychiatry 47: 260–268

Tow McD 1955 Personality changes following frontal leucotomy. Oxford University Press, London

Trimble M R 1981 Neuropsychiatry. Wiley, Chichester

Victor M, Adams R D, Collins G H 1971 The Wernicke–Korsakoff syndrome. Blackwell, Oxford

Walker A G 1957 Recent memory impairment in unilateral temporal lesions. Archives of Neurology and Psychiatry 78: 543–552

Walton J N 1953 The Korsakoff syndrome in spontaneous subarachnoid haemorrhage. Journal of Mental Science 99: 521–530

Wernicke C 1881 Lehrbuch Gehirnkrankheiten, vol II, Berlin

WHO 1978 Mental disorders: glossary and guide to their classification in accordance with the ninth revision of the international classification of diseases. World Health Organization, Geneva

Williams M 1979 Brain damage, behaviour and the mind. Wiley, Chichester

16. Epilepsy and psychiatric disorder

G. W. Fenton

INTRODUCTION

Epilepsy is a disorder of brain function characterised by recurring fits. Derived from the Greek, it literally means 'to be seized by forces from without'. It is a symptom of brain malfunction that can be caused by diverse disease processes, the final common pathway of expression being an intermittent, paroxysmal, excessive and disorderly discharge of cerebral neurones. This is due to instability of the cell membranes resulting from excessive depolarisation and repolarisation. Membrane stability and polarisation are maintained by ionic fluxes across the membrane. When this ionic balance is disturbed or when the intrinsic mechanisms for maintaining membrane stability are affected, there is a tendency for a seizure to occur. Individuals may have, by genetic determination or acquired condition, a lower threshold to spontaneous firing of certain neurones.

The disturbance may be restricted to a circumscribed population of neurones in a local area of brain within the cortical or subcortical structures and will therefore appear as transient electrical disturbances. When the disorderly discharges of a critical number of such 'epileptic' neurones synchronise, they are recorded by the scalp electroencephalogram (EEG) as interictal spikes, sharp waves (long duration spikes), slow waves or spike–wave complexes. Alternatively, the epileptogenic process can spread to recruit large populations of healthy nerve cells or even the whole of the cerebral cortex of both hemispheres. When the size of the discharging area is extensive, a clinical seizure occurs. The clinical phenomena manifest during the fit reflect the function of the area of brain affected due to excitation or inhibition of the population of neurones involved in the spread. The physiology of epilepsy is reviewed by Meldrum (1990)

CLASSIFICATION OF EPILEPSY AND EPILEPTIC SEIZURES

There are two classifications of epilepsy which are as follows:

1. *Epileptic seizures*: concerned with classifying each individual seizure as a single event.

2. *The epilepsies*: classifying the syndromes of epilepsy. In each syndrome there are often more than one seizure type and other factors such as aetiology, age of onset and evidence of brain pathology are taken into account, as in the proposed new international classification (ILAE 1989). The following is a simplified and abbreviated version.

Generalised epilepsies

The seizure discharge is generalised from the onset. Sudden unconsciousness without aura, with or without motor phenomena, is the usual mode of seizure onset though myoclonic jerks in clear consciousness may occur. Between attacks the EEG records generalised, bilaterally synchronous spike–wave complexes at 2–4 Hz. To account for the initial seizure generalisation, Penfield & Jasper (1954) introduced the concept of a system of neurones, located in the midline of the upper brain stem and projecting diffusely to all areas of the cerebral cortex which integrated the activities of both hemispheres (the centrencephalic system). Any seizure discharge arising from within the system or entering it from a local area of cortex rapidly generalises with diffuse and synchronous involvement of the cortex of both hemispheres. This centrencephalic model is no longer accepted. Clinical and experimental data indicate that cortical and subcortical structures clearly operate together in nearly all sustained epileptic processes but the evidence is not convincing that the midline thalamic nuclei are the initiators of generalised seizures. Based on findings obtained in feline penicillin-induced generalised epilepsy, Gloor (1978) has presented a new model. He postulates that in generalised epilepsy there is a diffuse and relatively mild state of chronic cortical hyperexcitability which increases the responsiveness of the cortical neurones. This leads to spike and wave discharges developing in the cortex in response to the afferent thalamocortical volleys

343

normally involved in the genesis of spindles and recruiting responses.

The generalised epilepsies are subdivided into the primary and secondary generalised epilepsies. The former are not the result of brain disease, genetic factors being dominant in the aetiology. The latter are due to acquired brain disease, usually of a diffuse or multifocal character. Those that cannot be classified into the primary and secondary classes because of insufficient information or lack of the necessary criteria are known as undetermined generalised epilepsies.

Partial (focal, local) epilepsies

The seizure discharge causing the epileptic attacks originates in a local area of cerebral cortex or related subcortical structures. This local epileptogenic lesion is usually the result of acquired focal brain damage and is manifest by local EEG spike and sharp wave interictal complexes. While the abnormal neuronal discharge that initiates the fits remains localised and involves only one hemisphere, it may elicit a conscious sensation or series of sensations that the patient learns to recognise as a warning or aura. The nature of the aura is determined by the function of the neuronal systems involved. Though the patient interprets the aura sensations as a warning heralding the fit, it is actually an initial seizure manifestation. Motor phenomena can also occur as the first event of the seizure. Partial attacks often spread bilaterally and develop into generalised seizures (secondary generalisation). The generalisation can occur so rapidly that no aura will be experienced. Partial seizures with onset in 'silent' areas of cortex like the frontal lobe have no aura and one in five patients with temporal lobe epilepsy presents with generalised convulsions without any aura.

Unclassifiable epilepsies

These are unclassifiable because of incomplete clinical and EEG data or the atypical nature of the epilepsy.

The international classification of epileptic seizures

Partial seizures

These begin in a local area of brain:

1. *Simple partial seizures.* Consciousness is not impaired, with symptoms appropriate to the function of the discharging area of brain: motor, sensory, autonomic, psychic or any combination of these.

2. *Complex partial seizures.* Consciousness is impaired.
   a. Simple partial features followed by brief clouding of consciousness or more prolonged automatism.
   b. Impaired consciousness at onset:
      (i) Clouding of consciousness only
      (ii) Automatism
3. *Partial seizures, evolving to secondarily generalised seizures (tonic–clonic, tonic or clonic):*
   a. Simple partial seizures evolving to generalised seizures
   b. Complex partial seizures evolving to generalised seizures
   c. Simple partial seizures progressing to complex partial seizures and then generalised seizures.

Generalised seizures (convulsive or non-convulsive)

1. Absence (petit mal) seizures
2. Myoclonic
3. Clonic
4. Tonic
5. Tonic–clonic (grand mal) seizures
6. Atonic.

Unclassified epileptic seizures

These are unclassifiable because of incomplete data.

PREVALENCE OF EPILEPSY

Estimates of the prevalence of all types of epilepsy vary from three to 20 per 1000, whereas figures for active epilepsy (those who have had two or more non-febrile seizures and have either had at least one fit within the previous 2 years or take antiepileptic treatment) are fairly consistent at 3–6 per 1000.

The onset of epilepsy occurs before the age of 5 years in nearly a quarter and before school-leaving age in more than half the cases. Community-based surveys indicate that epilepsy is usually a short-term problem in most patients with only 20% having intractable fits (Duncan & Shorvon 1986). This contrasts with the chronic nature of the disorder in patients attending hospital specialist clinics, only one-third of whom will have prolonged remissions. Therefore, it seems that epilepsy becomes a potentially handicapping condition in a minority of patients, possibly around one-fifth. Many of the latter are faced with a formidable array of potential epilepsy-related and psychosocial handicaps that may impair the individual's psychosocial adjustment (Tables 16.1 and 16.2).

CAUSES AND PRECIPITATING FACTORS

Genetic factors are predominant in the primary generalised epilepsies and also increase the susceptibility to symptomatic epilepsy. Chronic lesions, both diffuse and focal, involving the cerebral cortex, especially those involving the temporal lobe, are more likely to result in epilepsy.

These include heredofamilial diseases (e.g. tuberose sclerosis, the leucodystrophies, the lipoidoses, Lafora's disease and phenylketonuria), metabolic brain disease, brain damage due to antenatal and birth complications, severe infantile convulsions, cerebral infections (meningitis, encephalitis and brain abscess) and head injury, cerebrovascular disorders, cerebral tumours and degenerative diseases of the brain.

Around three-quarters of patients with epilepsy have no evidence of an underlying pathological lesion. The most complete data available are the thorough studies in Rochester, Minnesota, from 1935 to 1967 (Hauser

Table 16.2 Psychosocial handicaps

Type	Consequences
Family attitudes	
Parental overprotectiveness	Undue dependence on family Reduced peer group interaction Limited development of social skills Problems on becoming independent as a teenager Lifelong passive dependent attitudes
Altered perceptions of person's potential	Too low/too high, leading to problems at school and at work
Attitudes beyond the family	
Negative attitudes and expectations Peers Teachers Employers General public	Problems finding friends and appropriate educational, leisure and work opportunities, low self-esteem, depression/self-pity, paranoid, attitudes, stigma
Within the person	
	Low self-esteem Learned helplessness External locus of control Dependent attitudes Limited social skills Limited social orbit Depression/pessimism Paranoid attitudes

& Kurland 1975): 23% of their sample of 516 patients had epilepsy of known cause (2% birth injury, 4% congenital abnormalities, 4% postnatal head injuries, 3% infections, 5% vascular lesions, 4% cerebral tumours and 0.6% degenerative disorders).

The neuropathology of specimens taken from patients undergoing anterior temporal lobectomy for intractable temporal lobe epilepsy is of special interest to psychiatrists. About 50% show mesial temporal sclerosis, with loss of nerve cells in the amygdala and hippocampal areas accompanied by fibrosis, gliosis and atrophy, possibly due to hypoxia caused by severe infantile convulsions. Another 20% have small, circumscribed foci of abnormal tissue (hamartomas), probably of congenital origin. Of this group, ganglioglial lesions with an early age of first fit are strongly associated with the development of schizophrenia-like psychoses (Roberts et al 1990).

A number of precipitating factors may provoke a fit in susceptible people or exacerbate established epilepsy, for example sleep deprivation, hyperventilation, hypoglycaemia, antidepressant and neuroleptic drugs, alcohol and drug withdrawal, high fever, anoxia and

Table 16.1 Epilepsy related handicaps

Type	Consequence
Seizure occurrence	
Frequent fits	Trauma — body/brain Restriction of activities Anxiety and loss of internal locus of control with 'learned helplessness' Discrimination/ stigma by peers and general public
Cerebral dysfunction	
Diffuse brain damage	Low IQ Impaired impulse control
Focal temporal lobe damage	More severe epilepsy Specific learning deficits Reduced impulse control ?Enhanced sensory–limbic connections with altered interpretation of environmental stimuli
Frequent epileptic discharges Clinical	Restricted social, educational and work opportunities
Subclinical	Impaired information processing
Medication	Cognition impaired Dysphoria Reduced impulse control Low folate, calcium and sex hormone levels

the specific stimuli of reflex epilepsy. The reflex epilepsies occur in 1–6% of people with epilepsy. The most common modality is the visual one, though almost every sensory modality has been incriminated. Various types of mental and motor activity may also reflexly trigger fits. An excellent general introduction to the epilepsies is the textbook edited by Laidlaw et al (1988).

PSYCHIATRIC DISORDERS OF EPILEPSY: CLASSIFICATION AND CLINICAL FEATURES

Before classifying the psychiatric disorders of epilepsy it is necessary to exclude from consideration isolated fits that are a complication of mental illness or its treatment. In the past, single grand mal attacks were not an uncommon feature of acute catatonic schizophrenia. Generalised convulsions sometimes develop during drug and alcohol withdrawal (including benzodiazepine withdrawal) and single major seizures can occur as a consequence of neuroleptic or antidepressant medication due to the epileptogenic effects of these drugs (Chadwick 1981, Edwards 1985). Such patients should not be given the diagnostic label of epilepsy, since epilepsy is by definition a chronic brain disorder characterised by recurrent seizures which occur intermittently over an extended time period.

The psychiatric disorders of epilepsy can be divided into three main groups, the classification being introduced by Pond (1957) and elaborated by Fenton (1981; see Table 16.3). The main groups are as follows.

1. Disorders due to the brain disease causing the fits

a. *Mental handicap,* where the seizures and intellectual impairment are both a reflection of underlying cerebral pathology; between one-fifth and one-half of mentally retarded patients have epilepsy, the prevalence of fits increasing with the severity of mental handicap (Corbett 1981).

b. *The specific epileptic syndromes* of which seizures are a constant feature but are only one of a number of symptoms and signs of an organic brain syndrome, e.g. West's syndrome, Unverricht–Lundberg disease, subacute sclerosing panencephalitis (SSLE), the Lennox–Gastaut syndrome. These disorders are associated with global intellectual impairment, which in many cases is progressive.

c. *Organic brain syndromes,* in which fits may occur but are not a constant feature of the disease, e.g. Alzheimer's disease (major attacks are common in the terminal phase) and multi-infarct dementia (fits occur in 20% of patients).

Table 16.3 Psychiatric disorders of epilepsy: classification (Fenton 1981)

1. Disorders due to the brain disease causing the fits
2. Disorders time-locked to the occurrence of seizures:
   Preictal: (Prodromal)
   Ictal: Complex partial seizures
                  Absence status
                  Complex partial status
   Postictal: Automatism
                  Confusional/clouded states
3. Disorders unrelated in time to the seizure occurrence:
   Interictal
   Disorders of childhood and adolescence
   a.   Neurotic, antisocial and mixed
   b.   Childhood psychoses
   Disorders of adult life
   a.   Personality disorder
   b.   Personality change (from a 'normal' previous personality)
   c.   Neuroses
   d.   Behaviour disorder
   e.   Sexual dysfunction
   f.   Psychoses:
          Affective/schizoaffective
          Chronic schizophrenia-like
   g.   Dementia

d. *Focal brain disease,* especially that involving the frontal or temporal lobes. Dysfunction involving these local areas of cerebral cortex can cause organic brain syndromes with disorders of behaviour, personality and/or cognitive function; this is described in detail by Lishman (1987).

e. *Psychotic syndromes* of unknown or uncertain aetiology in which recurrent fits are not an uncommon finding and appear to be a manifestation of the underlying brain dysfunction causing the psychosis. These syndromes begin before puberty and fall into the ICD-9 category 'psychoses with origin specific to childhood', which, includes infantile autism, disintegrative psychosis and atypical childhood psychosis. Such psychotic syndromes are rare in children with epilepsy, apart from infantile autism in which fits occur in 29% of patients.

2. Disorders related in time to seizure occurrence

a. *Preictal.* Prodromal irritability and dysphoria for hours or days preceding the occurrence of a fit. This type of behaviour or mood change usually improves following seizures. Little is known about prevalence or pathogenesis.

b. *Ictal* (directly due to the seizure discharge). Paroxysmal disturbances of higher cerebral function during clinical seizures include the following:

(i) *Partial seizures with psychic manifestations.* Psychological symptoms such as illusions, hallucinations, alternations in affect or cognition as initial seizure phenomena, or automatic behaviour are the predominant features of the clinical fit. Such psychic phenomena are a common feature of partial seizures of temporal lobe or limbic system origin. Several types can be identified in terms of the origin and spread of electrical discharges, such as hippocampal or mesiobasal limbic, amygdalar, lateral posterior temporal and opercular. These anatomically defined seizure types tend to be associated with different groups of predominant symptoms. They may occasionally be generated from foci outside the limbic areas (posterior frontal or parietal) as a consequence of spread of the epileptic discharge from the latter primary areas of onset to involve the limbic structures. Psychic seizure phenomena include perceptive illusions (distorted perceptions of external stimuli), non-perceptive or agnosic illusions (an external object or internal event perceived normally but poorly understood), hallucinations of varying complexity, ictal affect, especially fear and cognitive symptomatology. The latter may be either ideational (forced thinking, dysphasia) or dysmnesic with disturbances of subjective memory (illusions of memory, e.g. *déjà vu* or *jamais vu* sensations; ecmnesic hallucinations in which previous experiences are recalled by the subject and 'relived' with great intensity — panoramic memories). These dysmnesic symptoms can be regarded as non-perceptive or agnosic illusions.

Many similar phenomena occur in functional psychiatric illness. Those of ictal origin are distinguished by a sudden onset, transient duration lasting minutes rather than hours or days, and relatively rapid resolution. They occur in brief attacks that are recurrent and stereotyped in quality, often associated with some degree of alteration of consciousness. In contrast, consciousness is clear in functional psychiatric syndromes.

Automatic behaviour due to partial seizure discharge is most commonly the result of temporal lobe epilepsy, due to an abnormal electrical discharge commencing in the periamygdaloid region. The degree of spread of this electrical disturbance determines whether or not the seizure discharge leads to automatic behaviour. For automatism to develop there must be spread to the midline upper brain stem structures and the contralateral areas of the opposite hemisphere with invariable clouding of consciousness (Jasper 1964, Fenton 1972). Lesions involving the frontal or parietal areas or the mesial surfaces of either hemisphere can occasionally cause ictal automatism due to spread of the discharge to involve the periamygdaloid structures of

both temporal lobes. A less common form of epileptic automatism is that due to prolonged generalised spike wave activity (absence or petit mal automatisms).

As well as being a manifestation of seizure discharge (ictal automatism), automatic behaviour can occur during the clouding of consciousness that commonly follows one or more generalised convulsions (postictal automatism): automatism is especially likely if the clouding persists for a period of minutes. In this situation, the clouded state is due to residual inhibition of cortical function due to neuronal fatigue following the period of intense neural activation by the seizure discharge. This impairment of cortical function is reflected in the appearance of diffuse EEG slow waves. If the clouding of consciousness lasts for hours, days or weeks, the condition is known as a postepileptic confusional state with symptoms identical to those of any organic confusional state.

Behaviour during epileptic automatism varies greatly from patient to patient and in the same individual on different occasions. Impairment of awareness and lack of responsiveness are usual. The complexity of behaviour manifest depends on the duration of EEG seizure discharge. Brief attacks (seizure discharge 10 seconds or less) merely cause cessation of on-going activity. Longer episodes (a discharge of 20–30 seconds) produce stereotyped repetitive movements, for example chewing, swallowing or clenching of fists. When the attack lasts several minutes or longer, there is more complex, variable and pseudopurposeful behaviour, e.g. undressing or wandering away. This involves an interplay with the environment and gradually merges into normal behaviour. The earlier stereotyped phenomena are a direct manifestation of the seizure discharge. In contrast, the later complex behaviour continues after the electrical discharge has ceased and is a manifestation of clouding of consciousness owing to temporary inhibition of neuronal function following the intense ictal activation.

The majority of automatisms are brief, lasting 5 minutes or less on 80% of occasions, and never last longer than 1 hour. The inevitable clouding of consciousness that is part of the epileptic automatism means that well-structured goal-directed behaviour is impossible to initiate and sustain. Hence, serious violence during epileptic automatism is rare. These clinical observations have been confirmed by detailed videotape EEG studies (Fenton 1986).

(ii) *Minor status epilepticus.* Absence (petit mal) status epilepticus due to continuous generalised spike–wave discharge is accompanied by clouding of consciousness and often slight clonic movements of the eyelids and hands and automatic movements of the face and hands. Impaired consciousness ranges from a mild subjective cognitive deficit to stupor from which the patient can be aroused only with difficulty and is characteristically variable over time. Attacks may last for hours or even days. Though most common in children, absence status may occur in adults and may even present for the first time in middle age.

Complex partial status epilepticus is continuous temporal lobe epileptogenic discharge leading to a state of clouding of consciousness, prolonged affective disturbance (anxiety or fear), hallucinosis or frequently occurring automatism, the latter occurring without recovery of consciousness between episodes of automatic behaviour. In contrast to absence status, which is not uncommon in generalised epilepsy, complex partial status is a rare event. The reasons for this are unclear but probably result from differences in the mechanisms of generalisation and maintenance of ictal processes in absence as opposed to complex partial seizures. The duration of complex partial status is similar to that of absence status, i.e. hours or days. The EEG during complex partial status may show continuous slow wave activity or temporal spike and slow wave complexes superimposed on a slow background.

c. *Postictal disorders (immediately on cessation of seizure discharge).* These are disorders which immediately follow one or more seizures, usually generalised convulsions. The common feature is clouding of consciousness due to postseizure depression of cortical function. Hence, the EEG is usually dominated by diffuse slow frequencies within the theta and delta range, no normal activity being present. If the disorder is brief (minutes only) automatic behaviour is manifest. When prolonged for hours or days the clinical picture is that of an acute confusional state. Complete recovery is the rule.

3. Interictal disorders unrelated in time to the seizures

Interictal symptoms are present between attacks and often in the absence of seizures. It is assumed that the epilepsy and/or the cerebral epileptogenic lesion have played a role in the genesis of the psychiatric disorder. Though the illness is unrelated in time to seizure occurrence the onset, intensity and course may be influenced by the fit frequency. This is commonly by an exacerbation of fits, less often and more controversially by a reduction in fit frequency so that there is an inverse relation between fits and mental state (Flor-Henry 1976).

The interictal disorders invariably occur in a setting of clear consciousness. The range and type of mental state phenomena and behaviour disturbance do not differ significantly from those found in psychiatric patients without epilepsy. In children they consist of neurotic, antisocial, mixed neurotic and antisocial disorder and, on very rare occasions, psychosis. Personality disorder (present from early life), organic personality change (as a consequence of the epilepsy, its treatment and/or the underlying brain lesion), neurotic and psychotic syndromes can occur as interictal manifestations in adults. Sexual dysfunction is not uncommon. Dementia is found in a small number of patients who require long-term hospital care because of severe epilepsy. Severe and frequent seizures, chronic anticonvulsant overdosage and recurrent head injury due to fits are thought to be contributory factors.

INTERICTAL BEHAVIOUR AND EPILEPSY: GENERAL COMMENTS

Both children and adults have a greater than expected prevalence of psychiatric disorder not directly related to seizure occurrence. In children this increased morbidity cannot simply be a reaction to the stress of coping with a chronic illness. Rutter et al (1970) in a community survey of schoolchildren with epilepsy found that epileptic children were five times more likely to have psychiatric disorder than children with chronic handicaps not affecting the brain. Children with epilepsy complicated by lesions above the brain stem had the maximum prevalence (more than eight times that of controls). The links between the epilepsy and behaviour were complex, organic brain dysfunction, temporal lobe disorder and adverse familial influences being important aetiological factors. A more recent hospital study by Hoare (1984) comparing epileptic and diabetic children has confirmed these earlier findings.

When disturbed children with epilepsy are selected by EEG criteria the site of origin of the epileptogenic process influences the symptom profile, children with temporal lobe spikes having high aggression and low neuroticism ratings and those with generalised spike–wave complexes showing the opposite trend (Nuffield 1961). Stores (1978) has reported that children selected because of left temporal lobe epileptogenic dysfunction are specially vulnerable to a range of behavioural difficulties, as are boys and children of both sexes on phenytoin.

The relation between epilepsy, EEG epileptogenic activity and behaviour in the adult is less clear. Certainly the presence of focal pathology, the extent of brain damage and the frequency of occurrence of the EEG epileptiform activity are important influences (Edeh and Toone 1987). Psychosocial predictors of psychopathology include increased perceived stigma, more adverse life events during the previous year, poor adjustment to epilepsy, vocational problems, external locus of control and an earlier onset of epilepsy (Hermann et al 1990). General practice surveys report that between one-third and almost a half of patients with active epilepsy suffer from minor psychiatric morbidity (Pond & Bidwell 1960, Edeh 1984). Further, a gender difference has been noted, males being more prone to anxiety, depressive and obsessional symptoms (Fenton 1986). However, the prevalence of such morbidity is not significantly higher than in adult patients with chronic diseases not affecting the nervous system (Hermann & Whitman 1984). The aetiological links involve biological, psychological and social factors, and cannot be accounted for by temporal lobe dysfunction alone.

The clinical features the patient develops are strongly influenced by age. Children and adolescents present with behaviour difficulties. In contrast, adults tend to develop mild affective symptoms, especially those with late-onset epilepsy. In unselected series psychosis is rare (Currie et al 1971) but suicide is five times more common amongst people with epilepsy than in the general population (Barraclough 1981). Personality disorder, unless a direct result of a focal brain lesion, is usually a reflection of lifelong disturbance with early onset of fits and a history of maladjustment with behaviour and/or neurotic problems in childhood.

At the turn of the century the concept of a specific epileptic personality of constitutional origin evolved as the result of observations made on long-stay patients. This view is no longer accepted. The characteristic 'epileptic' personality traits (e.g. slowness and circumstantiality in speech and thought, religiosity, unstable mood, irritability and impulsivity) do occur but are rare in pure culture (about 4%) and result from multiple acquired handicaps, biological, psychological and social.

More recently, a temporal lobe behavioural syndrome has been described (Geschwind 1979). Its characteristics are: an excessive tendency to adhere to each thought, feeling or action (viscosity); irritability and deepened emotionality (hyperemotionality); decreased sexual interest and arousal (hyposexuality). This is thought to be due to limbic system kindling with enhanced affective labelling of previously neutral stimuli, events or concepts due to induction of new synaptic connections between the primary sensory cortex and the mesial limbic structures. Subsequent attempts to identify this syndrome have not been particularly successful (Hermann & Whitman 1984), though a recent careful study reports trends in the predicted direction (Sorensen et al 1989).

The depressant effects of anticonvulsant drugs on cognitive function and emotional control also aggravate behaviour difficulties or mood disorder in both children and adults. Indeed, phenobarbitone may have a paradoxical exciting effect on children with a consequent increase in irritability and hyperkinetic behaviour.

EPILEPSY AND SEXUAL DYSFUNCTION

Complaints of reduced libido and impotence are common in male patients with epilepsy. As with other associations between epilepsy and behaviour, the relationships are complex. In many cases the poor sexual skills are a reflection of poor social skills in immature, dependent persons, who have led sheltered and restricted lives with little opportunity to relate to the opposite sex because of frequent fits, parental overprotection and/or too much medication.

Induction of liver enzymes by anticonvulsants leads to rapid metabolism of testosterone and low free testosterone levels in serum. The latter correlate with measures of low sex drive in epileptic patients.

An association between sexual deviation (fetishism and transvestism) and temporal lobe epilepsy has been reported. It is tempting to speculate on a relationship between the sexual abnormalities and limbic system dysfunction but it is difficult to draw firm conclusions from such a small and highly selected group of patients. In any event, temporal lobe dysfunction is rare among sexual deviants. The subject of sexual problems in epilepsy is reviewed by Toone (1986).

EPILEPSY AND VIOLENCE

In recent decades, interictal aggressive behaviour has come to be regarded as a specific manifestation of temporal lobe epilepsy. Though the prevalence of epilepsy amongst imprisoned male offenders is three times higher than in the general population, violent offences are no more common amongst epileptics than other offenders. Neither can any association between temporal lobe epilepsy and violence be found in an offender population (Gunn & Fenton 1969, Gunn 1977).

Gunn & Fenton (1969) have presented the following hypothesis to explain the higher prevalence of epilepsy in offenders: (1) in some, the brain damage causes fits and uninhibited antisocial behaviour; (2) some epileptics with psychosocial problems feel stigmatised by their fits and hit back at society by behaving in an antisocial manner; (3) a deprived early environment may provide the milieu both for acquiring brain damage and for learning an aggressive behavioural repertoire; (4) finally, brain damage and the resulting epilepsy can be the consequence of the person's basically disorganised and impetuous lifestyle that accompanies the criminality.

A critical review by Trieman & Delgado-Escueta (1983) reports that when unselected populations of patients with epilepsy are studied there is no increased incidence of violent behaviour. They comment that most studies linking temporal lobe epilepsy and violence have been heavily loaded with intractable forms of epilepsy complicated by an early onset of fits, organic brain disease, low IQ and personality and behaviour disorder. When such problem patients are excluded, there is no increased incidence of violence. Of course, such a total population approach excludes this small subset of patients whose habitual aggressive behaviour is such a problem. In such individuals one or more of a number of factors are likely to interact and predispose to violent behaviour. These include poor parenting, inappropriate social learning, resentment against the social isolation and stigma of being labelled 'epileptic', impaired cognition and poor impulse control due to organic brain disease and/or heavy anticonvulsant medication. In such patients, the possible influence upon the person's feeling state of transient, abnormal paroxysmal discharges from the amygdala should not be overlooked, in view of the implanted electrode studies of Heath (1986) and Weiser (1986).

CAUSATION OF INTERICTAL BEHAVIOUR AND PERSONALITY DISORDER IN EPILEPSY

The only aetiological model that can be plausibly applied to the interictal psychiatric disorders of epilepsy is a multifactorial one. In any one individual the disturbance of mental state or behaviour is the final manifestation of an interaction of factors. Some are merely predisposing in nature, increasing the individual's vulnerability to breakdown. Others may play an important role in precipitating or provoking breakdown of the vulnerable individual. The vulnerability and precipitating factors can be biological, psychological or social. Usually it is a complex interaction of all three, the relative importance of any one group of factors varying from one individual to another.

Vulnerability factors include the following: genetic loading for psychiatric disorder; an early onset of epilepsy with frequent fits in the first 15 years of life that may adversely influence parental and peer group attitudes and educational performance and the acquisition of social skills and personality maturation; diffuse cortical damage impairing IQ and impulse control; temporal lobe dysfunction (left sided and/or bilateral)

with its more intractable seizure pattern and potential to alter sensory–limbic connections and disrupt learning and memory processes; family psychopathology; the depressant effect of heavy anticonvulsant medication on cognitive function and folate metabolism and its disinhibiting effect on behaviour; and being male. Any combination of these factors may interact to make the individual vulnerable to breakdown.

Precipitating or provoking factors act on the vulnerable person and cause decompensation of his or her precarious psychosocial adjustment. This is manifest by psychiatric symptoms or behaviour disorder.

Provoking factors include crises in the person's life situation, adverse life events and social difficulties, emotional tension due to relationship problems or a role change, a marked change in seizure frequency, low folate levels and/or drug intoxication, and drug-induced folate deficiency.

As discussed previously, the resulting symptoms and signs will be determined by the age of the patient, conduct disorder in the child or adolescent and anxiety or depressive symptoms in the adult with late onset epilepsy. The adult with personality disorder may present a more complex picture with difficult behaviour or paranoid symptoms. Frequently, however, such floridly disturbed behaviour represents the immature person's process of coping with an underlying mood change of depression or anxiety.

INTERICTAL PSYCHOSES

In contrast to the ictal-related psychoses, the interictal psychoses occur in a setting of clear consciousness. In symptomatology they resemble affective, schizoaffective or schizophrenia-like psychoses and are thought to have a special relationship to temporal lobe dysfunction (Flor-Henry 1976). Such interictal psychotic states in clear consciousness take the following forms:

1. Short-lived psychotic episodes

These may last weeks or months with recovery as the usual outcome:

a. *Very transient schizophrenia-like psychoses* lasting a few days only and preceded by an exacerbation of seizures. Such brief psychoses remit quickly and are presumably due to subclinical electrical disturbance of limbic system function.

b. *Affective or schizoaffective states* lasting weeks or months. Complete remission is usual but, like classical bipolar or unipolar affective states, relapses and further episodes are not uncommon. Occasionally, pure paranoid symptomatology is predominant (Betts

1981, Pahla 1985). In contrast to the clouded states, the onset of these psychoses is rarely heralded by clinical seizures but is occasionally terminated by a generalised convulsion (Dongier 1959). Indeed, there may be a reduction in fit frequency immediately before the onset of the psychosis. In a series of 72 mental hospital epileptic admissions, a significant association between a 50% reduction in pre-admission seizure frequency and depressive illness was found. In contrast, a pre-admission exacerbation in fits was common in those admitted with either acute behaviour disturbance or clouded states (Betts 1981). Reports of a relationship between affective psychoses and non-dominant temporal lobe dysfunction (Flor-Henry 1976) have not been consistently replicated (Toone 1981, Robertson 1986). Their frequency of occurrence amongst epileptic admissions to psychiatric hospitals varies between one in five and one in three (Betts 1981, Pahla 1985).

2. Chronic schizophrenia-like psychoses

The mutual antagonism theory (i.e. that epilepsy protected against schizophrenia) led to the introduction of convulsive therapy to psychiatric practice in the 1930s, but more recently it has become apparent that a chronic schizophrenia-like psychosis occurs *more* often than can be accounted for by chance in patients with epilepsy. Slater et al (1963) published the first detailed study of the schizophrenia-like psychoses of epilepsy. They also provided some epidemiological evidence to suggest that the occurrence of the two conditions was not a coincidental finding. Two-thirds had temporal lobe dysfunction, the psychosis developing on average 14 years after the onset of the fits. The most characteristic clinical presentation was a paranoid schizophrenia-like state. Though the symptomatology was generally similar to that of non-epileptic schizophrenia, a number of differences were noted. Paranoid delusions and mystical delusional experiences were especially frequent, the patients feeling in communication with God or endowed with supernatural powers, or experiencing passivity phenomena with a mystical content. Visual hallucinations, often with a mystical content, were more common than in typical schizophrenia, and often experienced during dream-like states in the absence of confusion. The patients' affects were also warmer and better retained than is usual in schizophrenia. The progress of the disorder was more benign as well, with less personality and social deterioration. Finally, the patients showed no genetic loading for schizophrenia nor any excess of schizoid personality traits. This contrasts with non-epileptic schizophrenic patients where a family history is common and schizoid traits frequent.

Slater and his colleagues regarded this disorder as a symptomatic schizophrenia due to the temporal lobe dysfunction, a view generally accepted since. Though such psychoses have a high profile in the literature, they are rare in general psychiatric practice — 2% of a large temporal lobe epilepsy series (Currie et al 1971). Using a structured mental state assessment technique, Toone et al (1982) have partially confirmed Slater's findings. Delusions of persecution and of reference were more common in the schizophrenia-like psychoses of epilepsy and catatonic symptoms were less common than in a control group of non-epileptic patients with schizophrenia. Abnormal premorbid personalities were less often found in the epileptic psychotic patients. Another interesting observation was that there was an excess of females in the latter group. Toone (1981) and others have also reported an excess of left-handedness amongst psychotic epileptics.

The influence of the site and extent of the epileptic focus

The site and extent of the epileptogenic lesion in the brain and its role in the causation of such chronic schizophrenia-like psychoses is still the subject of much dispute. Both bilateral damage to the mesial temporal limbic structures and dysfunction of the dominant temporal lobe have been reported as predisposing to psychosis (Toone 1981). Flor-Henry (1969) was the first to report a link with left-sided foci. Toone (1991) has recently reviewed the literature on lateralization of epileptogenic focus and psychosis. In 265 patients with a schizophrenia-like psychosis, 129 (49%) had a left-sided focus, 58 (22%) a right-sided focus and 78 (29%) bilateral involvement. However, the data base from which these figures are calculated is seriously flawed, because of selection biases with heterogenous groups of patients from a wide range of treatment facilities and lack of uniform criteria for clinical diagnosis and EEG lateralisation.

A significant advance is the recent finding that only the small number of patients with a Catego diagnosis of nuclear schizophrenia (i.e. with Schneider's first-rank symptoms) have a significant excess of left temporal lobe epileptogenic lesions. Other psychotic syndromes (non-nuclear schizophrenia, etc.) associated with both temporal lobe and generalised epilepsy had a more diffuse organic process associated with an earlier age of onset of fits, longer duration between epilepsy onset and development of psychosis and a higher prevalence of cognitive deficit (Perez et al 1985). Given that more than half of the Schneiderian symptoms involve abnormal auditory perceptual or verbal processes, the assumption that they reflect an underlying disturbance of dominant temporal lobe function is plausible.

Change in fit frequency and the interictal psychoses

Change in seizure frequency, either a reduction or an exacerbation, has been demonstrated to herald the onset of psychosis, both with generalised convulsions and complex partial seizures (Flor-Henry 1976, Betts 1981, Toone 1981). These apparently conflicting observations can be reconciled if the following hypothesis is correct. An exacerbation in seizure occurrence may cause limbic system and/or global cortical dysfunction due to neuronal inhibition following the intense ictal activation. Such disturbances in brain function precipitate the psychosis, the extent of the neuronal disturbance within the brain determining the form of the psychotic state. Widespread involvement of the neocortex will cause a variable degree of clouding of consciousness confusion and disturbed behaviour (an acute organic reaction). Localisation to the deep mesial temporal–limbic structures will precipitate a psychosis in clear consciousness with schizophrenic, paranoid or depressive features. In contrast, the phenomenon of a reduced fit frequency leading to psychosis may reflect underlying neurotransmitter changes that cause both the seizure reduction and the abnormal mental state. Trimble (1977) has presented a dopamine hypothesis that accounts for these observations: increased dopaminergic activity being antiepileptic and schizophrenogenic, while diminution of such activity increases fits but ameliorates the psychosis. Other neurotransmitter systems may be involved in this process (Fenwick et al 1983).

'Forced normalisation', a concept introduced by Landolt (1958) and recently reviewed by Wolf (1991), refers to the electroclinical syndrome of an inverse relationship between fit frequency and mental state in recurrent epileptic psychoses; the psychosis being associated with fewer fits and EEG normalisation, and a normal mental state with more fits and EEG 'deterioration'. This syndrome is rare but its validity has been confirmed by intensive EEG video monitoring.

The causation of interictal psychoses: some comments

Although global cerebral dysfunction following major fits or due to absence status is almost invariably followed by clouding of consciousness, interictal psychosis in clear consciousness is a relatively rare association of temporal lobe epilepsy. Therefore a direct link between temporal lobe dysfunction and interictal psychosis is unlikely.

A more plausible hypothesis to account for the relatively small number of cases is that either an epileptogenic dysfunction localised to the dominant temporal lobe or extensive bilateral damage to the deep limbic system structures makes people more vulnerable to psychotic breakdown. In such a vulnerable individual, a florid psychosis will only develop when the patient is exposed to added pathogenic factors (biological, psychosocial). These may be either predisposing or precipitating and interact with the temporal lobe dysfunction to disrupt the person's capacity to deal with the environment. Hence the cerebral disorder caused by the epilepsy merely acts as one of a number of possible vulnerability or provoking factors in causing the psychosis.

CLINICAL INVESTIGATION

The investigation of a patient with seizures and psychiatric disorder requires a multidisciplinary approach. The neurological, psychological, psychiatric and social aspects of the problem must be considered separately during the initial assessment. However, the final diagnostic formulation will take account of the interaction between these various influences, all of which may contribute to the genesis of the person's problems. Of course, the relative importance of each of these groups of factors will vary from individual to individual.

Investigation of the seizures

The diagnosis of epilepsy should be made predominantly on clinical grounds from the seizure pattern description. This can be supplemented by EEG investigation. It is important to emphasise that a diagnosis of epilepsy should never be made on EEG grounds alone. A number of quite healthy people have brief bursts of generalised spike and wave activity during EEG recordings while some patients with epilepsy have relatively normal routine EEGs.

An isolated seizure can be the result of drug or alcohol withdrawal, medication with antidepressant or neuroleptic drugs, acute changes in the metabolic state of the brain, cerebral oedema due to acute fluid retention, structural brain disease and cardiac causes. It may also be the outcome of interaction between a genetically low convulsive threshold and certain provoking factors such as sleep deprivation, hypoglycaemia, high fever in infants, etc. The occurrence of an isolated seizure is an indication for further investigation to exclude such possible causes. However, a diagnosis of epilepsy should not be made unless there are recurrent seizures, that is, two or more separated by an interval of weeks or months. This is important since the label 'epilepsy' has social consequences as well as being a medical diagnosis.

When the diagnosis is made, full neurological investigation is required. This should include a detailed physical examination with special reference to the nervous system, a skull radiograph and EEG. If the patient is already on chronic anticonvulsant medication, full blood picture, serum folate and vitamin B_{12} estimations should be carried out since drug-induced bone marrow megaloblastic change is common and folate deficiency may contribute to depression. Similarly, serum calcium and alkaline phosphatase levels should be checked because of the risk of anticonvulsant induced osteomalacia. Serum anticonvulsant drug concentrations should be estimated if toxicity or non-compliance is suspected or if seizure control is a problem. When the epileptic nature of the fits is in doubt, postseizure serum prolactin levels are sometimes useful to distinguish tonic–clonic fits from pseudoepilepsy. The serum prolactin rises to 1000 munits/l 20 minutes after most, though not all, generalised convulsions and is not changed after pseudoepileptic fits or complex partial seizures.

EEG investigation assists the differential diagnosis between epileptic fits, hysterical pseudoseizures and other forms of transient unconsciousness and helps to classify the epilepsy. Correct classification is important since subjects with primary generalised epilepsy require no further investigation. The class of epilepsy also provides rough guidelines to the choice of antiepileptic medication and contributes to understanding the relationship between epilepsy and the patient's mental state. A normal routine waking EEG is common in the partial epilepsies, especially temporal lobe epilepsy. A sleep record, inducing sleep by oral quinalbarbitone, is always necessary for the investigation of the latter, since the temporal lobe spikes or sharp waves often appear only during light sleep. Spikes originating in the uncal and amygdaloid–hippocampal areas show phase reversal at the sphenoidal electrodes, inserted underneath the zygomatic arches so that their tips lie underneath the middle cranial fossae. Thiopentone sphenoidal records are required if conventional sleep EEGs are normal and when anterior temporal lobectomy is being considered. Foramen ovale electrode recordings in association with videotelemetry are useful as a means of identifying mesial temporal lobe epileptogenic activity not apparent at scalp electrodes and are valuable in lateralisation. The invasive nature of this investigation means that it should be restricted to those patients being considered for surgery. Continuous ambulatory EEG monitoring over 24 hours using a portable cassette tape recorder is useful in the differential diagnosis of pseudoepilepsy and as an accurate measure of the effect of medication on absence seizures. If a diagnosis of partial epilepsy is made on clinical and/or EEG grounds, computerised axial tomography (CT) should be carried out. CT scans show tumours in 11% of epileptic patients of all ages, but 22% in those with partial epilepsy. Some CT scan abnormality, usually atrophic changes, is shown in 50% of all patients. The lowest prevalence of abnormality is in patients with primary generalised epilepsy (10%). Magnetic resonance imaging, positron emission tomography, single-photon emission tomography and magnetoencephalography are proving useful for the localisation of epileptogenic foci, especially when epilepsy surgery is being considered.

Assessment of the relationship between the epilepsy and the psychiatric disorder

A conventional psychiatric diagnostic formulation should first be carried out. This will include diagnosis of the presenting psychiatric syndrome and an evaluation of the relative importance of genetic, organic, environmental and personality factors, and current situational problems in the illness. Then the following sequence of questions concerning the interaction between the fits and the mental state, which relate to the time relation between the seizure occurrence and mental state disturbance, must be considered:

1. If there is a direct relationship, then the mental state changes are a direct reflection of the cortical and subcortical dysfunction caused by the epileptogenic discharges:
Preictal — usually dysphoric symptoms
Ictal — complex partial seizures, absence or complex partial status
Postictal — automatisms or confusional states.
2. If there is no direct relationship in time to the fits, the phenomenology of the consequent interictal disorder is likely to resemble that of a functional psychiatric illness and the causation will be multifactorial. The respective roles of the following factors must be considered:
a. The influence of the underlying epileptogenic lesion on the subject's cognitive function, behaviour and emotional state because of its extent (diffuse), location (temporal lobe) or occurrence of frequent subclinical seizure discharges

b. The relation between seizure type and frequency and the mental state disturbance

c. The effects of anticonvulsant medication on the individual's behaviour, mental processes, and neurological, metabolic and haematological status

d. The effects of having fits and being labelled 'epileptic' on the subject's emotional development and acquisition of social, academic and vocational skills. The impact of all these personal and social factors on the development of the individual's social competence and capacity to cope with current life events should be evaluated. The subject's individual style of reacting to the problems of living with a chronic handicap should also be noted, for example adoption of the 'sick role', aggressive acting-out behaviour and the ego defence mechanisms of denial, projection, and reaction formation.

Of course, all the factors which influence the development of the interictal disorders may also play a role in determining the psychological adjustment of the person who presents with a mental disturbance directly related to seizure occurrence.

PRINCIPLES OF MANAGEMENT

After completing the diagnostic assessment of the patient with epilepsy, anticonvulsant medication should be commenced. The aim is to obtain the best possible control of seizure with minimum unwanted side-effects. It is estimated that current drugs completely control seizures in more than half of patients with epilepsy, though not without mild side-effects. Another 30–40% gain a varying degree of benefit. In such cases this often involves steering a narrow course between incomplete seizure control and side-effects that seriously impair the patient's cognitive and social functioning. A drug regime that permits a few seizures but clear cognition is infinitely preferable to absolute control and significant cognitive impairment. Treatment must continue for many years because the anticonvulsant medication merely raises the seizure threshold and does not cure the disease. The main indication for cessation of treatment is 3 years' freedom from attacks. However, it is well to remember that, even after a 3 year remission period, up to half of patients have a recurrence of seizures when the treatment is stopped.

The selection of the drug to be used depends on the type of seizure and the EEG findings (Table 16.4). Grand mal seizures of generalised origin respond best to phenytoin or carbamazepine. In resistant cases, both may be used together. When control is still not

Table 16.4 Recommended drugs (Duncan 1991)

Seizure type	Drugs
Generalized	*First-line drugs*
Tonic-clinic Tonic Clonic	Phenytoin Carbamazepine Sodium valproate
Simple absence	Ethosuximide Sodium valproate
Complex absence Atonic	Sodium valproate Clonazepam Clobazam
Infantile spasms	ACTH/steroids Clonazepam
Myoclonic	Sodium valproate Clonazepam
Partial	*First-line drugs*
Simple, complex and secondarily generalized	Phenytoin Carbamazepine Sodium valprate
	Second-line drugs
	Phenobarbitone Primidone Clonazepam Clobazam Vigabatrin Lamotrigine

possible with these drugs, it may be necessary to resort to phenobarbitone or primidone in combination with either phenytoin or carbamazepine. It is important to note that phenobarbitone and primidone tend to cause irritability and restlessness and aggravate behaviour problems, especially in children. Partial seizures tend to respond to the drugs of choice for generalised seizures. However, carbamazepine is now the drug of first choice for the treatment of temporal lobe epilepsy, one of the most difficult types to treat. This drug does not have the same degree of sedative effect as the barbiturates. Indeed it has been shown to have a psychotropic action. When the only type of seizure is absence attacks, the patient should be treated with sodium valproate or ethosuximide. Seizures due to secondary generalised epilepsy and the myoclonic epilepsies are notoriously resistant to treatment: sodium valproate is the drug of choice.

An important principle of anticonvulsant treatment is to avoid polytherapy and to use a single drug at one time if possible. Monotherapy is preferred because drug interaction is common with combinations of many antiepileptic drugs and this can lead to unpredictable side-effects (Table 16.5). Dosage should be adjusted

Table 16.5 Some important drug interactions involving antiepileptic drugs

Drugs causing interaction	Result
Interactions between antiepileptic drugs	
Sulthiame Pheneturide	Increase plasma levels of phenytoin with risk of intoxication
Carbamazepine Phenytoin	Reduce plasma levels of each other diminishing their effects
Sodium valproate	Increases plasma levels of phenobarbitone causing sedation
Interactions with other drugs	
Isoniazid Chloramphenicol Coumarin anticoagulants Phenothiazines Tricyclic antidepressants Chlorpheniramine	Increase plasma levels of phenytoin with risk of intoxication
Phenytoin Phenobarbitone Primidone Carbamazepine Pheneturide	Cause hepatic enzyme induction, increasing rate of metabolism and therefore reducing effectiveness of many drugs, e.g. oral anticoagulants, corticosteroids, contraceptive pill, tricyclic antidepressants, phenothiazines, benzodiazepines

From Richens (1977).

to keep the serum concentration of the drug within the range demonstrated to be the most therapeutically effective. Exceeding this level will only lead to toxic effects. If satisfactory control cannot be obtained with monotherapy, then it is permissible to try two drugs simultaneously. The therapist should always avoid getting into a position of using more than two drugs at one time because of the problem of drug interaction and its consequent side-effects. Chronic patients who have been taking a number of drugs concurrently for many years are difficult to manage; only a few are likely to be free of both fits and unwanted side-effects. Such patients are frequently amongst those presenting with psychiatric problems.

Recently two new anticonvulsants have been introduced as 'add on' drugs in refractory epilepsy. Vigabatrin is an inhibitor of GABA transaminase, the enzyme responsible for the catabolism of GABA, and increases brain GABA concentration. It is useful in partial seizures with or without secondary generalisation in doses of 0.5 g twice daily, increasing to a maximum of 3–4 g daily. A rare side-effect is psychosis. Lamotrigine acts by reducing the release of excitatory amino acids from presynaptic terminals and benefits refractory simple and complex partial seizures

when added to existing therapy. Skin rashes are sometimes a problem. Its elimination half life is prolonged by valproate and shortened by hepatic enzymeinducing drugs, i.e. carbamazepine, phenytoin, phenobarbitone and primidone.

The presence of a focal cortical lesion raises the possibility of surgical excision of the local area of epileptogenic cortex. Surgery is considered if the following criteria are fulfilled:

1. The patient is seriously handicapped by frequent seizures
2. An adequate trial of drug treatment over 3–5 years has failed
3. There is clinical and EEG evidence that the seizures arise consistently from a localised area of cortex that can be excised without causing the patient disability.

Temporal lobectomy, i.e. surgical removal of the anterior 6 cm of one temporal lobe, is the most commonly used surgical treatment and is very effective in some patients with drug-resistant temporal lobe seizures. About two-thirds of such patients are markedly improved after surgery, half becoming seizure-free. Surgical treatment can only be aimed at control of the fits. It usually has little effect on behaviour disturbance. The only exception to this rule is aggressiveness in young men with temporal lobe seizures due to unilateral temporal lobe pathology. Here the aggressiveness often responds to temporal lobectomy, but only if there is control of the seizures. It should be stressed that interictal aggressive behaviour in the absence of frequent seizures does not respond to surgery. Other types of operation used include amygdalohippocampectomy, extratemporal cortical excision, hemispherectomy and callosotomy (Oxbury and Adams 1989).

Once the initial diagnosis of epilepsy has been made, treatment commenced and any necessary social rehabilitation measures put into effect, the patient should be reviewed at regular intervals to make sure that he is taking his drugs and that they are effective; to sustain him in handling his life while the fits continue; to minimise the side-effects and toxic effects of the drugs, and to ensure that he benefits from advances in treatment.

PSYCHIATRIC MANAGEMENT

Management must never be restricted to the prescription of antiepileptic drugs even in patients without overt psychological difficulties. Coming to terms with the diagnosis and living with a chronic seizure disorder is a stressful experience both for the patient and the family. Counselling and support are needed at all stages in order to help the patients and those close to them with the series of potential psychological and social handicaps associated with recurrent fits. During the initial assessment, any handicaps must be identified and such rehabilitation measures as are appropriate undertaken.

Those organic mental states that are a direct result of seizure activity (complex partial seizures, absence and complex partial status) require energetic anticonvulsant therapy. Postictal confusional states, if prolonged, need a short period of hospital admission and treatment with adequate doses of chlorpromazine if behaviour is disturbed. Otherwise the principles of management of psychiatric disorder in the subject with epilepsy are essentially similar to that of non-epileptics with the same syndromes. The pharmacological, psychological and social measures appropriate to the individual patient's needs must be implemented. In the depressed person with epilepsy, the treatment indications, including electroconvulsive therapy, are no different to those for the patient without fits.

When prescribing psychotropic medication for a patient on anticonvulsant therapy, it is important to recall that the liver enzyme induction effects of the anticonvulsant drugs result in a much more rapid turnover and excretion of tricyclic antidepressants, neuroleptics and benzodiazepines. Hence, larger than standard doses may be required for therapeutic effect. Conversely, inhibition of antiepileptic drug metabolism caused by imipramine, viloxazine, chlorpromazine or thioridazine can lead to higher anticonvulsant serum levels, especially of phenytoin and carbamazepine.

The neuroleptics and antidepressants also have epileptogenic properties. However, an exacerbation of seizures is rarely a problem providing adequate anticonvulsant medication is given. Trimipramine, protriptyline and doxepin are the safest choices of antidepressant drugs (Luchins et al 1984). If seizures do increase in frequency during neuroleptic or antidepressant therapy, the antiepileptic drug dosage can be adjusted accordingly or a small dose of diazepam (5 mg three times a day) added. The psychotropic action of carbamazepine makes it the anticonvulsant of choice to use in epileptic patients with depressive or dysthymic states (Robertson 1986). A more detailed account of the assessment and management of the psychiatric disorders of epilepsy is given by Fenton (1983).

REFERENCES

Barraclough B 1981 Suicide and epilepsy. In: Reynolds E H, Trimble M R (eds) Epilepsy and psychiatry. Churchill Livingstone, Edinburgh

Betts T A 1981 Epilepsy and the mental hospital. In: Reynolds E H, Trimble M R (eds) Epilepsy and psychiatry. Churchill Livingstone, Edinburgh

Chadwick D W 1981 Convulsions associated with drug therapy. Adverse Drug Reaction Bulletin 87: 316

Corbett J 1981 Epilepsy and mental retardation. In: Reynolds E H, Trimble M R (eds) Epilepsy and psychiatry. Churchill Livingstone, Edinburgh

Currie S, Heathfield K W C, Henson R A, Scott D F 1971 Clinical course and prognosis of temporal lobe epilepsy. Brain 94: 173

Dongier S 1959 Statistical study of clinical and electroencephalographic manifestations of 536 psychotic episodes in 516 epileptics between clinical seizures. Epilepsia 1: 117

Duncan J S 1991 Modern treatment strategies for patients with epilepsy: a review. Journal of the Royal Society of Medicine 84: 159

Duncan J, Shorvon S 1986 Prognosis of epilepsy. British Journal of Hospital Medicine 35: 254

Edeh J 1984 Epilepsy in general practice. PhD Thesis, University of London

Edeh J, Toone B 1987 Relationship between interictal psychopathology and the type of epilepsy. Results of a survey in general practice. British Journal of Psychiatry 151: 95

Edwards J G 1985 Antidepressants and seizures: epidemiological and clinical aspects. In: Reynolds E H, Trimble M R (eds) The psychopharmacology of epilepsy. Wiley, Chichester

Fenton G W 1972 Epilepsy and automatism. British Journal of Hospital Medicine 7: 57

Fenton G W 1981 Psychiatric disorders of epilepsy: classification and phenomenology. In: Reynolds E H, Trimble M R (eds) Epilepsy and psychiatry. Churchill Livingstone, Edinburgh

Fenton G W 1983 Epilepsy. In: Lader M H (ed) Handbook of psychiatry, vol 2. Mental disorders and somatic illness. Cambridge University Press, Cambridge

Fenton G W 1986 EEG epilepsy and psychiatry. In: Trimble M R, Reynolds E H (eds) What is epilepsy? Churchill Livingstone, Edinburgh, pp 139-160

Fenwick P B C, Howard R C, Fenton G W 1983 Review of cortical excitability, neurohumeral transmission and the dyscontrol syndrome. In: Parsonage M, Grant R H E, Craig A G, Ward A A (eds) Advances in epileptology: XIVth International Symposium. Raven Press, New York

Flor-Henry P 1969 Psychosis and temporal lobe epilepsy: a controlled investigation. Epilepsia 10: 363

Flor-Henry P 1976 Epilepsy and psychopathology. In: Granville-Grossman K (ed) Recent advances in psychiatry. Churchill Livingstone, Edinburgh

Geschwind N 1979 Behavioural changes in temporal lobe epilepsy. Psychological Medicine 9: 217

Gloor P 1978 Generalised epilepsy with bilateral

synchronous spike and wave discharge. In: Cobb W A, Van Duijn H (eds) Contemporary clinical neurophysiology (EEG supplement 34). Elsevier, Amsterdam

Gunn J 1977 Epileptics in prison. Academic Press, New York

Gunn J, Fenton G W 1969 Epilepsy in prisons: a diagnostic survey. British Medical Journal iv: 326

Hauser W A, Kurland L T 1975 Epidemiology of epilepsy in Rochester, Minnesota 1935-1967. Epilepsia 16: 1

Heath R 1986 Depth electrode studies. In: Trimble M R, Reynolds E H (eds) What is epilepsy? Churchill Livingstone, Edinburgh

Hermann B P, Whitman S 1984 Behavioural and personality correlates of epilepsy: a review, methodological critique and conceptual model. Psychological Bulletin 95: 451

Hermann B P, Whitman S, Wyler A R, Anton M T, Vanderzwagg R 1990 Psychosocial predictors of psychopathology in epilepsy. British Journal of Psychiatry 156: 98

Hoare P 1984 The development of psychiatric disorder amongst school children with epilepsy. Developmental Medicine and Child Neurology 26: 2

ILEA 1989 Commission on Classification and Terminology of the International League against Epilepsy. Proposal for classification of seizures and epileptic syndromes. Epilepsia 30: 389

Jasper H H 1964 Some physiological mechanisms involved in epileptic automatism. Epilepsia 5: 1

Laidlow J, Richens A, Oxley J 1988 A textbook of epilepsy, 3rd edn. Churchill Livingstone, Edinburgh

Landolt H 1958 Serial electroencephalographic investigations during psychotic episodes in epileptic patients and during schizophrenic attacks. In: Lorentz de Haes A M (ed) Lecture on epilepsy. Elsevier, Amsterdam

Lishman W A 1987 Organic psychiatry, 2nd edn. Blackwell, Oxford

Luchins D J, Oliver A P, Wyatt R J 1984 Seizures with antidepressants: an in vitro technique to assess relative risk. Epilepsia 25: 25

Meldrum B S 1990 Epilepsy octet. Anatomy, physiology and pathology of epilepsy. Lancet 336: 231

Nuffield E G A 1961 Neurophysiology and behaviour disorders in epileptic children. Journal of Mental Science 107: 438

Oxbury J M, Adams C B T 1989 Neurosurgery for epilepsy. British Journal of Hospital Medicine 41: 372

Pahla A G P 1985 A epilepsia em psiquiatria. Doctoral thesis, University of Oporto

Penfield W, Jasper H 1954 Epilepsy and the functional anatomy of the brain. Little Brown, Boston

Perez M M, Trimble M R, Murray N F, Reider I 1985 Epileptic psychosis: an evaluation of PSE profiles. British Journal of Psychiatry 146: 155

Pond D A, Bidwell B H 1960 A survey of epilepsy in 14 general practices. II. Social and psychological aspects. Epilepsia 1: 285

Richens A 1977 Interactions with antiepileptic drugs. Drugs 13: 266

Roberts G W, Done D J, Bruton C, Crow T.J 1990 A "mock up" of schizophrenia: temporal lobe epilepsy and schizophrenia-like psychosis. Biological Psychiatry 28: 127

Robertson M 1986 Ictal and interictal depression in patients with epilepsy. In: Trimble M R, Bolwig I G (eds) Aspects of epilepsy and psychiatry. Wiley, Chichester

Rutter M, Graham P, Yule W 1970 A neuropsychiatric study of childhood. Heinemann, London

Slater E, Beard A W, Glithero E 1963 The schizophrenia-like psychoses of epilepsy. British Journal of Psychiatry 109: 95

Sorensen A S, Hansen H, Andersen R, Hogenhaven H, Allerup P, Bolwig T G 1989 Personality and epilepsy. Acta Psychiatrica Scandinavica 80: 620

Stores G 1978 School children with epilepsy at risk for learning and behaviour problems. Developmental Medicine and Child Neurology 20: 502

Toone B K 1981 Psychoses of epilepsy. In: Reynolds E H, Trimble M R (eds) Epilepsy and psychiatry. Churchill Livingstone, Edinburgh

Toone B K 1986 Hyposexuality among male epileptic patients: clinical and hormonal correlates. In: Trimble M R, Bolwig T G (eds) Aspects of epilepsy and psychiatry. Wiley, Chichester

Toone B K 1991 The psychoses of epilepsy. Journal of the Royal Society of Medicine 84: 457

Toone B K, Garralda M E, Ron M A 1982 The psychosis of epilepsy and the functional psychoses: a clinical and phenomenological comparison. British Journal of Psychiatry 141: 256

Trieman D M, Delgado-Escueta A V 1983 Violence in epilepsy: a critical review. In: Pedly I A, Meldrum B S (eds) Recent advances in epilepsy I. Churchill Livingstone, Edinburgh

Trimble M R 1977 The relationship between epilepsy and schizophrenia: a biochemical hypothesis: Biological Psychiatry 12: 299

Weisner H 1986 Monitoring of seizures. In: Trimble M R, Reynolds E H (eds) What is epilepsy? Churchill Livingstone, Edinburgh, pp 82–96

Wolf P 1991 Acute behavioral symptomatology at disappearance of epileptiform EEG activity. Paradoxical or "forced" normalization. Advances in Neurology 55:127

17. Dependence on alcohol and other drugs

E. B. Ritson   J. D. Chick   J. Strang

It is hard to think of any country which does not rely on some drug or other to facilitate social relations, mark festivals or enhance religious rituals. In Britain, alcohol is the most widely used and abused drug, but other forms of drug misuse are not a new phenomenon in this country. A 19th century reporter visiting Aberdeenshire noted:

Few people are aware to what a frightful excess the vice of opium eating has extended lately in this country and how rapidly it is increasing both in England and in Scotland. I could name one apothecary's shop where innumerable small packets, costing only a penny of this pernicious drug are prepared every night, and where a crowd of the wretched purchasers, many of them women, glide silently up to the counter, deposit the price, and without uttering a word, steal away like criminals, to plunge themselves into a temporary delirium, followed by those agonies of mind and body by which both are at last distorted and ruined. (Geikie 1904)

It is a 'curious fact that societies have at times been able to coexist with the more or less free use of drugs which, at other times or in different societies, have been considered so dangerous as to require strictest legal control' (Edwards 1971).

In considering the consequences of drug misuse, it is useful to differentiate between the pharmacology of the drug, the hazards inherent in the route of administration, the dose and frequency of use and the health and personality of the user. Finally, and perhaps more crucial, consider the setting in which the drug is taken, the immediate surroundings, the presence of friends, their attitudes and expectations, the culture and folklore surrounding the drug as well as the legal sanctions on its use.

Ethanol (ethyl alcohol) is a natural product of the breakdown of carbohydrates in plants. Its euphoriant and intoxicating properties have been known from prehistoric times and almost all cultures have had some experience of its use. Fermentation with yeast can achieve alcohol concentrations of approximately 10%. Higher strengths require distillation, which is thought to have been discovered by the Persian chemist Rhases in AD 800. The word 'alcohol' is Arabic in origin.

Early Egyptian and Greek writings make several references to alcohol and distinguish between its beneficial effects in moderation and the problem of drunkenness, for which severe penalties were often prescribed, particularly when it occurred amongst the young. Hippocrates recognised many of the medical complications of excessive drinking and Seneca introduced the idea of loss of control and habituation. Throughout the 17th century in Britain drunkenness was widespread. Positive incentives were given to produce cheap gin in an effort to promote agriculture. This liberating policy succeeded so completely that, by 1736, consumption of spirits was approximately a gallon a head per annum. Gradually, by means of licensing and taxation, consumption was reduced, only to rise again during the 19th century. The chief opponent of drunkenness at that time was the Temperance Movement. Initially it advocated moderate consumption but later moved to champion total abstinence. The prevailing view was that drunkenness was a vice or moral weakness. Some physicians, such as Benjamin Rush in the USA and Thomas Trotter in Scotland, pointed out both medical and psychological consequences of alcohol abuse, and moved towards the contemporary concept of alcohol addiction.

The Temperance Movement scored its greatest victory in the 18th Amendment of the US Constitution, which prohibited the manufacture and sale of alcohol except for therapeutic or sacramental purposes. The Amendment was difficult to enforce and led to gangsterism. Because of these social consequences and lack of public support, it was repealed in 1933. (It is noteworthy that cirrhosis mortality declined during the years of prohibition.)

The Temperance Movement never attained the political strength in Britain which it enjoyed in the USA or some Scandinavian countries. Nonetheless, it was a considerable force by the end of the 19th century and it facilitated the introduction of control measures which Lloyd George imposed during World War I. The government was deeply concerned at the drunkenness amongst munition workers and introduced taxation and licensing controls in an effective attempt to limit consumption.

There is nothing fixed or unchanging about a nation's drug or alcohol usage. Habits have changed dramatically in Britain during the past century, most often in response to economic and social influences. 'Dry' generations are often followed by those that are relatively 'wet', thus giving rise to the reinstatement of controls and the cycle repeats itself. New knowledge, such as the evidence concerning smoking and lung cancer or the association between intravenous drug usage and human immunodeficiency virus (HIV) infection, also has a demonstrable impact on practices and policies.

EPIDEMIOLOGY OF DRUG ABUSE

The extent and nature of abuse of different drugs change rapidly compared with most other behaviours which have such an intimate relationship with health sequelae. At any time there are three sources of relevant data which are routinely collected.

Firstly there are the data available from the Home Office Addicts Index which collects confidential information on the number of addicts to the opiates and cocaine who attend doctors. All doctors in the UK are under a statutory obligation to provide this information (for details see the summary in the *British National Formulary*): despite evidence of poor compliance by doctors, reviews have consistently concluded that the Addicts Index remains a valuable indicator of trends — especially in the relative absence of other sources of data (Edwards 1982, Advisory Council on the Misuse of Drugs 1991). Thus, the annual figures for 1970 were approximately 2000, increasing steadily through the late 1970s and early 1980s to reach 10 000 by the mid-1980s and to reach 17 756 by 1990. The vast majority of these individuals are addicted to heroin or another opiate with only 5% reported as addicted to cocaine (and only 1% reported as addicted to cocaine alone). The geographical distribution of these cases is not even, with 40% of notified addicts coming from the London area. Similarly, substance distribution is not even; for example, according to the Addicts Index, the recent increase in cocaine addiction is an almost exclusively English (and predominantly London) phenomenon with 243 out of 251 new cocaine addicts (addicted to cocaine alone) coming from England (112 from the London area) during 1990; and only four from Scotland and four from Wales (none from Northern Ireland). Since 1987 doctors have also been invited to provide additional information about whether the notified addict has been taking the drug by injection or by other routes (e.g. smoking or snorting the drug): levels of reported injectable drug use remained constant amongst Addicts Index cases and remain just as high for recently notified new addicts as in previous years. The sex ratio of individuals on the Addicts Index has remained remarkably constant, with men predominating, to result in a sex ratio of approximately 2:1.

The second source of routine information is from criminal statistics — including data on quantities, number and purity of seizures by Customs and also by police, as well as record of number of offences against the 1971 Misuse of Drugs Act. The striking feature about these data are the predominance of cannabis, with 85% of convictions relating to possession or attempt to supply cannabis: those found guilty of possession of cannabis for personal use are most usually dealt with on a non-custodial basis by fine (these data may become less comparable with previous years since the recent change in police practice to a much greater use of their cautioning authority).

The third source of routine information which became available at the beginning of the 1990s is data on health care activity recorded in the new *regional databases* introduced in all regional health authorities in England; and the equivalent national databases established in Scotland and Wales. These databases are due to report on aggregate data across their region with a more detailed set of information about the substances used, doses, routes of administration as well as recording initial treatment/management responses. It is intended that the data will be collected from voluntary agencies and non-medical services as well as National Health Service facilities. The extent or overlap or possible duplication with the Addicts Index will obviously be an area of future critical consideration (Advisory Council on the Misuse of Drugs 1991).

Further data are also available ad hoc as special studies are undertaken. Some of these have been studies of geographically defined populations such as the study of drug using networks in Cheltenham (Plant 1975), in the Wirrall (Parker et al 1987) or the study of opiate addicts in Oxford (Arroyave et al 1973), which was recently repeated (Pevelar et al 1988). More recent studies using social network or snowballing techniques include the studies of Hartnoll et al (1985) which report on the extent of illicit drug use in one area of North London.

Other geographical studies have used treatment agencies as the means of identification of cases, which give a different perspective on the local drug problem — a perspective which may have more relevance to the planning of services but is likely to be less sensitive to changes in new initiations into established or novel patterns of drug use. These treatment studies are necessarily geographically defined, such as the study from Bristol (Parker et al 1988). A different approach was used by Glanz and colleagues in their national survey of a 5% sample of general practitioners in England and Wales (Glanz & Taylor 1986) in which they gathered information on the extent of contact with opiate misusers by general practitioners over a 4 week period. From their findings they estimated that at least 30 000–44 000 cases of opiate misuse were seen by general practitioners in a 1 year period.

An alternative approach is to study populations defined in other ways — for example the study by Plant et al (1984) of schoolchildren in Lothian in 1980, and their follow-up in 1983. From this study Plant et al found consistently higher self-reported rates of drug use amongst boys than girls with levels of use increasing from 15 to 37% over the 3 year period for boys, and from 11 to 23% for girls (self-reported 'ever' use of illicit drugs). More recently, Swadi (1988) reported on the results of a self-report survey of 3333 school children in London, in which he found extensive evidence of use of solvents or illicit drugs at least once (prevalence rates rising from 13% in 11-year-olds to 26% in 16-year-olds), although only 2 and 16%, respectively, were using these drugs regularly. Wright & Pearl have published a series of studies on the knowledge and experience about drug use amongst school children in Wolverhampton, and they report on their data over a 20 year period (Wright & Pearl 1990).

EPIDEMIOLOGY OF DRINKING AND ALCOHOL-RELATED HARM

Influences on consumption

Government revenue statistics are the usual source of information about overall alcohol consumption in nations. Revenue on beer and spirits has been collected in the UK since the 17th century. The lowest point in per capita consumption of all forms of alcohol for three centuries was reached in the 1930s (Royal College of Psychiatrists 1986). The next four decades saw a steady rise in consumption of alcohol in most countries of the world (Table 17.1).

Since 1980, consumption has increased only slightly in many countries, including the UK. In France, Europe's heaviest consumer, alcohol consumption has fallen. Moderate patterns of drinking with less wine consumed evolved in the middle-class and metropolitan areas and then gradually percolated outwards (Sulkenen 1989). Low consumption in Japan and Iceland appears still to be rising. A world-wide homogenisation of drinking habits may be occurring with some exceptions; for example, 1988 saw severe restriction of official production and sales in the USSR.

Increased advertising and marketing, increasing numbers of outlets, extension of licensing hours and falling relative price have been shown in Britain (McGuiness 1980) and in other countries to contribute to rises in consumption. It has been unusual for alcohol not to be served at both private and public functions. 'Going out for a drink' is England's most popular leisure activity and the commonest reason men give for drinking is that it is 'what their friends do when they get together' (Wilson 1980).

The real cost of alcohol fell in the past decade in many countries. In the UK, the length of time necessary to work to pay for one large loaf of bread was 9 minutes in 1971 and 7 minutes in 1986, while for a bottle of whisky it reduced by half from 4.25 hours in 1971 to 2 hours in 1986 (HMSO 1988) (Fig. 17.1). If there was harmonisation of tax on alcohol within the European Community, it has been calculated by the Institute of Fiscal Studies that the proportion of drinkers in the UK exceeding 35 units* per week might increase by 12–20%.

Drinking amongst women

This has increased greatly, particularly when the second half of the 20th century is compared to the first half. Changes in the woman's role, with the result that she enters more male environments and has more income, have contributed. Advertising directed specifically at women has possibly played a part too. In the mid-1980s survey in England and Wales the risk-free level of drinking (up to 14 units per week) was exceeded by 18% of women in full-time employment, compared to 10% of women in part-time work and 8% of the economically inactive. Between 1978 and 1984/5 admitted alcohol consumption among young women rose by an average of 2 units per week.

---

* A single measure (1/5th gill) of 40% by volume spirits contains roughly the same amount of alcohol as half a pint of beer or lager (3–4% by volume), one glass of table wine (10%), one measure of sherry (20%), i.e. 8 g of ethanol or 1 'unit'. A bottle of spirits contains about 28 single measures.

Table 17.1 International comparison of alcohol consumption trends and liver cirrhosis deaths

	Consumption (pure ethanol) (litres/adult)					Liver cirrhosis (deaths/100 000)	
	1970	1975	1980	1984	1989	1974	1989
France	19.6	18.6	14.8	14.2	13.4	32.8	19.9
GDR	6.3	8.2	9.7	13.3	11.1	12.5	19.6
Portugal	9.9	13.3	11.0	12.9	10.4	31.3	24.1
FRG	11.2	12.3	12.7	11.9	10.4	26.9	23.7
Italy	14.4	13.2	13.0	11.5	9.5	31.9	26.8
Austria	11.9	11.7	11.0	11.0	10.3	32.7	28.5
Australia	8.2	9.7	9.8	9.3	8.5	8.3	7.0
Netherlands	5.7	8.9	8.8	8.6	8.3	4.5	5.4
USSR	5.0	5.3	6.2	8.4	3.6[a]	—	—
New Zealand	6.7	8.2	9.7	8.1	7.8	5.4	3.6
Canada	6.5	8.3	9.1	8.0	7.7[a]	11.6	8.0[a]
USA	6.8	7.9	8.7	7.9	7.5	15.8	10.8
UK	5.2	6.8	7.1	7.3	7.6	—	6.1
England and Wales[b]						3.6	6.0
Scotland[b]						6.3	8.5
Ireland	4.2	5.8	7.5	6.7	6.1	3.7	3.0
Finland	4.5	6.7	6.4	6.6	7.6	5.5	9.8
Japan	4.9	5.6	5.4	5.9	6.7	13.4	13.7
Norway	3.6	4.4	4.6	4.0	4.2[a]	4.1	6.6
Iceland	2.7	2.9	3.9	4.0	4.3[a]	3.3	1.2

From: Produktschap voor Gedistilleerde Dranken, Netherlands, 1991; and 'Deaths per 100 000 population, liver cirrhosis and chronic liver disease', WHO World Health Statistics Annual, 1991 and 1974–1983.
[a] 1988.
[b] Consumption data not available for England and Wales/Scotland separately.

Regional differences within the UK

Surveys show that, although the mean consumption and the proportion of drinkers who are heavy drinkers is the same in England and Wales in Scotland and Northern Ireland, a greater proportion (40%) of adult male drinkers in Scotland drink 8 units or more on one or more days a week than in England (27%) (Wilson 1980). The death rate for cirrhosis and chronic liver disease is higher in Scotland than in England and Wales — in 1989, 8.5 and 6.0 per 100 000 of the population, respectively.

Ethnic and religious minorities

Islam, Hinduism, Sikhism, Seventh Day Adventism and the Baptist Church oppose or prohibit consumption of alcohol. The percentage drinking over 36 units/week among Afro-Caribbean men is about half the national average for men of comparable age and social status. Some heavy drinkers are also to be found amongst Pakistanis and Indians, including some Muslims (Cochrane & Bal 1990).

North American Indians have a high rate of alcohol problems, and the Aborigines' drinking patterns cause great concern to the Australian authorities.

Occupation

Men in the drinks industry have the highest average per person consumption, while the construction industry has the highest proportion of men who drink 'heavily' (over 50 units per week). There are various reasons for the association of heavy drinking and certain occupations: availability of alcohol at work (the licensed trade): social pressure (e.g. the business lunch); separation from normal social and sexual relationships (e.g. seamen, servicemen). The drinks industry tends to recruit men who are already heavy drinkers, to which an 'availability' factor is added. Freedom from supervision may contribute to why doctors, lawyers and senior businessmen have an increased risk of being heavy consumers. The stress of medical life may have contributed to the once high rate of heavy drinking and alcoholism in doctors. The standardised mortality rate which used to be 300 or

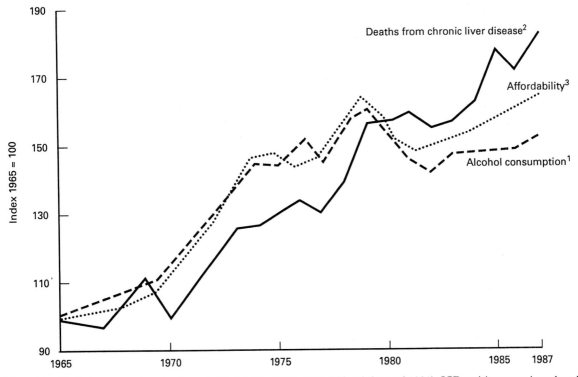

Fig. 17.1 Alcohol consumption, deaths and affordability, 1965–1987 (Humphries et al 1991). ICD revisions were introduced in 1968 and 1979. As a result there appears to be a discontinuity between 1978 and 1979 in the statistics of deaths and discharges from non-psychiatric hospitals with a main diagnosis of ICD-571 and the statistics of death may also be affected.

$$\text{Affordability} = \frac{\text{personal disposable income}}{\text{price of alcohol.}}$$

Sources: 1, Customs and Excise; 2, Office of Population, Censuses and Surveys; 3, Economics Adviser's Office.

more for cirrhosis amongst doctors was only 115 in the 1982–1983 mortality data (Chick 1992).

The prevalence of alcohol-related disorders

In the past, much effort was expended to derive prevalence estimates of 'alcoholism'. Epidemiologists nowadays choose to study the components of this conglomerate concept — alcohol dependence (see below), and the adverse health and social consequences of drinking (Fig. 17.2). Data on the prevalence of physical damage from alcohol are available in mortality records and hospital admissions statistics. Mortality from cirrhosis is greatest in the grape-growing countries of central and southern Europe where consumption is higher (see Table 17.1). The increase in cirrhosis deaths in the UK which has occurred since 1945 is accounted for by an increase in alcoholic cirrhosis (Saunders et al 1981). By 1980 a

peak had been passed in the USA, Canada and Sweden and a decrease noticed, the reasons for which remain to be clarified (Smart & Mann 1991), but getting more alcoholics into treatment and into mutual help groups may be a factor.

The number of admissions to general hospitals in which alcohol was recorded as one of the diagnoses increased nearly four-fold from 1968 to 1978 in Scotland. In general hospitals 20–30% of all male admissions and 5–10% of female admissions are deemed to be 'problem drinkers', the rate varying with the catchment area of the hospital and, of course, with the definitions of 'problem drinker' (Chick 1987).

Alcohol disorders account for approximately one-fifth of psychiatric first admissions, but admission figures are influenced by allocations for beds, and fashions in day patient and out-patient care versus in-patient care. This has been shown to be a partial explanation for the greater rate of alcoholism

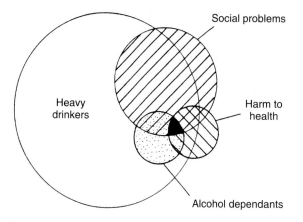

Fig. 17.2 The relationship between heavy drinking, alcohol dependence, social problems and harm to health. Drinkers who are dependent on alcohol are drawn from amongst 'heavy drinkers', but some social problems (e.g. family upsets, trouble with police) and some health problems (e.g. gastritis) are associated with sporadic, rather than regular consumption. 'Hazardous' drinking (the point at which the risk of harm begins to increase) is over 21 units per week for men and 14 units per week for women.

admissions in Scotland than in England and a trend towards out-patient treatment and detoxification may have contributed to the fall in Scottish admissions figures in the 1980s.

The general population survey permits a prevalence estimate that is not subject to the vagaries of hospital admission and referral policies or the defining processes of social agencies. However, the door-to-door interviewer has difficulty in finding the heavy drinker at home and when he is there he tends to under-report his consumption and his problems. The 1978 survey of England and Wales derived a point prevalence figure of 'problem drinking' of 5.3% in men and 1.6% in women.

Doorstep comments by refusers suggested that at least a further 0.77% might have been classified as problem drinkers (Wilson 1980). However, such estimates are very sensitive to alterations in the definition of a case, for example the number and severity of alcohol-related symptoms required to reach the criterion for inclusion, and whether or not past as well as present symptoms are counted.

In North America, DSM-III criteria have been applied in general population surveys. The St Louis sample revealed a lifetime prevalence of alcohol dependence of 16.1% for men and 3% for women. The same instrument (Diagnostic Interview Schedule, DIS) was translated for use in Korea and Taiwan where rates among men were 20 and 3%, respectively,

perhaps reflecting the less severe oriental flushing reaction in Koreans than Taiwanese as well as the high tolerance, indeed encouragement, of drinking in males in South Korean society (Helzer et al 1990).

The prevalence of alcohol-related problems in a population is linked to the alcohol consumption per person in that population. For example, when nations and regions are compared, there is a high correlation between consumption and cirrhosis mortality. Within countries, fluctuations in consumption over time are positively correlated with fluctuations in cirrhosis mortality (Table 17.1) (Skog 1980). Changes which increase consumption, such as more advertising or sales outlets or greater social permissiveness, also contribute to rising problem rates. Of course, overall consumption is not the only influence: different styles of drinking are linked to different problems. In cultures where people drink in very heavy sessions, interspersed by comparative abstinence there is a higher level of social harm than in cultures where heavy session drinking is rare. For example, in Scotland where average consumption per occasion is slightly higher than in England, there are correspondingly more social problems (Crawford et al 1985). The Nordic countries have higher rates of acute alcohol poisoning than southern European countries.

Level of consumption and adverse consequences

Community samples must be studied if estimates are to be made of the risk to health of drinking at particular levels. It has been shown for a particular district in France, by comparing what cirrhotics drink and what a sample from the rest of the population drinks, that the risk of cirrhosis increases logarithmically with increasing consumption starting at 6 units per day in women and 8 units per day in men. At 12 units per day the risk in men is increased 14-fold. The risk for delirium tremens begins at 12 units per day. This research is based on what people *admit* to drinking (in clinical practice, severe delirium tremens is usually associated with consumption of at least 24 units per day). The risk of being admitted to a medical ward for a variety of diagnoses (gastrointestinal, liver, cardiovascular disorders, myocardial infarction) is increased in men. In a Scottish study it began to rise at 21 units per week (Chick et al 1986). Stroke death in Chicago begins to be linked with alcohol when consumption reaches 42 units per week (Dyer et al 1980).

Although the greatest risk of experiencing or causing harm related to alcohol is incurred by the small percentage of the population who are the heaviest drinkers, the largest proportion of the total alcohol-related harm in a society is attributable to drinkers in more moderate consumption bands, simply because they are so much more numerous (Kreitman 1986). This means that to have most effect, public health preventive strategies should not concentrate only on high-risk groups. This conclusion has been called the 'preventive paradox'.

The term 'hazardous drinking' refers to levels of admitted drinking at or above the level at which the risk of adverse consequences — such as some forms of acute social or medical harm — begins to increase. For men this appears to be 21 units per week and for women 14 units per week.

Estimates have been made of the contribution of alcohol to the death rate, using data from follow-up studies where self-reports of alcohol consumption were obtained at entry to the study. Anderson (1988) arrived at a figure for England and Wales of 28 000 excess deaths (age range: 15–74 years). Those who drink 1–3 units of alcohol per day have a lower death rate than abstainers, but this is due partly to the light drinkers being over-represented and whose lifestyle is healthy in other ways, and partly because abstainers often turn out to be abstaining because of pre-existing ill-health (Shaper et al 1988, British Journal of Addiction 1990). There is growing evidence, however, that light alcohol consumption (1–3 units per day) may protect against coronary artery disease, and this may be partially mediated through higher high-density lipoprotein cholesterol levels (Jackson et al 1991).

Natural history of problem drinking

An important contribution of the epidemiologist has been to demonstrate that the problem drinker is not an individual irredeemably condemned, but rather that many people move into and out of problem drinking.

Surveys record low rates of drinking problems after the age of 50 years. An Australian study, examining the ages of alcoholics known to agencies, concluded that the prevalence of alcoholism in the population diminishes more rapidly with age than can be accounted for by mortality and successful treatment. One-half to one-third of respondents in several large US surveys who reported a given 'problem' no longer reported that problem when re-interviewed 4 years later. Though some of these had developed a different alcohol-related problem instead, others had stopped drinking or cut down considerably. Positive changes in social circumstances such as job and personal relationships were important in the history of these recovered individuals (see the section 'Evaluation of

treatment' below). In a Swedish general population cohort, re-interviewed after a 15 year interval, 41% of the 71 alcoholics identified originally and still alive were completely free of drinking problems (Ojesjo 1981). A similar proportion (45%) of 120 problem drinkers from the Boston inner-city sample (Vaillant et al 1982) followed during 20 years on average were no longer in difficulties. However, 10% had died and 40% had drinking problems still. At conscription to the Swedish armed forces, men who are drinking over 30 units per week have three and a half times the expected death rate in the coming 15 years (Andreasson et al 1988), which is similar to the excess rate shown by those who are discharged from hospital diagnosed as alcoholics.

DEFINITIONS OF DEPENDENCE ON PSYCHOACTIVE SUBSTANCES

'Alcoholism' still has currency amongst many clinicians and therapists in the field and is still used at times in this chapter. Though imprecise, the term carries the implication that the drinker is dependent and has incurred harm to himself or others.

In the forthcoming ICD-10 it is proposed that a diagnosis of dependence on drugs, of which alcohol is regarded as one among other psychoactive substances leading to disorder, should be made if three or more of the following have been experienced or exhibited at some time in the previous 12 months:

1. A withdrawal state
2. Drug use with the intention of relieving withdrawal symptoms and with awareness that this strategy is effective
3. Subjective awareness of an impaired personal capacity to control the onset, termination or level of drug use
4. A narrowing of the personal repertoire of patterns of drug use, e.g. a tendency to drink alcoholic beverages in the same way on weekdays and weekends and whatever social constraints
5. Progressive neglect of alternative pleasures or interests in favour of drug use
6. Persisting with drug use despite clear evidence of overtly harmful consequences
7. Evidence that return to drug use after a period of abstinence leads more or less rapidly to reinstatement of the dependence syndrome.

This definition leans on Edwards & Gross's (1976) paper on dependence on alcohol (see also Heather et al 1985).

The DSM-IIIR and ICD-10 definitions are similar

in many ways, but DSM-IIIR includes operational definitions of severity and remission (some clinicians find the term 'full remission' to be somewhat over-optimistic when defined as freedom from symptoms for only 6 months):

Diagnostic criteria for psychoactive substance dependence:

A. At least three of the following:
   (1)   substance often taken in larger amounts or over a longer period than the persons intended
   (2)   persistent desire or one or more unsuccessful efforts to cut down or control substance use
   (3)   a great deal of time spent in activities necessary to get the substance (e.g., theft), taking the substance (e.g., chain smoking), or recovering from its effects
   (4)   frequent intoxification or withdrawal symptoms when expected to fulfill major role obligations at work, school or home (e.g., does not go to work because hung over, goes to school or work "high", intoxicated while taking care of his or her children), or when substance use is physically hazardous (e.g., drives when intoxicated)
   (5)   important social, occupational, or recreational activities given up or reduced because of substance use
   (6)   continued substance use despite knowledge of having a persistent or recurrent social, psychological, or physical problem that is caused or exacerbated by the use of the substance (e.g., keeps using heroin despite family arguments about it, cocaine-induced depression, or having an ulcer made worse by drinking)
   (7)   marked tolerance: need for markedly increased amounts of the substance (i.e., at least a 50% increase) in order to achieve intoxification or desired effect, or markedly diminished effect with continued use of the same amount
   Note: the following items may not apply to cannabis, hallucinogens, or phencyclidine (PCP):
   (8)   characteristic withdrawal symptoms (see specific withdrawal syndromes under Psychoactive Substance-induced Organic Mental Disorders)
   (9)   substance often taken to relieve or avoid withdrawal symptoms

B. Some symptoms of the disturbance have persisted for at least one month, or have occurred repeatedly over a longer period of time.

Criteria for Severity of Psychoactive Substance Dependence:

Mild: Few, if any, symptoms in excess of those required to make the diagnosis, and the symptoms result in no more than mild impairment in occupational functioning or in usual social activities or relationships with others.
Moderate: Symptoms or functional impairment between 'mild' and 'severe'.
Severe: Many symptoms in excess of those required to make the diagnosis, and the symptoms markedly interfere with occupational functioning or with social activities or relationships with others.
In Partial Remission: During the past six months, some use of the substance and some symptoms of dependence.
In Full Remission: During the past six months, either no use of the substance, or use of the substance and no symptoms of dependence.

These recent definitions eschew components to do with the wish to feel the psychic effects of the drug — since these are common to most if not all drug users. The notion of 'compulsion' is also no longer included, perhaps because it begs the question of what 'compulsive' means. An individual can only experience a compulsion to do something if he has the intention not to do it and is struggling. He may have good reasons in his own view to desist from a rehearsed pattern of behaviour and intends not to repeat it; however, he finds himself again and again changing his mood (not sticking to that intention).

AETIOLOGY OF ALCOHOL DEPENDENCE AND ABUSE

From a public health perspective the availability of a substance is a powerful determinant of level of consumption, and culture and tradition are potent influences on the pattern and context. In addition to quantity and frequency of use other factors play a part in determining the development of dependence.

Heredity

It is becoming evident that while for some problem drinkers the causes are to be found principally in their environment, for others there is a major genetic contribution (dealt with in Ch. 9). Transmission may be of a greater propensity to dependence at a given dose of the drug, or a personality type (e.g. 'impulsive') that leads to a troublesome pattern of use, or a personality or constitution that leads to the individual obtaining particular rewards from the drug and/or absence of undesirable effects. Genetic transmission of alcohol dependence may well involve a mixture of these processes. It is likely on present evidence that alcohol dependence is a phenomenon that has many forms which, though phenotypically similar, are genotypically different, some with a fairly high environmental contribution, some with a fairly high genetic contribution. However, there is good epidemiological evidence that heavy drinking runs in families (see Ch. 9 and Marshall & Murray 1991).

Personality

Sufferers from alcohol- and drug-related problems who attend clinics contain a higher proportion of individuals with personality deviations and early family disturbance than is found in the general population. This is partly to be expected since clinics tend to be based in psychiatric services and thus attract psychiatrically disturbed cases. In the general population, follow-up studies of young men tend to find that the impulsive, rebellious, more extrovert individual is more at risk of developing alcoholism, particularly alcohol-related social problems. Childhood conduct disorder (itself related in general population studies, as well as in clinical work, to parental disharmony) also predicts alcoholism, typically of early onset and linked to criminality. A debate developed in the 1980s about whether there is a type of male alcoholic with early onset, severe problems (especially social problems) who is socially detached, distractable, confident and whose behaviour is linked to a similar pattern in the biological father ('type 2' — Cloninger 1987), which contrasts with a more dependent, anxious, rigid, less aggressive, more guilty alcoholic ('type 1') with either the biological mother or father an alcoholic. Some have felt that type 2 is best seen as alcoholism secondary to antisocial personality (ASP) (Shuckit & Irwin 1989). ASP (with alcohol-related items excluded from the ASP algorithm) greatly increases the risk that a man or a woman will have an alcohol problem in longitudinal and cross-sectional community studies. However, a majority of alcoholics have not had childhood conduct disorder (Wells et al 1991). In a large community study, having antisocial personality and/or a family history of alcoholism identified 48.1% of male alcoholics and 63.2% of female alcoholics (Lewis & Bucholz 1991). ASP (lifetime) in that study was diagnosed in 8.7% of the population.

Drake and Vaillant (1988), in a 33 year longitudinal study of 456 inner-city adolescent boys chosen as non-delinquent at that age, found that adolescent indicators of personality disorder were good predictors of adult personality disorder, but not alcoholism. (Having an alcoholic father was the best predictor — 28% of boys developed alcoholism as opposed to 12% of sons of non-alcoholic fathers.) Apart from the severe disturbance associated with childhood conduct disorders, community studies do not usually, especially in middle-class subjects, find evidence linking parenting styles — apart from parental drinking habits — to subsequent alcoholism (Vaillant et al 1983, Joyce et al 1992). Maternal over-protection is described, however, by some clinic attenders (Bernardi et al 1989).

Thus, there is no typical pre-alcoholic personality. Nevertheless, in clinical practice it is important to recognise those for whom drinking is a temporary solution to low self-esteem or a life difficulty, in self-assertion or anxiety. However, it must be emphasised that alcohol itself is a powerful cause of psychological disturbance because of its effects on mood, social relationships and even because of subtle brain damage.

Psychiatric disorder

As well as antisocial personality disorder in the community, alcohol dependence is found to be associated with phobic disorder, anxiety disorder, other psychotropic substance abuse (including tranquilliser dependence) and (especially in women) depression (e.g. Lewis & Bucholz 1991).

Alcohol may be used as an anaesthetic by the bereaved and may complicate pathological grief. Phobias, especially agoraphobia, are common in alcoholics attending psychiatric hospitals (Kushner et al 1990). Because it is a short-acting sedative causing rebound arousal, alcohol may exacerbate or even precipitate anxiety states. However, the phobia in some instances clearly predates the alcohol dependence. Manic–depressive illness, including the manic phase, may result in drinking to the point of physical dependence.

Psychological aspects of alcohol dependence in women

Women make up a third of alcoholics seen in psychiatric practice. There is often a male heavy drinker either in the family history, or the marriage. Women more often than men attribute the onset of problem drinking to a particular life stress. However, community surveys in both Scotland and North America have not shown that adverse life events predict whose drinking will increase during a follow-up period (Romelsjo et al 1991). Familial and interpersonal stress may precipitate a depressive episode. Depression in middle life following the departure of the children ('the empty nest'), or in the lonely spinster or widow, can lead to excessive drinking. Typically, this is at home and secret, and associated with considerable shame and denial. By the time she presents, the female alcoholic often holds herself in very low self-esteem, lacking the sense of control over her world. She may have come to believe that it is only with alcohol that she can appear confident, make decisions and assert herself.

Childhood experience of sexual abuse, when asked for in a research interview, is more commonly reported in women alcoholics than in the general population. It is not yet known if it is more common that in other psychiatric disorders (Hurley 1991).

Female patients, whether presenting with dependence, psychiatric or medical complaints, often give a shorter history of excessive drinking than men and tend to report a lower intake of ethanol, even after correction for body weight. This may partly be explained by the greater stigma attached to women's drinking, which might lead to their minimising their consumption. However, a given dose per kilogram of body weight of ethanol produces a higher peak blood level in a woman than a man. This may be due in part to the female body having a lower ratio of water to fat than the male body (alcohol dissolves more readily in water than in fat), and to a lower activity of alcohol dehydrogenase in the gastric mucosa.

Role of marital relationships

In an alcoholic's marriage, hostility, mistrust and attempts by one partner to control the other are common. Communication may be poor. Women problem drinkers sometimes have husbands whose energies are directed entirely towards their work or their hobbies, or husbands who make them feel worthless. It is difficult to disentangle cause from effect, and adequate research which would need to be longitudinal has not yet been conducted.

It is noted that people with personality problems tend to marry others with personality problems. When a marriage problem is linked with an alcohol problem, it is not easy for the clinician to know whether the marital disharmony results from the personality difficulties each brought to the marriage, or if it is a result of the drinking. However, some marital problems undoubtedly improve when the drinking ceases.

Psychobiology of alcohol dependence

Initiation and reinforcement

Drinking to reduce tension has been intensively researched, since it is an obvious route which might lead to dependence on a sedative drug such as alcohol, either by learning or by chemical tolerance/dependence, or both. The setting, the company and expectancy (what the subject believes the effects of alcohol to be) all contribute to whether alcohol has a relaxing effect or not as much as — and in some experiments more than — the pharmacological/dose action (Young et al 1990). In regular large daily doses alcohol can actually increase tension.

Use of alcohol to reduce tension, or the belief that it will, may be for some the initiation into alcohol use, though initiation is most often simply drinking for its social meaning.

Alcohol has an euphoriant effect for some individuals in some settings and this is a potent *reinforcer* of continued drinking. It is likely that genetic factors already touched on contribute at this point, since there is higher concordance in monozygotic than dizygotic twins in the general population for alcohol consumption, if not for alcohol problems, even when the greater social contact between monozygotic twins is controlled for (Kaprio et al 1987, Heath & Martin 1988, Heath et al 1989, Marshall & Murray 1991).

Orientals have varying degrees of acetaldehyde dehydrogenase deficiency, and the consequent 'flushing' reaction to alcohol is a deterrent to drinking for some (though alcohol dependence does develop in some Orientals despite flushing).

Sons of alcoholics, identified both from among sons of clinic attenders in a general population cohort and identified by questionnaire survey, for example in college students, have been compared with controls in numerous measures (Pihl et al 1990). Finding appropriate control subjects (especially if sons of clinic patients are being studied) is a crucial problem in this research, as is controlling for the effects of any alcohol already being consumed by teenagers and students. In sons of alcoholics, alcohol has a greater dampening effect on the physiological correlates of stress than is seen in controls. Expectancy has a role, though how much is debated. Children of alcoholics of school age tend to be distractable, quick to resort to aggression and often in trouble with authority. These traits may, of course, also be contributed to by parental separation and neglect. There is debate about whether some of the *cognitive abnormalities* seen in alcoholics such as rigidity of thought, poor abstracting and problem solving and impaired self-regulation and planning memory are to be found more than expected in children of alcoholics. Many studies have found such an association, those studies which do not tending to be those where either the affected parent was the mother, the subjects included daughters, or the samples were drawn from college students, which might have excluded people with cognitive impairment.

A twin study did not find cognitive impairment (or cortical atrophy) in the non-alcoholic monozygotic twins in discordant pairs and this also provides some evidence against the hypothesis that an inherited predisposing trait in alcoholism might be cognitive impairment. It points to aspects, at least, of cognitive impairment being a result rather than a precursor of the drinking (Gurling et al 1991).

Detoxified alcoholics have abnormalities in the *electroencephalogram (EEG) cortical evolved response measures.* In adolescent sons of alcoholics, the P300 wave amplitude is decreased and other wave abnormalities have been reported and replicated in several studies (Begleiter & Porjesz 1990). But when the sample is varied (e.g. college students recruited as reporting alcoholic parents rather than children of clinic patients), and the stimulus and attention conditions varied, findings are inconsistent (Pihl et al 1990). There is, of course, the need to control for the subject's own alcohol consumption. For the present, a somewhat complex working hypothesis has emerged that sons of alcoholics hyper-react to stimuli whose motivational significance is inherent or involuntary, and hypo-react during situations that require the voluntary maintenance of attention. There is a need to see if these findings are specific to certain alcoholic families or instead are associated with personality disorders.

A search is being made for *biochemical abnormalities* which occur in alcoholics and can also be demonstrated in their pre-drinking children. Decreased platelet monoamine oxidase (MAO) activity is suggested by some research, especially as linked to 'type 2' or more socially disturbed alcoholism, but this abnormality has also been associated with some other psychiatric disorders (Pihl et al 1990). It is highly likely that alcoholics' clinical heterogenicity will be reflected in any biological markers, for example it was in early onset 'type 2' alcoholics where Buydens-Branchey et al (1989) found evidence of diminished serotonin precursor availability.

Alcohol's reinforcing effects are modulated by dopamine, serotonin and γ-aminobutyric acid (GABA) neurotransmitter systems. Dopamine antagonists, serotonin uptake inhibitors, a GABA agonist, and an opioid antagonist have all been shown to reduce alcohol intake in strains of alcoholic-preferring animals, and sometimes in humans as well (Meyer 1989).

Tolerance and withdrawal

When drinking has become a regular habit — i.e. is in some sense regularly rewarding — there is a tendency for the dose to increase (tolerance); and if there is the intention to cut down, or stop, that may seem difficult.

There is a behavioural explanation of tolerance and withdrawal which is that, if an organism 'expects' the drug because it is confronted with signals that previously heralded the drug, 'drug compensatory conditional responses' act to cancel the effect of the drug, producing tolerance if the drug is administered,

or a 'withdrawal' state if the drug is withheld. Thus, animals may only display tolerance to alcohol in an environment where the alcohol was initially administered and not in a novel setting. There are also environmentally independent factors. These include dose, duration and frequency of alcohol administration and a variety of biochemical conditions. Several neurochemical systems are implicated in the development of alcohol tolerance including the noradrenaline, serotonin and GABA systems, and calcium channel activity. N-Methyl-D-aspartate (NMDA) receptors are 'up-regulated', perhaps increased in number, after chronic alcohol administration (US Department of Health and Human Services 1990).

The original demonstration that 'rum fits' and delirium tremens were withdrawal symptoms of alcohol dependence was made by Isbell et al (1955). In this experiment, recovered opiate addicts consumed between 1 and $1\frac{1}{2}$ bottles of spirits per day (250–370 g ethanol) for 7 weeks. On cessation all had withdrawal symptoms, and some had fits or delirium. Such a short history is unusual (but not unknown) in clinical practice. Usually the tendency to drink such large amounts over successive days takes years to develop. Nevertheless, traces of withdrawal phenomena (insomnia, restlessness, increased REM sleep) occur even after single large doses of a sedative such as alcohol. Hangover is in part a mild withdrawal state.

To our knowledge, genetic differences in propensity to withdrawal symptoms has not been shown in humans, but has been noted in strains of animal bred as alcohol-preferring.

Relapse and reinstatement

Some clinicians believe that there is a *protracted physiological withdrawal state* which outlasts the visible tremor, tachycardia, sweating and anxiety of the initial 3–10 days. Cognitive deficits are still improving several months after abstinence, cerebral atrophy also resolves in some patients, and cerebral blood flow improves (Chick et al, 1992). During this time, abnormalities in EEG evoked response and sleep architecture, and complaints of insomnia, persist; patients complain of anxiety and depressive symptoms diminishing proportionately with the length of abstinence; and there appears to be reduced suppression in the dexamethasone suppression test and blunted thyrotrophin response to thyrotrophin-releasing hormone (Meyer 1989, Garbutt 1991). The indications are that GABA receptors, their chloride channels and, perhaps, up-regulation of NMDA receptors continue to be abnormal.

During this time, some patients feel an urge to drink and they struggle with craving. There are *psychological and social processes* at work, as well as neurochemical ones. A drinker may weigh up the advantages and disadvantages of alcohol to him, perhaps based on new information he has about its harmful effects to him, or because of outside pressure (family, employee, legal) and may decide to stop drinking, and succeed for a time. Adhering to that decision may not be easy. The original precipitants of drinking, and memory of drinking's rewards, may still be present.

Then there is a range of cues to drinking that have been learnt over the years. Such cues may be environmental: social situations; his pub or club; the wine shop by the bus stop; the chair in which he customarily watches television. Cues may also be internal; for example, drinking may have become associated with feeling happy, sad, angry, tired, hungry, or all of these (Drummond et al 1990). Brain damage is likely to be important in impeding an alcoholic's intentions: he may have become inflexible in his thinking, impulsive and unable to plan ahead easily.

During these initial months, a sometimes contentious issue is that further — even slight — use of the drug may be powerful in eroding intentions about further consumption, i.e. leads to relapse. Many alcoholism recovery programmes recommend absolute abstinence. Clearly, after tolerance has been lost, five or six drinks may be sufficient to dissolve one's intention not to take a seventh. But there seems no obvious reason why that should lead to a return in the next day or so to heavy harmful drinking and, in the dependent drinker, reinstatement of craving and withdrawal symptoms. There is no evidence that one drink sets off a neurophysiological tripwire, but disposition to drink in alcoholics (measured objectively as work done to obtain alcohol or speed of drinking under standard conditions) has been shown in laboratory settings to increase after as little as three large measures of spirits. Increased disposition to drink in abstinent alcoholics has also been demonstrated on the morning after a dose of alcohol. Thus, in alcohol-dependent individuals who have been abstinent for some time the pattern of response to renewed drinking is 'carried over' from their previous drinking period. Carry-over has been demonstrated in monkeys and in rats: physical dependence (tendency to withdrawal phenomena) is more easily evoked in animals who have been previously made physically dependent even after 37 days of abstinence. 'Reinstatement' is also used to describe the carry-over phenomenon. It is interesting that prior severity of dependence in alcoholics may not predict relapse, but may predict severity of relapse.

As well as a learning theory/neurophysiological view of reinstatement, a cognitive explanation has also been put forward. It is said that abstinent alcoholics who relapse on recommencing drinking do so because they believe, as a result of treatment or attendance at Alcoholics Anonymous, that one or two drinks necessarily leads to harmful drinking — 'the self-fulfilling prophecy'. Of course, having a drink can also be seen as a stimulus with a long-ingrained conditional response — taking another drink. This view has led some to advocate cue exposure, including exposure to drinking environments, as a way of reducing severity of relapse (not as yet proven as a treatment method) (Drummond et al 1990).

Apart from the biological forces which may be operating, the alcoholic who has at one point decided to stop drinking experiences many mental processes which are completely conscious (well described by Ludwig 1988). Sometimes these are best seen as a way of justifying an urge to drink, for example thinking 'one won't harm me' or 'I'm not an alcoholic actually'. Sometimes it will be a feeling — self-pity, anger, guilt, frustration — which is followed by the thought 'a drink will get me over this'. By retraining his thinking, an alcoholic can free himself, sometimes completely, from the mental process that eventually leads to relapse (see below), despite biological abnormalities still unresolved. Otherwise, rationalisation, distortion of reality (minimising the harm alcohol has done to him), and projection (putting the blame on someone else) will allow the alcoholic to do what he wants (to drink alcohol) without a feeling of guilt or conflict.

AETIOLOGY OF DRUG USE AND DEPENDENCE

Environmental factors have appeared to be the dominant influence in determining the levels of drug use within society and the genesis of dependence. Whilst significant advances have been made in understanding the genetic and family influences on drinking behaviour and dependence, studies have not been undertaken with the same rigour with consideration of other drugs (see Mirin et al 1984). However, large-scale studies have now been commenced (e.g. see Rounsaville 1988) which should yield valuable data in the years ahead.

Classical conditioning and learning theory have been major theoretical contributions, influencing research and treatment models in the fields of both alcohol and drug dependence (e.g. see Wikler 1965, Bandura 1977, Marlatt & Gordon 1985).

More recently, significant advances have been made in our understanding of the neurobiological basis of drug use and drug dependence, and this has been accompanied by study of the neurobiological mechanisms of craving (e.g. see Wise 1988, Holman 1990) and of the neurobiological and cellular nature of the development of dependence (e.g. see Littleton & Harper 1990). Other predisposing factors have been postulated, including pre-existing psychopathologies such that the individual self-medicates (Khantzian 1985), or the pre-existence of definable conditions such as the attention deficit disorder (ADD) which leave the individual vulnerable to the development of dependence on cocaine, for example. Theories of disturbed personality have been put forward in which the use of the drug by the individual is seen as an attempt to cope with intrapersonal or interpersonal problems (e.g. see Khantzian 1985). However, several longitudinal studies have failed to identify any consistent relationship between personality traits and the subsequent development of problems of substance abuse (e.g. see McCord & McCord 1960, McCord 1972, Vaillant 1983).

CLINICAL FEATURES AND MANAGEMENT OF DRUG ABUSE

General principles

Whatever the specific treatment which may be considered for drug misuse or dependence, the doctor is in an excellent position to provide harm reduction advice to the drug user with whom he may come in contact. This may be in the form of advice about self-help strategies, or advice on key changes which the drug user may make in the nature of his continued drug use. Thus, even for the drug user who is determined to continue with their drug use, there may be important interventions which the doctor can deliver. If the drug user is injecting, advice may be given on safer injecting technique, the local availability of injecting equipment and treatment services, and advice on the benefits that may result from switching to less dangerous routes of administration (e.g. smoking heroin or snorting cocaine or amphetamines). Additionally, consideration should be given to hepatitis B and human immunodeficiency virus (HIV) counselling and screening; and hepatitis B immunisation may valuably be offered to those who have not yet been infected. It is probable in the years ahead that we will see specific early intervention strategies developed for use in the primary health care setting (similar to those already developed in the alcohol field — see review by Babor et al 1986, Anderson 1987), but as yet these are still at an early stage of development. Future practice is likely to include a similar more active approach with the counselling, testing and treatment of HIV status amongst drug injectors: there is already a dangerous tendency for work with drug users to lag behind advances which have occurred in the practice of care provision to the wider population.

Physical examination is an essential component of assessment of the drug taker. This should include examination for the presence of any venepuncture marks as well as a check for the presence of any drug – specific effects or drug withdrawal effects. It is important to remember that these separate lines of enquiry are necessary — one line of enquiry follows the particular substance or substances of use, whilst the other line of enquiry follows the route of administration and pattern of drug use. An extremely important laboratory aid to assessment and diagnosis is the drug screening of a urine sample: if a full screen is conducted this will indicate what drug or drugs the patient has been taking in the day or two preceding collection of the urine specimen — no amount of inspired retrospective speculation can replace the value of the urine specimen if collected at the point of diagnostic uncertainty (for a review, see Editorial 1987).

Clarifying the goals of treatment

Many doctors get into difficulty in their management of drug misusers because they fail to be clear in their own minds about the goals of their intervention. Clarification of treatment goals requires discussion and a degree of negotiation with the drug user himself about the feasibility of different possible goals at different points in the treatment process. Abstinence is not necessarily the most appropriate or feasible short-term goal for all drug misusers: the clinician who will only consider working with the drug misuser seeking immediate abstinence is likely to miss opportunities for constructive intervention in many of his patients. The recent report on the acquired immune deficiency syndrome (AIDS) and drug misuse from the Advisory Council on the Misuse of Drugs (1988) draws attention to the value which may result from identification of intermediate goals — staging posts in the longer journey of treatment, each of which constitutes a significant reduction in the harm to the individual and society which results from the continued drug use. Subsequent considerations of this approach (e.g. see Strang 1990) view the overall approach within treatment as working through a cascade of processes of change, with the identification of different treatment goals towards which progress may be made either sequentially or simultaneously.

Drug-free rehabilitation programmes

During the last two decades, a number of drug-free rehabilitation houses have been set up across the UK. These may conveniently be considered in four categories:

1. 'Concept houses' such as Phoenix House, in which great emphasis is placed on the power of the peer group influence of other ex-addicts and benefits that may arise from active group and individual confrontation of the problem within a supporting and strictly hierarchical structure
2. Christian houses, in which a gentler and more explicitly supportive environment allows for the gradual recovery of the individual either within a mandatory or optional Christian faith
3. Community integrated houses, in which an attempt is made to deliver residential care to recovering ex-addicts whilst maintaining close links with the local community, and most recently
4. Residential 12-step programmes (often known as Minnesota model or Narcotics Anonymous programmes), in which the underlying strategy is a faith in the principles of Narcotics Anonymous and Alcoholics Anonymous (see Cook 1988, Wells 1988).

Self-help strategies have been extensively developed for individuals who wish to change their use of alcohol or tobacco, although as yet there has been little systematic study or development of self-help manuals for users of illicit drugs. A recent UK study found extensive evidence of previous attempts at self-detoxification amongst patients at a London drug dependence unit, with a total of 212 previous attempts at self-detoxification being reported by 50 opiate addicts. Rates of short-term success were at least comparable with the results of many treatment programmes and it is likely that there may be an unexploited reservoir of benefit in this area. An extensive network of self-help programmes for recovering heroin addicts has been established during the 1980s with the growth of Narcotics Anonymous (mainly in the London area and in a few other towns and cities which have become Narcotics Anonymous strongholds) (for a review see Wells 1988).

Specific drugs and the treatment options

Opiates

Heroin remains the most widely used opiate on the black market, although a wide range of opiates have a significant place on the black market in the UK. These include Diconal (dipipanone and cyclizine mixture), dextramoromide (Palfium) as well as prescribed and diverted supplies of methadone. All forms of opiates command some price on the black market; it is particularly injectable forms of the opiates which command the highest prices, with ampoules being most valuable, followed by tablets (which can be crushed for injection) as the next most valuable, and uninjectable linctus preparations as the least valuable on the black market. In recent years the synthetic opioid buprenorphine (Temgesic) has been widely abused, with the sublingual tablets being frequently injected: the extent to which this has occurred has varied greatly from one city to the next, with Edinburgh and Glasgow being cities where abuse of buprenorphine was said to have become more widespread than abuse of heroin during the early 1990s. After repeated use of the opiates, the individual will become both physically and psychologically dependent on the drug, so that abrupt cessation of intake will result in a classic opiate withdrawal syndrome. The features of the withdrawal syndrome are broadly similar across all the natural and synthetic opiates, although the time-course of the withdrawal syndrome varies according to the duration of action of the particular opiate. For example, the heroin withdrawal syndrome is characterised by the development of abdominal cramps, nausea, diarrhoea, goose flesh, sweating, sleeplessness, irritability, rhinorrhoea, excessive lachrymation and uncontrollable yawning; and the severity of the withdrawal syndrome increases up to a peak at about 36–48 hours, following which there is a gradual decline in severity of symptomatology down to a baseline level of distress during the protracted withdrawal syndrome.

One of the distinctive trends within heroin use in the UK (and in several other countries in Europe) has been the increased variety of methods and routes of administration of the drug. During the late 1970s there was a brief fashion of taking heroin by snorting; but by the early 1980s this had been largely replaced by 'chasing the dragon', in which the heroin is heated on metal foil until it melts, runs and then sublimates so that it may be inhaled as it coils off the foil. Chasing the dragon is now a major route of administration of heroin in several regions in the UK (e.g. London, Mersey, Glasgow) whilst it remains rarer elsewhere (e.g. Edinburgh). The extent to which heroin chasing may be a robust behaviour or is merely a precursor of heroin injecting has recently been considered (Gossop et al 1988), as has consideration of the significance of transitions between routes in both directions (Des Jarlais et al 1992).

Detoxification, at its simplest, involves an approach similar to that seen with the alcohol- and benzodiazepine-dependent patient: steadily reducing doses of substitute drugs are prescribed according to a reducing schedule with the aim of keeping levels of withdrawal distress within manageable levels. The most widely used approach with opiate withdrawal is the provision of reducing doses of oral methadone (in linctus form such as mist. methadone 1 mg/ml), which is effective at moderating the severity of the withdrawal syndrome whilst having low levels of abuse potential. Recently, there has been interest in the use of non-opiate alternatives, in particular the anti-hypertension drug clonidine (for a review see Gossop 1988), although this drug is probably unsuitable for out-patient management due to the risk of postural hypotension. Attention is now increasingly turning to elements of care other than the detoxification, such as specific relapse prevention strategies (see Marlatt & Gordon 1985, Annis 1986), or behavioural approaches to interfere with craving (Childress et al 1987, Powell et al 1991) or the more general social and occupational rehabilitation of the recovering addict (Hawkins 1979, Anglin & McGlothlin 1984).

Extended withdrawal programmes are widely applied in the management of opiate addicts, in which the rate of reduction of dose of oral methadone on an out-patient basis is slow — so that the time-course of prescribing is likely to be at least many months. Little systematic study of this widespread approach in the UK has yet been undertaken: this is surprising as the US experience of such programmes (frequently known as Maintenance To Abstinence (MTA) programmes) did not indicate that the approach was particularly efficacious. Much importance is currently placed on the value of bringing about reduction in the harmful nature of continued drug use: if this is to be identified as the legitimate therapeutic goal of this approach, it is necessary for more rigorous examination of the extent to which these hoped-for reductions in risk behaviour are achieved — and whether these reductions are durable or transient.

Maintenance methadone programmes have become a dominant feature of the response to the heroin problem in the USA, where large-scale oral methadone maintenance programmes have now been running for a quarter of a century. Such an approach has never been applied in the UK. The original practice of prescribing injectable maintenance (initially heroin and subsequently injectable methadone) fell out of favour with many doctors and clinic staff when it became evident that the rate of 'maturing out' seemed much slower than had been hoped, and perhaps the continued availability of injectable maintenence might even be acting counter to the 'maturing out' process. As fashion and peer influence swung away from long-term injectable maintenance, some practitioners and clinics moved to programmes which relied heavily on oral methadone (as either maintenence or gradual withdrawal) whilst others moved to no-prescribing policies. A controlled study comparing addicts randomly assigned to either maintenance with oral methadone or maintenance with injectable heroin found that rates of continued attendance were poorest amongst those receiving oral drugs. However, larger numbers of the oral methadone group had become drug-free during the period, even though the injectable heroin group were less likely to have suffered severe adverse consequences. The findings seemed to indicate that injectable heroin maintenance consolidated the pre-existing levels of social physical and psychopathology, whilst oral methadone maintenance was more likely to result either in improvements along these parameters or deterioration — but with no pretreatment indications of which course would be followed by which patient (Mitcheson & Hartnoll 1978, Hartnoll et al 1980).

Naltrexone is an entirely new type of treatment approach in which an orally available long-acting antagonist can be administered to the detoxified addict, so that further use of the drug is not associated with any further drug effect. Thus, the addict who 'plans' to relapse must wait 2 or 3 days for the blocking action of naltrexone to pass. It may be that this approach is particularly valuable in ex-addicts whose relapses are precipitated by crisis situations or impulsive drug use, and there is some evidence to suggest that third-person naltrexone (in which the intake of naltrexone is linked to a probation order, for example) may be particularly effective (e.g. see Brahen et al 1984).

Stimulants

Amphetamines remain the most commonly abused stimulant in the UK, despite the recent increase in the extent of use of cocaine. Both amphetamines and cocaine may be taken either by snorting (like snuff) or by intravenous injection. Additionally, cocaine hydrochloride (the typical black market white powder) may be converted into 'freebase' cocaine by a simple backroom chemistry process which removes the hydrochloride: the drug may then be smoked, in which the application of heat results in the sublimation of the drug which is then inhaled and passes rapidly from the lungs to give a rapid-onset psychoactive effect comparable to intravenous use. The use of such 'crack' cocaine has been a major problem during the last decade in the USA, although at the time of writing it remains unclear about the extent to which the US problem will be transposed unaltered to a UK context (for a contemporary review, see Strang et al 1992). Recent reports from Hawaii and elsewhere in the USA draw attention to the possibility of a similar development with amphetamines, with adaptation of methylamphetamine to form a smokeable form, known as 'ice'.

At high doses both amphetamines and cocaine may result in amphetamine psychosis, in which paranoia and persecutory delusions may occur in clear consciousness, alongside ideas of reference and auditory or visual hallucinations. These will recover spontaneously with sedation and rest, and will not recur in the absence of further high-dose use of the drug. The differential diagnosis is schizophrenia, from which differentiation is difficult if the history of drug abuse is not known: urine analysis on admission is an invaluable aid to diagnosis and, in the presence of a negative urine result, abuse of amphetamines is not the cause of the psychosis.

Traditionally, management of the stimulant withdrawal syndrome has been entirely symptomatic. However, in recent years work has been undertaken on the acute management of the cocaine withdrawal syndrome with tricyclic antidepressants — in particular desipramine. It is postulated that desipramine exerts a moderating effect on the acute cocaine withdrawal syndrome via a different mechanism from its antidepressant effect (Gawin 1986). Some practitioners continue to prescribe desipramine beyond the immediate withdrawal phase in the hope of reducing the likelihood of postwithdrawal depression.

Cue exposure and response prevention methods (as described briefly in the section of opiates) have also been applied in recent years to the management of cocaine addiction and O'Brien and colleagues report more value and greater success with this approach in treatment of cocaine addiction than with opiate addiction (O'Brien & Childress 1991).

Hypnotics and tranquillisers

The clinical effects and syndromes of central nervous system depressants such as barbiturates and benzodiazepines are similar to those of alcohol. Intravenous barbiturate abuse is now rare, and is an example of a drug epidemic which largely passed by the early 1980s after several years of high morbidity and mortality. A particularly disturbing feature was the rapid development of dependence on the drug; and the slowness with which tolerance developed to the effect of respiratory depression whilst tolerance to the psychoactive effect developed rapidly — so that the dependent barbiturate injector would increase the dose to obtain the psychoactive effect to a point where the therapeutic margin of safety became dangerously narrow.

During the latter part of the 1980s, the intravenous abuse of benzodiazepines (almost exclusively temazepam gel capsules) became more widespread (see Hamersley et al 1989, Farrell & Strang 1989) and it may be that some of the particular problems associated with high-dose intravenous abuse of barbiturates may be recreated in a new generation of intravenous benzodiazepine abusers.

Adolescents may abuse sedatives such as benzodiazepines in order to enhance the disinhibiting and relaxed effect of alcohol — either in addition to or as a replacement for alcohol. Burr (1984) has described how use of such sedative drugs represents a deliberate choice by some groups, such as the choice of barbiturates by punks and skinheads who were attracted to the nihilistic properties of the drug.

Iatrogenic benzodiazepine dependence is extremely widespread, with an estimated 2 million adults taking benzodiazepines each day in the UK. Withdrawal symptoms are diverse (see Ashton 1987, Lader 1989), and may have a superficial similarity to the anxiety state for which they were originally prescribed. One of the diagnostic challenges is to identify the extent to which continued pathology relates to the persistence of the original psychopathology or the side-effects of treatment. Increased sensory arousal, photophobia, headaches, paraesthesiae, muscle spasms, vertigo, disturbed sleep, and gastrointestinal upsets are all described. Symptoms may persist for months or even years after withdrawal from benzodiazepines. Abrupt withdrawal may precipitate fits or confusional states: consequently, a gradual reduction regime is necessary — especially in cases of severe and high-dose dependence. Frequently, the rate of withdrawal is titrated against the patient's response and will often take at least 4 weeks (for further details, see Higgitt et al 1985). Regular support and reassurance are essential during the withdrawal phase, and self-help groups are becoming increasingly common and provide a useful source of additional support.

Hallucinogens (including LSD and 'ecstasy')

LSD (lysergic acid diethylamide) is undoubtably the most famous synthetic hallucinogen and is widely abused in the UK. There is also extensive seasonal use of 'magic mushrooms' (*Psilocybe semilanceata* — 'liberty caps') which grow across most of the UK in the early Autumn. These hallucinogens are taken specifically for the effect they have on perception and mental events. The subject may seek treatment after experiencing a 'bad trip', in which intake of a regular dose results in perceptual distortions, visual hallucinations and intense emotions of a frightening and unpleasant nature — in contrast to the usual 'good trip'. At such a time the threat and distress are very real to the user and there is a risk of attempted suicide. Codes of practice frequently develop amongst drug users, with caution against solitary use of LSD, so as to ensure that a friend is on hand to provide reassurance and a link to reality (as well as a link to back-up services) in the event of an unanticipated bad trip. A minor tranquilliser may be useful to allay panic and to await spontaneous recovery. There have been anecdotal reports of aggravation of the phenomena by the administration of phenothiazines.

Long after the use of the drug the user may experience a 'flashback' — a recurrence of part or all of the original LSD experience. This may occur months or years after the original use of the drug and is frequently characterised by distress associated with the phenomenon, which in many ways is similar to a panic attack. Such flashbacks pass within minutes or at most a few hours and rarely require pharmacotherapy.

Recently, a synthetic amphetamine analogue (MDMA, 'ecstasy') has become available and is used for its mixed stimulant/hallucinogenic effects. Consideration of the presenting features and management of use of this drug should be guided by joint consideration of management of both amphetamines and the hallucinogens. (For further detail of this and other hallucinogens see Strang & Shapiro (1991).)

Cannabis

Cannabis is the most widely used illicit drug in the UK. Smoking is the most frequent method of use and may involve either smoking a mixture of tobacco with the dried leaves (marijuana) or with the resin (hashish, hash). The main active constituent is Δ^9-tetrahydrocannabinol (Δ^9-THC).

The effects of cannabis depend greatly on the circumstances in which it is taken, on the user's expectations of the drug effect, and on previous experience with the drug. (For further descriptions, see Johnson (1991).)

Effects on motor performance. These have been studied in simulated driving situations (e.g. see Rafaelson et al 1973, Hindmarch 1980, also reviewed by Chesher 1985) and in simulated air pilot flying situations (Blaine et al 1976, Janowsky et al 1976, Yesavage et al 1985), and use of cannabis is found to have a pronounced effect on estimations of time and distance, and impairment of attention and short-term memory; and these effects are still well discernible 24–48 hours after use of the drug.

Short-term adverse reactions. These include anxiety states and panic attacks which are apparently brought on by the episode of use of cannabis — especially in novice users. Panic attacks certainly occur even in the absence of prior psychopathology, but are time limited (Pillard 1970).

Short-term psychotic reactions. Although such reactions may occur, it remains unclear whether there is a risk of development of such acute reactions in all cannabis smokers or whether there are individuals who are at particular risk. Anxiety, depersonalisation and confusion are often prominent features (Tennant & Groesbeck 1972). Seizures have been reported in individuals with pre-established epilepsy (Feeney 1977). In general, the condition is adequately treated by general measures and by reassurance, although on occasions antipsychotic medication may briefly be required.

Chronic psychosis. A causal link between cannabis use and chronic psychotic illness has been postulated, but the evidence remains inconclusive and unsubstantiated (Edwards 1976). Use of cannabis has also been identified as a precipitating factor with recurrence of psychosis in schizophrenics (Treffert 1978) and the recurrence of dysphoric reactions in depressed patients (Ablon & Goodwin 1974). There have also been descriptions of a specific 'amotivational syndrome' resulting from long-term exposure to cannabis, with apathy, loss of effectiveness and reduced drive and ambition as prominent features (McGlothlin & West 1968). Although major reviews have cast doubt on the likely causal relationship between the drug and clinical syndromes (Graham 1977, Ghodse 1981), the concept of the 'burnt out' chronic cannabis smoker lives on in both the general public and amongst drug users themselves.

Other drugs

Many other substances are also used as psychoactive drugs and their popularity in society as a whole, and in particular amongst youth culture, will wax and wane over time. Thus, use of various volatile substances (volatile substance abuse, VSA; 'glue sniffing') came to be identified in the late 1970s and 1980s as an extensive problem amongst adolescents (Watson 1977, Black 1982), and continues to be associated with morbidity (King et al 1981, Ron 1986) and mortality (Oliver & Watson 1977). However, strategies for management include harm minimisation approaches, education about avoidance of particularly risk-laden practices (e.g. placing head in plastic bag to inhale, or solitary sniffing on canal banks or rooftops, etc.), accompanied by general measures of psychiatric care and resuscitation (ISDD 1980). Various other drugs are abused, including prescribed medications (e.g. antiparkinsonian drugs, benzodiazepines, appetite suppressants) and over-the-counter products (e.g. antihistamines, antidiarrhoea preparations, minor analgesics), for which management must similarly include reliance on general principals of prevention and treatment.

CLINICAL FEATURES AND MANAGEMENT OF PATIENTS WITH ALCOHOL-RELATED PROBLEMS AND DEPENDENCE

Identification and assessment

Alcohol may contribute to a variety of presenting complaints. The sickness certificates of people eventually diagnosed as alcohol-dependent reveal, for example, anxiety states, depression, injuries, 'gastritis', and 'debility'. The general practitioner may have been aware of frequent absences from work for minor symptoms, or stress symptoms in other members of the family.

Patients may not appreciate the contribution which alcohol makes to their presenting complaint, or deny it because of shame, or dislike or fear of being advised to abstain. They may be evasive because they are sensitised to criticism about their behaviour. Sometimes it is better to avoid focusing the whole interview on the drinking, taking instead a problem-oriented approach, beginning with trying to understand what led them to seek advice at this stage. With respect to the drinking, enquire about a recent period (e.g. the past 7 days) by asking in detail about work, leisure activities, the company kept, and the amount and type of beverage consumed. Spirits, wines and beers should be enquired into separately. Reconstruct the cues which have been important in the patient's drinking: the situations and moods that trigger drinking, the benefits that he experiences from

alcohol, and what has helped to control drinking on occasions in the past.

Severity of dependence is assessed as follows. Mildly dependent patients will regularly notice restlessness at certain times of the day or in certain situations and at these times wish to have alcohol or seek out their drinking companions. They may have tried to cut down, and have found this to be difficult. If they occasionally have very heavy sessions, they may relieve the next morning's hangover with a drink, but this will not be more than once or twice a week at most. More severely dependent patients report that the restlessness they feel without a drink is noticeable at times to colleagues or family, or prevents them from getting on with other matters. They organise their day to ensure that they are able to have a drink at times when they predict they will need one, such as the salesman who plans his morning's calls so that he is with a customer who drinks at around 11.30 a.m. when he is beginning to feel tense. There may be times when he finds himself unable to think of anything but getting a drink. Morning nausea, sweating and relief drinking may be reported for periods of many days consecutively. Insomnia becomes frequent unless late-evening intake relative to daytime drinking is very heavy. Wakefulness in the small hours of the night, like daytime tenseness and anxiety in the dependent drinker, can of course be an effect of a falling blood alcohol level. A widely used rating scale is the Severity of Alcohol Dependence Questionnaire (Stockwell et al 1979).

Adverse consequences in the areas of health, work, family, friends and the law should be explored. Excessive overall consumption may be the cause of damage to health, while drinking to intoxication is usually the cause of social problems. These aspects of drinking may or may not be related to dependence (see Fig. 17.2).

An epileptic fit for the first time in an adult should raise the suspicion of alcohol dependence. A withdrawal fit may occur without other gross signs. Tremor of the outstretched fingers or tongue, injected conjunctivae and sclerae, stigmata of liver disease, excessive facial skin capillarisation, and alcohol on the breath are valuable clues.

The mean cell volume is raised (without anaemia) in 30–50% of patients, probably due to a direct toxic action of alcohol on the marrow. The γ-glutamyltranspeptidase and/or other liver enzymes are elevated in 60–70% of patients, due to enzyme induction and/or liver damage. A specimen for blood alcohol or a reading on a portable breathalyser may help, remembering that, roughly speaking, in a 70 kg man 1 unit of alcohol produces a peak blood alcohol concentration of 15 mg after about half an hour, and takes an hour to be metabolised.

Assessment of brain damage, important in planning future treatment, should be left until the patient has been free of alcohol for 3 weeks. It is vital that the spouse or other relatives should be interviewed, to add objectivity and to assess the quality of their relationship with the drinker. These relationships are important in predicting outcome. The spouse often feels both angry and guilty and feels relieved when these feelings are acknowledged and understood.

Great emphasis should not be put on assessing 'motivation'. A moment's introspection shows that our own motivation to change familiar habits varies greatly. Problem drinkers are no exception. On some occasions they feel strongly motivated to change their way of life, perhaps to save their job or their marriage. On other occasions the attraction of the pub, the relief from daily worries and the familiar comfort of that first drink are overwhelming. We have to work with fluctuating levels of motivation. Probably the psychiatrist's most important step is to acquire the trust of the patient and to establish an atmosphere in which frankness prevails and confrontation is seen as caring. Patients will then be able to start making decisions about themselves and their drinking.

Psychiatric complications of alcohol abuse

Delirium tremens

Although often taken as the hallmark of alcoholism, it is not a common condition, with only about 5% of alcoholics attending clinics having experienced it. It occurs when an individual who is severely dependent on alcohol stops or reduces drinking. The full syndrome is characterised by marked tremor of the limbs, body and tongue, restlessness, loss of contact with reality, disorientation and illusions progressing to terrifying hallucinations, which are most commonly visual, but may be auditory or tactile. Delusions, often of a paranoid kind, may arise out of the hallucinations. Fever, sweating and tachycardia are pronounced. The disturbance usually develops out of milder withdrawal symptoms 1 day after cessation of drinking and rarely persists for more than 4 days. Symptoms are often worse at night. There is a significant mortality in this condition (approximately 10%), partly because it often complicates other medical emergencies like appendicitis, infections or injuries. The development of fever, dehydration and signs of shock are ominous prognostic signs. It is important to remember that concomitant infection, Wernicke's encephalopathy, metabolic disturbance, hypoglycaemia, or head injury may complicate the clinical features and prognosis. Withdrawal fits may occur at any time from the first to the 14th day (Isbell et al 1955).

Admission to hospital will usually be necessary unless nursing can be arranged at home. The patient's environment should be uncluttered and uniformly lit to avoid ambiguities. Parenteral multivitamin preparations (Parentrovite) may be given, provided resuscitation equipment is available. Electrolytes and plasma glucose should be checked. An oral benzodiazepine, such as chlordiazepoxide, starting at 100–150 mg/day and reducing after the second or third day, will usually be sufficient to contain the patient's agitation. It is important that the dosage should be progressively reduced, and should not be continued after, at most, 14 days.

Alcoholic hallucinosis

As well as in delirium tremens, hallucinations in alcohol dependents may occur in clear consciousness. Sometimes these are a continuation of hallucinations first experienced during withdrawal from alcohol. However, hallucinations may also start de novo in a patient who is still drinking. Usually these experiences begin as fragmentary sounds. For example:

> A woman, of previously stable personality, who had begun drinking heavily in her job as a motor trade representative and hostess, was surprised to hear the clinking of glasses and sounds of merriment from a neighbour's flat. Though the flat was in fact empty most of the time, she began to believe that continuous parties were taking place and heard people coming to and fro with bottles.

In such cases the sounds gradually become formed and voices are heard, often making unpleasant remarks: 'She ought to be ashamed of herself', 'He's a lush', etc. The voices give commands to do things against the subject's will and delusions of imagined persecutors may develop. The experiences may be very compelling and distressing, occasionally resulting in violent suicide. Visual hallucinations are a less common feature of this syndrome.

In the two large published series of cases (Bendetti 1952; Victor & Hope 1958) only a few cases (5–10%) continued to have symptoms for 6 months or more if abstinence was maintained. Renewed drinking, however, tends to bring about a return of hallucinations.

Despite the close resemblance of the hallucinations to those of acute schizophrenia, only a few go on to show typical schizophrenic deterioration (four out of 76 in Victor and Hope's series and 13 out of 113 in

Bendetti's series). Furthermore, in the initial presentation there is no disturbance of volition or experience of interference with thinking. Premorbid adjustment in the social and sexual spheres tends to be normal. A family history of schizophrenia is usually absent (Bendetti 1952) except in the cases where hallucinations persist and schizophrenic personality deterioration occurs. There is no close relationship with gross cognitive impairment, though both may be present in some patients.

Management commonly requires admission to hospital, withdrawal from alcohol and, if the hallucinations still continue, phenothiazines. It is usually possible to stop the phenothiazines after 2 or 3 months. Thereafter the patient usually has full insight into the illness and the experience may have been so frightening that he never drinks again.

The basis of alcoholic hallucinosis is presumably subtle alcohol-induced damage or dysfunction, perhaps of the temporal lobes, though this has not been formally demonstrated.

Pathological jealousy (Othello syndrome)

Firmly held delusions of infidelity are not uncommon in alcohol abuse. They may be precipitated by the patient's feeling of inadequacy stemming from alcohol-induced impotence and further aggravated by the spouse's growing indifference towards her drunken partner. The patient's accusations become repetitive and aggressive demands for proof are reinforced by violence. No amount of contrary evidence will dispel the delusion and cases sometimes end in tragic assault or murder. Alcohol abuse is not the only cause of this syndrome. Treatment is of the underlying condition. Sometimes it may be advisable for the couple to separate permanently.

Depression and alcohol

Symptoms of depression are common amongst excessive drinkers. This understandably reflects the lifestyle of dependent drinkers, who frequently wake with a hangover facing a day overshadowed by the problems caused by their drinking. Biological changes induced by excessive drinking may also contribute to depressed mood.

Alcohol abuse may mask the symptoms of depressive illness, an association commonly observed in females. Menninger (1938) described alcoholism as chronic suicide, alcoholics being in his view depressive personalities who seek temporary oblivion in drinking. Alcohol also releases inhibitions, which make it easier

to express feelings of sadness and to give way to self-destructive impulses. It is therefore hardly surprising that alcohol figures so prominently in studies of parasuicide and successful suicide. Kessel (1965) found amongst suicides that 56% of men and 23% of women were alcoholics. Factors increasing risk are previous attempts, a history of depression, evident physical and social problems, male sex and older age.

The clinician should discriminate between those patients whose alcohol abuse is symptomatic of depression and the much larger number who have become depressed because of their drinking. In the latter, improvement usually follows cessation of drinking and appropriate therapy, whereas the former may require antidepressant medication, combined with a period of abstinence.

Nakamura et al (1983) studied 88 alcoholics in a treatment programme. Although 75% had depressive symptoms at the onset, only 5% had any after 4 weeks of abstinence. Depression is a primary factor in a relatively small number of alcohol-dependent individuals. This is more commonly the case in women.

There is now believed to be no genetic link between affective disorder and alcoholism (Schuckit 1986).

Cognitive impairment and brain damage

Some 50–60% of alcoholics presenting to psychiatrists perform worse on cognitive testing than would be predicted from their verbal intelligence, educational level and age. There is: impairment of memory, visual more than verbal; narrowing and rigidity of thought processes, i.e. difficulty changing from one way of construing and categorising to another; difficulty learning new material; and impairment of visuospatial and visuoperceptive skills. Heavy alcohol consumption, particularly heavy consumption on single occasions, is the main cause, although malnutrition and folate and vitamin deficiency play a part (Guthrie & Elliot 1980). That some of these deficits might predate the heavy drinking has support from cognitive research in sons of alcoholics and in the accounts that alcoholics give of their patterns of behaviour when they were children. But in monozygotic twins discordant for alcohol dependence, there is also discordance for cognitive deficits, emphasising the effect of the heavy drinking itself (Gurling et al 1991). There is also improvement of many cognitive deficits with long-term abstinence. Social functioning is of paramount importance and good outcome has been observed in abstinent alcoholics despite significant impairment on formal testing (Lennane 1988).

Imaging techniques show cortical atrophy and

ventricular enlargement in 50–70% of admissions for alcohol dependence. There are modest correlations between atrophy and cognitive impairment. Magnetic resonance imaging, T_1 relaxation time and brain density measured during computerised tomography are altered in proportion to lifetime consumption (Chick et al 1989). The shrinkage is mainly in white matter. In liver cirrhosis, hepatic encephalopathy is an additional factor. Repeated head injury further complicates the clinical picture. Cognitive impairment occurs in females after a shorter duration and lower alcohol consumption than in men.

Cognitive functioning improves most in the first few days after detoxification and in many cases continues to improve for at least a year, if further drinking is avoided. It is prudent to give thiamine-containing vitamin supplements for at least 4 months. Small bowel malabsorption, in addition to poor intake and excessive utilisation, contributes to vitamin deficiency in alcoholics. Since this may take some weeks to recover, parenteral vitamins despite their small risk of allergic reaction are necessary initially. (For further reading, see US Department of Health and Human Services (1990).)

Korsakoff's psychosis

This late consequence of alcoholism is characterised by impairment of short-term memory with a tendency to confabulate. Although these are the classic features which, along with peripheral neuropathy, first attracted the attention of the Russian pathologist Korsakoff to the condition and led him to link it to alcoholism, the defects are less clear cut than at one time thought and a wide range of other memory and cognitive defects may be also present. Total recovery, even after abstinence and treatment with thiamine, is rare but gradual improvement is often observed over many months. Observed pathological changes are chiefly necrosis and gliosis in the mamillary bodies.

Physical complications of alcohol abuse

Cancer (oesophageal and oropharyngeal), cardiovascular disease, cirrhosis, pancreatic and gastrointestinal disease, accidental death and suicide all contribute to the raised mortality amongst excessive drinkers (see also the section on epidemiology).

Gastrointestinal complications

Gastritis, presenting as upper abdominal pain and haematemesis, perhaps accompanied with acute gastric erosions, is very often related to alcohol. However, peptic ulcer, though it occurs in 10% of alcoholics, is as common in the general population, so it is unlikely that alcohol is a cause. Alcohol nevertheless provokes the symptoms of an ulcer and probably delays healing. Severe diarrhoea sometimes occurs in excessive drinkers and small bowel damage leading to malabsorption exacerbates dietary vitamin deficiency. Chronic relapsing pancreatitis is characterised by recurring acute abdominal pain with inflammation, fibrosis and, eventually, calcification of the pancreas. It is usually associated with an alcohol intake of over 20 units per day. A protein-deficient diet and hyperlipidaemia are believed to contribute.

Deaths from cancer of the mouth, pharynx, oesophagus and liver are elevated in heavy drinkers. Some, but not all, studies have also found a relationship between alcohol and cancer of the pancreas and rectum.

Alcohol and liver disease

Over 90% of ingested alcohol is converted by an obligatory oxidative process in the hepatocytes to acetaldehyde, thence to acetate and finally to carbon dioxide and water. The redox state of the cell is altered with wide-ranging potential effects on fat, carbohydrate and nitrogen metabolism. Fat deposition in liver cells (steatosis) almost invariably accompanies heavy drinking and may be present even though liver function tests are normal. Less fortunate drinkers go on to develop hepatitis or cirrhosis. Cirrhosis of the liver is nowadays amongst the five commonest causes of death in those under 60 years of age in most industrial countries.

Liver injury is related to volume and duration of alcohol consumption and not to type of beverage. The fact that wine-drinking nations such as France, Italy or Portugal have the highest cirrhosis rates is because they have the highest per capita consumption of alcohol. Cirrhosis can be induced in the individual who has drunk moderately for years and then rapidly escalates consumption for 1 or 2 years. Women are more vulnerable than men and there are indications that progression to cirrhosis depends on immune responses and also, from studies of the human leucocyte antigen system, that heredity contributes.

Modern treatments, despite being expensive, do not appear to have been very successful in reversing the complications of cirrhosis (hepatic failure, variceal bleeding, ascites and primary liver cancer) and there have not been improvements in recent years in the survival of patients with alcoholic cirrhosis. About one-third of patients will still be alive after 5 years, though with abstinence the survival rate doubles, so that those with compensated cirrhosis at presentation have a 90% 5-year survival (Saunders et al 1981).

Death from variceal haemorrhage and hepatic or renal failure may also result from alcoholic hepatitis in the absence of cirrhosis.

Metabolic complications

Life-threatening hypoglycaemia occasionally follows 6–8 hours after heavy alcohol consumption in previously fasting individuals. It may follow imperceptibly from alcoholic stupor. Treatment is urgent intravenous glucose. Insulin-dependent diabetics who ingest moderate to large amounts of alcohol with little carbohydrate may become hypoglycaemic, as may well-fed normal subjects who undertake vigorous exercise in the cold. Chronic alcoholics are prone to reactive hypoglycaemia following a carbohydrate-rich meal, perhaps related to their known accelerated gastric emptying.

A condition closely resembling Cushing's syndrome sometimes occurs in alcoholics. It remits spontaneously over 1–3 weeks.

Acute renal failure after a beer-drinking binge has been reported in Britain and several other countries.

Cardiovascular disease

Drinking 1–3 units per day is associated with reduced risk of coronary disease, and the reasons for this are debated (see p.365). Heavier consumption is related to increased morbidity and mortality from this cause. Drinking more than 6 units per day is associated with rising blood pressure and an increased risk of cerebrovascular accidents.

Alcohol is a cause of supraventricular arrhythmias, and of cardiomyopathy leading to congestive cardiac failure.

Sexual impairment

High blood alcohol levels impair penile erection by a direct pharmacological effect. Heavy drinkers who repeatedly fail to maintain an erection become anxious about their sexual performance, which itself leads to further failure. Alcohol also has direct toxic effects on the Leydig cells of the testis, resulting in reduced testosterone production, impaired spermatogenesis and testicular atrophy.

Fetal alcohol syndrome

This syndrome has been observed in children born to mothers who have severe alcohol problems. It is characterised by developmental and growth retardation, facial abnormalities and neurological abnormalities. Lesser degrees of the syndrome have been observed after moderate consumption. It may be that there are critical developmental stages when alcohol is most likely to do damage. It is also likely that other drugs used, particularly smoking (Plant 1987), are confounding factors.

Forrest et al (1991) could not detect any effect of moderate maternal consumption on the development of their offspring at 18 months and concluded that pregnant mothers could safely consume 70–85 g of alcohol per week. Women are now advised either to abstain or confine their drinking during pregnancy to one or two drinks once or twice a week.

Neurological complications

The triad of confusion, ataxia and ocular palsy known as Wernicke's encephalopathy was described by Wernicke in 1881. Patients dying of this condition show haemorrhages in the brain stem and hypothalamus. Identical lesions have been produced in thiamine-deficient animals. The condition responds to urgent treatment with intravenous thiamine and withdrawal of alcohol, but even with such measures there is often a residual dementia or Korsakoff psychosis (Victor et al 1971).

Disturbance of consciousness in the alcoholic must also raise the suspicion of traumatic subdural haematoma, though unilateral signs will then probably be present. Cognitive impairment is described above. Occasionally dementia is marked and accompanied initially by incontinence, generalised weakness, tremor persisting long after withdrawal from alcohol, slurred speech and ataxia. Alcoholic cerebellar degeneration presents as ataxia of stance and gait.

Polyneuropathy, contributed to by vitamin deficiency, is common in alcoholics in at least a mild form, with asymptomatic absence of ankle jerks and calf tenderness. In the established condition the patient complains of muscular cramps and unpleasant paraesthesiae in the feet and calves and unsteadiness of gait. All forms of sensation are impaired in a stocking distribution. Flaccid weakness in the limbs may progress to wrist drop. The cranial nerves are spared. Incontinence, if admitted to, is usually not due to nerve damage but to intoxication to the point of stupor.

Alcoholic myopathy presents as chronic weakness with wasting, punctuated by exacerbation during bouts of drinking.

Alcohol-related social harm

As alcohol comes to play an increasingly salient part in the drinker's life, he often experiences a number of distressing social consequences. Frequently these have their first impact on family and work. Most of the social disabilities which arise are easier to list than quantify. They include those discussed below.

Disruption of family relationships.

Alcohol abuse contributes to as many as one-third of divorces, and various forms of domestic suffering and violence are commonplace. The relatives of the problem drinker may pass through stages of anguish and frustration as they struggle, sometimes fruitlessly, to bring about change in the drinker. The drinker breaks promises and perhaps lies. Disappointments may lead to depression in the parent, child or spouse, or to a numbed state in which the drinker is disowned. The children of problem drinkers are specifically at risk of developing behaviour problems and alcohol problems later in life. A fellowship of support groups formed by adult children of alcoholics has been prominent in the USA in recent years.

Economic factors

Alcohol is expensive and the family budget suffers accordingly. Earning power is usually reduced, which compounds the disability. Debts may accumulate. The quality of accommodation which he can sustain may decline, leading to homelessness.

Employment problems

Alcoholic employees usually develop a poor work record with frequent absences due to sickness, erratic time-keeping, low productivity and a greatly increased risk of accidents, involving both themselves and others. The cost of all this to the employer has persuaded many companies to set up programmes to encourage employees with drinking problems to seek early treatment (see below).

Crime

As many as 60% of prisoners report significant alcohol problems. Heather (1981) found 15% of young offenders physically dependent on alcohol and a further 48% had alcohol problems. Young offenders whose crimes are alcohol related have been shown to benefit from attendance at alcohol education courses designed to promote sensible drinking practices (Baldwin 1991).

Although it affects a different social stratum, drink–driving offences are common amongst dependent drinkers. One in three of all drivers killed have more than the legal limit of alcohol in their blood. Offenders whose blood alcohol is found to be exceptionally high (over 150 mg%), or who have previous drink–driving convictions, are likely to be alcohol–dependent. Many drink-driving offenders have an elevated serum γ-glutamyltranspeptidase level, indicating that they are regular heavy drinkers. Conversely, drink–driving offences are common in patients with other alcohol-related problems.

Drunkenness offences

The majority of men and women charged by the police with drunkenness offences have been shown to be alcohol-dependent, and 60% are homeless or living in hostels. The *Report on the Habitual Drunken Offender* (Home Office 1974) recognised that processing these unfortunate people through the courts was wasteful and even dangerous, as alcoholics sometimes died in police custody. Concern about the 'revolving door' for these habitual offenders passing in and out of the penal system gave rise to a number of alternative approaches. In some countries such as Finland, parts of Canada and the USA, public drunkenness was decriminalised, while in Britain the approach has been to divert the habitual drunken offender out of the courts into a medicosocial system. The Criminal Justice Acts in both England and Wales and Scotland now allow the police to take a man charged with simple drunkenness to a 'designated place' for detoxification and rehabilitation. Very few of these places exist in Britain. It has been shown that severe withdrawal symptoms are rare and that non-medical detoxification is often sufficient, providing nursing and medical help is available to the 5% who become seriously disturbed. Many of these men and a few women are homeless and socially deteriorated. Their primary needs are often to use the detoxification service as an entrée to a more stable lifestyle (Orford & Wawman 1986). Policy in Britain has recently moved away from detoxification towards police cautioning, which takes no account of rehabilitation.

Vicious circles

The problems discussed above may create a misleading sense of a number of discrete social disabilities, whereas in most cases they are interrelated. It is helpful to think of a number of 'vicious circles' which interconnect. For example, drinkers' debts may be the focus of domestic rows which provoke assault, arrest and marital breakdown. The problem drinker then finds himself unemployed, divorced and living alone in a hostel with other who drink heavily, and so on. The circularity of social disability is replicated in worsening physical problems and personality deterioration. In Britain the social cost of alcohol misuse was estimated as £1846 million a year at 1985 prices — this figure included the costs to industry and the Health Service, damage due to road traffic accidents and the cost of criminal activities (Maynard et al 1987).

Psychiatric responses to alcohol-related problems

General principles

1. *Exploit the moment of decision.* The patient has made the decision to seek advice but this is rarely securely founded. At first it is often fleeting and characterised by ambivalence about change. The psychiatrist can help him be clear about reasons for changing, for example by drawing up a balance sheet of the benefits versus the harm of drinking in this way. (This avoids a fruitless argument about whether or not he is 'an alcoholic'.) The psychiatrist helps the patient complete a balance sheet by explaining the physiology of symptoms that may be due to physical dependence and the role of alcohol in other presenting symptoms, be it sleep disturbance, tension, depression or family disharmony. The status and role of a physician is a powerful persuasive force. Often, patients respond to a more Socratic, less directive, interview style (motivational interviewing) which results in the patient arguing their own case for a change in drinking habits (Miller 1983).

2. *Set goals.* Goals should be detailed, attainable, short-term, immediately rewarding and ones which the patients defines. For example: no alcohol for 4 weeks; rewards — better physical health and a better family atmosphere. Abstinence is often immediately rewarding and is an easier target for many than reduction of drinking. However, some see abstinence as totally inappropriate. For them a goal might be: reduce intake by half; or reduce γ–glutamyltranspeptidase to below 50 units, when the reward is the satisfaction of watching the abnormal blood result improve over the next 2 or 3 months.

3. *Involve the family.* Family distress is common and advice on being firm with the drinker, not entering into fruitless struggles, but remaining caring and positive, may be necessary. Without information from those near at hand, the clinician may not get the full picture from the patient.

4. *Enhance self-esteem.* Often patients feel powerless to change their lives. The doctor should convey hope and encourage patients to believe in their own ability to change things. Help them to recognise their own strengths.

5. *Review impediments* that the patient may meet in sticking to decisions, such as former cues and triggers to drinking. Such cues may be subjective, for instance the feelings of anxiety or depression which experience suggests will be relieved by a drink, or external, like the atmosphere among friends in the pub in which it is so tempting to accept just a single pint. Encourage substitute activities.

6. *Identify associated conditions* such as depressive illness or phobias that might respond to specific treatment.

7. *Consider other agencies* such as voluntary councils on alcohol which may provide a counselling service or a social programme, such as Alcoholics Anonymous (see below), or hostels for recovering alcoholics.

8. *Follow-up.* Active follow-up is one of the ingredients of successful treatment. Relapse is common in the first 6–12 months after treatment. Brief but regular appointments are for the following: to remind the patient of goals; to give encouragement and praise; perhaps to repeat a blood test for blood alcohol, mean corpuscular volume or serum γ–glutamyltranspeptidase. It is important to be prepared to confront the patients when necessary and risk anger, while at the same time offering continued support. The spouse should usually be encouraged to attend follow-up sessions. Relapse, if and when it occurs should be viewed as an opportunity for further learning, not as an irrevocable catastrophe.

Close study of the precipitants of relapse shows that they have a lot in common across a range of addictions. Marlatt & Gordon (1984) analysed 311 relapses amongst patients with a variety of addictive behaviours (problem drinking, smoking, heroin addiction, gambling and overeating). They identified three high-risk situations which accounted for three-quarters of all relapses: negative emotional states, interpersonal conflicts and social pressure. Litman and colleagues (1983), in a study of 256 hospitalised alcoholics, found that unpleasant mood states, external events and euphoria, and lessened cognitive vigilance commonly presaged relapse. In therapy, the patient should learn to identify cues to relapse and develop strategies for handling them.

9. *Faith and hope.* Faith in the therapist, faith in the treatment, and the warmth, empathy and authenticity displayed by the therapist have often been termed non-specific ingredients of therapy. In the treatment of smokers by the specific techniques of rapid smoking (puffing cigarettes every 6 seconds, until the subject can take no more and feels sick), the success rate after 3 months of treatment was 6% for a 'cold' therapist and 72% for a 'warm' therapist who gave encouragement, communicated enthusiasm and talked about his own experience of giving up and his success with the treatment.

In a 2 year follow-up study of out-patient treatment of problem drinkers, low-empathy therapists were associated with the same or even a worse outcome compared to patients given a booklet only, while high-empathy therapists improved on the booklet-only outcome (Miller & Baca 1983). Non-specific factors in therapy need to be transformed into clearly defined specifics.

Medical aspects of treatment

Medication to minimise withdrawal symptoms makes stopping drinking easier, but is only essential when delirium threatens or there is a history of fits. A long-acting benzodiazepine such as chlordiazepoxide (starting at 80–100 mg/day and reducing to nil over 5–7 days) is usually adequate. It should not be continued for more than 14 days at the most. If there is a history of fits, greater initial doses of the benzodiazepine should be given. Chlormethiazole is probably more addictive than long-term benzodiazepines. Fatal alcohol/chlormethiazole interactions have occurred. Chlorpromazine is less effective and may increase the risk of withdrawal fits. When the patient is reasonably well intentioned and there is someone at home, or a nurse or family doctor who can call, where there is no history of fits and no confusion, withdrawal can be undertaken at home (Stockwell 1987). The patient is advised to take time off work, to rest, and to drink fruit juices and other soft drinks, but avoid large quantities of caffeine-containing tea and coffee.

In view of the frequency of cognitive impairment in heavy drinkers and its probable relation to vitamin depletion, vitamin supplements should be given to most patients and, in cases whom cognitive impairment or neuropathy is clinically demonstrable, for several months.

Drug treatments

There has been understandable resistance to the use of psychotropic drugs in the treatment of alcohol problems; one of the reasons for this is concern that individuals who have abused alcohol as a means of coping with life are very likely to become reliant on any other drug offered as a substitute. The addictive properties of many of the tranquillisers used in detoxification have been a further deterrent. Nonetheless, drug treatments of various kinds do seem to have a significant place in the management of alcohol problems. Drugs which have specific effects on neurotransmitters have been shown to reduce alcohol consumption in animal experiments. Serotonin re-uptake inhibitors are being actively investigated in clinical populations. Drugs such as these have been described as effect-altering drugs, reducing the reinforcing properties of alcohol. Further research into appetitive mechanisms seems likely to lead to new pharmacological treatments for drug and alcohol dependence (Meyer 1989, Liebowitz et al 1990).

Antidepressant and other antipsychotic medication are of benefit to those problem drinkers who have associated psychiatric disorders.

Disulfiram (Antabuse) (200–400 mg/day) is a useful adjunct in the follow-up phase until a new lifestyle has developed. After disulfiram has been taken in a sufficient dosage over several days, consumption of alcohol leads to an extremely unpleasant reaction of flushing, headache, nausea, tachycardia, laboured breathing and hypotension. Patients who realise they need to abstain are glad to take disulfiram as an insurance that they will not drink, and may report that knowing that they cannot drink stops all craving. Disulfiram's actions lasts for a variable number of days after the last dose. When doses over 500 mg/day have been used, the hypotensive reaction with alcohol can be dangerous. Tiredness and halitosis are sometimes noted, although other side-effects only occur at the same rate as with placebos. Reversible neuropathies and confusional states have been reported. It should not be given to patients with recent heart disease, suicidal impulses or who are taking potent hypotensive drugs; and it should be used with caution if liver disease is marked. To ensure success, the patient will often agree to the nomination of a supervisor, for example the spouse, the clinic or, in cases with employment problems, a representative of the employer. These measures improve compliance. The supervisor ensures that the compound is dispersed in water and swallowed.

Social skills training

Many excessive drinkers are influenced by social cues. Many report that they feel deficient in social skills. Refusing drinks, buying non-alcoholic drinks, applying for jobs, being firm with subordinates, expressing affection to loved ones and expressing annoyance without being insulting are some of the items of interpersonal behaviour that alcoholics find it useful to role play in social skills training groups.

Identifying triggers to drinking and learning new methods to cope with such triggers are common parts of these behaviour-based programmes.

Group therapy

The comradeship of others who have similar difficulties greatly enhances the self-esteem of some alcoholics. Participating in treatment in a group carries other advantages. Fellow problem drinkers are quick to expose the rationalisations and self-deception of their peers, but often do so most sympathetically and with great tolerance. If a member recommences drinking, it can be difficult to retain him in the group;

but others will be able to empathise with his once again turning to alcohol as a response to, for example, rejection or disappointment.

Conjoint and family therapy (see also Ch. 40)

Cohesiveness of marriage and family life is a predictor of recovery (Orford & Edwards 1977). Bitterness, mistrust and fear in the spouse and children may take many months to subside even when the patient has achieved abstinence. Family interviews enable members to have their views heard, without the discussion spiralling into denials, accusations and counter-accusations. The patient can be helped to see that family members are bound to feel hesitant at first but that this need not imply that they do not care or appreciate the efforts that are being made. The man who has opted out of married and family life, or who has gradually been extruded because of his drinking, may suddenly want to resume his roles of husband and father, ignoring the fact that others in the family now have their own way of doing things (Chick & Chick 1992).

Other members of the family sometimes fear that

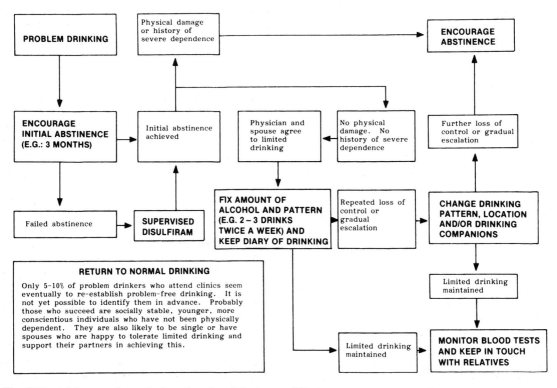

Fig. 17.3 Advice to patients who have found total abstinence difficult.

the therapist is going to blame them for the patient's drinking and so refuse to be involved in discussions. The psychiatrist's invitation to them might be 'to hear their views of how things have been, and to have their opinions on how X can best be helped'.

To drink or not to drink

The best advice to all who have sustained physical damage from alcohol or who have been physically dependent, and to patients aged 40 years and over, is lifetime abstinence. However, in young people, particularly those who have not been severely physically dependent, return to limited drinking after a few months of abstinence is sometimes appropriate. Therapist and patient can work out appropriate strategies together (Fig. 17.3): stick to drinks that are low in alcohol (e.g. lager at 3% rather than beer at 4%, or low-alcohol beers); avoid buying rounds; intersperse drinks with non-alcoholic drinks; go to the pub at 9.30 p.m. instead of 7.00 p.m.; sip rather than gulp; no lunch-time drinking; eat while drinking; completely avoid situations or company where heavy drinking is likely; set a limit (e.g. never more than 6 units per day). Keeping a daily record of consumption sometimes helps (Heather & Robertson 1981). Controlled studies on clinic attenders aimed at demonstrating the efficacy of controlled drinking training are few and in need of replication (Chick 1986).

Specialist services

Units for the treatment of alcohol problems.

These units offer a specialised service in most regions of Britain. They have a responsibility for treatment, training and research, and facilities of a similar kind are to be found in many parts of the industrial world. Traditionally, they have offered in-patient treatment of 6–8 weeks in duration with an emphasis on group psychotherapy. In recent years there has been a shift away from this devotion to in-patient treatment towards offering out-patient therapy combined with brief in-patient or day patient treatment. In response to evaluation studies which have cast doubts on the importance of very intensive forms of therapy, these units have become more flexible, offering a range of approaches, including behaviour therapy, marital and family therapy as well as more familiar group and individual psychotherapy.

Glaser (1980) has criticised the tendency for specialist services to act as if the alcoholic population were homogeneous and to offer a single form of treatment for all. He has proposed a careful assessment of each patient's needs and matching these to range of treatment options (US Department of Health and Human Services 1990).

Councils on alcohol and alcohol advice centres

Many developed countries now have counselling services separate from psychiatric or medical clinics. Problem drinkers or their families may initiate the contact and referrals will be accepted from doctors. In some countries drink–driving offenders will be directed by the court to seek help from these or other agencies.

Employment policies

Employers who are prepared to face the issue of drinking problems amongst their workforce may arrange with their employees and trade unions for affected employees to be encouraged to seek help at an early stage. Such firms usually realise the cost to the industry of absenteeism, accidents and inefficiency due to alcohol. When drinking has led to a breach of work regulations, the employee may be offered the opportunity of attending a treatment service rather than facing dismissal. The outcome of problem drinkers identified and treated in the work context tends to be good.

Alcoholics Anonymous (AA)

Since the meeting of its two founder members, Dr Bob and Bill W. in Akron, Ohio, in 1935, AA has spread to most countries of the world. It grew particularly in the 1960s and 1970s in the USA and the UK, and is currently growing at a rate of 15% per annum. Members meet regularly and share a common faith that, as alcoholics, they are powerless where alcohol is concerned and that total abstinence is the only route to recovery.

The principles on which AA was founded are open self-scrutiny, the giving of aid to others, and fellowship. The AA programme offers hope and clear, simple advice (e.g. avoid the first drink, attend meetings, take life a day at a time, 'stay sober for yourself', etc.). A prayer is said at every meeting, 'God give me the detachment to accept those things which I cannot alter; the courage to alter those things which I can alter; and the wisdom to distinguish the one from the other'. However, each member may have his own conception of God and potential affiliates should not be put off by AA's spiritual language.

AA groups usually offer to meet and introduce a new affiliate personally, though they will also make the new member welcome simply by attending the local meeting. Records are not kept and all members are anonymous. Observation shows that AA helps large numbers of regular attenders (Robinson 1979). Those most likely to adhere to AA tend to have suffered much harm from their drinking, but this is by no means always the case.

Al-Anon is a parallel organisation for the partners, relatives and friends of alcoholics, to whom it offers an opportunity for mutual support and understanding. Membership does not require the partner to attend AA or even admit he is an alcoholic. Affiliated to their organisation is Al-ateen for the teenage children of alcoholics. This offers them a chance to share some of the tensions and problems which they commonly experience.

Services for the homeless alcoholic

The homeless alcoholic usually finds abstinence unattainable unless he can be helped out of the 'skid row' environment of lodging houses or sleeping in the open. Hostels are an important part of rehabilitation. Most hostels for alcoholics require abstinence as a condition of residence, and they usually provide a therapeutic programme in which the residents help each other to find a new lifestyle. After a residence of up to 1 year, many find the transition to independent life extremely difficult and some areas provide half-way houses and supported accommodation as the next stage.

Hostels need not be the exclusive domain of the homeless. They are often valuable for alcoholics who live in unsatisfactory accommodation, or in a domestic setting which is so tense that a period of separation is a necessary prelude to a return to the family. Most hostels are managed by church or other voluntary organisations. In some cities they are also provided by the social work department.

Evaluation of treatment

During the past 20 years, there have been a large number of studies evaluating the effectiveness of treatment for alcoholism (Miller & Hester 1986, Saunders 1989). Most have shown that patient characteristics, particularly social and marital stability and, to a lesser extent, severity of dependence are better predictors of outcome than specific features of therapy. Those features of therapy which have been shown to have some importance are involvement of

spouse, community reinforcement strategies, social skills training and active follow-up.

Specific approaches for which controlled studies have demonstrated efficacy are few. Disulfiram, when dispensed by spouse as part of a contract, or by a clinic as part of an arrangement with the patient's employer, is of proven efficacy in maintaining abstinence for substantial periods (Azrin et al 1982, Chick et al 1992), reducing absenteeism at work (Robichaud et al 1979), and is also of proven value with socially deteriorated clients (Bourne et al 1966). Controlled studies of AA have not been conducted, but follow-up studies in the USA indicate strongly its value. For example, Vaillant et al (1983) followed 100 patients at regular intervals for 8 years. Of the 39 men attaining stable abstinence, two-thirds did so through AA. In the same city, 120 problem drinkers identified in the community and not at clinics, who were followed for between 10 and 30 years, yielded 34% who became stable abstainers. Of those, a third were regular AA attenders and many had commenced abstinence through that route (Vaillant & Milofsky 1982). Group treatment programmes teaching 'problem-solving' and 'social skills' (see above) proved effective in a controlled study (Chaney & O'Leary 1978) which has not yet been replicated.

There is considerable instability in the drinking status of samples of patients followed up in the first 2–4 years after commencing treatment (Polich et al 1981). Six studies have been published where follow-up was at least 8 years and objective as well as subjective data are available on outcome. A fifth of subjects died (a mortality two to three times greater than expected). Of the survivors, half to two-thirds were still in some difficulty with their drinking. Of those who were well, most were abstainers. Some 5-10% had been drinking without problems for a year or more. Whether treatment improves on the natural history of the condition over such a time span is impossible to evaluate (see above), because it is not possible or always ethical to withhold treatment. It is clear, however, from following problem drinkers identified in the community that many change their habits without professional help (Vaillant 1983).

In large samples of patients, in-patient treatment has not shown clear advantages over out-patient treatment. There have even been difficulties in demonstrating superiority of standard treatments over very brief one-session interventions, as was the case in the London study of Orford & Edwards (1977). This study randomly allocated 100 married male alcoholics to two treatment groups: one was offered intensive therapy, including admission to hospital when indicated; the other was assessed and given carefully chosen advice in a single session. The two groups were followed closely for 1 year. A total of 60% improved but no difference was found between the two groups, although 2 year follow-up suggested that severely dependent patients did better if given intensive treatment.

McLachlan & Stein (1982) compared day treatment with in-patient treatment and found no significant difference in outcome. More than a dozen controlled studies have examined the influence of duration and intensity of treatment on prognosis. With remarkable consistency these studies have failed to demonstrate any relationship (Institute of Medicine 1990). Chick et al (1988) compared very minimal treatment with a broad package of treatments, including for some in-patient and group therapy, along with a systematic follow-up for those patients who accepted it. This research showed that the stable abstinence rate was no higher after 2 years in the more intensively treated group; however, the intensive group had experienced less total problems related to their drinking than the advice only group. Before concluding that there are no advantages inherent in more intensive treatment, it is worth recording that relatively few studies have adequately characterised the clinic populations, and there are indications that more severely dependent patients do have a better outcome if offered somewhat more intensive treatment.

Such studies have cast doubt on the need for prolonged and expensive therapies for all problem drinkers and have intensified the search for careful matching of patients and resources. Relatively little is yet known about optimal matching, but alcoholics are not a homogeneous group and require a wide range of different rehabilitation strategies.

Organisation of services

Alcohol-related problems vary enormously in character and severity. An appropriate community response requires a range of services that reflects this diversity. Emphasis should be placed on early recognition and help at primary level, for instance by general practitioners, occupational health services, general hospitals and courts.

The problem drinker experiences a series of crises. For example:

Mr X regularly spent his wages on drinking with his friends. His wife consulted the Social Work Department about rent arrears and complained to the priest about her husband's behaviour. He was attending his general practitioner on account of recurrent gastritis, and repeated absences from work led to complaints from his supervisor. His daughter finally broke down at school and told the guidance teacher about the terrible conditions at home and help was obtained for the family.

This typical case illustrates the range of agencies encountered by the problem drinker. There is an opportunity for change inherent in each crisis, provided the problem is recognised and the primary level agency has received adequate training and feels competent in coping with the problem and giving advice.

Front-line services will require support from agencies, such as councils on alcohol, AA and specialised treatment units. It is generally acknowledged that the majority of alcohol problems can be managed in the community while a smaller number will require some initial residential hostel care or in-patient treatment. Community alcohol teams have evolved as a means of providing support to the primary level and linkage with specialist resources. (For a discussion see Stockwell & Clement (1987).) A comprehensive range of services will require planning coordination by health, social work and voluntary services. Their joint plan for each district should be concerned with both prevention and treatment (Faculty of Public Health Medicine 1991).

There is evidence that only 10% of alcoholics are in contact with an appropriate agency, yet they are regularly in contact with other potential care givers, as described above. The Department of Health and Social Security (1978) has recommended that 'treatment and care should be provided at a primary level' and identified the main tasks of the primary level worker as:

1. To recognise problem drinking, its causes and effects
2. To have adequate knowledge of the help required by the problem drinker and the family
3. To give this help as far as lies within their scope
4. To know where and when to seek more expert help
5. To provide continuing care and support before, during and after any period of specialist treatment
6. To provide adequate follow-up.

Primary level workers are often ill-equipped to provide this kind of service unless they received adequate training and have continuing support from a specialist team. It seems likely that the role of the specialist in alcohol problems will increasingly involve providing this kind of support. He will work with a community alcohol team in which psychiatrist, social worker, nurse and psychologist combine to form a resource for the primary level worker.

PREVENTION

Primary prevention of both drug and alcohol abuse has focused on restricting availability, or strengthening the resistance of the individual by education and persuasion. Health promotion is most effective when all sectors of government recognise its importance and give due consideration to health in the policies of departments as diverse as agriculture, trade, foreign affairs, penal policy and finance. Healthy public policy is the key to prevention (WHO 1988).

Prevention of drug abuse

The prevention report from the Advisory Council on the Misuse of Drugs (1984) identified two legitimate goals of prevention: the prevention of drug use, and the prevention of harm consequent upon drug use. Evangelical fervour surrounding anti-drugs campaigns are in danger of blinding the practitioner to the value of strategies dealing with the second goal (that of reducing harm) as well as the first goal.

Reducing harm

During the late 1980s, with increasing recognition of the risks of HIV transmission amongst drug injectors and their sexual partners, strategies for harm-minimisation were considered more actively and gained greater public and political acceptance (Buning 1990, Dorn 1990, Strang & Farrell 1991, Stimson 1992). The most publicised aspect of this approach has probably been the establishment of the original experimental needle exchange schemes (Stimson et al 1988) and the subsequent extensive expansion of this approach (Lart & Stimson 1990); whilst little attention has been paid to the adaptations in the practice of high street pharmacists, many of whom now sell needles and syringes to presumed addicts (Glanz 1990), in accordance with new advice from their professional association (Pharmaceutical Society of Great Britain 1986, National Pharmaceutical Association 1986). The adoption of a harm-minimisation perspective has implications for the practice of the general practitioner as well as the drug specialist. In different ways, both are in a position to assist in identification of valuable changes which may be made to the continued drug use (if the drug user is unable or unwilling to refrain from further drug use); and this practice may be seen as similar to other secondary prevention approaches such as advice to cigarette smokers on reducing the harm resulting from their continued smoking (e.g. switching to low-tar cigarettes, smoking less, altering the diet).

Reducing drug use

Health educators and politicians have generally been more comfortable with the more obvious goal of preventing drug use in the first instance: irrespective of the extent to which it is achievable, it is certainly politically safer. In recent years, UK national advertising campaigns have called on the expertise of the market research and advertising industry in an attempt to apply the experience of industry to this new area. Thus, the 'heroin screws you up' campaign represented an attempt to remove the glamour associated with the 'alternative' and anti-hero nature of drug use: this was perhaps achieved most effectively with the poster of the weary-looking teenage girl with mild acne above the simple message of 'skin care by heroin' — as with so much product advertising, the validity of the claim is almost irrelevant as the goal is to build up a new association in the minds of the prospective purchaser.

Secondary prevention approaches have also featured in national advertising campaigns, where particular attention has been paid to patterns of use (e.g. injecting and the sharing of equipment). Implicit in this approach is the recognition that some individuals will continue with the behaviour, but that it may be possible for them to alter the nature of their continued drug use in such a way that it constitutes less of a risk to personal and public health (e.g. by ceasing to share injecting equipment, or by moving from injecting to smoking or snorting their drugs).

Prevention of alcohol abuse

For alcohol-related problems, prevention should be better than cure because the efficacy of treatment is uncertain and the problem is endemic in most industralised countries. Unfortunately, prevention is often seen to imply prohibition and interference with the liberty of the individual.

Prevention is most efficient when a specified effect can be traced to a cause which is readily amenable to influence. For example, the association between drink–driving and road accidents is clear-cut and the 1967 legislation imposing penalties on those driving with a raised blood alcohol level had an immediate effect in reducing the number of road fatalities by 15%, although the effect diminished as drivers began to realise that the risk of detection was low. There is good evidence that the introduction of random breath testing would lead to a further decline in alcohol-related accidents.

Primary prevention in alcohol abuse relies on three

strategies: control of availability, education about sensible use, and providing alternative pursuits (Table 17.2).

These are not alternatives but approaches which are interdependent. For instance, it would be politically unwise to introduce controls which did not enjoy a measure of public acceptance, an aim which would have to be pursued first by an active public education programme. There is considerable scope for local action aimed, for instance, at licensing practices, road safety or providers of alternative leisure pursuits (Robinson et al 1989).

Controls

Prohibition is an extreme form of control. It proved effective in reducing mortality from liver cirrhosis in the USA in the 1920s, but these gains were outweighed by other social problems which arose. The limitations of prohibition and similar restrictive endeavours include the public resentment which they may generate, difficulties with enforcement, loss of tax revenue (currently over £6000 million per annum in the UK), and the growth of smuggling and illicit production of what may prove to be lethal brews. Recent experience with restrictive policies in Russia illustrates all of these issues. Most countries now endeavour to restrict rather than prohibit availability. (An exception is within Islam where cultural tradition sustains prohibition.)

Legislation restricting times of sale and the number, type and location of premises probably influences consumption, but such legislation is usually introduced at times when other attitudes are changing, making it difficult to pinpoint its effectiveness. The major restrictions on permitted hours in Britain were introduced by Lloyd George in 1915 in an effort to ensure that the workforce was sufficiently sober to meet the demands imposed by the war effort. Consumption certainly dropped at that time and remained low for more than a decade.

Most countries impose a minimum age at which young people are allowed to drink in public. Most will drink in a clandestine way before that age, but there is some evidence that the real age at which drinking commences is further reduced by lowering the permitted age. In the USA and Canada, experience has shown that states or provinces which lowered the permitted age experienced a rise in motor accidents and drink–driving offences amongst the young.

Advertisers argue that they are simply concerned with promoting or sustaining brand loyalties amongst drinkers. There is conflicting evidence about the extent to which they influence overall consumption. Research suggests that they also stimulate overall consumption (McGuiness 1980). In Britain there is now pressure from the health lobby to restrict alcohol advertising. There is already a voluntary code of practice governing the ethics of alcohol advertising, and breaches of this agreement should be referred to the Advertising Standards Authority.

Over the past 300 years, alcohol consumption in Britain has shown marked fluctuations. Every time the price of alcohol relative to disposable income has fallen, as it has almost continuously since 1945, consumption has risen. While it is simplistic to consider that price is the only important variable, an increase in the excise duty on alcohol is probably the most effective way of reducing the per capita consumption of the population. In 1981 an increase in the excise duty on beer and spirits caused their price to rise faster than the retail price index and average disposable incomes. These economic changes were associated in Edinburgh with a decline in alcohol consumption of 18% and a reduction in alcohol-related harm of 16%. Contrary to predictions, heavy

Table 17.2 Primary prevention strategy

Strategy	Method	Aim
Controls	Fiscal Legislative	To reduce availability
Education	1. The general public 2. Young people and at risk groups	Aim: to foster moderate informed drinking
Provision of alternatives	Promoting alternative leisure activities, facilitating sensible drinking, e.g. with meals, ensuring that inexpensive non- or low-alcohol beverages are readily available	Promote sensible drinking

drinkers and even dependent drinkers reported a disproportionate reduction in their consumption (Kendell et al 1983).

The health lobby is but one competing interest group in the debate about controlling the availability and consumption of alcohol. Other groups argue in favour of continuing growth in the alcohol market. There is, for instance, the employment argument (the drink trade in Britain employs 750 000 people), the desire to expand overseas trade (a viewpoint which ignores the probably harmful effect on health in developing countries), and the needs of the tourism and advertising industries.

Education

Education needs to take into account the medium, the audience and the message. In the past, education has often been woolly in focus and content, but even with carefully considered campaigns the lasting impact may be minimal (Plant et al 1979). Education in schools should recognise that children know about alcohol from the age of 6 years onwards and that their attitudes towards drinking change markedly between 11 and 14 years, as the peer group begins to exert more influence than parents or teachers. The style of presentation should be consonant with the child's developmental stage. Information about the alcohol content of various alcoholic beverages, sensible drinking practices and safe limits for consumption are facts which should be part of a young person's knowledge of the world so that his choices are well informed. Skill and confidence in coping with drinking situations should be part of education.

Public education can have a number of objectives. It can be concerned with informing the public about alcohol problems along with specific advice about where to seek help. Campaigns of this kind have not influenced drinking habits but have often produced an increase in utilisation of treatment and counselling facilities.

Other campaigns may be directed towards specific high-risk groups, for instance education for employees in the brewing trade, young males in social class V, or towards populations who are unusually vulnerable to alcohol, such as pregnant women. Television advertisers can, for example, highlight the immediate consequences of drinking too much, such as fights or embarrassment, and illustrate alternative models of moderate problem-free drinking. Recent campaigns have disseminated information about sensible drinking, along with booklets describing self-help strategies for limiting consumption.

Provision of alternatives

Many communities are heavily dependent on drinking places as a principal source of entertainment. Clearly the pub has a significant social role in its neighbourhood, but those concerned with planning should ensure that other leisure pursuits are encouraged and that non-alcoholic beverages are also readily available. The promotion of low-alcohol beers and wine has proved helpful. Alternative choices for relieving tension and facilitating social contacts can be taught, for instance relaxation training, meditation and social skills training. These alternative styles of living could be explored within schools, if the curriculum were thoughtfully redrawn.

Secondary prevention

Secondary prevention aims to prevent the further progression of a condition by identifying and treating cases at an early state. Symptom-free excessive drinkers see little reason to change their habits. However, a primary care worker, consulted perhaps for some other reason, might educate and persuade him to cut down. The general practitioner, occupational health physician, social worker, nurse and health visitor are all in a position to do this, provided they understand alcohol problems sufficiently.

Primary health care physicians can use the mean corpuscular volume (MCV) and γ-glutamyltranspeptidase in screening, since about 60% of heavy drinkers will show an elevation of one or other test (Chick et al 1981).

There are a number of questionnaires available which facilitate early recognition of hazardous drinking (Babor et al 1986). A sensible policy which would immeasurably enhance recognition would be to follow the Royal College of Physicians (1987) recommendation that every person seen in general practice or in hospital should be asked about his or her alcohol intake as a matter of routine, along with questions about smoking and medication and the answers recorded.

A number of studies have shown that simple advice given by a suitably trained doctor or nurse can produce a significant decline in hazardous drinking with demonstrable benefit to health. For example, Wallace et al (1988) randomly allocated heavy drinkers (men reporting drinking at least 35 units a week and women drinking at least 21 units) to treatment or control groups. Treatment involved simple advice from the general practitioner about reducing consumption and follow-up at 3-monthly intervals. After 1 year, 44% fewer men were drinking excessively in the treatment group compared with 26% fewer amongst controls, and 48% fewer women were drinking heavily in treatment compared with 29% in controls. Chick et al (1985) demonstrated that a significant reduction in consumption followed one session of advice and counselling given by a trained nurse to male patients in a general hospital who had been identified as drinking in a hazardous way. Self-help manuals have proven benefits (Miller & Taylor 1980) and show the importance of individuals taking responsibility for changing their habits to develop a less harmful way of drinking.

REFERENCES

Ablon S L, Goodwin F K 1974 High frequency of dysphoric reactions of tetrahydrocannabinol among depressed patients. American Journal of Psychiatry 131: 448–453

Anderson P 1987 Early intervention in general practice. In: Stockwell T, Clements S (eds) Helping the problem drinker: new initiatives in primary care. Croom Helm, London

Anderson P 1988 Excess mortality associated with alcohol consumption. British Medical Journal 297: 824–826

Andreasson S, Alleback P, Romelsjo A 1988 Alcohol and mortality among young men: longitudinal study of Swedish conscripts. British Medical Journal 296: 1021–1025

Anglin M D, McGlothlin W H 1984 Outcome of narcotics addict treatment in California. In: Tims F, Ruchman N (eds) Drug abuse treatment evaluation: strategies, progress and prospects. NIDA research monograph series. US Government Printing Office, Washington, DC

Annis H M 1986 A relapse prevention model for treatment of alcoholics. In: Miller W E, Heather N (eds) Treating addictive behaviours: processes of change. Plenum Press, New York, pp 407–434

Arroyave F, Little D, Litendia F, De Alarcon R 1973 Misuse of heroin and methadone in the city of Oxford. British Journal of Addiction 68: 129–135

Azrin N H, Sisson R W, Meyers R, Godley M 1982 Alcoholism treatments by disulfiram and community reinforcement therapy. Journal of Behavior Therapy and Experimental Psychiatry 13: 105–112

Babor T F, Ritson E B, Hodgson R J 1986 Alcohol related problems in the primary health care setting: a review of early intervention strategies. British Journal of Addiction 81: 23–46

Baldwin S 1991 Alcohol education and young offenders. Springer–Verlag, Berlin

Bandura A 1977 Self efficacy: towards a unifying theory of behavioural change. Psychological Review 84: 191–215

Begleiter H. Porjesz B 1990 Neuroelectric processes in individuals at risk for alcoholism. Alcohol and Alcoholism 25: 251–256

Bendetti G 1952 Die Alkoholhalluzinosen. Thieme, Stuttgart

Bernardi E, Jones M, Tennant C 1989 Quality of parenting in alcoholics and narcotic addicts. British Journal of Psychiatry 154: 677–682

Black D 1982 Misuse of solvents. Health Trends 14: 27–28

Blaine J D, Meecham M P, Janowsky D S et al 1976 Marijuana smoking and simulated flying performance. In: Braude M C, Szara S (eds) Pharmacology of marijuana. Raven Press, New York

Bourne P G, Alford J A, Bowcock J Z 1966 Treatment of skid row alcoholics with disulfiram. Quarterly Journal of Studies on Alcohol 27: 42–48

Bowers M B 1972 Acute psychosis induced by psychotomimetic drug abuse. Archives of General Psychiatry 27: 437

Bozarth M 1990 Drug addiction as a psychobiological process. In: Warburton D M (ed) Addiction controversies. Harwood Academic, London

Brahen L S, Henderson R K, Capone T, Kordal N 1984 Naltrexone treatment in jail work-release program. Journal of Clinical Psychiatry 49: 49

Brill L 1972 The de-addiction process. Charles C Thomas, Illinois

British Journal of Addiction 1990 A series of papers on alcohol and mortality: prospective studies British Journal of Addiction 85: 837–861

Burr A 1984 The ideology of despair: a symbolic interpretation of punks and skinheads usage of barbiturates. Social Science and Medicine 19: 929–938

Buydens-Branchey L, Branchey M H, Noumair D, Lieber C S 1989 Age of alcoholism onset: relationship to serotonin precursor availability. Archives of General Psychiatry 46: 231–236

Cahal D A 1974 Misuse of drug regulations. British Medical Journal i: 73

Chaney E F, O'Leary M R Marlatt G A 1978 Skill training with alcoholics. Journal of Consulting and Clinical Psychology 46: 1092–1104

Chester G B 1985 The influence of analgesic drugs in road crashes. Accident Analysis and Prevention 17: 305–309

Chick J 1986 Treatment of alcohol dependence: abstinence or controlled drinking? British Journal of Hospital Medicine 36: 241

Chick J 1987 Early intervention in the general hospital. In: Stockwell T, Clement S (eds) Helping the problem drinker. Croom Helm, London, pp 105–117

Chick J 1992 Doctors with emotional problems: how can they be helped? In: Hawton K, Cowen P (eds) Dilemmas in the management of psychiatric patients, vol 2. Oxford University Press, Oxford

Chick J, Chick J 1992 Drinking problems: information and advice for the individual, family and friends 2nd edn. MacDonald Optima Press, London

Chick J. Kreitman N, Plant M 1981 Mean cell volume and gamma glutamyl transpeptidase as markers of drinking in working men. Lancet i: 1249–1251

Chick J. Lloyd G, Crombie E 1985 Counselling problem drinkers in medical wards: a controlled study. British Medical Journal 290: 965–967

Chick K, Duffy J, Lloyd G, Ritson B 1986 Medical admissions in men: the risk among drinkers. Lancet ii: 1380–1383

Chick J, Ritson B, Connaughton J et al 1988 Advice versus extended treatment for alcoholism; a controlled study. British Journal of Addiction 83: 159–170

Chick J, Smith M A et al 1989 Magnetic resonance imaging of the brain in alcoholics: cerebral atrophy, lifetime alcohol consumption, and cognitive deficits. Alcoholism: Clinical and Experimental Research 13: 512–518

Chick J, Gough K, Falkowski W et al 1992 Disulfiram treatment of alcoholism. British Journal of Psychiatrists (in press)

Cloninger C R 1987 Neurogenetic adaptive mechanisms in alcoholism. Science 23: 410–415

Cochrane R, Bal S 1990 The drinking habits of Sikh, Hindu, Muslim and white men in the West Midlands: a community survey. British Journal of Addiction 85: 759–769

Connell P H 1958 Amphetamine psychosis. Oxford University Press, London

Cook C C H 1988 The Minnesota model in the management of drug and alcohol dependency: miracle, method or myth? British Journal of Addiction 83: 625–634

Crawford A, Plant M A, Kreitman N, Latcham R W 1985 Self-reported alcohol consumption and adverse consequences of drinking in three areas of Britain: general population studies. British Journal of Addiction 80: 421–428

de Alarcon R, Noguera R 1974 Clinical effects on drug abuse of a conviction for a drug offence. Lancet ii: 147

de Alarcon R, Rathod N H 1968 Prevalence and early detection of heroin abuse. British Medical Journal ii: 549

Department of Health and Social Security 1978 The pattern and range of services for problem drinkers. Her Majesty's Stationery Office, London

Dorn N 1990 Substance abuse and prevention strategies. In: Ghodse H, Maxwell D (eds) Substance abuse and dependence: an introduction for the caring professions. Macmillan, London

Drake R E, Vaillant G E 1988 Predicting alcoholism and personality disorder in a 33-year longitudinal study of children of alcoholics. British Journal of Addiction 83: 799–807

Drummond D C, Cooper T, Glautier S P 1990 Conditioned learning in alcohol dependence: implications for cue exposure treatment. British Journal of Addiction 85: 725–743

Dyer A R, Stamler J, Oglesby P et al 1980 Alcohol consumption and 17-year mortality in the Chicago Western Electric Company study. Preventive Medicine 9: 78–90

Edwards G 1971 Unreason in an age of reason. Royal Society of Medicine, London

Edwards G 1974 Cannabis and the criteria for legislation of a currently prohibited recreational drug. Acta Psychiatrica Scandinavica suppl 251

Edwards G 1976 Cannabis and the psychiatric position. In: Graham J D P (ed) Cannabis and health. Academic Press, London, pp 341–342

Edwards G, Gross M 1976 Alcohol dependence: provisional description of a clinical syndrome. British Medical Journal i: 1058

Feeney D M 1977 Marujana and epilepsy. Science 197: 1301–1302

Forrest F, Florey C de V, Taylor D, McPherson F, Young J A 1991 Reported social alcohol consumption during pregnancy and infant development at 18 months. British Medical Journal 303: 22–25

Ganwin F, Riordan C E, Kleber H 1985 Methylphenidate treatment of cocaine abusers without attention deficit disorder: a negative report. American Journal of Drug and Alcohol Abuse 2: 193–197

Garbutt J C, Mayo J P, Gillette G M et al 1991 Dose-response studies with thyrotropin-releasing hormone (TRH) in abstinent male alcoholics: evidence for selective thyrotropin dysfunction? Journal of Studies on Alcohol 52: 275–280

Gawin F H 1986 New uses of antidepressants in cocaine abuse. Psychosomatics 27 suppl: 27–29

Geikie A 1904 Scottish reminiscences. Maclehose, Glasgow

Ghodse A H 1981 Mortality and morbidity. In: Edwards G and Busch C (eds) Drug problems in Britain: a review of 10 years. Academic Press, London, pp 171–215

Ghodse A H 1987 Cannabis psychosis. British Journal of Addiction 81: 473–478

Glanz A, Taylor C 1986 Findings of a national survey on the role of general practitioners in the treatment of opiate abuse – extent of contact with opiate misusers. British Medical Journal 293: 427–430

Glaser F B 1980 Anybody got a match? Treatment research and the matching hypothesis. In: Edwards G, Grant M (eds) 1980 Alcoholism treatment in transition. Croom Helm, London

Goldstein D 1979 Some promising fields of inquiry in biomedical alcohol research. Journal of Studies on Alcohol suppl 8: 204

Gossop M 1988 Clonidine and the treatment of the opiate withdrawal syndrome. Drug and Alcohol Dependence 21: 253–259

Graham J D P 1977 Cannabis now. H M & M, London

Gurling H M D, Curtis D, Murray R M 1991 Psychological deficit from excessive alcohol consumption: evidence from a co-twin control study. British Journal of Addiction 86: 151–155

Guthrie A, Elliot W A 1980 The nature and reversibility of cerebral impairment in alcoholism. Journal of Studies on Alcohol 41: 147–155

Hartnoll R L, Mitcheson M C, Lewis R, Bryer S 1985 Estimating the prevalence of opioid dependence. Lancet i: 203–205

Hawkins J.D 1979 Reintegrating street drug abusers: community roles in continuing care. In: Brown B S (eds) Addicts and aftercare. Sage, Beverley Hills, pp 25–79

Heath A C, Martin N G 1988 Teenage alcohol use in the Australian Twin Register: genetic and social determinants of starting to drink. Alcoholism: Clinical and Experimental Research 12: 735–741

Heath A C, Jardine R, Martin N G 1989 Interaction effects of genotype and social environment on alcohol consumption in female twins. Journal of Studies on Alcohol 50: 38–48

Heather N 1981 Relationship between delinquency and drunkenness among Scottish young offenders. British Journal of Addiction 16: 50–61

Heather N, Robertson I 1981 Controlled drinking. Methuen, London

Heather N, Robertson I, Davies P (eds) 1985 The misuse of alcohol: crucial issues in dependence, treatment and prevention. Croom Helm, London

Helzer J, Canino G, Yeh E-K et al 1990 Alcoholism — N America and Asia. Archives of General Psychiatry 47: 313–319

Higgit A C, Lader M H, Fonagy P 1985 Clinical management of benzodiazepine dependence. British Medical Journal 291: 688–700

Hindmarch I 1972 Drugs and their abuse, age groups particularly at risk. British Journal of Addiction 67: 209

Hindmarch I 1980 Psychomotor function and psychoactive drugs. British Journal of Clinical Pharmacology 10: 189–209

HMSO 1988 Social trends, vol 18. Her Majesty's Stationary Office, London

Hodgson R J 1980a The alcohol dependence syndrome: a step in the wrong direction? British Journal of Addiction 75: 255

Hodgson R J 1980b Treatment strategies for the early problem drinker. In: Edwards G, Grant M (eds) 1980. Alcoholism treatment in transition. Croom Helm, London

Holman R B 1990 Physical dependence on alcohol and other sedatives. In: Warburton D M (ed) Addiction controversies. Harwood Academic, London

Home Office 1974 Report on the habitual drunken offender. Her Majesty's Stationery Office, London

Humphries T, Bennet M, Ray C 1991 Alcohol can damage your health. Alcohol Concern, London

Hurley D L 1991 Women, alcohol and incest: an analytical review. Journal of Studies on Alcohol 52: 253–268

Interdepartmental Committee on Drug Addiction 1965 Her Majesty's Stationery Office, London

Institute of Medicine 1990 Prevention and treatment of alcohol problems: research opportunities. National Academy Press, Washington, DC

Isbell H, Fraser H F, Wikler D W et al 1955 An experimental study of the etiology of 'rum fits' and delirium tremens. Quarterly Journal of Studies on Alcohol 16: 1–23

ISDD 1980 Teaching about a volatile situation – suggested health education strategies for minimizing casualties associated with solvent sniffing. Institute for the Study of Drug Dependence.

Janoswky D S, Meacham M P, Blaine J D, Schoor M, Bozetti L 1976 Marijuana effects on simulated flying ability. American Journal of Psychiatry 133; 384–388

Jones R T 1984 The pharmacology of cocaine. Cocaine: pharmacology, effects and treatment of abuse. Research monograph 50 Department of Health and Human Services, Washington, DC

Johnson B A 1991 Cannabis. In: Glass I B (ed) International handbook of addiction behaviour. Routledge, London, pp 69–76

Jackson R, Scragg R, Beaglehole R 1991 Alcohol consumption and risk of coronary heart disease. British Medical Journal 303: 211–216

Joyce P R, Sellman J D, Wells J E et al 1992 Parental bonding in alcoholic men: a relationship with conduct disorder but not alcoholism. British Journal of Psychiatry (in press)

Judd L L, Huey L Y 1984 Lithium antagonises ethanol intoxication in alcoholics. American Journal of Psychiatry 141: 1517

Kaprio J, Koskenvuo M, Langinvaino H, Romanov, K, Sarna S, Rose R J 1987 Genetic influences on use and abuse of alcohol. Alcoholism Clinical and Experimental Research 11: 349–356

Kendell R E, de Roumanie M, Ritson E B 1983 Effect of economic changes on Scottish drinking habits 1978–1982 British Journal of Addiction 78: 365–379

Kessel N 1965 Self poisoning. British Medical Journal 2: 1265–1336

Khantzian E J 1985 The self medication hypothesis of addictive disorders: focus on heroin and cocain dependence. American Journal of Psychiatry 142: 1259–1264

King M D, Day R E, Oliver J S, Lush M, Watson J M 1981 Solvent encephalopathy. British Medical Journal 283: 663–665

Kreitman N 1986 Alcohol consumption and the preventive paradox. British Journal of Addiction 81: 353–363

Kushner M G, Sher K J, Beitman B D 1990 The relation between alcohol problems and anxiety disorders. American Journal of Psychiatry 147: 685–695

Lancet 1980 Treatment of opiate withdrawal symptoms. Lancet ii: 349

Editorial 1987 Screening for drugs of abuse. Lancet i: 365–366

Lennane K J 1988 Patient with alcohol related brain damage: therapy and outcome. Australian Drug and Alcohol Review 7: 89–92

Lewis C E, Bucholz K K 1991 Alcoholism, antisocial behaviour and family history. British Journal of Addiction 86: 177–194

Lebowitz N R, Kranzler H R, Meyer R E 1990 Pharmacologic approaches to alcoholism treatment. Alcohol Health and Research World 14: 144–153

Littleton J, Harper C 1990 Biological models of alcohol dependence. In: Edwards G, Lader M (eds) The nature of drug dependence (Society for the Study of Addictions monograph 1). Oxford University Press, Oxford

Littman G, Stapleton J, Oppenheim A N et al 1983 Situations related to alcoholism relapse. British Journal of Addiction 78: 381–390

Ludwig A M 1988 Understanding the alcoholic's mind: the nature of craving and how to control it. Oxford University Press, Oxford

McCord J 1972 Etiological factors in alcoholism. Quarterly Journal for the Study of Alcohol 33: 1020–1027

McCord W, McCord J 1960 Origins of alcoholism. Stanford University Press, Stanford

McGlothlin W H, West L J 1968 The Marijuana problem: an overview. American journal of Psychiatry 125: 126–134

McGuiness I 1980 An econometric analysis of total demand for alcoholic beverages in the UK 1956–1975. Journal of Industrial Economics 29: 85–109

McLachlan J F C, Stein R L 1982 Evaluation of a day clinic for alcoholics. Journal of Studies on Alcoholism 43: 262–272

Marlatt G A, Gordon J R 1984 Relapse prevention: maintenance strategies in addictive behaviour. Guildford, New York

Maynard A, Hardmann G and Whelan A 1987 Measuring the social cost of addictive substances. British Journal of Addiction 82: 701–706

Marshall E J, Murray R M 1991 Familial alcoholism: inheritance and initiation. British Medical Journal 303: 72–73

Menninger K A 1938 Man against himself. Harcourt Brace, New York

Meyer R E 1989 Prospects for a rational pharmacotherapy of alcoholism. Journal of Clinical Psychiatry 50: 403–412

Miller W R 1983 Motivational interviewing with problem drinkers. Behavioural Psychotherapy 11: 147–172

Miller W R, Baca L 1983 Two year follow-up of bibliotherapy and therapist-directed controlled drinking training for problem drinkers. Behaviour Therapy 14: 441–448

Miller W R, Hester R K 1986 The effectiveness of alcoholism treatment methods, what research reveals. In: Miller W, Heather N (eds) Treating addictive behaviours; process of change. Plenum Press, New York

Miller W R Taylor C A 1980 Relative effectiveness of bibliotherapy, individual and group self-control training in the treatment of problem drinkers. Addictive Behaviours 5: 13–24

Mirin S M, Weiss R D, Sollogub A, Michael J 1984 Psychopathology in families of drug abusers. In: Mirin S M (ed) Substance abuse and psychopathology. American Psychiatric Press, Washington, DC

Mitchison M, Hartnoll R 1980 Evaluation of heroin in a maintenance controlled trial. Archives of General Psychiatry 37: 877

Murray R. Ghodse H, Harris C et al 1981 The misuse of psychotropic drugs. Gaskell, London

Murray R M 1974 Analgesic abuse. British Journal of Hospital Medicine 11: 772

Nakamura H, Overall J, Hollister L, Radcliffe E 1983 Factors affecting outcome of depressive symptoms in alcoholics. Alcoholism: Clinical and Experimental Research 7: 188–193

National Pharmaceutical Association 1986 The dilemma — drug addicts and AIDS. The Supplement 1–2: 690

O'Brien C P, Childress A R 1991 Behaviour therapy of drug dependence In: Glass I B (ed) The international handbook of addiction behaviour. Routledge, London

Ogborne A C, Melotte C 1977 An evaluation of a therapeutic community for former drug users. British Journal of Addiction 72: 75–83

Ojesjo 1981 Long-term outcome in alcohol abuse and alcoholism among males in the Lundby general population. British Journal of Addiction 76: 391–400

Oliver J S, Watson J M 1977 Abuse of solvents for kicks: a review of 50 cases. Lancet i: 84–86

Orford J, Edwards G 1977 Alcoholism. Oxford University Press, London

Orford J, Wawman T 1986 Alcohol detoxification services: a review. Department of Health and Social Security, London

Parker H, Newcome R, Bakx K 1987 The new heroin users prevalence and characteristics in Wirrell, Merseyside. British Journal of Addiction 8: 147–157

Parker J, Pool Y, Rawle R, Gay M 1988 Monitoring problem drug use in Bristol. British Journal of Psychiatry 152: 214–221

Patursson H, Lader M H 1981 Benzodiazepine dependence. British Journal of Addiction 76: 133

Pevelar C, Green R, Mandelbrote R 1988 Prevalence of heroin abuse in Oxford City. British Journal of Addiction 83: 513–518

Pharmaceutical Society of Great Britain 1986 Statement: sales of hypodermic syringes and needles. Pharmaceutical Journal, 15 Feb

Pihl R, Peterson J, Finn P 1990 Inherited predisposition to alcoholism: characteristics of sons of male alcoholics. Journal of Abnormal Psychology 99: 271–301

Pillard R C 1970 Marijuana. New England Journal of Medicine 283: 292–304

Plant M A 1975 Drug takers in an English town. British Journal of Criminology 15: 181–186

Plant M A 1981a Drugs in perspective. Hodder & Stroughton. London

Plant M 1981b What aetiologies? In Edwards G, Busch C (eds) Drug problems in Britain, a review of 10 years. Academic Press, London

Plant M 1987 Women drinking and pregnancy. Tavistock, London

Plant M A, Pirie F, Kreitman N 1979 Evaluation of the Scottish Health Education Unit's 1976 campaign on alcoholism. Social Psychiatry 14: 11–24

Plant M A, Peck D F, Samuel E 1985 Alcohol, drugs and school leavers. Tavistock, London

Polich J M, Armor D J, Braiker H 1981 The course of alcoholism four years after the treatment. Wiley, New York

Priest R, Montgomery S 1988 Benzodiazepines and dependence: a college tutorial. Bulletin of the Royal College of Psychiatrists 12: 107

Rafaelsen L, Christrup H, Bech P, Rafaelsen O J 1973 Effects of cannabis and alcohol on psychological tests. Nature 242: 117

Report of the Departmental Committee on Morphine and Heroin Addiction (Rolleston Committee) 1926. His Majesty's Stationery Office, London

Reported social alcohol consumption during pregnancy and infant development at 18 months. British Medical Journal 303: 22–25

Robichaud C, Strickler D, Bigelow G, Liebson I 1979 Disulfiram maintenance alcoholism treatment: a 3-phase evaluation. Behaviour Research and Therapy 17: 618–621

Robins L N, Davis D H, Goodwin D W 1974 Drugs used by US army enlisted men in Vietnam. American Journal of Epidemiology 99: 235

Robinson D 1979 Talking out of alcoholism: the self help process of Alcoholics Anonymous. Croom Helm, London

Robinson D, Tether P, Teller S 1989 Local action on alcohol problems. Routledge, London

Romelsjo A, Lazarus N B, Kaplan G A, Cohen R D 1991 The relationship between stressful life situations and changes in alcohol consumption. British Journal of Addiction 86: 157–169

Ron M 1986 Volatile substance abuse: a review of possible long-term neurological intellectual and psychiatric sequelae. British Journal of Psychiatry 148: 235–246

Rose G, Day S 1990 The population mean predicts the number of deviant individuals. British Medical Journal 301: 1031–1034

Rounsaville B J 1988 The role of psychopathology in the familial transmission of drug abuse. In: Biological vulnerability to drug abuse (NIDA research monograph No 89). National Institute of Drug Abuse, Rockville. MD

Royal College of Physicians 1987 A great and growing evil. Tavistock, London

Royal College of Psychiatrists 1986 Alcohol our favourite drug. Tavistock, London

Russell M A H, Wilson C, Taylor C, Baker C D 1979 Effect of general practitioners' advice against smoking. British Medical Journal ii: 231

Saunders J B 1989 The efficacy of treatment for drinking problems. International Review of Psychiatry 1: 121–138

Saunders J B, Walters J R F, Davies P, Paton A 1981 A

20–year prospective study of cirrhosis. British Medical Journal 282: 263–266

Shaper A G, Wannamethee G, Walker M 1988 Alcohol and mortality in British men: explaining the U-shaped curve. Lancet ii: 1267–1273

Schuckit M A 1986 The genetic and clinical implication of alcoholism and affective disorder. American Journal of Psychiatry 143: 140–147

Schuckit M A, Irwin M 1989 An analysis of the clinical relevance of type 1 and type 2 alcoholics. British Journal of Addiction 84: 869–876

Siegel S 1979 The role of the conditioning in drug tolerance and addiction. In: Keehn J D (ed) Psychopathology in animals: research and clinical applications. Academic Press, New York

Skog O J 1980 Liver cirrhosis epidemiology: some methodological problems. British Journal of Addiction 282: 263

Smart R G, Mann R E 1991 Factors in recent reductions in liver cirrhosis deaths. Journal of Studies on Alcohol 52: 232–240

Stimson G V 1973 Heroin and behaviour. Irish Universities Press, Dublin

Stockwell T 1987 The Exeter home detoxification projects In: Stockwell T and Clement S (eds) Helping the problem drinker. Croom Helm, London

Stockwell T, Clement S (eds) 1987 Helping the Problem Drinker: New Initiatives in Community Care. Croom Helm, London

Stockwell T, Hodgson R, Edwards G et al 1979 The development of a questionnaire to measure severity of alcohol dependence. British Journal of Addiction 73: 79–87

Strang J 1990 Intermediate goals and the process of change. In: Strang J, Stimson G (eds) AIDS and drug misuse: the challenge for policy and practice in the 1990s. Routledge, London

Strang J, Johns A R, Caan W 1992 Cocaine in the UK. British Journal of Psychiatry (in press)

Sulkunen P 1989 Drinking in France 1965–79: an analysis of household consumption data. British Journal of Addiction 84: 61–72

Swadi H 1988 Drug and substance use among 3 333 London adolescents. British Journal of Addiction 83: 935–942

Tarter R E, Hegedus A M, Goldstein G et al 1984 Adolescent sons of alcoholics: neuropsychological and personality characteristics. Alcoholism: Clinical and Experimental Research 8: 216

Tennant F S, Groesbeck C J 1972 Psychiatric effects of hashish. Archives of General Psychiatry 27: 133

Thorley A 1981 Longitudinal studies in drug dependence. In: Edwards G, Busch G (eds) Drug problems in Britain. Academic Press, London

Treffert D 1978 Marujana use in schizophrenia: A clear hazard.

US Department of Health and Human Services 1990 Alcohol and health: 7th special report to congress, Department of Health and Human Services, Washington, DC

Vaillant G E 1983 The natural history of alcoholism: causes, patterns and paths to recovery. Harvard University Press, Boston

Vaillant G E, Milofsky E S 1982 Natural history of male alcoholism IV. Paths to recovery. Archives of General Psychiatry 39: 127–133

Vaillant G E, Clark W, Cyrus C et al 1983 Prospective study of alcoholism treatment – 8 years follow-up. American Journal of Medicine 75: 455–463

Victor M 1962 Alcoholism. In: Baker A B (ed) Clinical neurology, vol 2. Hoeber-Harper, New York

Victor M, Hope J M 1958 The phenomenon of auditory hallucinations in chronic alcoholism. Journal of Nervous and Mental Disease 126: 451–481

Wallace P, Cutler S, Haines A 1988 Randomized controlled trial of general practitioners in patients with excessive alcohol consumption. British Medical Journal 297: 663–668

Watson J 1981 Solvent abuse: a review. British Journal of Addiction 75: 27

Watson J M 1977 Glue sniffing in profile. The Practitioner 218: 255–259

Wells B 1987 Narcotics Anonymous (N.A.): the phenomenal growth of an important resource. British Journal of Addiction 82: 581–582

Wells F O 1970 Voluntary restriction on amphetamine prescribing. British Medical Journal ii: 361

Wells J E, Bushnell J H, Joyce P R, Oakley Browne M A, Hornblow A R 1991 Preventing alcohol problems: the implications of a case-finding study in Christchurch, New Zealand. Acta Psychiatrica Scandinavica 83: 31–40

WHO 1988 Towards healthy public policies on alcohol and other drugs. Consensing statement proposed by WHO Expert Working Group, Sydney, Canberra. March 1988. World Health Organization, Geneva

Wilson P 1980 Drinking in England and Wales. Her Majesty's Stationery Office, London

Wikler A 1965 Conditioning factors in opiate addiction and relapse. In: Willner D I, Kassenbaum G G (eds) Narcotics. McGraw-Hill, New York, pp 85–100

Wise R A 1988 The neurobiology of craving: implications for the understanding and treatment of addiction. Journal of Abnormal Psychology 2: 118–132

Wright J D, Pearl L 1990 Knowledge and experience of young people regarding drug abuse 1969–1989. British Medical Journal 300: 99–103

Yesavage J A, Leirer V O, Denari M, Hollister L E 1985 Carry-over effects of marijuana intoxication on aircraft pilot performance: a preliminary report. American Journal of Psychiatry 142: 1325–1329

Young R M, Oei T P S, Knight R G 1990 The tension reduction hypothesis revisited: an alcohol expectancy perspective. British Journal of Addiction 85: 31–40

18. Schizophrenia

R. E. Kendell

Schizophrenia is the heartland of psychiatry and the core of its clinical practice. Every layman knows that the term means 'split mind' and his concept of madness is largely based on the oddities and abnormalities of those who suffer from this enigmatic illness. Because it is a relatively common condition, which often cripples people in adolescence or early adult life, it probably causes more suffering and distress and blights more lives than any cancer; and because it cripples people in their youth without greatly reducing their life expectancy it constitutes a huge burden on health services. In Britain some 10% of all hospital beds are still occupied by schizophrenics and a generation ago the proportion was even higher.

HISTORICAL INTRODUCTION

Although brief descriptions of an illness resembling schizophrenia are to be found in the Hindu *Ayurveda* as long ago as 1400 BC, and in the writings of the Cappadocian physician Arataeus in the 2nd century AD, recognisable descriptions of schizophrenia are historically considerably less common, in medical texts or literature generally, than those of melancholia or mania. The earliest unambiguous descriptions date only from the end of the 18th century and it was a further 100 years before the syndrome was defined with any clarity. That crucial step was achieved by Emil Kraepelin, professor of psychiatry at the University of Munich, in the fifth (1896) edition of his *Psychiatrie, ein Lehrbuch für Studierende und Ärzte*. Throughout the 19th century psychiatrists had struggled, with scant success, to develop a satisfactory classification of insanity. In 1856 Morel had coined the term *démence précoce* to describe an adolescent patient, once bright and active, who had slowly lapsed into a state of silent withdrawal. In 1868 Kahlbaum had described the syndrome of *Katatonie* and 3 years later Hecker had described *Hebephrenie*. But it was Kraepelin who first succeeded in going beyond straightforward clinical description by his division of the myriad and shifting forms of insanity into two great groupings on the basis of their long-term course. The first, which he called manic–depressive insanity, pursued a fluctuating course with frequent relapses but full recovery after each. The second, for which he used Morel's term dementia praecox, embraced Kahlbaum's catatonia, Hecker's hebephrenia and his own dementia paranoides and was a progressive disease which either pursued a steady downhill course to chronic invalidism or, if improvement did occur, resulted only in partial recovery. Initially, Kraepelin was criticised for introducing yet another classification without any aetiological or pathological basis, but it was not long before the force and utility of his unifying concepts impressed themselves on his contemporaries and they started to come into general use. In 1911, however, while acceptance of this new classification was still incomplete, the Swiss psychiatrist Eugen Bleuler published his *Dementia Praecox or the Group of Schizophrenias*, which was to be at least as influential as Kraepelin's *Lehrbuch*. Although Bleuler regarded himself as confirming and developing Kraepelin's concept of dementia praecox in fact he changed it fundamentally, and it was his term schizophrenia which eventually won universal adoption. Kraepelin had assumed, in the tradition of German academic psychiatry, that dementia praecox was a disease of the brain, and speculated that it might be an endocrine disorder of some kind. Bleuler, influenced by the writings of Sigmund Freud and the infant school of psychoanalysis, thought of schizophrenia in psychological rather than in neuropathological terms. He coined the term schizophrenia, meaning 'split mind', because he believed that the disorder was due to a 'loosening of associations' between different psychic functions, affecting both the transition from one idea to the next in thought and speech and the coordination between emotional, volitional (conative) and intellectual (cognitive) processes in general. He also drew a distinction between the thought disorder, the blunting or incongruity of affect, the autism and the pervasive ambivalence of the disorder, which he regarded as the 'fundamental symptoms' and the more obvious hallucinations, delusions and catatonic phenomena which for him were accessory phenomena of less importance. This led him to conclude that schizophrenia could develop and be diagnosed in the absence of hallucinations and delusions, and so to add a fourth type, simple schizophrenia, to the hebephrenic, catatonic and paranoid forms recognised by Kraepelin.

Although Bleuler's term schizophrenia eventually displaced Kraepelin's dementia praecox and his assumptions about the nature of the disorder became very influential, particularly in the USA, Kraepelin's original concept remained dominant in many European centres. This failure to resolve the incompatibility of the Kraepelinian and Bleulerian approaches, together with the inherent ambiguities of each, resulted in considerable confusion and seriously hindered fruitful research for the next half century.

The crucial characteristic of Kraepelin's dementia praecox — what distinguished it from manic–depressive insanity — was its prognosis. The illness progressed to a state of permanent dementia, and if recovery did occur it was either temporary or incomplete. However, it soon came to be recognised that some patients with the typical clinical characteristics of the condition did recover, and remained well indefinitely without any detectable defect. Kraepelin himself eventually accepted that this occurred in 13% of his own cases. Unfortunately, the implications of this were never properly faced. Kraepelin and most of his contemporaries had assumed that dementia praecox was a 'disease entity' with its own characteristic symptomatology, aetiology, pathology and course. But the aetiology and neuropathology remained a mystery and here was evidence that the course was variable and inconstant. Understandably, the predominant reaction to this quandary was to assume that this variable prognosis was an artefact, occurring because patients with a superficially similar psychosis of good prognosis were being confused with those suffering from real dementia praecox schizophrenia. Determined efforts were therefore made to distinguish the two. In Europe the Norwegian psychiatrist Langfeldt sought to distinguish between schizophrenia and what he called schizophreniform psychosis on the basis of a detailed study of the symptomatology of the illness and presented evidence to suggest that the two had quite different outcomes, and that

electroconvulsive therapy (ECT) and insulin coma therapy were ineffective in schizophrenia itself (Langfeldt 1960). Although his results owed a good deal to retrospective adjustments to the original diagnoses his claim was initially widely accepted because it was so welcome. In the USA similar efforts were made by clinical psychologists and a series of rating scales — the Elgin, Phillips and Kantor Scales — were developed to discriminate between what they called process and non-process schizophrenia, mainly on the basis of the premorbid personality and psychosexual adjustment. Both Langfeldt and these American workers assumed that true process schizophrenia was endogenous and hereditary and that schizophreniform or non-process psychoses were psychogenic, but neither succeeded in demonstrating a clear demarcation between the two. The cardinal defect of Bleuler's concept of schizophrenia was its lack of clear boundaries. Although he provided little empirical evidence to justify his belief that his 'fundamental symptoms' were indeed fundamental his assumptions were widely accepted, particularly in the USA, and as a result the diagnosis of schizophrenia came to be based on the presence of one or more of the so-called 'four As' (loosening of associations or thought disorder, blunting or incongruity of affect, autism and ambivalence), whether or not the patient was psychotic. Unfortunately, all four of these phenomena are intangible qualities which with a little imagination can be detected in most psychiatric patients and in some healthy people, particularly when under stress. Their use as diagnostic criteria therefore led to a marked expansion of the concept of schizophrenia, to the point at which it was degenerating into a vague synonym for severe mental illness.

Between 1920 and 1960 the confusion increased steadily. With the partial exception of French psychiatry, which pursued its own traditions untroubled by outside influences, the term 'schizophrenia' was used throughout the world, but in a bewildering variety of different ways which were rarely made explicit. Some authorities, like Kleist and Leonhard in Germany and Langfeldt in Norway, insisted that the term should be restricted to illnesses resulting in permanent damage to the personality; others were prepared to use it freely regardless of outcome. Some psychiatrists would only make the diagnosis in adolescents or young adults; others were willing to do so at any age. Some insisted on the presence of certain key symptoms; others were prepared to make a confident diagnosis on the basis of indefinable subjective impressions, the so-called 'praecox feeling'. In the USA Bleuler's views predominated, largely because his concept of schizophrenia as a psychological, and possibly psychogenic, disorder was readily compatible with the prevailing psychoanalytic orientation. The overuse of the term was therefore most marked in that country, particularly in centres where the popularity of terms like pseudoneurotic schizophrenia and borderline state extended its application even further. In most of Europe, on the other hand, Kraepelin's concepts still held sway. In most of the German-speaking world schizophrenia was regarded as an endogenous and hereditary psychosis and the diagnosis restricted to patients exhibiting certain cardinal symptoms, mainly hallucinations and delusions of particular kinds. Kleist in Frankfurt and Leonhard in Berlin developed very detailed classifications of different forms of schizophrenia, mainly on the basis of a meticulous study of the chronic stage of the illness. Of greater influence, however, were the teachings of Kurt Schneider, who focused attention on the earlier acute stage of the illness and described a number of 'symptoms of the first rank' (see Table 18.1) which he considered to be diagnostic of schizophrenia in the absence of overt brain disease (Schneider 1959).

Many of these hallucinations and delusions can be interpreted as the result of a failure to distinguish

Table 18.1 Kurt Schneider's 'symptoms of the first rank'

1. Auditory hallucinations taking any one of three specific forms:
   a. Voices repeating the subject's thoughts out loud (*Gedankenlautwerden* or *écho de la pensée*), or anticipating his thoughts
   b. Two or more hallucinatory voices discussing the subject, or arguing about him, referring to him in the third person
   c. Voices commenting on the subject's thoughts or behaviour, often as a running commentary
2. The sensation of alien thoughts being put into the subject's mind by some external agency, or of his own thoughts being taken away (thought insertion or withdrawal)
3. The sensation that the subject's thinking is no longer confined within his own mind, but is instead shared by, or accessible to, others (thought broadcasting)
4. The sensation of feelings, impulses or acts being experienced or carried out under external control, so that the patient feels as if he were being hypnotised, or had become a robot
5. The experience of being a passive and reluctant recipient of bodily sensations imposed by some external agency
6. Delusional perception — a delusion arising fully fledged on the basis of a genuine perception which others would regard as commonplace and unrelated

between ideas and impulses arising in the patient's own mind and perceptions arising in the external world, a so-called 'loss of ego boundaries'. However, they had no particular theoretical significance for Schneider himself; he regarded them simply as convenient diagnostic aids which were pathognomonic of schizophrenia in the absence of brain disease. He accepted that some patients with otherwise typical schizophrenic illnesses never exhibited any of these symptoms, and that all of them could occur at times in epileptic and other organic psychoses, but he regarded them nonetheless as sufficiently characteristic to be worth distinguishing from what he called 'second rank' symptoms like perplexity, emotional blunting and hallucinations and delusions of other kinds.

DEFINITIONS OF SCHIZOPHRENIA

The confusion caused by the unresolved differences between Kraepelin's and Bleuler's concepts of schizophrenia, and the subsequent development of other differences in usage as well, have been referred to already. These differences were at their worst in the 1950s and the best known and most extensively studied were Anglo-American. Spurred by the observation that the first-admission rate for schizophrenia was considerably higher in the USA than in England and Wales, and that for manic–depressive illnesses the difference was the other way about, detailed studies were mounted of series of consecutive admissions to mental hospitals in the two countries, using identical interviewing methods and diagnostic criteria (Cooper et al 1972). These comparisons showed that the symptoms of patients admitted to public mental hospitals in New York and London were virtually identical. But the proportion of patients given a diagnosis of schizophrenia was nearly twice as high in New York as in London because the New York psychiatrists' concept of schizophrenia embraced many patients who in London would have been regarded as suffering from depressive or manic psychoses, or even from neurotic illnesses or personality disorders. Shortly after this the International Pilot Study of Schizophrenia confirmed that psychiatrists in Washington — and also, for rather different reasons, in Moscow — had a considerably broader concept of schizophrenia than their counterparts in the other seven countries involved, namely Colombia, Czechoslovakia, Denmark, India, Nigeria, Taiwan and the UK (WHO 1973).

Increasing awareness of the scale and consequences of international differences of this kind, and of the low reliability of psychiatric diagnoses generally, led in the 1970s to a widespread realisation that key terms like schizophrenia must be operationally defined in order to make it quite clear what criteria had to be satisfied to establish the diagnosis. Because schizophrenia, like most other psychiatric disorders, is still recognised by its syndrome and its aetiology is still obscure this means that it must be defined either by the presence of particular symptoms or combinations of symptoms, or by its course, or some combination of the two. In the last 20 years many different operational definitions of schizophrenia have been proposed and this has inevitably led to comparisons of their relative merits. High reliability and a reasonable concordance with traditional usage are obviously important qualities, but not sufficient by themselves. What we are really trying to do when faced with a choice between alternative definitions is to decide which is likely to be more useful in predicting response to treatment or long-term course, or which is likely to correspond most closely with the putative biological abnormality underlying the disorder. Because the syndrome of schizophrenia appears to merge into neighbouring syndromes, because we have not yet identified the underlying biological abnormality, and because political considerations are also involved, there is not yet any single agreed definition, or any immediate prospect of a consensus. Areas of agreement are emerging all the same. Bleuler's fundamental symptoms, and thought disorder in particular, have lost their former influence, mainly because they are too intangible, and therefore incapable of being reliably identified. Schneider's first-rank symptoms are still influential in Britain and Germany, partly because their presence can be reliably rated, but several studies have demonstrated that they have little significance for long-term prognosis. The presence of first-rank symptoms in the acute illness does not predict either incomplete recovery or the development of a schizophrenic defect state (Kendell et al 1979) and it is not uncommon for these symptoms to develop in the course of what are in other respects typical manic illnesses (Brockington et al 1980). In fact, it is increasingly apparent that none of the symptoms of the acute illness is as good a predictor of the long-term course as the duration and mode of onset. If the initial illness starts insidiously and lasts for several months a poor long-term prognosis is much more likely than if it starts acutely in response to obvious stress and lasts only a few weeks, regardless of the detailed symptomatology.

Currently, the most widely used definitions of schizophrenia, at least for research purposes, are the St Louis criteria (Feighner et al 1972), the Research Diagnostic Criteria (RDC; Spitzer et al 1975) and the American Psychiatric Association's (DSM-III and DSM-IIIR) criteria. They all require clear evidence of psychosis, currently or in the past, and all but the Feighner criteria specify particular kinds of hallucinatory experience or delusional ideation. All four stipulate that affective symptoms must not be prominent and all require a minimum duration of illness, but this is only 2 weeks for the RDC definition and 6 months for the Feighner, DSM-III and DSM-IIIR definitions. From 1993 onwards all of these definitions are likely to be replaced by the new definitions of ICD-10 and DSM-IV, but at the time of writing neither of these was in its final form.

It is, of course, very confusing for everyone, not merely for students, to have several alternative definitions of a single disorder, particularly when it is commonplace for a patient to fulfil one set of criteria but not others. Under present circumstances, however, for the reasons described above, this is inevitable; and it is better for differences of this kind to be overt than to be concealed and unsuspected. The existence of a number of alternative definitions also helps to emphasise that all definitions are arbitrary, justified only by their usefulness, and liable to be altered or supplanted. The St Louis, DSM-III and DSM-IIIR definitions, which require a 6-month symptom duration, are the most restrictive but have the merit of defining a group of patients with a poor long-term prognosis akin to Kraepelin's original dementia praecox. The Schneiderian concept of schizophrenia and the criteria incorporated in the computer program Catego derived from it (Wing et al 1974) are broader, and because no account is taken either of symptom duration or of the presence of affective symptoms the outcome is more variable in both the short and the long term.

CLINICAL PRESENTATION AND SYMPTOMATOLOGY

It follows from what has been said above about the definition of schizophrenia that the symptoms and other characteristics of the condition will vary some-what, according to the way in which the syndrome is defined. There is, nonetheless, a core group of patients who fulfil most definitions, and international comparisons using films or videotapes of diagnostic interviews confirm that psychiatrists throughout the world will confidently identify these as schizophrenics.

The premorbid personality

Although schizophrenia can develop in personalities of all kinds it is more likely to develop in people of some kinds than others. The most typical premorbid personality traits are those of emotional and social detachment. Such people have few friends, often appear cold and aloof, and seem bored or ill at ease in social situations. They have a preference for solitary occupations and pastimes and their behaviour may be mildly eccentric. They are also indifferent to praise or criticism, tend to avoid competition and seek refuge in fantasy. These characteristics are also over-represented in the close relatives of schizophrenics and are designated by the epithet 'schizoid' in recognition of their association with the illness. These abnormalities can often be traced back to early childhood. Prospective studies of the children of schizophrenic mothers and other 'high-risk' children (e.g. see Parnas et al 1982) have established that future schizophrenics tend to have lower scores on intelligence tests and poorer educational attainments at school than other children, and also to have more interpersonal difficulties and more disturbed behaviour as a result of poor affective control and defective emotional rapport. None of these characteristics is constant enough, or sufficiently specific, however, for it to be feasible to identify individuals at high risk of developing schizophrenia in advance. They may well, though, be responsible for the overprotective behaviour often shown by the mothers of schizophrenics.

The acute illness

Although schizophrenia can occur at any age from 7 to 70 the onset is usually in adolescence or early adult life. Often it develops insidiously. A youth whose previous behaviour had been unremarkable slowly becomes more withdrawn and introverted. He may acquire a new interest in religion, psychology or the occult and drift away from his friends. He also loses his drive and determination and may fail to complete a university degree or an apprenticeship which had previously seemed well within his grasp. His parents may be worried by his failures, his apparent lack of interest in achievement and his progressive estrangement from them but they do not suspect that he is ill until one day, months or even years later, it suddenly becomes apparent that he is entertaining delusional ideas, or hearing voices. In other cases the onset is acute. Often in the aftermath of some obvious stress, perhaps being spurned by a girlfriend or failing an exam, or while in the unfamiliar environment of a foreign country, the subject becomes obviously and sometimes floridly ill over the course of a few days. He becomes convinced that he is being watched or followed, may attach great significance to the colours of clothes or postage stamps, talk of Martians, laser beams or hypnosis, or suddenly be found, mute and inaccessible, kneeling on the floor.

The delusions of the acute illness are very variable in type and even more so in their detailed content. Delusions of reference and persecutory, grandiose, religious and hypochondriacal ideas of various kinds are all common but most characteristic are a variety of *passivity phenomena*. The subject feels that he is no longer in control of his own thoughts, feelings or will and that he is being influenced or controlled by some mysterious, alien force. Thoughts which are not his own are put into his mind (*thought insertion*), or his own thoughts are taken away (*thought withdrawal*), or somehow have become accessible to other people (*thought broadcasting*). Or he may be convinced that someone is trying to hypnotise him or impose their will on his. The subject's interpretation of these phenomena, which lie beyond the bounds of normal experience, depends of his cultural background. Our forefathers attributed them to God or the Devil; most Africans and West Indians attribute them to spirits or witchcraft; and the inhabitants of modern industrial countries attribute them to electricity, X-rays, television, laser beams and satellites. In short, the subject endeavours to make an unintelligible experience intelligible by attributing it to some powerful, invisible force with which he is conversant but does not fully understand.

The hallucinations are equally varied and may involve any of the five senses. Auditory hallucinations in the form of voices are the most common, however, and visual, olfactory, gustatory and tactile hallucinations are all uncommon in the absence of hallucinatory voices. Although Schneider and others have drawn attention to particular types of hallucinatory voices that are characteristic of schizophrenia (see Table 18.1) it is commonplace for schizophrenics to hear voices talking to them as well as about them and their content is very variable. Indeed, from a diagnostic point of view their duration is probably more important than their detailed perceptual characteristics or their content, because hallucinatory voices do not often continue all day long, week after week, in other psychoses. Traditionally, psychiatrists have distinguished between true hallucinations, which have all the characteristics of normal perceptions and are therefore treated as genuine, and pseudohallucinations, which are sufficiently different for the subject to realise that he is 'hearing voices'. Although the distinction may have considerably practical significance — a man who hears a voice threatening to murder him behaves very differently from a man who realises he is hearing things — it rarely has much diagnostic significance. Indeed schizophrenic hallucinations frequently have a quality intermediate between that of a genuine auditory perception and a thought. Although the subject speaks spontaneously of a 'voice' he will often admit on questioning that he does not really hear it out loud or with his ears. It is in the mind, a 'silent voice', which none the less is insistent, troublesome and sometimes frightening. Often too the subject has difficulty describing what it says. Doubtless this is often due to embarrassment, or reluctance to divulge what the subject suspects his questioner will regard as evidence of insanity, but it does sometimes seem that the patient has genuine difficulty in describing the content of the hallucination, perhaps because the normal link between perception and memory is only partly established.

The patient's affect during the acute illness is as variable as his thought content but is nearly always disturbed in some way. Perplexity is a common and characteristic feature of acute schizophrenic illnesses. The subject suspects that something strange is going on around him but is not sure what, and ideas of reference and persecutory and grandiose ideas may come and go in rapid succession as he seeks to integrate his changing perceptions and affective state with his premorbid experience (*delusional mood*). At other times the subject may be depressed, elated or angry and it is sometimes difficult to tell whether the content of his delusions and hallucinatory voices is derived from the prevailing mood or vice versa. The most characteristic emotional abnormality, however, is either a general flattening or blunting of all affective responses, or incongruity. The former refers to a loss of the ability to feel, or at least to express, any deep or profound emotion, and a matching inability to evoke a sympathetic response in other people. The latter refers to a mismatch between the subject's emotional responses and the setting or the topic of conversation, silly giggling while important or distressing events are taking place being the most common example.

Finally, the patient's global behaviour is affected. Again the nature of the change is variable but characteristically involves withdrawal from contact with and interest in other people, and actions which seem bizarre or inexplicable to the onlooker. Occasionally, the patient displays the particular behavioural abnormalities of Kahlbaum's catatonia, becoming mute, or stuporose, or adopting strange postures, sometimes for hours on end. Catatonic phenomena of this kind used to be common and figured prominently in Kraepelin's original descriptions of dementia praecox. Indeed, for an earlier generation of psychiatrists it was an important part of the clinical examination of any psychotic patient to determine which of a variety of other catatonic behaviours they exhibited, including automatic obedience (a wooden, robot-like response to all requests or commands however silly or pointless), negativism (a similarly wooden response, but the opposite of that required by the request) and waxy flexibility (a curious disturbance of muscle tone in which the patient's limbs could be moved only slowly into new positions, but would then remain exactly as placed for minutes on end). Although catatonic phenomena of this kind are still common in developing countries they are rarely seen nowadays in industrial countries, and then mainly in immigrants or isolated rural areas. The reason why this should be so is a mystery, but it serves to emphasise that the clinical features of the illness are not inherent and predetermined, but the product of an interaction with the subject's personality and cultural background.

The chronic stage

Sooner or later, even without treatment, the hallucinations and delusions of the acute illness die down. Often they disappear completely, and if they do persist for months or years on end their influence on the patient's behaviour usually wanes. Unfortunately, the disappearance of hallucinations and delusions does not always betoken recovery, even temporarily. Recovery may be, and often is, complete after one or two short-lived episodes of illness. But the more episodes a patient has had, and the more insidiously developing and longer lasting these have been, the more likely it is that some residual damage will remain. This 'defect state' is much less conspicuous than the florid symptoms of the acute illness and may not be apparent at all to those who did not know the patient well before his illness. But in the long run it is far more handicapping. In its mildest form it involves nothing more than a subtle loss of vivacity, enthusiasm and emotional responsiveness. More commonly, however, the patient's drive and determination are affected. He becomes apathetic, no longer strives, no longer cares. At the same time, and perhaps fundamentally for the same reason, he loses interest in other people. He talks much less ('paucity of speech') and his capacity to form enduring emotional relationships is greatly reduced. He is no longer capable of falling in love or even developing new friendships, and if unmarried is likely to remain so. It is this apathy and emotional blunting which make schizophrenia the terrible illness it is, because they are permanent changes in the personality which handicap the subject in every sphere — his ability to get and keep a job, to be an effective husband, wife or parent, to achieve anything, to fully enjoy anything.

Most patients with chronic schizophrenia have recurrent psychotic episodes with hallucinations and delusions, usually taking much the same form on each occasion, or faded remnants of earlier delusional systems, as well as this characteristic apathy and emotional blunting. Depression is also a common and important feature of chronic schizophrenia. Indeed, ICD-10 recognises post-schizophrenic depression as a distinct subtype of schizophrenia (F20.4). Some patients become depressed in the immediate aftermath of their original psychotic episode, others make an apparently full recovery only to return weeks or months later with widespread depressive symptoms. It is sometimes suggested that this lowering of mood is induced by neuroleptics, but there is no convincing evidence from controlled trials that this is so. More likely, it is partly inherent in schizophrenia and partly an understandable psychological reaction to its dire effects and implications. Although the depression of chronic schizophrenia is rarely as severe, or accompanied by such a widespread disturbance of sleep, appetite and concentration as primary depressive disorders often are, it is nonetheless an important cause of suffering and disability. Many schizophrenics, at least in the early stages of their illness, are well able to appreciate that it has deprived them of their capacity to enjoy or feel deeply about anything and some 10% die by suicide, usually in the early years of the illness (Miles 1977).

Frank Fish, and indeed Hughlings Jackson in the 19th century, used to distinguish between positive and negative symptoms, the former being based on some active disturbance of cerebral function, the latter reflecting a reduction or loss of normal function. Crow has suggested distinguishing between what he calls the type I and type II syndromes of schizophrenia, the former being characterised by positive symptoms (delusions, hallucinations and thought disorder) which are well controlled by neuroleptics and the latter by negative symptoms (affective flattening, apathy and poverty of speech) which resemble the sequelae of frontal lobe damage and are usually not controlled by neuropleptics (Crow

1980). His main purpose in advocating this distinction was to suggest that the two syndromes had different aetiologies, the type I syndrome being associated with a disturbance of dopaminergic transmission in the mesolimbic system and the type II syndrome with cognitive impairment and structural changes in the brain. These ideas have been a fertile stimulus to research even though it now seems unlikely that Crow's original hypothesis is correct. Andreasen has developed separate structured interviews for eliciting positive and negative symptoms, and shown that schizophrenics with predominantly negative symptoms tend to have a poor premorbid adjustment, poor educational and occupational attainments, an early age of onset and a poor response to treatment. However, most patients have positive and negative symptoms simultaneously and the evidence that the latter are associated with enlarged lateral ventricles is weak (Andreasen et al 1990). What matters, though, is the temporal rather than the cross-sectional relationship between positive and negative symptoms and the evolution of each over time. Positive symptoms are characteristic of the acute illness and negative symptoms of the chronic illness or defect state, and if the one tends to follow the other in a fairly predictable sequence they are likely to have important determinants in common.

In his original monograph Bleuler had maintained that intelligence, and cognitive function in general, was unimpaired in schizophrenia and this view was generally accepted until recently. It was well known, of course, that many schizophrenics performed poorly on formal tests of intelligence. But it was assumed that this could usually be explained as a secondary consequence of apathy, or of the subject's preoccupation with hallucinatory experiences or delusional ideas. There was no doubt too that chronic schizophrenia was compatible at least in some people with high intellectual achievement, and that some of the patients who scored badly on an intelligence test on one occasion performed far better on retesting. This view was challenged by the demonstration by computerised tomography (CT) that many chronic schizophrenics had abnormally large lateral ventricles (Johnstone et al 1976). For if schizophrenia was accompanied by some form of atrophic cerebral pathology cognitive decline was to be expected. Members of the same MRC research group at Northwick Park quickly showed that many chronic schizophrenics were disoriented in time and did not even know how old they were (Crow & Stevens 1978) and, when the cognitive abilities of chronic schizophrenics were examined in detail, evidence of widespread impairments was soon found.

Thought disorder

Thought disorder is a characteristic feature of schizophrenia. This rather unsatisfactory term has traditionally been applied to a variety of ill-defined abnormalities of the subject's speech and writing which are assumed — and it is an assumption — to be secondary to a more fundamental disturbance of thinking. (The term formal thought disorder is sometimes used to emphasise that it is an abnormality of the form rather than of the content of speech, i.e. thought disorder does not embrace delusional ideation.) These abnormalities were first noted by Hecker in 1871 ('a peculiar departure from normal logical sentence structure, with frequent changes in direction that may or may not lose the train of thought . . . '), and then by Kraepelin, but they were studied and described in much more detail by Bleuler who regarded them as a direct consequence of the 'loosening of associations' which he assumed to be the fundamental deficit of schizophrenia. It is therefore to Bleuler that we owe the long-lived assumption that thought disorder was of cardinal importance, aetiologically and diagnostically, and that it was exhibited by all schizophrenics and by no-one else. These were unfortunate assumptions for several reasons. No-one has ever succeeded in producing a satisfactory definition of the term thought disorder, or in identifying any fundamental psychological or linguistic deficit capable of accounting for the various observable abnormalities of schizophrenic speech. Worse still, few of the abnormalities Bleuler and his successors identified have proved to be specific to schizophrenia, and none to be manifested by more than a proportion of patients with what in other respects are typical schizophrenic illnesses.

The most obvious abnormality in the early stages of the illness is the subject's inability to give a straight answer to any but the simplest of questions, so that the interviewer suddenly realises, after talking to his patient for 5 or 10 minutes, that he has not yet learned anything useful. Usually none of the patient's statements or replies has been obviously non-sensical or bizarre, but almost every one has been vague or irrelevant, and as a result little useful information has been transmitted. Metaphorical terms like 'derailment' and 'Knight's move thinking' have been coined to describe the sudden changes of topic sometimes observed in schizophrenic speech but gross abnormalities of this kind are comparatively rare, at least in the acute illness. More commonly there is a gradual slippage in which a sequence of minor shifts eventually produces a major change of theme. Rochester had drawn attention to another important cause of the listener's difficulty in comprehension — the subject's failure to provide normal cohesive links between one sentence and the next, with the result that the listener is uncertain which of several previously mentioned nouns subsequent pronouns refer to. The problem is often compounded by the subject's preoccupation with abstruse themes and also by his failure to appreciate his listener's difficulties. Quite unlike the aphasic, who is usually distressed by his inability to make his meaning clear, the schizophrenic either fails to appreciate his listener's difficulties, or is indifferent to them.

It is sometimes said that thought disorder involves the semantic content rather than the syntactic structure of speech and that the latter remains intact until a very late stage. This is not so. It has been demonstrated by detailed linguistic analysis that the syntactic structure of schizophrenics' speech is quite different from both that of manics and of normal controls (Morice & Ingram 1982); and also that these abnormalities progress with the passage of time. Schizophrenic speech may be harder to comprehend in the acute illness, partly because the patient is often excited, and preoccupied with abstruse themes and delusional ideas. But its structure is more abnormal in the chronic stage. Sentence structure becomes more primitive with fewer and less deeply embedded subordinate clauses and grammatical errors of varied kinds become more frequent. Above all, the total quantity of speech is reduced.

Bleuler and Kretschmer regarded thought disorder as a result of a generalised 'dissociation' of psychic functions. Subsequently, Babcock suggested that it was simply due to a slowing of all intellectual processes, but later work showed that, although schizophrenics were indeed slower than normals, so too were depressives and psychotics in general. In the 1930s Goldstein suggested that the fundamental disturbance was an inability to make abstract generalisations and it is to him that we owe the rather pointless tradition of asking suspected schizophrenics to explain the meaning of proverbs. It is true that schizophrenics often confuse the different meanings of words like 'fall' and 'sweet' and assume the concrete meaning ('tasting of sugar') when it should have been clear from the context that the abstract one ('charming') was intended, but this may simply be because for most such words the concrete meaning is the common or dominant one. Certainly, formal tests of abstract reasoning capacity indicate that this is primarily a function of intelligence and unrelated to schizophrenia. In the 1940s Cameron suggested that 'over-inclusiveness' was the fundamental disability, by which he meant an inability to maintain conceptual boundaries because of a failure to exclude irrelevant associations. This has some empirical support from object sorting tests, and has interesting parallels with the psychophysiological evidence that schizophrenics have difficulty discriminating between relevant and irrelevant sensory information. Both, in other words, might be due to the breakdown of some hypothetical filtering or attentional focusing mechanism. In the 1960s it was claimed, though never fully confirmed, that schizophrenic speech tended to be less 'redundant' than normal speech so that, if every fourth or fifth word was deleted (the Cloze technique), naive readers were less successful at guessing the identity of the missing words. It is established, however, that schizophrenics tend to use a more restricted range of words, and hence to have a lower 'type/token ratio' than normal people, and that this tendency to repetition applies to syllables as well as to words and phrases, indicating that the cause is something more fundamental than simply having a limited vocabulary. Bannister has also shown that, in terms of Kelly's personal construct theory, schizophrenics' constructs are less stable and more idiosyncratic than other people's.

Unfortunately, none of these observations has yet proved to be of much practical use and none of these various hypotheses has illuminated the fundamental nature of thought disorder. At present it seems that, however thought disorder is defined, a significant proportion of schizophrenics do not exhibit the phenomenon at all. Worse still, it is also exhibited by patients with other psychiatric disorders, particularly mania, and by several revered dramatists and poets. For this reason, interest in thought disorder has waned in the last 20 years and its diagnostic importance has been downgraded. Andreasen (1979) attempted to define 20 of the terms most widely used to describe different facets of thought disorder, including derailment, tangentiality, clanging and illogicality. She succeeded in demonstrating that most of these terms can be defined and rated with reasonable reliability, and showed which were relatively specific to schizophrenia and which equally or more common in mania. She also suggested replacing the term thought disorder with the less ambiguous but more cumbersome phrase 'disorders of thought, language and communication'. These are valuable achievements, but a more radical approach is needed. Seventy years of research into thought disorder has achieved little, not because Bleuler was

wrong in believing that there was something very odd about the speech of many schizophrenics, but because that research was conducted, often without adequate controls, by psychiatrists and psychologists who knew nothing of linguistics. It remains to be seen whether modern linguistic analysis will be any more successful, but future research is more likely to illuminate the fundamental nature of thought disorder if it is based on linguistic concepts like cohesion, lexical density and dysfluency rather than on ancient clinical metaphors like derailment.

Varieties of schizophrenia

Kraepelin recognised three varieties of schizophrenia — hebephrenic, catatonic and paranoid — and Bleuler added a fourth — simple schizophrenia. He also said that, although he assumed schizophrenia to be a group of allied conditions rather than a single disease, he regarded these subdivisions as purely provisional, like a classification of tuberculosis into cases with and without haemoptysis, or with and without amyloidosis. It is ironical, therefore, that his four varieties have figured in most classifications of schizophrenia ever since. Although several additional varieties have often been added to them no schema which attempted to supplant them has ever won more than local acceptance. The expansion of the concept of schizophrenia which took place in the 1940s and 1950s was partly due to the emergence of a series of new concepts, like residual schizophrenia, latent schizophrenia, schizoaffective psychosis (Kasanin 1933) and pseudoneurotic schizophrenia (Hoch & Polatin 1949), which were added to the original four and had the effect of bringing new types of patients under the schizophrenic rubric.

The new (10th) revision of the ICD recognises seven varieties — Bleuler's original four (paranoid, hebephrenic, catatonic and simple) plus undifferentiated schizophrenia, residual schizophrenia and post-schizophrenic depression. Schizoaffective states are classified separately from both schizophrenic and affective disorders and latent schizophrenia has been dropped completely. Its demise was overdue, for it allowed the label of 'schizophrenia', with all its medical and social implications, to be attached to people who had never exhibited schizophrenic symptoms simply on the suspicion that they might do so in future. It is replaced by schizotypal disorder (F21), 'a disorder characterised by eccentric behaviour and anomalies of thinking and affect which resemble those seen in schizophrenia, though no definite and characteristic schizophrenic anomalies have occurred at any stage.' Although schizotypal disorder does sometimes evolve into overt schizophrenia it is usually a stable and enduring personality disorder which is relatively common in the close relatives of schizophrenics and assumed to be part of the genetic 'spectrum' of schizophrenia.

In day-to-day clinical practice most British psychiatrists content themselves with a plain diagnosis of schizophrenia and only use the subcategories for the minority of patients whose symptomatology corresponds closely to one of the subcategory stereotypes. If the illness starts early and insidiously and is dominated by thought disorder and disturbance of affect it is called hebephrenic; if motor abnormalities like posturing or stupor are present it is called catatonic; if hallucinations and delusions are prominent and the personality relatively well preserved it is called paranoid; if progressive deterioration and increasing eccentricity develop in the absence of overt psychotic symptoms it is called simple; and if the original psychotic symptoms have died away, leaving only the apathy, emotional blunting and eccentricity of the defect state, it is called residual. Although the hebephrenic and catatonic forms tend to have the worst prognosis and the paranoid form the best there are no consistent differences in response to treatment or prognosis between the various categories and patients may show the characteristic symptoms of different varieties at different stages in their careers. Nor is there convincing evidence from family studies that the different varieties 'breed true'. Partly for these reasons contemporary interest is focused primarily on how schizophrenia should best be defined rather than on how it should be subdivided. The current American classification (DSM-IIIR), for example, recognises only five varieties — disorganised (hebephrenic), catatonic, paranoid, undifferentiated and residual — and emphasises that the distinction between them is based only on 'the predominant clinical picture that occasioned the most recent evaluation or admission to clinical care'.

THE EPIDEMIOLOGY OF SCHIZOPHRENIA

In most of the industrial countries in which population surveys have been carried out the lifetime risk of schizophrenia is about 1% and the incidence of the order of 15 new cases per 100 000 population per annum. In the American Epidemiologic Catchment Area (ECA) survey, for example, which was based on over 18 000 interviews with random population samples in five sites, the lifetime risk for schizophrenia

using DSM-III criteria was 1.3% (Regier et al 1988). Studies in Africa and Asia are less numerous and have tended to produce somewhat lower estimates. The International Pilot Study of Schizophrenia established that substantial numbers of schizophrenics were admitted to psychiatric hospitals in all the countries involved (Colombia, Czechoslovakia, Denmark, India, Nigeria, Russia, Taiwan, the UK and the USA) and that their symptoms were remarkably similar in all nine despite major differences in language, religion, culture and degree of urbanisation (WHO 1973). The main findings of an even larger cross-cultural comparison by the World Health Organization, based on nearly 1400 patients from 12 centres in ten countries, have been reported since then (Sartorius et al 1986). This study attempted to identify all schizophrenics making a first contact with any treatment agency, including religious institutions and traditional healers, within a defined geographical area, and so was able to generate incidence or inception rates. Although affective symptoms (mainly depressive) were commoner in the industrial countries and visual and auditory hallucinations and catatonic symptoms commoner in the developing countries, the core symptoms of schizophrenia were again remarkably similar in all centres. So too were the inception rates, and also the reasons for admission or referral. When the same operational definition (Catego class S+, which effectively identifies patients with Schneiderian first-rank symptoms) was applied in all centres the inception rate ranged only from seven per 100 000 population per year in Aarhus (Denmark) to 14 in Nottingham with both the urban and rural areas in Chandigarh (India), Dublin, Honolulu, Moscow and Nagasaki in between. This suggests rather strongly that the incidence of schizophrenia is fairly stable across a wide range of cultures, climates and ethnic groupings. Although Torrey (1987) has argued that there may be a ten-fold variation in prevalence from one geographical area to another, with the highest rates in the Arctic and the lowest in the tropics, there appears to be far less variation in the incidence of schizophrenia than for most other common diseases, apart from mental handicap and epilepsy.

It used to be assumed, mainly on the strength of the historical studies of Goldhamer & Marshall (1953) in Massachusetts and Astrup & Ödegaard (1960) in Norway, that the incidence of schizophrenia had not changed since the first decades of the 19th century despite the profound social and cultural changes that have taken place since that time. Recently, however, Hare (1988) has marshalled a mass of historical data to support the view that schizophrenia either arose de novo, or at least became much commoner, towards the end of the 18th century, and that its prevalence increased steadily for the next 100 years. It is also generally accepted that the presentation of the illness has changed, at least in Europe and North America, since the beginning of the 20th century, the hebephrenic and catatonic forms having become much less common and the paranoid form considerably more common since Kraepelin and Bleuler wrote their classical descriptions. These changes have been accompanied by a gradual improvement in prognosis and a rise in the average age of onset. There have also been several reports of declining hospital first-admission rates for schizophrenia in industrial countries in the last 25 years. Eagles & Whalley (1985) drew attention to a 40% fall in the first-admission rate in Scotland between 1969 and 1978, and similar declines have since been reported in Denmark, England and New Zealand. Although the consistency of these reports is impressive it seems likely that the observed decline is due either to changing diagnostic criteria, or to an increasing reluctance to admit schizophrenics to hospital, or some combination of the two (Kendell et al 1993).

The onset of the disease is characteristically between the ages of 15 and 45 years, but it may be before puberty, or delayed until the seventh or eighth decades. Although schizophrenia is equally common in men and women, male schizophrenics are consistently admitted to hospital 4 or 5 years earlier than females, and this appears to reflect a genuine and unexplained difference in the age of onset in the two sexes (Häfner et al 1989). The incidence is considerably higher in the unmarried than the married in both sexes and both also have a considerably reduced fertility (see below).

The first-admission rate for schizophrenia is generally higher in urban than in rural areas, and much higher from the central areas of large cities than from the surrounding suburbs. Faris & Dunham (1939) first drew attention to this striking phenomenon in Chicago and it has since been confirmed in several other American and European cities. The highest admission rates are consistently from the poor working class areas adjacent to the business district and the railway stations and the lowest rates from the middle-class suburbs. This geographical gradient is accompanied by an equally impressive social class gradient, the admission rate of social classes IV and V (unskilled and semiskilled manual workers) being consistently higher than that of other occupational groupings. These findings were originally regarded as evidence that being brought up in a working class family, or in the central slum areas of a big city, created a predisposition to develop schizophrenia, and indeed a recent study of Swedish conscripts found a raised incidence of schizophrenia in those with an urban upbringing (Lewis et al 1992). Even so, it is generally believed that both phenomena are mainly due to selective migration and that the excess of schizophrenic admissions from city centres is largely due to the high admission rate of people who have moved there relatively recently, into bedsitters, hostels or lodging houses. Similarly, Goldberg & Morrison (1963) were able to show, by examining the birth certificates of a series of 672 young male schizophrenics, that although they themselves were predominantly from social classes IV and V, their fathers' social class had not differed from that of the general population, and that the disparity between the two was due to a 'downward drift' of the sons a few months or years before their admission to hospital. The young man, for example, who had started at university or became apprenticed had drifted away before finishing and was working as a labourer (and probably living in lodgings as well) at the time he was eventually admitted to hospital.

Migration has also long been associated with an increased risk of schizophrenic breakdown. Ödegaard (1932) found that Norwegians who had emigrated to Minnesota had a higher risk of schizophrenic breakdown than those who had remained in Norway, and Malzberg & Lee (1956) showed that immigrants to New York had a much higher hospital admission rate than native born Americans, with their children half-way between. More recently, Cochrane (1977) has shown that most immigrant groups to England and Wales, particularly West Indians, Asians and Poles, have higher hospital admission rates for schizophrenia than the English and the Scots. Similar findings have been reported from other countries, but the relationship is not invariable. Jaco (1960), for example, failed to find any increased risk of schizophrenia in Spanish-speaking immigrants to Texas. At times the cause of this increased risk has had considerable political as well as scientific significance, with the host country or community being tempted to attribute the phenomenon to a selective migration of unstable undesirables, and the immigrants themselves and their fellow countrymen back home attributing it to the stresses of living in a foreign and sometimes hostile land. In reality, it is not yet firmly established that the incidence of schizophrenia is increased in immigrants. Most studies have been based on hospital admissions, and psychiatrically disturbed immigrants are more likely to be admitted to mental hospitals than other people. Once admitted they are also at greater risk of being labelled as schizophrenic, particularly if their behaviour is unusual and the examining doctor has difficulty communicating with them. Moreover, most comparisons between immigrant and native populations have not matched the two for age, a crucial omission because most immigrants are young adults and schizophrenia is a disease of young adults.

It has recently been reported that the Afro-Caribbean populations of several English cities have extremely high hospital admission rates for schizophrenia, perhaps ten times as high as that of their white neighbours (McGovern & Cope 1987, Harrison et al 1988). Although it seems unlikely that differences of this magnitude could be generated by racial biasing of diagnostic criteria, inaccurate demographic assumptions (there were no questions about ethnicity in the 1981 census) or ethnic differences in contact rates with psychiatric services, these findings, which are largely generated by people born in the UK rather than first-generation immigrants, are bound to be controversial and politically sensitive until rigorously designed epidemiological comparisons have been carried out. No adequate explanation for this very high hospital admission rate has yet been offered, partly because at present it is unclear whether Afro-Caribbeans have a similarly high incidence of schizophrenia in the Caribbean. The widespread use of cannabis may be a partial explanation.

The fertility of schizophrenics has been studied many times and there is general agreement that they marry less often than other people, remain childless more often even when they do marry, and have fewer children than other people in or out of wedlock. In the past this was usually attributed to their confinement in sexually segregated asylums. However, it is now apparent that their fertility is low even before admission to hospital, and studies carried out in the 1960s and 1970s after the introduction of 'open door' policies confirm that, despite the increased opportunities for marrying and conceiving thus provided, schizophrenics still have far fewer children than other people.

Schizophrenics also have a raised mortality. Studies in Europe and North America suggest that their relative risk of death is increased two-fold and most of this increased risk is accounted for by the first few years after diagnosis or hospital admission. Although this raised mortality is shared by other forms of mental illness there have been repeated claims of associations,

both positive and negative, between schizophrenia and other physical illnesses (Baldwin 1979). The only one of these relationships that seems well established at the present time is a negative, and as yet unexplained, association between schizophrenia and rheumatoid arthritis. Despite many conflicting claims it is not established that schizophrenics are either more or less likely to develop cancers in general, or any particular form of cancer, than other people. Nor is the claimed association between schizophrenia and coeliac disease supported by convincing evidence.

One of the most important reasons for studying the epidemiology of a disease is to obtain clues to its aetiology. At one time the striking relationships found between schizophrenia and the central areas of big cities, low social class, being unmarried and being a migrant all seemed capable of providing that vital clue. But the relationship with migration is still in doubt and the other three have turned out to be consequences rather than causes of the disorder. There is, however, one important relationship which is safe from this risk and must have some aetiological significance: the relationship between schizophrenia and season of birth. It has been found in virtually every country in the temperate latitudes of the Northern hemisphere that schizophrenic first admissions are more likely to have been born in the early months of the year than the rest of the population, and correspondingly less likely to have been born in July to September. This relationship is not shared by other diagnostic categories and, although the excess of births in January to March is only about 8%, it is consistent and highly significant statistically (Bradbury & Miller 1985). In Australia and South Africa the excess of births is July to September (i.e. the winter months, as in Europe). Preliminary evidence also indicates that the siblings of schizophrenics show the same distribution of birth dates as the general population and that the excess of winter births of schizophrenics is greater the colder the winter. This suggests that the incidence of schizophrenia is influenced by some widely distributed seasonal variable, probably infective or dietary, acting either in utero or in the early months of life. Current interest is focused on intrauterine viral infection, for many viral infections have a well-defined seasonal variation and rubella demonstrates that an inconspicuous infection in a young woman may cause permanent damage to the fetal nervous system if she is pregnant at the time. There have been several reports in recent years, from Finland, Denmark, England and Scotland, that fluctuations in the birth dates of schizophrenics can be related to fluctuations in the incidence of influenza 2 or 3 months beforehand (e.g. see Sham et al 1992), suggesting that damage to the fetus in the sixth or seventh month of pregnancy may be aetiologically important. Until the mechanism involved is established, however, these potentially important findings are likely to remain controversial.

THE AETIOLOGY OF SCHIZOPHRENIA

Endogenous factors

The evidence summarised in Chapter 12 establishes beyond reasonable doubt that schizophrenia, or a liability to develop schizophrenia, is genetically transmitted. The evidence of family, twin and adoption studies all points in the same direction, though the mode of transmission remains obscure, and may well be polygenic (see Ch. 12 for details). This evidence of genetic transmission establishes that there must be an innate biological difference — qualitative or quantitative — between schizophrenics and other people. So far that difference has not been identified, though there is an emerging consensus that schizophrenia is a neurodevelopmental disorder and that the crucial abnormalities are situated in the deep structures of the temporal lobes.

The most obvious clue to the putative biological abnormality is provided by the mode of action of neuroleptic drugs. Most of the chemical substances with proven antipsychotic activity — phenothiazines, butyrophenones and thioxanthenes — have multiple pharmacological actions. The only action common to them all is that of inhibiting transmission in dopaminergic, and particularly D_2, neurone systems. The likelihood that this effect on dopaminergic transmission is responsible for their therapeutic effects is strengthened by other evidence. For most neuroleptics other than clozapine there is a direct relationship between their potency as inhibitors of postsynaptic D_2 receptors in experimental animals and their clinical efficacy as antipsychotic agents. Amphetamine, which facilitates dopaminergic transmission, can produce an acute psychosis indistinguishable from paranoid schizophrenia. It is also claimed that amphetamine infusions often exacerbate schizophrenic hallucinations and delusions, and that this temporary deterioration predicts the likelihood of future relapse.

This evidence has led to many attempts to demonstrate an abnormal dopaminergic neurone system in the brains of schizophrenics. Whalley et al (1984), for example, claimed that drug-free patients with Schneiderian first-rank symptoms had a greater growth hormone response to the dopamine agonist apomorphine than other psychotic patients. It is well established that the density of postsynaptic D_2 receptors is increased in the caudate nucleus (part of the nigrostriatal dopaminergic system) and the nucleus accumbens (part of the mesolimbic dopaminergic system) of schizophrenics' brains at post mortem compared with those of matched controls (Owen et al 1978, Mackay et al 1982). This might have been the crucial biological abnormality underlying the clinical syndrome, and the explanation of the therapeutic efficacy of neuroleptics. Alternatively, it might have been a mundane consequence of previous neuroleptic administration, for it is known that chronic administration of neuroleptics to experimental animals leads to a proliferation of postsynaptic dopamine receptors in much the same way as section of a motor nerve leads to proliferation of the motor endplate. For a long time the issue remained unresolved because it was so difficult to find schizophrenics who had died without ever receiving antipsychotic drugs. Recently, however, it has become possible to measure D_2 receptor density in the brains of young live schizophrenics who have never received neuroleptics using positron emission tomography (PET) (see Ch. 21). It is claimed by Wong et al (1986) in Baltimore, using $[^{11}C]N$-methylspiperone as their D_2 receptor ligand, that drug-naive chronic schizophrenics have a two- to three-fold increase in dopamine receptor densities in their basal ganglia. However, neither Sedval's research group in Stockholm, who use $[^{11}C]$raclopride as the ligand (Farde et al 1990), or a French team using $[^{76}Br]$bromolisuride as the ligand (Martinot et al 1991), have been able to find any difference in D_2 receptor density between schizophrenics and normal controls.

At present, therefore, the balance of evidence suggests that there is no primary abnormality of either the nigrostriatal or the mesolimbic dopamine systems in schizophrenia. There are also clinical reasons for suspecting that neuroleptics probably exert their beneficial effects indirectly, like diuretics in heart failure, rather than counteracting any fundamental abnormality. In the first place, their therapeutic action is not specific to schizophrenia, but extends to mania and most other psychoses. Secondly, not all schizophrenics respond to neuroleptics even in the acute phase of their illness, and even in those who do the time-course of clinical response extends over several days or weeks, whereas the effects on dopaminergic transmission are fully developed within hours.

The fact that schizophrenics have enlarged lateral and third ventricles is the other important evidence of a biological abnormality. Ventricular enlargement was first demonstrated by air encephalography in the 1950s but firm evidence had to await the introduction of CT in the 1970s. Since the original CT study by Johnstone et al (1976) over 50 blind controlled comparisons of the ventricle/brain ratio (VBR) in schizophrenics and matched controls have been published and 75% of these show a significant increase in VBR in the schizophrenics (Andreasen et al 1990). The enlargement is modest, however, and only about a third of patients have a VBR more than 1 standard deviation above the control mean. Schizophrenics with enlarged ventricles tend to be male and to have a poor premorbid adjustment, early age of onset, poor cognitive performance and poor prognosis, but in most respects they differ little from those with normal ventricles. In particular, contrary to earlier assumptions and predictions, they are no more likely to have negative symptoms or less likely to have a family history. Moreover, no study in which a group of schizophrenics has been rescanned after an interval of several years has succeeded in demonstrating any further increase in VBR, which suggests that ventricular enlargement probably precedes the onset of the illness rather than, as was originally assumed, developing as the illness progressed.

Magnetic resonance imaging (MRI; see Ch. 21) is now confirming and extending the CT findings and comparisons have been carried out with both techniques between pairs of monozygous (MZ) twins discordant for schizophrenia in order to eliminate the confounding influence of genetic variation on cerebral morphology and ventricular size. Suddath et al (1990) compared the MRI scans of 15 pairs of MZ twins and found that in at least 13 of the 15 both lateral ventricles and the third ventricle were larger in the schizophrenic twin and both hippocampi smaller. As Reveley et al (1982) had previously found similar differences in the CT scans of discordant twins this suggests that subtle anatomical changes may be present in nearly all schizophrenics, but not be demonstrable unless an MZ twin is available for comparison.

This evidence of radiological abnormalities has led to a renewed interest in the neuropathology of schizophrenia, and to a re-examination of schizophrenic brains collected long ago. Bogerts et al (1985) at the Vogt Institute in Dusseldorf carried out a detailed quantitative comparison of the brains of 13 schizophrenics and nine controls who had died between 1928 and 1953 without receiving phenothiazines, insulin or ECT. The amygdala, hippocampus, parahippocampal gyrus and globus

pallidus (but not the putamen, caudate or nucleus accumbens) were found to be significantly smaller in the schizophrenics. Similar differences emerged from a comparison of the brains of 41 schizophrenics and 29 patients with affective disorder from Runwell Hospital (Brown et al 1986). The schizophrenics' brains weighed about 6% less, their lateral ventricles, particularly the temporal horns, were larger in cross-section, and the cortex of their left parahippocampal gyrus, but not that of the cingulate gyrus or the insula, was much thinner. Crow et al (1989) compared the brains of 22 schizophrenics with those of matched non-psychiatric controls. They delineated the lateral ventricles of their formalin-fixed half brains with X-ray photographs after filling them with radio-opaque dye and found that dilatation of the ventricle was greatest in the temporal lobe (82% larger than controls) and much more prominent on the left than the right. Like Brown et al (1986) they found the schizophrenics' brains to be significantly lighter and shorter than their controls. They also failed to find any evidence of gliosis accompanying the structural changes they found, either by Holzer staining or using immunological techniques. Finally, there are now reports of abnormalities of the detailed cellular architecture of specific cerebral structures in schizophrenia. Pakkenberg (1990) in Denmark used an objective stereological technique to demonstrate a substantial reduction in the number of cells (neurones, astrocytes and oligodendroglia) in the mediodorsal nucleus of the thalamus and the nucleus accumbens in schizophrenics' brains. Conrad et al (1991) in California have also demonstrated, by laboriously measuring the axis of orientation of tens of thousands of pyramidal cells in the hippocampus, that in the cornu amonis the normal parallel orientations of these cells are disturbed, both on the left and the right.

Although we are not yet in a position to define a characteristic neuropathology for schizophrenia, still less to ask neuropathologists to confirm or refute the clinical diagnosis, 13 of the 16 controlled studies carried out in the last decade have found pathological changes in the medial temporal lobe. In addition, there is an emerging consensus that schizophrenics' brains are smaller and lighter, and the temporal horns of their lateral ventricles larger, than those of matched controls, that abnormalities are often present in the basal ganglia, the hippocampus and parahippocampal gyrus and other temporal lobe structures, and that these abnormalities are usually more prominent on the left side of the brain. There is also general agreement that these changes are not accompanied by gliosis, which implies either that they represent developmental abnormalities or, if they are the result of a pathological process, that the damage occurred before birth.

Many other biological differences have been reported in the last 20 years between schizophrenics and matched controls. In normal people, cerebral blood flow and cerebral oxygen and glucose utilisation are greater in the frontal lobes than in other parts of the brain, indicating that metabolic activity is higher in the frontal lobes. Ingvar & Franzen (1974) showed by intracarotid injection of ^{133}Xe that schizophrenics were different; that, although their overall cerebral blood flow was normal, there was a relative deficiency over the frontal lobes. This 'hypofrontality' has since been confirmed by other workers using more sophisticated technologies. DeLisi et al (1985), for example, used PET to measure the metabolism of ^{18}F-labelled deoxyglucose by different parts of the brain and found hypofrontality both in schizophrenics and in patients with bipolar disorders. Other American researchers have claimed that chronic schizophrenics show a selective failure to increase regional cerebral blood flow to the dorsolateral prefrontal cortex while performing the Wisconsin Card Sorting Test, an abstract reasoning task widely used as a specific test of frontal lobe functioning (Weinberger et al 1986). There are also intriguing indications that the division of function between the two halves of the brain may be abnormal in schizophrenics. For example, Gur et al (1983) found that while the increase in regional cerebral blood flow generated by thinking is greater in normal right-handed people over the left hemisphere during a verbal task and over the right hemisphere during a spatial task, the pattern was different in schizophrenics. In them, verbal tasks were associated with an equal increase in cerebral blood flow on both sides and spatial tasks with a greater increase on the left than on the right.

Murphy & Wyatt (1972) reported that platelet monoamine oxidase (MAO) activity was reduced in schizophrenics and, because the assay involved is relatively straightforward, many attempts have been made to replicate this finding. Several groups confirmed their results but others failed to do so, or found low platelet MAO activity to be a general characteristic of all chronic psychoses. The explanation of these conflicting findings is still unclear, but they are unlikely to have any fundamental significance. Indeed, there is no evidence that platelet MAO activity correlates with MAO activity in the brain (Young et al 1986).

The eye-tracking movements of schizophrenics have also been shown to be abnormal (Holzman et al 1974). When normal people watch a rhythmically moving object like a pendulum their eyes follow it with a smooth sinusoidal movement that keeps the moving object focused on the macula with remarkable accuracy. Holzman's observation that schizophrenics and many of their first-degree relatives do so less accurately than other people has been confirmed several times. Abnormal eye-tracking movements have also been reported in a high proportion of manic subjects, both ill and in remission, though this may be attributable to lithium. Finally, there is accumulating evidence that the cortical potentials evoked by repetitive sensory stimuli — auditory, visual or tactile — are abnormal in schizophrenics. Blackwood et al (1987) studied the latency of the P300 wave (i.e. the positive potential occurring about 300 ms after the stimulus) during a two-tone discrimination task in both schizophrenia and depression. Latency was increased in both, but in the depressives it returned to normal after recovery whereas in the schizophrenics it remained prolonged and was also unaffected by medication. Although this increased P300 latency is not specific to schizophrenia (it has also been reported in Alzheimer's disease and Down's syndrome) it does suggest the presence of a stable abnormality of auditory information processing. Siegel et al (1984) in Colorado have also claimed that if experimental subjects are exposed to two loud clicks half a second apart and the amplitudes of the P50 waves (i.e. the positive potentials about 50 ms after the stimulus) evoked by these two clicks are then compared, schizophrenics and many of their first-degree relatives do not show the same reduction in amplitude in response to the second click as normal people.

Although several of the abnormalities described above are very intriguing, it is important to realise that there are considerable technical difficulties in the detection or measurement of all of them. None is invariably present, none has been shown to be specific to schizophrenia and few have been confirmed often enough to be regarded as established fact. Nor do they fit together to form a coherent whole. Even so, it is difficult to believe that some of these abnormalities will not eventually prove to be important clues to the fundamental biological dysfunction underlying the clinical syndrome.

Environmental influences

Although the twin and adoption studies described in Chapter 12 prove beyond reasonable doubt that schizophrenia is genetically transmitted, this evidence also establishes that environmental influences must play a major role as well, for estimates of the concordance rate in MZ twins derived from whole populations are consistently less than 50%. In other words, someone whose genetically identical twin develops schizophrenia has less than a 50:50 chance of doing the same, and whether or not he does so must depend on his past or present environment. We still know little of the nature or time of action of these environmental influences, through the CT and MRI studies of discordant MZ twins described above strongly suggest that they result in hippocampal damage and ventricular enlargement.

The association between schizophrenia and winter/spring births described previously points strongly to the influence of some environmental agent, either in utero or early in postnatal life. So too does the observation that when MZ twins are discordant for schizophrenia it is usually the twin of lower birth weight who subsequently becomes psychotic. There is currently much interest in the possibility that an intrauterine viral infection may be at least partly responsible for the season of birth effect, and some epidemiological evidence to incriminate the influenza virus (Sham et al 1992). There is also evidence of an increased incidence of obstetric complications in schizophrenics, thus raising the possibility that anoxic or other injury at or near the time of birth may contribute to aetiology. Most of these studies are based on the mothers', or in some cases the patients' own, memories of the circumstances of their birth and these are obviously liable to be biased in different ways in schizophrenics and controls. There is one substantial Swedish study, however, based on blind rating of the original birth records of 100 schizophrenics and 100 controls from the same obstetric unit, which found a significant excess of obstetric complications in the 'process' schizophrenics (McNeil & Kaij 1978).

In the last 40 years the possibility that pathological relationships or patterns of communication within the nuclear family may lead, at least in genetically vulnerable children, to the eventual development of schizophrenia has received a great deal of attention, particularly in the USA. In the 1940s Freda Fromm-Reichmann coined the phrase 'schizophrenogenic mother' and later workers supported the concept with claims that the mothers of schizophrenics were both overprotective and hostile to their children. A few years later Bateson at Palo Alto (Bateson et al 1956) suggested that schizophrenia was produced by the constant reception of incongruent messages from a key relative — to take a trite example, the verbal message 'You know that Mummy loves you'

accompanied by non-verbal behaviour implying something quite different — and this 'double-bind hypothesis' remained in vogue for a decade or more. Shortly afterwards, Lidz and his colleagues at Yale carried out a series of intensive studies of 17 upper middle-class families with what they regarded as schizophrenic children. They described several highly abnormal relationships within these families which differed with the sex of the schizophrenic child and which they suggested were associated with the development of schizophrenia in this son or daughter (Lidz et al 1965). Their work aroused great interest and their terms 'marital schism' and 'marital skew' obtained the same wide currency as Bateson's 'double bind'. Unfortunately, these studies all had serious methodological defects and owed their influence more to their catch phrases and the prevailing climate of opinion than to objective evidence. They were not conducted blind, had no adequate control groups, involved a very diffuse concept of schizophrenia and were retrospective, so that it was difficult to tell which of the observed abnormalities had preceded the onset of schizophrenia in the child, and might therefore have some aetiological significance, and which were merely reactions to the child's illness.

Alongside these global studies of parental personalities and family interactions a series of more limited and better designed studies of communication patterns in schizophrenic and non-schizophrenic families was carried out. The most influential of these were by Singer & Wynne (1965) who gave Rorschach tests to the parents of schizophrenics and claimed that they consistently produced more deviant responses (i.e. that they were more 'thought disordered') than control parents. However, when Hirsch & Leff (1975) repeated this work they were unable to confirm Wynne's findings. Although there was a significant difference between the average deviance scores of the parents of schizophrenics and the parents of neurotic controls, the overlap was considerable and the higher deviance scores of the former were entirely due to the fact that they spoke at greater length, i.e. there was no difference in the rate at which the two groups made deviant responses.

What then survives from all this? It is reasonably well established that the parents of schizophrenics are psychiatrically disturbed more often than the parents of normal children and that more of the mothers have schizoid personality traits. Moreover, the parents of schizophrenics do seem to be in conflict with one another more often than the parents of other psychiatric patients, and the mothers more concerned about and protective towards their children even before the onset of the psychosis. There is plenty of scope in all this for baneful influence on the preschizophrenic child but as yet there is no convincing evidence that any of these influences do in fact contribute to the development of schizophrenia. Furthermore, all the well-substantiated parental abnormalities are easily explicable in genetic terms, and none is invariably present.

Events in the weeks or months immediately prior to the onset of illness have received less attention than the events of childhood but there is some evidence that they may be important. Steinberg & Durrell (1968) showed in the 1960s that the schizophrenic breakdown rate of recruits to the US army was much higher in their first month of military service than at any time in the next 2 years, suggesting that the transition from civilian life to recruiting barracks was contributing to the genesis of these illnesses. The effect was the same in volunteers as in enlisted men and they were able to produce fairly convincing evidence that the illnesses presenting in the first month of service were indeed new and not merely newly detected. Further evidence was provided by Brown & Birley (1968) who obtained detailed information about the events of the previous 12 weeks from 50 patients with schizophrenic illnesses of recent onset and 400 controls from the same neighbourhood. They found that the schizophrenics had experienced significantly more life events than the controls in the 3 weeks immediately prior to the onset of illness, but only in those 3 weeks. The difference between schizophrenics and controls remained even when all events which might have been a consequence of incipient illness (i.e. losing a job by being sacked as opposed to the closure of the firm) were eliminated. It has to be borne in mind, however, that the concept of schizophrenia employed in both these studies was a broad one. In Brown & Birley's study, 24 patients were only 'probably schizophrenic' and, furthermore, only 24 of the 50 were first admissions.

More attention has been paid to the determinants of relapse in those who have already had one episode of schizophrenia, mainly because the comparatively high probability of a further episode makes it feasible to mount prospective studies. Brown et al (1972) showed that the relapse rate over the next 12 months in young men who had just recovered from a first episode of schizophrenia was far higher (58% versus 16%) in those who returned to live with a relative, usually a parent or wife, who was prone to make critical comments about them than in those who lived with a relative who was more tolerant and accepting. The difference between the two was not simply due to

a difference in the initial severity of illness or frequency of antisocial behaviour. Moreover, the ill effects of what the authors called 'high expressed emotion' or high EE were mitigated to some extent if the patient was receiving phenothiazines, and also if patient and relative were in contact with one another for less than 35 hours a week, i.e. social withdrawal seemed to be protective. These very interesting findings have subsequently been confirmed by Vaughn & Leff (1976) and by Vaughn et al (1984) in California. This led to widespread interest in the phenomenon and Parker & Hadzi-Palovic (1990) were recently able to review 12 published studies assessing the capacity of EE status to predict schizophrenic relapse in a total of 908 subjects, including one study in a rural Indian village. Overall, high EE patients were 3.7 times more likely to relapse within 9–12 months of leaving hospital than low EE patients, so there can be no doubting the importance of schizophrenics' emotional environment. The mechanism by which a critical or emotionally over-involved relative precipitates relapse is also unknown, though there is some evidence to suggest that it is mediated by an effect on physiological arousal (Tarrier et al 1988a).

Psychological theories

Innumerable psychological theories of both the aetiology and the pathogenesis of schizophrenia have been proposed in the past. Many were derived from psychoanalysis, others from behavioural or cognitive psychology. Apart from the defective filter theory of sensory overload, few were backed by any substantial empirical data and most are now of only historical interest. Recently, however, some new and more promising hypotheses have been propounded.

Frith (1987), like Kraepelin, assumes that schizophrenia is a disorder of volition. He suggests that the brain maintains a fundamental distinction between actions occurring in response to perceptual stimuli (stimulus intentions) and those occurring in response to internal goals (willed intentions). He also proposes that there is a central monitoring system (corollary discharge) informing the subject what action has been selected and why (i.e. in response to which intention), independently of visual and proprioceptive feedback from the action itself. He then suggests that 'positive' symptoms (delusions of control, hearing voices, etc.) are due to faulty central monitoring of willed intentions and negative symptoms (paucity of speech, apathy, etc.) to a failure to translate willed intentions into actions, and that neuroleptics work by inhibiting all willed intentions, thereby diminishing the misinterpretations arising from their faulty central monitoring. Much of this is speculation. Frith has shown, however, that when drug-free schizophrenics perform a motor task (a videogame) designed to elicit errors those with delusions of control perform strikingly worse if they are deprived of visual feedbacks, whereas the performance of schizophrenics without such delusions, and that of other controls, is hardly affected (Frith & Done 1989).

Latent inhibition is a phenomenon readily demonstrable in animals and man whereby repeated exposure to a stimulus without consequence retards subsequent conditioning to that stimulus. (For example, a rat repeatedly exposed to a particular odour will take longer to learn the significance of that odour if the odour is subsequently paired with a rewarding or punishing stimulus.) Gray & Hemsley have recently shown that although schizophrenics in remission display latent inhibition in the same way as normal controls, acutely ill schizophrenics do not (Baruch et al 1988). Quite apart from the intrinsic interest of a simple and widely applicable paradigm in which schizophrenics perform better than normals, latent inhibition is known to be abolished in rats by amphetamine, and to be strengthened by neuroleptics. It has the makings, therefore, of a promising animal model of schizophrenia, and the potential to link the neurochemical dopamine hypothesis with the cognitive evidence that schizophrenics are unable to filter out, or ignore, irrelevant sensory information.

Summary

The most plausible synthesis of the genetic, neuropathological and epidemiological evidence described above and in Chapter 12 is that schizophrenia is a neurodevelopmental disorder as Weinberger (1987) has suggested. The architecture of the hippocampus and other temporal lobe structures, and the connections between these and the frontal lobes, are abnormal in at least a substantial proportion of schizophrenics. These abnormalities may either be genetically determined, or produced by injury to the developing brain (mediated perhaps by disruption of the normal sequence of neuronal migrations) either in utero or at the time of birth. This would account for the enlarged lateral ventricles of schizophrenics, the changes in their brains found at post mortem and the subtle intellectual and social disabilities of schizophrenic children before the overt onset of their illness. The 20–30 year delay before the onset of the psychosis could be explained in maturational terms.

Myelination and synaptic pruning are not complete in the frontal lobes until or after puberty, and it has been shown that the behaviour of infant monkeys with surgical lesions of their dorsolateral prefrontal cortex does not become overtly abnormal until they are adult (Weinberger 1987). A model of this kind could explain most of the established facts about schizophrenia, including the role of stress in precipitating onset and subsequent relapses, the therapeutic effects of neuroleptics and the very variable course of the disorder. There are, of course, major speculative elements in the model but it does at least provide, almost for the first time, a plausible conceptual framework to guide future research.

THE COURSE AND PROGNOSIS OF SCHIZOPHRENIA

Although Kraepelin's original concept of dementia praecox was founded on the belief that such illnesses all progressed to a state of global deterioration, or at least resulted in permanent damage to the personality, the outcome of schizophrenic illnesses, as Kraepelin himself eventually came to realise, is in fact very variable however the syndrome is defined. Some resolve completely, with or without treatment, and never recur (pattern A). Some recur repeatedly with full recovery every time (pattern B). Others recur repeatedly but recovery is incomplete; that is, there is a persistent defect state that characteristically becomes more pronounced after each successive relapse (pattern C). Finally, some illnesses pursue a progressive downhill course from the beginning (pattern D). The relative frequency of these different outcomes depends a great deal on how schizophrenia is defined. If it is defined in such a way as to exclude those with prominent affective symptoms, the proportion of patients making a full recovery (patterns A and B) is reduced; and if the diagnosis is also restricted, as it is by the Feighner, DSM-III and DSM-IIIR definitions, to patients with a 6 month history the proportion recovering without permanent defect is reduced still further. Despite this variability of outcome there is firm agreement on the characteristics of the initial illness predicting good or bad outcome. Vaillant (1964) demonstrated, 25 years ago, first retrospectively and then prospectively, that a simple rating scale based on the presence or absence of the following seven items predicted outcome with 80% accuracy:

● Acute onset (i.e. within the previous 6 months)
● A stressful event or situation at the time of onset

- A family history of depressive illness
- No family history of schizophrenia
- No schizoid traits in the premorbid personality
- Confusion or perplexity
- Prominent affective symptoms.

Subsequently, Stephens et al (1966) studied two groups of 50 patients in Baltimore, one composed of patients who had all remained well for at least 5 years after their initial illness, the other of patients who had all spent at least 5 years in hospital. The original case notes of these patients were rated, blind to the follow-up findings, for 54 items of potential prognostic significance and 11 of these were found to distinguish the good and bad prognosis groups at the 5% level. Like Vaillant, they were able on this basis to predict good or bad outcome in individual patients with over 80% accuracy. Most of their indices were the same as his, though they also found that being married was associated with a good outcome and low intelligence and emotional blunting with a bad outcome. One can see, therefore, that definitions of schizophrenia which exclude patients with affective symptoms or a symptom duration of under 6 months have a poor prognosis at least partly because they exclude from the schizophrenic fold patients for whom Vaillant's and Stephens' prognostic scales would have predicted a good outcome. (Alternatively, looking at the problem from the perspective of DSM-III or DSM-IIIR, most of the patients whom Vaillant and Stephens would have regarded as having good prognosis schizophrenia were actually suffering from affective or schizophreniform disorders misdiagnosed as schizophrenia.) But however schizophrenia is defined the most characteristic, though not necessarily the most frequent, outcome is the development of a 'defect state' characterised by emotional blunting and apathy, and often accompanied by the faded remnants of previous delusions and hallucinations (patterns C or D above). And however the term is defined a sizeable proportion of patients do not develop any defect state, whether or not they have further psychotic episodes (patterns A or B above). In recent years several long-term follow-up studies of schizophrenics have been published and most have concluded that the eventual prognosis is relatively good (i.e. patterns A or B without the development of lasting damage to the personality) in about 50%. For example, Ciompi and Muller in Lausanne followed up a series of 289 schizophrenics for 37 years and found complete or almost complete recovery in 49% (Ciompi 1980). Manfred Bleuler in Zurich followed 208 patients for 22 years and found a 'favourable end state' in 53%

(Bleuler 1972). And Huber in Bonn followed 502 patients for 21 years and found a favourable end state in 57% (Huber et al 1980). Although none of these authors employed operational diagnostic criteria, the results of a more recent American study using DSM-III criteria were surprisingly similar. Eighty-two patients referred from the Vermont State Hospital to a rehabilitation programme in 1955–1960 were interviewed in 1980–1982. Two-thirds were found to have few or no symptoms and 40% had been employed in the previous year (Harding et al 1987). This was in a rural area, however. Similar follow-up studies in large American cities have suggested a much poorer outcome.

Outcome seems to be determined more by the circumstances under which the illness develops and the premorbid personality than by the symptomatology of the illness itself. Illnesses that develop acutely in response to stress have a much better prognosis than those that develop insidiously for no apparent reason. And if the patient has prominent schizoid personality traits, particularly if he is also young, of low intelligence, and has a poor work record, the outlook is much bleaker than if he is married, more mature, and with a more normal personality. Several studies have also reported a worse prognosis, at least where hospital discharge rates are concerned, in men than in women. Social considerations are partly responsible for this difference. Women are more likely to possess the basic housekeeping skills needed for survival outside hospital, and also pose less threat of violence to others. But the fact that women also have a considerably later age of onset than men suggests that there are intrinsic differences between the sexes as well.

Illnesses, of course, do not have an outcome in vacuo, or even a natural history. Outcome is always affected for good or ill by treatment and other environmental influences, and there is little doubt that the outcome of schizophrenia has improved considerably in the last 50 years. Follow-up studies conducted in the 1920s and 1930s, before any effective treatments were available, only reported full recovery in about 12% of patients, and at least 70% were either unimproved or dead at the time of assessment (Stalker 1939). Since the 1950s all comparable follow-up studies have shown much better results. Wing's (1966) 5 year follow up of 111 schizophrenic first admissions to three mental hospitals in southern England is as representative as any. Only 7% of these patients remained in hospital as long as 2 years, only 28% spent any part of the last 2 years in hospital, and at the time of final follow-up 63% of the men were employed and 69% of the women either employed or successfully running a household. To what extent this improvement was due to the phenothiazine drugs introduced in 1953 and to what extent it was due to the changes in the milieu of mental hospitals and in public attitudes to mental illness taking place simultaneously is difficult to determine, but the combination certainly produced a dramatic change. In most industrial countries the number of mental hospital beds fell by at least 50% between 1950 and 1990, and although financial and political considerations played an important role in many places the major cause of this massive reduction was the changed outlook and management of schizophrenia. There is little doubt, though, that the effects of neuroleptics on the long-term prognosis of schizophrenia are less impressive than the short-term effects. Although contemporary patients spend less time in hospital than their predecessors, and are far less likely to end their days as permanent hospital invalids, a disturbingly high proportion still remain chronically handicapped by defect states or recurring hallucinations and delusions and still require repeated admissions to hospital despite long-term drug therapy.

The follow-up studies described so far were all carried out in the industrialised countries of western Europe and North America. There is, however, fairly substantial evidence that the prognosis of schizophrenia is considerably better in so-called underdeveloped countries, despite their meagre psychiatric services. The most important evidence to this effect comes from the International Pilot Study of Schizophrenia. In that study a large series of psychotic patients, the majority of whom were schizophrenics, were studied in nine different centres in different parts of the world. The same structured interviewing methods were used in all nine centres and the patients were re-interviewed at 2 years and 5 years, again using the same methods and criteria throughout. Quite unexpectedly, the average outcome was considerably better in the underdeveloped countries (Colombia, India and Nigeria) than in the industrialised countries (Czechoslovakia, Denmark, the UK, the USA and Russia) (Sartorius et al 1977). The difference did not lie in the proportion of patients pursuing a steady downhill course (pattern D); this was much the same throughout. It lay in the proportion suffering recurrent relapses. Despite the much more extensive follow-up treatment available in the industrial countries, a high proportion of their patients had further psychotic episodes, whereas Colombian, Nigerian and Indian patients did not. The same finding had emerged from an earlier comparison of the outcome of schizophrenia in London and Mauritius. Although careful comparisons of the initial symptomatology and other characteristics of the patients from the nine study centres did not reveal any important differences between them, the possibility that these differences in outcome were due to unrecognised differences in the types of patients admitted to hospital in the nine centres can obviously not be excluded. Certainly people with acute behavioural disturbances are more likely to come to medical attention in settings where psychiatric services are novel and thinly spread than those with insidiously developing disorders that do not cause the same alarm, and the former are, of course, likely to have a better prognosis than the latter. Partly to elucidate these intriguing differences in outcome the WHO mounted a further international comparison, involving 12 centres in 10 countries, known as the Determinants of Outcome of Severe Mental Disorders programme. The preliminary results of this major study confirm that, at follow-up 2 years after their initial inception into treatment, schizophrenic illnesses have a better prognosis in developing than in developed countries (Sartorius et al 1986). Part, but only part, of this difference is attributable to a higher proportion of illnesses in the developed countries having a relatively insidious onset. It seems likely, therefore, that there is something about the social organisation of contemporary industrial societies, or their family structure or attitude to mental illness, which has a profoundly deleterious effect on the course of schizophrenic disorders. Lack of tolerance on the part of other family members is one obvious possibility which receives some support from the finding that the proportion of schizophrenics' relatives obtaining a rating of 'high expressed emotion' is substantially lower in Chandigarh than in London or Denmark (Wig et al 1987).

Schizophrenia used to be regarded as a steadily progressive disease with a poor prognosis. It is now clear that this is not so, or perhaps no longer so. Not only is the long-term prognosis much better than we used to believe, the course of the illness is very variable, and its outcome worse in industrial than in developing countries, and probably worse in urban than in rural areas within industrial countries. On the whole, patients do not deteriorate further after the first 5–10 years, and even chronic patients may show surprising changes, either improvement or deterioration, after many years of apparent stability. These facts are incompatible with the assumption that schizophrenia is a steadily progressive brain disease;

they force us to consider aetiological hypotheses of quite different kinds. Schizophrenia also seems to have a better prognosis now than it had at the beginning of the century and, at least in industrial countries, its clinical presentation has changed. The catatonic and hebephrenic forms have become much less frequent and paranoid forms more frequent. These changes and differences are usually attributed to advances in treatment and to the pathoplastic effects of cultural differences and social changes. It is possible, however, that they are actually due to a slowly progressive change in the nature of the disease, as occurred with general paresis during the 19th century and with scarlet fever in the 20th.

If such a change has indeed taken place, it is likely to be due to some change in the environmental factors contributing to the aetiology of the condition.

THE TREATMENT OF SCHIZOPHRENIA

Physical methods

Before the 1930s there was no effective treatment for any of the so-called functional psychoses and the prime function of mental hospitals was to keep their patients in tolerable comfort and physical health in the hope that spontaneous remission would take place. Regimes were essentially custodial, with whatever occupational, recreational and spiritual accompaniments local custom and resources allowed. The introduction of Sakel's insulin therapy in 1933, Moniz' prefrontal leucotomy and von Meduna's convulsive therapy in 1935 and Cerletti's electroconvulsive therapy in 1938, and the possibilities of cure which these dramatic new therapies seemed to offer, had a profound effect on the atmosphere and morale of mental hospitals throughout the world. ECT and insulin coma therapy were both widely used throughout the 1940s and thousands of patients were enthusiastically subjected to prefrontal leucotomy. The discovery of the tranquillising effects of chlorpromazine by Charpentier and Laborit in 1953 had an even more profound effect and within a few years of the introduction of these new phenothiazine drugs the insulin coma regime and leucotomy both passed into a rapid decline. ECT remained in widespread use much longer, but mainly in combination with phenothiazines, or as a second-line treatment for patients who had failed to respond to these drugs.

There is no doubt that the phenothiazines, butyrophenones and thioxanthenes have a major effect on the symptoms of acute schizophrenic illnesses. Their efficacy has been demonstrated in dozens of double-blind placebo comparisons and they have been used routinely throughout the world for the last 40 years. The best known large-scale clinical trial was the collaborative trial organised by the National Institute of Mental Health (1964) in the USA. There were four treatment groups — chlorpromazine, fluphenazine, thioridazine and placebo — with 90 patients in each, and overall clinical state and 14 different symptoms were rated, blind, before and after the 6 week treatment period. Patients receiving the three active drugs improved far more than those on placebo and the only significant differences between them were in their side-effects, fluphenazine with its piperazine side-chain producing the highest incidence of extrapyramidal disturbances and chlorpromazine and thioridazine the highest incidence of drowsiness and dizziness. All three drugs produced a generalised improvement across all 14 symptom areas, thus disposing of the claim that phenothiazines merely 'tranquillised' patients without affecting their underlying psychosis.

The efficacy of neuroleptics in chronic schizophrenia is less certain, though several well-designed studies have demonstrated a significant drug/placebo difference. The American Veterans Administration, for example, conducted a double-blind discontinuation trial on 350 patients who had been in hospital for an average of 10 years (Caffey et al 1964). For 16 weeks a third of these patients received placebo, a third remained on their previous regime (chlorpromazine or thioridazine in an average dose of 350–400 mg/day) and a third received placebo 4 days a week and their previous medication on the other 3 days. Of the placebo patients, 45% relapsed in the course of the 16 weeks, compared with only 5% of those who remained on their previous medication and 15% of those on the placebo/active medication combination. Other well-designed trials, however, have failed to demonstrate any drug/placebo difference. The explanation of these contradictory results is not entirely clear. It is clear, though, that neuroleptics are generally less effective in chronic than in acute schizophrenia, and that whether they are beneficial in any given individual depends on the chronicity of the illness, the dosage employed and how stressful their social environment is at the time. It is also clear that all neuroleptics have less effect on the negative symptoms (apathy and blunting of affect) than on the positive symptoms (hallucinations and delusions) of the illness, and the former usually predominate in the chronic stage.

It is equally important to know whether neuroleptic drugs are effective in preventing relapses in patients who have had one or more acute episodes and recovered. The most interesting evidence on this score is provided by Leff & Wing (1971). These authors conducted a double-blind trial of maintenance treatment over 12 months in patients who had recovered from an acute schizophrenic illness and remained stable for 6 weeks after leaving hospital. Of the patients who actually entered the trial, 35% of those receiving active medication (chlorpromazine in an average dose of 150 mg/day or trifluoperazine in an average dose of 12 mg/day) relapsed in the course of the year compared with 80% of those on placebo, a highly significant difference. (Similar results were also obtained over a 2 year period by Goldberg et al (1977)). However, Leff and Wing also followed up three other groups of patients who had qualified to enter the trial but had not done so, either because the clinician responsible believed the risk of relapse too remote to justify medication, or because he believed the risk too high to justify placebo medication, or because the patients themselves refused to take drugs after leaving hospital. The relapse rates in these three groups were, respectively, 27, 67 and 67%. The results of the trial suggest, therefore, that phenothiazines are effective in preventing relapse at least for the first 12 months and in patients in the 'middle third' of the range. But some good-prognosis patients will remain well without any drugs, and other poor-prognosis patients will relapse despite receiving regular medication, and clinicians are able to identify these two groups fairly successfully.

The results of these clinical trials provide the basis of a rational prescribing policy. Acute schizophrenic illnesses should almost invariably be treated with neuroleptics and it is probably wise to try to keep most patients on a maintenance dose for a year or two thereafter even if their recovery is complete and rapid. With so many similar preparations to choose from, the choice of drug is largely a matter of personal preference and relative costs. Many psychiatrists still use chlorpromazine in the acute phase, and if the patient is overactive or frightened its sedative effects are valuable. However, the hypotensive effects of chlorpromazine (and of thioridazine) may be dangerous in the elderly or in patients with a history of heart disease and in them a drug like trifluoperazine or droperidol is preferable. Usually the drug can be given orally, but intramuscular injection may be necessary initially if the patient is violent or refusing to take tablets, and an elixir is preferable if there are doubts about their compliance. Except in the first 48 hours there is no point in giving any phenothiazine, orally or intramuscularly, more frequently than twice a day. All these drugs have a half-life of 12 hours or more, so three times a day or 6-hourly prescribing is simply a waste of valuable nursing time in in-patients and a pointless imposition on out-patients. Moreover, there is good evidence that the more frequently patients are asked to take tablets the more likely they are to forget, or get fed up.

Partly because of individual differences in absorption and metabolism, the dose required to bring psychotic symptoms under control varies considerably from one patient to another, in chlorpromazine equivalents from 150 mg/day to as much as 1000 mg/day. Some clinicians use massive doses — up to 100 mg/day — of potent piperazine side-chain phenothiazines like fluphenazine, or of butyrophenones like haloperidol, and claim that some patients who do not respond to conventional dosages do respond to this massive assault. There is no convincing evidence that this is so, however. PET suggests that 80–90% blockade of dopamine D_2 receptors is produced by quite modest doses of neuroleptics and a recent clinical trial failed to find any difference in the response of newly admitted schizophrenics to oral haloperidol in doses ranging from 10 to 80 mg/day (Rifkin et al 1991). Baldessarini et al (1988) reviewed all published comparisons of different neuroleptic dosages in the treatment of schizophrenia. They concluded that in the acute illness moderate doses (chlorpromazine 300–600 mg/day, or equivalent doses of other neuroleptics) are most effective, and that quite low doses (chlorpromazine 50–100 mg/day or equivalent) often provide adequate maintenance therapy. They also suggest that if a patient does not respond to moderate doses of neuroleptics it is as logical to decrease the dose as to increase it.

Because they also affect the dopamine receptors of the nigrostriatal system, all conventional neuroleptics tend to produce troublesome extrapyramidal side-effects and the liability of any individual drug to do so is, with one or two exceptions, proportional to its potency as an antipsychotic agent. For this reason some clinicians prescribe antiparkinsonian drugs routinely whenever they want to use more than a small dose of a neuroleptic. This is not good practice, for a variety of reasons. Akathisia and parkinsonism are the most common and troublesome extrapyramidal side-effects and there is little evidence that the routine prescribing of antiparkinsonian drugs reduces them to any worthwhile extent (e.g. see Mindham et al 1972). There is also some evidence that the use of these drugs may impair the efficacy of neuroleptics, particularly in controlling positive symptoms (e.g. see

Singh et al 1987), and increase the incidence of tardive dyskinesia; and because they have mild stimulant properties some patients abuse them or become dependent. In general, therefore, antiparkinsonian drugs should only be used if the patient actually develops troublesome akathisia or parkinsonism and it is not feasible to reduce the dose of neuroleptic. And even if this is necessary, and successful, an attempt should be made to withdraw the antiparkinsonian agent after a couple of months because it will often be possible to do so without the extrapyramidal symptoms returning. Some patients develop severe akathisia or parkinsonism on quite small doses of neuroleptics which are not adequately controlled by antiparkinsonian drugs even in maximum dosage. Thioridazine is probably the best drug to use under these circumstances because it has anticholinergic actions of its own and so has a more favourable antipsychotic action/extrapyramidal side-effect ratio than other neuroleptics.

The case for giving neuroleptic drugs to chronic schizophrenics year in year out is much less compelling than the case for using them during acute episodes or exacerbations. The disadvantages of doing so are also substantial. Many patients are seriously distressed by chronic akathisia or muscular rigidity and others who are fortunate enough not to suffer in this way are understandably reluctant to continue 'taking drugs' indefinitely. There is also the long-term risk of tardive dyskinesia to consider. It used to be believed that the risk of developing persistent dyskinesias depended on the magnitude of the dose and the length of time for which it had been taken, but more recent studies suggest that increasing age and female sex are the most important risk factors. Certainly, it is well established that indistinguishable involuntary movements are not uncommon in elderly schizophrenics who have never received neuroleptics of any kind (e.g. see Owens et al 1982) and that persistent chewing movements and other dyskinesias were observed in chronic schizophrenics long before neuroleptics existed (Farran-Ridge 1926). It is also important to realise that stopping a patient's maintenance medication may, paradoxically, result in their receiving an increased rather than a decreased total dose over the next year or two, because they relapse and then require a substantially larger dose to bring their hallucinations or other symptoms back under control (Johnson et al 1983). Only rarely is it appropriate to give patients two or more different neuroleptics simultaneously. Sometimes there are good reasons for temporarily increasing the effective dose in a patient on an injectable depot preparation by

giving a second drug orally as well; and some patients cannot tolerate an adequate dose of one drug because of its hypotensive or sedative effects, or an adequate dose of another because of its extrapyramidal effects, but can tolerate a mixture of the two. But most polypharmacy, like prescribing phenothiazines or tricyclic antidepressants three times a day, is simply a public display of pharmacological ignorance.

Schizophrenics are notoriously unreliable at taking tablets once their acute symptoms have subsided and they have left hospital. There are several reasons for this. They may not accept that they have been ill in the first place, and even if they do may not accept that there is any risk of the illness recurring. And the drugs often cause akathisia and other unpleasant side-effects which are more obvious than their antipsychotic effect. For these reasons 'depot' preparations capable of producing adequate serum levels when administered at intervals of 2 weeks or more have been developed. Most of these preparations, like fluphenazine decanoate (Modecate) and flupenthixol decanoate (Depixol), are phenothiazines or thioxanthenes esterified with a long-chain fatty acid from which they are slowly released in vivo, though some orally administered drugs like pimozide have a sufficiently long half-life for adequate serum levels to be maintained by doses at 2–3 day intervals. The introduction of these injectable depot preparations 20 years ago was hailed as a great advance and they are now very widely used, often with special clinics and elaborate follow-up arrangements to ensure that patients do not miss their regular injection every 2, 3 or 4 weeks. Probably they are a significant advance, but it is important not to forget that no trial comparing long-term relapse rates on daily tablets and fortnightly injections has demonstrated any clear advantage for the latter (e.g. see Falloon et al 1978).

Some psychiatrists treat their patients' acute psychoses in hospital with daily tablets and then change to a depot injection, starting with a small test dose, when they become out-patients. However, if the patient is to be treated with a depot injection in the long term — and in most cases this is probably sensible despite the results of the trials referred to above — there is much to be said for giving them a full dose (i.e. Modecate 25 mg or Depixol 40 mg) straight away. The traditional test dose rarely serves any useful purpose as the most troublesome side-effects take 2 or 3 weeks to develop anyway; if the depot injection is initially inadequate to control the psychosis it can always be augmented with an oral preparation; and if the patient departs or absconds before his psychotic symptoms have resolved he will continue to receive appropriate medication for at least a week or two.

Concern about the extrapyramidal side-effects of neuroleptics has led in recent years to several attempts to maintain chronic patients on very small doses of neuroleptics, or to give these drugs only at the first sign of impending relapse. The results have been disappointing. Johnson et al (1987), for example, found that if chronic schizophrenics who were well controlled on relatively low doses of Depixol (up to 40 mg i.m. fortnightly) were transferred double blind to half that dose their relapse rate over the next 3 years was significantly increased. Jolley et al (1990) were more ambitious. They attempted to maintain schizophrenic out-patients in stable remission off all medication, but to ensure that they received oral haloperidol at the first signs of relapse by warning both patients and their relatives what those signs were likely to be and providing both monthly follow-up appointments and a 24 hour telephone contact. Unfortunately, the experiment failed, partly because only 50% of relapses were preceded by any prodromal symptoms at all. And although the drug-free patients had fewer extrapyramidal symptoms than their controls this was not accompanied by any improvement in social functioning.

The most interesting recent pharmacological innovation in the treatment of schizophrenia has been the come-back of the atypical neuroleptic clozapine, a drug which was originally introduced in the 1970s, but abandoned after several deaths from agranulocytosis. A large multicentre trial in the USA based on 268 chronic schizophrenics who had failed to respond to at least three different neuroleptics, and also to a 6 week trial of haloperidol 60 mg/day, found clozapine (in doses up to 900 mg/day) to be significantly more effective than chlorpromazine (in doses up to 1800 mg/day) in a 6 week double-blind comparison (Kane et al 1988). Not only did more of the clozapine patients meet a priori criteria for improvement (30 versus 4%), both negative and positive symptoms improved. As well as being effective in many patients resistant to other neuroleptics, clozapine has an unusual and puzzling pharmacological profile, for it has a low affinity for both D_1 and D_2 dopamine receptors, thus raising the possibility that it works either in some entirely novel way, or by binding to the recently described D_4 receptor (Van Tol et al 1991). For both these reasons it is currently attracting great interest. Its disadvantages are its very high cost, and the fact that very frequent neutrophil counts are necessary in order to detect incipient marrow depression and prevent deaths from agranulocytosis.

Although neuroleptics have been the mainstay of the treatment of acute schizophrenia for the past 40 years, ECT and analytically oriented psychotherapy have been extensively used in some centres, though less so now than in the past. The results of May's (1968) trial in California indicated quite unequivocally that psychodynamic psychotherapy was valueless in the active phase of the illness. The only detectable effects, whether psychotherapy was given alone or in combination with a phenothiazine, were on the duration and cost of hospital treatment, both of which were substantially increased. Patients treated with ECT fared significantly better, though less well than those receiving phenothiazines. Two more recent English trials of ECT, both comparing real and dummy ECT under double-blind conditions, found it to have genuinely beneficial effects in acute schizophrenia, though these were no longer detectable 3 or 4 months later (Taylor & Fleminger 1980, Brandon et al 1985). For this reason the only strong indications for using ECT in the treatment of schizophrenia nowadays are schizoaffective illnesses (whose relationship to schizophrenia is uncertain) and rare cases of catatonic stupor. Tricyclic and other antidepressants are frequently given to schizophrenics in an attempt to relieve their associated depressive symptoms. Usually they are given in combination with a neuroleptic after the acute phase of the illness is over, and a convincing response is not often obtained. Sometimes this is because apathy and flattening of affect are mistakingly interpreted as depressive symptoms. More fundamentally it is probably because tricyclic drugs are ineffective in relieving post-schizophrenic depression (Johnson 1981).

Social and psychological measures

Although in the short run neuroleptics have a much more dramatic effect on the symptoms of schizophrenia than any other therapeutic measure there is a great deal more to treatment than prescribing neuroleptics, and it may well be that in the long run other less tangible social and psychological influences have a more powerful influence on outcome than any drugs. There is abundant evidence that the course of schizophrenic illnesses and the resulting social handicaps can be affected, for good or ill, by the patient's social environment and it has been known for 30 years that many of the most obvious behavioural abnormalities of chronic schizophrenics, like posturing and talking to themselves, are not intrinsic or inevitable, but are to a considerable extent the product of a monotonous, unstimulating environment. This was well illustrated by Wing & Brown's (1961) comparison of three mental hospitals in southern England. In their hospital C, patients had few if any personal possessions, little liberty, spent much of the time unoccupied in the wards, and were generally treated as 'inmates'; whereas in hospital A they had their own clothes and other personal possessions, spent most of the day actively employed and generally lived as free and normal a life as possible. The incidence of social withdrawal (underactivity, lack of conversation, neglect of hygiene and personal appearance) and socially embarrassing behaviour (incontinence, mannerisms, purposeless overactivity, threats of violence, talking to self) was much higher in hospital C than it was in A (B was intermediate in all respects), despite the fact that their patients' initial type and severity of illness appeared to have been the same, and there were no important differences in the prescribing and discharge policies of the two hospitals.

Too much stimulation, or stimulation of the wrong kind, can also be harmful. There is, for example, the evidence that schizophrenic illnesses may be precipitated by events in the previous few weeks, pleasant or unpleasant, which disrupt the subject's normal lifestyle (Brown & Birley 1968). There is also the evidence that returning to live with a critical or hostile relative after a schizophrenic illness greatly increases the relapse rate over the next 12 months (Vaughn & Leff 1976, Parker & Hadzi-Pavlovic 1990). The overall management of schizophrenia is based, therefore, on an attempt to avoid both extremes. As Dyer says in Chapter 42, psychiatrists are 'constantly walking the dividing line between under- and overstimulation'. To this end, attempts are made to get the patient out of hospital and into an occupation and a domestic setting in which they have some real but limited responsibilities, in which they have a daily routine which is ordered and predictable without being too monotonous, and in which they are protected from emotional demands they cannot meet. It is often easier said than done.

For the last 40 years, partly because of the realisation that mental hospitals themselves could have profoundly harmful effects on their patients if they stayed too long, and partly for straightforward financial reasons, intensive efforts have been made to discharge schizophrenics as soon as their psychotic symptoms have resolved and to keep them 'in the community' as much as possible thereafter. To be successful, or for the patient to be better off, such a policy requires the provision of a range of hostels, day centres, 'half-way houses' and sheltered workshops in the community. Unfortunately, for reasons which are discussed in Chapter 42, these facilities have not yet materialised in anything like adequate numbers. For this reason many psychiatrists (though not hospital managers) are increasingly questioning whether early discharge is always in the patient's interests, and whether mental hospitals have not been too eager to discard their traditional 'asylum' role. A back bedroom can be just as deprived and harmful an environment as a back ward, and a park bench even more so. Discharging patients from hospital when adequate community facilities are not available may also place a heavy burden on relatives, a burden which psychiatrists and social workers do not fully comprehend and often do little to relieve (National Schizophrenia Fellowship 1974).

Although many patients have a home and a job to return to, or succeed in obtaining accommodation and employment without the aid of any formal rehabilitative measures, others are too badly handicapped, and the effects of illness on their drive, initiative and demeanour, by the social stigma of having been mentally ill, and often too by their previous lack of education and marketable skills, to be capable of obtaining a job without assistance. In the past it was one of the primary functions of rehabilitation programmes to help people who had had schizophrenic illnesses to obtain suitable paid employment subsequently. However, in the last decade or so this has become increasingly difficult, partly because the general level of unemployment has risen (and whenever the level rises above about 6% it become increasingly difficult to obtain jobs for handicapped people of any kind), and partly because fundamental industrial changes have resulted in a substantial reduction in the need for unskilled or semiskilled workers. As a result, rehabilitation programmes are increasingly geared to help patients with defect states or recurring psychotic episodes to cook and shop for themselves, to obtain temporary or unpaid employment and to use their leisure time productively. (These issues are discussed in more detail in Chapter 42.)

Some schizophrenics have become homeless by the time they are first admitted to hospital and others become so later on after a series of further relapses and re-admissions. Accommodation has to be found for most such patients if they are ever to leave hospital and many of them are incapable of surviving in ordinary rented accommodation even if landladies can

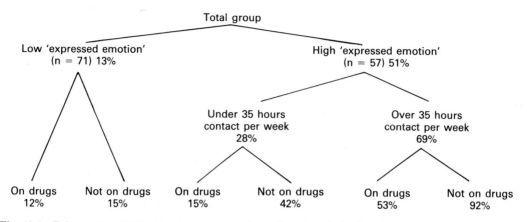

Fig. 18.1 Relapse rates of 128 schizophrenics over a 9 month study period (after Vaughn & Leff 1976; reproduced by kind permission of *The British Journal of Psychiatry*).

be persuaded to take them. So other types of accommodation geared to their needs have to be provided. In the past hostels were often provided by psychiatric hospitals themselves, either on the hospital site or elsewhere, and supervised to varying extents by nurses. Now hostels, group homes, flats and bedsitters reserved for former psychiatric patients are increasingly provided by local authority social work departments and voluntary organisations. The amount and quality of supervision provided is very variable, but the greater quantity and variety of protected housing available increases the likelihood that individual patients will eventually find a suitable niche.

A more difficult situation arises when the patient is living with a relative, usually a spouse or parent, who is willing to have him back, but it becomes clear while the patient is in hospital that this relative cannot accept and adapt to the change that has come over him and remains angry, frightened and critical. There are various ways of trying to deal with this potentially hazardous situation. It may be possible to arrange for the patient to move into a hostel instead of returning home; but suitable accommodation is not always available, and even if it is it may be impossible to persuade either the patient or the relative that this is preferable to returning home. Indeed, it is often the mothers who are most critical of their schizophrenic son's or daughter's behaviour who are least willing to be parted from them. An alternative strategy in such circumstances is to mitigate the ill effects of the relative's emotional involvement by reducing the time the two spend in one another's company. A fulltime job is, of course, the best way of doing this, but if this

is impossible regular attendance at a day hospital or day centre of some kind may achieve the same ends. Regular neuroleptic medication also mitigates the ill effects. Figure 18.1 illustrates the striking effect of the quality of the emotional relationship with the key relative, as well as medication and reduced contact, on the relapse rates observed in the two series of patients studied by the MRC Social Psychiatry Unit. Patients returning to live with a 'low expressed emotion' relative had a relapse rate over 12 months of 15% or less, whether or not they were taking medication. The relapse rate was no higher in patients living with a 'high expressed emotion' relative, provided they received neuroleptics regularly and were in contact with the relative for less than 35 hours a week. However, if either of these protective influences was missing the relapse rate was much higher, and if both were missing the relapse rate was an alarming 92%.

A fourth preventive strategy is to try to alter the attitudes and behaviour of the relatives, and the development of various forms of family therapy to this end has been the most interesting development in the treatment of schizophrenia in the last decade. Several small-scale but important clinical trials have now been reported. In the first, 24 schizophrenics who were all living in a 'high expressed emotion' environment, and therefore at high risk of relapse, were randomly allocated either to routine out-patient care or to receive a special package of social interventions consisting of factual talks to their relatives about schizophrenia, fortnightly group meetings for the relatives designed to help them share experiences, discharge emotions and learn new coping techniques, and regular family therapy sessions in the patient's home designed to lower expressed emotion and face-to-face contact (Leff et al 1982). All 24 patients received depot neuroleptics throughout. After 9 months the relapse rate was 50% in the controls but only 9% in the treatment group (*p* = 0.40) and the only patients in the treatment group to relapse were the two in whom no reduction in expressed emotion or face-to-face contact was achieved. The results of this trial therefore add to the evidence that high expressed emotion does provoke relapse and that reduced face-to-face contact is protective. They do not, of course, reveal which elements of the treatment package were most important.

A similar trial was carried out in Los Angeles by Falloon et al (1985). Thirty-six newly discharged schizophrenics returning to stressful parental households were stabilised on neuroleptics and then randomly assigned to individual or family therapy. Both regimes consisted of 25 sessions of 1 hour over 9 months, and both were predominantly problem oriented and behavioural rather than interpretative, but the family sessions were held at home and involved the whole family, whereas the individual sessions were in the clinic, and if relatives were seen they were usually seen separately from the patient. After 9 months of family therapy patients had had fewer schizophrenic relapses and fewer hospital admissions (11 versus 50%) despite receiving rather less medication. They also had fewer schizophrenic symptoms, positive and negative, and these differences in outcome were maintained at 2 year follow-up. A more recent trial by Tarrier et al (1988) in Salford has confirmed that the relapse rate in schizophrenics living with 'high expressed emotion' relatives can be reduced to that of schizophrenics living with 'low expressed emotion' relatives if the key relatives are given about a dozen sessions of information and advice about schizophrenia, coping with stress and coping with the patient's frustrating behaviour. It seems clear, therefore, that there needs to be a substantial shift in emphasis in the management of schizophrenia with far more attention being given to patients' families than in the past.

The effect of social casework on the patients themselves in this post-psychotic, post-hospital phase of the illness had previously been explored in a large American trial (Goldberg et al 1977). Four hundred newly discharged schizophrenics were randomly allocated to one of four groups and followed up for 2 years. The first group received maintenance chlorpromazine plus what the authors called 'major role therapy' (a combination of intensive psychoanalytically oriented social casework and vocational rehabilitation); a second group received maintenance chlorpromazine but only minimal contacts with a social worker, a third group received placebo tablets and 'major role therapy'; and a fourth group placebo tablets and minimal social contacts. As expected, the relapse rate was much lower in patients on maintenance chlorpromazine than in those on placebo (48 versus 80%). Overall, 'major role therapy' had no effect on the relapse rate. But more detailed analysis showed that in patients who might have been expected to have a good prognosis the relapse rate was reduced by this treatment, and in those who might have been expected to have a relatively poor prognosis the relapse rate was increased. In other words, as other trials of the efficacy of psychotherapy have demonstrated in other settings, some patients benefited but others were harmed and the two tended to cancel each other out. What the mechanism of harm is we can only speculate, but it is easy to imagine how an intensive relationship with a keen social worker might create something akin to a 'high expressed emotion' situation. The moral is clear. Would-be psychotherapeutic relationships and other emotional pressures may be positively harmful to those who have recently had a schizophrenic illness, and so should only be offered if it is quite clear that the patients are capable of responding. Emotional withdrawal is not merely a symptom; it is also a valuable protective strategy.

REFERENCES

Andreasen N C 1979 Thought, language and communication disorders. Archives of General Psychiatry 36: 1315–1321, 1325–1330

Andreasen N C, Swayze V W, Flaum M, Yates W R, Arudt S, McChesney C 1990 Ventricular enlargement in schizophrenia evaluated with computed tomographic scanning. Archives of General Psychiatry 47: 1008–1015

Astrup C, Ödegaard Ø 1960 The influence of hospital facilities and other local factors upon admission to psychiatric hospitals. Acta Psychiatrica et Neurologica Scandinavica 35: 289–301

Baldessarini R J, Cohen B M, Teicher M H 1988 Significance of neuroleptic dose and plasma level in the pharmacological treatment of psychoses. Archives of General Psychiatry 45: 79–91

Baldwin J A 1979 Schizophrenia and physical disease. Psychological Medicine 9: 611–618

Baruch I, Hemsley D R, Gray J A 1988 Differential performance of acute and chronic schizophrenics in a latent inhibition task. Journal of Nervous and Mental Disease 176: 598–606

Bateson G, Jackson D D, Haley J, Weakland J H 1956 Toward a theory of schizophrenia. Behavioral Science 1: 251–264

Blackwood D H R, Whalley L J, Christie J E, Blackburn I M, St Clair D M, McInnes A 1987 Changes in auditory P3 event-related potential in schizophrenia and depression. British Journal of Psychiatry 150: 154–160

Bleuler E 1911 Dementia praecox or the group of schizophrenias. English translation by Zinkin J 1950. International Universities Press, New York

Bleuler M 1972 Die schizophrenen Geistesstorungen im Lichte langjähriger Kranken-und Familiengeschichten. Thieme, Stuttgart

Bogerts B, Meertz E, Schonfeldt-Bausch R 1985 Basal ganglia and limbic system pathology in schizophrenia. Archives of General Psychiatry 42: 784–791

Bradbury T N, Miller G A 1985 Season of birth in schizophrenia: a review of evidence, methodology and etiology. Psychological Bulletin 98: 569–594

Brandon S, Cowley P, McDonald C, Neville P, Palmer R, Wellstood-Eason S 1985 Leicester ECT trial: results in schizophrenia. British Journal of Psychiatry 146: 177–183

Brockington I F, Wainwright S, Kendell R E 1980 Manic patients with schizophrenic or paranoid symptoms. Psychological Medicine 10: 73–83

Brown G W, Birley J L T 1968 Crises and life changes and the onset of schizophrenia. Journal of Health and Social Behaviour 9: 203–214

Brown G W, Birley J L T, Wing J K 1972 Influence of family life on the course of schizophrenic disorders: a replication. British Journal of Psychiatry 121: 241–258

Brown R, Colter N, Corsellis N et al 1986 Postmortem evidence of structural brain changes in schizophrenia. Archives of General Psychiatry 43: 36–42

Caffey E M, Diamond L S, Frank T V et al 1964 Discontinuation or reduction of chemotherapy in chronic schizophrenics. Journal of Chronic Diseases 17: 347–358

Ciompi L 1980 The natural history of schizophrenia in the long term. British Journal of Psychiatry 136: 413–420

Cochrane R 1977 Mental illness in immigrants to England and Wales: an analysis of mental hospital admissions, 1971. Social Psychiatry 12: 25–35

Conrad A J, Abebe T, Austin R, Forsythe S, Scheibel A B 1991 Hippocampal pyramidal cell disarray in schizophrenia as a bilateral phenomenon. Archives of General Psychiatry 48: 413–417

Cooper J E, Kendell R E, Gurland B J, Sharpe L, Copeland J R M, Simon R 1972 Psychiatric diagnosis in New York and London. Maudsley Monograph 20. Oxford University Press, London

Crow T J 1980 Molecular pathology of schizophrenia: more than one disease process? British Medical Journal 280: 66–68

Crow T J, Stevens M 1978 Age disorientation in chronic schizophrenia: the nature of the cognitive deficit. British Journal of Psychiatry 133: 137–142

Crow T J, Ball J, Bloom S R et al 1989 Schizophrenia as an anomaly of development of cerebral asymmetry. Archives of General Psychiatry 46: 1145–1150

DeLisi L E, Buchsbaum M S, Holcomb H H et al 1985 Clinical correlates of decreased anteroposterior metabolic gradients in positron emission tomography of

schizophrenic patients. American Journal of Psychiatry 142: 78–81

Eagles J M, Whalley L J 1985 Decline in the diagnosis of schizophrenia among first admissions to Scottish mental hospitals from 1969–78. British Journal of Psychiatry 146: 151–154

Falloon I, Watt D C, Shepherd M 1978 A comparative controlled trial of pimozide and fluphenazine decanoate in the continuation therapy of schizophrenia. Psychological Medicine 8: 59–70

Falloon I R H, Boyd J L, McGill C W et al 1985 Family management in the prevention of morbidity of schizophrenia. Archives of General Psychiatry 42: 887–896

Farde L, Wiesel F A, Stone-Elander S et al 1990 D_2 dopamine receptors in neuroleptic-naive schizophrenic patients. Archives of General Psychiatry 47: 213–219

Faris R, Dunham W 1939 Mental disorders in urban areas. Reprinted 1960 Hafner, New York.

Farran-Ridge C 1926 Dementia praecox and epidemic encephalitis. Journal of Mental Science 72: 513–523

Feighner J P, Robins E, Guze S B, Woodruff R A, Winokur G, Munoz R 1972 Diagnostic criteria for use in psychiatric research. Archives of General Psychiatry 26: 57–63

Frith C D, 1987 The positive and negative symptoms of schizophrenia reflect impairments in the perception and initiation of action. Psychological Medicine 17: 631–648

Frith C D, Done D J 1989 Experiences of alien control in schizophrenia reflect a disorder in the central monitoring of action. Psychological Medicine 19: 359–363

Goldberg E M, Morrison S L 1963 Schizophrenia and social class. British Journal of Psychiatry 109: 785–802

Goldberg S C, Schooler N R, Hogarty G E, Roper M 1977 Prediction of relapse in schizophrenic outpatients treated by drug and sociotherapy. Archives of General Psychiatry 34: 171–184

Goldhamer H, Marshall A 1953 Psychosis and civilisation. Free Press, Illinois

Gur R E, Skolnick B E, Gur R C et al 1983 Brain function in psychiatric disorders 1. Regional cerebral blood flow in medicated schizophrenics. Archives of General Psychiatry 40: 1250–1254

Häfner H, Riecher A, Maurer K, Löffler W, Munk-Jørgensen P, Strömgren E 1989 How does gender influence age at first hospitalisation for schizophrenia? Psychological Medicine 19: 903–918

Harding C M, Brooks G W, Ashikaga T, Strauss J S, Breier A 1987 The Vermont longitudinal study of persons with severe mental illness. American Journal of Psychiatry 144: 718–726, 727–735

Hare E H 1988 Schizophrenia as a recent disease. British Journal of Psychiatry 153: 521–531

Harrison G, Owens D, Holton A, Neilson D, Boot D 1988 A prospective study of severe mental disorder in Afro-Caribbean patients. Psychological Medicine 18: 643–657

Hirsch S R, Leff J P 1975 Abnormalities in parents of schizophrenics. Maudsley monograph 22. Oxford University Press, London

Hoch P, Polatin P 1949 Pseudoneurotic forms of schizophrenia. Psychiatric Quarterly 23: 248–276

Holzman P S, Proctor L R, Levy D L et al 1974 Eye-tracking dysfunctions in schizophrenic patients and their relatives. Archives of General Psychiatry 31: 143–151

Huber G, Gross G, Schüttler R, Linz M 1980 Longitudinal

studies of schizophrenic patients. Schizophrenia Bulletin 6: 592–605

Ingvar D H, Franzen G 1974 Distribution of cerebral activity in chronic schizophrenia. Lancet ii: 1484–1486

Jaco E G 1960 The social epidemiology of mental disorders: a psychiatric survey of Texas. Russell Sage Foundation, New York

Johnson D A W 1981 A double-blind trial of nortriptyline for depression in chronic schizophrenia. British Journal of Psychiatry 139: 97–101

Johnson D A W, Pasterski G, Ludlow J M, Street K, Taylor R D W 1983 The discontinuance of maintenance neuroleptic therapy in chronic schizophrenic patients: drug and social consequences. Acta Psychiatrica Scandinavica 67: 339–352

Johnson D A W, Ludlow J M, Street K, Taylor R D W 1987 Double-blind comparison of half-dose and standard-dose flupenthixol decanoate in the maintenance treatment of stabilised out-patients with schizophrenia. British Journal of Psychiatry 151: 634–638

Johnstone E C, Crow T J, Frith C D et al 1976 Cerebral ventricular size and cognitive impairment in chronic schizophrenia. Lancet ii: 924–926

Jolley A G, Hirsch S R, Morrison E, McRink A, Wilson L 1990 Trial of brief intermittent neuroleptic prophylaxis for selected schizophrenic outpatients: clinical and social outcome at two years. British Medical Journal 301: 837–842

Kane J, Honigfeld G, Singer J et al 1988 Clozapine for the treatment-resistant schizophrenic. Archives of General Psychiatry 45: 789–796

Kasanin J 1933 The acute schizoaffective psychoses. American Journal of Psychiatry 90: 97–126

Kendell R E, Brockington I F, Leff J P 1979 Prognostic implications of six alternative definitions of schizophrenia. Archives of General Psychiatry 36: 25–34

Kendell R E, Malcolm D E, Adams W 1993 The problem of detecting changes in the incidence of schizophrenia. British Journal of Psychiatry 162: (in press).

Kraepelin E 1896 Psychiatrie, ein Lehrbuch für Studierende und Ärzte, 5th edn. Barth, Leipzig

Langfeldt G 1960 Diagnosis and prognosis of schizophrenia. Proceedings of the Royal Society of Medicine 53: 1047–1052

Leff J P, Wing J K 1971 Trial of maintenance therapy in schizophrenia. British Medical Journal iii: 599–604

Leff J, Kuipers L, Berkowitz R, Eberlein-Vries R, Sturgeon D 1982 A controlled trial of social intervention in the families of schizophrenic patients. British Journal of Psychiatry 141: 121–134

Lewis G, David A, Andréasson S, Allebeck P 1992 Schizophrenia and city life. Lancet 340: 137–140

Lidz T, Fleck S, Cornelison A R 1965 Schizophrenia and the family. International Universities Press, New York

McGovern D, Cope R V 1987 First psychiatric admission rates of first and second generation Afro-Caribbeans. Social Psychiatry 22: 139–149

Mackay A V P, Iversen L L, Rossor M et al 1982 Increased brain dopamine and dopamine receptors in schizophrenia. Archives of General Psychiatry 39: 991–997

McNeil T F, Kaij L 1978 Obstetric factors in the development of schizophrenia. In: Wynne L C, Cromwell R L, Matthysse S (eds) The nature of schizophrenia. Wiley, New York, pp 401–429

Malzberg B, Lee E S 1956 Migration and mental disease: a study of first admissions to hospitals for mental disease, New York, 1939–1941. Social Science Research Council, New York

Martinot J L, Paillère-Martinot M L, Loc'h C et al 1991 The estimated density of D_2 striatal receptors in schizophrenia. British Journal of Psychiatry 158: 346–350

May P R A 1968 Treatment of schizophrenia. Science House, New York

Miles C P 1977 Conditions predisposing to suicide: a review. Journal of Nervous and Mental Disease 164: 231–246

Mindham R H S, Gaind R, Anstee B H, Rimmer L 1972 Comparison of amantadine, orphenadrine and placebo in the control of phenothiazine induced parkinsonism. Psychological Medicine 2: 406–413

Morice R D, Ingram J C L 1982 Language analysis in schizophrenia: diagnostic implications. Australian and New Zealand Journal of Psychiatry 16: 11–21

Murphy D L, Wyatt R J 1972 Reduced monoamine oxidase activity in blood platelets from schizophrenic patients. Nature 238: 225–226

National Institutes of Mental Health Psychopharmacology Service Centre Study Group 1964 Phenothiazine treatment in schizophrenia. Archives of General Psychiatry 10: 246–261

National Schizophrenia Fellowship 1974 Living with schizophrenia — by the relatives. National Schizophrenia Fellowship, Surrey

Ödegaard Ø 1932 Emigration and insanity: a study of mental disease among Norwegian-born population in Minnesota. Acta Psychiatrica et Neurologica Scandinavica suppl 4

Owen F, Cross A J, Crow T J et al 1978 Increased dopamine-receptor sensitivity in schizophrenia. Lancet ii: 223–226

Owens D G C, Johnstone E C, Frith C D 1982 Spontaneous involuntary disorders of movement. Archives of General Psychiatry 39: 452–461

Pakkenberg B 1990 Pronounced reduction of total neuron numbers in mediodorsal thalamic nucleus and nucleus accumbens in schizophrenics. Archives of General Psychiatry 47: 1023–1028

Parker G, Hadzi-Pavlovic D 1990 Expressed emotion as a predictor of schizophrenic relapse: an analysis of aggregated data. Psychological Medicine 20: 961–965

Parnas J, Schulsinger F, Schulsinger H, Mednick S, Teasdale T 1982 Behavioral precursors of schizophrenia spectrum. Archives of General Psychiatry 39: 658–664

Regier D A, Boyd J H, Burke J D et al 1988 One-month prevalence of mental disorders in the United States. Archives of General Psychiatry 45: 977–986

Reveley A M. Reveley M A, Clifford C A, Murray R M 1982 Cerebral ventricular size in twins discordant for schizophrenia. Lancet i: 540–541

Reveley A M, Reveley M A, Murray R M 1984 Cerebral ventricular enlargement in nongenetic schizophrenia: a controlled twin study. British Journal of Psychiatry 144: 89–93

Rifkin A, Doddi S, Karajgi B, Borenstein M, Wachspress M 1991 Dosage of haloperidol for schizophrenia. Archives of General Psychiatry 48: 166–170

Sartorius N, Jablensky A, Shapiro R 1977 Two-year follow - up of the patients included in the WHO International Pilot Study of Schizophrenia. Psychological Medicine 7: 529–541

Sartorius N, Jablensky A, Korten A et al 1986 Early manifestations and first contact incidence of schizophrenia in different cultures. Psychological Medicine 16: 909–928

Schneider K 1959 Klinische Psychopathologie. English translation by Hamilton M W. Grune & Stratton, New York

Sham P C, O'Callaghan E, Takei N et al 1992 Schizophrenia following pre-natal exposure to influenza epidemics between 1939 and 1960. British Journal of Psychiatry 160: 461–466

Siegel C, Waldo M, Mizner G et al 1984 Deficits in sensory gating in schizophrenic patients and their relatives. Archives of General Psychiatry 41: 607–612

Singer M T, Wynne L C 1965 Thought disorder and family relations of schizophrenics. Archives of General Psychiatry 12: 187–212

Singh M M, Kay S R, Opler L A 1987 Anticholinergic-neuroleptic antagonism in terms of positive and negative symptoms of schizophrenia: implications for psychological subtyping. Psychological Medicine 17: 39–48

Spitzer R, Endicott J, Robins E 1975 Research Diagnostic Criteria. Instrument 58 New York State Psychiatric Institute, New York

Stalker H 1939 The prognosis in schizophrenia. Journal of Mental Science 85: 1224–1240

Steinberg H R, Durrell J 1968 A stressful social situation as a precipitant of schizophrenic symptoms: an epidemiological study. British Journal of Psychiatry 114: 1097–1105

Stephens J H, Astrup C, Mangrum J C 1966 Prognostic factors in recovered and deteriorating schizophrenics. American Journal of Psychiatry 122: 1116–1121

Suddath R L, Christison G W, Torrey E F, Casanova M F, Weinberger D R 1990 Anatomical abnormalities in the brains of monozygotic twins discordant for schizophrenia. New England Journal of Medicine 322: 789–794

Tarrier N, Barrowclough C, Poiceddu K, Watts S 1988a The assessment of psychophysiological reactivity to the expressed emotion of the relatives of schizophrenic patients. British Journal of Psychiatry 152: 618–624

Tarrier N, Barrowclough C, Vaughn C et al 1988b The community management of schizophrenia. British Journal of Psychiatry 153: 532–542

Taylor P, Fleminger J J 1980 ECT for schizophrenia. Lancet i: 1380–1382

Torrey E F 1987 Prevalence studies in schizophrenia. British Journal of Psychiatry 150: 598–608

Vaillant G E 1964 Prospective prediction of schizophrenic remission. Archives of General Psychiatry 11: 509–518

Van Tol H H M, Bunzow J R, Guan H-C et al 1991 Cloning of the gene for a human dopamine D_4 receptor with high affinity for the antipsychotic clozapine. Nature 350: 610–614

Vaughn C E, Leff J P 1976 Influence of family and social factors on the course of psychiatric illness. British Journal of Psychiatry 129: 125–137

Vaughn C E, Snyder K S, Jones S et al 1984 Family factors in schizophrenic relapse. Archives of General Psychiatry 41: 1169–1177

Weinberger D R 1987 Implications of normal brain development for the pathogenesis of schizophrenia. Archives of General Psychiatry 44: 660–669

Weinberger D R, Berman K F, Zec R F 1986 Physiologic dysfunction of dorsolateral prefrontal cortex in schizophrenia. Archives of General Psychiatry 43: 114–124

Whalley L J, Christie J E, Brown S, Arbuthnott G W 1984 Schneider's first-rank symptoms of schizophrenia, Archives of General Psychiatry 41: 1040–1043

WHO 1973 Report of the International Pilot Study of Schizophrenia. World Health Organization, Geneva

Wig N N, Menon D K, Bedi H et al 1987 Distribution of expressed emotion components among relatives of schizophrenic patients in Aarhus and Chandigarh. British Journal of Psychiatry 151: 160–165

Wing J K 1966 Five year outcome in early schizophrenia. Proceedings of the Royal Society of Medicine 59: 17–18

Wing J K, Brown G W 1961 Social treatment of chronic schizophrenia: a comparative survey of three mental hospitals. Journal of Mental Science 107: 847–861

Wing J K, Cooper J E, Sartorius N 1974 Description and classification of psychiatric symptoms. Cambridge University Press, Cambridge

Wong D F, Wagner H N, Tune L E et al 1986 Positron emission tomography reveals elevated D_2 dopamine receptors in drug-naive schizophrenics. Science 234: 1558–1563

Young W F, Laws E R, Sharbrough F W et al 1986 Human monoamine oxidase: lack of brain and platelet correlation. Archives of General Psychiatry 43: 604–609

19. Mood (affective) disorders

R. E. Kendell

The term mood disorder (ICD-10, DSM-IIIR) or affective disorder (DSM-III) is applied to a large group of related conditions in which a disturbance of mood — either depression or elation — is prominent, and believed to be fundamental. Although mania and melancholia were two of the five types of madness recognised by Hippocrates in the 4th century BC, and continued to figure in most classifications and treatises on insanity for the next 2000 years, the meaning of these terms varied from author to author and century to century almost as much as the noxae to which they were attributed and the therapeutic measures advocated for their relief. Recognisable descriptions of depressive illnesses, and even the suggestion of a relationship with elation, can be found as far back as the 2nd century AD in the writings of the Cappadocian physician Aretaeus. However, the concept of mood disorder can best be said to have originated in 1845 with Baillarger's description of *folie à double forme* and Falret's very similar description of *folie circulaire*, both of them detailed and unmistakable accounts of alternating manic and melancholic mood swings, separated by intervals of perfect lucidity. But it is to Kraepelin that we really owe our present concept of affective illness. In the fifth (1896) edition of his *Psychiatrie, ein Lehrbuch für Studierende und Ärzte* he divided the functional psychoses into two broad categories — dementia praecox and manic–depressive insanity — the latter embracing not only Falret's folie circulaire and all melancholic and manic illnesses, single or recurrent, but also a variety of other morbid fluctuations of mood, intermittent or enduring.

Illnesses in which the prevailing affect is depression are much commoner than those based on an elevation of mood, and people who suffer from manic illnesses almost invariably suffer from depressions as well at some stage. As the classification of these illnesses is unsatisfactory and controversial, and has been since the 1920s, it seems sensible to describe the main syndromes first, before embarking on a discussion of their relationship to one another and the many competing nomenclatures and classifications this involves.

BASIC SYNDROMES

Mania

The core of the syndrome is not elation so much as a subjective sense of well-being accompanied by increased activity. The patient has abundant energy. He says that he feels fine, is superbly healthy and can think more clearly than ever before. His head is full of exciting plans and ideas and he is more talkative than normal (*pressure of speech*). He stays up till long after midnight or rises in the early hours of the morning, not because he is troubled by insomnia but because he feels no need for sleep or is too busy to waste precious hours in bed. But despite this energy and expansive enthusiasm he achieves little. He is too distractable, constantly dropping one scheme to take up another, and his judgement of what is feasible or desirable is badly impaired. As a result large sums of money may be squandered on expensive luxuries or hare-brained business ventures. He is also uninhibited. He flouts normal social conventions, asks personal questions of the doctor trying to interview him, and behaves in other ways that are normally considered impolite, indecorous or indecent. Sexual behaviour is most obviously affected, perhaps because it is normally under the greatest restraint. Women are promiscuous, and may become pregnant as a result, and respectable middle-aged men get involved in public escapades which may be a source of great embarrassment to them on recovery. Grandiose ideas are very characteristic, varying from an exaggerated view of genuine talents or assets to delusional convictions of being the prime minister, or the son of God, or having solved the country's economic problems.

The patient's mood may well be elated, but is not always obviously so. Irritability is often more prominent, particularly if he is thwarted, as he generally has to be; and sometimes the only obvious abnormality of mood is an uncharacteristic equanimity, or a failure to be alarmed or disconcerted by bad news. Sometimes, in addition to the pressure of speech referred to above, there is a characteristic *flight of ideas*, the subject's train of thought changing repeatedly in mid-sentence in response to distracting stimuli, words with double meanings or new but related ideas. ('I'm fine, doc, how are you? Are you a real doctor or just a trick cyclist off on the Tour de France or the Round Britain Quiz? I've whizzed round Britain more than once myself in an old Ford car but an old Ford car don't get that far. Tra la la. Ha ha. What's the next question?')

Despite the general air of hilarity and grandiosity, however, depression lurks like an iceberg just beneath the surface. It is commonplace for the patient to be in tears and prey to gloomy thoughts at times and suicide is by no means rare. Moreover, something like 25% of manic illnesses are preceded by a period of mild depression lasting for days or weeks. A similar percentage are followed by depression, which may be exacerbated by the patient's awareness of the damage he did to himself while manic — the money he squandered or the embarrassing escapades he will have to live down.

Severe, untreated mania is a dangerous condition. The subject's defective judgement and loss of normal inhibitions expose him and others to the risk of serious accidents, and in the days before effective treatments were available a long period of sustained overactivity and sleeplessness sometimes ended in sudden cardiovascular collapse and death. Mild mania, so called *hypomania*, on the other hand, may in some circumstances be positively advantageous. If they are not outweighed by the effects of defective judgement and disinhibition the subject's increased energy, heightened creativity and greater self-confidence may enable him to achieve things he would not normally be capable of, particularly in the artistic and social spheres.

Melancholia

This syndrome is known variously as endogenous, endogenomorphic, psychotic, retarded, vital and manic–depressive depression. None of these terms is satisfactory and in the writer's view the old word 'melancholia', revived in DSM-III and DSM-IIIR, is preferable.

The essence of the condition is a lowering of mood, accompanied by a marked reduction in energy and activity. The subject is no longer able to enjoy anything (*anhedonia*) and as a result loses interest in

and abandons his normal recreations and pastimes. He takes a gloomy view of himself, of the world about him and of the future, and undervalues his abilities and achievements. He may describe himself as sad or unhappy but often he insists that the feeling is different from, and worse than, normal sadness, the so-called 'special quality' of the melancholic mood. Libido and appetite are lost as part of the general anhedonia and as a result of the latter there is often a substantial loss of weight, perhaps 5–10 kg over a few weeks or months. Sleep is severely disturbed and what sleep the patient does get tends to be in the first half of the night. Often this is associated with a characteristic diurnal variation in mood, the patient feeling at his worst in the morning, or on first wakening, and improving as the day goes on. Indeed, sometimes by the evening he may look and feel almost normal.

Retardation is another characteristic feature. The patient's movements are slowed and the play of facial expression and the gestures that normally accompany social interactions and speech are restricted or lost. At the same time the voice becomes quiet, dull and monotonous and speech restricted in quantity and limited in range to a few themes of immediate personal concern. These changes may be so slight that they are only recognised in retrospect on recovery, or so marked that the patient is mute and almost motionless for hours on end. Agitation is also common. The patient is restless, pacing aimlessly to and fro, wringing his hands, plucking at sleeves or buttons, and often asking the same importunate questions over and over again. Retardation and agitation used to be regarded as alternatives, but in reality they commonly coexist, though of course the grosser manifestations of agitation are incompatible with severe retardation.

The patient's thoughts, like his speech, are restricted to a few gloomy themes. As a result there is a characteristic, and diagnostically important, impairment of attention and concentration. When he tries to read a book or a newspaper, or even to watch television, he finds he cannot take it in for his worries keep intruding. This difficulty concentrating prevents the patient from registering current events normally, and this impairment of registration he often wrongly interprets as a failing memory. Guilt feelings are very characteristic, though, like complaints of constipation, they are probably less common than they were 50 years ago. Like the grandiose ideas of mania they vary greatly in severity, from a justifiable but novel guilt over genuine misdemeanours, to a quite unwarranted preoccupation with peccadilloes committed long ago, or an entirely delusional conviction of having committed heinous crimes. Sometimes there are hallucinations, usually in the form of accusatory or condemnatory voices, and sometimes persecutory delusions as well as, or instead of, delusions of guilt.

Perhaps the most distressing of all the patients' thoughts concern the future, for often they are convinced that there will be no end to their suffering, that they will never recover. As a result suicide is an ever-present risk. Few patients with melancholia fail to think of ending their lives, or at least to wish that they could die, and many make serious suicidal attempts. It is commonly believed that the risk of suicide is greater during recovery than at the height of the illness, but this is only really so in those who are so retarded at the height of their illness that they lack the energy or initiative to put their thoughts into action.

As with mania the severity of the illness varies greatly, though there is no convenient term, corresponding to hypomania, to denote a mild disturbance. The patient may be deluded and deeply retarded for weeks or months on end and may make desperate attempts at suicide whenever an opportunity arises. Other episodes, however, may be so mild that the subject is able to remain at work and continue to fulfil most of his normal responsibilities despite sleeping badly, eating little, finding everything an effort and being unable to relax or enjoy anything.

Other depressions

Most depressive illnesses do not possess the characteristic features of melancholia described above, or at least only a few of them. They are also less severe, and do not cause such profound incapacity. For this reason, most of the people who fulfil criteria for a depressive episode (ICD-10) or a major depressive episode (DSM-IIIR) never enter psychiatric care and many never seek treatment of any kind. Nevertheless, their mood is depressed, their self-esteem low, their view of the future gloomy or despairing and their ability to cope with the demands of everyday life impaired. They have little energy and they complain that everything is an effort, but they do not have the severe impairment of concentration or the total loss of capacity for enjoyment that is so characteristic of melancholia. Sleep is usually disturbed but some patients exhibit hypersomnia rather than insomnia and regular early morning wakening is infrequent. Similarly, there is usually a disturbance of appetite, but severe loss of weight is unusual and 'comfort eating', despite reduced enjoyment of food, may result in an increase rather than a decrease in weight, particularly in women. The depression of mood is usually accompanied by irritability and, almost invariably, by anxiety, which may take the form of a constant feeling of tension, foreboding and inability to relax, or of intermittent attacks of panic, or of phobic symptoms. As a result it is often extremely difficult to decide whether a given illness is better regarded as a depression or an anxiety state. (See Chapter 22 for further discussion of this issue.)

The duration of the mood change is very variable. It may last only a few days or be so long lasting or oft recurring that it is difficult to distinguish between illness and personality disorder. Some variation from day to day or week to week is common, usually in response to life events, but a consistent diurnal variation in mood is rare. Guilt is variable, and resentment at the behaviour of others often more prominent. Many patients withdraw from social contact with others, either because they have lost interest in company, or because they are ashamed to be seen as they are, or because they have developed true phobic anxiety. Others become clinging and demanding. Suicidal behaviour of various kinds (parasuicide) is common but death by suicide is not, though the risk can never be ignored.

It is clear from this description that these 'other depressions' are very variable in symptomatology, severity and duration as well as being extremely common. They are also characterised more by the *absence* of the characteristic features of melancholia than by the *presence* of characteristic features of their own. It is unclear, and much debated, whether the difference between the two syndromes is primarily quantitative (i.e. melancholic illnesses are simply severe depressions) or whether there are qualitative differences also.

CLASSIFICATION OF MOOD DISORDERS

There is no satisfactory classification of mood disorders. Indeed, the majority of psychiatrists have never been agreed on how these disorders should best be classified, and controversy has been continuous since the 1920s. The problem is the depressions. The concept of depressive illness embraces a wide variety of disorders differing considerably in severity, symptomatology, course and prognosis. It also spans the historical distinction between neurosis and psychosis. On the other hand, the prevailing mood of sadness, helplessness and hopelessness tends to provide a common core, a unifying theme, to all depressions. So detailed subdivision and refusal to subdivide are both invested with a certain justification. The reasons why it has been so difficult to develop a generally acceptable classification and several of the alternative classifications that have been used or advocated in recent years have been discussed in some detail elsewhere (Kendell 1976). It is only appropriate here to consider some of the major issues and concepts involved.

Manic–depressive illness

This was Kraepelin's concept and it embraced all illnesses with the symptomatology of either mania or melancholia or some mixture of the two. Whether the patient had had one illness or many, whether these were brief or prolonged, mild or severe, and whether the patient suffered from depression alone, mania alone, or both, he was regarded as being afflicted with the same disorder, manic–depressive insanity. Kraepelin's reasoning was based on detailed observation of many patients over 20 or 30 years and remained unchallenged for half a century (Kraepelin 1921). Although some patients had episodes of both depression and mania, while others suffered from depressions alone and a few from mania alone, Kraepelin was impressed by the fact that there were no consistent differences in symptomatology or course between the depressions of those who only became depressed and the depressions of those who became manic as well. He was also impressed by the fact that several of his patients' relatives had regular fluctuations in mood (*cyclothymia*) which, though striking and unmistakable, were not severe enough to be labelled as illness. He also observed a great variety of mixed states in which manic and depressive symptoms were present simultaneously.

The concept had two weaknesses, however, and these were responsible for much subsequent confusion. Because manic–depressive insanity was regarded as an *endogenous* psychosis, illnesses of identical symptomatology developing in response to stress had to be classified separately. So too did other depressions which lacked the characteristic symptoms of melancholia despite the fact that, to equally careful observers like Lewis (1934), there appeared to be no clear boundary between the two. Despite these problems, and the difficulties in classifying other depressions to which they contributed, it was not until the 1960s, when Angst and Perris drew attention to the many differences between patients who suffered from both mania and depression and those who suffered only from depression, that the concept of manic–depressive psychosis was seriously challenged. Since then the term has slowly been replaced by Leonhard's terms unipolar and bipolar (see below). As a result the adjective 'manic–depressive' has changed its meaning and become a synonym for bipolar illness.

Unipolar and bipolar affective disorders

The proposal to divide Kraepelin's manic–depressive psychosis into separate bipolar (alternating mania and depression) and unipolar (recurrent depression or recurrent mania) disorders was first made by Leonhard, but it was Angst (1966) and Perris (1966) who first produced convincing evidence in support of the distinction. Perris studied 138 patients with at least one episode of depression and one of mania (bipolar illness), 139 patients with at least three episodes of depression without mania (unipolar depression), and a small group of 17 patients with at least three episodes of mania without depression (unipolar mania). He showed that bipolar illness started on average 15 years earlier than unipolar depression and recurred more frequently. Individual episodes of illness were shorter, and the morbidity risk in first-degree relatives was higher. There were also personality differences between the two, the bipolar patients tending to be warm, energetic and extraverted, the unipolar patients retiring, tense and anxious. Moreover, both bred true; the first-degree relatives of bipolar patients had bipolar illnesses and the relatives of unipolar depressives had unipolar illnesses.

Many of these findings have since been confirmed by others, though the distinction between the two is not quite so neat as Perris originally suggested. In particular, although the risk of bipolar illness in the relatives of unipolar patients does seem to be no higher than in the general population, several more recent studies have found that the relatives of bipolar patients have a higher risk of developing unipolar illness than bipolar illness (see Table 12.4). Moreover, between 10 and 20% of bipolar patients start off with three consecutive episodes of depression, and so qualify at that stage as unipolar, thereby making some degree of misclassification inevitable. And despite a number of claims, no consistent differences have yet been demonstrated between unipolar and bipolar depressions either in symptomatology or in their response to electroconvulsive therapy (ECT) or tricyclic antidepressants. Nor have the personality differences reported by Perris been found in more recent studies in which pains were taken to ensure that all patients were fully recovered at the time of testing (Hirschfeld et al 1986). Finally, it is still unclear whether patients who only develop mild, short-lived hypomanic swings (sometimes called bipolar II patients), or who only become manic briefly in the aftermath of a depressive illness successfully treated with ECT or a tricyclic drug, are fundamentally unipolar or bipolar.

Despite these problems the unipolar/bipolar distinction is incorporated into both the international (ICD-10) and American (DSM-III and DSM-IIIR) classifications, though not quite in the way that Leonhard proposed. The first-degree relatives of the rare patients who have recurrent manic illnesses without depression suffer not from mania alone but from bipolar illness or unipolar depression. For this and other reasons, recurrent mania is regarded as bipolar illness which has not yet manifested its first episode of depression, i.e. the important distinction is not whether the illness manifests itself in two forms or one, but whether or not the patient has ever had a manic episode. The validity of the unipolar/bipolar distinction is supported by a study of 110 pairs of Danish twins with Kraepelinian manic–depressive psychoses (Bertelsen et al 1977). Eleven of 32 pairs of monozygotic twins concordant for manic–depressive psychosis were concordant for unipolar illness and 14 concordant for bipolar illness. There were only seven pairs in which one twin was bipolar and the other unipolar, though the existence of these seven discordant pairs does, of course, indicate that unipolar and bipolar illness are not genetically distinct. The fact that both lithium and tricyclic antidepressants reduce the risk of future relapse in unipolar illness, whereas only lithium does so in bipolar illness (see below), provides further support for the validity of the distinction between the two.

The endogenous/reactive and psychotic/neurotic dichotomies

For most of this century many psychiatrists have been convinced that there are two fundamentally different kinds of depressive illness, one — described above under the heading of 'Melancholia' — usually being called endogenous or psychotic depression, and generally being regarded as the depressive phase of a manic–depressive illness, the other — described above under the heading 'Other depressions' — usually being called reactive or neurotic depression. These dichotomies have always been controversial, partly because of the terminology employed and partly because of doubts about the validity of the distinction between the two syndromes.

The terms endogenous and reactive are unsatisfactory because there is much evidence to suggest that life events and constitutional factors both contribute to the aetiology of both syndromes. In the 1960s several studies found a weak relationship between melancholic symptoms and absence of environmental precipitants, but this was at least partly due to failure to control for the effects of age. Melancholic symptoms become more and life events less common with increasing age. Since then several studies of representative samples of patients with depressive illnesses have failed to find any relationship between melancholic symptoms (anhedonia, retardation, diurnal mood variation, etc.) and either the morbid risk of depression in first-degree relatives or the incidence of life events and difficulties shortly before the onset of illness (Paykel 1974, Bebbington et al 1988). Twin studies also suggest that there is a substantial genetic component to neurotic or reactive depressions (Englund & Klein 1990). Andreasen et al (1986) investigated the incidence of depressive illnesses in 2942 first-degree relatives of the 566 subjects in the US National Institute of Mental Health (NIMH) collaborative programme on the psychobiology of depression with a Research Diagnostic Criteria (RDC) diagnosis of definite unipolar major depressive disorder. Of these relatives, 40% were personally interviewed and, for the remainder, information was available from the proband and at least one other family member. Four alternative definitions of endogenous depression were investigated — the DSM-III melancholia criteria, and the RDC, Newcastle and Yale criteria. Although the Newcastle criteria (Carney et al 1965) did generate a significantly higher rate of recurrent unipolar depression in the relatives of endogenous than of non-endogenous probands (26 versus 17%) the authors of this large multicentre study still concluded that 'in general, no matter which definition was used, the relatives of the patients with endogenous illness did not have higher rates of depressive illness than those of the non-endogenous group'.

The psychotic/neurotic dichotomy is equally objectionable. Bowman & Rose (1951) pointed out long ago that the distinction between psychosis and neurosis reflected nothing more fundamental than a rule of thumb judgement about the severity of the illness and the need for hospital admission. Although this was a heretical view at the time, the persistent inability of those who regarded the distinction as fundamental and crucial to provide either term with a viable definition resulted eventually in their exclusion from both the international (ICD-10) and American (DSM-III and DSM-IIIR) classifications. A further source of confusion is that American writers have usually reserved the term psychotic for illnesses accompanied by hallucinations, delusions or gross loss of insight while many British writers, following the usage of ICD-6 to ICD-9, have used the term as a synonym for endogenous depression or melancholia. To the former, therefore, an illness could be psychotic without being endogenous, or vice versa, whereas to the latter such distinctions were meaningless.

The question of the validity of the distinction between the two syndromes is, however, more important than any matter of terminology. This issue was a source of continuous controversy amongst British psychiatrists for 50 years. Fundamentally, it was a dispute between a Kraepelinian tradition, represented by Mayer Gross and Roth, which regarded the identification and delineation of disease entities as one of the major tasks of scientific psychiatry, and a Meyerian tradition, represented by Mapother and Lewis at the Maudsley Hospital, which regarded reaction types simply as convenient abstractions. In a series of papers published in the 1960s and 1970s, Roth and his Newcastle colleagues attempted to prove that what they called 'endogenous' and 'neurotic' depressions were distinct illnesses, and that there was a similar clear-cut boundary between depressive illnesses as a whole and anxiety states. In order to demonstrate a valid boundary it has to be shown that interforms between the two conditions are comparatively rare — that the 'greys' are outnumbered by the 'blacks' and the 'whites' — and the strongest evidence put forward by the Newcastle school was essentially a demonstration that this was the case. Clinical ratings from a series of 129 depressed in-patients, diagnosed clinically as 'endogenous' or 'neurotic', were subjected to multiple regression analysis and the distribution of scores on the resulting function shown to be bimodal rather than unimodal (Carney et al 1965). Subsequently, an analogous study of 145 patients suffering from depressive illnesses or anxiety states produced a similar bimodal distribution of scores on a discriminant function separating these two (Gurney et al 1972). Taken in isolation this was strong evidence for the validity of the distinctions in question. However, many other investigators have tried to obtain a bimodal distribution of scores on a discriminant function derived from consecutive series of depressions, some using the items and weights of the Newcastle scales and others their own independently derived discriminant functions. Almost invariably they failed to obtain a bimodal distribution (e.g. see Kendell 1968, Ni Bhrolchain et al 1979, Abou-Saleh & Coppen 1984, Zimmerman et al 1987). As a result it is now generally agreed that the symptomatology of depressive illnesses forms a continuous spectrum and that patients with a mixture of endogenous and reactive (or psychotic and neurotic) symptoms are commoner than pure forms of either kind.

The underlying relationships between the constituent symptoms of depressive illnesses have also been explored by factor analysis. Countless factor-analytic studies of depressive symptomatology have been published in the last 30 years and the majority have either generated a factor corresponding to the traditional concept of endogenous depression, or a bipolar factor expressing the distinction between the endogenous/reactive or psychotic/neurotic stereotypes. More recently, clustering techniques have been applied to similar clinical data. Despite many differences in the patient populations and clinical ratings involved, and in the clustering programs employed, most of these have produced a cluster corresponding to endogenous depression or melancholia. But none has produced a convincing second cluster corresponding to reactive or neurotic depression. They have either produced two or three different clusters incorporating different elements in the reactive/neurotic stereotypes, or no other depressive cluster at all.

The most important recent attempts to elucidate the classification of depressions by multivariate analysis of symptom ratings have been based on the extensive data generated by the NIMH collaborative study of the psychobiology of depression. Young et al (1986) investigated the patterning of symptoms in the Schedule for Affective Disorders and Schizophrenia (SADS) ratings of 788 patients fulfilling the RDC for major depression by latent class analysis. They found that neither the symptoms of DSM-III melancholia nor those of RDC endogenous depression identified an underlying dichotomous classification. Instead their material suggested the presence of two other overlapping dichotomies — the presence or absence of anhedonia (pervasive loss of enjoyment, depression of mood with a 'distinct quality' and no 'reactivity') and the presence or absence of vegetative symptoms (especially early morning wakening and weight loss). Retardation, guilt and diurnal mood variation appeared to be unrelated to either of these dichotomies, or to one another. The 5 year follow-up of these patients also provided an opportunity to compare the symptomatology of successive episodes of depression in the 201 subjects who had at least two further episodes during those 5 years (Young et al 1990). There was little evidence of syndromal stability. Although much of the variation was attributable to differences in severity, what consistency there was 'was largely that to be expected by chance'.

The field remains, therefore, as confused as it was 30 years ago despite a great deal of large-scale and increasingly sophisticated research. No valid boundaries or subgroups have been demonstrated, but most psychiatrists still baulk at the idea of lumping together all depressive illnesses, with their great variation in symptomatology, severity and outcome. This is one of the reasons why, despite the failure of many attempts at validation, the concept of melancholia or endogenomorphic depression retains its appeal. The same is not true, though, of neurotic depression and for most purposes that term is now obsolete. The cluster analyses referred to above suggest that, although melancholia may be a valid grouping, neurotic depression is not and this accords with most psychiatrists' clinical experience. Akiskal (1983) has suggested, partly on the basis of a 4 year follow-up of a personal series of 100 patients and partly on the basis of measurements of REM sleep latency, that so-called neurotic depression embraces four fairly distinct subgroups — primary depressions with residual chronicity, chronic dysphoric states secondary to other non-affective psychiatric disorders or physical illness, fluctuating characterological depressions starting in adolescence, and mild subthreshold unipolar and bipolar disorders.

Primary and secondary depressions

This dichotomy originated in St Louis and is used mainly in the USA. To be primary a depression must not be preceded chronologically by any other psychiatric disorder, other than mania. Secondary depressions are either *preceded* by another psychiatric illness (anxiety disorder, alcohol dependence, etc.) or *accompany* a serious physical illness. As a research strategy the distinction is sensible. It can be made reliably and provides a convenient means of separating out all those illnesses whose symptoms and antecedents are complicated and obscured by drug misuse, physical illness and lifelong personality disorder. Despite claims that dexamethasone fails to suppress cortisol secretion in nearly 50% of primary depressions but almost never in secondary depression (Schlesser et all 1980), and that REM latency is greatly reduced in primary depression but within the normal range in secondary depression (Akiskal et al 1982), it is not established that there is any fundamental difference between the two. It is said that about 40% of all depressions are secondary. On average these patients are younger than those with primary depressions and a higher proportion are male. In community surveys the commonest antecedent diagnosis is alcohol dependence, but this varies with the setting and sociopathy, hysteria, drug abuse and anxiety disorders are also common. According to Clayton & Collins (1981) the search for differences in symptomatology between primary and secondary depressions has been unrewarding. Retardation may be genuinely commoner in primary depressions but most of the reported differences are attributable to contamination of secondary depressions by the symptoms or behaviours of the antecedent disorder. Surprisingly little is known about differences in treatment response and prognosis between the two. Secondary depressions tend to be treated with antidepressants and ECT less frequently, but often respond well when they are.

According to Winokur et al (1988), depressions secondary to medical illnesses differ in several respects from those secondary to other psychiatric disorders and have many of the characteristics of pure 'reactive depressions'. They have a later age of onset, respond better to treatment (provided the underlying illness is not fatal), are less likely to relapse and less likely to be associated with depression or alcoholism in first-degree relatives.

Mood disorders in contemporary classifications

The American Psychiatric Association's classifications

DSM-III had several salutary effects on the classification of affective disorders when it was introduced in 1980. It brought them all together as a coherent group. Every category and subcategory was provided with an operational definition. The term manic–depressive, and other ambiguous epithets like psychotic, neurotic, endogenous and reactive, were all discarded. The two basic categories of DSM-III were designated as 'manic episode' and 'major depressive episode' and a fundamental distinction was drawn between unipolar and bipolar disorders (based on whether or not a manic episode had ever occurred). Major depressive episode was defined rather broadly, but could be subdivided in a number of alternative ways, for example as with or without melancholia (reintroduced as a less objectionable synonym for endogenous depression) and with or without mood-congruent or mood-incongruent psychotic features. The term depressive neurosis survived only as a synonym for *dysthymic disorder*, defined as recurrent depressive episodes lasting for at least 2 years which were not severe or long lasting enough to meet the criteria for a major depressive episode. The only relic of Kraepelin's terminology was *cyclothymic disorder*, defined as a combination of depressive and hypomanic mood swings lasting for at least 2 years which were not sufficiently severe or enduring to meet criteria for either manic or major depressive episodes.

DSM-IIIR differs only in minor ways from its predecessor. The detailed criteria for a major depressive episode are different and now make it possible for the diagnosis to be made in the absence of a depressed mood, provided there is anhedonia. The criteria for melancholia are also changed, with diagnostic weight now given to a good previous response to antidepressants or ECT and to full recovery from a previous episode. There is also a new set of criteria for seasonal mood disorders (see below).

The distinction between mood-congruent and mood-incongruent psychotic features was one of several important innovations in DSM-III. The concept of an affective illness accompanied by persecutory delusions or other mood-incongruent psychotic features greatly enlarged the American concept of affective disorder, and simultaneously restricted that of schizophrenia. It also produced an awkward and unresolved overlap with the concept of schizoaffective illness (see Ch. 20). Kendler (1991) has recently reviewed the literature of the last decade on mood-incongruent psychotic affective illness and concludes that its status as a distinct subtype of affective illness is supported. He is forced to concede, however, that it could equally well be regarded as a form of schizoaffective illness.

The international classification

The classification of depressive disorders in ICD-9 was widely regarded as unsatisfactory, mainly because there were no less than ten widely scattered three-digit categories and 19 four-digit categories under which illnesses with prominent depressive symptoms could be classified. It was a hotch potch with no coherent structure. ICD-10 is much better, mainly because it incorporates most of the important features of DSM-III. In particular, all mood disorders are brought together in one section (F3); the two basic syndromes — *manic episode* and *depressive episode* — are adequately described and defined; a distinction is drawn between unipolar and bipolar disorders; and terms like manic depression, melancholia, reactive, endogenous and psychogenic are relegated to the status of inclusion terms. The preamble is also notably tentative, even apologetic. After observing that 'affective disorders are not yet sufficiently understood to allow their classification in a way which is likely to meet with universal approval' it concludes: 'Nevertheless a classification must be attempted, and the one presented here is put forward in the hope that it will at least be acceptable, since it was the result of widespread consultation'.

Most of the distinctions drawn are explicitly based on differences in severity or duration rather than assumed differences in aetiology. For example, a distinction is drawn between single, recurrent and persistent disorders (cyclothymia and dysthymia). There are then two gradations of mood elevation (mania and hypomania) and three of depression (mild depressive

episode, moderate depressive episode and severe depressive episode). Mild and moderate depression can be recorded as with or without somatic symptoms (which correspond to the 'melancholic type' of DSM-IIIR) and manic and severe depressive episodes can be recorded as with or without psychotic symptoms. Seasonal affective disorder remains unrecognised but there is a category for *recurrent brief depressive disorder* in recognition of the evidence (see Angst et al 1990) that recurrent episodes of depression lasting only a few days but recurring many times a year are common in young adults of both sexes. In summary, the classification of mood disorders in ICD-10 is quite complicated, and makes provision for a wide range of detailed distinctions, but is singularly free of assumptions about disease entities and causation.

EPIDEMIOLOGY OF MOOD DISORDERS

Until recently our knowledge of the epidemiology of mood disorders was largely derived from three sources: the questionnaire responses of population samples, mostly North American; population surveys, mostly Scandinavian, in which psychiatrists personally interviewed entire populations but made their diagnoses to unspecified criteria (e.g. see Hagnell et al 1982); and psychiatric case registers which, of course, only record those in contact with psychiatric services. Only in the last decade have structured interviews designed to elicit affective symptoms been administered to representative population samples and diagnoses been derived from the ratings thus obtained using operational criteria. As a result of this new generation of studies we are now much better informed, but several problems remain.

The most important problem is that there is no evidence of any boundary or discontinuity between unhappiness, or what Kraepelin called 'the well founded moodiness of health', and clinical depression. Whatever criterion is examined — subjective distress, social impairment, illness behaviour, duration, or the distribution of particular symptoms or groups of symptoms — the variation appears to be continuous. All attempts to measure the prevalence of depressive disorders are therefore comparable to attempts to measure the prevalence of stupidity; the answer largely depends on how stupidity, or depression, is defined in the first place. It has also become clear that apparently minor differences between one definition of depression and another may result in major differences in the incidence and prevalence values obtained.

There is no doubt, however, that depressive disorders are extremely common and are responsible for a high proportion of total psychiatric morbidity. In the Epidemiologic Catchment Area (ECA) programme in the USA, in which representative samples of over 3000 adults aged 18 years or over were interviewed in each of five centres, the lifetime prevalence for all DSM-III affective disorders varied from 6.1% in Baltimore to 9.5% in New Haven. Major depression was responsible for the bulk of this morbidity with a lifetime prevalence ranging in women from 4.9 to 8.7% and in men from 2.3 to 4.4% (Robins et al 1984). These values must be regarded as minimum estimates, if only because episodes of illness in the distant past are often forgotten and remain unreported. Indeed, estimates of the 6 month prevalence of affective disorder in the same three centres were not much lower, ranging from 6 to 8.3% in women and 2.7 to 4.6% in men. In women aged 25–44 years the range was from 8.9 to 11.4%, i.e. about one woman in ten in that age range had had a diagnosable affective disorder within the previous 6 months. After allowing for differences in the structured interviews and diagnostic criteria employed, community surveys in Britain have yielded very similar rates (Surtees & Sashidharan 1986).

Epidemiology of depression

All estimates of the incidence or prevalence of depression, whether based on population surveys, psychiatric contact rates or hospital admission rates, find depressions to be twice as common in women as in men. The cause of this female predominance is much debated. Most authorites regard it as a genuine difference (Weissman & Klerman 1977) though Angst & Dobler-Mikola (1984) have argued that it is largely due to the greater reluctance of men to admit to having depressive symptoms and to their forgetting previous symptoms quicker. The difference is maximal in young adults and considerably reduced in old age, mainly because women have a very high incidence of depression in the reproductive years while men do not. It is uncertain to what extent the difference is rooted in biological differences between the sexes (hormonal differences perhaps, plus the biological effects of childbirth) and to what extent differences in the social roles of men and women are responsible, though most contemporary research and speculation are concerned with the latter. Jenkins (1985) tried to elucidate the problem by comparing men and women carefully matched for a variety of social variables. All were executive-grade civil servants, aged 20–35 years and working in the same government department in London. Psychiatric morbidity was measured with

the 30-item General Health Questionnaire and the Structured Clinical Interview (see Ch. 9 for details of these). Overall the prevalence of minor psychiatric morbidity was the same in both sexes, though somatic symptoms were significantly commoner in women and they consulted their doctors more frequently. Although this study was carefully designed it does not provide compelling evidence that the observed difference between the sexes is socially determined. The criterion of psychiatric morbidity adopted was very low, embracing over a third of a healthy population, and many depressive symptoms (depressed mood, fatigue, irritability, excessive concern) were somewhat commoner in women. And as 99% of the women were childless, biological sequelae of childbirth were necessarily eliminated.

Brown & Harris (1978) found a higher prevalence of depression in working class than in middle class women in south London and this social class difference has been confirmed, at least in women, in other surveys (e.g. see Surtees et al 1986). There is also general agreement that, for reasons which are still obscure, the prevalence of depression is higher in urban than in rural areas. In the North Carolina sample of the ECA study major depressive disorder was twice as common in the urban as in the rural area even after controlling for the effects of differences in age, sex, ethnic group, education and migrant status (Blazer et al 1985). Brown & Harris also found a higher prevalence of depression in south London than in the Hebrides. Unemployment is also associated with an increased prevalence of depressive symptoms (Melville et al 1985). Differences between ethnic groups, at least in North America, appear to be secondary to social class differences, and to disappear when the latter are controlled.

Before the 1960s it was widely believed, on the testimony of hospital-based psychiatrists, that depressive illnesses were rare throughout Africa and Asia. Almost every study since that time has refuted this view and there is now little doubt that depressive symptoms and severe depressive illnesses both occur with similar frequency in most races and cultures (Prince 1968). Nor is there any evidence of major differences in symptomatology between different cultures. A comparative study by the World Health Organization of series of patients attending psychiatric facilities in Basle, Montreal, Teheran, Nagasaki and Tokyo revealed no important differences (Jablensky et al 1981). Somatic symptoms do, however, often dominate and obscure the clinical picture in rural communities in Africa and Asia, and guilt is rarely prominent in non-Judaeo-Christian cultures.

Recent evidence suggests that the incidence of depression may be increasing rapidly, at least in industrial countries. Essen Möller and Hagnell surveyed all the inhabitants of Lundby in Southern Sweden on three occasions — in 1947, 1957 and 1972. The incidence of severe depression did not change over this 25 year period but the incidence of illnesses of mild or medium severity increased steadily between 1947 and 1972 in both men and women (Hagnell et al 1982). More recently, the NIMH psychobiology of depression programme has generated some intriguing data which also suggest a steadily increasing incidence (Klerman et al 1985). Ratings on the lifetime version of the Schedule for Affective Disorders and Schizophrenia-L (SADS-L) administered to 523 probands with affective disorders and 2289 first-degree relatives reveal a striking birth cohort effect. For six successive birth decades — from before 1910 to the 1950s — the risk of RDC major depressive disorder was higher at every age in each successive cohort and the mean age of the first episode younger. Similar findings have been reported from New Zealand (Joyce et al 1990).

It is important to appreciate, however, that there are other plausible explanations for these dramatic findings. An increasing willingness to admit to having psychiatric symptoms may be at least a partial explanation in both cases, and changing diagnostic criteria cannot be ruled out as a contributory cause of the Lundby findings. It is also likely that the failure of the elderly to remember earlier episodes of depression contributes to the birth cohort effect observed by Klerman and his colleagues. If the incidence and the lifetime risk of depression are really increasing at the rate these studies suggest the public health implications are profound.

Personality and depression

Most studies of the personalities of depressives have concluded that they tend to be introverted, obsessional, dependent, unassertive and prone to worry. Similarly, comparisons of the personalities of patients with unipolar and bipolar illnesses have generally concluded that the latter are more energetic, more gregarious and less inhibited. These conclusions are suspect, for two main reasons. Almost all have been based on personality assessments, usually by self-report questionnaire, in the aftermath of an episode of illness, and may well have been influenced by that illness even after apparent recovery. Ratings of neuroticism and dependency in particular are susceptible to the influence of quite minor mood changes, and the mere fact of having experienced a depressive illness

may influence peoples' self concepts in subtle ways. Secondly, nearly all studies have been based on patients, and as it is known that only a minority of those with depressive illnesses ever enter psychiatric care the personality traits identified may be those associated with consulting behaviour rather than with depression per se.

More recent and better designed studies find fewer personality differences between depressives and controls, and between unipolar and bipolar patients, than earlier comparisons. Paykel et al (1976) studied 185 patients from a variety of in-, out- and day patient facilities in New Haven. All 185 completed the Maudsley Personality Inventory (MPI) and the Lazare Klerman Armor Scale (LKAS) weeks or months after 'substantial clinical improvement'. Ratings on the LKAS were also obtained from relatives. The most prominent correlation — one reported in several previous studies — was between a high neuroticism (N) score on the MPI and a 'neurotic' as opposed to an 'endogenous' symptom pattern. Patients with 'endogenous' symptoms were also more likely to have obsessional personality traits, and less likely to have neurotic, 'oral' or hysterical traits. This was largely an age effect, however. Patients with endogenous symptoms are generally older than those without and obsessional personality traits become more prominent with advancing age, whereas neurotic and hysterical traits do the reverse. After the effect of age had been partialled out the most striking finding was the weakness and paucity of the remaining relationships between symptoms and personality attributes.

More recently, Hirschfeld et al (1986) have compared the ratings on a battery of self-report questionnaires, including the MPI and LKAS, of 45 patients with bipolar affective disorders, 78 with unipolar affective disorders and 1172 of their first-degree relatives with no history of mental illness. The patients' ratings were obtained a year after their illness and only those 'fully recovered' were included. Both patient groups scored lower than their relatives on 'emotional strength' (i.e. higher on neuroticism) but the personality profiles of the unipolar and bipolar patients were almost identical.

It seems likely, therefore, that the personalities of depressives differ from those of the general population, and that patients with different kinds of mood disorder differ from one another less than we once thought. Firm conclusions, however, will have to await the completion of prospective studies of the kind that Angst and Clayton are currently pursuing, in which personality assessments of large populations of healthy young adults are carried out with the intention, many years later, of comparing those who have developed mood disorders in the interim with those who have not.

Epidemiology of mania

Most of those who suffer from manic illnesses also suffer sooner or later from depressions and, for the reasons described above, a single episode of mania is regarded in both ICD-10 and DSM-IIIR as sufficient to establish a diagnosis of bipolar disorder. In most respects, therefore, the epidemiology of mania is the same as that of bipolar disorder.

Bipolar disorder is considerably less common than unipolar disorder. Recent American estimates using DSM-III criteria give a lifetime prevalence of 1.2%, compared with 4.4% for major depression and 3.1% for dysthymia (Weissman et al 1988). In sharp contrast to unipolar disorder the risk is the same in men and women. Nor is there any lower social class predominance; indeed, the risk may be somewhat higher in upper social classes. The mean age of onset is earlier than that of unipolar disorder with the first episode occurring before the age of 30 years in over 60%. It is important to appreciate, though, that bipolar illness can still present for the first time in the sixth or seventh decade; and also that manic illnesses in adolescence are often atypical, and wrongly diagnosed as schizophrenia.

The ratio of manic to depressive illnesses in consecutive series of hospital admissions is consistently higher in developing countries than in industrial countries. Whether this is simply because depressions are less likely to be admitted to hospital in Africa or Asia, or because there is a genuine difference in the relative incidence of mania and depression in different parts of the world remains uncertain, though the first explanation is probably at least partly responsible for the reported ratios.

AETIOLOGY

The biological substrate of mood disorders

The evidence that genetic factors make a major contribution to the aetiology of both bipolar and unipolar disorders (see Ch. 12) implies that there must be innate differences between those who suffer from these illnesses and other people. These differences may be either qualitative or quantitative and the imperfect concordance between monozygous twins establishes that environmental factors must also play a significant role, particularly in unipolar disorders (see Table 12.5).

So far, however, the innate biological abnormalities have not yet been identified, though there are many clues to their identity.

Cerebral amine metabolism

For the last 30 years the 'amine hypothesis' of affective disorder has occupied the centre stage, mainly because of the indirect pharmacological evidence pointing to a close association between cerebral amine metabolism and mood. Since the early 1960s it has been known that both tricyclic antidepressants (TCAs) and monoamine oxidase inhibitors (MAOIs) facilitate transmission in aminergic neurone systems, the TCAs by inhibiting amine re-uptake from the synaptic cleft by the presynaptic neurone, the MAOIs by inhibiting the oxidation of amine in presynaptic storage vesicles. Conversely, drugs like reserpine and tetrabenazine which deplete these storage vesicles may precipitate severe depressions. The original hypothesis (Schildkraut 1965) suggested that depression was associated with a functional deficit and mania with a functional excess of a transmitter amine at some crucial site in the brain. Because both the original TCAs and the MAOIs affected several different amines there were three plausible candidates: the catecholamines dopamine and noradrenaline, and the indoleamine 5-hydroxytryptamine or serotonin (5-HT). In the brain, serotonin is mainly metabolised to 5-hydroxyindoleacetic acid (5-HIAA), dopamine is mainly metabolised to homovanillic acid (HVA) and noradrenaline mainly converted to 3-methoxy-4-hydroxyphenylglycol (MPHG) (see Ch.7 for details).

Several lines of evidence suggest that serotoninergic pathways are involved in the genesis of depression. It was established at an early stage that 5-HIAA levels are low in the cerebrospinal fluid (CSF) of depressed subjects (Ashcroft et al 1966) and that the rate at which 5-HIAA accumulates in CSF after probenecid blockade is reduced (van Praag 1977). The serotonin precursor tryptophan has been shown to have antidepressant activity, both on its own (Thomson et al 1982) and in combination with an MAOI. It has also been shown that acute tryptophan depletion leads to a rapid return of depressive symptoms in people who have recently recovered from depression (Delgado et al 1990). Suicides have been reported to have lowered serotonin levels in their brain stems and a low CSF 5-HIAA level has been found to predict subsequent suicide, particularly by violent means (Träskman et al 1981).

Other studies appear to implicate dopaminergic neurones. It has been shown that the dopamine precursor L-dopa enhances the antidepressant activity of

MAOIs and may precipitate hypomania in bipolar patients. And although the resting level of the dopamine metabolite HVA in CSF is the same in depressives as in controls, the rate at which it accumulates after probenecid blockade is lowered (van Praag et al 1970), suggesting that dopamine turnover is reduced.

Other evidence suggests that noradrenergic neurones have a major role. Depressive have lower levels of urinary MHPG than normal controls, and bipolar depressives have been reported to have lower levels than unipolar depressives (Goodwin & Potter 1979). It has also been claimed that the activity of catechol-*o*-methyl transferase, the enzyme responsible for inactivating noradrenaline released into the synaptic cleft, is increased in erythrocytes from patients with primary affective disorders and their first-degree relatives (Gershon & Jonas 1975). There are at least four different kinds of adrenoceptor, known as α_1, α_2, β_1 and β_2 adrenoceptors, and there is evidence to implicate at least two of these. Several investigations have found that the growth hormone (GH) response to both insulin-induced hypoglycaemia and clonidine is impaired in depression (e.g. see Checkley et al 1981), and there is some evidence that the impaired response to clonidine persists after recovery (Mitchell et al 1988). The GH response to clonidine depends on stimulation of α_2 adrenoceptors but, as the hypotensive effect of clonidine is normal in depressives and this also depends on α_2 adrenoceptors, it is unlikely that any generalised abnormality of α_2 receptor activity is involved. Wright et al (1984) have also claimed that lymphoblastoid cell lines from members of families with early onset bipolar disorder (created by culturing their lymphocytes with Epstein–Barr virus) show a persistently reduced binding to β adrenoceptors.

Although many of these findings seem important and convincing in isolation the overall picture is extremely confusing. Several of the claims referred to above have not been substantiated even by their original authors, and the technical problems involved are formidable. It is still uncertain, for example, whether 5-HIAA and MHPG in lumbar CSF come from the cerebral ventricles or mainly from the spinal cord, and equally uncertain what proportion of urinary MHPG is of central rather than peripheral origin. In the 1980s it was repeatedly claimed that the binding of tritiated imipramine or yohimbine (^{3}H is simply a convenient isotopic label) to platelets from depressed subjects was reduced (lower B_{max} values, indicating a reduced number of binding sites). As these binding sites for ^{3}H imipramine are believed to be serotonin receptors and similar sites are found on neurones, this was potentially important. However, although several, but not all, antidepressants increase ^{3}H imipramine binding it seems increasingly doubtful whether platelets from drug-naive depressives do after all have fewer binding sites than properly matched controls (Healy et al 1990). Similar claims have been made that the binding of ^{3}H clonidine to platelets from depressed subjects is increased, indicating an increased density of α_2 adrenoceptors. But, even though it is established that long-term administration of either TCAs or MAOIs to experimental animals results in a decrease in cerebral α_2 adrenoceptors, the aetiological significance of this finding is still unclear (Kafka & Paul 1986). Positron emission tomography (PET) has so far done little to clarify the complexities of cerebral amine metabolism in depression, mainly because of a lack of positron-emitting ligands for noradrenergic and serotonergic receptors.

Several comparisons have been made of the antidepressant efficacy of selective noradrenaline uptake inhibitors like desipramine and selective serotonin uptake inhibitors like zimelidine and trazodone. Frustratingly, most of these trials have failed to demonstrate any difference between the two, either in efficacy or in speed of action.

For these and other reasons it seems increasingly doubtful whether antidepressants do act by facilitating transmission in aminergic neurone systems. Mianserin and iprindole have no significant effect on amine re-uptake yet both are effective antidepressants. Conversely, drugs like cocaine and amphetamine which do inhibit amine re-uptake do not have antidepressant properties. The original amine hypothesis does not explain why the therapeutic effects of both the TCAs and the MAOIs are delayed for 10 days or more when their effects on amine metabolism are fully developed within hours. Nor does it account for the puzzling fact that so many antidepressants are strikingly similar in their efficacy and speed of action despite major differences in chemical structure and pharmacological profile.

It is now recognised that most neuroceptors slowly adapt to changes in the transmitter concentration to which they are exposed. For example, antidepressants which increase intrasynaptic noradrenaline concentrations subsequently produce a compensatory reduction, or *down regulation*, in the density or functional activity of β adrenoceptors, and some do the same to α adrenoceptors. Most antidepressants seem to produce a cascade of secondary changes of this kind, including changes in the density or sensitivity of serotonin, dopamine, γ-aminobutyric acid (GABA) and benzodiazepine receptors, and it is unclear which of these are primary and which are therapeutically important

(Garrattini & Samanin 1988). At present it seems likely that down regulation of adrenergic β receptors, and possibly of $5\text{-}HT_2$ receptors also, is the crucial therapeutic change, partly because increased β receptor and $5\text{-}HT_2$ receptor density is consistently found in the brains of suicides at post mortem.

Endocrine abnormalities

Cortisol secretion. It has been known for 30 years that most patients with depressive illnesses have an abnormally high cortisol output and that this usually falls to normal on recovery. In the 1970s this was usually assumed to be a non-specific reaction to stress, analogous to the raised cortisol secretion of normal people before examinations or sporting contests. Subsequently, however, the development of accurate methods of measuring 24 hour urinary cortisol, and methods of plotting diurnal changes in plasma cortisol by sampling every 20 minutes from an indwelling venous catheter, suggested that the two were different. In normal people cortisol is secreted mainly between 4 a.m. and noon, and serum cortisol levels are low at other times of the day. In depressives this morning peak is more pronounced, starts earlier and lasts longer (Sachar et al 1980). This abnormal pattern cannot be reproduced in normal people by subjecting them to stress or sleep deprivation, and occurs in apathetic as well as anxious depressives. It is not, however, an invariable accompaniment even of severe depression.

The dexamethasone suppression test (DST) has been widely used as an indirect index of cortisol hypersecretion. Dexamethasone is a potent synthetic steroid which inhibits the secretion of corticotrophin (adrenocorticotrophic hormone, ACTH), and hence of cortisol, by its action on cortisol feedback receptors in the brain. In normal people, but not those with Cushing's syndrome, it suppresses cortisol secretion for up to 24 hours and the primary use of the test is in the diagnosis of Cushing's syndrome. Extensive trials by Carroll et al (1981) suggested that, if dexamethasone 1 mg was given at 11.30 p.m. and a plasma cortisol greater than 5 mg/dl at 4 p.m. or 11 p.m. the following day was taken as the criterion of non-suppression, the test had a specificity for melancholia of 96% and a sensitivity of 67%. The DST was hailed as a 'specific laboratory test for the diagnosis of melancholia' and came into widespread use throughout the USA. Unfortunately, only a minority of attempted replications have been successful. For example, a detailed investigation of hypothalamic/pituitary/adrenal activity, including a DST, was carried out on 132 depressives from six cen-

tres in the NIMH psychobiology of depression programme. Virtually no endocrine differences were found between 'endogenous' and non-endogenous depression, however endogenous was defined, or between psychotic and non-psychotic depressions (Kocsis et al 1985). Another major study, based on 231 patients from the Max Planck Institute in Munich produced similar results (Berger et al 1984). Berger and his colleagues also found many instances of non-suppression in mania, schizophrenia, dementia, non-endogenous depressions and obsessional illnesses and concluded that 'neither our data nor several other recent reports ... support the utility of the DST for diagnostic decisions in psychiatry'. Claims that non-suppression predicts a good response to ECT or TCAs, and that persistent non-suppression despite apparent recovery predicts early relapse, also remain unconfirmed.

Several factors have contributed to the downfall of the DST, including technical problems affecting the radioimmunoassay of cortisol, the dose of dexamethasone and the optimum time interval before measuring the serum cortisol. It also appears that non-suppression may sometimes be a secondary consequence of weight loss or insomnia rather than of melancholia per se (Mullen et al 1986), or of impaired absorption or accelerated metabolism of dexamethasone itself. All the same, the central finding that a high proportion of depressed patients have an abnormally high cortisol output, and an abnormal diurnal pattern of output, remains and recent work is starting to clarify the underlying mechanisms. Increased cortisol production is accompanied by, and presumably secondary to, increased output of ACTH and the hypothalamic corticotrophin-releasing hormone CRH-41 (Pfohl et al 1985). Computerised tomography (CT) scanning suggests that this endocrine hyperactivity is accompanied by hypertrophy of the adrenal glands (Amsterdam et al 1987) and magnetic resonance (MRI) scanning now suggests that the pituitary is also larger in depressives than controls, presumably as a result of hyperplasia of corticotrophic cells (Krishnan et al 1991).

Other endocrine abnormalities. Although thyroid function seems to be normal in melancholia there is evidence that small doses of tri-iodothyronine potentiate, or at least speed up, the clinical response to TCAs (Prange et al 1976). It is also established that the thyroid-stimulating hormone (TSH) response to thyrotrophin-releasing hormone (TRH) is impaired in some depressives, but although this finding has been confirmed several times its significance it still unclear (Loosen & Prange 1982). The impaired response persists after recovery in some patients, but not all, and has also been reported in alcoholism and mania. It does seem unlikely, though, that an impaired TSH response to TRH is simply a secondary consequence of increased cortisol production. For one thing it does not correlate well with failure of dexamethasone suppression.

Mania has been studied less often than melancholia and the pattern of endocrine responses is even more confused. Some investigators have reported that dexamethasone suppression is almost invariable; others that non-suppression is as common and as characteristic as in melancholia. The most interesting finding reported so far is that plasma levels of luteinising hormone are raised in young men with mania (Whalley et al 1985).

Neuropeptides

There have been several reports that CSF levels of somatostatin are low in depression (e.g. see Doran et al 1986) and that low CSF somatostatin correlates with dexamethasone non-suppression. Increased output of corticotrophin and CRH in depression have been referred to already. The normal nocturnal increase in GH production is also lost or reduced. Nemeroff et al (1991) have recently measured CSF levels of several peptides in psychotic depressives before and after ECT and found that concentrations of CRH and β-endorphin fell significantly on recovery while that of somatostatin rose, suggesting that the reported abnormalities are state dependent.

In view of the role of neuropeptides in modulating aminergic transmission in the central nervous system it is likely that the next few years will see a blossoming of interest in their potential role in the pathogenesis of mood disorders.

Sleep and the electroencephalogram (EEG)

Insomnia is a frequent and characteristic depressive symptom. Although the association between early morning wakening and melancholia is not so invariable as an earlier generation of psychiatrists believed, insomnia in the second half of the night is certainly common in severe depression. Together with the evidence that the diurnal pattern of cortisol secretion is abnormal in depression, and that sleep deprivation for 36 hours often produces a temporary alleviation of depression, this suggests that the diurnal rhythms underlying the alternation between sleep and wakefulness may be disturbed in some fundamental way in depression. All-night EEG recordings of depressed and control subjects appear to confirm that this is so. Several different abnormalities have been reported (see Ch. 24 for details), the most characteristic and the best established being a reduction in the total quantity of deep (slow wave) sleep and a shortened REM latency, i.e. a shortened interval between the onset of sleep and the start of the first period of REM sleep. Normally this is about 90 minutes but in depression it is characteristically reduced to about 40 minutes (Kupfer & Foster 1978). It has been claimed, however, that REM latency can be reduced in normal people simply by waking then regularly at 5 a.m. suggesting that the phenomenon may simply be a consequence of lack of sleep (Mullen et al 1986).

Light and darkness

Melatonin secretion by the pineal is inhibited by light and melatonin appears to act as the *Zeitgeber* (time-keeper) for several diurnal rhythms as well as controlling the onset of the annual cycle of sexual activity in many herbivores. The evidence referred to above that there may be a fundamental disturbance of diurnal rhythms in depression, and the existence of stable seasonal fluctuations in the incidence of both suicide and mania, suggest that some mood disorders may be precipitated by a loss of synchronisation of circadian rhythms. In the 1980s Lewy et al (1981) claimed that exposing euthymic manic–depressives to bright light in the middle of the night produced a much larger reduction in serum melatonin than in controls. It was subsequently claimed by Rosenthal et al (1985) that the depressive symptoms of people with recurrent winter depressions could be relieved by lengthening the winter photoperiod by exposing them to bright light for several hours in the early morning and evening. This led to a flurry of interest in what came to be known as seasonal affective disorder, and a series of clinical trials of the effects of exposure to light of various kinds for varying periods on depressive symptoms. It now seems clear that *seasonal affective disorder* does exist, in the sense that people who experience recurrent winter depressions can be found in appreciable numbers (Thompson & Isaacs 1988). Most are women, their depressions tend to be accompanied by irritability, hypersomnia, hyperphagia and social withdrawal, and many also become hypomanic in the spring. But their symptoms are rarely severe enough to come to medical attention and there is little evidence that the syndrome becomes commoner as latitude increases. Although several clinical trials have confirmed that exposure to bright light (about 2500 lux) does relieve the depressive symptoms of such people more effectively than dim or red light it is difficult to be sure that this is not a placebo effect, particularly as it does not seem to matter whether or not the photoperiod is lengthened or whether melatonin levels are altered. Nor has Lewy's original claim that melatonin secretion is more light-sensitive in manic–depressives or people with seasonal affective disorder been confirmed. It seems likely, therefore, that interest in seasonal affective disorder will soon wane. It is recognised in DSM-IIIR but not in ICD-10.

Water and electrolyte metabolism

In the 1960s, sodium and water metabolism were extensively investigated in manic–depressives, often in individuals with regular, predictable alternations in mood. The most interesting of many reported abnormalities was that *residual sodium* (an approximate measure of total intracellular sodium) was increased by 50% in depression and 200% in mania (Coppen 1967). Eventually interest waned, because different investigators were unable to confirm one another's findings and because it was suspected that the observed abnormalities were merely consequences of the changes in diet, physical activity and cortisol secretion accompanying depression. The possibility remains, however, that there is a fundamental abnormality of sodium metabolism in mood disorders and some British investigators are still pursuing this possibility. Naylor has claimed that the sodium content of erythrocytes falls on recovery from both depression and mania, and that this is due to increased sodium/potassium-dependent adenosine triphosphatase (Na^+/K^+ ATPase) activity, and hence to increased sodium transport across cell membranes. He also claims that the lymphocytes of manic–depressives are unable to produce new 'pump sites' in response to a rise in intracellular sodium (Naylor & Smith 1981). More recently, Wood and his colleagues, using the rate of rubidium uptake by erythrocytes as a measure of Na^+/K^+ ATPase activity, have claimed that the activity of this enzyme is increased in acute mania (the opposite of Naylor's finding). They also claim that lymphocytes from manic depressives in remission do not show the normal increase in Na^+/K^+ ATPase sites when they are incubated in lithium or ethacrynate and that this is an enduring trait marker for bipolar illness (Wood et al 1991).

Anatomical and psychophysiological abnormalities

Much less attention has been paid to the neuropathology and psychophysiology of mood disorders than of schizophrenia. It is an uncomfortable fact, however, that many of the abnormalities reported in schizophrenics, and initially assumed to be specific to schizophrenia, have been found in patients with mood disorders as well. There have, for example, been several reports of an increased ventricle/brain ratio, indicating enlargement of the lateral ventricles, in both unipolar and bipolar disorders (e.g. see Dolan et al 1985). 'Hypofrontality' (relatively low oxygen and glucose utilisation by the frontal lobes of the brain) has also been reported in bipolar patients (Buchsbaum et al 1986). So too have abnormal eye tracking movements.

The environmental contribution to aetiology

Environmental influences must play a part in the aetiology of mood disorders. If they did not the concordance between monozygotic twins would be close to 100% and the illness would develop at a similar age, and pursue a similar course, in both. In the past the continental European concept of endogenous psychosis, and that of endogenous depression in particular, tended to focus attention on genetic and constitutional factors and it was tacitly assumed that social and psychological influences were only important in the genesis of so-called neurotic or reactive depressions. An increasing interest in the milder mood disorders encountered in general population surveys, together with a realisation that no distinction could be drawn between endogenous and reactive illnesses, has led in the last 20 years to a blossoming of interest in environmental influences, particularly in Britain.

Of all the exogenous influences which might play a part in the causation of mood disorders, three have attracted particular interest: parental loss in childhood; life events of various kinds shortly before the onset of illness; and social or emotional isolation. All three have usually been studied with respect to depressive illnesses and their possible role in the genesis of mania largely ignored. It is, of course, true that the concordance between monozygotic twins is higher for bipolar than for unipolar illnesses (see Table 12.5). The morbid risk in first-degree relatives is also higher in bipolar illness. Nevertheless, clinical experience strongly suggests that in many patients life events play as important a role in the genesis of manic episodes as they do for depressions. Enforced lack of sleep may also be an important factor in some cases. What formal evidence there is is conflicting. Most studies have found a raised incidence of life events preceding the onset of manic illnesses but one recent, well-designed study failed to confirm this (Sclare & Creed 1990).

Parental loss in childhood

Interest in parental loss, either by death or separation, stems from psychoanalytic theory. Freud (1917) and

Abraham (1924) both regarded melancholia as a reaction to the loss of a 'love object', and Abraham believed that losses of various kinds later in life precipitated depression by re-opening the wounds originally inflicted by a crucial loss in early childhood. This theoretical background has inspired many studies of the relationship between parental loss and subsequent depression, and in the last 30 years there have been over 20 comparisons of depressives and control populations of various kinds. Unfortunately, the results are very confusing, largely because of the methodological problems involved.

Because of the progressive increase in life expectancy that has taken place this century, and the influence of two world wars, the incidence of childhood bereavement varies considerably from one generation to another, and also with geographical location and social class. Divorce rates vary even more than mortality rates. This makes accurate matching of controls all important. A further problem is that until recently the depressives in most studies were all patients, thus making it impossible to distinguish between an association between parental loss and the *occurrence* of depression, and an association with subsequent help-seeking behaviour. (This is important because there is some evidence that loss of a parent in childhood may lead to dependency or hypochondriasis later in life.) To compound the problem some studies do not distinguish between loss of a parent by death and loss by separation; some distinguished between mothers and fathers while others distinguished between same- and opposite-sexed parents; some looked at particular kinds of depressive illness, others at depressions as a whole.

Most studies comparing the incidence of early parental death in depressive and general population controls have found a higher incidence of parental death in the depressives (e.g. Dennehy 1966, Birtchnell 1970). However, studies in which depressives were compared with medical controls or other psychiatric patients (including those of Dennehy and Birtchnell) have generally found no significant differences. This suggests that the relationship is not specific to depression; either there is a non-specific relationship between childhood bereavement and psychiatric illness, or parental death in childhood simply makes people more dependent, and so more likely to consult doctors. Even in those studies in which a relationship was found between childhood bereavement and depression there is no agreement which parent is more important, or at which stage in childhood the effect of bereavement is most pronounced.

The evidence for an association between depression and parental loss for reasons other than death (the commonest being breakdown of the parental marriage by divorce or desertion) is stronger. Roy (1985) compared 300 patients with non-endogenous depressions and 300 medical controls with no history of depression and found a considerably higher incidence in the former of permanent separation from one or other parent before the age of 17 years, but not of parental death. In a carefully designed community-based study in north London, Brown and Harris have also demonstrated, in women, a relationship between loss of their mother by death or separation before the age of 17 years, but not of their father, and depression in the previous 12 months (Harris et al 1986). Further analysis of the sequelae of loss suggested that it was subsequent 'lack of care' rather than the loss itself that mattered, and that the reason why paternal loss was not related to subsequent depression was that it was less likely to lead to 'lack of care'. Neither is the relationship specific to depression. Psychopaths, delinquents, alcoholics and drug abusers have an even higher incidence of parental loss through divorce or desertion than depressives. The observed relationship may also be genetically mediated to some extent; that is, the genetically determined personality traits which predispose to marital breakdown may also predispose to depression, alcoholism and delinquency.

Even if one assumes that there is a relationship between parental loss and depression it is unclear whether the relationship holds for all depressions or only for particular subgroups. Gregory (1966) found no difference between psychotic and neurotic depressives after allowing for the age difference between them and Perris (1966) found no difference between unipolar and bipolar psychoses. Both Brown and Birtchnell, however, found a higher incidence of early bereavement in severe depressions. Brown has also claimed, somewhat improbably, that there is a strong relationship between melancholic or psychotic symptoms and 'past lost by death', which he defined as the loss of either parent or a sibling before the age of 17 years, or the loss of a child or husband at any age (Brown & Harris 1978).

In summary, the literature on the relationship between depression and parental loss is large, conflicting and inconclusive. It seems unlikely that childhood bereavement does predispose to subsequent depressive illness. There is much better evidence for a relationship between *separation* from a parent in childhood and subsequent depression; but the relationship is not specific to depression and it is probably the poor and unstable care which ensues that matters rather than parental loss itself.

The quality of a child's relationship with his parents is a related issue of obvious potential importance. Parker in Sydney, Australia, has developed a self-report questionnaire, the Parental Bonding Instrument (PBI), for assessing this retrospectively. He claims that neurotic depressives are far more likely than matched controls to report their parents as uncaring and over-protective and that there is no comparable difference between endogenous depressives and their controls (Parker et al 1987). Although an American study has yielded similar results (Plantes et al 1988), these relationships cannot yet be regarded as established. It is doubtful whether people in late middle age can produce valid ratings of their childhood relationships 40 years before, the controls were not well matched in either the Australian or the American studies, and there was an 18 years difference in the mean ages of Parker's neurotic and endogenous depressives.

Recent life events

In the last 25 years much interest has been taken in the role of *life events* in the genesis of depressive illnesses. Until recently, most of this research was retrospective. People with depressive symptoms were questioned about events in their lives in the weeks or months prior to the onset of their symptoms and the same questions asked of non-depressed controls. This raises a number of methodological problems. Anyone who becomes depressed tries to understand why they have done so and this 'search after meaning' may cause them to remember events controls would forget, or to magnify their significance. Moreover, controls are usually questioned about the last *x* months, whereas patients are questioned about a more distant time period, the *x* months before they became ill. A further problem is that some events, like the breakup of a relationship or failure to pass an exam, may be either a cause or a consequence of illness. For this reason several investigators have concentrated their attention on 'independent events', such as losing a job because of closure of the firm, which of their nature could hardly have been the result of illness. Most important of all, the impact of many events will vary greatly with the context. A stillbirth, for example, would probably be more stressful to a childless woman who had been trying to conceive for years than to a mother of four who had unintentionally become pregnant once more. Early investigators ignored this issue on the assumption that differences of this kind would affect both patients and controls and tends to cancel out. Brown, however, developed a technique for rating the *contextual threat* of each event for the individual concerned

without that rating being contaminated by knowledge of its sequelae (Brown & Harris 1978).

Comparisons of the incidence of life events in depressives and general population controls have shown that depressives report more events before the onset of illness than controls. Paykel et al (1969), for example, found that depressives referred to a variety of psychiatric facilities in New Haven reported three times as many events in the 6 months before onset as matched controls. Brown & Harris (1978), in an influential community-based study in south London, found that depressed women only had a raised incidence of events of all kinds in the 3 weeks before onset, though they had experienced more events rated on the basis of their contextual threat as 'markedly threatening' over the whole of the previous year. Paykel found that the majority of events preceding the onset of depression involved losses from the subject's social field (e.g. death of a parent, divorce or a child leaving home) or were undesirable in other ways, and found no excess of desirable events or additions to the subject's social field (e.g. marriage, or the birth of a child or grandchild). It is clear from other studies, though, that events of very varied kinds may precede the onset of depression and, although most can be interpreted as stressful, the majority do not involve losses, or at least not unless a very broad concept of symbolic loss is invoked. Brown & Harris studied chronic problems like poor housing, friction with in-laws or worry about a child's behaviour (situations which they referred to as *major difficulties* if they lasted for at least 2 years) and showed that these were also commoner in depressives than controls, and so probably of similar aetiological significance.

In their original community study in south London, Brown & Harris claimed to have identified a number of *vulnerability factors* which do not lead to depression in the absence of *provoking agents* (i.e. the threatening life events or chronically stressful major difficulties described above) but do increase the risk of depression if a provoking agent is present. They listed four such vulnerability factors — loss of the mother before the age of 11 years, having three or more children at home below the age of 14 years, the lack of a confiding relationship with a husband or other intimate, and lack of a full- or part-time job. This claim, and the painstaking interviewing procedures used in the survey, both aroused widespread interest and stimulated much further research, including several attempted replications.

Some but not all of the elements of the Brown & Harris model have been replicated. Their claim that some 15% of urban women have depressive symptoms which are as severe and extensive as those of the patients seen by psychiatrists in their clinics has been confirmed. So has their finding of a higher prevalence in working-class than in middle-class women. Their concept of vulnerability factors which only lead to depression in the presence of a provoking agent remains more contentious, partly because the issue is complicated by a disagreement about whether the appropriate statistical technique for testing the model is additive (i.e. the simple χ^2 comparisons which Brown & Harris used) or multiplicative (i.e. the log linear analysis advocated by Tennant & Bebbington (1978)). Costello (1982) in Alberta, and Campbell et al (1983) in Oxford, found that lack of an intimate, confiding relationship did act as a vulnerability factor, but both failed to find any convincing evidence that loss of the mother in childhood, lack of paid employment or having three or more young children at home had any comparable effect. Hallstrom (1986) in Gothenburg failed to find any significant interaction between provoking agents and any of Brown & Harris' four vulnerability factors despite using their additive model. Lack of intimacy did, however, increase the risk of depression in its own right, i.e. it acted as Tennant & Bebbington (1978) had suggested as a provoking agent rather than as a vulnerability factor.

Two major prospective surveys have since been reported, one in Islington in north London (Brown et al 1986), the other in Edinburgh (Surtees et al 1986). In both, community samples of women were interviewed on two occasions a year apart, thus making it possible to examine the relationship between ratings of vulnerability and stress made at the first interview and onsets of depression during the following 12 months, thereby avoiding the shortcomings of the retrospective studies referred to above. The Islington survey was based on 400 working-class women aged 18–50 years who all had at least one child under 18 years living at home. In this study, low self-esteem emerged as the most important vulnerability factor. Of the women rated as having low self-esteem at the first interview, 33% of those who were exposed to a provoking agent in the following year became depressed compared with only 13% of those without low self-esteem ($p<0.01$). A confiding relationship with a husband, lover or other confidant at the time of the first interview provided relatively poor protection, mainly because what mattered was whether support was provided at the time of need. Women who were exposed to a provoking agent and then 'let down' by their confidant had as high an incidence of depression as those with no confidant in the first place. The Edinburgh study was based on a random population sample of 576 women aged 18–65 years. The prevalence of depressive symptoms was high, and higher in working-class than in middle-class women. However, many of the crucial elements in Brown's model were not replicated. An onset of depressive symptoms was not significantly commoner in the 12 months between the two interviews in women with one or more putative vulnerability factors than in those without (12% versus 10%). Nor were independent life events significantly commoner in women who experienced an onset of depression than in those who did not. The most potent stresses were major difficulties (i.e. chronically stressful situations) and dependent events.

In summary, the majority of depressive episodes — Brown would say over 90% — are either preceded by a stressful event or occur in the setting of a chronically stressful situation. However, many of these events and situations are at least partly self-generated and the majority of women exposed to them do not become depressed; the relative risks even of severe events and major difficulties are only of the order of 2 to 4 (Surtees et al 1986). Although the evidence is still conflicting it seems likely that *vulnerability factors* which only increase the risk of depression in the presence of a *provoking agent* do exist. However, the only vulnerability factor which is reasonably well established is a confiding relationship with a spouse or other intimate, and this probably exerts its influence by an effect on self-esteem. There is therefore a common thread between the social theory of Brown & Harris and Beck's cognitive theory referred to below and in Chapter 41.

Social support

The confiding relationship of Brown & Harris is obviously a form of social support and the work of Miller & Ingham (1976) in general practice suggests that more diffuse relationships may also have a protective role. The potential role of social supports in general in protecting against life stresses or *adversity* has been investigated by many people, notably by Henderson in Canberra using a specially developed Interview Schedule for Social Interaction. There is general agreement that those who are dissatisfied with the number and quality of their friendships have a higher psychiatric morbidity than other people. But dissatisfaction, or loneliness, does not necessarily mean that they really have fewer social supports than those who are not dissatisfied. There are two other problems as well. First, the loss of a friend or relative may be construed both as a reduction in social support and as a stressful life event, which makes it difficult to test the value of social support in protecting against adversity. Second, an individual's personality is a major determinant of the social supports available to him; he has to be likeable and responsive to have friends. This means that it is almost impossible to prove that the relationship between lack of social support and depression is not simply a secondary consequence of the subjects' personality characteristics. Partly because of these problems and partly because none of the social support indices in Henderson's prospective study (Henderson et al 1981) predicted the subsequent onset of symptoms, at least in those exposed to relatively low levels of adversity, research in this area has reached something of an impasse.

Relatives and friends can, of course, be either supportive or destructive. It is well established that living with a hostile or critical relative increases the risk of relapse in schizophrenia (see Ch. 18). Vaughn & Leff (1976) showed that this high *expressed emotion* (EE) also increased the risk of relapse in depression, but that the critical EE threshold was lower. Hooley et al (1986) in Oxford subsequently confirmed Vaughn & Leff's findings in a group of 39 married depressives. A high EE score (defined as two or more critical comments during the Camberwell Family Interview) was associated with a high risk of relapse during the 9 month follow-up period and the effects of this adverse emotional climate were not mitigated, as they are in schizophrenia, by a reduction in the number of hours of contact per week.

Other aetiological factors

Childbirth is a major influence. Although only about one woman in 500 become psychotic after childbirth this represents a 20-fold increase in incidence (Kendell et al 1987). The majority of these illnesses are depressive or manic, albeit with some atypical features, and most start within 2 or 3 weeks of parturition. Women with a history of previous affective illnesses are particularly at risk. It is possible that childbirth acts as it does by virtue of being a particularly potent life event, but it is more likely that its influence is largely due to the associated endocrine and other metabolic changes. Milder depressive illnesses may also be particularly common in the early months after childbirth. Both phenomena are discussed in more detail in Chapter 26.

It has often been suggested that, because of its symbolic connotations of loss of femininity, *hysterectomy* is more likely than other surgical procedures to be followed by depression. Richards (1973) found that 36% of 200 women were treated for depression by their general practitioners at some stage in the first 3 years after operation, four times the rate of matched controls. The risk was higher in women with no significant pelvic pathology at operation, with a past history of depression and under the age of 40 years, but parity and oophorectomy had no influence. Barker (1968) found that psychiatric referral was much commoner in the 3 years after hysterectomy than after cholecystectomy and found the same relationships as Richards with previous psychiatric disorder and the absence of pelvic pathology. This suggests that the observed relationship is due, not to the effects of the operation, but rather to the liability of psychiatrically vulnerable women to have hysterectomies. A prospective study of 156 women with menorrhagia of benign origin confirms that this is the case (Gath et al 1982). The overall level of psychiatric symptomatology in these women was higher *before* hysterectomy than it was either 6 or 18 months after operation, and higher than that of general population controls on all three occasions.

Drugs of various kinds have often been blamed for causing depression. The list of suspects is a long one and includes reserpine and tetrabenazine, methyldopa and other hypotensive drugs, steroids, the contraceptive pill, L-dopa and neuroleptics, particularly intramuscular depot preparations. There is no doubt that the large doses of reserpine used as a tranquilliser in the 1950s were liable to provoke quite severe depressions. For most of the other drugs listed above, including the much lower doses of reserpine used in the treatment of hypertension, the evidence is much weaker, and consists of little more than a number of reports of depression developing in people taking the drug in question. This is unsatisfactory, particularly when one considers that in many cases the population concerned (young women on 'the pill', schizophrenics on phenothiazines, Parkinsonian patients on L-dopa) would be likely to have a relatively high incidence of depression anyway. A common symptom like depression can only be confidently attributed to a drug if there is a consistent temporal relationship between starting and stopping the drug and becoming depressed, or if depression is found in a random allocation drug trial to be commoner in one group than another. This has not been shown in any trial of a neuroleptic, oral or intramuscular, and the only placebo controlled trial of the contraceptive pill showed no excess of depressive symptoms in women receiving the active preparation. This does not mean, of course, that it may not sometimes be wise to change or withdraw the medication of someone who becomes depressed while taking one of these drugs.

Several *viral infections*, including influenza, infectious mononucleosis and hepatitis A, have a reputation for often being followed by depressive symptoms which may be severe and last for several weeks. The same is true of brucellosis. These postinfective depressions have rarely been systematically studied and their pathogenesis is obscure.

Over the years there have been several reports of a high incidence of *cancer*, usually of the lung or pancreas, developing in middle-aged people with pre-existing depressive illnesses, and on this basis it has been suggested that depression might be the presenting symptom of an initially occult neoplasm. Probably these are all chance relationships, for when the association between cancer and depression is examined within the framework of a record-linkage system no statistically significant relationship is found (Evans et al 1974).

Several *endocrine disorders*, including hypothyroidism, Cushing's syndrome and hypo- and hyperparathyroidism, are associated with depression, though all are capable of inducing other psychiatric disorders as well. The relationship is strongest in the case of Cushing's syndrome. Haskett (1985) described a consecutive series of 30 patients with Cushing's syndrome who were all rated using the SADS-L. All but five (i.e. 83%) met the RDC for some kind of affective disorder during the course of their endocrine disturbance even though only one had a family history of affective disorder. Two-thirds of the whole series met the RDC for endogenous depression and eight (27%) also met criteria for mania or hypomania. Why the endogenous overproduction of cortisol should usually be associated with depression when the therapeutic administration of steroids is more commonly associated with euphoria is unknown, but the symptom relief often provided by therapeutic steroids may be part of the explanation.

Finally, there is evidence that gross physical and psychological stresses, such as those to which political prisoners and prisoners of war are sometimes subjected, may be followed by a lifelong liability to anxiety states and depressive illnesses (e.g. Tennant et al 1986). *Sexual abuse in childhood* may well have similar consequences. Although its true prevalence is still unknown, clinical experience suggests that women who have been sexually abused as children are subsequently at increased risk of depression and bulimia as well as of specifically sexual difficulties. Bifulco et al (1991) recently found that 9% of 286 working class mothers in Islington in north London admitted to sexual abuse involving physical contact in childhood or adolescence, and no less than 64% of these women had an episode of depression during the 3 year study period. Unemployment is also associated with an increased prevalence of depressive symptoms (Melville et al

1985). A lowering of self-esteem may be the mediating variable in each of these situations.

COURSE AND OUTCOME OF MOOD DISORDERS

'The prognosis of manic-depressive insanity is favourable for the individual attack... On the other hand in every case... we must reckon with the possibility that the disease will be repeated several times or even very frequently.' This statement by Kraepelin, made in 1921 before any effective therapies were available, is still true, particularly of bipolar disorders.

Chronic mania was always uncommon and is now almost unknown. The duration of individual episodes of mania varies but is usually 1–3 months and rarely longer than 6 months. The risk of recurrence is high, particularly if the first episode occurs before the age of 30 years, which it does in over 60% of cases. Once someone has had a manic illness in adolescence or early adult life they are almost certain to have further illnesses, and in the long run some of these further illnesses are almost certain to be depressions.

Episodes of depression tend to last longer but are somewhat less likely to recur. Although the duration of individual episodes varies considerably it is generally between 3 and 8 months and, as with mania, many patients have repeated episodes which are all of very similar duration. Occasionally, even with energetic treatment with a variety of antidepressants and ECT, an episode of depression will last for 2 years or more. It is also quite common, particularly in the elderly, for the patient to be left with a residue of mild symptoms, not severe enough to be incapacitating but preventing them coping with the routine tasks of daily life, or enjoying its pleasures, as well as before.

Less is known about the long-term course of mood disorders than of schizophrenic illnesses, because fewer long-term follow-up studies have been carried out and because a much larger proportion of illnesses never result in hospital admission, or even come to medical attention. Lewinsohn et al (1989) obtained retrospective information from 1130 community respondents interviewed with the SADS who had fulfilled RDC for unipolar depression (major, minor or intermittent) at some time in their lives. The majority had never received treatment and 55% had only had a single episode. In the 45% who had had at least two episodes the mean interval between them was 15 years, and in the 33% who had had at least three episodes the mean interval between the second and third episodes was 10.5 years. Later episodes tended to be more severe and women tended to have more episodes with shorter intervals between them than men. However, people who were depressed at the time of interview were more likely to report previous depressions than those who were euthymic, and this highlights the major shortcoming of retrospective studies of this kind — the risk that the findings may be biased, and biased differently in men and women, or in the young and the old, by respondents' failure to remember or unwillingness to admit previous episodes. Prospective studies do not suffer from this problem but so far all have been based on hospital in-patients.

A 40-year follow-up of a large cohort of patients admitted to the Iowa Psychopathic Hospital in 1934–1945 provides useful information about the comparative outcome of different mood disorders, and of mood disorders and schizophrenia. Rather surprisingly, Tsuang et al (1979) found no difference in outcome between patients whose index illness had been manic and those in whom it had been depressive, but their only indices of outcome were four simple scales measuring marital, occupational, residential and psychiatric status at the time of follow-up and they made no attempt to study the course of the illness during the intervening years. Coryell & Tsuang (1985) subsequently demonstrated that when DSM-III criteria were applied, blind to family history and outcome data, to the same cohort, non-psychotic depressions had the best outcome on all four scales, followed by depressions with mood-congruent psychotic features and then by depressions with mood-incongruent psychotic features. All three groups of depressions had a better outcome than schizophreniform disorders, which in turn had a better outcome than schizophrenic illnesses.

Lee & Murray (1988) followed up a consecutive series of 89 in-patient depressives the writer had originally studied at the Maudsley Hospital in 1965–1966 (Kendell 1968), and succeeded in reinterviewing 94% of those still alive 18 years later. Although 61% had been first admissions the overall outcome was poor despite the availability, and frequent use, of tricyclic antidepressants and lithium throughout the follow-up period. Only 11 of 89 patients had a good outcome (i.e. no further admissions, no suicide attempts and good social functioning at follow-up) and 25 had a very poor outcome (suicide or other unnatural death, repeated episodes of illness and poor social functioning at follow-up). There was also a striking relationship between the symptomatology of the index illness and outcome, those with the most psychotic or endogenous symptoms having the worst outcome. A 15

year follow-up of 145 Australian patients (Kiloh et al 1988) produced rather similar findings. Although the overall prognosis was rather less gloomy, only 20% had no further episodes of depression and 9% committed suicide.

There is some evidence that the interval between one episode and the next gets progressively shorter as time goes on, in both unipolar and bipolar disorder (Angst et al 1973). Post has suggested that this is due to a mechanism analogous to kindling, i.e. that each episode of illness produces enduring cerebral changes which increase the likelihood of further episodes (Post et al 1984). Whether or not this is so, the risk of recurrence, and the duration and spacing of successive episodes, vary greatly from one patient to another, and in any given individual the best estimate of the future is provided by his own past history. Chronic illnesses and incomplete recoveries are more common in the elderly; and in bipolar patients manic episodes tend to become less frequent and depressive episodes more frequent with the passage of time. On the other hand it is not rare for mania to develop for the first time in the seventh or eighth decade. Brain disease may play a part in the genesis of such illnesses which have not been studied as closely as they deserve.

Some patients have a regular sequence of illnesses, of either uni- or bipolar type, their mood changing predictably every few days, weeks or months. Although they fascinate research workers they are very rare and the regular sequence does not usually last for more than a few years.

On average, affective disorders carry a considerably better prognosis than schizophrenia. It has been shown many times that patients with affective illnesses are more likely to make a full recovery from their original illness, spend less time in hospital both in the short and the long run, and experience less social deterioration than those with schizophrenia. (See, for example, the comparison by Coryell & Tsuang described above). However, these averages obscure considerable individual variation. Just as some schizophrenics make a full and lasting recovery, so some patients with affective disorders have their lives totally disrupted by illness and some become chronic invalids, either because their episodes of illness are too frequent and too long-lasting for them to re-establish themselves outside hospital in the intervals, or because they become chronically depressed.

The risk of suicide is high in both uni- and bipolar illness. The consensus of several studies suggests that the lifetime risk in Kraepelinian manic–depressive illness is at least 15% and that it is greatest in the early years of illness (Guze & Robins 1970). With milder depressions the risk is much less. Before the 1940s, mood disorders carried other risks as well. Patients with mania died of exhaustion after weeks of sustained overactivity and sleeplessness, and those with melancholia died of inanition or intercurrent infections after long months of severe retardation or agitation, with refusal to eat and progressive weight loss. Although there is evidence that this immediate mortality was greatly reduced by the introduction of ECT (Slater 1951) there is, as yet, little firm evidence that the long-term outlook of mood disorders has been improved by any of the therapeutic measures at our disposal. Despite the undoubted efficacy of ECT and tricyclic antidepressants in the acute treatment of depression there is little evidence that either treatment has reduced the suicide rate. And despite the proven ability of maintenance treatment with lithium or tricyclic antidepressants to reduce the risk of further episodes no-one has yet demonstrated a reduction in the incidence of non-first episodes of either depression or mania in any geographically defined population.

TREATMENT OF MOOD DISORDERS

Treatment of mania

Usually it is advisable to admit the patient to hospital, for the risks of attempting to treat even hypomania on an out-patient basis are considerable. Because he feels fine, and cannot be convinced that he is ill, the patient rarely takes medication regularly. He may also squander money he can ill afford, get himself into all manner of embarrassing situations which may jeopardise his job or his position in the community, and endanger himself and other people by reckless behaviour. Often, therefore, it is necessary to compel the patient to enter hospital whether he wants to or not. Relatives are sometimes unconvinced of the need for prompt admission if this is the first manic episode they have witnessed, but on subsequent occasions they usually need no persuasion.

There is considerable skill in the nursing of mania. The patient's boisterous overactivity, sudden whims and capacity for causing mayhem have to be restrained. An experienced nurse can often do this by distracting his energies into other and less dangerous channels, or by winning his cooperation by entering his mood of playful good humour. A less skilful nurse tries to forbid or physically restrain, which annoys the patient and easily provokes him to violence. Three different drugs are widely used in treatment — chlorpromazine, haloperidol and lithium — and because most of the clinical trials comparing them have involved compa-

ratively small numbers their relative merits are still uncertain. Johnson et al (1971) found no significant difference between lithium and chlorpromazine and Shopsin et al (1975) found no significant difference between lithium, chlorpromazine and haloperidol. Garfinkel et al (1980), on the other hand, found haloperidol significantly more effective than lithium in the treatment of severe mania.

Lithium acts in quite a different way from neuroleptics. Its side-effects are much less unpleasant and, if it works, it controls all the symptoms of the illness, including the racing thoughts, instead of simply sedating the patient and slowing him down. However, it takes several days to act, which is a serious disadvantage if the patient is aggressive and disruptive. If lithium is used in the acute episode it should be started quickly and in full dosage. In young adults with no history of renal disease there is no need to wait for the results of detailed tests of renal function. Indeed, those which involve collecting an accurate 12 or 24 hour urine are usually impracticable until the patient has become more cooperative. The serum level usually needs to be at least 1.0 mmol/l to control manic behaviour. The dose needed to sustain this serum level may produce some toxic effects but there is little risk involved when the patient is under constant observation and the serum level can be checked at any time.

Under steady state conditions the lithium concentration in erythrocytes is only about a third that in plasma because of an active lithium/sodium exchange across the erythrocyte membrane. The erythrocyte/plasma ratio is under genetic control and there are reports that it is abnormally high in bipolar patients, and also that the distribution of erythrocyte/plasma ratios in their first-degree relatives is bimodal, suggesting the presence of a genetically distinct subgroup (Dorus et al 1983).

Although lithium may be the best treatment for hypomania, and has the added advantage of minimising the risk of a swing into depression, its delayed action is a serious disadvantage, and in severe illnesses chlorpromazine (in doses up to 1000 mg/day) or haloperidol (in doses up to 40 mg/day) are preferable because they have a more immediate effect on overactivity. Although the matter has not been demonstrated by controlled trial, haloperidol and droperidol are widely believed to control motor overactivity more effectively than chlorpromazine, though this may be at the cost of severe extrapyramidal side-effects. A combination of lithium and haloperidol has obvious attractions in severe mania but there are two problems: there is no evidence that the combination is more effective than haloperidol alone (Garfinkel et al 1980);

and there are reports of patients developing an acute brain syndrome, followed in some cases by lasting extrapyramidal and cognitive deficits, on large doses of the two drugs together.

In the past mania was frequently, and effectively, treated with ECT (McCabe 1976). It is rarely employed nowadays but still has a role in patients with severe manic illnesses which do not respond, or not quickly enough, to medication and a recent random allocation trial has demonstrated that bilateral ECT given three times a week is more effective than lithium (Small et al 1988). Carbamazepine also has antimanic activity and may be useful in some patients.

As the patient's mood returns to normal and his overactivity abates he must still be kept under observation, for the risk of a relapse, or of a sudden swing into depression, are both considerable. The need for long-term lithium prophylaxis must also be considered (see below).

Treatment of depression

Depressive illnesses are common and the majority can be, and are, successfully treated by general practitioners. Depressions which are referred to psychiatrists tend to be those which are severe, chronic, recurrent or accompanied by a high risk of suicide.

Tricyclic antidepressants

The tricyclic and tetracyclic antidepressants are the mainstay of the treatment of depressive illness and their efficacy in the treatment of both 'endogenous' and 'reactive' illnesses has been demonstrated in numerous controlled trials. A bewildering variety of these drugs is available and their pharmacology and the broad principles governing their administration are described in Chapter 36. In the writer's view, amitriptyline is still the best drug for most patients. The evidence for its efficacy is strong, and although it has a number of troublesome side-effects and is dangerous in overdose it is free of the serious complications that have resulted in several more recently developed antidepressants having to be withdrawn. It is also cheap. It has often been demonstrated that a high proportion of out-patients do not take the antidepressants they are prescribed but this does not have to be so. If the doctor explains to the patient that they will not start to feel better until they have been taking their tablets for a fortnight or so, and warns them of the common side-effects, they will usually persevere, particularly if the doctor has also taken a sufficiently detailed history to convince the patient that he does understand their problems.

The normal adult dose of most tricyclic antidepressants is 150 mg/day, taken either as a single dose at bedtime or in two doses, say 100 mg at night and 50 mg in the morning. The elderly will usually only be able to tolerate half this amount and it is important to start with a maximum of 75 mg/day in everyone to minimise the impact of sedative and anticholinergic side-effects. Amitriptyline and several other antidepressants have pronounced sedative as well as antidepressant actions. In most patients these are valuable. Anxiety and tension are reduced and insomnia relieved, and as these actions are immediate the patient gets some benefit straight away, which helps persuade him to persevere. Some patients complain, however, that they feel drugged and in them a less sedative preparation like imipramine is preferable. Tetracyclic drugs like mianserin are valuable for patients who are likely to attempt to kill themselves, or who develop intolerable anticholinergic side-effects on amitriptyline or imipramine. They are also useful in patients with ischaemic heart disease, though it is important to realise that, provided the patient does not have a bundle branch block or other conduction defect, a history of myocardial infarction or heart failure is not in itself a reason for avoiding amitriptyline or other tricyclic drugs (Glassman & Bigger 1981, Veith et al 1982).

Because of their delayed action no patient under the age of 60 years should be deemed to have failed to respond to a tricyclic drug until they have taken 150 mg/day for at least 3 weeks. If there is no improvement within this time it is usually better to increase the dose still further (i.e. to 200 or 250 mg/day of amitriptyline) than to change to a different drug, unless side-effects have prevented an adequate dose being taken or poor compliance is suspected. This probably applies to the newer tetracyclic drugs as well, though at present there is little evidence either way. It is well known that the steady state plasma produced by a given dose of antidepressant varies considerably from one person to another, which suggests that estimating the plasma level would facilitate more rational and more effective prescribing. In fact, although plasma assays have been available for several years they have not come into widespread use, despite the fact that for at least one drug, nortriptyline, there is good evidence that both high and low plasma levels are associated with lower efficacy than a level between 50 and 150 ng/ml. An American Psychiatric Association Task Force concluded in 1985 that blood level estimations could be 'unequivocally useful in certain situations' for imipramine, desmethylimipramine and nortriptyline, but that for amitriptyline the relationship between plasma level and efficacy was still hopelessly confused.

Other physical treatments

Several drugs which inhibit the re-uptake of serotonin from the synaptic cleft without any significant effect on noradrenaline or dopamine have become available in the last few years. The available evidence suggests that these selective serotonin re-uptake inhibitors are all as effective as amitriptyline, do not have anticholinergic side-effects, do not stimulate appetite, and are comparatively safe in overdose. However, they are expensive and have troublesome side-effects of their own (nausea, vomiting and sometimes increased agitation). At present they are probably best reserved for patients at high risk of suicide, or who gain weight alarmingly on tricyclic drugs.

For tricyclic non-responders whose illnesses are 'reactive' or 'neurotic' in character the best alternative treatment is usually either an MAOI (see Chapter 36) or cognitive psychotherapy (see Chapter 41). For those with the characteristic symptoms of melancholia, ECT is more likely to be effective. At present there is no evidence that patients who fail to respond to a full dose of a tricyclic antidepressant are likely to respond to a selective serotonin re-uptake inhibitor, but patients who cannot tolerate a full dose may well do so.

There is a long tradition that the MAOIs are effective in patients with 'atypical' depressions, and although some investigators (e.g. Rowan et al 1982) have been unable to distinguish between the clinical characteristics of tricyclic and MAOI responders there is good evidence that phenelzine and other MAOIs are effective antidepressants in anxious or 'atypical' depressions (Robinson et al 1973, Quitkin et al 1991). Like the tricyclic drugs, however, they have to be given for several weeks and in adequate dosage. In the case of phenelzine this usually means 60–90 mg/day, or whatever dose is needed to provide 80–90 % inhibition of platelet MAO activity if the assay is available.

There is quite strong evidence that the amino acid L-tryptophan, given in a dose of about 3 g/day, is an effective antidepressant in relatively mild illnesses (Thomson et al 1982) and that it potentiates the antidepressant activity of MAOIs. At present, however, its use is restricted because of an outbreak of eosinophilia and myalgia, probably caused by some unidentified contaminant. Phenothiazines like thioridazine may also be useful in patients with severe agitation or widespread delusions. American claims that the triazolobenzodiazepine alprazolam is as effective as

amitriptyline have not been substantiated (Goldberg et al 1986).

The indications for ECT are discussed in detail in Chapter 37. In summary, a severe depressive illness with retardation, diurnal variation, or other typical melancholic features which has failed to respond to a tricyclic drug, or has generally failed to respond in previous episodes, is the commonest indication. Prominent depressive or paranoid delusions are another, for there is much evidence that deluded depressives respond poorly to tricyclic drugs (Hordern et al 1963, Glassman et al 1975). Refusal to eat or drink, or any situation in which rapid improvement is imperative, is a further indication, particularly in the elderly, as ECT acts more quickly than any drug (Medical Research Council 1965).

Psychological treatments

Although psychotherapies of various kinds have long been employed in the management of depressions there was until recently little evidence that any of them was effective. Now, however, there is good evidence that at least two well-defined forms of psychotherapy, Beck's cognitive behaviour therapy (see Ch. 41) and Klerman's interpersonal psychotherapy, are effective, though probably less so than the tricyclic drugs. The most convincing evidence is provided by a multicentre trial organised by NIMH (Elkin et al 1989). Two hundred and fifty out-patients with major depressive disorders were randomly allocated to one of four treatments for 16 weeks — imipramine in an average dose of 185 mg/day, cognitive behaviour therapy, interpersonal psychotherapy and imipramine placebo. Both psychotherapies involved one 50 minute session every week. At the end of treatment, outcome was best in the imipramine group and worst in the placebo group with the two psychotherapies in between. Overall, there were few significant differences between the four groups, partly because patients with mild depressions did well with all treatments, including placebo. For severe depressions, however, imipramine was by far the most effective treatment. There were no significant differences between the two psychotherapies but there were unexplained differences between centres, suggesting that the skills of individual therapists were important.

Although cognitive behaviour therapy is probably less effective than drug therapy, and also more expensive, and there is no evidence that the combination of the two is particularly efficacious (e.g. see Murphy et al 1984), there are suggestions from several trials that the relapse rate after cognitive therapy is lower than after drug treatment. If true this might well justify the additional time and expense involved, but so far no adequately designed trial has been carried out to determine whether this is really so.

There is little evidence that social casework increases the efficacy of the predominantly pharmacological treatment provided by general practitioners (Corney 1984).

General measures

Although antidepressant drugs and ECT are the mainstay of the treatment of severe depressions this does not mean that other measures can be ignored. The risk of suicide must never be forgotten. Although surveillance should be as unobtrusive as possible, people who are deeply depressed should not be left alone for long and everyone — doctor, nurse and relatives — must be alert to any hint that they are contemplating an attempt on their life. It is also important to try to boost patients' morale and lowered self-confidence and to reassure them firmly and repeatedly that they will eventually recover. Various forms of occupational therapy, formal and informal, can also be very useful, though it is important to recognise that some patients need undemanding companionship rather than enthusiastic 'therapy'.

Depressed patients often talk of resigning their jobs, selling their homes, or taking other major decisions which at the time seem sensible or even unavoidable. Even if the psychiatrist shares the patient's view that the job or financial problems in question played a part in precipitating the illness, it is usually a mistake to make irreversible decisions at a time when the subject's whole view of himself, his talents and his future is gravely distorted. Things often look very different after the depression has lifted and it is so difficult to predict the effect of recovery on the patient's outlook that it is best to try to persuade him not to make major decisions until he is well.

Hospital admission

Just as the majority of depressions are treated by general practitioners rather than being referred to psychiatrists, so the majority of patients treated by psychiatrists are treated as out-patients. The decision whether or not to admit the patient to hospital, or to try to persuade them to come into hospital, is largely governed by three considerations — the risk of suicide, the need for ECT, and whether or not the patient is still at work. The most important of these is the risk of suicide, and the patient should always be questioned about this. Merely having had thoughts about suicide, or having wished not to have to wake up in the morning, are not necessarily cause for alarm, for they are almost invariable in severe depressions. But if the patient is preoccupied with thoughts of suicide, planning how he might kill himself, or frightened that he might do so, he probably needs to be under observation in hospital. So too does anyone who is seriously depressed and living alone. Age, sex, previous suicidal attempts and alcohol intake are other important determinants of risk. Whether the patient is still at work is important partly as an indication of the severity of the illness and partly because anyone who is already unable to work has much less to lose by coming into hospital. And in the writer's view anyone who is ill enough to need ECT needs to be either an in-patient or a day patient.

'Resistant' depressions

The most appropriate treatment for patients with severe depressions which have failed to respond both to a tricyclic drug in full dosage and to ECT is very uncertain. Partly because such patients are uncommon, few adequately designed clinical trials have been carried out and our ignorance of how the many antidepressants available to us really work adds to our difficulties. Although controlled trials suggest that MAOIs are relatively ineffective in melancholia, occasional patients undoubtedly respond to an MAOI if it is given in sufficiently high dosage. If the drug is ineffective on its own its efficacy can be enhanced by the addition of tryptophan 3 g/day, or by combining it with lithium. There are also a number of reports of patients responding within days to the combination of lithium and a tricyclic drug when they had not responded to the tricyclic alone. Some psychiatrists are convinced that the combination of a tricyclic drug and an MAOI is peculiarly potent, while pharmacologists insist that the combination is dangerous. In fact there is little evidence that this combination is particularly potent, but it does seem to be safe to give the two drugs together provided they are started simultaneously and only given in moderate doses (Razani et al 1983).

Sometimes depressed patients respond rapidly to a second course of ECT a few months after failing to respond to an apparently identical regime. For this reason a second course is always worth considering after a gap of several months if two or three of the drug combinations referred to above have been tried without success. This is particularly true if the first course of ECT was unilateral.

Prophylactic treatment

Short-term

All affective illnesses are prone to recur and the risk is greatest in the early months after recovery. In patients with depressive illnesses which have responded to imipramine or amitriptyline there is good evidence from controlled trials that remaining on the antidepressant for a further 6 months considerably reduces the relapse rate during that time (Mindham et al 1973, Klerman et al 1974). For this reason all recovered depressives should be kept on whichever drug they responded to, including MAOIs, for several months after recovery. For the same reason patients who have responded to ECT should be given a maintenance dose of a tricyclic antidepressant for 6 months or so. In the past it was customary to use a relatively low dose (e.g. amitriptyline 75–100 mg/day) during this maintenance period. Recent evidence suggests, however, that higher doses are more effective (Frank et al 1990), so it is probably advisable to keep most patients on their original therapeutic dose if this does not produce troublesome side-effects.

The risk of relapse is highest in those whose recovery was incomplete and Prien & Kupfer (1986) have produced evidence suggesting that maintenance treatment needs to be continued for 4 months, but no longer, after *full* recovery. Changing to placebo before then was associated with a considerably increased risk of relapse, but beyond 4 months the relapse rates on drug and placebo were the same.

Long-term

In patients who have already had more than one episode of illness, particularly those who have had several episodes within a few years, there is evidence from a number of controlled trials that long-term maintenance treatment reduces the risk of relapse both in bipolar and unipolar disorders. In bipolar illness maintenance on lithium is effective but maintenance on a tricyclic antidepressant is not, mainly because of the continuing and possibly increased risk of manic episodes (Baastrup et al 1970, Prien et al 1984). In unipolar illness a large multicentre British trial found lithium and amitriptyline to be equally effective (Medical Research Council Drug Trials Subcommittee 1981); a similar American trial under the aegis of the NIMH found imipramine to be more effective than lithium and a combination of the two to be only marginally more effective than imipramine alone (Prien et al 1984).

A more recent trial in Pittsburgh, based on patients who had had at least three episodes of major depression in the previous $2\frac{1}{2}$ years, compared the prophylactic effects of psychotherapy with those of medication over 3 years (Frank et al 1990). Patients received either maintenance imipramine in an average dose of 200 mg/day, or a monthly session of interpersonal psychotherapy, or both. In this dose imipramine was highly effective in preventing relapse. Interpersonal psychotherapy was associated with a significantly lower relapse rate than placebo but did not add significantly to imipramine alone. The overall pattern, therefore, was rather similar to that obtained for the immediate treatment of depression (Elkin et al 1989).

Despite the strength of the evidence it is not a straightforward decision to put someone with a recurrent mood disorder on long-term prophylactic medication. If the patient has had, say, three incapacitating illnesses in the last 2 years the decision is clear enough because the risk of further episodes in the next year or two is obviously high. But what of the patient who has had three depressive illnesses at intervals of 5–10 years, or a single manic illness? Obviously the patient's willingness to remain on long-term medication, and one's own estimate of the likelihood of their persevering conscientiously for years on end, are important considerations. As a general rule it is only sensible to try to persuade a patient to take long-term medication if the pattern of their previous illnesses suggests that they are likely to have another incapacitating illness within the next 2 or 3 years. In an adolescent or young adult, however, the risk of recurrence is so high that it may be sensible to try to persuade them to take prophylactic lithium even after a single manic illness. In theory, prophylactic medication, once started, is for life, and Schou's patients certainly relapsed alarmingly quickly when they were transferred to placebo after several years on lithium (Baastrup et al 1970). In practice, most patients want to try stopping sooner or later. As the memory of their previous illnesses fades they become increasingly confident of remaining well and the proportion of patients who remain on prophylactic medication for longer than 5 years in the absence of any relapse is small.

Is there any point in keeping a patient on lithium or a tricyclic antidepressant if they have already relapsed once despite this medication? At present there is no clear answer to this important question, partly because in most clinical trials patients were excluded as soon as they had had their first relapse. The fact that a patient relapses while on prophylactic medication does not prove that the drug is ineffective; without it the relapse might have come sooner, or been more severe. In practice the best policy is probably to persevere with the drug until it is clear that the frequency and severity of episodes are both as bad as they were beforehand.

Even in bipolar patients the efficacy of prophylactic lithium is limited. It does not abolish mood swings so much as damp them down to the point at which they are no longer incapacitating. Nor is it very effective at preventing overt illness. In the NIMH collaborative trial only a third of the patients on lithium remained well throughout the 2 years (Prien et al 1984). In general, prophylactic lithium is least effective in 'rapid cyclers', i.e. patients who have very frequent and short-lived episodes. Conversely, its beneficial effects are often most convincing in those whose mood was previously unstable from day to day and week to week. Indeed, some people refuse to take lithium because it abolishes the 'highs' which they enjoy and look forward to, or in some cases which they feel they need for creative work.

Because the gastric absorption and renal excretion of lithium are both fairly rapid the serum level is constantly rising and falling, and may be altered by changes in water and sodium intake as well as by missed doses. And, of course, an inadequate dose may not lead to relapse for months or years. For these reasons it is difficult to determine what serum level is needed for optimal prophylactic effect and all statements about the 'therapeutic range' have a rather fragile empirical basis. In the 1970s it was usually assumed that the therapeutic range was 0.8–1.2 mmol/l (measured 10–12 hours after the last dose) but the target range was subsequently lowered because of anxieties about renal damage. There is some evidence that a serum level as low as 0.4 mmol/l may be adequate in many patients (Hullin 1980) and in view of the side-effects and possible long-term risks (see Ch. 36) it is probably best to aim for between 0.6 and 1.0 mmol/l. If the patient

relapses at this level the dose can always be raised subsequently. A single daily dose of lithium produces less polyuria and other renal effects than divided doses, despite the temporarily higher serum level it involves (Plenge et al 1982). For this reason lithium is best taken as a single night-time dose. There is no advantage in using so-called delayed absorption preparations.

The dose of tricyclic antidepressant needed for successful long-term prophylaxis is also uncertain. The clinical trials referred to above both used a dose close to the therapeutic dose; in Prien's trial the average dose of imipramine was 125 mg/day but in the more recent Pittsburgh trial (Frank et al 1990) it was 200 mg/day and the relapse rate was lower. In practice, of course, patients will not tolerate troublesome side-effects for long when they are well, so in effect the prophylactic dose is often determined by them.

The management of patients who continue to have frequent episodes of illness despite long-term lithium or amitriptyline is extremely difficult. In unipolar patients it is always worth trying both drugs together despite the lack of objective evidence for the efficacy of the combination. In bipolar patients carbamazepine is always worth a trial, either alone or in combination with lithium. There have been several reports in recent years that carbamazepine and other anticonvulsants like sodium valproate have both antimanic and antidepressant properties, and that they prevent further episodes in some patients who have not responded to lithium. Although no adequate clinical trial has yet been published there are indications that the prophylactic efficacy of carbamazepine in bipolar illness is comparable to that of lithium (e.g. see Lusznat et al 1988). Depot phenothiazines are also worth a trial in patients with recurrent mania despite the lack of formal evidence that they are effective.

REFERENCES

Abou-Saleh M T, Coppen A 1984 Classification of depressive illnesses: clinico-psychological correlates. Journal of Affective Disorders 6: 53–66

Abraham K 1924 Neue Arbeiten zur ärzlichen Psychoanalyse. In: Selected papers of Karl Abraham (1927). London

Akiskal H S 1983 Dysthymic disorder: psychopathology of proposed chronic depressive subtypes. American Journal of Psychiatry 140: 11–20

Akiskal H S, Lemmi H, Yerevanian B et al 1982 The utility of the REM latency test in psychiatric diagnosis: a study of 81 depressed outpatients. Psychiatry Research 7: 101–110

American Psychiatric Association Task Force 1985 Tricyclic antidepressants — blood level measurements and clinical outcome: an APA task force report. American Journal of Psychiatry 142: 155–162

Amsterdam J D, Martinelli D L, Arger P, Winokur A 1987 Assessment of adrenal gland volume by computed tomography in depressed patients and healthy volunteers: a pilot study. Psychiatry Research 21: 189–197.

Andreasen N C, Scheftner W, Reich T et al 1986 The validation of the concept of endogenous depression: a family study approach. Archives of General Psychiatry 43: 246–251

Angst J 1966 Zur Atiologie und Nosologie endogener depressiver Psychosen. In: Monographen aus der Neurologie und Psychiatrie 112. Springer-Verlag, Berlin

Angst J, Dobler-Mikola A 1984 The Zurich study III. Diagnosis of depression. European Archives of Psychiatry and Neurological Sciences 234: 30–37

Angst J, Baastrup P, Grof P, Hippius H, Pöldinger W, Weis P 1973 The course of monopolar depression and bipolar psychoses. Psychiatria Neurologia Neurochirurgia 76: 489–500

Angst J, Merikangas K, Scheidegger P, Wicki W 1990 Recurrent brief depression: a new subtype of affective disorder. Journal of Affective Disorders 19: 87–98

Ashcroft G W, Crawford T B B, Eccleston D 1966 5-Hydroxyindole compounds in the cerebrospinal fluid of patients with psychiatric or neurological diseases. Lancet ii: 1049–1050

Baastrup P C, Poulson J C, Schou M, Thomsen K, Amidsen A 1970 Prophylactic lithium: double-blind discontinuation in manic–depressive and recurrent depressive disorders. Lancet ii: 326–330

Barker M G 1968 Psychiatric illness after hysterectomy. British Medical Journal ii: 91–95

Bebbington P E, Brugha T, MacCarthy B et al 1988 The Camberwell depression study. British Journal of Psychiatry 152: 754–765, 766–774, 775–782

Berger M, Pirke K M, Doerr P, Krieg J C, von Zerssen D 1984 The limited utility of the dexamethasone suppression test for the diagnostic process in psychiatry. British Journal of Psychiatry 145: 372–382

Bertelsen A, Harvald B, Hauge M 1977 A Danish twin study of manic–depressive disorders. British Journal of Psychiatry 130: 330–351

Bifulco A, Brown G W, Adler Z 1991 Early sexual abuse and clinical depression in adult life. British Journal of Psychiatry 159: 115–122

Birtchnell J 1970 Depression in relation to early and recent parent death. British Journal of Psychiatry 116: 299–306

Blazer D, George L K, Landerman R et al 1985 Psychiatric disorders: a rural/urban comparison. Archives of General Psychiatry 42: 651–656.

Bowman K, Rose M 1951 A criticism of the terms "psychosis", "psychoneurosis" and "neurosis". American Journal of Psychiatry 108: 161–166.

Brown G W, Harris T 1978 Social origins of depression. Tavistock, London.

Brown G W, Andrews B, Harris T, Adler Z, Bridge L 1986 Social support, self esteem and depression. Psychological Medicine 16: 813–831

Buchsbaum M S, Wu J, DeLisi L E et al 1986 Frontal cortex and basal ganglia metabolic rates assessed by positron emission tomography with ^{18}F 2–deoxyglucose in affective illness. Journal of Affective Disorders 10: 137–152

Campbell E A, Cope S J, Teasdale J D 1983 Social factors and affective disorder: an investigation of Brown and Harris's model. British Journal of Psychiatry 143: 548–553

Carney M W P, Roth M, Garside R F 1965 The diagnosis of depressive syndromes and the prediction of ECT response. British Journal of Psychiatry 111: 659–674

Carroll B J, Feinberg M, Greden J F et al 1981 A specific laboratory test for the diagnosis of melancholia. Archives of General Psychiatry 38: 15–22

Checkley S A, Slade A P, Shur E 1981 Growth hormone and other responses to clonidine in patients with endogenous depression. British Journal of Psychiatry 138: 51–55

Clayton P J, Collins E J 1981 The significance of secondary depression. Journal of Affective Disorders 3: 25–35

Coppen A 1967 The biochemistry of affective disorders. British Journal of Psychiatry 113: 1237–1264

Corney R H 1984 The effectiveness of attached social workers in the management of depressed female patients in general practice. Psychological Medicine Suppl 6

Coryell W, Tsuang M T 1985 Major depression with mood-congruent or mood-incongruent psychotic features: outcome after 40 years. American Journal of Psychiatry 142: 479–482

Costello C G 1982 Social factors associated with depression: a retrospective community study. Psychological Medicine 12: 329–339

Delgado P L, Charney D S, Price L H, Aghajanian G K, Landis H, Heninger G R 1990 Serotonin function and the mechanism of antidepressant action. Archives of General Psychiatry 47: 411–418

Dennehy C M 1966 Childhood bereavement and psychiatric illness. British Journal of Psychiatry 112: 1049–1069

Dolan R J, Calloway S P, Mann A H 1985 Cerebral ventricular size in depressed subjects. Psychological Medicine 15: 873–878

Doran A R, Rubinow D R, Roy A, Pickar D 1986 CSF somatostatin and abnormal response to dexamethasone administration in schizophrenic and depressed patients. Archives of General Psychiatry 43: 365–369

Dorus E, Cox N J, Gibbons R D et al 1983 Lithium ion transport and affective disorders within families of bipolar patients. Archives of General Psychiatry 40: 545–552

Elkin I, Shea T, Watkins J T et al 1989 National Institute of Mental Health treatment of depression collaborative research program. Archives of General Psychiatry 46: 971–982

Englund S A, Klein D A 1990 The genetics of neurotic-reactive depression: a reanalysis of Shapiro's (1970) twin study using diagnostic criteria. Journal of Affective Disorders 18: 247–252

Evans N J R, Baldwin J A, Gath D 1974 The incidence of cancer among in-patients with affective disorders. British Journal of Psychiatry 124: 518–525

Frank E, Kupfer D J, Perel J M et al 1990 Three-year outcomes for maintenance therapies in recurrent depression. Archives of General Psychiatry 47: 1093–1099

Freud S 1917 Trauer und Melancholie. In: Standard edition of the complete psychological works of Sigmund Freud (1957), vol 14. Hogarth Press, London, p 243

Garattini S, Samanin R 1988 Biochemical hypotheses on antidepressant drugs: a guide for clinicians or a toy for pharmacologists? Psychological Medicine 18: 287–304

Garfinkel P E, Stancer H C, Persad E 1980 A comparison of haloperidol, lithium carbonate and their combination in the treatment of mania. Journal of Affective Disorders 2: 279–288

Gath D, Cooper P, Day A 1982 Levels of psychiatric morbidity before and after hysterectomy. British Journal of Psychiatry 140: 335–342

Gershon E S, Jonas W Z 1975 Erythrocyte soluble catechol-o-methyl transferase activity in primary affective disorder: a clinical and genetic study. Archives of General Psychiatry 32: 1351–1356

Glassman A H, Bigger J 1981 Cardiovascular effects of therapeutic doses of tricyclic antidepressants. Archives of General Psychiatry 38: 815–820

Glassman A H, Kantor S J, Shostak M 1975 Depression, delusions and drug response. American Journal of Psychiatry 132: 716–719

Goldberg S C, Ettigi P, Schulz P M, Hamer R M, Hayes P E, Friedel R O 1986 Alprazolam versus imipramine in depressed out-patients with neurovegetative signs. Journal of Affective Disorders 11: 139–145

Goodwin F K, Potter W Z 1979 In: Usdin E, Kopin I J,

Barchas J (eds) Catecholamines: basic and clinical frontiers, vol 2. Pergamon Press, New York, pp 1863–1865

Gregory I 1966 Retrospective data concerning childhood loss of a parent: category of parental loss by decade of birth, diagnosis and MMPI. Archives of General Psychiatry 15: 362–367

Gurney C, Roth M, Garside R F, Kerr T A, Shapira K 1972 Studies in the classification of affective disorders: the relationship between anxiety states and depressive illnesses. British Journal of Psychiatry 121: 162–166

Guze S B, Robins E 1970 Suicide and primary affective disorders. British Journal of Psychiatry 117: 437–438

Hagnell J, Lanke J, Rorsman B, Öjesjö L 1982 Are we entering an age of melancholy? Depressive illness in a prospective epidemiological study over 25 years: the Lundby study, Sweden. Psychological Medicine 12: 279–289

Hallstrom T 1986 Social origins of major depression: the role of provoking agents and vulnerability factors. Acta Psychiatrica Scandinavica 73: 383–389

Harris T, Brown G W, Bifulco A 1986 Loss of parent in childhood and adult psychiatric disorder: the role of lack of adequate parental care. Psychological Medicine 16: 641–659

Haskett R F 1985 Diagnostic categorization of psychiatric disturbance in Cushing's syndrome. American Journal of Psychiatry 142: 911–916

Healy D, Theodorou A E, Whitehouse A M et al 1990 ^{3}H Imipramine binding to previously frozen platelet membranes from depressed patients, before and after treatment. British Journal of Psychiatry 157: 208–215

Henderson S, Byrne D G, Duncan-Jones P 1981 Neurosis and the social environment. Academic Press, Sydney

Hirschfeld R M A, Klerman G L, Keller M B, Andreasen N C, Clayton P J 1986 Personality of recovered patients with bipolar affective disorder. Journal of Affective Disorders 11: 81–89

Hooley J M, Orley J, Teasdale J D 1986 Levels of expressed emotion and relapse in depressed patients. British Journal of Psychiatry 148: 642–647

Hordern A, Holt N F, Burt C G, Gordon W F 1963 Amitriptyline in depressive states: phenomenology and prognostic considerations. British Journal of Psychiatry 109: 815–825

Hullin R P 1980 In: Johnson F N (ed) Handbook of lithium therapy. Medical and Technical Publishing, Lancaster, p 243

Jablensky A, Sartorius N, Gulbinat W, Ernberg G 1981 Characteristics of depressive patients contacting psychiatric services in four cultures. Acta Psychiatrica Scandinavica 63: 367–383

Jenkins R 1985 Sex differences in minor psychiatric morbidity. Psychological Medicine suppl 7

Johnson G, Gershon S, Burdock E I, Floyd A, Hekimian L 1971 Comparative effects of lithium and chlorpromazine in the treatment of acute manic states. British Journal of Psychiatry 119: 267–276

Joyce P R, Oakley-Browne M A, Wells J E, Bushnell J A, Hornblow A R 1990 Birth cohort trends in major depression: increasing rates and earlier onset in New Zealand. Journal of Affective Disorders 18: 83–89

Kafka M S, Paul S M 1986 Platelet α_2 adrenergic receptors in depression. Archives of General Psychiatry 43: 91–95

Kendell R E 1968 The classification of depressive illnesses.

Maudsley monograph 18. Oxford University Press, London

Kendell R E 1976 The classification of depressions: a review of contemporary confusion. British Journal of Psychiatry 129: 15–28

Kendell R E, Chalmers J C, Platz C 1987 Epidemiology of puerperal psychoses. British Journal of Psychiatry 150: 662–673

Kendler K S 1991 Mood-incongruent psychotic affective illness. Archives of General Psychiatry 48: 362–369

Kiloh L G, Andrews G, Neilson M 1988 The long-term outcome of depressive illness. British Journal of Psychiatry 153: 752–757

Klerman G L, Dimascio A, Weissman M, Prusoff B, Paykel E S 1974 Treatment of depression by drugs and psychotherapy. American Journal of Psychiatry 131: 186–191

Klerman G L, Lavori P W, Rice J et al 1985 Birth-cohort trends in rates of major depressive disorder among relatives of patients with affective disorder. Archives of General Psychiatry 42: 689–693

Kocsis J H, Davis J M, Katz M M et al 1985 Depressive behavior and hyperactive adrenocortical function. American Journal of Psychiatry 142: 1291–1298

Kraepelin E 1896 Psychiatrie, ein Lehrbuch für Studierende und Ärzte, 5th edn. Barth, Leipzig

Kraepelin E 1921 Manic–depressive insanity and paranoia. Translation of Psychiatrie, ein Lehrbuch für Studierende und Ärzte, 8th edn. by Barclay R M. Livingstone, Edinburgh

Krishnan K R R, Doraiswamy P M, Lurie S N et al 1991 Pituitary size in depression. Journal of Clinical Endocrinology and Metabolism 72: 256–259

Kupfer D J, Foster F G 1978 EEG sleep and depression. In: Williams R L, Karacan I, Frazier S H (eds) Sleep disorders, diagnosis and treatment. Wiley, New York, pp 163–204

Lee A S, Murray R M 1988 The longterm outcome of Maudsley depressives. British Journal of Psychiatry 153: 741–751

Lewinsohn P M, Zeiss A M, Duncan E M 1989 Probability of relapse after recovery from an episode of depression. Journal of Abnormal Psychology 98: 107–116

Lewis A J 1934 Melancholia: a clinical survey of depressive states. Journal of Mental Science 80: 277–378

Lewy A J, Wehr T A, Goodwin F K, Newsome D A, Rosenthal N E 1981 Manic-depressive patients may be supersensitive to light. Lancet i: 383–384

Loosen P T, Prange A J 1982 Serum thyrotropin response to thyrotropin-releasing hormone in psychiatric patients: a review. American Journal of Psychiatry 139: 405–416

Lusznat R M, Murphy D P, Nunn C M H 1988 Carbamazepine vs lithium in the treatment and prophylaxis of mania. British Journal of Psychiatry 153: 198–204

McCabe M S 1976 ECT in the treatment of mania: a controlled study. American Journal of Psychiatry 133: 688–691

Medical Research Council 1965 Clinical trial of the treatment of depressive illness. British Medical Journal i: 881–886

Medical Research Council Drug Trials Subcommittee 1981 Continuation therapy with lithium and amitriptyline in unipolar depressive illness: a controlled clinical trial. Psychological Medicine 11: 409–416

Melville D I, Hope D, Bennison D, Barraclough B 1985 Depression among men made involuntarily redundant. Psychological Medicine 15: 789–793

Miller P McC, Ingham J G 1976 Friends, confidants and symptoms. Social Psychiatry 11: 51–58

Mindham R H S, Howland C, Shepherd M 1973 An evaluation of continuation therapy with tricyclic antidepressants in depressive illness. Psychological Medicine 3: 5–17

Mitchell P B, Bearn J A, Corn T H, Checkley S A 1988 Growth hormone response to clonidine after recovery in patients with endogenous depression. British Journal of Psychiatry 152: 34–38

Mullen P E, Linsell C R, Parker D 1986 Influence of sleep disruption and calorie restriction on biological markers for depression. Lancet ii: 1051–1054

Murphy G E, Simons A D, Wetzel R D, Lustman P J 1984 Cognitive therapy and pharmacotherapy. Archives of General Psychiatry 41: 33–41

Naylor G J, Smith A H W 1981 Defective genetic control of sodium-pump density in manic depressive psychosis. Psychological Medicine 11: 257–263

Nemeroff C B, Bissett G, Akil H, Fink M 1991 Neuropeptide concentrations in the cerebrospinal fluid of depressed patients treated with electroconvulsive therapy. British Journal of Psychiatry 158: 59–63

Ni Bhrolcháin M, Brown G W, Harris T O 1979 Psychotic and neurotic depression: clinical characteristics. British Journal of Psychiatry 134: 94–107

Parker G, Kiloh L, Hayward L 1987 Parental representations of neurotic and endogenous depressives. Journal of Affective Disorders 13: 75–82

Paykel E S 1974 Recent life events and clinical depression. In: Gunderson E K E, Rahe R H (eds) Life stress and illness. Charles C Thomas, Springfield, pp 134–163

Paykel E S, Myers J K, Dienelt M N et al 1969 Life events and depression: a controlled study. Archives of General Psychiatry 21: 753–760

Paykel E S, Klerman G L, Prusoff B A 1976 Personality and symptom pattern in depression. British Journal of Psychiatry 129: 327–334

Perris C 1966 A study of bipolar (manic–depressive) and unipolar recurrent depressive psychoses. Acta Psychiatrica Scandinavica suppl 194

Pfohl B, Sherman B, Schlechte J, Stone R 1985 Pituitary–adrenal axis rhythm disturbances in psychiatric depression. Archives of General Psychiatry 42: 897–903

Plantes M M, Prusoff B A, Brennan J, Parker G 1988 Parental representations of depressed outpatients from a USA sample. Journal of Affective Disorders 15: 149–155

Plenge P, Mellerup E T, Bolwig T G et al 1982 Lithium treatment: does the kidney prefer one daily dose instead of two? Acta Psychiatrica Scandinavica 66: 121–128

Post R M, Rubinow D R, Ballenger J C 1984 Conditioning, sensitization and kindling: implications for the course of affective illness. In: Post R M, Ballenger J C (eds) Neurobiology of mood disorders, vol 1. Williams & Wilkins, Baltimore, pp 432–466

Prange A J, Wilson L C, Breese G R et al 1976 Hormonal alteration of imipramine response. In: Sachar E J (ed) Hormones, behaviour and psychopathology. Raven Press, New York, pp 41–67

Prien R F, Kupfer D J 1986 Continuation drug therapy for major depressive episodes: how long should it be maintained. American Journal of Psychiatry 143: 18–23

Prien R F, Kupfer D J, Mansky P A et al 1984 Drug therapy in the prevention of recurrences in unipolar and bipolar affective disorders. Archives of General Psychiatry 41: 1096–1104

Prince R 1968 The changing picture of depressive syndromes in Africa. Canadian Journal of African Studies 1: 177–192

Quitkin F M, Harrison W, Stewart J W et al 1991 Response to phenelzine and imipramine in placebo nonresponders with atypical depression. Archives of General Psychiatry 48: 319–323

Razani J, White K L, White J et al 1983 The safety and efficacy of combined amitriptyline and tranylcypromine antidepressant treatment. Archives of General Psychiatry 40: 657–661

Richards D H 1973 Depression after hysterectomy. Lancet ii: 430–433

Robins L N, Helzer J E, Weissman M M et al 1984 Lifetime prevalence of specific psychiatric disorders in three sites. Archives of General Psychiatry 41: 949–958

Robinson D S, Nies A, Ravaris C L, Lamborn K R 1973 The monoamine oxidase inhibitor phenelzine in the treatment of depressive-anxiety states. Archives of General Psychiatry 29: 407–413

Rosenthal M E, Sack D A, Carpenter C J et al 1985 Antidepressant effects of light in seasonal affective disorder. American Journal of Psychiatry 142: 163–170

Rowan P R, Paykel E S, Parker R R 1982 Phenelzine and amitriptyline: effects on symptoms of neurotic depression. British Journal of Psychiatry 140: 475–483

Roy A 1985 Early parental separation and adult depression. Archives of General Psychiatry 42: 987–991

Sachar E J, Asnis G, Nathan R S et al 1980 Dextroamphetamine and cortisol in depression. Archives of General Psychiatry 37: 755–757

Schildkraut J J 1965 The catecholamine hypothesis of affective disorders: a review of supporting evidence. American Journal of Psychiatry 122: 509–522

Schlesser M A, Winokur G, Sherman B M 1980 Hypothalamic–pituitary–adrenal axis activity in depressive illness. Archives of General Psychiatry 37: 737–743

Sclare P, Creed F 1990 Life events and the onset of mania. British Journal of Psychiatry 156: 508–514

Shopsin B, Gershon S, Thompson H, Collins P 1975 Psychoactive drugs in mania: a controlled comparison of lithium carbonate, chlorpromazine and haloperidol. Archives of General Psychiatry 32: 34–42

Slater E T O 1951 Evaluation of electric convulsion therapy as compared with conservation methods of treatment in depressive states. Journal of Mental Science 97: 567–569

Small J G, Klapper M H, Kellam J J et al 1988 Electroconvulsive treatment compared with lithium in the management of manic states. Archives of General Psychiatry 45: 727–732

Surtees P G, Miller P McC, Ingham J G, Kreitman N B, Rennie D, Sashidharan S P 1986 Life events and the onset of affective disorder: a longitudinal general population study. Journal of Affective Disorders 10: 37–50

Surtees P G, Sashidharan S P 1986 Psychiatric morbidity in two matched community samples: a comparison of rates and risks in Edinburgh and St Louis. Journal of Affective Disorders 10: 101–113

Tennant C, Bebbington P 1978 The social causation of depression: a critique of the work of Brown and his colleagues. Psychological Medicine 8: 565–575

Tennant C, Goulston K, Dent O 1986 Clinical psychiatric illness in prisoners of war of the Japanese: forty years after release. Psychological Medicine 16: 833–839

Thompson C, Isaacs G 1988 Seasonal affective disorder — a British sample. Journal of Affective Disorders 14: 1–11

Thomson J, Rankin H, Ashcroft G W et al 1982 The treatment of depression in general practice: a comparison of L-tryptophan, amitriptyline and a combination of L-tryptophan and amitriptyline with placebo. Psychological Medicine 12: 741–751

Träskman L, Åsberg M, Bertilsson L, Sjöstrand L 1981 Monoamine metabolites in CSF and suicidal behavior. Archives of General Psychiatry 38: 631–636

Tsuang M T, Woolson R F, Fleming J A 1979 Long-term outcome of major psychoses. Archives of General Psychiatry 36: 1295–1301

van Praag H M 1977 Significance of biochemical parameters in the diagnosis, treatment and prevention of depressive disorders. Biological Psychiatry 12: 101–131

van Praag H M, Korf J, Puite J 1970 5 Hydroxyindoleacetic acid levels in the cerebrospinal fluid of depressive patients treated with probenecid. Nature 225: 1259–1260

Vaughn C E, Leff J P 1976 Influence of family and social factors on the course of psychiatric illness. British Journal of Psychiatry 129: 125–137

Veith R C, Raskind M A, Caldwell J H et al 1982 Cardiovascular effects of tricyclic antidepressants in depressed patients with chronic heart disease. New England Journal of Medicine 306: 954–959

Weissman M M, Klerman G L 1977 Sex differences in the epidemiology of depression. Archives of General Psychiatry 34: 98–111

Weissman M M, Leaf P J, Tischler G L et al 1988 Affective disorders in five United States communities. Psychological Medicine 18: 141–153

Whalley L J, Christie J E, Bennie J et al 1985 Selective increase in plasma luteinising hormone concentrations in drug free young men with mania. British Medical Journal 290: 99–102

Winokur G, Black D W, Nasrallah A 1988 Depressions secondary to other psychiatric disorders and medical illnesses. American Journal of Psychiatry 145: 233–237

Wood A J, Smith C E, Clarke E E, Cowen P J, Aronson J K, Grahame-Smith D G 1991 Altered in vitro adaptive responses of lymphocyte Na+, K+ ATPase in patients with manic depressive psychosis. Journal of Affective Disorders 21: 199–206

Wright A F, Crichton D N, Loudon J B, Morten J E N, Steel C M 1984 Adrenoceptor binding defects in cell lines from families with manic depressive disorder. Annals of Human Genetics 48: 201–214

Young M A, Scheftner W A, Klerman G L, Andreasen N C, Hirschfeld R M A 1986 The endogenous sub-type of depression: a study of its internal construct validity. British Journal of Psychiatry 148: 257–267

Young M A, Fogg L F, Scheftner W A, Fawcett J A 1990 Concordance of symptoms in recurrent depressive episodes. Journal of Affective Disorders 20: 79–85

Zimmerman M, Coryell W, Pfohl B, Stangl D 1987 An American validation study of the Newcastle diagnostic scale. British Journal of Psychiatry 150: 526–532

20. Paranoid and other psychoses

R. E. Kendell

Since the early years of this century most patients with psychotic illnesses which were not accompanied by overt brain pathology have been regarded as suffering either from schizophrenia or from an affective psychosis. But a proportion, varying greatly from country to country, have been regarded as suffering from other unrelated psychoses of very varied kinds. In Britain, and also in the USA before the introduction of DSM-III, such patients were few. Although terms like paranoia and paraphrenia were described in textbooks they were rarely used in practice. For most practical purposes psychoses that were not organic were either schizophrenic or affective and no other possibility was considered. Since the 1970s the situation has been changed a little by the increasing recognition of, and interest in, patients exhibiting a mixture of schizophrenic and affective symptoms, but these are still designated as 'schizoaffective' and regarded either as interforms between, or as a mixture of, the major syndromes. In other parts of the world, however, the situation has been, and to some extent still is, very different.

In Scandinavian countries up to a third of all psychotic illnesses used to be regarded as 'reactive' or 'psychogenic' psychoses, and therefore fundamentally different from the 'endogenous' disorders schizophrenia and manic–depressive illness. In France many acute psychoses were designated as *bouffées délirantes* and many chronic paranoid illnesses as chronic hallucinatory psychoses, both of which were regarded as diagnostic entities quite unrelated to either of Kraepelin's concepts. And in many African and Asian countries there is general agreement that the florid psychoses of good prognosis that are so conspicuous a feature of psychiatric practice in the third world are different from both schizophrenic and affective psychoses. Broadly speaking, two types of illness are excluded from the affective and schizophrenic rubrics. The first consists of acute psychoses which often develop in response to stress and have a good prognosis but a tendency to recur. The second consists of chronic paranoid illnesses which usually start insidiously in middle age but do not develop the progressive personality deterioration of dementia praecox. Both groups have been designated by a variety of different labels, and until recently the German, French, Scandinavian and Anglo-American schools retained their own terminologies and pursued their separate traditions quite independently of one another. As a result we do not know to what extent, for example, the French term *bouffée délirante*, the Scandinavian term psychogenic psychosis, the Anglo-American term schizoaffective illness and Leonhard's term *zycloide Psychose* all refer to the same group of patients. And insofar as the patient populations to whom these terms apply are different we do not know which is the most useful of these concepts or which the most soundly based theoretically. Indeed, it is striking how little basic clinical research has been done in the last 50 years on psychoses falling outside the affective and schizophrenic rubrics. The best the writer can do in this situation is to describe these various concepts, emphasising that they are derived from quite different, and in some respects incompatible, conceptual traditions.

SCHIZOAFFECTIVE PSYCHOSES

The term schizoaffective was coined in the 1930s by an American psychiatrist, Kasanin, to describe the illnesses of a group of nine young adults who had all become floridly psychotic at a time of obvious emotional turmoil (Kasanin 1933). Their illnesses all had a strong affective colouring and they recovered completely within a few weeks or months, though they showed a marked tendency to recur later on. Since that time the term has been widely used as a convenient label for the many patients who exhibit both schizophrenic and affective symptoms, either simultaneously or sequentially.

It is commonplace for patients to have ill-defined depressive symptoms, and even to be diagnosed and treated for a depressive illness, over a period of weeks or months before developing overt schizophrenia. It is equally common for patients to have persistent or recurrent depressive symptoms in the aftermath of a schizophrenic illness — post-schizophrenic depression (F20.4) in ICD-10. Such patients complain of depression, lack of energy and interest, and difficulty concentrating and sleeping. They may also have serious suicidal thoughts and hear voices urging them to kill themselves, but they do not usually have diurnal variation in mood, guilt, marked loss of weight or appetite, or other characteristic melancholic symptoms. Both these sequences are well known and accepted as part of the normal course of schizophrenia. It is also quite common to encounter patients in their 20s or 30s with typical affective illnesses who give a history of an earlier illness which was diagnosed as schizophrenia at the time, but from which they made a full recovery. In such cases the notes of the original illness usually describe either fairly typical manic symptoms or a florid psychosis with no clearly differentiating features. Either way, it seems likely with hindsight that the original illness was manic and the diagnosis of schizophrenia incorrect.

None of these situations or sequences of events justifies the epithet 'schizoaffective'. There are, however, descriptions in the literature of patients having one or more typical and sometimes prolonged schizophrenic illnesses, eventually making a full recovery, and subsequently having a series of equally typical affective illnesses without any return of their original schizophrenic symptoms (Sheldrick et al 1977). Such patients are probably rare but the evidence that such a metamorphosis is possible does carry implications for the assumptions we make about disease entities.

The term schizoaffective is most commonly and usefully applied to acute psychotic illnesses in which schizophrenic and affective symptoms are present simultaneously and are equally prominent. In ICD-10, for example, schizoaffective disorders are defined as 'episodic disorders in which both affective and schizophrenic symptoms are present within the same episode of illness'. The affective element may be depressive or manic, or alternate between the two, and ICD-10 recognises distinct manic (F25.0) and depressive (F25.1) types of schizoaffective disorder. The schizophrenic symptoms are also very variable, though they are usually 'positive' rather than 'negative' symptoms, if only because apathy and blunting of affect are hardly compatible with depression or elation. Most commonly they are hallucinations or delusions, like voices discussing the patient in the third person or delusions of control, which are normally regarded as characteristic of schizophrenia. Sometimes, though, they consist of catatonic phenomena or evidence of thought disorder. Typically both sets of symptoms, the schizophrenic and the affective, develop together and wane together in the course of recovery. In DSM-IIIR, however, criteria for schizoaffective disorder require not only the simultaneous presence of a major depressive or manic syndrome and the typical positive symptoms of schizophrenia but also, for reasons which are not explained, a period of at least 2 weeks in which delusions or hallucinations were present in the absence of any prominent mood disturbance.

The relationship of schizoaffective illnesses to schizophrenic and affective disorders

Before the 1970s patients with both schizophrenic and affective symptoms, the patients Kurt Schneider called *Zwischen-Fälle* ('cases in between'), received little attention. Because their existence was an embarrassment to the general assumption that schizophrenia and manic–depressive illness were separate disease entities, they were usually either set aside and ignored, or else lumped in with one or other of their neighbours and their atypical features glossed over. Most of the literature on the subject is therefore fairly recent. It is also confusing, because there is no agreement on the kinds of patients to whom the label 'schizoaffective' should be applied. This is because the proportion of all psychotic illnesses regarded as schizoaffective and their detailed symptomatology are both at the mercy of varying concepts of schizophrenia and affective illness. If broad concepts of both schizophrenia and affective illness are employed, the term schizoaffective will be needed much less often, if at all, than if narrow definitions of schizophrenia and affective illness are employed. And the kinds of patients regarded as schizoaffective in a centre using a narrow definition of schizophrenia and a broad one of affective illness will be different from those so regarded in a centre using a narrow definition of affective illness and a broad one of schizophrenia.

Most recent research has been concerned to elucidate the relationship of schizoaffective patients to typical schizophrenics and typical affectives. In principle, patients with mixed symptomatology might be:

1. Schizophrenics with some incidental affective symptoms

2. Affectives with some incidental schizophrenic symptoms
3. Suffering from schizophrenia and an affective psychosis simultaneously
4. Suffering from a third unrelated psychosis
5. Genuine interforms between schizophrenia and manic–depressive illness
6. A mixture of 1 to 5 above.

A rather fanciful analogy may help to clarify the difference between these possibilities. If one equates schizophrenics and affectives with two related but distinct animal species, horses and donkeys, then hypothesis 1 above implies that schizoaffective illnesses are horses, hypothesis 2 that they are donkeys, hypothesis 3 that they are donkeys and horses harnessed in pairs, hypothesis 4 that they are zebras and hypothesis 5 that they are mules.

If hypothesis 1 were true, schizoaffective patients should have the same response to different therapies and the same course and prognosis as typical schizophrenics. There should also be a raised incidence of schizophrenia, but not of affective illness, in their first-degree relatives. Similar considerations would apply with respect to typical affective illnesses if hypothesis 2 were true. Hypothesis 3 requires schizoaffective illnesses to be rare (the chance coincidence of two illnesses each affecting around one person in 100 is one in 10 000), and also to have a prognosis at least as bad as that of schizophrenia, the more serious of the two separate illnesses. The implications of hypothesis 4 — the 'zebra hypothesis' — are less certain. The putative third psychosis might have a quite distinctive response to some therapeutic agent, or a distinctive course; and if it were genetically transmitted there should be a raised incidence of schizoaffective illness in first-degree relatives. Either way, there should not be a raised incidence of typical schizophrenic or affective illnesses in the relatives. Finally, hypothesis 5 — the 'mule hypothesis' — requires both treatment response and prognosis to be intermediate between those of typical schizophrenic and affective psychoses, and also requires a somewhat raised incidence of schizophrenic, affective and schizoaffective illness in the relatives.

Although for the reasons referred to above there are a number of puzzling discrepancies in the literature the facts appear to be as follows:

1. Most of the studies which have compared the medium- or long-term outcome of schizoaffective disorders with that of typical schizophrenic and affective illnesses have found it to be intermediate, i.e. better than that of schizophrenia but worse than that of affective illness (e.g. Tsuang & Dempsey 1979, Brockington et al 1980a, b, Maj & Perris 1990). There is a difference, however, between the manic and depressive types of schizoaffective disorder. The prognosis of the former is very similar to that of bipolar illness. The prognosis of the latter is more variable and the risk of a typically schizophrenic outcome is higher.

2. Although the ratio of schizoaffective to schizophrenic and affective psychoses varies with the diagnostic criteria used, the former are too common to be explained by the chance coincidence of separate schizophrenic and affective illnesses.

3. Although there are reports of individual family pedigrees in which several members have had virtually identical schizoaffective psychoses (e.g. Wålinder 1972) almost all studies of the first-degree relatives of schizoaffectives have found a raised incidence of schizophrenia and/or typical affective illness and comparatively little schizoaffective illness (Angst et al 1979, Scharfetter 1981, Baron et al 1982, Gershon et al 1988). In most of these studies the incidence of affective illness in the relatives was higher than that of schizophrenia.

4. Although most family and follow-up studies suggest that schizoaffective illnesses are more closely related to affective illness than to schizophrenia some recent American studies suggest the opposite. This is probably because their diagnostic criteria have either required schizophrenic symptoms to be present in the absence of significant affective symptoms (as in DSM-IIIR), or required the index illness to be chronic (e.g. Williams & McGlashan 1987, Gershon et al 1988).

5. Although the most characteristic outcome of schizoaffective illness is full recovery followed by further episodes, and electroconvulsive therapy (ECT) and phenothiazines are generally more effective than tricyclic antidepressants, there is nothing about the course or treatment responses of these illnesses to distinguish them clearly from typical schizophrenic and affective illnesses.

This evidence is sufficient to eliminate hypotheses 3 and 4 above. Occasional schizoaffective patients may be suffering from both schizophrenia and an affective illness, or from a third psychosis unrelated to either, but neither hypothesis can account for the majority of cases. Most of the facts summarised above could be explained equally well by hypothesis 5, or by a combination of hypotheses 1 and 2, i.e. schizoaffective patients could be a mixture of schizophrenics and affectives, or genuine interforms ('mules'), or a combination of all three. Most authors reject the 'mule' hypothesis either because they believe that schizophrenic and affective psychoses have been shown to be distinct conditions, or simply because the possibility is not one they are prepared to entertain. They therefore assume that schizoaffective populations must be a mixture of schizophrenics and affectives. The writer's view is that the persistent failure to demonstrate, by discriminant function analysis or other means, that schizoaffective illness *does* consist of a mixture of two quite different kinds of patients, and the related failure to demonstrate any discontinuity between the symptomatology of unselected populations of schizophrenics and affectives, mean that the possibility has to be taken seriously. In other words, schizoaffective illnesses may be intermediate between schizophrenic and affective illness in their aetiology just as they are intermediate in symptomatology and outcome. For this to be so, of course, the genetic basis of both schizophrenic and affective psychoses would have to be polygenic.

These persisting uncertainties are reflected in ICD-10 and DSM-IIIR. Both classify schizoaffective disorders separately from both schizophrenic and affective disorders. ICD-10 states that 'their relationship to typical mood disorders and to schizophrenic disorders is uncertain. They are given a separate category because they are too common to be ignored.' DSM-IIIR describes schizoaffective disorder as 'one of the most confusing and controversial concepts in psychiatric nosology'.

Patients with both schizophrenic and depressive symptoms usually respond either to ECT or to neuroleptics, but do not often respond to tricyclic antidepressants. Regardless of what treatment is used both sets of symptoms tend to improve simultaneously, i.e. there is no evidence that schizophrenic or affective symptoms respond selectively to particular therapies. If the patient has further episodes of illness, as the majority do, these are equally likely to be typically schizophrenic, typically depressive or a mixture of the two once more. Patients with both schizophrenic and manic symptoms are less common and appear to respond equally well to chlorpromazine and lithium. This is part of the reason for believing that they have more in common with mania than with schizophrenia. If they have further episodes, as they almost invariably do, these are usually either typical depressions or schizomanic once more.

ACUTE PSYCHOSES OF GOOD PROGNOSIS

As indicated above, it is widely believed that some acute psychoses, particularly illnesses developing in response to obvious stress, are unrelated to both schizophrenic and affective disorders, and have a better prognosis than either. Such illnesses appear to be commoner in underdeveloped countries than in industrialised countries. This may be partly due to coincidental infections, anaemia or malnutrition, and partly due to higher levels of stress, but such patients have not yet been studied in sufficient detail for firm conclusions to be possible. The paucity of information about these acute psychoses is reflected by ICD-10. There is a single category (F23) for 'acute and transient psychotic disorders' which is subdivided simply according to whether or not the onset of the illness is acute (within 2 weeks), whether or not it was related to obvious stress, and whether the psychotic symptoms are polymorphic or typical of schizophrenia. The American classification DSM-IIIR, on the other hand, recognises *brief reactive psychoses* (brief psychotic episodes accompanied by emotional turmoil developing shortly after major stress and resulting in complete recovery within a month) and *schizophreniform* disorders (schizophrenic illnesses with a duration of less than 6 months) in addition to schizoaffective disorders and a residual group of atypical psychoses. Several of the European schools of psychiatry, however, have recognised acute psychoses unrelated to schizophrenic and affective illnesses for most of this century, and the more well known of these are described below.

Psychogenic or reactive psychoses

The concept of psychogenic or reactive psychosis was most strongly developed in Scandinavia and derived from the writings of August Wimmer, Professor of Psychiatry in Copenhagen from 1921 to 1937, and the 1945 monograph of his pupil Faergeman. The best account in English is by Strömgren (1974). The essence of the concept is expressed by the title. The psychosis is assumed to be the result of psychic trauma, often an event or situation to which the subject's past experience or constitution rendered him particularly vulnerable. Psychogenic psychoses are therefore fundamentally different from schizophrenic and manic–depressive illnesses, which used to be regarded in Scandinavia and continental Europe generally as endogenous disorders, even if, as was often the case, the illness developed in the aftermath of some obvious mental trauma.

This unambiguous theoretical position was, however, rather less straightforward in practice. Although psychic trauma is by definition the cause of the psychosis, constitutional factors 'play a predisposing role' and, according to Strömgren, except in time of war the majority of cases are neurotics and psychopaths. Indeed, the Norwegian term for psychogenic psychosis is constitutional psychosis. What is more, failure to identify any important stresses affecting the patient immediately prior to the onset of the illness did not preclude the diagnosis, provided the clinical presentation was sufficiently characteristic in other respects. The popularity of the diagnosis varied considerably even within Scandinavia. In Denmark, 15–20% of all functional psychoses used to be regarded as psychogenic, in Norway 30%, but in Sweden only 5%. As one might expect, the majority of these illnesses ended in recovery and overall their prognosis was considerably better than that of the so-called endogenous psychoses. However, up to a third of those originally diagnosed as having psychogenic psychoses were subsequently, in a later episode of illness, rediagnosed as suffering from schizophrenia or a manic–depressive illness. Jørgensen (1985), for example, re-examined a series of 41 Danish patients 10 years after their original admission with a diagnosis of acute reactive psychosis. Thirteen were psychotic at the time of re-interview and only seven were symptom-free and well adjusted. The current diagnosis was schizophrenia in 12, an affective psychosis in three and a paranoid psychosis in five. Even allowing for the likelihood that a diagnosis of reactive psychosis was sometimes made in order to avoid the socially damaging consequences of a schizophrenic or manic–depressive label, changes in diagnosis on this scale obviously weaken the case for maintaining that psychogenic psychoses are fundamentally distinct. As Jørgensen said of his own findings, they 'show the need for circumspection in predicting a favourable prognosis and handling the group as a nosological entity.'

According to Strömgren, 65% of psychogenic psychoses are *emotional reactions*, mainly depressions but sometimes states of elation or inappropriate apathy. A further 15% are *disorders of consciousness*, i.e. delirious reactions, oneiroid states and episodes of depersonalisation, and the remaining 20% are *paranoid types*. The disorders of consciousness are typically very short-lived, lasting only hours or days. Emotional reactions usually last a few weeks, sometimes a few months, while the paranoid types may persist for years. Although no formal comparisons were ever carried out it seems likely that patients regarded in Scandinavian countries as having psychogenic psychoses would have attracted a variety of different diagnoses in Britain. Many would have been said to have depressive illnesses, or acute schizophrenic illnesses arising in response to stress, and therefore likely to have a relatively good prognosis. Others might have attracted such labels as acute stress reaction, adjustment disorder and paranoid psychosis.

Cycloid psychoses

Although the term cycloid psychosis (*zykloide Psychose*) was coined by Leonhard (1957) the idea of an endogenous psychosis with a sudden onset, polymorphous symptomatology and phasic course which was unrelated to the dementia praecox and manic–depressive psychosis of Kraepelin goes back to the 'degeneration psychoses' of Wernicke and Kleist. The concept is known to English-speaking psychiatrists largely from the work of Perris (1974) in Sweden who described 60 patients identified by a retrospective study of case notes. Cycloid psychoses are illnesses of sudden onset in which there are fluctuations in mood — from depression to elation or from either to normality — during the course of the illness. In addition, according to Perris, at least two of the following five symptoms must be present:

1. Perplexity or confusion
2. Delusions of reference, influence or persecution and/or hallucinations not syntonic with mood
3. Hypo- or hyperkinesia
4. Episodes of ecstasy
5. Overwhelming fear of some catastrophe (pananxiety)

The majority of Perris' 60 cases were young adults and a high proportion were women. Their premorbid personalities were unremarkable and in only a third did the onset of the first episode appear to be related to stress. A high proportion of their first-degree relatives (20% of their parents and 9% of their siblings) had had similar illnesses, whereas few had had typical schizophrenic or manic–depressive illnesses, and this was an important part of the evidence that cycloid psychoses constituted a distinct entity. The course of the illness was characteristically phasic with a high risk of recurrence — an average of 4.5 episodes in 10 years. Subsequently, Cutting et al (1978) showed that 8% of psychotic admissions to the Maudsley Hospital met Perris' criteria and that such patients, who again were mostly women, did have a good immediate outcome and an unusually high relapse rate. More recently, Perris himself identified 30 (12%) of the 242 patients in two other English series of psychotics as having cycloid psychoses (Brockington et al 1982). Again, these 30 patients had a strikingly good short-term outcome but a high relapse rate. Despite this impressive homogeneity of outcome these 30 patients were not drawn from any particular British or American diagnostic category. The computer program Catego classified 60% of them as schizophrenics, largely on the basis of Schneiderian first-rank symptoms, but according to Spitzer's Research Diagnostic Criteria the majority were schizoaffective disorders.

The concept of cycloid psychosis is clearly an interesting one, and worthy of further study. In the writer's view, however, the prominent affective disturbance and mood changes, the phasic course, the fact that puerperal psychoses quite often have cycloid symptomatology, and Perris' own evidence that the relapse rate is reduced by prophylactic lithium (Perris 1978) all suggest that cycloid psychoses are a variant of manic–depressive illness rather than an independent psychosis, and that they probably owe their distinctive features mainly to their unusually sudden onset.

Bouffées délirantes aiguës (acute delusional psychoses)

Like other French concepts this has no exact equivalent in other nosologies and is not easily comprehended by those unfamiliar with the subtle complexities of the French tradition. The term *bouffée délirante* (literally, a 'puff' of madness) was coined by Magnan who regarded these short-lived psychoses as the stigma of a constitutional weakness. As described by Ey (1954) the illness starts with dramatic suddenness, often in someone who is 'more or less unbalanced or psychopathic' but usually *not* in response to any obvious stress. The central feature is a polymorphous delusional state. There may be ideas of persecution, of grandeur, of sexual transformation, of possession or poisoning, of influence, riches or fabulous power, blending with each other and changing in kaleidoscopic succession. The patient is totally absorbed by these vivid ideas, at times utterly convinced of their reality, at others able to stand back from them as a bewildered onlooker. The mood is constantly changing too, from exaltation to terror and from terror to perplexity, as the delusional ideas ebb and flow. Hallucinations of various kinds may also be present.

The psychosis usually lasts a few weeks, though sometimes only a matter of days and occasionally several months. Full recovery is the commonest outcome but there may be recurrences, and not infrequently the psychosis is the herald to a more ominous schizophrenic development. This suggests that *bouffées délirantes* have much in common with oneiroid states or acute schizophrenic episodes with a prominent delusional mood. Indeed, it is said that the majority fulfil DSM-III or DSM-IIIR criteria for schizophreniform disorder.

Hysterical psychoses

Although this term does not occur in any contemporary glossary it has been used intermittently throughout this century, mainly in countries which did not possess any official concept corresponding to that of psychogenic psychosis, and so had no ready means of categorising transient psychotic states which the psychiatrist believed to be a response to emotional stress unrelated to schizophrenia. Hollander & Hirsch (1964) are among the few authors to define their meaning with any clarity. As they described it, the illness is most commonly seen in women with prominent histrionic personality traits. It begins suddenly and dramatically in the immediate aftermath of some profoundly upsetting event, but seldom lasts longer than 3 weeks and usually recedes as suddenly and dramatically as it began. Its manifestations may take the form of hallucinations, delusions, depersonalisation or grossly abnormal behaviour of very varied kinds. There is no thought disorder and the subject's mood is either unaltered or simply more changeable than normal.

To designate a psychosis as hysterical, rather than simply as psychogenic or reactive, presumably implies that the illness is purposive and not merely a spontaneous reaction to a stressful situation. It implies that the subject is, without conscious simulation, behaving in a psychotic fashion at least in part because of the temporary advantages of being regarded as psychotic by others. A special type of hysterical psychosis was described by the German psychiatrist Ganser. He described three men who had developed auditory hallucinations and other symptoms suggestive of psychosis while in prison awaiting trial or execution (Ganser 1898). As this state was short-lived and followed by retrospective amnesia he was convinced it was a hysterical phenomenon rather than a conscious attempt to subvert the course of justice. The term 'Ganser syndrome' has subsequently been used by some writers for any behaviour simulating madness or dementia which is thought to have a hysterical basis. Others restrict the term to cases occurring in a forensic setting. The latter are rare, and sometimes the patient was already psychotic or brain-damaged before the onset of the Ganser symptoms, e.g. a psychotically depressed widower with a delusional belief that he was responsible for his wife's death and therefore about to face trial.

Ganser's name is also associated with the phenomenon of *vorbeigehen*, i.e. giving absurd answers to questions which nevertheless make it clear that the question has been understood, like saying 'five' when asked how many legs a horse possesses. As with other hysterical phenomena, the speech and behaviour of a patient simulating madness or dementia vary greatly with their sophistication and cultural background. *Vorbeigehen* may also be the product of aphasia or acalculia.

CHRONIC PSYCHOSES

There is considerable variation in different parts of the world in the way in which chronic psychoses which are not obviously schizophrenic or affective in nature are conceived and classified. In Britain most chronic paranoid psychoses tend to be regarded as an attenuated form of schizophrenia and their failure to develop apathy and flattening of affect is attributed to their comparatively late age of onset or to 'diminished penetrance' of schizophrenic genes. In other countries this is not so, however. In France, for example, the diagnosis of *délire chronique*, which embraces that of chronic hallucinatory psychosis referred to above, used to be made more frequently than that of paranoid schizophrenia; and in the USA the DSM-III definition of schizophrenia restricted that diagnosis to illnesses starting before the age of 45 years, so that all psychoses presenting after that age had to be categorised separately. The main reason for this unsatisfactory state of affairs is, as was said above, that too little straightforward clinical research has been done on these chronic psychoses. If series of patients meeting defined diagnostic criteria were examined in two or three different centres, the illnesses of their first-degree relatives studied without knowledge of the probands' diagnoses, and the probands themselves followed for 5 or 10 years, the situation would be much clearer. Other problems are created by the adjective 'paranoid'. In its original German meaning — and much of the literature on paranoid disorders is German — the term paranoid embraces all delusions relating to the subject himself. So persecutory, grandiose, somatic and hypo-chondriacal delusions are all paranoid. But many English-speaking writers, including the authors of DSM-III, have used the term in the restricted persecutory sense it has acquired in everyday speech without realising that they were changing the meaning of a technical term by doing so.

Although the German meaning of the term will be retained here the largest and most important group of these illnesses do involve persecutory ideas. The patient may be convinced that he is being watched or followed and that programmes on television or articles in the newspaper refer to him. People signal to one another as they pass him in the street, cars flash their lights on his windows at night, he hears people talking about him or God's voice addressing him. Middle-aged spinsters experience unfamiliar genital sensations in bed at night and attribute them to the amorous advances of a well-known newscaster or the gentleman next door. Middle-aged men become convinced that they are under surveillance by the CIA or MI5, and that their homes and offices are bugged and laser beams directed at them. Usually these unfamiliar attentions are interpreted as persecution. The neighbours are hostile and trying to drive them out of their home. Unknown malefactors are trying to drive them insane. Ungrateful relatives or the government are trying to poison them in order to inherit their wealth. Less commonly the interpretation is grandiose, or at least involves no danger. The flashing lights and the signals in the street are evidence that other people recognise their extraordinary gifts and achievements. The voice is a message from God telling the subject of his divine mission. Or the whole thing is an elaborate experiment 'for the sake of science' in which the patient has, by chance, been chosen as the human guinea-pig.

Other patients have hypochondriacal or somatic delusions. They are convinced that they have cancer or some other illness which a series of negligent or insufficiently skilful doctors have failed to detect, or perhaps that their skin is infested with parasites. Others are convinced that their body is misshapen in some way and that this must be corrected, surgically if need be, before they can give any thought to the future, or even appear in public. Many of those with hypochondriacal delusions are suffering from depressive illnesses in which typical depressive symptoms are relatively inconspicuous, and some of the adolescents and young adults who present with insistent and increasingly bizarre somatic complaints subsequently develop clear-cut schizophrenic symptoms. But some retain their isolated delusional ideas unchanged for years on end.

Differential diagnosis of paranoid illnesses

Persecutory delusions and delusions of reference have little diagnostic significance. They may occur in schizophrenic illnesses, in manic and depressive illnesses and in organic states. They may also occur in isolation. Anyone living in a foreign or unfamiliar cultural setting is likely to develop persecutory ideas if he develops a psychotic illness of any kind. For this reason, ideas of persecution have even less diagnostic significance in immigrants than they do in other people. Indeed, in some cases their suspiciousness and sense of being under threat are justified. They are indeed living in a potentially hostile setting and their awareness of this may have played a part in the development of the illness.

Partly for this reason, patients with paranoid symptoms often pose diagnostic problems. Perhaps the commonest dilemma is a middle-aged patient who presents with delusions of persecution and reference, perhaps accompanied by ill-defined auditory hallucinations, but with no other symptoms. In these circumstances all one can do is make a provisional diagnosis of paranoid psychosis and treat the patient with neuroleptics. In doing this, however, it is important to appreciate that the nature of the underlying illness has not yet been recognised. If such patients are followed for long enough, the majority have other symptoms in subsequent episodes which clarify the situation. Some develop classical schizophrenic symptoms like thought broadcasting and delusions of control, others develop typical depressive symptoms, with or without the return of their original paranoid ideas. A few are elated and overactive as well as paranoid in a subsequent episode. It is, of course, the belief that most patients with isolated paranoid symptoms later develop schizophrenic or affective symptoms as well which justifies the British tradition of regarding the great majority of psychoses as schizophrenic or affective. Not all patients do so, however. Some maintain their original persecutory ideas and auditory hallucinations, with or without periods of remission, for years on end without any other symptoms appearing. There are also occasional patients who present over a series of years with a sequence of different illnesses which defy classification. On one occasion, perhaps, they have persecutory delusions in isolation, on another they present with a fairly typical agitated depression, a year later they have an acute illness with perplexity and widespread schizophrenic symptoms which fade away after a few weeks to be replaced by depressive symptoms accompanied by vague persecutory ideas, and so on.

Aetiology of paranoid illnesses

Although the aetiology of illnesses presenting with ideas of persecution is very diverse they do have a number of identifiable predisposing characteristics in common. Immigrant status, or being a member of any minority ethnic group, has been mentioned already.

Deafness is another predisposing factor and the high proportion of elderly patients with paranoid illnesses who are hard of hearing has been commented on many times (Post 1966, Cooper et al 1974). Characteristically these patients have long-standing and severe bilateral deafness, usually middle-ear disease resulting from chronic mastoiditis rather than perceptual deafness present from birth. Severe bilateral deafness impairs communication with other people and so tends to produce social isolation, and it is generally believed that it is this social isolation which predisposes them to feel threatened, though tinnitus may well play a part in producing or potentiating the accompanying auditory hallucinations. Certainly the blind do not appear to be predisposed to the same extent as the deaf, perhaps because blindness acts as a barrier between the subject and the inanimate world rather than between them and other people.

Many of those who develop paranoid illnesses in middle or old age have long-standing predisposing personality traits. They are sensitive and wary in all their relationships, quick to take offence or to suspect that a slight is intended, and as a result often avoid social gatherings and group activities and have few friends. Sometimes this sensitivity is associated with some obvious physical abnormality, perhaps a disfiguring naevus, a hare lip or a club foot. More often, the abnormality is social or cultural rather than physical; they come from a different social class or ethnic group from the majority of their neighbours and associates and, rightly or wrongly, have never felt fully accepted by them. Genetic factors are probably also involved, for these sensitive personality traits tend to run in families without any obvious physical or social justification. Marital status is another important influence, for a strikingly high proportion of those with paranoid illnesses are single, divorced or widowed. This is not because marriage in some way protects against the development of ideas of persecution, but rather because the personality traits which predispose to social isolation and subsequent paranoid illness also make those concerned comparatively unlikely to marry, or for their marriages to survive if they do.

Classical syndromes

It will be clear from what has been said above that most British psychiatrists regard the great majority of psychoses as schizophrenic or affective and doubt whether a sufficiently good case has been made for the existence of most of the other independent syndromes that have been described. This view may be correct, though in some areas there is insufficient evidence to justify firm opinions either way. Even if it is correct, however, some concepts have exercised so important an influence in the past, or are referred to so often in the literature, that every psychiatrist needs to be familiar with them. The more important of these are therefore described in outline below.

Paranoia

This ancient Greek word for madness was resurrected by Kahlbaum in 1863 who used it in preference to Heinroth's term *Verrücktheit* to describe a form of insanity affecting intellectual activity in relative isolation from other psychic functions. Subsequently Kraepelin incorporated the term into his classification to denote a group of psychoses characterised by 'the insidious development of a permanent and unshakeable delusional system resulting from internal causes, which is accompanied by perfect preservation of clear and orderly thinking, willing and acting' (Kraepelin 1921). He described separate persecutory, grandiose and jealous forms, and a tentative hypochondriacal form as well. The French psychiatrist Magnan had earlier developed a similar concept under the title *délire chronique à évolution systematique*.

The concept of paranoia has remained controversial ever since, for two main reasons. Some psychiatrists doubt whether such patients — with chronic systematised delusions but no other disturbance of cognition or affect — exist at all; and if they do their independence from schizophrenia remains uncertain. Doubts on the latter score were first raised by the German psychiatrist Kolle who followed up 66 cases of paranoia in the 1930s, including 19 of Kraepelin's own patients, and found that with the passage of time the majority had developed primary delusions, one of the hallmarks of schizophrenia. For these reasons the diagnosis of paranoia is rarely made in the English-speaking world. It only figured twice, for example, in a representative sample of 4000 in-patient diagnoses made by English psychiatrists between 1968 and 1980. It has, however, lingered on in textbook descriptions and kept its place in the ICD, and recent American research suggests that it may be premature to discard the concept. Winokur (1977) identified 29 patients admitted to the Iowa Psychopathic Hospital between 1920 and 1975 who met rigorous criteria for what he called *delusional disorder* — non-bizarre delusions developing before the age of 60 years in the absence of hallucinations, flattened or inappropriate affect, overt brain disease or symptoms of depression

or mania. Only two of these patients subsequently attracted other diagnoses and although there were some schizophrenics and paranoid personalities amongst their first-degree relatives, raising the possibility of a relationship with paranoid schizophrenia, there was no raised incidence of affective disorder.

Kendler (1980) subsequently reviewed the English and French literature bearing on the nosological independence of paranoia. He found few studies that were methodologically sound by modern criteria but concluded that 'although some data suggest that simple delusional disorder might be a mild form of schizophrenia the bulk of the evidence suggests that the two are distinct syndromes.' This conclusion has been reinforced by two more recent studies. The first of these was based on independent interviews with 329 relatives of the Danish schizophrenic adoptees studied by Kety and Schulsinger (Kendler et al 1981). Eleven of the 14 relatives given blind diagnoses of schizotypal personality disorder proved to be biologically related to a schizophrenic proband, but this was not so for any of the five relatives given blind diagnoses of delusional disorder. The second study was based on blind interviews with the relatives of 62 schizophrenics meeting Feighner criteria, 18 medical controls and 18 patients meeting (somewhat modified) criteria for delusional disorder (Kendler et al 1985). The morbid risk for schizophrenia and schizoid/schizotypal personality was raised in the first-degree relatives of the schizophrenics but not of the patients with delusional disorder. Conversely, the morbid risk for paranoid personality was raised in the relatives of the patients with delusional disorder, but not in the schizophrenics' relatives.

The concept is, therefore, worth retaining. It seems clear, though, that patients fitting Kraepelin's original description are quite rare. Winokur's 29 cases were only obtained by searching the records of 21 000 consecutive admissions, and this rarity makes it difficult to collect a sufficiently large series to determine how often the syndrome evolves into schizophrenia and whether the two are genetically related. Partly for this reason the concept of delusional disorders has been expanded both in ICD-10 and DSM-IIIR to include patients who also experience intermittent hallucinations or mood disturbances, provided these are relatively inconspicuous.

Paraphrenia

In 1920 Kraepelin classified some of the patients he had previously placed within the rubric of dementia praecox separately under the new title of paraphrenia. The patients in question had relatively chronic illnesses with persecutory or grandiose delusions which usually developed in middle age and did not develop, or so he thought, the characteristic flattening of affect, loss of volition and other stigmata of dementia praecox. These characteristic they shared, of course, with paranoia. What distinguished them was that their delusions were accompanied by prominent auditory hallucinations. The independence of paraphrenia was, however, cast in doubt even sooner than that of paranoia. In 1921 Mayer followed up the 78 patients Kraepelin had used to establish the new concept and found that several had relatives with dementia praecox and that no less than 40% had themselves developed clear signs of dementia praecox within a few years. He was also unable to detect any difference in the initial symptomatology of those who later developed personality deterioration and those who did not. Since then it has been the general view that paraphrenia is simply a variant of schizophrenia which owes its relatively good prognosis and personality preservation to its comparatively late age of onset.

The term *late paraphrenia* is sometimes used as an omnibus term to describe paranoid illnesses presenting for the first time in middle or old age (e.g. see Roth 1955). Some of these patients have persecutory delusions and auditory hallucinations in isolation; others have delusions of control and other Schneiderian first-rank symptoms as well. Although there are no obvious differences between those with and without schizophrenic symptoms these paranoid patients differ in a number of ways from those developing affective illnesses for the first time in old age (Post 1966). A high proportion are unmarried, divorced or widowed and many have life-long personality traits which have prevented them from forming easy relationships with other people. They are sensitive, jealous, opinionated, puritanical or self-centred. Deafness is also common, though in other respects their physical health is often remarkably good.

Erotomania (délires passionels)

This comparatively rare syndrome was best, if not first, described by the French psychiatrist de Clerambault in 1942. The patient, usually a woman, is unshakeably but quite unjustifiably convinced that someone else, usually a man of higher social standing, is in love with her. She believes that the unsuspecting object of her affections can never be happy without

her and that his marriage is invalid. She endows him with comprehensive and sometimes miraculous powers and maintains that he communicates his love for her in a variety of oblique ways — by making remarks of special significance, by causing particular songs to be played on television, and by protecting her from dangers. Eventually the patient develops an elaborately systematised set of delusions which represent a sort of mirror image of the persecutory form of paranoia. The course is similarly chronic. In the early stages the patient is usually buoyed up with hope but the rebuffs which her repeated attempts to contact her loved one inevitably provoke may eventually convert her amorous expectations to spite and resentment.

In practice, most of these patients have other more typical schizophrenic or paranoid symptoms as well.

Delusional jealousy

Jealousy can take many forms, and which of these are considered morbid varies considerably with the cultural setting. So probably does the incidence of the phenomenon. At all events, jealousy seems to loom larger in Mediterranean cultures than it does in northern Europe, perhaps because of their greater tendency to regard wives as prized possessions or indices of status rather than as equal partners in a marriage. It is also very striking that men are far more prone to jealousy than women, despite the fact that wives often have more realistic grounds than husbands to suspect their partner's fidelity. The common morbid forms of jealousy are well described by Shepherd (1961). Many men, and some women, resent their wives or husbands indulging in any social activity alone and try to prevent their doing so. Others worry constantly lest their spouse or sexual partner should be attracted by someone else, and seek by constant questioning to reassure themselves that their fears are groundless. By doing so, of course, they make these fears more rather than less likely to be realised. A few pass beyond this stage to one of delusional conviction. They are unshakeably convinced that their wife is being unfaithful to them and devote their energies to obtaining proof of this. The unfortunate woman is cross-examined, accused and followed. A smudge of lipstick on a handkerchief or a rumpled pillow is pounced upon as proof. Handbags are rifled, underclothes searched for seminal stains and any sexual refusal interpreted as proof of prior satiation. Characteristically, the jealous husband does not abandon or divorce the wife whose behaviour he is convinced is so infamous. Instead he seeks desperately to obtain proof or a confession and he may, in a frenzy of passion, seriously assault his wife, not to punish her but in an attempt to obtain a confession, or in exasperation at her refusal to provide one. Indeed, jealous husbands not infrequently murder their wives, though they usually do so unintentionally and may be so stricken with remorse that they commit suicide immediately afterwards.

Jealous men are often inferior to their wives in some way and in that sense have some grounds for their fears. They are less intelligent, from a humbler social background, or simply less talented and attractive. Some are alcoholics, some have long-standing paranoid personality traits, some only become jealous in the context of a depressive or schizophrenic illness. Some, however, appear perfectly normal, reasonable and rational outside this limited sexual context. Management is often very difficult. If the jealous ideas are held with delusional intensity neuroleptics should always be tried, but may well have little effect. Sometimes all that can be done is to warn the wife of the risks involved, and help her to escape from an intolerable and dangerous relationship.

Monosymptomatic hypochondriacal psychosis

Hypochondriacal delusions of various kinds are common features of schizophrenic or depressive illnesses, and are sometimes the presenting symptom of an incipient schizophrenic illness. The term monosymptomatic hypochondriacal psychosis, popularised by Munro (1980), is reserved for disorders in which a firmly held and isolated hypochondriacal delusion persists in the absence of any mood disturbance or other psychotic phenomena. The content of the delusion is very variable though there are several common themes, including a conviction that the subject's skin is infested with insects, that his bowel contains worms or other parasites, and that he emits a foul smell. It is uncertain how common the syndrome is, partly because the patients tend to pester specialists of several different kinds — skin complaints being seen by dermatologists, bowel complaints by gastroenterologists and so on — without ever being seen by a psychiatrist. Often the development of the delusion can be related to some minor physical disorder which once produced relevant symptoms. The course is usually very chronic. Typically the patient takes his complaints, which remain remarkably unchanged over many years, to an endless series of doctors, seeking confirmation of his diagnosis and a cure which he never obtains. Sometimes the complaint is buttressed by evidence, a matchbox containing a few particles of debris being produced time after time as a sample of dead parasites, for example. Treatment is unrewarding both to the patient, who resents any suggestion that he is psychiatrically ill, and to the doctor. A minority benefit from neuroleptics, and Munro makes the improbable claim that the syndrome responds specifically to pimozide.

Dysmorphophobia

A misleading and inappropriate term, coined by Morselli in the 19th century, which is used to describe patients with an unshakeable and unjustified conviction that some part of their body is misshapen or deformed and who have no other psychotic symptoms and no relevant bodily abnormality. By convention the term is not applied to anorexic patients unshakeably convinced that they are too fat or overweight, though the similarities are compelling. Dysmorphophobia usually develops in adolescence or early adult life, often in apparent response to some casual comment on the subject's appearance. Although the delusion commonly involves the face or head, or some part of the body endowed with sexual significance, almost any part of the body can be involved, being too large, too small, asymmetrical or misshapen in some other way. If the supposed abnormality is susceptible to surgical treatment — a misshapen nose or breasts that are too big or too small — the subject may make insistent requests for surgical correction, but often he or she realises that this is impossible. Some of these patients slowly develop schizophrenic symptoms, but the majority do not. Almost always, however, there is an underlying 'sensitive' personality disorder and a failure to develop normal relationships with other people. Often the delusion is accompanied by a profound social phobia. The patient is convinced, for example, that his face is asymmetrical or his hair line in the wrong place and that passersby in the street are instantly aware of this. He therefore refuses ever to appear to public, or can only bring himself to do so after dark, and may live as a recluse for years on end. Treatment is always difficult but cognitive and behavioural forms of psychotherapy are more likely to be effective than interpretive psychotherapy or neuroleptics.

In the absence of schizophrenic symptoms or an underlying disturbance of mood, erotomania, delusional jealousy, monosymptomatic hypochondriacal psychosis and dysmorphophobia are all best regarded as variants of paranoia or delusional disorder, and they are classified in this way in both ICD-10 and DSM-IIIR. In the former they are called persistent delusional disorders (F22) and in the latter delusional (paranoid) disorder. Both are defined in such a way as to allow patients who also experience auditory, olfactory or tactile hallucinations and mood disturbances to be included, provided these phenomena are intermittent and less conspicuous than the delusions. No convincing explanation, psychological or somatic, has ever been adduced for any of these delusional syndromes and their comparative rarity makes them difficult to study effectively in isolation. Understanding is likely to be helped rather than hindered, therefore, by grouping them together.

Capgras' syndrome (illusion des sosies)

This was described by the French psychiatrist Capgras in 1923 and has since received more attention than it deserves. The patient, usually a woman, is convinced that someone who is familiar and emotionally important to her has been replaced by a double (*sosie*), someone who closely resembles him in appearance but is in fact an imposter. The phenomenon is never seen in isolation, only in the setting of a paranoid psychosis of some kind. It is therefore a symptom rather than a syndrome and has no particular diagnostic significance, though the underlying illness is most commonly schizophrenia. The conviction that the person in question no longer looks as he should is usually based either on derealisation or on his reappearance after a period of separation. Often, too, the so-called imposter is no longer behaving towards the subject in the way he or she would like and the underlying conviction is 'you cannot be X because he would never treated me like this'.

Cotard's syndrome (délire de négation)

The patients Cotard described in 1880 under the title *délire de négation* were convinced that they had lost everything, not only their wealth, their social status and their families but also their hearts, their brains, their intestines. The world beyond was also reduced to nothingness. Other people, even animals and trees, no longer existed any more and time had ceased. They were exhibiting particularly extensive and florid nihilistic delusions, and there is no more to the syndrome than that, despite the grandiose element

involved in the belief that they themselves were responsible for this worldwide destruction. Usually such patients are suffering from melancholia, sometimes from overt brain disease.

Folie à deux (induced delusional disorder)

This intriguing phenomenon was first described by Lasègue & Falret in 1877 and subsequent writers have added little to their beautiful description. Normally delusions and hallucinations are not contagious, either from the psychotic to the healthy or from one patient to another. But a sane person may acquire delusional beliefs from someone else if the two are living in a unusually close relationship in which they are relatively isolated from other people, particularly if the 'healthy' member of the pair is less intelligent than or dependent on the other. Typically the sick partner has a paranoid schizophrenic illness and the 'healthy' partner is a close relative, usually a child, a younger sibling, or a spouse. They may be isolated from other people by distance, cultural barriers or language. Sometimes more than two people are involved so that one may speak of a *folie à trois* or *folie à quatre*, but the mechanism is the same and all concerned are usually members of the same family. The morbid ideas transmitted to the healthy patients are usually persecutory or grandiose delusions which are not utterly implausible. Once transmitted they are shared and reinforced by both partners, and may persist for many years if the relationship remains undisturbed.

As Lasègue & Falret observed, if the two people concerned are physically separated the originally healthy partner usually loses his symptoms and separation should always be the basis of management for that reason. But recovery does not always follow separation, even after several months. If the emotional relationship is very close, as it often is, the dependent 'healthy' partner may be unable to abandon their morbid ideas, because to do so would endanger and perhaps destroy a relationship which is vitally important to them. For this reason separation usually needs to be combined with psychotherapy. There is no place for neuroleptics or ECT in the treatment of induced delusional disorders unless one suspects that the illness is not induced at all, but coincidental and independent — *folie simultanée* rather than *folie imposée*.

REFERENCES

Angst J, Felder W, Lohmeyer B 1979 Schizoaffective disorders: results of a genetic investigation. Journal of Affective Disorders 1: 139–153, 155–165

Baron M, Gruen R, Asnis L, Kane J 1982 Schizoaffective illness, schizophrenia and affective disorders: morbidity risk and genetic transmission. Acta Psychiatrica Scandinavica 65: 253–262

Brockington I F, Kendell R E, Wainwright S 1980a Depressed patients with schizophrenic or paranoid symptoms. Psychological Medicine 10: 665–675

Brockington I F, Wainwright S, Kendell R E 1980b Manic patients with schizophrenic or paranoid symptoms. Psychological Medicine 10: 73–83

Brockington I F, Perris C, Kendell R E, Hillier V E, Wainwright S 1982 The course and outcome of cycloid psychosis. Psychological Medicine 12: 97–105

Cooper A F, Curry A R, Kay D W K, Garside R F, Roth M 1974 Hearing loss in paranoid and affective psychoses of the elderly. Lancet ii: 851–854

Cutting J C, Clarke A W, Mann A H 1978 Cycloid psychosis: an investigation of the diagnostic concept. Psychological Medicine 8: 637–648

Ey H 1954 Les bouffées délirantes et les psychoses hallucinatoires aiguës. Études psychiatriques, vol 3. Desclée de Brouwer, Paris

Ganser S J M 1898 A peculiar hysterical state. Archiv für Psychiatrie und Nervenkrankheiten 30: 633. Translation by Schorer C E, 1965 British Journal of Criminology 5: 120

Gershon E S, De Lisi L E, Hamovit J, Neuberger J I et al 1988 A controlled family study of chronic psychoses. Archives of General Psychiatry 45: 328–336

Hollander M H, Hirsch S J 1964 Hysterical psychosis. American Journal of Psychiatry 120: 1066–1074

Jørgensen P 1985 Long-term course of acute reactive paranoid psychosis. Acta Psychiatrica Scandinavica 71: 30–37

Kasanin J 1933 The acute schizoaffective psychoses. American Journal of Psychiatry 90: 97–126

Kendler K S 1980 The nosologic validity of paranoia (simple delusional disorder). Archives of General Psychiatry 37: 699–706

Kendler K S, Gruenberg A M, Strauss J S 1981 The relationship between paranoid psychosis (delusional disorder) and the schizophrenia spectrum disorders. Archives of General Psychiatry 38: 985–987

Kendler K S, Masterson C C, Davis K L 1985 Psychiatric illness in first degree relatives of patients with paranoid psychosis, schizophrenia and medical illness. British Journal of Psychiatry 147: 524–531

Kraepelin E 1921 Manic–depressive insanity and paranoia. Translation of Psychiatrie, ein Lehrbuch für Studierende und Ärtze, 8th edn by Barclay R M. Livingstone, Edinburgh

Lasègue C, Falret J 1877 La folie à deux ou folie communiquée. Translation of the original paper in American Journal of Psychiatry October 1964 suppl: 121

Leonhard K 1957 Aufteilung der endogenen Psychosen. Akademie Verlag, Berlin

Maj M, Perris C 1990 Patterns of course in patients with a cross-sectional diagnosis of schizoaffective disorder. Journal of Affective Disorders 20: 71–77

Munro A 1980 Monosymptomatic hypochondriacal psychosis. British Journal of Hospital Medicine 24: 34–38

Perris C 1974 A study of cycloid psychoses. Acta Psychiatrica Scandinavica suppl 253

Perris C 1978 Morbidity suppressive effect of lithium carbonate in cycloid psychosis. Archives of General Psychiatry 35: 328–331

Post F 1966 Persistent persecutory states of the elderly. Pergamon Press, Oxford

Roth M 1955 The natural history of mental disorder in old age. Journal of Mental Science 101: 281–301

Scharfetter C 1981 Subdividing the functional psychoses: a family hereditary approach. Psychological Medicine 11: 637–640

Sheldrick C, Jablensky A, Sartorius N, Shepherd M 1977 Schizophrenia succeeded by affective illness: catamnestic study and statistical enquiry. Psychological Medicine 7: 619–624

Shepherd M 1961 Morbid jealousy: some clinical and social aspects of a psychiatric symptom. Journal of Mental Science 107: 687–753

Strömgren E 1974 Psychogenic psychoses. In: Hirsch S R, Shepherd M (eds) Themes and variations in European psychiatry. Wright, Bristol, pp 97–117

Tsuang M T, Dempsey M G 1979 Long term outcome of major psychoses: schizoaffective disorder compared with schizophrenia, affective disorders. Archives of General Psychiatry 36: 1302–1304

Wålinder J 1972 Recurrent familial psychosis of the schizoaffective type. Acta Psychiatrica Scandinavica 48: 274–283

Williams P V, McGlashan T H 1987 Schizoaffective psychosis 1. Comparative long term outcome. Archives of General Psychiatry 44: 130–137

Winokur G 1977 Delusional disorder (paranoia). Comprehensive Psychiatry 18: 511–521

21. Neuroimaging techniques

Eve C. Johnstone

INTRODUCTION

The view that psychiatric illnesses were the result of disorders of the brain gained support during the 18th century (Hunter & MacAlpine 1963) and was later developed by Griesinger, Professor of Psychiatry and Neurology in Berlin. He considered that normal mental processes are dependent upon the integrity of the brain and that lesions of some parts of the brain are more likely than those of others to be associated with mental disorders (Griesinger 1857). This idea that the brain was the seat of insanity led to the view that psychiatric illnesses could be investigated in a similar way to other illnesses and in Germany there were extensive and sometimes successful attempts by Alzheimer, Wernicke and others to correlate psychiatric conditions with neuropathology. Although neuropathological techniques were limited, replicable findings could be made both in relation to gross postmortem change and to histology. There was, however, at that time, no means of examining the structure or function of the brain until after death. A variety of imaging techniques have since been developed which have allowed the brain to be examined during life. Although they are sometimes used in the investigation of individual psychiatric patients, as far as psychiatry is concerned their greatest application until now has been in research. They have been used to compare groups of patients with groups of controls, to demonstrate the nature and progress of the changes found in organic disorders; and they have been used to study patients with disorders of uncertain aetiology, such as schizophrenia and bipolar affective disorder, in the hope of identifying underlying changes in anatomy or physiology. The findings of studies of this kind have given rise to hypotheses concerning the organic basis of the disorders formerly known as the functional psychoses.

IMAGING TECHNIQUES WHICH EXAMINE THE STRUCTURE OF THE BRAIN

Pneumoencephalography (PEG; air encephalography)

This technique was introduced by Dandy 1919. It involves introducing air into the subarachnoid space by lumbar puncture and allowing it to rise to outline the ventricular system and the basal cisterns of the brain. This technique clearly demonstrates ventricular dilatation and may also reveal cortical atrophy as the pooling of air in dilated sulci over the convexity of the brain or around the cerebellar hemispheres may be shown. Such atrophy was, for example, demonstrated in some hypothyroid patients by Jellinek in 1962. Investigations of schizophrenic patients using PEG date back to 1927, when Jacobi & Winkler claimed that 18 of 19 schizophrenic patients showed 'unquestionable' internal hydrocephalus. A number of other early studies were reported with similar conclusions (Crow & Johnstone 1987), but the interpretation of some of these findings is made difficult by lack of blindness, inadequate diagnostic criteria or inadequate controls. PEG is not a pleasant procedure for the subject. Headache is usual and may persist for 48 hours or longer, with nausea and meningeal irritation. The procedure may also involve serious risks in certain situations. Where intracranial pressure is raised the alteration of cerebral hydrodynamics following the introduction of air may lead to the development of tentorial herniation or a medullary pressure cone and patients with degenerative brain disease may show at least temporary clinical deterioration after the procedure. In the light of these problems it is not surprising that in 1929 the American Roentgen Ray Society declared that it was unethical to use normal controls in pneumoencephalographic studies. The propriety of this declaration is indisputable, but it did place limitations on the methodology of subsequent studies. Furthermore, it was later shown that with PEG (Le May 1967) variation in the amount and nature of the injected gas and the length of time between gas injection and radiography could affect the result obtained. These difficulties are not likely to be of great relevance in the interpretation of individual pneumoencephalograms carried out for the investigation of particular patients, but should be borne in mind when considering comparative studies of groups of patients.

Echoencephalography (ultrasound)

This technique involves transmitting ultrasonic frequencies through the skull and recording echoes, the pattern of which reflects midline structures such as the third ventricle. This is a rapid procedure without risk or discomfort to the patient, but unfortunately there is a high incidence of false positive and negative results. The technique is therefore rarely now used for the investigation of individual patients. Although it has been used by several groups of workers (Kruger et al 1967, Holden et 1973, Daum et al 1976) to compare third ventricular size in schizophrenic patients and normal controls, it has been superseded for such purposes by computerised tomography (CT) or magnetic resonance imaging (MRI).

Computerised tomography (CT scan, CAT Scan, EMI scan)

The introduction of CT by Hounsfield (1973) represented a major advance in the investigation of the structure of the brain. Essentially, CT is a procedure in which X-ray transmission readings are taken through the head at many angles by means of a narrow beam of X-rays: from these data absorption values of the material contained within the head are calculated and presented as a series of pictures of transverse slices of the cranial contents (Fig. 21.1). The system exposes the patient to no greater radiation dosage than a standard series of ordinary skull X-rays. There is no need for anaesthesia or any invasive procedure. When this procedure was first introduced it involved the patient lying still with the neck hyperextended for periods of half an hour or more, but this is no longer the case and now a CT scan involves no more discomfort and requires little more time than standard skull X-rays.

Gawler et al (1975) have described the CT findings in the normal brain and the range of structures identified. The ventricular system is clearly shown along with the basal cisterns and the cortical sulci. Within the cerebral substance, the thalami, the heads of the caudate nuclei, the internal capsule and optic radiations are generally identifiable. A number of pathological processes are readily visualised, including tumours, abscesses, haematomas and local cerebral oedema. Intravenous injections of contrast material can be used in doubtful cases to enhance the differences between tumour and surrounding brain tissue. The technique is highly effective in the demonstration of most tumours, but those in the posterior fossa are not well visualised by techniques dependent upon the use of X-rays because of the radiopacity of bone.

The CT measure which has gained the widest acceptance in the psychiatric literature is the ventricular brain ratio (VBR) (Weinberger et al 1983). The first CT scan study in schizophrenia (Johnstone et al 1976) found the lateral ventricular area to be increased in a group of chronically institutionalised schizophrenic patients in comparison with an age-matched group of normal controls. Numerous subsequent studies of lateral ventricular size have been conducted, and many, although not all, have confirmed the finding (Crow & Johnstone 1987). These findings have been extensively reviewed (Weinberger et al 1983, Gattaz et al 1991).

It is often difficult to separate the effects of physical treatments of long-standing illnesses from those of the disorders they are used to treat, but the opportunity to make this separation in the case of the treatment of schizophrenia was available in a study conducted at Northwick Park Hospital (Owens et al 1985) in which a sample of 112 patients was selected from a total in-patient schizophrenic population of 510 cases who had been treated in accordance with a variety of policies. This meant that some patients had received a full range of physical treatments while others had received little or none, and it was possible to match groups of treated and untreated cases. These comparisons showed that neither the fact of treatment with electroconvulsive therapy (ECT), insulin coma therapy or neuroleptics, nor the extent of treatment with each, was related to lateral ventricular size. It may thus be concluded that physical treatments are not the cause of the ventricular enlargement associated with schizophrenia. From the findings of CT studies (and indeed they are supported by those of pneumoencephalographic and echoencephalographic studies) it appears that reduction of brain substance occurs in schizophrenia more often than in controls and is not due to treatment. This ventricular enlargement is not a necessary concomitant of

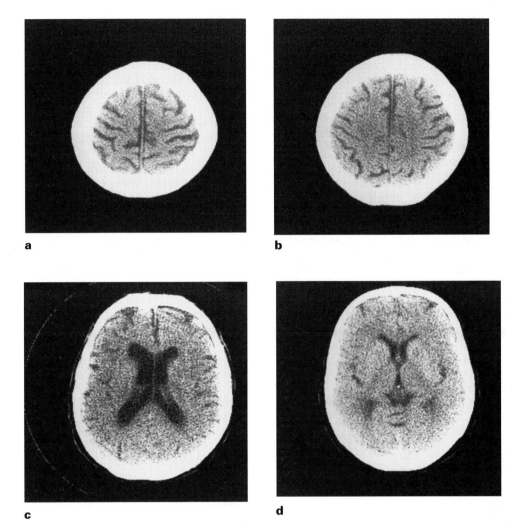

Fig. 21.1   a CT scan (apical cut) showing generalised cortical atrophy. **b** CT scan (lower cut) showing generalised cortical atrophy. **c** CT scan showing generalised atrophy with enlarged ventricles. **d** CT scan showing normal anterior horns of lateral ventricles and third ventricle.

schizophrenia, even in its most severe and chronic forms, as many patients show normal appearances on imaging studies. Nor indeed is ventricular enlargement sufficient for the development of schizophrenia, as it has been found in manic–depressive illness (Rieder et al 1983), in long-term benzodiazepine users (Lader et al 1984) and as a reversible phenomenon in association with alcoholism (Carlen et al 1978) and anorexia nervosa (Heinz et al 1977). This reversible enlargement raises the possibility that changes in ventricular size may reflect fluid, electrolyte and nutritional status. It is

implausible that such factors underlie the consistent findings in schizophrenic patients, as these have been demonstrated in out-patients as well as in the institutionalised and in young patients in their first episode of illness (Gattaz et al 1991). The temporal relationship of the ventricular enlargement to the development of schizophrenia is an important issue which is not yet fully resolved, but the body of evidence currently available suggests that the structural abnormalities probably occur before the onset of the psychosis and remain stable over time (Gattaz et al 1991). This information has been incorporated into hypotheses regarding a possible neurodevelopmental aetiology for schizophrenia (e.g. see Lewis 1989) and this area of work has been further developed using MRI. Nuclear magnetic resonance (NMR) may be used for imaging or for spectroscopy. Imaging is in clinical use but to date spectroscopy remains essentially a research technique.

Nuclear magnetic resonance (NMR; MRI scanning)

When the nuclei of certain atoms are placed in a magnetic field they can be made to absorb or emit electromagnetic radiation. The observation of this phenomenon — NMR — was first reported in 1946 by the groups of Bloch and Purcell. The spectrum of absorbed or emitted electromagnetic radiation depends upon the nature of the nucleus of interest and its local chemical environment. Only asymmetric nuclei with an odd atomic number (number of protons + neutrons) are NMR-responsive and this, of course, restricts the possibilities of the technique. The available nuclei of biological interest include hydrogen nuclei (protons), phosphorus, sodium and carbon. Of the nuclei responsible to NMR, hydrogen nuclei (each of which consists of a single proton) are by far the most abundant in the human body in the form of water.

NMR imaging

Clinical NMR imaging as it currently exists is based on hydrogen nuclei. The first published NMR image was produced by Lauterbur in 1973 and clinical trials of proton tomographic imaging began about 1980. As with CT, MRI uses advanced computer technology to form images from tissue signals. Neither CT nor MRI could have become a reality without the computer revolution. MRI scans, however, do not involve ionising radiation but are formed by directing non-ionizing pulsed radio waves at brain tissue. In a strong magnetic field asymmetric nuclei align in the same direction and resonate at the same frequency as the radio frequency that stimulates them. A receiver and a computer complete the process of transforming signals into a visible scan. Proton tomographic imaging of the brain actually depicts water distribution in the brain. Tissues that contain very little water, such as bone, return little or no signal. For this reason tissues which on CT (or any imaging dependent on X-ray) remain hidden within a heavy bony structure (e.g. the contents of the posterior fossa) will show up clearly on MRI.

In a typical MRI system a large and very powerful cryogenic magnet is used to produce a uniform static magnetic field of 0.1–2.5 T. Cooling apparatus is required to keep the magnet at an appropriate temperature and steel shielding is used to confine the magnetic field to the area of the magnet. In modern scanners this is built into the machine, but when it is not the shielding is incorporated into the walls of the building where it is housed. In the absence of any externally applied magnetic field, hydrogen nuclei (protons) are randomly positioned. But they behave like little bar magnets, and in the presence of the static magnetic field produced by the magnet in the NMR machine the protons line up in the direction of the field, producing a net nuclear magnetisation in the long axis of the patient. Additional radio frequency pulses are applied by means of a coil which surrounds the patient. These pulses are used to rotate the nuclear magnetisation, which returns to its original position between the pulses.

For example, if a 90° pulse is applied the nuclear magnetisation is rotated from the longitudinal into the transverse plane. Following this rotation, the component of the magnetisation in the long axis of the patient recovers from zero to its original amplitude in an exponential way. This recovery is called longitudinal or spin–lattice relaxation and is characterised by the time constant T_1. Relaxation of the component in the transverse direction back to its original amplitude of zero is termed transverse or spin–spin relaxation and is characterised by the time constant T_2. T_1 depends upon the interaction of protons with surrounding nuclei and molecules (the 'lattice'), while T_2 depends upon the interaction of protons with each other. Both T_1 and T_2 are sensitive indices of the local molecular environment. By using a variety of pulse sequences it is possible to produce images with varying dependence on proton density, T_1 and T_2. It is necessary to specify these sequences before the image is made (Bydder 1983).

No adverse effects of NMR have yet been reported. The only known potential hazard of serious practical significance is the possibility that ferromagnetic aneurysm clips might be dislodged by the magnetic fields (New et al 1983), and patients with these in situ should not be examined. Some theoretical risks of the procedure, most of which relate to overheating, have been described and are discussed by Budinger (1981) and Godlee (1991). The procedure does involve the patient being enclosed in a narrow metal tube, where his attendants cannot really see him and cannot touch him. The duration of the examination is variable, depending on the number of sites to be examined, but

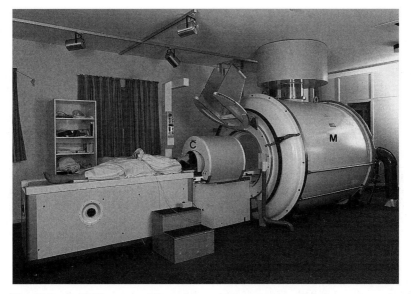

Fig. 21.2   An MRI scanner without the usual external casing: M is the magnet and C is the coil which applies the radio frequency pulses.

may be as much as an hour. A few patients (and normal controls) become so anxious in this situation that the procedure has to be abandoned. Because it is difficult to observe the patient adequately during the procedure, it is not usually appropriate to use sedation to overcome such problems. An MRI scanner without its external casing is shown in Figure. 21.2. This allows the component parts to be visualised. The table on which the patient is lying is mobile and slides into the magnet, so that during the head-scanning procedure the patient's head is within the coil, which is then slid right into the magnet.

Table 21.1   Advantages and disadvantages of MRI as compared with CT

Advantages of MRI	Disadvantages of MRI
Better resolution and better grey/white matter contrast	Expensive and therefore available in few centres
Ease of axial, sagittal and coronal imaging	Scanning time is longer than with CT
Visualisation of posterior fossa because bone returns little signal	Abnormalities of bone are not visualised
Does not involve ionising radiation and therefore multiple rescanning even of controls is possible	The enclosed environment of MRI is unpleasant and 5-10% of subjects cannot tolerate it

The introduction of MRI has been a significant advance and the procedure offers several advantages in comparison with CT, but there are disadvantages as well. The 'pros and cons' of the two types of imaging in relation to the investigation of psychiatric patients are shown in Table 21.1.

MRI provides a high degree of contrast between grey and white matter, and this displays considerable anatomical detail which is not defined with CT (Fig. 21.3). Vascular lesions such as intracerebral or subdural haemorrhages are readily visualised with MRI and cerebral infarction produces a loss of grey–white contrast which is readily seen. MRI is particularly useful in demonstrating brain stem infarcts because of the absence of bone artefacts. Abscesses are clearly displayed and herpes encephalitis is associated with regions of prolonged T_1 and T_2 values and may give a strikingly abnormal picture. The high level of grey–white matter contrast seen on MRI provides the basis of the application of this technique to demyelinating disease. In an initial study of ten patients with multiple sclerosis Young et al (1981) found many more lesions with MRI than with CT. Since then the value of the technique in demonstrating the lesions of multiple sclerosis has been shown repeatedly, and rarer disorders of white matter such as radiation damage and Binswanger's disease can also be demonstrated. The ventricular system is well visualised with MRI, as it is with CT. MRI may offer the advantage of showing

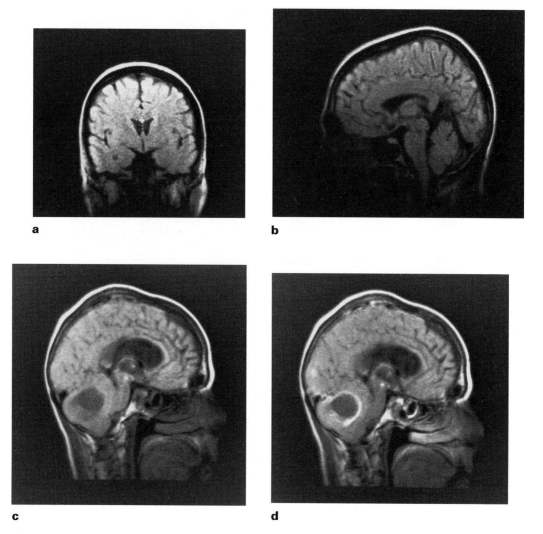

a

b

c

d

Fig. 21.3   a MRI scan, coronal, normal. **b** MRI scan, sagittal, normal. **c** MRI scan, sagittal, showing posterior fossa tumour. **d** MRI scan, sagittal, showing posterior fossa tumour with contrast enhancement.

periventricular oedema, which is sometimes of value in the recognition of acute ventricular shunt problems. Tumours are well demonstrated and the lack of bone artefacts is a significant advantage in posterior fossa lesions. It may be difficult with MRI to differentiate the tumour edge from surrounding oedema and in some cases this is more clearly defined with contrast enhanced CT scans. Paramagnetic contrast agents have, however, been developed for MRI and may be valuable in this context (Fig. 21.3).

MRI has been extensively used in research investigations comparing groups of psychotic, principally schizophrenic, patients with controls

(Table 21.2). The main findings of these studies of schizophrenic patients may be summarised as showing that: (1) there is confirmation on the coronal and midsagittal planes of the increased size of the cerebral ventricles described in CT studies; (2) abnormalities of temporal lobe size and symmetry in both grey and white matter are found, tending to suggest that schizophrenia may be associated with left temporal lobe pathology; (3) hypoplasia of the hippocampus and amygdala in some cases, confirming the suggestion of some post mortem studies that the development of some limbic structures may be impaired in some schizophrenics; (4) inconsistent

Table 21.2   Findings of MRI studies of schizophrenia.

Smith et al (1984)	9 schizophrenics 4 controls	No differences in structural measures
Johnstone et al (1986)	27 schizophrenics 12 controls	No difference in periventricular signal intensity
Andreasen et al (1986)	38 schizophrenics 49 controls	Reduction in various brain areas in schizophrenia
Nasrallah et al (1986)	38 schizophrenics 41 controls	Differences between schizophrenics and controls in corpus callosum structure
Besson et al (1987)	23 schizophrenics 15 controls	50% of schizophrenics had dilated ventricles. Greater abnormalities in negative-symptom cases
Nasrallah et al (1988)	35 schizophrenics	Smaller cerebral areas in schizophrenic patients with family history of schizophrenia
Johnstone et al (1989)	21 schizophrenics 20 bipolars 21 controls	Temporal horns of lateral ventricles larger in schizophrenics than others. Left temporal lobe area reduced in schizophrenia
Stratton et al (1989)	20 schizophrenics 20 controls	Greater ventricular size and greater cerebral asymmetry in schizophrenics
Suddath et al (1990)	15 sets of discordant monozygotic schizophrenic twins	14 of 15 affected twins had smaller left hippocampi and larger left lateral ventricles than their well twin

differences between schizophrenic and control populations in the area, length and thickness of the corpus callosum.

So far most MRI studies have been small-scale and not all have been well controlled. It is, however, increasingly well established that at least a subgroup of schizophrenic patients present subtle structural brain abnormalities which can be demonstrated by imaging techniques. The relationship between such abnormalities and the aetiology of the disease is not yet clarified. The detail shown by MRI and the safety of the technique for repeated use, including control subjects, provides possibilities for illuminating these issues. Much work remains to be done, but the study of Suddath et al (1990) in which MRI was used to demonstrate that in monozygotic twins discordant for schizophrenia the abnormal twin almost always can be identified from the scan is an example of the value of the technique. It was appropriately concluded from this study that subtle abnormalities of cerebral anatomy (namely small anterior hippocampi and enlarged lateral and third ventricles) are consistent neuropathological features of schizophrenia and that their cause is, at least in part, not genetic. It is clear that imaging studies are playing a major role in unravelling the complexities of the organic basis of 'functional' psychoses.

NMR spectroscopy

Independently of proton tomography it has been shown that NMR spectroscopy has substantial potential as a non-invasive, analytical tool for measuring quantitatively in vivo levels of certain biochemicals. It is possible, at least in principle, to obtain high-resolution spectra from any defined volume within the human body. A number of commonly occurring nuclides, ^1H, ^{13}C, ^{19}F, ^{23}Na and ^{31}P, can be detected by NMR. Of the exogenous nuclides, ^{19}F is much the most sensitive (Hall et al 1986). Much of the pioneering work for in vivo NMR spectroscopy was performed in Oxford by the groups of Radda and Richards and by the Oxford Research Systems Group. These developments enabled a number of valuable studies to be conducted and the work of Ross et al (1981) demonstrated the potential value of measurements of the ^{31}P NMR resonances of the principal storage compartments of the energy cycle, adenosine triphosphate and phosphocreatine. From the standpoint of brain research, probably the most important results stem from the studies of neonates (Cady et al 1983). Unfortunately, the early successes with neonates did not lead to equivalent progress in adults. A number of problems have persisted. In particular, although NMR spectroscopy can detect very small changes in concentrations of relevant substances, problems of localisation remain, so that the technique is essentially measuring very small changes in concentration within a volume of perhaps 1–2 cm^3. The limitations of this are obvious, but if these difficulties can be overcome NMR spectroscopy — which, like NMR imaging, is associated with no known hazard in patients without ferromagnetic aneurysm clips or pacemakers — is likely to have great potential in the investigation of psychiatric disorders, for it provides the possibility of examining the function rather than the structure of the brain. (Because it is not yet in clinical use, it has been included in the NMR section, although it might be appropriately placed in the section which follows.)

IMAGING TECHNIQUES WHICH EXAMINE THE FUNCTION OF THE BRAIN

Assessment of regional cerebral blood flow (rCBF) by the ^{133}Xe inhalation technique

The ^{133}Xe inhalation technique is non-invasive and said to be reliable and reproducible (Obrist et al 1975, Meyer et al 1978). ^{133}Xe, a chemically inert and diffusible gas which emits γ activity, is mixed with ambient air and inhaled through a face mask. After a 1 minute period of inhalation, the decreasing activity of the isotope is monitored for 10 minutes by 16 collimated probes mounted in a helmet and applied to the scalp. The end-tidal ^{133}Xe activity is also measured. The values of rCBF are calculated by two compartmental analyses of the recorded curves, by a computer, during the 10 minute desaturation period. The end-tidal ^{133}Xe curves recorded from the face mask are used for correction of the ^{133}Xe recirculation to the brain.

The procedure is non-invasive and exposes the patient to minimal doses of radiation. Xenon is an inert, freely diffusible gas, and as such exchanges readily between blood and tissue with no known effect on physiological or biochemical processes in man. Problems with the technique include poor spatial resolution and interference from the contralateral hemisphere, reducing the sensitivity, especially for detecting asymmetries between the two sides of the brain. Haemoglobin values (given the affinity of xenon for haemoglobin) as well as the arterial carbon dioxide tension (carbon dioxide being a potent vasodilator) need to be taken into account when evaluating data. The assessment of cerebral blood flow by xenon inhalation is used in research rather than in routine clinical practice. Studies have been conducted in depressive illness (e.g. see Mathew et al 1980, Uytdenhoef et al 1983), but results have been inconsistent. Most studies have concentrated on schizophrenia. An early study (Ingvar & Franzen 1974) showed that although patients had a normal mean hemisphere flow when compared to controls, higher levels were less common in frontal structures and more common postcentrally. This 'hypofrontality' was noted especially in elderly and deteriorated schizophrenics. This finding has not always been replicated. Attempts have been made to activate the brain with cognitive tasks during cerebral blood flow studies. A decrease in anterior left hemisphere activity during spatial tasks, a pattern rarely found in normal people, has been reported in unmedicated schizophrenic patients (Gur et al 1985), together with a higher resting left hemisphere flow. Frontal lobe tasks, such as the Wisconsin Card Sorting Test, have shown that the increases in frontal lobe activity seen in normals are not found in schizophrenics (Weinberger et al 1986). Regional cerebral blood flow studies localised the changes to the prefrontal association cortex and there has been some replication of these findings (Berman et al 1986).

Positron emission tomography (PET scan, ECAT scan)

PET represents the most complex and ambitious method of brain imaging to date. It is restricted to special centres since a cyclotron must be close at hand for the manufacture of the short-lived isotopes involved. Certain compounds are radiolabelled with short-lived positron-emitting isotopes, which are injected or inhaled. After being allowed to reach a steady state in the tissues, their distribution within the body is measured tomographically. Isotopes of biological elements such as ^{15}O, ^{11}C, ^{13}N or ^{18}F are frequently used. These isotopes have an excess of protons over neutrons and so they emit positrons (positively charged particles with the same mass as electrons) to achieve stability. The positrons quickly encounter electrons (which are negatively charged) in the tissues, and the two annihilate each other with the simultaneous production of two photons (γ rays) of equal energy, but emitted in opposite directions. These are detected by a scanner and a computerised reconstruction of the image is performed by a similar method to that used in CT scanning. The two techniques contrast with each other, however, in that while CT radiation is passed through the patient's brain, in PET radiation is emitted from the brain, detected and quantified. The reconstructed image based upon mathematical models of tissue tracer distributions is essentially functional rather than structural.

The isotopes most widely used to date are ^{15}O$_2$ and ^{18}F. ^{15}O$_2$ is inhaled and the arterial blood sampled to yield quantitative measurements of regional cerebral blood flow and regional cerebral oxygen utilisation (Frackowiak et al 1980). ^{18}F is incorporated into 2-deoxy-D-glucose (^{18}FDG), which is injected to measure local glucose metabolic rates (Phelps et al 1979). The compound enters the brain as though it were glucose but cannot be degraded for some time (half-life 110 minutes). Estimates of regional glucose utilisation can therefore be made by repeated venous sampling in conjunction with the scan. Using such a technique it has been possible to demonstrate severely impaired cerebral glucose utilisation in Alzheimer's disease in proportion to the severity of the dementia (Benson et al 1982). PET has been used fairly widely in studies of schizophrenia. These have generally concentrated on the issues of hypofrontality, laterality and the effects of treatment (Reveley & Taylor 1990), and so far results are not entirely consistent. PET has also been used to assess the density and affinity of neuroreceptors, most often dopamine receptors. These are estimated using ligands such as 3-N-[^{11}C]methylspiperone (Wong et al 1986) or [^{11}C]raclopride (Farde et al 1986, 1990). Results from these two groups are contradictory but the balance of the evidence at present is that there is no difference in dopamine receptors between schizophrenic patients and controls. The interest of PET scan studies can be enhanced by linking the investigations to the recent advances in neuropsychology described, for example, by Posner et al (1988). Posner postulates that fundamental cognitive operations are specifically localised in the brain and suggests plans of investigation which assume that every task calls upon a number of basic cognitive operations, each of which has a specific brain localisation. It is therefore possible that appropriate choice of tests could reveal, and with the concomitant use of PET (or SPET, see below) localise, the dysfunctional cognitive processes specific to a disorder. This type of investigation is obviously relevant to a wide range of psychiatric disorders.

Single-photon emission computerised tomography (SPECT scan; SPET scan)

This procedure is in many ways similar to PET scanning, but it is simpler and does not require a cyclotron. It employs radiochemicals which emit a single photon (γ ray), e.g. ^{123}I, ^{133}Xe or ^{99}Tc, and are present in the brain long enough to allow imaging by a rotating γ camera. Recently, new radiochemicals, e.g. ^{99}Tc-HM-PAO, have been developed which bind immediately to brain tissue in close proportion to, and thus accurately reflecting, blood flow. Relatively slow clearance rates allow tomographic images of consecutive slices of brain to be made. Image resolution with SPET is not as good as that with PET. PET can quantify tracer concentrations in absolute units, which means that the measurement of the physiological or other variable can be expressed in absolute terms so that measurements made within patient groups are comparable. This is not possible with the simpler and less expensive SPET, which is used to measure relative cerebral blood flow or metabolism within different areas of the brain in one individual. The disadvantage of both PET and SPET relate to radiation risks. These are small, but limitations are set upon the number of investigations which can be conducted in any individual, so repeated scans of patients in different clinical states and on and off different treatments are not really possible.

Use of these new imaging techniques has provided findings of considerable value in the investigation of individual psychiatric patients and in psychiatric research. Their full potential has yet to be realised.

REFERENCES

Andreasen N C, Nasrallah H A, Dunn V et al 1986 Structural abnormalities in the frontal system in schizophrenia: a magnetic resonance imaging study. Archives of General Psychiatry 43: 136–144

Benson D F, Kuhl D E, Phelps M E et al 1982 Positron emission computed tomography in the diagnosis of dementia. Transactions of the American Neurological Association 106: 68–71

Berman K F, Zec R F, Weinberger D R 1986 Physiological dysfunction of dorsolateral prefrontal cortex in schizophrenia: role of neuroleptic treatment, attention and mental effort. Archives of General Psychiatry 43: 126–135

Besson J A, Corrigan F M, Cherryman G R, Smith F W 1987 Nuclear magnetic resonance brain imaging in chronic schizophrenia. British Journal of Psychiatry 150: 161–163

Bloch F, Hansen W W, Packard M E 1946 Nuclear induction. Physiological Reviews 70: 460–473

Budinger T F 1981 Nuclear magnetic resonance (NMR) in vivo studies: known thresholds for health effects. Journal of Computer Assisted Tomography 5: 800–811

Bydder G M 1983 Clinical aspects of NMR imaging. In: Steiner R (ed) Recent advances in radiology and medical imaging. Churchill Livingstone, Edinburgh, pp 15–33

Cady E B, de L Costello A M, Dawson M J et al 1983 Non-invasive investigation of cerebral metabolism in newborn infants by phosphorous nuclear magnetic resonance spectroscopy. Lancet i: 1059–1062

Carlen P L, Workman G, Holgate R C, Wilkinson D A, Rankin J C 1978 Reversible cerebral atrophy in recently abstinent chronic alcoholics measured by computed tomography scans. Science 200: 1076–1078

Crow T J, Johnstone E C 1987 Schizophrenia: the nature of the disease process and its biological correlates. In: Plum F (ed) Handbook of physiology; the nervous system V. American Physiological Society, Bethesda, pp 843–869

Dandy W E 1919 Roentgenography of the brain after injection of air into the cerebral ventricles. American Journal of Roentgenology 6: 26

Daum C H, McKinney W M, Proctor R C 1976 Echoencephalographs of 100 consecutive acute psychiatric admissions. Journal of Clinical Ultrasound 4: 329–333

Farde L, Hall H, Ehrin E, Sedvall G 1986 Quantitative analysis of D_2-dopamine receptor binding in the living human brain by PET. Science 231: 258–261

Farde L, Wiesel F A, Halldin C, Stone-Elander S, Nordstrom A L 1990 D_2 dopamine receptor characteristics in neuroleptic-naive patients with schizophrenia. Archives of General Psychiatry 47: 213–219

Frackowiak R S J, Lenzi G L, Jones T, Heather J D 1980 Quantitative measurement of regional cerebral blood flow and oxygen metabolism in man using ^{15}O and positron emission tomography theory procedure and normal values. Journal of Computer Assisted Tomography 14: 727–736

Gattaz W F, Kohlmeyer K, Gasser T 1991 Computer tomographic studies in schizophrenia. In: Häfner H, Gattaz W F (eds) Search for the causes of schizophrenia, Vol II. Springer-Verlag, Berlin

Gawler J, Bull J W D, Du Boulay G H, Marshall J 1975 Computerized axial tomography: the normal EMI scan. Journal of Neurology, Neurosurgery and Psychiatry 38: 935–947

Godlee F 1991 Warning over magnetic resonance imaging. British Medical Journal 303: 205

Griesinger W 1857 Mental pathology and therapeutics. Translated by Lockhart Robertson C and Rutherford J. New Sydenham Society, London

Gur R E, Gur R C, Sholnik B E et al 1985 Brain function in psychiatric disorder. Archives of General Psychiatry 44: 126–129

Hall L D, Luck S L, Norwood T, Rajanayagam V, Schachter J 1986 Nuclear magnetic resonance spectroscopy — future technical prospects. In: New brain imaging techniques and psychopharmacology. British Association for Psychopharmacology monograph 9. Oxford University Press, Oxford

Heinz R, Martinez J, Haenggli A 1977 Reversibility of cerebral atrophy in anorexia nervosa and Cushing's syndrome. Journal of Computer Assisted Tomography 1: 415–418

Holden J M C, Forno G, Itil T, Hsu W 1973 Echoencephalographic patterns in chronic schizophrenia. Biological Psychiatry 6: 129–141

Hounsfield G N 1973 Computerised transverse axial scanning (tomography) Part I Description of the system. British Journal of Radiology 46: 1016–1022

Hunter R, McAlpine I 1963 Three hundred years of psychiatry 1535–1860. Oxford University Press, London

Ingvar D H, Franzen G 1974 Abnormalities of cerebral blood flow distribution in patients with chronic schizophrenia. Acta Psychiatrica Scandinavica 50: 425–462

Jacobi W, Winkler H 1927 Encephalographische studien an chronisch schizophrenien. Archiv für Psychiatrie und Nervenkranzen 81: 299–332

Jellinek E H 1962 Fits, faints, coma and dementia in myxoedema. Lancet ii: 1010–1012

Johnstone E C, Crow T J, Frith C D, Husband J, Kreel L 1976 Cerebral ventricular size and cognitive impairment in chronic schizophrenia. Lancet ii: 924–926

Johnstone E C, Crow T J, Macmillan J F, Owens D G, Bydder G M, Steiner R E 1986 A magnetic resonance study of early schizophrenia. Journal of Neurology, Neurosurgery and Psychiatry 49: 136–139

Johnstone E C, Owens D G C, Crow T J et al 1989 Temporal lobe structure as determined by nuclear magnetic resonance in schizophrenia and bipolar affective disorder. Journal of Neurology, Neurosurgery and Psychiatry 52: 736–741

Kruger H, Zumpe V, Veltin A 1967 Das Echoencephalogram des III ventrikels bei Gesunden und Schizophrenen. Nervenarzt 38: 412–414

Lader M H, Ron M, Petursson H 1984 Computed axial tomography in long-term benzodiazepine users. Psychological Medicine 14: 203–206

Lauterbur P C 1973 Image formation by induced local interactions: examples employing NMR. Nature 242: 190–191

Le May M 1967 Changes in ventricular size during and after pneumoencephalography. Radiology 88: 57–63

Lewis S W 1989 Congenital risk factors for schizophrenia. Psychological Medicine 19: 5–13

Matthew R J, Meyer J S, Francis D J, Semchuk K M, Mortel K, Claghorn J L 1980 Cerebral blood flow in depression. American Journal of Psychiatry 137: 1449–1450

Meyer J S, Ishiara N, Deshmukh V D et al 1978 Improved method for noninvasive measurement of regional cerebral blood flow by ^{133}Xenon inhalation Part I. Stroke 9: 195–204

Nasrallah H A, Andreasen N C, Coffman J A et al 1986 A controlled magnetic resonance imaging study of corpus callosum thickness in schizophrenia. Biological Psychiatry 21: 274–282

Nasrallah H A, Olsen S C, Coffman J A et al 1988 Magnetic resonance imaging, perinatal injury and negative symptoms in schizophrenia. Schizophrenia Research 1: 171–172

New P F J, Rosen B R, Brady T J et al 1983 Potential hazards and artefacts of ferromagnetic and non-ferromagnetic surgical and dental materials and devices in nuclear magnetic resonance imaging. Radiology 147: 139–148

Obrist W D, Thomson H K, Wang H S, Wilkinson W E 1975 Regional cerebral blood flow estimated by ^{133}Xenon inhalation. Stroke 6: 245–256

Owens D G C, Johnstone E C, Crow T J, Frith C D, Jagoe J R, Kreel L 1985 Lateral ventricular size in schizophrenia: relationship to the disease process and its clinical manifestations. Psychological Medicine 15: 27–41

Phelps M E, Huang S C, Hoffman E J, Selin E J, Sokoloff L, Kuhl D E 1979 Tomographic measurement of local cerebral glucose metabolic rate in humans with (F-18) 2-fluoro-2-deoxy D glucose: validation of method. Annals of Neurology 6: 371–388

Posner M I, Peterson S E, Fox P T, Raichle M E 1988 Localisation of cognitive operations in the human brain. Science 240: 1627–1631

Purcell E M, Torrey H C, Pound R V 1946 Resonance absorption by nuclear magnetic movements in a solid. Physiological Review 69: 37

Reveley M A, Taylor C J A 1990 Recent advances in brain imaging. In: Dinan T G (ed) Principles and practice of biological psychiatry, vol 1. Clinical Neuroscience Publishers, London, pp 183–199

Rieder R O, Mann L S, Weinberger D R, van Kammen D P, Post R M 1983 Computed tomographic scans in patients with schizophrenia, schizoaffective and bipolar affective disorder. Archives of General Psychiatry 40: 1735–1739

Ross B D, Radda G K, Rocker G, Esiri M, Falconer J 1981 Examination of a case of suspected McArdle's syndrome by ^{31}P nuclear magnetic resonance. New England Journal of Medicine 304: 1338–1342

Smith R C, Calderon M, Ravichandran G K et al 1984 Nuclear magnetic resonance in schizophrenia: a preliminary study. Psychiatry Research 12: 137–147

Stratton P, Rossi A, Galluci M, Amicarelli I, Passanello R, Cassacchia M 1989 Hemispheric asymmetries and schizophrenia: a preliminary magnetic resonance imaging study. Biological Psychiatry 25: 275–284

Suddath R L, Christison G W, Torrey E F, Casanova M F, Weinberger D R 1990 Anatomical abnormalities in the brains of monozygotic twins discordant for schizophrenia. New England Journal of Medicine 322: 789–794

Uytdenhoef P, Charles G, Jacquy J, Portelange P, Linkowski P, Mendlewicz J 1983 Regional cerebral blood flow and lateralised hemispheric dysfunctional in depression. British Journal of Psychiatry 143: 128–132

Weinberger D R, Wagner R L, Wyatt R J 1983 Neuropathological studies of schizophrenia: a selective review. Schizophrenia Bulletin 9: 193–212

Weinberger D R, Berman K R, Zec R F 1986 Physiological dysfunction of dorsolateral prefrontal cortex in schizophrenia 1. Regional cerebral blood flow evidence. Archives of General Psychiatry 43: 114–125

Wong D F, Wagner H N, Tune L E et al 1986 Positron emission tomography reveals elevated D_2 dopamine receptors in drug naive schizophrenics. Science 234: 1558–1563

Young I R, Hall A S, Pallis C A, Legg N J, Bydder G M, Steiner R E 1981 Nuclear magnetic resonance imaging of the brain in multiple sclerosis. Lancet ii: 1063–1066

22. Neurotic disorders

C. P. L. Freeman

INTRODUCTION

The term neurosis was introduced by the Edinburgh physician William Cullen in 1769. By neurosis he meant 'disorders of sense and motion' caused by a 'general affectation of the nervous system'. He included a wide range of conditions in which he felt there was some pathological deficiency in the nervous system but in which fever was absent, so that — as well as hysteria, hypochondriasis, melancholia and palpitations — epilepsy, mania, chorea, asthenia and diabetes were included.

One hundred years later the concept had been refined so that by the end of the 19th century it had come to mean psychiatric disorders which were neither organic nor psychotic.

We owe to Freud the term *psychoneurosis*. He used it to mean three specific syndromes: anxiety hysteria (now called phobic anxiety); obsessive–compulsive neurosis and hysteria proper. He distinguished the 'psychoneuroses' from the 'actual' neuroses which were neurasthenia and anxiety neurosis. He saw the actual neuroses as being predominantly physical and chemical in nature and not due to underlying conflict. In contrast he saw the psychoneuroses as resulting from unconscious conflicts, either between opposing wishes or between wishes and prohibitions. He saw such conflicts leading to unconscious perception of anticipated danger which evokes defence mechanisms that become manifest as personality disturbances or symptoms or both. Freud used the term neurosis in at least two ways. Firstly to indicate an aetiological process, viz. unconscious conflict arousing anxiety and leading to maladaptive use of defence mechanisms that result in symptom formation; and secondly as a descriptive term to indicate a painful symptom in an individual with intact reality testing.

As this century has progressed the use of the term has widened again so that if many current definitions of neurosis were taken literally all forms of non-psychotic non-organic distress would be included. For example, the World Health Organization (WHO 1974) international glossary definition is as follows:

Mental disorders without any demonstrable organic basis in which the patient may have considerable insight and has unimpaired reality testing in that he usually does not confuse his morbid subjective experiences and fantasies with external reality. Behaviour may be greatly affected, although usually remaining within socially acceptable limits, but personality is not disorganized. The principal manifestations include excessive anxiety, hysterical symptoms, phobias, obsessional and compulsive symptoms and depression.

In this chapter the term neurosis is used in three distinct but related ways:

1. As a global term to indicate all non-psychotic syndromes. The use here is synonymous with the term minor psychiatric morbidity and it is in this sense that the term has been used in most epidemiological research. The majority of such disorders are states of depression or anxiety or a mixture of the two. They have been called dysthymic states by some authors, but the term dysthymic disorder now has a more precise meaning in both DSM-III and ICD-10.

2. As a term to indicate specific neurotic disorders such as anxiety, depressive, obsessional and phobic neuroses.

3. As a term to describe assumed underlying mental mechanisms, so-called neurotic processes leading to the production of defence mechanisms.

The American (DSM-III; APA 1980) definition of neurotic disorders is as follows and encompasses the use of neurosis in the first and second sense above:

A symptom or group of symptoms that is distressing to the individual, or recognised by him/her as unacceptable and alien (egodystonic). Reality testing is grossly intact, behaviour does not actively violate gross social norms though functioning may be markedly impaired. The disturbance is relatively enduring or recurrent and is not noted to be a transitory reaction to stressors. There is no demonstrable organic aetiology or factor.

What is clear is that definitions which stress only the minor, transitory or minimally incapacitating nature of neurotic disorder cannot encompass all types of neuroses, for example the crippling nature of severe obsessional states, or the lifelong pattern of disability in Briquet's syndrome, or the poor response to treatment that many neurotic disorders show. In contrast, many psychoses are brief and respond dramatically to treatment.

Neurosis: should we retain the term?

DSM-III has abandoned the category of neurosis almost completely, but ICD-10 is likely to retain it. The three main justifications for discarding the term are: (1) that it groups together conditions which could be classified better in other ways; (2) that it involves aetiological assumptions which are unjustified; and (3) that it is a redundant adjective, which we can do without.

The first argument is illustrated by the reclassification of minor depressive disorders or 'neurotic depressions'. In both DSM-III and ICD-10 these are now grouped with other affective (mood) disorders. Rather than just reduce the types of neuroses by one, DSM-III has tried to find new homes for all the other 'neurotic disorders' and in doing so has created as many problems as it has solved. Obsessional states are now classified as a type of anxiety disorder and depersonalisation syndromes are included under dissociative disorders. ICD-10, on the other hand, will retain the general class of neurotic disorders under the title 'neurotic, stress-related and somatization disorders'.

The second argument is that the term neurosis is a confusing one and with multiple meanings. It is used to refer to specific syndromes, to a variety of psychopathological process and to a general class of non-psychotic non-organic psychological disorders. Gelder (1986) suggested that this problem can be solved by a more exact use of terms such as neurotic process and neurotic mechanism to distinguish these concepts from neurotic disorders.

The third argument is that the term is redundant. Adding the term neurosis to anxiety disorder or obsessional disorder adds nothing to the meaning and the concept of a broad grouping of neurotic disorders is so vague that it is not worth using.

The most cogent reasons for retaining the term relate to this latter point. Although there have been advances in the classification of neurotic disorders such as separate recognition of panic disorder and somatization disorder, there are still many cases which

do not fit neatly into any existing category. There are patients who exhibit mixtures of anxiety, depressive, hypochondriacal and obsessional symptoms without any one cluster appearing to dominate. No satisfactory term for this group has emerged, though minor psychiatric disorder, subclinical neurosis and minor affective disorder have been suggested. It is unlikely that all these conditions represent variants of affective disorder, and the term minor is misleading as some are serious and disabling. Until this problem is resolved it seems sensible to retain the term neurosis, or preferably neurotic disorder, to embrace this whole class of disorders.

A second weaker argument has been proposed by Sims (1985). He suggests that the shared clinical features and to some extent the common methods of treatment justify retention of the term. Although this is partly true, features such as bodily symptoms without organic cause and anxiety are not exclusive to the neuroses and frequently occur in other non-neurotic conditions.

In this chapter the term neurosis has been retained in the sense that it is used by ICD-10, though, as mentioned in the introduction, other uses of the term are not ignored.

NEUROSIS AS MINOR PSYCHIATRIC MORBIDITY

This section deals with investigations which have regarded neurosis as a global concept synonymous with minor psychiatric morbidity. Most studies of the nature and causes of neurosis have considered neurosis in a global sense rather than describing individual clinical syndromes, so factors in the aetiology of neurosis are conveniently described here.

Epidemiology of neurosis

Figures for the prevalence, incidence and lifetime risk of neurotic disorder are virtually meaningless unless one has some idea of the criteria that were used for case identification. Two extreme examples will serve to illustrate the problem. The mid-town Manhattan survey (Srole et al 1962), in which a random sample of New Yorkers were asked by non-medical interviewers about the presence of psychiatric symptoms, found them to be present in 81.5% of that population. However, Fremming (1951), studying a Danish population and using a clinical interview, found a lifetime prevalence of only 1.3% for men and 3.7% for women. Clearly, with such disparity, widely differing concepts of mental illness or minor

Table 22.1 Prevalence of all psychiatric disorder and of depressive illness and depressive symptoms in the general population. Results from five surveys.

Reference	Place	Method	Period	Depression (%)			All psychiatric morbidity (%)		
				Male	Female	Total	Male	Female	Total
Weissmann et al (1978)	New Haven, CT 1975–1976	SADS + RDC	Point	6	7	7	16	19	18
Wing (1979)	Camberwell	PSE-10	1 month	5	7	6	6	12	9
Orley & Wing (1979)	Ugandan villages	PSE-10	1 month	14	23	18	19	29	24
Brown & Harris (1978)	Camberwell	PSE	1 year	—	15	—	—	17	—
Brown et al (1977)	North Uist, Outer Hebrides	PSE	1 year	—	8	—	—	12	—

[a]Prevalence expressed as a whole number percentages for clarity

psychiatric morbidity are being used. One major advance has been the introduction of standardised interviews with clearly stated diagnostic criteria. With the aid of such instruments it is possible to produce some sort of definition of what is a psychiatric case. Unfortunately the border between a case and a non-case is blurred and most researchers have had to introduce some intermediate concept such as a probable case, borderline or threshold category, or subclinical disturbance. Despite the imprecise and vague nature of such terms there is considerable agreement amongst researchers that such subclinical disturbance consists largely of symptoms such as fatigue, irritability, insomnia and dysthymia. Table 22.1 shows the results of five studies and gives percentage figures for definite and probable cases combined. Four of the studies used the Present State Examination (PSE — see Ch. 9) and are therefore

roughly comparable. Figures are given for all psychiatric morbidity and for depressive illness alone. In all studies psychotic disorders formed a very small proportion of cases and therefore these figures can be regarded as representing the prevalence of minor psychiatric morbidity. We see that depression and depressive symptoms form a large part of the total in all studies. There is a marked sex difference in all studies in which both sexes have been examined, females outnumbering males in a ratio of between 3:2 and 2:1. It will be noted that, in the four studies which used the PSE, depression forms a greater part of the total psychiatric morbiditiy than in the American study which used the Schedule for Affective Disorders and Schizophrenia (SADS — see Ch. 12). This is in part because the PSE tends to group together cases which show both anxiety and depression and call them depression and in part because the PSE does not

Table 22.2 Two-stage prevalence studies

Area	Reference	Size of study	Screening instrument	Case confirmation	Prevalence		Total
					Male	Female	
Spain (rural)	Vasquez-Barquero et al (1981)	1156	GHQ-60	CIS	19.1	28.3	23.8
Australia (urban)	Henderson (1981)	756	GHQ-30	PSE	7.1	11.1	9.0
England (urban)	Bebbington et al (1981)	800	PSE-40	PSE	6.1	14.9	10.9
Holland (urban)	Hodiamont et al (1987)	3282	GHQ-60	PSE	7.2	7.5	7.3
Spain (rural)	Vasquez-Barquero et al (1987)	1232	GHQ-60	PSE	8.1	20.6	14.7

Table 22.3 Point prevalence rates for neurotic disorders from 1975 to 1976 (New Haven study)

	Prevalence (%)
All psychiatric morbidity	18
Major depressive disorder	4.3
Minor depressive disorder	2.6
Any anxiety disorder	4.3
Generalised anxiety disorder	2.5
Phobic disorder	1.4
Panic disorder	0.4
Obsessive compulsive disorder	0.0
Personality disorder definite	15.1
Personality disorder probable	2.7

From Weissmann et al (1978)
[a] Rates for all disorders except personality are definite and probable combined with probable cases comprising a very small proportion of the total.

regard alcoholism, organic states or personality disorders as psychiatric illness, whereas when the SADS is used approximately 25% of diagnoses are either alcoholism or drug abuse. Strictly speaking, studies which report results in terms of point prevalence, 1 month period prevalence and 1 year period prevalence cannot be compared. However, differences due to such factors are probably small when compared with the variability in case-finding techniques between studies. We can see that, as well as marked sex differences, there appears to be greater morbidity in an urban (Camberwell) than a rural (North Uist) setting and that the figures for the Ugandan villages are staggeringly high and that much of this is due to depressive disorders.

Table 22.2 gives the results of five large community studies which have used mainly the General Health Questionnaire as a screen and then confirmed cases with the PSE.

It would appear that, using the criteria of these investigators, between 17 and 24% of a Western population can be said to be a psychiatric case or a borderline case at any one point in time. Table 22.3 gives results of the New Haven study by diagnosis in greater detail.

Two other studies are worthy of note. Hagnell (1966), studying a Swedish population, found a lifetime expectancy rate for neurosis alone of 13% (7.5% for males and 17% for females). Very similar figures were found by Helgason (1964), who intensively studied a cohort of 5395 Icelanders born between 1895 and 1897 and followed up over 60 years. He found a lifetime risk for neurosis of 8% for males and 16% for females.

Community studies looking at point prevalence

rates on a single day (Finlay-Jones & Burvill 1977), using the General Health Questionnaire (GHQ) as a screening measure and defining a case as anyone scoring 12 or more on that questionnaire, have shown point prevalence rates of 13.5% for men and 18.7% for women. The lowest rates were in the married and the highest in the widowed, with the single, the separated and the divorced in between. Rates in social classes I and II were 50% of those in social class V.

The Epidemiologic Catchment Area (ECA) study

The ECA programme was a massive collaborative study designed to apply common diagnostic and health utilisation instruments at 6 month intervals to large general population samples in the USA. It included both people at home and those in institutions. Lifetime and 6 month prevalence rates are available for 15 DSM-III diagnoses. Estimates have been derived from responses to the Diagnostic Interview Schedule (DIS), an instrument constructed to provide lifetime DMS-III, Research Diagnostic Criteria and Feighner diagnoses (Robins et al 1984). The total sample size was over 15 000 with over 3000 interviewed in each of the five sites. Details are given in Table 22.4. The five areas were New Haven (Connecticut), Baltimore, St Louis, Los Angeles and North Carolina.

Six month prevalence rates

These are detailed in Table 22.5 and will be discussed more fully under the sections on each specific diagnosis.

The most common disorder in the three communities studies were phobias, alcohol abuse and/or dependence, dysthymia and major depression. The most common diagnoses for women were phobias and major depression, whereas for men the main disorder was alcohol abuse and/or dependence. In no site was the total rate of disorders higher in women than in men. This contrasts with previous findings and probably reflects the fact that earlier studies neglected to enquire systematically about male-predominant diagnoses such as alcoholism, drug dependence and antisocial personality.

Lifetime prevalence

The most striking finding and one that was replicated in all five sites was that most disorders have their peak occurrence in the 25–44-year-old age group. Panic disorder, obsessive–compulsive disorder, agoraphobia and simple phobias all showed a drop in prevalence over the age of 45 years. It is not yet clear what the explanation is for this finding. It may be due

Table 22.4   ECA study sample characteristics

	New Haven	Baltimore	St Louis
Survey date	1980–1981	1981	1981–1982
Sample population size	298 000	175 000	277 000
Sample age range (years)	18+	18+	18+
Completed interviews	3058	3481	3004
Completion rate (%)	75.3	78	79.1

From Myers et al (1984).

to an absence of affected older people because of death, emigration or institutionalisation or due to older persons forgetting their symptoms or being less willing to disclose them. There is also the possibility that there has been a true historical increase in neurotic disorders over the last 50 years. If so, then the current generation of 44 years of age and under will report even higher lifetime rates as they age.

Surprisingly racial differences were small and non-significant. For most disorders in all five sites, rates were no higher in blacks than non-blacks. Rates were higher in blacks for simple phobias in two of the five sites. For psychiatric disorders as a whole, an inner-city environment was associated with higher lifetime rates, but this did not apply to any of the neurotic disorders studied. In fact the rate for panic disorder was significantly higher in a rural setting. In general, higher levels of education were associated with lower levels of disorder but this was most marked for non-neurotic disorders.

Neurosis in general practice

This is dealt with in more detail in Chapter 33. Shepherd et al (1966) found that 8.9% of patients on a general practitioner's list consulted in 1 year with a diagnosis of neurosis (11.7% for women and 5.6% for men), and that neuroses formed 63% of all psychiatric cases seen in general practice whereas psychoses and character disorders formed only 4% each. This is in contrast to the approximate figures for out-patient referrals where neuroses account for 40%, character disorders 35% and psychoses 25%. Cooper (1972) studied eight general practices in the London area and found that depression and anxiety neuroses accounted for approximately 80% of all psychiatric cases. Most showed a mixed picture and specific neurotic syndromes such as phobias, obsessions and hypochondriases were rare, accounting for only 2.8% of cases.

Outcome

In a study of non-psychotic illness presenting to general practitioners Mann et al (1981) found that after one year 24% had improved, 52% showed a variable course through the year and 25% a chronic course. Good outcome was associated primarily with the patient having a stable, supportive family life. Being younger, male, without physical illness and not

Table 22.5   Six month and lifetime prevalence rates (%) from the ECA study

	6 month prevalence			Total lifetime prevalence
	Men	Women	Total	
Panic disorder	0.6	1.0	0.8	1.4
Obsessive–compulsive	1.2	1.9	1.6	2.5
Somatisation disorder	0	0.2	0.1	0.1
Simple phobia	4.3	9.4	7.0	—
Social phobia	1.3	2.0	1.7	—
Agoraphobia	1.8	5.4	3.8	—
Total phobia[a]	4.9	11.1	8.2	13.5
Total for any DSM-III diagnosis	17.7	18.3	18.1	32.6

From Myers et al (1984) and Robins et al (1984).
[a] Subjects may have more than one phobic diagnosis.

receiving psychotropic medication were also significant factors. A chronic course was associated with being older, having more psychiatric disturbance at onset, having concomitant physical illness and receiving psychotropic medication. Social measures and severity of illness rather than type of neurosis or personality assessment appeared to be the most effective means of predicting outcome. A study of Huxley et al (1979) in psychiatric out-patient practice showed similar percentage figures for improvement and also found the best predictor of final outcome to be the initial severity of a neurotic illness rather than any particular diagnosis.

Life events

It may seem self-evident that major happenings in a person's life, especially stressful events and losses, will predispose them to neurotic illness. In fact this area has only been looked at in a systematic way over the past 25 years and it has proved exceedingly difficult to define causal relationships between life events and the onset of illness.

Much of the work has been on depressed patients, particularly depressed women. Life events, usually loss events, have been shown to cluster before the onset of depressive episodes. Occurrences such as increasing arguments with a spouse, marital separation, starting a new type of work, departure from home of a family member, severe illness and illness or death of a family member are classed as life events. The sociologist George Brown has proposed that three factors operate: what he calls *vulnerability factors*, *long-term difficulties* and *provoking agents*. He has isolated four such influences. Three of them are long-term difficulties: having three or more children who are under the age of 14 years; being unemployed; and lacking an intimate or confiding relationship with a spouse or boyfriend. The fourth is a vulnerability factor: loss of the mother before the age of 11 years. Such long-term difficulties and vulnerability factors do not in themselves cause depression but make the onset of a depressive episode more likely in the presence of a provoking factor, particularly a life event causing loss.

Life event research is difficult and requires meticulous methodology. It is often hard to define a clear-cut onset of a neurotic episode or a well-defined exacerbation. So far most research has been retrospective and therefore subject to errors of omission, distortion and falsification. It is also difficult to decide whether events that do occur are independent of the patient's mental condition or related to it in some way. In other words, are events causes or consequences of illness? For example, if an executive loses his job and then becomes depressed what is the direction of causality? Did losing his job precipitate a depression or did the insidious onset of depressive symptoms cause him to function poorly at work, resulting in his dismissal? In much of Brown's work, events are only counted if they are clearly independent of the illness.

Cooper & Sylph (1973) looked at the relationship of life events to the onset of new episodes of neurotic illness in general practice. They found an increase in the total number of events in the 3 months prior to onset when cases were compared with controls, with a marked tendency for events to cluster in the weeks immediately prior to consultation. The type of event reported also differed in the two, cases reporting more unexpected crises and more failures to attain life goals. Only a quarter of cases reported no events at all.

It may be that whereas major events or multiple events can provoke neurotic illness in previously stable individuals, minor events have a small contributory effect which becomes decisive only when the risk of breakdown is already great because of lack of social supports, personality variables or both. It is still to be established whether life events precipitate the onset of illness or precipitate the decision to seek medical help. What evidence there is suggests the former.

Much of the criticism of life event research has been directed towards the methodology involved. What is perhaps more important to the clinician is the power of life events to precipitate illness. Though 85% of depressions are preceded by life events, there is a sizeable minority where no events are detected. Conversely, the majority of events (90%) are not followed by illness. The term *relative risk* of an event — the rate of disease amongst those exposed to the event in question divided by the rate amongst those not exposed — is a measure of the power of the event to cause illness. Using this index and counting any exit event in the previous 6 months, Paykel found increased relative risks of 6.5 for depressive illness, 6.7 for attempted suicide and 3.9 for schizophrenia.

(The role of life events and other stresses in the genesis of depressive illnesses is discussed in more detail in Chapter 19.)

Social class

Most studies show a definite association with low social class and psychological disturbance and this holds whether the studies have been done in the community, general practice, patients referred to psychiatrists or patients admitted. In Brown's original study (Brown & Harris 1978) there was a four times greater rate of caseness amongst working class women compared with middle-class women (23 versus 6%). In a similar Edinburgh study these social class differences only appeared for working-class women who had children (Surtees et al 1983). However, not all studies have shown this. Bebbington et al (1981) in their study in Camberwell found a non-significant difference between middle- and working-class women (11.1% versus 17.5%, respectively).

Social relationships

In a series of papers from Australia, Scott Henderson has looked at the interplay between social relationships and neurotic illness. He has produced evidence that a lack of social relationships is associated with neurotic illness and that the former probably produces the latter. It may not be the lack of such relationships that is aetiologically important, however, so much as the way they are perceived by the individual. In other words, those who view their relationships as inadequate have an increased risk of developing neurotic symptoms under conditions of adversity. Neurotic symptoms then emerge in individuals who consider themselves deficient in care, support or concern from those around them. In this sense neurotic symptoms can be seen as care-eliciting behaviour.

Housing

Several studies have shown a relationship between housing and psychiatric morbidity. As early as 1957 when the rehousing of families due to slum clearance was just beginning, Martin et al (1957) showed higher rates of 'neurosis' and of psychiatric admissions among adults living in high-rise flats when they were compared with those still living in traditional houses on the same estate. Other studies have shown similar findings and confirmed that it appears to be the stress of living in such buildings rather than moving to them that contributes to psychiatric disorder. More recent studies in Newcastle and Northern Ireland (Byrne et al 1986, Blackman et al 1989) have confirmed the relationship but shown that there is probably an interaction between area of residence and type of residence. In other words, there is an additive effect of type of housing, quality of housing and the facilities and general environment of a housing estate. In the recent study by Platt et al (1991) on a group of 1220 households, carried out in Edinburgh, Glasgow and London, housing conditions were the most powerful predictor of GHQ caseness. The families all came from areas of public housing where families with young children predominated. Despite the fact that the study was on a fairly homogenous population, social and economic factors were still powerful predictors of psychiatric caseness. Women living in poor housing conditions (damp and mouldy dwellings), living on very low incomes, being unemployed themselves or living in a household where no one was employed, and bringing up children without the support of a partner all had higher risks of psychological disturbance.

Marriage and family

The prevalence of psychiatric disorders in both the husband and wife is greater than would be expected by chance. Most of this morbidity is neurotic illness and/or personality disorders. This could be because neurotics selectively marry other neurotics, but studies which have looked at the length of marriage and the time of onset of neurotic symptoms in the spouses of neurotic patients have found that a more important explanation is that neurotic illness in one partner creates stresses under which the spouse sooner or later breaks down. If assortative mating of neurotic individuals was the explanation for the excess of neurotic marriages, it would be expected that the recently married would show the same or greater concordance for neurosis as more long-standing marriages. This is not the case. The longer a marriage continues the more likely it is for both rather than one partner to be neurotic.

Male patients have sick wives more often than female patients have sick husbands, though it is not simply that marriage is a protective factor for men and a vulnerability factor for women. Neurotic couples spend more time alone together, are less socially integrated and have more conflict over roles than non-neurotic couples. All these factors may contribute to the onset of neurosis in the spouse.

Employment versus non-employment

There is now a confirmed relationship between unemployment and psychiatric status which applies for both men and women. Although most studies have concentrated on the unemployment status of men, there is a relationship between rates of attempted suicide and of completed suicide and unemployment in both men and women. The Edinburgh study (Surtees et al 1983) did find a relationship between psychiatric disorder and employment status for women but other studies have not found a striking relationship between paid employment and mental health for women. It is likely there is a complex interaction between many factors and that employment for women, particularly women with young children, may bring benefits in terms of social contact, extra money, variety of lifestyle and feelings of personal identity but these may only be important if such factors are not met within their domestic role.

It is of considerable interest that all published studies on psychological disorder in employment also show higher rates than in the general population. These studies include teachers, journalists, factory workers and health professionals. Sometimes there are groups of individuals who must have lower than average risks of disorder. As yet they remain to be clearly identified and studied.

Culture

Many of the factors discussed above may not translate to different cultures. Most of the studies have been carried out not just in western but in northern European populations. One of the studies summarised in Table 22.2 carried out in rural Spain (Vazquez-Barquero et al 1987) did not show any relationship between psychiatric morbidity and unemployment, low social class or child care, though it continued to find much higher rates amongst women than men. It also found different patterns of symptom presentation with much higher rates of phobic disorders and for women a reversal of the usually found excess of depressive as opposed to anxiety symptoms. Similar cultural variations in the ratio between presentation of depression versus anxiety have been found in another study which compared Greeks, Greek-Cypriots living in the UK and Londoners (Mavreas & Bevington 1988). It may be that cultural factors are the most powerful factors in determining which vulnerability and which stress factors increase the risk of minor psychiatric morbidity.

Mortality

Neurosis does not cause death, but those with neuroses do appear to die prematurely. Hospitalised neurotics have about 1.5 times the risk of death of normal controls. This is partly due to suicide, and partly to accidental death (which may not always be accidental). Alcoholism and drug abuse account for other deaths. Whether a neurotic mental state can precipitate a potentially fatal physical illness is still uncertain. It is possible, though, that the association of the 'type A' behaviour pattern and coronary artery disease may be an example of this. Type A behaviour is characterised by striving, an intense commitment to vocational goals, impatience and ambition. More relaxed people who do not display these goals are labelled as type B (see Ch. 27). A recent study followed up 3302 patients from Stockholm County, Sweden. These patients had all been discharged with a diagnosis of anxiety disorder between 1973 and 1986. They found a definite excess mortality with a ratio of observed-expected deaths amongst men of 2.21 and amongst women of 2.49. This excess was nearly all due to suicide. Lower rates of death from other causes such as malignancy and cardiovascular disorders were found but this may have been because of the strong influence of premature death by unnatural causes and the relatively short follow-up period. An interesting subsidiary finding of the study was the lack of any influence of drug treatment. Within the sample just over 500 had been treated in units with an express policy of not prescribing anxiolytic drugs. They were compared with a similar-sized group who were treated in units with a more positive attitude and practice of anxiolytic drug therapy. No differences in mortality were found. The authors concluded that the risk of suicide for patients with anxiety disorders severe enough to warrant admission may be as high as patients with depressive illness who require in-patient care.

Physiological factors

It is well established that increase in heart rate, increase in forearm blood flow, decrease in finger pulse volume, decrease in salivation and augmentation of sweat gland and electromyogram (EMG) activity are physiological responses associated with arousal. The electroencephalogram (EEG) shows a more alert pattern with diminished alpha and increased beta activity. These changes occur in aroused individuals whether or not arousal is accompanied by anxiety and there are no physiological changes which are pathognomonic of anxiety. One possible exception is the different pattern of habituation of the galvanic skin response (GSR) to a standard stimulus in patients with thyrotoxicosis and with anxiety states. Both groups are aroused but the thyrotoxic group show a normal habituation pattern whereas in anxiety states increased arousal is associated with decreased habituation. It has also been shown that an intravenous infusion of sodium lactate produces attacks of panic much more frequently in patients with a diagnosis of anxiety disorder than in controls. Infusions of glucose of normal saline do not have this effect. (This phenomenon is discussed more fully under the heading 'Panic disorder'.)

Childhood behaviour and adult neurosis

The relationship between behaviours in childhood and neurotic illness in adult life has been reviewed by Rutter (1972). He concluded that although there was some continuity between child and adult neurosis, most neurotic children become normal adults and most neurotic adults develop their neurosis only in adult life. Most of the evidence of a positive relationship comes from retrospective assessments of adult neurotic populations, and even when these are compared with carefully matched controls the possibility of retrospective distortion makes firm conclusions difficult to draw. Robins (1966) followed up a group of 5000 child psychiatric patients for a 30 year period and compared them with a matched control group of 100 normal children. She found that most of the children who were referred for neurotic problems did not suffer from neurosis as adults and that those adults who did show neurotic symptoms were just as likely to have been in the control group as children as in the child psychiatric clinic group. Mellsop (1972) followed up a group of 3000 children who had presented to an Australian child psychiatric clinic 20 years earlier. He found that child psychiatric patients were three times as likely as controls to receive psychiatric treatment as adults but that there was little correlation between particular symptom patterns in childhood and adult life.

One interesting and consistent finding is that whereas in adults there is a preponderance of females with neurosis, in children there is an excess of boys. This change in sex distribution takes place during adolescence. Its significance is not clear. It may be that adult female neurotics are more likely to seek and accept treatment from doctors than their male counterparts, or that neurotic symptoms evaporate during adolescence in males, or that males cope with stresses and anxieties with different behaviours such as alcohol and drug abuse in adult life. The so-called 'neurotic traits' of childhood such as thumb sucking, nail biting, food fads, stammering and bed wetting seem to have little association with either childhood or adult neurosis. There are all quite common phenomena and are usually not indicative of maladjustment or psychiatric disorder.

So far only the relationship between child and adult neurosis has been considered. Very little is known about other childhood behaviours or personality traits in children that may be associated with adult neurosis, and there is a need for prospective developmental studies continuing into adult life. One exception to this is a small study by Wolff & Chick (1980) who followed up a group of 22 young men diagnosed in childhood as having schizoid personalities. Ten years later, 18 out of 22 were still diagnosed as schizoid, compared with only one out of 22 controls. Clearly, there was still something distinctive about these formerly diagnosed schizoid individuals despite the vicissitudes of the intervening years from childhood to adulthood. Studies which have looked at non-neurotic adult populations who are high achievers, such as top-grade jet fighter pilots, show that there is an excess of first-born children, and that such people tend to have had unusually close father–son relationships.

SPECIFIC NEUROTIC SYNDROMES

CLASSIFICATION: ICD-10 AND DSM-IIIR

ICD-10 represents a considerable change from ICD-9. Unlike DSM-III the term neurosis is retained but only to cover the whole group of syndromes, viz. 'neurotic, stress-related and somatisation disorders'. Individual syndromes are referred to as disorders, so generalised anxiety neurosis became generalised anxiety disorder. Several new terms are introduced, mostly derived from DSM-III; these include panic disorder and somatisation disorder. The term neurasthenia is retained but it is recognised that in many if not most countries such cases would be diagnosed as depressive or anxiety disorder.

Table 22.6 compares the classification of pathological anxiety as described by ICD-9, ICD-10, DSM-III and DSM-IIIR. There seems to be agreement that panic disorder justifies separate status but ICD-10 has not taken the view that panic disorder should take precedence in a hierarchical sense over agoraphobia and that the latter should become a subtype of panic disorder. ICD-10 keeps obsessive compulsive disorder as a separate category of neurosis but DSM-IIIR includes it under the anxiety disorders. A new category of organic anxiety syndrome has also been included in DSM-IIIR. Organic factors include such stimulants as amphetamine-containing products and caffeine. This parallels the similar category in DSM-III of organic affective syndrome.

Both ICD-10 and DSM-IIIR include the category of generalised anxiety disorder. This is a residual

Table 22.6 Classification of pathological anxiety

ICD-9	Proposed ICD-10	DSM-III	DSM-IIIR	Main diagnostic features
	Post-traumatic stress disorder	Post-traumatic stress disorder — acute 308.3 Post-traumatic stress disorder — chronic or delayed 309.81	As DSM-111	Time-limited anxiety linked to marked stressful events
Acute stress reaction 308.0	Acute stress reaction			
Adjustment reaction 309.2	Adjustment disorder			
Anxiety states 300.0	Generalised anxiety disorder	Generalised anxiety disorder 300.02	As DSM-111	Not situational anxiety
	Panic disorder	Panic disorder	Panic disorder uncomplicated	Acute attacks of anxiety
Phobic state 300.2	Agoraphobia	Agoraphobia 300.22 Agoraphobia with panic 300.21	Panic disorder with limited phobia avoidance Panic disorder with agoraphobia Agoraphobia without panic	
	Social phobias Specific (isolated) phobias Illness phobias (nosophobia)	Social phobia Simple phobia	Social phobia Simple phobia	Situational anxiety
		Somatisation disorder 300.81		Somatic anxiety with fears of physical disease
Hypochondriasis 300.7	Hypochondriacal syndrome			
OCD classified separately		Obsessive–compulsive disorder	Obsessive–compulsive disorder	
			Organic anxiety syndrome	Anxiety specifically secondary to organic factors eg caffeine, amphetamines

category for patients with anxiety symptoms but no panic or agoraphobic symptoms. The DSM-IIIR criteria are stricter than those of DSM-III used to be.

PANIC DISORDER

This syndrome was first given separate status by DSM-III, and ICD-10 also has a separate category of panic disorder subtitled 'episodic anxiety'. The decision is still a controversial one and the boundaries between panic disorder and generalised anxiety disorder and panic disorder and agoraphobia are by no means clear.

Clinical picture

The essential features are recurrent attacks of severe anxiety (panic) which are not restricted to any particular situation or set of circumstances and are therefore unpredictable. The dominant symptoms vary from individual to individual, but include the sudden onset of palpitations, sweating, trembling and feelings of unreality (depersonalisation and/or derealisation). There is almost always a secondary fear of dying, losing control or going mad. Typically, individual attacks last only for a few minutes, though they may last longer.

A common complication is the development of anticipatory fear of helplessness or loss of control during a panic attack, so that the individual may become reluctant to be alone or in public places away from home. Similarly, a panic attack occurring in a specific situation — e.g. on a bus — may lead to the development of a specific phobia of that setting.

Panic disorder may in this way result in the development of agoraphobia or specific phobias.

When taking the history it is important to ask about subthreshold panic attacks. As well as full-blown episodes, patients may have near-panic attacks which do not quite meet the full criteria but may still be markedly handicapping and lead to definite avoidance.

Diagnostic guidelines

Both DSM-III and ICD-10 require the occurrence of at least three panic attacks within a 3 week period, in circumstances where there is no objective danger. The same clinical picture occurring during marked physical exertion or during a life-threatening situation is not regarded as a panic attack. There is also a requirement that the individual must be relatively free of anxiety between attacks, though phobic avoidance secondary to the attacks may be quite marked. If the patient has extensive depressive symptomatology around the time the attacks start, or if there is a history of recurrent depressive disorder, then it is likely that the panic attacks are symptomatic of a depressive illness and this diagnosis should take precedence.

Epidemiology

Figures from the ECA study show consistent findings across the five sites, with a 6 month prevalence of DSM-III panic disorder of between 0.6 and 1.0 per 100 of the population. The rates are slightly higher in women; and there is no strong relationship with race, education or age. The age range 25–44 years was the highest period of risk and the rates were generally lower in persons over the age of 65 years. These findings support earlier data. The 1975 New Haven study found a current prevalence rate for panic disorder of 0.4 per 100. In this study 17% of the subjects with panic disorder had at some time in their life had a diagnosis of some other anxiety disorder. The New Haven study also showed that only about one-quarter of subjects with any current anxiety disorder had received treatment specifically for that disorder in the past year, though in fact they were high utilisers of health facilities for non-psychiatric reasons. In particular, subjects with panic disorders were the highest users of psychotropic drugs, especially minor tranquilisers. The 1979 National Survey of Psychotherapeutic Drug Use (Uhlenhuth 1983) used different diagnostic groupings, and agoraphobia and panic were considered together. Annual prevalence rates were 0.5 per 100 for males and 1.8 per 100 for females, giving a total of 1.2%. Again, use of antianxiety agents was highest in the agoraphobic–panic group.

Family studies

There is increasing evidence of a familial transmission of panic disorder. Crowe et al (1983) found a morbidity risk for panic disorder in the first-degree relatives of panic disorder patients of 17.3% definite and an additional 7.4% probable. These rates were significantly higher than control relatives at 1.8 and 0.4%. The risk of panic disorder was twice as high in female as in male subjects. The rate of generalised anxiety disorder was the same in both groups of families and no other psychiatric disorders were increased in the families of patients with panic disorder.

The sex ratio findings are important because sex differences are difficult to interpret in clinical populations as they may simply reflect one sex preferentially seeking treatment. These findings are from a family study and represent an unselected population, suggesting that the sex ratio is characteristic of the disorder and not a result of selection bias. The finding of no excess of relatives with generalised anxiety disorder, alcoholism or primary depression supports the separation of panic from other disorders by DSM-III and ICD-10.

Biological aspects of panic disorder

Since 1967 it has been known that the intravenous infusion of 0.5 mol/l sodium lactate induces clinical panic attacks in some individuals. Recently there has been renewed interest in this area because of the finding that patients with panic disorder, but not normal controls, become panicky with sodium lactate infusion. The mechanism of this effect is unclear. It has been suggested that it may be secondary to hypocalcaemia, the induction of metabolic alkalosis, peripheral catecholamine release and/or central noradrenergic stimulation. It has also recently been demonstrated that breathing carbon dioxide produces panic in clinically vulnerable patients and does so with about the same frequency as sodium lactate. Both lactate and carbon dioxide increase cerebral blood flow and it has been postulated that there may be a hypersensitivity of the 'suffocation alarm mechanism' to rising levels of carbon dioxide and that central chemoreceptor hypersensitivity may explain both carbon dioxide- and lactate-induced panic. At present there is no definitive hypothesis for this phenomenon but it seems more likely that it is a centrally induced experience rather than due to peripheral catecholamine effects, depression of ionised calcium or induction of metabolic alkalosis.

Clinically, the importance of this phenomenon is that it provides further evidence of a biological susceptibility to panic attacks in some individuals.

Reiman and his group in St Louis, using positron emission tomography (PET), have found abnormalities in the right parahippocampal area of panic disorder patients vulnerable to lactate-induced panic. They have observed asymmetry in blood flow, blood volume and oxygen metabolism, suggestive of abnormal increases in the right side. These are the first documented brain changes in such patients. They may represent an increase in neuronal activity or a relative or absolute increase in permeability of the blood–brain barrier in that area. The changes were observed in the basal non-panic state. The parahippocampal area receives input from all sensory modalities and has efferent connections to the septum, amygdala, hypothalamus and brain stem. These connections suggest that it functions to integrate sensory information and could initiate complex behavioural responses, especially those of a defensive nature.

Ambulatory monitoring of patients with panic disorder has shown that panic attacks are accompanied by an abrupt increase in heart rate of approximately 40 beats per minute and that these changes begin 4–5 minutes after the onset of a panic attack and last about 20 minutes.

Neurotransmitters in panic disorder

Functioning of the noradrenergic, serotonergic and γ-aminobutyric acid (GABAergic) systems have all been found in panic disorder. Some studies have implicated α_2 adrenoreceptor function. Serotonergic re-uptake blockers such as fluvoxamine and fluoxetine appear to be effective antipanic agents whereas serotonin (5-HT) receptor agonists such as Ritanserin are ineffective or may even exacerbate panic symptoms. It has also been found that there is enhanced nocturnal production of melatonin in panic patients and that this disappears with antipanic drug treatment. 5-HT is the direct precursor of melatonin and this study provides further evidence of the role of 5-HT in panic. At present it is difficult to see how all the above biological and neuroendocrine abnormalities are linked; many changes have been found but there is no coherent neurobiological view of panic disorder.

The treatment of panic disorder

Drug treatment

A similar confusion is mirrored in the treatment for panic disorder. Many drugs with quite different properties all appear to be effective antipanic agents.

Benzodiazepines do reduce the frequency of panic attacks but they have to be given in relatively high doses. Clinically they appear to work quite quickly, reducing the frequency of attacks within a week. Alprazolam has developed a reputation as an antipanic drug, particularly in the USA, but there is no reason to suppose that it has a more powerful antipanic action than other benzodiazepines given in high dosage. Given that these drugs appear to only suppress panic attacks and therefore need to be given over long periods the risk of dependency is high and benzodiazepine drug treatment is not the treatment of choice.

Antidepressants. Imipramine, phenelzine and clomipramine have all been shown to be effective in the treatment of panic disorder. At present it is not possible to say which, if any, of these drugs is superior, or that they have any differential effects on the syndrome. The largest study, by Klein et al (1980), compared imipramine with placebo, and in addition all patients received either behaviour therapy or supportive therapy. Imipramine was significantly better than placebo in blocking recurrence of panic attacks and the addition of either form of psychotherapy to imipramine significantly reduced the avoidance behaviour associated with the anticipation of panic.

Selective serotonin re-uptake inhibitors (SSRIs) are effective in panic disorder. Several different drugs in this group have been shown to be effective and as yet there is little to choose between them. They are probably better tolerated than tricyclic antidepressants but as with all drug treatments the evidence appears to be that panic attacks are reduced or suppressed whilst the drug is being taken but return when the drugs are discontinued. What evidence there is suggests that antidepressant drugs should be given in full antidepressant doses and that their antipanic effects develop over 2–3 weeks and that the effects are independent of initial levels of depression. With regard to SSRI drugs there is some evidence of a biphasic response, with the panic attacks and background anxiety somewhat increasing in the first week of treatment before subsequent reduction.

Psychological treatment

The key ingredient to psychological treatment is exposure, particularly if the panic is situational and/or includes phobic avoidance. Many patients are helped by breathing exercises and can easily learn to control the hyperventilation which is associated with most panic attacks. Cognitive therapy appears to be effective with the patient being taught the bodily sensations with panic attacks. The cognitive theory of panic predicts that panic disorder patients are more likely to interpret bodily sensations in a catastrophic fashion and that this interpretation leads to anxiety, which leads to further somatic symptoms. The patient then gets into a downward spiral of increasing panic. If the patient can learn to recognise the early signs of a panic attack and to reassign these symptoms to a less stressful cause then panic attacks may be aborted.

GENERALISED ANXIETY DISORDER (GAD)

Introduction

Now that both DSM-III and ICD-10 have separated panic disorders from anxiety states, generalised anxiety disorder has become a residual category containing patients who have anxiety symptoms without panic attacks, agoraphobia or other marked phobic symptoms. What used to be called anxiety neurosis has now become a much narrower concept. Much of the research in this area carried out before 1980 relates to the older, wider definition and studies of patients with anxiety states or anxiety neurosis included patients with panic attacks and significant phobic symptoms. Even before DSM-III, most classifications separated anxiety neurosis from phobias despite the large areas of overlap. The majority of patients with phobias have some degree of generalised anxiety and many with anxiety states find that their anxiety wells up into panic attacks from time to time. The biggest area of overlap would appear to be with agoraphobia, which seems in many respects identical to anxiety neurosis, and the term phobic anxiety neurosis has been proposed as an alternative to agoraphobia. The rest of the phobias are sufficiently distinct on clinical, prognostic and therapeutic grounds to justify separate diagnostic categories.

The second problem is the relationship between normal and abnormal anxiety. Anxiety disorder is not synonymous with anxiousness, which is a symptom rather than a syndrome. Anxiety symptoms and attacks can occur as a part of any psychiatric illness. It is only when they occur in the absence of other significant psychiatric symptoms that a diagnosis of anxiety disorder should be made. The third problem is the differentiation of anxiety states from minor depressive disorders and this is dealt with later in this chapter.

In 1869 an American physician, Beard, described the condition of *neurasthenia* or nervous exhaustion. It was a global term probably more inclusive than our present concept of anxiety neurosis. We owe the latter term to Freud (1894; *Angstneurose*), who separated the syndrome of anxiety neurosis from neurasthenia in a description which has stood the test of time.

Clinical picture

Two clinical pictures predominate, acute and chronic. Acute anxiety states are of sudden onset, often occurring as a reaction to severe external stress and sometimes occurring in apparently stable personalities with low trait anxiety. They generally have a short course with a good prognosis, resolving completely. Such episodes are rarely seen by psychiatrists and are usually dealt with by general practitioners. They can to some extent be considered as a normal reaction to stress. Chronic anxiety states run a prolonged course, waxing and waning, and may or may not be associated with events or circumstances which the patient perceives as stressful. Such individuals are often described by relatives as 'always having been a bit nervous' or 'tending to worry a lot', indicating previous high trait anxiety.

The symptoms of the two syndromes are essentially the same; it is the course that is different. Attacks of anxiety are the central feature of both. These usually begin suddenly. The patient feels afraid, perhaps about the future, perhaps about his sudden change in state. He may feel he is about to die or lose control and there may be subjective feelings of depersonalisation and/or derealisation. Pure psychic anxiety without accompanying somatic symptoms is unusual but a few patients complain only of feelings of dread, foreboding, an impending panic or marked depersonalisation. On examination, there will be tachycardia, tachypnoea, tremor, hyperactive deep reflexes, dilated pupils, and coarse bilateral tremor present at rest but worse on intention. Over-breathing may lead to hypocapnia and tetany. The somatic symptoms of anxiety may occur without psychic ones and there is some evidence that less intelligent patients are rather more prone to somatise their anxiety.

The frequency with which different symptoms occur in anxiety states is listed in Table 22.7. Points worthy of note are the large and varied number of somatic symptoms and the frequency of symptoms such as chest pain, nausea/vomiting and loss of weight.

Table 22.7 Symptoms of anxiety (modified from Noyes et al 1980). All figures are percentages

Symptom	Psychological anxiety states	Normal controls	Symptom	Mixed anxiety states	Normal controls	Symptom	Somatic anxiety states	Normal controls
Attacks of nervousness	88	15	Fatigue, tiredness	75	22	Palpitations	73	17
Persisting nervousness	80	16	Restlessness	71	23	Headaches	69	37
Poor concentration	54	12	Irritability	69	9	Muscle aches, tensions	68	23
Fear of nervous breakdown	43	6	Dyspnoea, choking sensations	64	14	Sweating, flushing, chilly sensations	68	17
Fear of death or dying	42	11	Insomnia	64	14	Dizziness, vertigo	63	10
			Abdominal pain, discomfort	63	21	Paraesthesias	62	22
			Chest pain, discomfort	62	14	Trembling, shaking	57	12
			Fainting lightheadedness	62	9	Nausea, vomiting	53	12
			Weakness	55	7	Tinnitus	50	13
			Loss of libido	52	14	Dry mouth	44	9
						Loss of weight	41	6
						Urinary frequency	42	12
						Blurred vision	40	7

Symptom pattern

To some extent this appears to depend on where and by whom such patients are seen. The classic study of Wheeler et al (1950) using specific diagnostic criteria was carried out in a cardiologist's private practice. Only 18% of patients in that study had consulted a psychiatrist. Not surprisingly, very high rates of cardiovascular symptoms were reported. Wheeler also found that the course was usually chronic and that other psychiatric syndromes did not appear when patients were followed up. Anxiety neurotics who present to psychiatrists may be atypical. Such a group was described by Woodruff et al (1972). They found that less than half their patients had an uncomplicated anxiety neurosis and suggested that other problems, particularly secondary depression and the development of alcohol dependency, were important in bringing patients with anxiety neuroses to a psychiatrist.

Mitral valve prolapse

A number of studies have shown that up to a third of patients with anxiety disorders have structural and functional mitral valve lesions. This has led to the suggestion that this physical finding may be of aetiological importance in the development of anxiety disorders and that palpitations induced by mitral valve prolapse might lead to panic attacks. However, when a group of unselected patients with mitral valve prolapse are examined, one finds no excess of patients with anxiety symptoms. Mazza et al (1986), in a controlled study, found no difference between valve prolapse patients and controls with respect to anxiety symptoms. They suggest that if any hypothesis is tenable it is that there are a group of patients suffering from anxiety disorders who develop prolapse because of the increased demands placed on their cardiovascular systems by anxiety.

Diagnostic criteria

DSM-III requires persistent anxiety of at least 1 month's duration and at least three symptoms from a group of four categories which are broadly labelled motor tension, autonomic hyperactivity, apprehensive expectation and problems with vigilance and scanning. ICD-10 is very similar but stipulates that symptoms should have been present on most days for several weeks on end. In DSM-IIIR symptoms have to be present for 6 months and at least six from an 18-item list of commonly associated symptoms have to be present. Finally, GAD is no longer a residual category.

Patients with simple and social phobias frequently do not have generalised anxiety: when they do, recognition of an associated GAD may have important treatment implications. Under DSM-IIIR it is possible to make concurrent diagnoses of phobic disorder and GAD.

Tyrer's (1984) review of the classification of anxiety suggests that a formal category of mixed states with both anxiety symptoms and other neurotic symptoms should be introduced, as anxiety–phobic states, anxiety–depression and anxiety–depersonalisation all occur commonly. Barlow et al (1986) have provided some support for this view. On examining a cohort of

108 anxiety disorder patients, they found that nearly all met the vague criteria for GAD as well as meeting criteria for panic disorder or agoraphobia, and that a group of GAD patients could not be distinguished by severity or chronicity. They suggest that the nature of the anticipatory anxiety is crucial. In other words, what are the patients worrying about? If they are worrying about their next panic attack or social encounter then this generalised anxiety can be seen as part of the panic disorder or social phobia. If, however, the focus of their apprehensive expectation is multiple life circumstances, then a separate diagnosis of GAD may be considered. They suggest that there is a group of chronic worriers who worry about all sorts of past and future events and that these events may be quite unrelated to the primary diagnosis of panic or phobic disorder. Such patients would warrant the additional diagnosis of GAD.

Differential diagnosis

Physical illnesses which produce similar symptoms include thyroid disease (particularly hyperthyroidism), parathyroid disease, phaeochromocytoma, and cardiac conditions such as angina pectoris, paroxysmal atrial tachycardia and mitral valve prolapse. The latter may affect up to 5% of the population but is easily diagnosed by auscultation and ultrasound scan.

Anxiety is a common symptom of many psychiatric disorders and diagnosis of anxiety disorder should only be made in the absence of evidence for other psychiatric diagnoses. The most difficult decision to make is to distinguish anxiety disorder from depression. It is important not to miss a treatable condition such as primary depressive disorder. Mixed states are common and it is often impossible to decide whether anxiety or depression is primary. DSM-III has a hierarchical relationship between depression and anxiety, with depression taking precedence. In much the same way that they have claimed to distinguish between neurotic and endogenous depression, the Newcastle group (Roth et al 1972) have distinguished between anxiety states and reactive depression. Their studies were based entirely on an in-patient population and were distorted by the inclusion of some endogenous depressives. They therefore tell us little about the validity of such a differentiation in general practice where these conditions are most commonly encountered. On present evidence there is no satisfactory way of separating out which is the primary disorder in patients with a mixed anxiety depression syndrome unless one set of symptoms clearly precedes the other. Nor it is possible to say

whether anxiety and depression should be placed on opposite ends of a continuum or regarded as dichotomous categories.

Tyrer (1979) has suggested the following steps in the assessment of the significance of anxiety as a symptom:

1. Is the anxiety pathological? A complaint of anxiety without any evidence of physiological or behavioural abnormality suggests that the anxiety may be normal.
2. What is causing the anxiety and to what extent is the anxiety a normal reaction to the degree of stress?
3. Is any other psychiatric disorder present and if so is the anxiety primary?
4. Are both psychic and somatic symptoms present?
5. Is the anxiety situational, internally focused or free-floating?
6. What is the premorbid personality of the patient?

Outcome of anxiety disorders

Noyes et al (1980) followed up a group of patients with a diagnosis of 'anxiety neurosis' over a period of 6 years. They found that the diagnosis remained relatively stable and that the commonest change in diagnosis was to alcoholism. About 50% of subjects had brief secondary episodes of depression. At follow-up 12% were completely symptom-free, 17% had mild symptoms with no real impairment, 39% had mild symptoms, 22% had moderate impairment and 9% had severe impairment. Thus, approximately 68% were mildly impaired or not impaired at all. Factors which predicted poor outcome were increasing age, long duration of illness so far, and lower social class.

Syndromes related to anxiety disorders

Table 22.8 lists a large group of disorders, all of which are closely related to or part of anxiety disorders. There is no justification for any of these clusters of symptoms being regarded as a separate diagnostic category. A full discussion of each is beyond the scope of this book.

There has been considerable interest recently in the hyperventilation syndrome (HVS) and good review is provided by Garrsen & Rijken (1986). Respiration is characterised by an irregular sighing pattern or by rapid, shallow regular breathing. High-thoracic rather than diaphragmatic breathing is common. The syndrome is of interest because it can be provoked by voluntary respiration and because specific breathing regulation and relaxation exercises have been developed to control it.

Table 22.8 Syndromes synonymous with or closely related to anxiety disorders

Syndrome	Investigator
Neurasthenia	Beard (1869)
Cardiac neurosis	
Neurosis of the heart	William Osler
Irritable heart	Da Costa (1871)
Da Costa syndrome	
Soldier's heart (men)	Lewis
Effort syndrome (women)	Wood (1941)
Mitral valve prolapse syndrome	Wooley
Neurocirculatory asthenia	Freidländer (1918)
Disorderly action of the heart	
Hyperdynamic β-adrenergic circulatory state	Frolich (1966)
Hyperventilation syndrome (HVS)	Burns & Howell (1969)
Irritable bowel syndrome	
Irritable colon	Liss (1973)

PHOBIC DISORDERS

These are a group of disorders in which anxiety is evoked only, or predominantly, in certain well-defined situations which are not inherently dangerous. Phobic anxiety is indistinguishable subjectively and physiologically from other types of anxiety and may vary in severity from mild unease to terror.

Marks (1969) gives the following classification of adult fears:

1. Normal fears
2. Abnormal fears (phobias)
   a. Phobias of external stimuli
      (i)   Agoraphobia
      (ii) Social phobias
      (iii) Animal phobias
      (iv) Miscellaneous specific phobias
   b. Phobias of internal stimuli
      (v)   Illness phobias (much overlap with hypochondriasis)
      (vi) Obsessive phobias (usually classified with obsessional neurosis).

Normal fears occur in most young children and in many adults in some form. Mild fears of heights, lifts, darkness, aeroplanes, spiders, moths, mice, etc., are within cultural norms and do not usually lead to total avoidance of such objects. When fears become sufficiently intense to handicap the individual in his everyday life, then they can be said to amount to phobias.

Phobias can therefore be defined by the following four criteria:

1. A fear out of proportion to the objective risks of the situation
2. The fear cannot be reasoned or explained away
3. The fear is beyond voluntary control
4. The fear leads to avoidance of the feared situation.

Phobic disorders range from isolated fears in otherwise completely healthy persons to extensive fears occurring in the presence of other psychiatric symptoms. Phobias can also be symptoms of other psychiatric disorders and when this is the case (e.g. in depressions) treatment is usually that of the underlying disorder.

Epidemiology

Phobic disorders are not commonly seen in psychiatric practice. They account for only about 3% of psychiatric out-patient referrals and Agras et al (1969) found a total prevalence of all sorts of phobias of 7.7% of the population. Only 2% of those were considered to be severely disabling, giving a 1 year period prevalence of 0.22%. In that North American community sample, the commonest fears were of illness or injury, storms, animal phobias and agoraphobia, in that order. In a community survey from Zurich, Angst et al (1982) found a 1 year prevalence of all phobias, including agoraphobia of 3.0%. The ECA study found much higher rates, however. Details are given in Table 22.9. The much higher rates for Baltimore are probably due to a longer list of specific phobias being asked about in this centre.

Table 22.9 The rates of phobia by sex in three sites of the ECA study (6 month prevalence)

Site	Men	Women	Total
Social phobia[a]			
Baltimore	1.7	2.6	2.2
St Louis	0.9	1.5	1.2
Simple phobia			
New Haven	3.2	6.0	4.7
Baltimore	7.3	15.7	11.8
St Louis	2.3	6.5	4.5
Agoraphobia			
New Haven	1.1	4.2	2.8
Baltimore	3.4	7.8	5.8
St Louis	0.9	4.3	2.7
Total phobia			
New Haven	3.4	8.0	5.9
Baltimore	8.5	17.5	13.4
St Louis	2.8	7.7	5.4

[a]Data not collected on social phobia for New Haven.

Agoraphobia (synonym: phobic anxiety state, phobic anxiety depersonalisation)

Agoraphobia (literally fear of market places) is a misleading term. Although fear of open spaces is common this syndrome, the central features of the disorder are multiple phobic symptoms and a generalised high level of anxiety. There is considerable overlap with anxiety neurosis and some authors have suggested that the two syndromes should be combined. Pragmatically, a diagnosis of anxiety neurosis is made when symptoms of generalised or free-floating anxiety appear to predominate over phobic symptoms, and a diagnosis of phobic anxiety state when the converse is true.

The main fears are of open spaces, closed spaces, shopping, crowds, travelling on buses or trains and of social situations. In clinical practice it is more common than all other phobias put together. Women comprise 75% of sufferers, the symptoms usually developing between the late teens and the mid-30s. There is often much generalisation from specific phobias to other situations. Associated symptoms such as dizziness, depersonalisation, panic attacks and depression are common. Sufferers tend to be somewhat introverted and score highly on neuroticism questionnaires. The condition is probably much commoner than the frequency of clinical presentation would suggest, many sufferers not reaching treatment. Agras et al (1969) found the prevalence to be 6.3 per 1000 of the population.

There is little evidence of specific precipitating factors, though in retrospect most patients can recall some incident which they feel may have triggered their symptoms. The onset of symptoms often seems to coincide with life changes which required the assumption of adult responsibilities, such as leaving home, marriage, the birth of a child or the loss of a close maternal relationship. Such individuals tend to have exhibited marked dependency traits before the onset of symptoms. Symptoms fluctuate markedly and the course is usually prolonged. Bluglass et al (1977) found that one-third of their patients could vary within a month from being virtually house-bound to being able to move around with only minimal discomfort. This study compared married agoraphobics with normal controls on a large number of measures and, surprisingly, found that they were strikingly similar in terms of domestic organisation, social relationships and symptomatology in children and husbands. On one important point agoraphobics did differ — they had a history of having more unstable home backgrounds.

Noyes et al (1986) compared the first-degree relatives of agoraphobics and panic disorder patients. The risk of panic attacks in relatives was roughly equal; 19.9% in the agoraphobic and 19.2% in the panic disorder relatives, suggestive of a common fundamental disturbance in the two disorders. There was an increased risk of agoraphobia in the relatives of agoraphobic patients but not in the relatives of panic disorder patients. This finding is consistent with the view that agoraphobia is a more severe form of panic disorder. This has been incorporated in DSM-IIIR where agoraphobia has been eliminated as a separate category and panic disorder is qualified as uncomplicated or complicated by limited or extensive phobic avoidance. ICD-10 retains separate categories for agoraphobia and panic disorder.

Animal phobias

These are the rarest variety of phobia in clinical practice (though not, of course, in the general population) and the most clearly defined in their presentation. Women comprise 95% of complainants and the phobias are isolated with little generalisation. There are few other symptoms, no generalised anxiety and sufferers are not neurotic as measured by personality tests. Adult animal phobics appear to be childhood animal phobics who for some reason have not lost their fears as they grew up. Interestingly, animal phobias in children occur equally in the sexes, boys apparently losing their fears around puberty whereas a few girls seem to maintain theirs. Despite their chronicity, animal phobias respond well to systematic desensitisation.

Social phobias

These consist of a diffuse group of fears of meeting people or of eating, drinking, blushing or behaving oddly in public. Whereas agoraphobics who are afraid of crowds are usually afraid of the mass of people around them, social phobics are more afraid of personal interactions in a social setting. The core feature appears to be a fear of seeming ridiculous to others. Social phobics can often cope well with shopping, or travelling on buses or trains, provided they are on their own and do not meet someone they know. Unlike most other phobias the sex ratio is equal. There are usually few associated symptoms but sufferers score as neurotic and somewhat introverted on personality measures. Marked anticipatory anxiety often occurs to the extent that performance may be impaired, thus providing apparent justification for the phobic avoidance. The onset is usually in the teens or early adulthood and rarely after the age of 30 years. The course is a continuous one and abuse of alcohol or anxiolytic drugs is a common complication. Specific 6 month prevalence rates are given in Table 22.9.

The term primary social phobia is sometimes used to indicate patients who have the disorder in the absence of any other psychiatric condition. When social phobia is secondary, it is nearly always secondary to a depressive illness. Studies have shown that 20–40% of patients who develop a major depressive disorder develop some degree of social phobia whilst they are depressed and that these symptoms may persist long after the depressive symptoms have resolved. Secondary social phobia may be missed unless it is specifically asked about and this underlines the importance of asking about social functioning at follow-up after depressive illness.

It has been suggested that the term social phobia should be restricted to specific social fears of speaking, eating or performing in public and not include more general forms of social anxiety such as fears of initiating conversations or going to parties, this latter group being classified separately as avoidant personality disorder. At present, there is no empirical evidence for this distinction and it seems unwise to label such socially fearful patients as personality disordered. It is important to differentiate social phobia from paranoid ideation. The social phobic realises that his concerns are exaggerated and does not feel persecuted. A comprehensive review is provided by Liebowitz et al (1985).

Interest in social phobia is likely to increase over the next few years because of the possibility of drug treatments. In a study by Liebowitz et al (1988) it was suggested that phenelzine was a more effective drug treatment that the β blocker atenolol or placebo. In the most recently published study (Gelernter et al 1991) cognitive behaviour therapy, phenelzine and alprazolam were all more effective than a pill placebo plus exposure treatment. Both these studies were short-term and longer-term follow-up results have not been published to date.

Miscellaneous specific phobias

These are a group of monosymptomatic fears of specific situations such as heights, air travel, thunderstorms, darkness, etc. They can occur at any time of life. About 5% of adults have a specific fear of going to the dentist which is severe enough for them to avoid dental treatment. Other specific fears include fear of vomiting, of incontinence or of defecation. Sufferers who come to treatment are predominantly female and the course is usually continuous. There are few associated symptoms and low levels of general anxiety. Response to treatment is usually good but desensitisation may need to be prolonged.

Phobias of internal stimuli

In both illness phobias and obsessive phobias, the feared situation is internal and there is no external setting which has to be avoided to reduce anxiety. It is therefore doubtful whether this is an appropriate use of the term phobia, and illness phobias are described under hypochondriasis, and obsessive phobias under obsessional neurosis.

Aetiology of phobias

Phobias occur to certain stimuli much more frequently than to others and the age of onset varies with different types of fears. Infants are not born with fears but acquire them. These facts suggest that, at least for some phobias, humans have innate tendencies to form fearful links with some objects or situations, like snakes, spiders, the dark, and being alone or in an enclosed space, and that there may be critical times when these links are forged. It has also been suggested that these fears may have been acquired by natural selection, i.e. that they were advantageous to our distant ancestors. Little is known about why childhood fears become fixed in some people and progress into adulthood.

Natural history

Agras et al (1972) looked at the response of phobias to treatment. They found that childhood phobias were invariably improved 5 years later (40% were symptom-free and 60% improved). In adults, however, 37% were worse, 20% unchanged and 37% improved 5 years later. For childhood fears, then, the prognosis is good. For adults without treatment the prognosis appears poor and the majority of fears remain static or get worse. This is one of the few studies which has found a substantial proportion of those with a neurotic syndrome getting worse with time.

RELATIONSHIP BETWEEN ANXIETY AND DEPRESSION

Anxiety and depression commonly occur together and in community studies such mixed syndromes appear to be the commonest type of psychiatric disorder. We must first consider whether anxiety and depression as normal human moods can be distinguished from each other. The topic has been reviewed by Klerman (1977), who argues that four basic propositions are fundamental to an understanding of anxiety and depression as clinical symptoms:

1. The fundamental or basic emotions, such as happiness, sadness, anger and fear, are differentiated psychobiological states consisting of subjective mood, psychophysiological (neuromuscular and autonomic) and behavioural components.

2. Combinations and patterns of fundamental or basic emotions may occur to form stable complexes similarly distinguished from each other by mood, physiological and behavioural components.

3. Normal, anxious and depressive states are differentiated complexes of fundamental emotions in which the predominant basic emotions are fear and sadness, respectively.

4. Clinically, anxious and depressive symptom patterns are similar to the corresponding states in normals but are greater in intensity and more prolonged, and may in some instances have qualitatively different patterning. Simply stated, the major component of clinical anxiety is the fundamental emotion of fear, whereas the major component of depression is the fundamental emotion of sadness. However, anxiety is more than just fear, and depression is more than just sadness.

At the level of disorder at which many patients are seen in general practice it may be impossible to distinguish between anxiety and depressive disorders, either because the patient complains of both emotions equally, or because there are so few other associated symptoms that it is impossible to make a syndrome diagnosis at all.

As with the distinction between neurotic and psychotic depressions, psychiatrists can be divided into two conflicting camps on the basis of their views about the distinction between anxiety and depressive states. The separatists believe that anxiety and depressive disorders are basically discreet conditions, whereas the dimensionalists consider that no true separation exists and that a continuum from anxiety through mixed states to depression is a better working model. The validity of each view can be assessed by looking at three areas.

Clinical features

The Newcastle group headed by Roth have published a series of papers supporting the view that there is a definite distinction between anxiety states and depressive disorders (Roth et al 1972). They concluded that the two syndromes could be separated on the basis of clinical features, past history and personality. Unfortunately, these studies add little weight to the separatist argument. All the patients studied were in-patients, and therefore not typical of patients in whom mixed states are said to be common, and the bias of the observers towards a separatist view may have affected the recording of clinical data. Prusoff & Klerman (1974) used a self-report symptom check list to study female out-patients diagnosed as suffering either from anxiety neurosis or neurotic depressions. They found a large overlap of 25–40% between the two groups. They also found that depressed patients scored as more disturbed on all the subscales used except that measuring somatic symptoms. Thus, depressed patients scored themselves as more anxious than patients diagnosed as having anxiety neuroses. However, within the groups, depressed patients scored themselves as more depressed than anxious and anxious patients scored themselves as more anxious than depressed. A number of other studies have found similar extensive overlaps.

Outcome studies

The Newcastle group followed up their patients and found that those with an original diagnosis of anxiety neurosis had more persistent symptoms, particularly of anxiety, and a generally poor outcome. However, Clancy et al (1978) followed up a group of 112 patients with a clear initial diagnosis of anxiety neurosis and found that 44% subsequently suffered from clear-cut depressive episodes.

Treatment studies

An important study by Johnstone et al (1980) was based on a group of 240 neurotic out-patients. They found that depression and anxiety could not be separated either by patients' self-ratings or by ratings derived from psychiatric interviews. They compared treatment with (1) amitriptyline, (2) diazepam, (3) placebo and (4) a combination of amitriptyline and diazepam. All four groups did well, including the placebo-treated group. The added improvement due to an active drug was small and the initial severity of symptoms and the number of life events predicted outcome better. The only significant drug effects were for amitriptyline. The authors concluded that: (1) drugs may not be necessary for such conditions at all;

(2) as far as treatment is concerned a distinction between depression and anxiety is unimportant; and (3) if a drug is to be given, amitriptyline is preferable to benzodiazepines both in depressions and anxiety states.

Conclusions

There appears to be evidence for both points of view. Much of the confusion may have arisen because research has largely been carried out on patients who present to psychiatrists when the syndromes have reached such a degree of severity that some separation is possible. It may be that anxiety and depressive states early in their respective courses have similar symptom complexes but, as the severity of each condition increases, secondary symptoms appear which allow a distinction between the two to be made. Unfortunately, it may also be that the reverse is the case, and that anxiety and depressive disorders start as relatively discreet syndromes but that gradually chronically anxious patients become depressed and chronically depressed patients become anxious. Perhaps both conditions represent the same sort of reaction to either internal or external stress and the symptom pattern is determined by the personality structure of the individual or by the nature of the external events. Finally, it may be that anxiety and depressive states can be differentiated by age of onset, natural history or treatment outcome but that much of the symptomatology of the two conditions is similar.

What is clear is that mixed states are common in general practice and in the community and that no general practitioner or psychiatrist should feel ashamed of making such a diagnosis. ICD-10 has recognised this view with a new category of mixed anxiety/depressive disorder. It is likely that DSM-IV will follow suit. It is also clear that pure anxiety states are uncommon in psychiatric practice compared with depressive or mixed states. Finally, if anxiety and depression coexist and drug treatment is required, antidepressant treatment is preferable to anxiolytics and the combination of the two has no advantage. A good review is provided by Stavrakaki & Vargo (1980).

OBSESSIVE–COMPULSIVE DISORDER (OCD)
(synonym; obsessional neurosis, compulsive neurosis, obsessional state, psychasthenia)

The last 10 years have seen an enormous increase in the interest in this disorder and major changes have occurred in our understanding of its aetiology and treatment. Of all the disorders in this chapter, it is the one that has been most intensively investigated in the last 5 years.

Epidemiology

Until recently the prevalence of OCD in the general population was generally accepted to be low at around 0.05%. The incidence in patients presenting to psychiatric outpatient clinics varied from 0.1 to 4% (Black 1974). The disorder was thought to begin in early adulthood (< 25 years) with an onset after the age of 35 years being relatively uncommon. Data from the ECA study and other recent studies using the DIS show that OCD is much more prevalent than previously believed. The lifetime prevalence according to the ECA study ranges from 1.9 to 3.1%. This has been confirmed by other DIS studies with the exception of a study from Taiwan which showed lower prevalence rates of 0.3–0.9%. In a study from Edmonton, 6 month prevalence rates for OCD were calculated by age and sex. The authors found that the age prevalence curves were different for the two sexes. Both curves confirmed that OCD is more common in adults, but the peak for women occurs in the 24–35-year-old age group whereas that for men occurs later. So far this finding has not been explained or replicated in other studies.

An interesting finding is that the lifetime prevalence of OCD by age does not show a gradual increase. One would expect that, if OCD is such a chronic disorder, cumulative prevalence would slowly increase, whereas this has not been found. One explanation is that OCD is actually getting more common and that patients in older age groups have lived through the risk period before this increase in prevalence began. Another is that patients in the older age cohorts have suffered previous episodes of OCD but have forgotten about them.

The DIS studies all show that the female to male ratio is between 1.2:1 and 2.3:1 with the exception of the Canadian study where the ratio is 1.0:1. It is clear from these studies that many patients who have significant degrees of OCD pathology do not seek treatment. As yet, similar studies using other diagnostic instruments in other cultures have not replicated these findings.

Clinical features

OCD symptoms tend to fall into one of several groups: these may be checking rituals, cleaning rituals, obsessional thoughts alone, obsessional slowness or mixed rituals. Table 22.10 summarises how frequently these patterns occur. Obsessional thoughts may have a number of different presentations. The characteristic features are:

1. They come repeatedly into the subject's consciousness against his will

Table 22.10   Frequency of obsessive phenomena

1   Obsessive–compulsive symptoms on admission ($n = 250$)

Obsessions	Rate (%)	Compulsions	Rate (%)
Contamination	45	Checking	63
Pathologic doubt	42	Washing	50
Somatic	36	Counting	36
Need for symmetry	31	Need to ask or confess	31
Aggressive impulse	28	Symmetry and precision	28
Sexual impulse	26	Hoarding	18
Other	13	Multiple compulsions	48
Multiple obsessions	60		

2   Course of illness ($n = 250$)

	Age of onset (years)	Type	Rate (%)	Precipitant	Rate (%)
Male	17.5 ± 6.8	Continuous	85.0	Not present	71
Female	20.8 ± 8.5	Deteriorative	10.0	Present	29
Total	19.8 ± 9.6	Episodic	2.0		

2. They are usually unpleasant and often abhorrent
3. They are always recognised by the patient as his own thoughts in spite of features 1 and 2, and he often protests that his mind should function in such silly and senseless fashion
4. They cannot be accepted as harmless and inevitable; the subject feels compelled to try and push them out of his mind and resist them.

The commonest obsessions are of contamination and pathological doubting. The majority of patients have multiple thoughts though one particular pattern may predominate at any given time. The thoughts may have a ruminative quality with a repetitive inconclusive patterns such as 'What is the meaning of life?' or 'What is God really like?'. Other patients have fears of being unable to resist certain aggressive or sexual impulses so that they fear harming a family member, committing suicide or murdering a child. Sometimes instead of thoughts the patient is preoccupied with vivid images. These can be clearly distinguished from visual hallucinations. The patient sees clear pictures inside his head which he knows are a product of his own mind. These are often violent or sexual in nature. It is important when taking a history to ask about intrusive pictures or images as well as intrusive thoughts.

Obsessional acts or rituals (compulsions)

These are repetitive actions based on obsessional thoughts. Their performance is never directly pleasurable. At most they relieve some tension and anxiety. They often have an important symbolic quality, like Lady Macbeth's hand washing.

Obsessional ritual is a better term than compulsive behaviour because the latter is a feature of all obsessional phenomena, be they thoughts or actions. It is important to include in the definition of rituals the stipulation that they should not be inherently enjoyable. Without this it would be possible to classify some people who have urges to drink, gamble, masturbate or take drugs as obsessional, though clinically this makes little sense.

Obsessional rituals may consist of repeating, checking, cleaning, avoiding, slowness, striving for completeness, being meticulous or a mixture of these. Rituals of checking, cleaning and avoiding are the commonest, each occurring in over 50% of those diagnosed.

Typical examples are counting up to certain predetermined numbers in order to ward off feared consequences, counting all the cracks on the pavement or all the shoes in a shop window. Such rituals may have to be performed many times until the subject is certain he has carried them out correctly. Ritual hand washing is the commonest form of cleaning behaviour and is usually a response to fear of contamination. Rituals concerning personal hygiene may result in an individual taking several hours to get ready for work each morning.

It is probably a mistake to attribute a fundamental role to the concept of *resistance* so firmly stated by Aubrey Lewis in the 1930s and repeated in most

Table 22.11 Outcome in obsessional neurosis

	Condition at follow-up (%)		
Sample	No symptoms	Improved	No improvement
In-patient only			
6 studies ($n = 285$)	19	41	39
Mixed in- and out-patients			
5 studies ($n = 385$)	19	34	34
Out-patients only			
2 studies ($n = 146$)	40	26	35

Modified from Goodwin et al (1969).

textbook definitions ever since. Stern & Cobb (1978) found that 46% of their subjects showed little or no resistance to carrying out their rituals and only 30% made a great effort to resist. These authors suggest that Schneider's criterion of *recognition of senselessness* is more important than Lewis' criterion of resistance. Another important finding was that 31% of their patients performed their rituals either exclusively or predominantly in one place, and that the majority of such patients confined their rituals to home. This challenges the widely assumed view that obsessional rituals continue regardless of the environment.

Obsessional slowness

Patients who exhibit this pattern are not common, representing only 3 or 4% of referred cases. These patients have to do everything in an exactly correct manner. Their whole behaviour appears to be one slow ritual. They do not repeat behaviour unless their behaviour is interrupted in which case they may start the whole 'ritual' again. The majority of cases probably do have marked obsessional thought patterns and may be engaging in silent checking. The uniqueness of primary obsessional slowness has recently been questioned by Ratnasuriya et al (1991), who found that such patients could not readily be distinguished from other cases of OCD. Patients who did exhibit slowness nearly always did so in response to mental or overt rituals. It was of interest that 90% of such cases were male and similar high male predominance has been found for OCD cases concerned with symmetry and exactness.

Natural history

The syndrome can begin in childhood but this is unusual. It was infrequent in Rutter's series of 10- and 11-year-old children (Rutter et al 1970). Larger collections of childhood OCD cases are now being published showing an excess of boys, with long histories of symptoms before presentation often going unrecognised as disorder by either parents or child. More commonly it begins in adolescence or early adulthood and may be tolerated for many years before the sufferer seeks treatment.

The largest collection of cases so far published is from Rasmussen & Tsuang (1986). The mean age of onset was 20 years and the mean age of first seeking treatment 27.5 years. The distribution of age of onset appeared to be bimodal, with peaks at 12–14 and 20–22 years of age. Men had an earlier onset than women and only 75 of this cohort of 250 experienced an onset of symptoms after the age of 35 years.

Goodwin (1969) reviewed 13 studies whose results are summarised in Table 22.11. They show that outcome is more favourable than was thought from earlier work based on in-patient samples. The commonest course for patients with symptoms so severe that hospital in-patient treatment was required was a steady one, with occasional exacerbations often related to physical illness or fatigue and with a tendency for the symptoms to gradually wane in severity over many years. Approximately 40% of out-patient samples were symptom-free at follow-up. Only between 5 and 10% were worse and their course seemed to show a progressive decline.

The mode of onset may be acute or insidious and most studies show no clear precipitants in about 30% of cases. Depression is the most common complication but suicide is rare.

Even in out-patients the commonest course is a continuous one and episodic obsessive–compulsive neurosis in the absence of an underlying affective disorder is unusual. About 10% of patients have a chronic deteriorating course. Such patients have often completely given up resisting their obsessions. Those patients with a continuous course do experience exacerbations of their symptoms at times of stressful life events. There is a tendency for patients whose illness runs a deteriorating course to be more likely to be men and to have an early age of onset. A need for symmetry or exactness also appears to predict a poor prognosis.

Family history

Studies of family history are sparse. There appears to be a slight excess of first-degree relatives with depressive disorders, but no excess of relatives with anxiety or obsessive–compulsive states. Brown et al (1942) found a rate of obsessive–compulsive disorder of 6.9% in first-degree relatives. Although a number of concordant monozygotic twin pairs have been reported, there are no systematic twin studies large enough to justify any clear conclusions.

Biological basis

There are three main areas that have contributed to our understanding of the biological basis of OCD: neuroimaging, psychometric testing and neuro-pharmacological studies.

PET scanning has shown abnormalities of glucose metabolism in the orbital frontal cortex and left caudate nucleus when compared with controls. More recent evidence shows that these abnormalities resolve with successful drug treatment. Computerised tomography (CT) scanning has demonstrated decreased caudate nucleus size. Other studies using CT scanning or magnetic resonance imaging (MRI) have shown more diverse abnormalities. Those regions implicated in PET scan studies are also areas of high serotinergic innervation. Other lines of investigation have implicated serotonin as an important factor in OCD. Low levels of platelet serotonin and cerebrospinal fluid 5-hydroxyindoleacetic acid (5-HIAA) have been found and these appear to reverse with treatment response. mCPP (a serotinergic agonist) may produce an exacerbation of symptoms whereas metergoline (a serotinergic antagonist) produces a corresponding decrease. Treatment with a wide range of serotonin re-uptake blockers have definite anti-obsessional effects. All these findings point to hypersensitivity of postsynaptic serotonin receptors. Whether this is in response to low synaptic serotonin concentrations has yet to be determined but it may be that serotonin re-uptake blockers exert their action by down-regulating postsynaptic receptors.

Neuropsychological studies of OCD have not identified specific deficits but several studies have shown abnormalities suggestive of organic damage when compared with controls. Further large studies are needed in this area.

Differential diagnosis

Obsessional behaviour may occur as a normal phenomenon in all age groups. Rituals and superstitions may be less conspicuous in Western society than they used to be but in many cultures they still form a major part of life. Avoiding walking on pavement cracks, laying out toys in certain ways and rituals at bedtime are all normal behaviour in children. Though such behaviour may resemble obsessional rituals it is different in that children find it natural and it produces little or no distress. Many adult obsessionals give a history of obsessional behaviour in childhood. This may be due to the universality of such phenomena, retrospective distortion, or a real relationship between the two; it is not known which. However, a history of tantrums, stealing or truancy in childhood is unusual, indicating that obsessionals may have been unusually good or quiet as children.

Relationship to depression

Obsessional phenomena and depression commonly occur together. Such depressions may be secondary to prolonged obsessional illness, coincidental with it or the primary aetiological factor. In one large series, 31% of severe depressives developed obsessional symptoms. Such patients tend to have normal premorbid personalities and when their depression is treated the obsessional symptoms subside. Their rate of attempted suicide is less than one-sixth that of depressives without obsessions. Depressive illness occurring in a person of obsessional personality may exacerbate obsessional traits to the level of symptoms. It is clear, however, that OCD is not simply a complication of depressive illness. Marks has reported depressive mood swings occurring frequently in obsessional patients before, during and after treatment and that such depressive episodes continue after successful behavioural treatment for obsessional symptoms. Millar (1980) showed that obsessionals could be differentiated from other neurotics and normals by their markedly negative cognitive set. In other words, they had a negative, isolated and very low opinion of themselves, similar to that found in depressive states. He suggested that obsessional symptoms may represent a neurotic coping device defending against depression.

Perhaps the most powerful evidence is that in all the large recent controlled drug studies the anti-obsessional effects of drugs such as fluvoxamine and fluoxetine has not been dependent on an initial level of depression and the time-course of response appears to be a steady but gradual one over 12–16 weeks. Some drugs which are effective antidepressants such as desimipramine appear to be ineffective antiobsessional drugs.

Relationship between obsessional fears and phobias

Phobics have fears which are irrational but which are only evoked by the phobic situation. For example, a patient with a fear of hospitals will feel relaxed and not anxious away from hospitals, though he may get anticipatory anxiety prior to a hospital visit. His behaviour would be characterised by avoidance of hospitals and he certainly would not continuously search for them. In contrast, an obsessional who says that he is phobic of dirt and disease will in fact spend much of his time scanning his environment, seeking the very features which alarm him. He will continually look for dirt even in the cleanest of environments. A further distinguishing feature has been described by Marks (1969), who states that an obsessional fear is not a direct fear of an object or situation but rather of the imagined consequences thereof. Thus a person with a phobia of dogs will experience extreme anxiety at the sight of a dog whereas an obsessional will engage in prolonged anxious concern about contamination from the dog. He is also more likely to worry about the dogs he does not see than those he does.

Organic brain disease

Obsessional symptoms can be signs of intracerebral pathology but classical obsessional symptoms are rare in organic states. The obsessional-like manifestations associated with organic brain disease are usually motor, and usually simple stereotyped movements; and often the movement precedes the compulsive thought, if any. A typical example is the OCD symptoms that occur in Sydenham's chorea, again pointing to caudate nucleus involvement.

There is an association between OCD and Gilles de la Tourette's syndrome. Between 11 and 80% of Tourette's patients have obsessional symptoms. Pedigree studies show an unusually high number of cases of Tourette's and OCD in affected families. Conversely, 20% of OCD patients suffer from tics. These findings would fit with the common involvement of the frontal lobes, corpus striatum and caudate nucleus as suggested from the neuroimaging studies.

Treatment

Simple reassurance may be needed and may have to be given in abundance. It is important not to endorse the patient's unrealistic ideas and behaviour in any way. The chronic nature and fluctuating course of many obsessional illnesses means that long-term supportive psychotherapy is often indicated. Explorative and interpretative psychotherapy seldom help and may make ruminations worse. Offering continuing support and hope, supporting the family and particularly the spouse, and monitoring the patient's mood for signs of depressive illness are all important aspects of management.

Special behavioural treatments

These are discussed more fully in Chapter 41.

Vicarious learning or modelling. In this technique the therapist demonstrates 'fearless' behaviour by, for instance, handling 'contaminated' objects. In subsequent sessions the patient is asked to do likewise. It would appear that, in the majority of patients, modelling has little advantage over exposure alone but it may help in some cases.

Response prevention (synonym: in vivo exposure, real-life exposure). Observation shows that for many people the frequent performing of rituals does not relieve anxiety but rather increase it. This suggests the possibility that interrupting compulsive behaviour might be therapeutic. Control may be achieved in a variety of ways — by verbal persuasion, continuous monitoring, or engaging in alternative behaviour. Force is counterproductive; it only produces an angry uncooperative patient. Spouses and other family members may be enlisted as co-therapists. Such treatment can be relatively short (3–8 weeks) and seems to have enduring effects.

Relaxation. This does not in itself produce improvement and does not seem to be necessary for improvement during in vivo exposure. Research reports indicate that cognitive behaviour therapy may be an effective treatment for some patients.

Other psychotherapies. There is general agreement that dynamically oriented psychotherapies are ineffective for OCD.

Antidepressants

Claims have been made for the efficacy of

clomipramine in obsessional disorders over the past 10 years. Initially it was not clear whether clomipramine had a specific anti-obsessional effect or whether any antidepressant would work as well. Nor was it resolved whether clomipramine primarily relieved depressive rather than obsessional symptoms. Work from Sweden by Thoren et al (1980) has clarified the problem. He and his colleagues found that clomipramine, but not nortriptyline, was significantly superior to placebo in relieving obsessional symptoms. The effect took 5 weeks to develop and could not be predicted from the severity of duration of the illness, from the sex or age of the patient, or from the presence or absence of primary or secondary depressive symptoms. They also found that obsessional symptoms returned when clomipramine was stopped. Clomipramine is a potent (serotonin) re-uptake inhibitor, though its most potent active metabolite, n-desmethylclomipramine, is a nor-adrenaline re-uptake inhibitor. Amelioration of obsessional symptoms was positively correlated with reduction of 5-HIAA cerebrospinal fluid concentrations, perhaps reflecting potent 5-HT uptake blockade. Some support for this possibility comes from Stern et al (1980), who found that outcome for obsessional behaviour was related to plasma clomipramine levels whereas outcome for depressive symptoms was related to plasma n-desmethylclomipramine levels.

It is clear that a robust anti-obsessional effect may require more than 4 weeks to develop. In a recent trial by Mavissakalian et al (1985), symptomatic improvement continued throughout the 12 week trial period. It is also clear that in the absence of significant depressive symptomatology antidepressant drugs are not curative. They ameliorate symptoms and studies report 30–60% pretreatment to post-treatment reduction in symptomatology.

The newer more specific serotonin re-uptake blockers such as fluvoxamine, fluoxetine and paroxetine all appear to be clearly anti-obsessional drugs. At present it is not possible to recommend one drug over others in the group.

Longer-term and follow-up studies following drug treatment are still needed. At present the evidence is that when drugs are discontinued the obsessional symptoms return and that this may occur even after several years of continuous treatment. It may well be that patients with severe OCD need very long-term drug treatment. A sensible clinical alternative is to gain some control over the behaviours using drugs and then to add in specific behavioural and cognitive techniques to help the patient control his behaviour.

Physical treatment

Electroconvulsive treatment (ECT) is only indicated for the treatment of depression within this syndrome; there is no evidence that ECT has a specific anti-obsessional effect. Severe and crippling obsessional neurosis is always quoted as one of the indications for psychosurgery and techniques such as bimedial leucotomy, restricted orbital undercutting and stereotactic limbic leucotomy have been advocated (see Ch. 37). Reported studies are either retrospective, uncontrolled or both. They were also carried out before the advent of modern behavioural therapies. Psychosurgery should only be considered in patients with a history of several years of continuous, crippling symptoms and in whom all other treatments have failed. Postoperatively, an intensive therapy programme should be planned.

Aetiology

Neither learning theory nor psychoanalytic theory provides comprehensive explanations for obsessional phenomena.

Psychoanalytic views

Freud believed that obsessional neurosis was more common in men. In his early writings he saw it as the result of early aggressive sexual trauma, obsessional symptoms being conceptualised as disguised self-reproach for some sexual act performed in childhood. Later came the idea that obsessional neurosis represented a regression to the pregenital and sadistic stage of development, obsessional neurotics being seen as individuals concerned with conflicts between aggressiveness and submissiveness, cruelty and gentleness, dirt and cleanliness, order and disorder.

Learning theory views

It is clear that obsessional rituals are not simply an avoidance response to some supposed noxious stimulus, since they frequently result in increased rather than decreased anxiety. Teasdale (1974) has suggested that conflict arises because performance and non-performance of rituals have equally aversive consequences for the individual. In other words, the obsessional is constantly having to make a choice between two responses, both of which are negatively reinforced. Whichever choice the individual makes he feels anxious, and this anxiety may in a circular fashion lead to further repetitive behaviour. This may explain in part the intractable nature of obsessional rituals but it does not explain their original appearance.

Personality and OCD

It has traditionally been thought that the link between obsessional personality and frank OCD is a strong one and that most patients will show previous obsessional personality traits. Recent studies have challenged this view. Although high levels of previous personality disorder have been found, only a minority have been of the DSM-IIIR compulsive type. In terms of more general personality characteristics, individuals with OCD are said to be characterised by feeling that they constantly fail to live up to perfectionistic ideals, that magic rituals can prevent catastrophies and of having abnormally high expectations of unpleasant outcomes of events. They tend to give single events undue credence and may have deficiencies in the ability to link concepts and integrate them. The problem with these ideas is that they may be beliefs that are a result of having OCD rather than in any way being causative.

SOMATOFORM DISORDERS

This section deals with a wide range of syndromes that have one central feature in common: the association of physical symptoms, which mimic physical illness, with psychological stress. For clarity each syndrome is briefly described but the separation into so many different subtypes does not necessarily imply separate or differing aetiologies. Many of these syndromes are closely related and it seems likely that common aetiological processes are involved and that symptom choice may be determined by fairly mundane factors.

Somatoform and dissociative disorders

This group of disorders includes hysterical and hypochondriacal syndromes as well as a group of other related disorders where symptoms are produced without adequate physical cause. Both DSM-III and ICD-10 have abandoned the term hysteria because of its confused and vague meanings. The term functional somatic symptoms (FSS) has also been suggested to cover this group of disorders. ICD-10 has made a clear distinction between dissociative and somatisation disorders and includes all conversion symptoms under the former.

The concept of hysteria

Perhaps one of the few things that is certain in psychiatry is that no two psychiatrists can agree on what the terms hysteria and hysterical convey. As individuals we may all think we know what we mean and can recognise a hysteric when we see one. Such confidence is ill-founded.

The term hysteria is currently used in a number of different senses:

1. A pattern of behaviour habitually exhibited by certain individuals who are said to be hysterical personalities or hysterical characters
2. To indicate the presence of a physical symptom (usually neurological) produced by the mental mechanism of conversion, viz. conversion hysteria or conversion reaction
3. To indicate that a similar mechanism occurs in dissociative states such as amnesias and fugues
4. As in Briquet's syndrome or 'St Louis hysteria', to describe a syndrome occurring mainly in women with multiple somatic complaints in the absence of bodily disease and running a chronic course (somatisation disorder)
5. As a psychoanalytic term, 'anxiety hysteria' used to describe phobic states
6. As in 'epidemic hysteria', a term used to describe the apparently infectious spread of somatic symptoms or odd or disturbed behaviour from individual to individual
7. As a term used by doctors, both physicians and psychiatrists, to indicate that a patient, usually female, is exaggerating or simulating symptoms, or when a doctor feels manipulated by such a patient
8. As a diagnosis in general medicine when all laboratory tests and examinations have proved negative and the symptom cannot be explained
9. As a lay term to indicate the sudden onset of severe distress or tantrums in an individual
10. The term 'hysterical psychosis' is used by some authors to describe syndromes such as latah or amok which occur in specific cultures; and by others to refer to an acute psychotic syndrome, occurring mainly in women in Western cultures, starting and ending abruptly and lasting only a few days.

Whilst the links between some of these uses are obvious, the only thing that others appear to have in common is the term hysteria or hysterical itself.

The concept of somatisation

The central feature of somatisation is that symptoms are produced for which there is insufficient or no underlying physical cause. The symptoms are then used for psychological purposes or for personal gain.

This broad definition includes both normal and abnormal behaviour and stresses that somatisation is a universal phenomenon.

The gains from somatisation are not mutually exclusive; one or more may operate. None of the mechanisms is exclusive to non-organic illness — all may apply to genuine illness and all of us somatise at times. The gains include:

1. The displacement of unpleasant emotions into a physical symptom
2. The use of a symptom to communicate an idea or emotion symbolically, e.g. hysterical paraplegia symbolising helplessness
3. The alleviation of guilt through suffering, e.g. physical pain experienced after the death of an ambivalently regarded individual
4. To manipulate personal relationships, e.g. the spouse who says 'Not tonight dear I've got a headache' when refusing sexual advances
5. To obtain release from duties and responsibilities, e.g. absence from work or a parental role
6. For financial gain, e.g. compensation after an accident or premature retirement on medical grounds
7. To obtain attention or sympathy

What follows is an account of the main syndromes that have been described. Essentially, the diagnosis of all these disorders involves a value judgement made by the doctor in deciding that the individual is behaving abnormally; or that the patient is complaining too much, or too long, or complaining of pain or other symptoms without adequate justification.

Somatisation disorder

Multiple somatisation disorder (synonym: Briquet's syndrome or St Louis hysteria)

In a series of papers over the past 20 years the St Louis group of Guze, Perley, Woodruff and Clayton has tried to refine and clarify one particular syndrome to which they have given the eponym 'Briquet's syndrome' after the French physician who wrote a monograph on the subject in 1859. This syndrome was included in DSM-III and is now in ICD-10 under the rather ugly title of somatisation disorder. This is a significant advance and the term somatisation disorder should be retained, partly because it separates the syndrome from hysteria and partly because the syndrome originally described by Briquet is not the same as that described by the St Louis group.

Somatisation disorder is characterised principally by multiple physical complaints in various different parts of the body and appearing to affect different organ systems. The multiple somatic complaints are often dramatically described and almost any symptom can occur, but the commonest are chest and cardiac complaints such as dyspnoea, palpitations and chest pain, followed by back and joint pains and by menstrual symptoms such as dysmenorrhoea, irregular periods, excessive bleeding and dyspareunia. Conversion symptoms can occur but they are not essential to the diagnosis. Whether the syndrome is really confined to the female sex as the St Louis group suggest is not yet clear.

Such patients usually present first to their general practitioner or to a physician with multiple vague complaints. It is often difficult to get a clear history of onset, or of why the patient has come for help now. Such patients tend to be extensively investigated medically and surgically and there is evidence that they eventually undergo three times as many surgical operations as either sick or healthy controls. As well as their physical complaints they have psychiatric symptoms, such as nervousness, anxiety, episodes of depression, moodiness or irritability. Menstrual symptoms, sexual indifference and frigidity are said to be so characteristic that the diagnosis should be made with caution if menstrual and sexual histories are normal. Histories given to different doctors tend to show inconsistencies. It is often a pointless task to try and decide if such patients are deliberately malingering or whether their behaviour is under unconscious control. Marked depression and anxiety are frequently present and may need to be specifically treated.

Symptoms usually begin in adolescence and probably run a life-long but fluctuating course. The picture is thus very different to conversion disorders with their sudden onset and often quite brief course. The same authors (Woerner & Guze 1968) have found that the syndrome runs in families. The prevalence in the general population of the USA was once thought to be about 1% of females but the ECA study has found a much lower figure. It occurs in about 20% of the first-degree female relatives of index cases. There is also an excess of psychopathic personality and alcoholism in first-degree male relatives. As yet there is no evidence of a true genetic transmission of this disorder, only that it runs in families. It may well be that having a mother who herself continually complained of, and sought treatment for, physical symptoms may be a potent determinant of similar behaviour in the daughter.

Multiple somatisation disorder and undifferentiated somatoform disorder

The ICD-10 concept of multiple somatisation disorder is looser than the DSM-IIIR category: the patient does not have to have a specific number of symptoms nor is there a need to have the onset below a certain age. Symptoms do have to be present in the absence of an organic explanation and the essential criteria are 'at least two years of multiple and various physical symptoms for which no adequate physical explanation has been found'. Thus, the ICD-10 concept is likely to include a large number of cases who in DSM-IIIR would fall into the category of 'undifferentiated somatoform disorder'. ICD-10 has a further category of undifferentiated somatoform disorder where cases have 'less striking symptom patterns and the duration of symptoms of less than two years'. The validity and reliability of these concepts have yet to be tested but they probably represent a much larger group of patients than the narrower definition, particularly that of DSM-IIIR.

Differential diagnosis

The duration of multiple and varying physical symptoms should be at least 2 years. There should have been many contacts with doctors and negative results from numerous investigations, often including invasive procedures and surgery.

It is important to remember that individuals with somatisation disorder have the same chance of developing genuine physical disorders as any other person of that age and they may also suffer from iatrogenic disease. Vigilance is required to ensure that such developments are not overlooked.

Depression and anxiety are common. These are usually secondary to the underlying disorder but may be severe enough to warrant separate treatment. The onset of the syndrome after the age of 40 years is unusual and particular care should be taken not to miss underlying primary affective disorders.

The disorder is differentiated from hypochondriasis because the emphasis is on the symptoms themselves and not on the underlying disease or fear of disease.

Hypochondriasis

Just as the term hysteria has multiple meanings so does the term hypochondriasis. Again the word is used both by clinicians and by the lay public and there is overlap of the meanings:

1. It can mean a morbid concern with health and with protecting one's healthy status. Such people may be preoccupied with health foods, patent medicines and remedies to delay ageing and prolong life. Many such people do not complain at all of ill health. In fact they protest their healthiness, linking it to the measures they have taken to protect it.

2. It can be used to describe a group of individuals who seem to pursue ill health as a way of life. They appear to enjoy bad health, collecting new symptoms and shedding others as they progress through life.

3. It can describe a conviction of the actual presence of disease or fear of developing a serious disease. It is the latter sense which forms the care of the psychiatric syndrome of hypochondriasis.

Clinical picture

The essential feature is a persistent preoccupation with the possibility of having one or more serious and progressive physical disorders. This abnormal attitude to health may take the form of a phobia, an obsession, an overvalued idea (morbid preoccupation) or a delusion.

The unrealistic fear, or belief, of having a disease persists despite medical reassurance and causes impairment in social and occupational functioning. The patient interprets minor symptoms as evidence of major disease. In Kenyon's (1964) series of 512 patients seen over a 10 year period at the Maudsley Hospital with a diagnosis of hypochondriasis, the most common regions of the body involved were the head and neck, abdomen and chest, in that order. The bodily systems most affected were musculoskeletal, gastrointestinal and the central nervous system. Where symptoms were unilateral they were predominantly left sided.

The hypochondriacal reaction may present as a phobia. The patient fears that at some time they may develop breast cancer, have a heart attack or a stroke. Such individuals make repeated requests for examination and reassurance. In ICD-10 these are classified as illness phobias though few patients indulge in any avoidance behaviour. In fact there is often an obsessional quality to the presentation. For example the patient suffering with a fear of developing acquired immune deficiency syndrome (AIDS), watching and reading more and more on the subject. Unlike the true obsessional, however, the thoughts are not usually recognised as ego alien and there is little attempt to resist them.

When hypochondriasis presents as a morbid preoccupation it must be distinguished from delusional states. The delusional forms which are usually part of a depressive or schizophrenic disorder are discussed in Chapters 18 and 19 and monosymptomatic hypochondriacal psychosis is described in Chapter 20.

Differential diagnosis

The reader may rightly question the difference between somatisation disorder and hypochondriasis. In somatisation disorder there tends to be a preoccupation with the symptoms rather than fear of having a specific disease or diseases. The patient with hypochondriacal concern will want constant reassurance that he does not have cancer or heart disease. In contrast, the patient with somatisation disorder may never enquire at all about the pathology behind the symptoms and be concerned only with symptom relief. Clearly the overlap between hypochondriacal and hysterical syndromes is great, but it is simplistic merely to regard hypochondriasis as hysteria in the male.

Kenyon (1976) in a persuasive review article recommended that the terms hypochondria and hypochondriasis should be dropped altogether and that hypochondriacal should be retained only as a descriptive term. The great majority of hypochondriacal symptoms appear to be secondary to other disorders, particularly depressive illness, paranoid psychosis, schizophrenia and anxiety states. Neither Kenyon (1964) nor Lader & Sartorius (1968) in two large comprehensive enquiries could isolate a clear-cut primary state of hypochondriasis. In both studies the heterogeneous group of hypochondriacal states could on close inspection be allocated to other psychiatric syndromes of which hypochondriasis was simply a symptom.

In Kenyon's study, primary hypochondriasis, where the admission diagnosis was one of hypochondriasis only, represented 1% of all admissions. The sex ratio was equal and the peak age range was 30–39 years. Even in this group, depression, anxiety and paranoid symptoms were common. In contrast, Pilowsky (1967) described 66 patients with primary and 88 with secondary hypochondriasis. The distinction was an important one, for at follow-up 50% of the primary group described their symptoms as unremitting or continuous compared with only 17% of the secondary group. The latter were nearly always secondary to an affective disorder.

Unlike multiple somatisation disorder, the sex ratio in hypochondriasis is equal and there is no evidence of a familial tendency.

Psychogenic pain disorder

The complaint of severe and prolonged pain which is inconsistent with anatomical patterns of innervation and for which no organic pathology or pathophysiological mechanisms can be detected is the central feature of this syndrome. Patients usually reach psychiatrists after much fruitless investigation. The onset of pain may have some temporal relationship to an emotionally stressful event, may enable the patient to avoid certain activities, and may enable them to get considerable sympathy, at least initially, from friends and relatives.

We must remember that individual pain thresholds vary greatly and that what may not seem painful to one may be very painful to another. Hence the exaggerated or dramatic complaints of pain that come from some patients with minimal organic disease. If we exclude patients in whom there could be some organic aetiology (e.g. some cases of backache), these patients seem to fall into two groups; those in whom the onset of pain precedes depressive symptoms, often by many years, and those in whom pain and depression start together (Bradley 1963). In the latter group successful treatment with antidepressants or ECT removes both pain and depression. In the former, depression may be relieved but the pain remains, though it is often reported to be more bearable. The same study showed that the previous personality and background of such patients were notable for orderliness, obsessionality, overconscientiousness and anxiety and rigidity, but with no past history of hysterical conversion symptoms, hysterical personality traits or any evidence of gain. The course is very variable, but in some cases the complaints may persist for many years if suitably reinforced by relatives and medical attention.

Dissociative disorders

In ICD-10 this diagnosis has been much expanded to include not just amnesia and fugues but all conversion disorders in which definite physical and not just psychological symptoms are produced. The onset of these disorders is characteristically sudden, but rarely observed and associated with a traumatic life event or chronic, apparently insoluble life stresses.

Conversion and dissociative disorders are often considered together, presumably because the underlying psychogenic mechanisms are thought to be similar, in that 'conversion' occurs in both, the emotional conflict being converted into a physical symptom in one disorder and into an amnesia or personality change in the other. In our present state of knowledge, it is rash to invoke such an aetiological mechanism and use it to define the syndrome. However, the term conversion disorder has been retained here because it is so commonly used.

Conversion disorders (synonym: conversion hysteria)

The central feature of this syndrome is a loss or impairment of function which appears to be due to a physical cause but is in fact a manifestation of some underlying psychological conflict or need. Almost any physical symptom can be produced but the most common are those that suggest neurological disease, e.g. paralyses, aphonias, seizures, anaesthesias and paraesthesias. Other senses are often impaired, leading to apparent blindness, tunnel vision, loss of smell or deafness. The syndrome is not very common and such patients often present to neurologists rather than psychiatrists. The more dramatic forms described a century ago by Charcot are now unusual.

The syndrome should not be diagnosed just because no organic cause for the physical symptoms can be found, or because all medical investigations have been negative. Follow-up studies by Slater & Glithero (1965) and Merskey & Buhrish (1973) have both shown high rates of overt organic disease in those previously diagnosed as having conversion symptoms. Slater & Glithero studied 85 patients given a diagnosis of hysteria at the National Hospital, Queen Square. At follow-up 9 years later only 39% had no significant organic disease and some of these had received other psychiatric diagnoses such as schizophrenia and endogenous depression. Hysterial pain had been rediagnosed as trigeminal neuralgia, hysterical fits as epilepsy and bizarre paraesthesiae and weakness as Takayasu's disease. Similarly, Merskey & Buhrish examined 89 patients attending a neurology clinic and found that 67% had some organic diagnosis, and in 48% the organic pathology affected the brain. Lewis (1975) found a very different picture when psychiatric patients diagnosed as having hysteria were followed up. Out of 98 subjects 57% were well and working and in those with residual symptoms the pattern of symptomatology was similar to that when the patient was first diagnosed. Relatively few had had a change in diagnosis. Thus, it would seem that a diagnosis of hysteria, when made in a psychiatric hospital, does have some validity and that the clinical picture remains fairly uniform over time.

Conversion hysteria is characterised by the sudden onset of symptoms in clear relation to stress. *La belle indifference* is not often present and is of little diagnostic value. Lader & Sartorius (1968) found that most such patients were highly aroused and anxious. Conversion hysterics were found to be more anxious than either normal controls or patients with phobic and anxiety states. They concluded that conversion was not occurring in the classic psychoanalytic sense, or if it was it was a very imperfect mechanism. There is no definite information available on the sex ratio, but conversion symptoms clearly do occur in men. One particular symptom, globus hystericus, is apparently more common in women.

The course is most often of short duration with sudden onset and complete resolution. The syndrome while it lasts is usually incapacitating. It has recently been suggested that conversion symptoms are now beginning to be less common in non-Western countries, mirroring the gradual decline that has occurred in the West (Nandi et al 1992).

Psychogenic amnesia. This uncommon syndrome consists of the sudden onset of memory impairment, usually the forgetting of important personal information. It should only be diagnosed where there is no organic cause for the symptom. The most common type is a failure to recall all events during a circumscribed period. An example might be an individual who walks away unscathed from a major road traffic accident but appears to have no memory for the events surrounding the incident. Less common is a generalised amnesia in which the individual cannot recall anything about his past life. A picture of total personal amnesia, but with preservation of cognitive skills such as reading, writing, and knowing what a telephone is and how to use it is practically diagnostic of psychogenic amnesia. Such complete memory impairment without any other cognitive deficits is very rarely caused by intracranial pathology.

Psychogenic amnesias usually begin and end suddenly. They tend to follow markedly stressful episodes, recovery is usually complete and with no residual memory impairment. Recurrence is unusual. The syndrome is probably commoner in the young. The differential diagnosis is from organic causes, alcoholic amnesia, epilepsy and postconcussional syndromes.

Psychogenic fugue. A fugue involves a sudden travelling away from home or work during an amnesic episode. Unlike the vague wandering that may occur during a period of psychogenic amnesia, an individual's behaviour during a fugue is often purposeful. A new identity may be briefly assumed during the fugue. Such states usually last for just a few hours or at most a few days and involve limited travelling. Occasionally more dramatic pictures are seen with a fugue lasting many weeks. In an extreme case an individual may move away from home, adopt a new identity and live as such for several weeks. Again, fugues are usually precipitated by severe personal stress such as quarrels at home, or the break-up of a relationship. They may be symptomatic of alcohol misuse or depressive illness. The wandering that occurs in temporal lobe epilepsy is usually less complex and there is no tendency to assume a new identity. Recovery from fugue states is usually abrupt and complete. It is probably impossible to distinguish amnesias from conscious malingering unless the patient confesses.

Psychogenic stupor. The patient appears to be stuporose in that they lie or sit motionless for long periods but muscle tone, posture and eye movements indicate that the patient is not asleep or unconscious. The onset is sudden and stress related, unlike manic and depressive stupor which develop more slowly. There should be no evidence of trauma, alcohol or drug abuse.

Multiple personality. This syndrome is extremely rare and some doubt its existence outside literature and psychoanalysis. Essential features are the assumption of one or more new and different personalities which the individual switches into at various times. Each personality is separate from the others and appears to have no knowledge of its rivals. The assumed personality is characteristically widely different from the subject's own. Whereas fugues and amnesias are limited to a single, brief episode, multiple personality may run a prolonged course. The most dramatic cases have been described during the course of psychoanalytic treatment. The well-published case of Kenneth Bianchi, the Californian 'Hillside Strangler' who faked multiple personality and hypnosis to avoid the death penalty and completely fooled many 'expert' psychiatrists and psychologists was a salutory lesson to supporters of this concept.

Syndromes related to somatoform and dissociative disorders

Compensation neurosis (accident neurosis)

The central feature is the seeking of financial compensation after sustaining a relatively trivial injury. The term compensation neurosis implies that the patient is not faking disability but is suffering from a mental disorder. In an influential paper Miller (1961) showed that men seeking compensation following head injury had more prolonged complaints than those with more serious injuries who were not involved in compensation and that 90% improved after the claim was settled. Claimants were characterised by being unskilled or semiskilled, employed by large impersonal corporations and usually middle aged. Miller's view has held great sway in the courts despite the fact that nearly every subsequent study has obtained contradictory findings.

In fact, return to work is unusual and complete recovery rare. Improvement tends not to occur after the financial settlement. Tarsh & Royston (1985) found that family influences were important in that the more firmly the relatives believed the claimant to be physically ill, the more they relapsed into chronic illness. All authorities agree that the lengthy legal process with its long delays and multiple medical examinations and reports exacerbates the situation and that legal liability should be decided early, or a 'no fault' system of compensation introduced.

Ganser syndrome

This disorder, named after the German psychiatrist who first described it in 1897, is rare and probably not a dissociative or hysterical disorder. Ganser described a small group of prisoners who developed short-lived, florid, psychotic episodes with subsequent retrograde amnesia. The term Ganser syndrome has subsequently been used to apply to any behaviour where dementia or psychosis is simulated or to a similar presentation but restricted to a forensic setting. It has also been used in a more restricted sense to refer to cases of simulated madness or dementia characterised by approximate and absurd answers to questions (*Vorbeireden*). Subjects may say, for example, that a horse has five legs or a camel three humps, making it clear that they understand the question they were being asked. *Vorbeireden* can occur, however, in association with organic brain disease and is not always psychogenic.

Epidemic hysteria (synonym: mass hysteria, communicable hysteria)

There are dramatic accounts from history of dancing manias, nuns mewing like cats and biting each other which spread from convent to convent, and each year several minor outbreaks occur in the UK and are reported by the media. They have a number of common features: they tend to occur in women, often schoolgirls; they usually arise in an atmosphere of stress or constraint such as a boarding school or other institution; they frequently begin in an individual of high status, with a peer group then developing the same symptoms, and which thereafter spread down the status hierarchy, and from older to younger. New cases appear at times of social contact rather than during classes and those who initially deal with the outbreak are often indecisive and anxious.

A typical example occurred at the National Young Brass Band Championships held in the open air near Northampton. The conductor and leader of the favourite all-girls band had left hospital after giving birth to her first child, especially to conduct her band in this prestigious event. During the pre-performance rehearsal she felt faint and ill and these symptoms were transmitted to a few players in the band. Several announcements were made over the loudspeakers about not sitting on damp grass, and rumours spread about the toilets being contaminated and, as a result of crop-spraying in the adjacent fields the previous day, the grass being poisoned. More and more girls became ill with nausea, diarrhoea, fainting and skin rashes until eventually the competition had to be abandoned. There was no evidence of any viral, bacterial or toxic aetiology and all affected individuals recovered.

There are some reports of the same individual initiating more than one outbreak when moved from school to school.

Combat hysteria (synonym: shell-shock, war neurosis)

Overt 'hysterical' symptoms occurred on an unparalleled scale during the trench warfare in World War I and have probably occurred to some extent in every theatre of war before and since. Although the civilian psychiatrist may have little contact with this syndrome, it is important for a number of reasons. The cases of mutism, paraplegia and blindness that occurred in the trenches spread infectiously from soldier to soldier. They affected men from very differing backgrounds with differing levels of intelligence and men who had already shown great bravery. This suggests that, given sufficient stress and sufficient secondary gain, all of us may be liable to such conversion disorders. The life expectancy of a soldier in trench warfare was only a few weeks, but popular opinion fiercely condemned those who would not fight whilst the wounded were praised and esteemed.

The aetiology of somatoform and dissociative disorders

Freud introduced the term *conversion*, by which he meant the rendering innocuous of a dangerous or threatening idea by its conversion into a physical

symptom. The conflict itself was said to be unconscious and the resultant physical symptom to have symbolic meaning (e.g. a wife who has murderous impulses towards her husband finds her right arm paralysed so that she cannot attack him). The relief of emotional conflict achieved thereby is called primary gain. Secondary gain refers to the more direct advantages that being ill bring to the patient, such as sympathy, attention and the avoidance of everyday obligations. Whilst such mechanisms may make certain hysterical behaviours in some patients understandable it is doubtful if they have general applicability.

Two sociological concepts provide us with a better understanding of these syndromes. Talcott Parsons in 1951 described the *sick role* and pointed out that in our society it carried with it many privileges. The person who is sick is exempt from normal social obligations. They no longer have to work, or go to school, they are treated with sympathy and understanding by those around them, they are allowed to show weakness and distress. The only obligation on such a sick person is to seek appropriate help and accept the treatment that is offered. Children are particularly adept at prolonging the sick role after minor childhood illnesses and this behaviour is often tolerated for a few days by mothers. Most of us can probably remember the pleasures of being treated as sick whilst feeling quite well, after the toxic phase of a childhood illness had passed.

The second concept is that of *illness behaviour* (Mechanic 1962). This term refers to the ways in which given symptoms may be differentially perceived, evaluated and acted (or not acted) upon by different kinds of persons. Illness behaviour, therefore, describes the actions of the patient. This includes his behaviour when ill. He may be stoical and restrained or histrionic and dramatising. His communication may be entirely verbal or may take the form of physical dysfunction which is displayed for the doctor to see with a minimum of verbal description. It also includes his attitude to those involved in his diagnosis and treatment. He may be hostile, suspicious, fearful, flirtatious, pleading, aloof, or excessively cooperative and agreeable. There are marked cultural and ethnic differences in illness behaviour. Most workers have compared Mediterranean and Anglo-Saxon cultural groups and found that the former are more likely to show hypochondriacal concern, manifest more conviction as to the presence of serious physical illness and take a more somatic view of illness. Pain thresholds are reported as 'painful' by subjects of Italian or Jewish backgrounds but described as 'warm' by subjects of north European origin.

Illness behaviour may be a learned phenomenon. People's behaviour when ill may depend as much on their previous experience of illness, illness behaviour they have observed in others and the rewards their previous behaviour has received as on the severity of the illness itself.

If we combine these two concepts we can see much hysterical and hypochondriacal behaviour as a resort to the 'sick role' at times of stress. To a few people the normal demands of life are so onerous that the sick role is preferable most of the time. Such people, because of lack of ability, feelings of vulnerability, insecurity or low self-esteem, may feel that only when ill do they receive sufficient love, sympathy or attention from other people. To others the sick role only becomes attractive at times of particular stress. Stresses may include the impending break-up of relationships, or fear of debt or imprisonment. A good example is what used to be called 'shell-shock' or 'combat neurosis' and was reported from many theatres of war. Presumably the advantages of the sick role are greatly increased if you are in active combat where either fighting or deserting may mean that you get shot.

Neither of these concepts involves any judgement by the doctor as to whether the processes involved are conscious or unconscious. Nor is such a decision particularly helpful in the management of patients with these syndromes.

Management of somatoform and dissociative disorders

Doctors, like other people, do not like to feel they are being manipulated or 'conned' by patients and have a tendency when they feel this is happening to confront patients with their views about the basis of their symptoms. Patients are usually very sensitive to any insinuation that their symptoms are not genuine, so such confrontations often end in disaster, with the patient angry and resentful and often discharging himself from treatment. The doctor usually sees such behaviour as a vindication of his point of view and feels content that he has made the right diagnosis. The patient, though, is left with his symptoms and by the very nature of the disorders under discussion will continue to complain and suffer and probably seek help from other specialists. One of the great weaknesses of the psychoanalytic view of such disorders is that a distinction has to be made between conscious and unconscious motivation. The former is

malingering and is therefore strongly disapproved of; the latter is illness, viz. hysteria, which is worthy of concern and treatment. In clinical practice it is usually impossible to make any such clear distinction. It is likely in the majority of cases that the patient's awareness and insight into his behaviour varies with time and with the degree of stress or threat he feels subject to.

The best approach is not confrontation but to emphasise that the symptoms are familiar, that serious physical illness has been excluded and that full recovery can be expected. It is usually unwise to get into arguments about the cause of the symptoms or underlying disorder. Physical, radiological and laboratory examinations should be completed as quickly as possible with the minimum of drama and attention and the symptoms should then be ignored. A team approach to such problems is vitally important: all members of staff and family members who have contact with the patient should adopt the same approach. It is common for such patients to seek out the most junior nurse or medical student who will innocently take great interest in their fascinating symptoms. The main aim is to minimise the advantages of the sick role and to try and ensure that the patient receives no attention or rewards for sick behaviour. Conversely, he should receive praise and interest from staff and family for healthy behaviour. It is important that the patient be allowed to discard his symptoms without losing self-esteem, so gradual recovery should be the aim. With such an approach the relief of conversion symptoms can be confidently expected.

An added advantage of this approach is that it is unlikely to prolong symptoms or create secondary handicaps. Even in more intractable disorders where recovery seems less likely it will often allow a partial recovery of function and will help relatives to deal more firmly and appropriately with the 'sick' member in the family. For example, a bed-ridden patient with weak or paralysed legs would be given a gradual programme of tasks to achieve. Starting with passive leg exercises in bed, gradually moving to active ones 'to build up the muscles', then sitting on the bed with his feet on the floor, standing by the bed with support, standing with a Zimmer frame, walking a few steps with the frame, etc. All complaints of muscle aches and pains should be ignored or answered only briefly and much praise and attention should be given for each task the patient achieves. This may not sound a very 'psychological' treatment but it is likely to be much more effective than attempting to explore the unconscious meaning of the patient's bed-ridden state. This approach, then, concentrates on the patient's adoption of the sick role rather than on the actual symptoms or their psychodynamic significance.

Pilowsky (1983) has suggested that in the management of these disorders it is important to distinguish between illness experience, illness statements and illness behaviours. A patient who makes multiple illness statements may manifest few illness behaviours and be leading a reasonably active and productive life. Hypochondriasis, for example, may be a coping, defensive style and sympathetic listening and reassurance may be what is required. In contrast, a patient with much illness behaviour as well may require different management.

ABNORMAL STRESS REACTIONS AND ADJUSTMENT DISORDERS

The proposed ICD-10 classification has three categories: acute stress reaction, post-traumatic stress disorder and adjustment disorder. DSM-III has only post-traumatic stress disorder, acute and delayed.

Acute stress reaction

After a major stressful event, some individuals develop a characteristic pattern of symptoms. These include a dazed state, with some degree of disorientation and perhaps an impaired ability to comprehend and answer questions. Autonomic signs of severe anxiety, such as tachycardia, sweating or flushing occur. There may be apparently purposeless overactivity or agitation or the subject may lapse into stupor, or wander away from the stressful situation in a fugue-like state. Characteristically these symptoms start within a few minutes or at most hours of the stress. There is usually complete resolution within 2–3 days of termination of the stress, or removal from the threatening situation. To make the diagnosis there must be no evidence of a psychiatric disorder immediately prior to the stressful event. Characteristically these reactions follow events, such as natural catastrophes, major accidents, assaults or rape. As yet they have been the subject of little systematic enquiry.

Post-traumatic stress disorder (PTSD)

This is a new category for ICD-10, but was included in DSM-III. It has received much interest because of studies of American Vietnam War veterans and because of a series of major civilian disasters occurring in the mid- and late 1980s. It differs from acute stress reactions in that the onset is usually delayed. In other words, there is a latency period which may range from a few weeks to several months, following the stress. Both ICD-9 and DSM-III suggest that the stressful event must be exceptionally threatening or catastrophic in nature, and likely to cause pervasive distress in almost anyone. For example, a natural disaster, combat, serious accident, witnessing the violent death of someone or being the victim of torture or rape. However, in a study by Horrowitz et al (1980) the same distinctive syndrome of re-experiencing the trauma is often present even when the traumatic event is not outside the normal range of experience. The typical features of the syndrome include repeated reliving of the trauma, intrusive memories or flashbacks, and vivid nightmares. These occur against the background of a persisting sense of numbness and emotional blunting. There is usually a marked avoidance of any situation which might resemble that in which the original trauma occurred. Hyperarousal, hypervigilance, insomnia, anxiety and depression are associated features.

Stimuli that resemble or symbolise the original traumatic event may cause exacerbations of the symptoms. Cases have been described where even fairly non-specific changes may cause this, such as hot, humid, thundery weather in Pacific war veterans.

There is debate as to whether the clinical features of PTSD sufficiently separate it from generalised anxiety disorder. Clearly the disorders overlap considerably but at the severe end of PTSD the constant intrusive thoughts, the flashbacks, hypervigilance and marked social withdrawal produce a quite different clinical picture to that usually seen in generalised anxiety disorder. PTSD may coexist with major depressive disorder, may present as a combination of the above symptoms and typical grief and often leads to drug and alcohol overuse.

Epidemiology

Relatively few studies have looked at the prevalence in the general population but a description of those exposed to the Mount St Helen's explosion in Washington State in the early 1980s showed a level of 1% in men and 3% in women in those who had not been exposed to any danger from the volcano at all. Presumably this background rate is a combination of individuals exposed to previous mass trauma such as the Vietnam War and to individual tragedies. Rates following major disasters vary depending on the nature of the disaster, the degree of exposure to it and whether it is natural or manmade. In circumstances such as the Piper Alpha oilrig explosion in 1988 where only a quarter of the men survived and all survivors had horrific and life-threatening experiences, virtually every survivor had severe PTSD. In most of the major disasters in the UK over the past 10 years the incidents have been sudden, but short lived. This was not true of the Lockerbie air disaster where a Pan American 747 jet fell on a small Scottish town. There were no survivors from the plane. The local community had to live with the acute effects of the disaster for many weeks as wreckage was sifted through and bodies and bits of bodies removed from the area. In this situation the threat of danger lasts only a few seconds but the continued exposure to the disaster scene and its consequences also produced a high rate of PTSD. In general, manmade disasters appear to produce higher rates than natural ones. It has been suggested that PTSD is a particularly Western disorder and that the high rates following civilian disasters are in part a consequence of the increasing lack of exposure to death and disaster in Western society. Disasters in Third World countries have been much less studied but recent reports from studies in Nicaragua and Sri Lanka do not support this view and show equally high rates and very similar symptom patterns.

The duration of the disorder may be very long. European psychiatrists frequently see patients with 40–50 years of continuous symptoms following concentration camp experiences. In MacFarlane's study of firefighters dealing with Australian bush fires, 50% of firefighters had some sort of PTSD reaction, a surprisingly high rate in a group of trained men used to dealing with disaster. MacFarlane followed this cohort at 4, 11 and 23 months, showing that the commonest type of reaction was a delayed onset with symptoms not being present at 4 months, but occurring subsequently. It is difficult to know to what extent such later-onset cases represent the first emergence of PTSD symptoms at this time or whether sufferers tolerate symptoms for several months because they appear understandable and only when they do not begin to wane do they see themselves as having a disorder.

Treatment

Most recent disasters have been followed by hurriedly set up post-disaster counselling services and there is now an expectation that such services should be available following a major disaster. Treatment of this type is difficult to evaluate and although it seems both humane and sensible to provide it, there is no evidence that it protects against the longer-term consequences of the disaster. Several studies are currently underway comparing different types of treatment for well-established PTSD with structured psychotherapies such as cognitive behaviour therapy being the current psychological treatment of choice. Antidepressant drugs may be of help in chronic, well-established PTSD. They seem particularly useful in coping with the persistent overarousal that may make the disorder self-sustaining.

Finally, it is important that our preoccupation with major disasters does not deflect attention from those individuals who have clear symptoms from an individual catastrophe. It is much more likely that a typical psychiatrist will have to deal with such individuals who have been raped, assaulted or involved in car crashes.

Adjustment disorder. This category is used in the ICD, though not in DSM-III, to describe the mild and transient states of distress that arise following life changes or stressful life events. These events are such situations as changing school, emigrating, retirement, becoming a parent, etc. The symptoms — which usually consist of depressed mood, anxiety, worry and irritability — are mild and usually develop within 3 months of the event in question. Other symptoms of more serious depression such as anhedonia, loss of appetite and weight, and loss of drive or interest are not present.

MISCELLANEOUS SYNDROMES

Dysmorphophobia

This rather clumsy term describes a condition in which an individual insistently complains about some presumed defect in physical appearance which he is convinced is noticeable to others, although in reality their appearance is quite normal. For example, the patient who complains that his nose is too big, too small, hooked or turned up at the end when in fact it looks quite normal is said to be suffering from dysmorphophobia. Plastic surgeons deal with large numbers of patients who wish to have their appearance altered and it is becoming increasingly possible to have such treatment on the National Health Service, especially if the patient is genuinely distressed by his appearance. A psychiatrist will sometimes be asked by the plastic surgeon to help in the selection of patients for surgery. From the few rather poorly designed follow-up studies published it would appear that such psychiatric screening is worthwhile. In some individuals, particularly if their appearance is essentially normal, the complaint of bizarre dysmorphophobia is an ominous symptom, for dislike of a bodily part may be the first symptom of a developing psychotic illness.

In others, intractable emotional and interpersonal difficulties have become focused on one particular physical attribute and the patient has entirely unrealistic expectations of how surgery will change his life. A psychiatrist's role in such a consultation is firstly to screen for overt psychiatric illness and secondly to make some assessment of how realistic the patient's expectations of operation are. Where a deformity is obvious surgery is often indicated even though the patient may have unrealistic ideas about the changes to his life that surgery will produce.

Depersonalisation syndromes

Depersonalisation is a quite common experience which occurs in both healthy and ill individuals. A lengthy but clear definition is as follows (Leading article 1977):

> Depersonalisation is a strange, complex and essentially private experience, one characteristic of which is the individual's difficulty in communicating a comprehensible account of it. A prominent feature of the experience is a feeling of change involving either or both the inner and the outer worlds and carrying with it a vague but uncomfortable sense of unfamiliarity. The description 'unreal' or 'detached' is usually accepted, but the experience varies greatly between individuals and between attacks. These phenomena, which occur intermittently, always have the quality of unfamiliarity and discomfort, and are recognised as changes in experience rather than in reality itself. The patient always uses an 'as if' qualification in his often bizarre descriptions of the experience, and one of the serious risks of the condition is it may be misunderstood and a more malign significance attributed to it.

The term derealisation is employed to describe the feeling that changes appear to have occurred in the environment. The patient may say that things appear smaller, larger, closer or further away, or that the room around him appears to have gone flat or two-dimensional. Depersonalisation is sometimes restricted to changes in the individual's perception of himself such as feeling dead, hollow, detached from his surroundings or puppet-like.

When it occurs in normal individuals, depersonalisation may be associated with recent emotional disturbance, fatigue or anxiety. It can occur as a symptom in anxiety states, depressive illness and schizophrenia and may be induced by drugs such as LSD. It may also be a symptom of organic brain disease. Mild depersonalisation without significant impairment of function is estimated to occur at some time in 30–70% of young adults. Depersonalisation and derealisation are usually normal phenomena, or symptoms of some other psychiatric or physical illness. Occasionally, though, attacks of depersonalisation lasting from a few seconds to a few hours form the central feature of a troublesome disorder. In such cases a primary diagnosis of depersonalisation disorder may be justified and DSM-III contains such a category.

In eliciting the symptom it is probably not sufficient to ask only about feelings of unreality as this may often produce a positive response. Closer questioning is needed to establish the exact nature of the experience. Depersonalisation can be frightening and distressing but reassurance that the experience is a common one and not a sign of impending madness may be all the treatment that is required. There is no specific treatment for the symptoms, but they generally subside when levels of anxiety are reduced.

NEUROTIC DEFENCE MECHANISMS

One of the greatest debts we owe to psychoanalysis and to Freud in particular is the description of a set of mental mechanisms which have helped to make some aspects of human behaviour more readily understandable. The use of such mechanisms seems to be universal and is not limited to sufferers from neurotic illness. Nor is it true to say they are necessarily signs of disturbance or underlying unhappiness, or that they indicate some preneurotic state. They are demonstrated most clearly and dramatically in certain types of neurotic illness but may in fact be indicative of health rather than disease. For instance, there is recent evidence that women diagnosed as having breast carcinoma and told of that fact but who then deny it have a better long-term outcome than those who fail to use denial. In a fascinating recent study, Valliant et al (1986) studied the defence mechanisms of 307 healthy middle-aged men followed up for 40 years and described the defence styles associated with coping and success. Defence mechanisms, then, are universal phenomena which all of us use at times to limit and constrict awareness so that threatening cues, either from the inner or outer environment, can be excluded.

They appear to be invoked automatically and not under conscious control and are psychological measures which allow stressful situations to be coped with by distorting reality. Psychoanalytic theory maintains that excessive use of defence mechanisms leads to eventual neurotic breakdown. However, there is no objective evidence for this and the theory could easily be turned around to suggest that inadequate or inappropriate use of defence mechanisms leads to overt anxiety and neurotic breakdown. These concepts can be usefully invoked to help in the understanding of certain patients. They are certainly extremely useful when trying to help medical students understand psychological problems and it may sometimes be useful for the patient to understand his behaviour in such terms. However, like masturbation, their excessive use may lead to blindness, and they should not be regarded as an all-embracing or comprehensive explanation of neurotic behaviour. Behavioural and learning theory approaches have as much if not more to offer in this regard and have certainly led to more effective forms of treatment. What follows is a brief description of the more common defence mechanisms which have been described.

Repression. Freud considered this to be the central and basic defence mechanisms and that other defence mechanism only come into operation when repression starts to fail. Thoughts or feelings which the conscious mind finds unacceptable are repressed from consciousness; thus repression is a way of dealing with unbearable aspects of inner life, so that aggressive or sexual feelings, fantasies or desires are thrust out of consciousness. Freud saw repression as a mental process arising from conflict between the 'pleasure principle' and the 'reality principle', indicating that when impulses and desires are in conflict with enforced standards of conduct painful emotions arise and the conflict is resolved by repression. It has been suggested that the term suppression should be used for this automatic process and that repression should be employed in its ordinary sense of 'actively thrusting out of the mind', but generally repression is still used to mean an unconscious process.

Denial. Repression and denial are sometimes confused but, whereas the former refers to internal feelings, denial is the involuntary and automatic distortion of an obvious aspect of outer reality. Thus, when a patient is told by a doctor that he has cancer this fact may be denied at subsequent interviews even though a clear and concise explanation was given which the patient obviously registered and understood. Denial is not the same as lying, which is also a common human habit. (Incidentally, the widespread use of denial is often given as a reason for not explaining such things to patients, whereas in fact it should encourage us to do this more often. Patients have a right to know what a doctor thinks they are suffering from and, should the reality prove too painful, denial offers a solution.)

Projection. This occurs when an individual unconsciously disowns an attitude or attribute of his own and ascribes it to somebody else. Children when they are angry or afraid commonly ascribe such feelings to inanimate objects or pets so that 'Be careful, the dog will bite you' or 'The table is very cross with you, mummy' are used instead of 'I would like to bite you' or 'I am cross with you'. A husband who is unfaithful, or wishes to be, may project such attributes on to his wife and then become intensely jealous of her, constantly suspecting her infidelity. A person with latent homosexual tendencies may be quick to notice homosexual traits in others.

Reaction formation. This term describes the process of developing the opposite attitude to the one being defended against. The obsessional traits of orderliness, neatness and punctuality can be seen as a reaction formation against inner feelings of squalor, dirt and chaos. Similarly, some very needy individuals who really desire to be cared for and cosseted cope with these feelings by caring and cosseting others, sometimes very successfully.

Displacement. This is the transfer of affect, usually fear or anger, from one person, situation or object to another to which it does not really belong. In psychoanalytic terms phobias are explained in this way, the phobia representing an unconscious fear of some other situation or person. Freud's case of Little Hans, who developed a phobia of horses which in fact represented a fear of his father, is well-known. Freud's explanation of phobias is almost certainly wrong and, as has been discussed earlier, a simple learning model is more appropriate. A more everyday example of displacement might be the wife who, furious and irritated with her husband for always coming home late or giving her no support with the children, vents her anger not on her husband but on the children instead. Actions such as kicking the cat or smashing plates when angry are not displacements in the analytic sense as these are usually quite conscious and deliberate actions.

Rationalisation. This is the process of justifying reasoning after the event. An individual tries to provide logical and believable explanations for his behaviour to persuade himself and others that his irrational behaviour is justified and therefore should not be criticised. A patient who consistently and repeatedly arrives late for out-patient appointments but always has a plausible excuse, and assures you that he always tries to get to your sessions on time, may really be expressing his resentment at your failure to cure him, or devote more time to him, but he tries to conceal this from himself, and you, with talk of slow watches and missed buses.

Undoing. Unconsciously motivated acts, which

magically or symbolically counteract, cancel out or otherwise reverse a previous act or thought motivated by an unacceptable, unconscious impulse. This is the main mechanism that operates in obsessional thoughts and compulsive rituals.

Regression. Reversion to modes of psychological functioning, characteristic of earlier life stages, especially childhood phases. This occurs when the individual is faced by some serious conflict in the present. A simple example is when an elder sibling becomes more infantile in his behaviour at the time of the birth of a younger sibling. Regressive behaviour occurs frequently in the context of psychiatric treatment and some treatment regimes encourage the development of such behaviours.

Turning against the self. The process through which the subject deflects hostile aggressiveness and directs it onto himself, perhaps injuring himself physically or deliberately putting himself at a social or financial disadvantage. Examples are the destruction of one's valued possessions when one is distressed or depressed and self-damaging behaviour, such as hair pulling, self-mutilation, etc.

Sublimation. Is one of the least harmful of the defensive formations. Urges particularly harmful to the person are given socially acceptable expression, for example an extremely aggressive person may select the occupation of a butcher or a latent homosexual can put his tendencies to social use by becoming a Scout master. Thus, sexual or aggressive impulses instead of being given free expression are sublimated to other activities, which are carried out with great vigour and often great success. Sometimes the term is used loosely to indicate any substitution of what appears to be a higher satisfaction for a more basic or instinctual one. Sublimation is the most effective of the defence mechanisms in that no symptoms or odd behaviour are produced and the impulses or fears in question find unconscious expression in activities which fulfil the subject and benefit others.

Compensation. This is the development of abilities to an unusual degree, to conceal or make up for a defect. The childhood stammerer who eventually becomes a great orator is a classical example.

REFERENCES

Agras W S, Sylvester D, Oliveau D 1969 The epidemiology of common fears and phobias. Comprehensive Psychiatry 10: 151

Agras W S, Chapin H N, Oliveau D 1972 The natural history of phobia. Archives of General Psychiatry 26: 315

Allgulander C, Lavori P W 1991 Excess mortality among 3302 patients with 'pure' anxiety neurosis. Archives of General Psychiatry 48: 599

Angst J, Dobler-Mikola A, Scheidegger P 1982 A panel study of anxiety states, panic attacks and phobias among young adults. Paper at Research Conference on Anxiety Disorders, Panic Attacks and Phobias. Key Biscayne Florida, 9 December

A P A 1980 Diagnostic and statistical manual, 3rd edn. American Psychiatric Association, Washington, DC

Barlow D H, Blanchard E B, Vermilyea J A, Vermilyea B B, Dinardo I A 1986 Generalised anxiety and generalised anxiety disorder: description and reconceptualization. American Journal of Psychiatry 143: 40

Bebbington P, Murray J, Tennant C, Stewart E, Wing J K 1981 Epidemiology of mental disorders in Camberwell. Psychological Medicine II: 556

Black A 1974 The natural history of obsessional neurosis. In: Beech H R (ed) Obsessional states. Methuen, London

Blackman P, Evason E, Melaugh M, Woods R 1989 Housing and health: a case study of two areas in West Belfast. Journal of Social Policy 18: 1

Bluglass D, Clarke J, Henderson A S, Kreitman N, Presley A S 1977 A study of agoraphobic housewives. Psychological Medicine 7: 73

Bradley J J 1963 Severe localized pain associated with the depressive syndrome. British Journal of Psychiatry 109: 741

Brown F 1942 Heredity in the psychoneuroses. Proceedings of the Royal Society of Medicine 35: 785

Brown G M, Harris T O 1978 Social origins of depression: a study of psychiatric disorders in women. Tavistock, London

Byrne D S, Harrison S P, Keithley J, McCarthy P 1986 Housing and health. The relationship between housing conditions and the health of council tenants. Gower, Aldershot

Clancy J, Noyes R, Hoenk P R, Slymen D J 1978 Secondary depression in anxiety neurosis. Journal of Nervous and Mental Disease 166: 846

Cohen M E, Badel D W, Kilpatrick A 1951 The high familial prevalence of neurocirculatory asthenia (anxiety neurosis, effort syndrome). American Journal of Human Genetics 3: 126

Cooper B 1972 Clinical and social aspects of chronic neurosis. Proceedings of the Royal Society of Medicine 65: 509

Cooper B, Sylph J 1973 Life events and the onset of neurotic illness: an investigation in general practice. Psychological Medicine 3: 421

Crowe R R, Noyes R, Paul D L, Slymen D 1983 A family study of panic disorders. Archives of General Psychiatry 40: 1065

Finlay-Jones R A, Burvill D W 1977 The prevalence of minor psychiatric morbidity in the community. Psychological Medicine 7: 474

Fremming K H 1951 The expectation of mental infirmity in a sample of the Danish population. Occasional Papers on Eugenics 7

Freud S 1894 The justification for detaching from neurasthenia a particular syndrome, the anxiety neurosis. In: Early papers Freud S, vol 1. Hogarth Press 1924, London, p 76

Freud S 1896 The aetiology of hysteria. In: Strachey J (ed) Collected papers, vol I. Hogarth Press 1946, London, p 183

Garssen B, Rijken H 1986 Clinical aspects and treatment of the hyperventilation syndrome. Behavioural Psychotherapy 14: 46

Gelder M G 1986 Neurosis: another tough old word. British Medical Journal 292: 972

Gelernter C S, Uhde T W, Cimbulic P, Arnkoff OB et al 1991 Cognitive, behavioural and pharmacological treatments of social phobia. Archives of General Psychiatry 48: 938

Goodwin D W, Guze S B, Robbins E 1969 Follow-up studies in obsessional neurosis. Archives of General Psychiatry 20: 182

Hagnell O 1966 Incidence and duration of episodes of mental illness in a total population. In: Hare E M, Wing J K (eds) Psychiatric epidemiology. Oxford University Press, Oxford

Helgason T 1964 Epidemiology of mental disorders in Iceland. Acta Psychiatrica Scandinavica suppl 173

Henderson A S, Duncan Jones P, Byrne D G, Scott R, Adcock S 1979 Psychiatric Disorders in Canberra. Acta Psychiatrica Scandinavica 60: 355

Hodiamont P, Peer N, Sybe N 1987 Epidemiological aspects of psychiatric disorders in a Dutch health area. Psychological Medicine 17: 495

Huxley P J, Goldberg D P, Maguire P, Kincey V 1979 The prediction of the course of minor psychiatric disorders. British Journal of Psychiatry 135: 535

Johnstone E C, Cunningham D, Owens D G et al 1980 Neurotic illness and its response to amitriptyline and antidepressant treatment. Psychological Medicine 10: 321

Kenyon F E 1964 Hypochondriasis: a clinical study. British Journal of Psychiatry 110: 478

Kenyon F E 1976 Hypochondriasis: a clinical study. British Journal of Psychiatry 129: 1

Klein D F, Gittelman R, Quitkin F H, Rifkin A 1980 Diagnosis and drug treatment of psychiatric disorders: adults and children. Williams & Wilkins, Baltimore

Lader M, Sartorius N 1968 Anxiety in patients with hysterical conversion symptoms. Journal of Neurology, Neurosurgery and Psychiatry 31: 490

Leading article 1977 Depersonalisation syndromes. British Medical Journal iv: 378

Lewis A 1975 The survival of hysteria. Psychological Medicine 5: 9

Liebowitz M R, Gorman J M, Fyer A J, Klein D F 1985 Social phobia. Archives of General Psychiatry 42: 729

Liebowitz M R, Gorman J M, Fyer A, Campias R et al 1988 Pharmacotherapy of social phobia; an interim report of a placebo-control comparison of phenelzine and atenolol. Journal of Clinical Psychiatry 49: 252

Mann A H, Jenkins R, Belsey E 1981 The twelve-month outcome of patients with neurotic illness in general practice. Psychological Medicine 11: 535

Marks I M 1969 Fears and phobias. Heinemann Medical, London

Mazza D L, Martin D, Spacavento L, Jacobsen J, Gibb J H 1986 Prevalence of anxiety disorders in patients with mitral valve prolapse. American Journal of Psychiatry 143: 349

Mavissakalian M, Turner S M, Michelson L, Jacob R 1985 Tricyclic antidepressants in obsessive compulsive disorder: antiobsessional or antidepressant agents. American Journal of Psychiatry 142: 572

Mechanic D 1962 The concept of illness behaviour. Journal of Chronic Disease 15: 189

Mellsop G W 1972 Psychiatric patients seen as children and adults: childhood predictors of adult illness. Journal of Child Psychology and Psychiatry 13: 91

Merskey H, Buhrish N A 1973 Hysteria: organic brain disease. British Journal of Medical Psychology 48: 359

Millar D G 1980 A repertory grid study of obsessionality: distinctive cognitive structure or distinctive cognitive element? British Journal of Medical Psychology 53: 59

Miller H 1961 Accident neurosis. British Medical Journal i: 919

Myers J K et al 1984 Six month prevalence of psychiatric disorders in three communities. Archives of General Psychiatry 41: 959

Nandi DN, Banerjee G, Nandi S, Nandi P 1992 Is hysteria on the wane: a community survey in West Bengal, India. British Journal of Psychiatry 160: 87

Noyes R, Clancy J, Crowe R, Hoenk P R, Slymen D 1978 The familial prevalence of anxiety neurosis. Archives of General Psychiatry 35: 1057

Noyes R, Clancy J, Hoenk P R, Slymen D J 1980 The prognosis of anxiety neurosis. Archives of General Psychiatry 37: 173

Noyes R, Crowe R R, Harris E L, Hamra B J, McChesney C H, Chavomry D R 1986 Relationship between panic disorder and agoraphobia. Archives of General Psychiatry 43: 227

Parsons T 1951 The social system. Free Press, New York

Pilowsky I 1967 Dimensions of hypochondriasis. British Journal of Psychiatry 113: 89

Pilowsky I 1983 Hypochondriasis. In: Russell G F M, Hersov L A (eds) The neuroses and personality disorders. Handbook of Psychiatry Vol 4. Cambridge University Press

Platt S, Martin G, Hunt S 1991 The mental health of women with children living in deprived areas of Great Britain. The role of living conditions, poverty and unemployment. In: Goldberg D, Tantam D (eds) The public health impact of mental disorders. Hogrefe and Huber, Ch. 12

Prussoff B, Klerman G L 1974 Differentiating depressed from anxious neurotic patients. Archives of General Psychiatry 30: 302

Rasmussen R A, Tsuang M T 1986 Clinical characteristics and family history in DSM-III obsessive–compulsive disorder. American Journal of Psychiatry 143: 317

Ratnasuriya R H, Marks I M, Forshaw D M, Hymas M F S 1991 Obsessive Slowness Revisited. British Journal of Psychiatry 159: 273

Reiman E M et al 1986 The application of positron emission tomography to the study of panic disorder. American Journal of Psychiatry 143: 469

Robins L N 1966 Deviant children grown up. Williams & Wilkins, Baltimore

Robins L N et al 1984 Lifetime prevalence of specific psychiatric disorders in three sites. Archives of General Psychiatry 41: 949

Roth M, Gurney C, Garside R F, Kerr T A 1972 Studies in the classification of affective disorders. British Journal of Psychiatry 121: 147

Rutter M L 1972 Relationships between child and adult psychiatric disorders. Acta Psychiatrica Scandinavica 48: 3

Rutter M, Tizard J, Whitmore K (eds) 1970 Education, health and behaviour. Longmans, London

Schwab J J 1979 Social order and mental health. Brunner-Mazel, New York

Shepherd M, Cooper B, Kelton G W, Brown A C 1966

Psychiatric illness in general practice. Oxford University Press, London

Sims A 1978 Hypotheses linking neuroses with premature mortality. Psychological Medicine 8: 255

Sims A C P 1985 Neurotic illness: conserving a threatened concept. British Journal of Clinical Pharmacology 19: 95

Slater E, Shields J 1969 Genetical aspects of anxiety. In: Lader M M (ed) Studies of anxiety. World Psychiatric Association & Royal Medico-Psychological Association, London, p 62

Slater E T O, Glithero E 1965 A follow-up of patients diagnosed as suffering from 'hysteria'. Journal of Psychosomatic Research 9: 9

Srole L, Langner T, Michael S, Opler M, Rennie T 1962 Mental health in the metropolis. McGraw-Hill, New York

Stavrakaki C, Vargo B 1980 The relationship of anxiety and depression: a review of the literature. British Journal of Psychiatry 149: 7

Stern R S, Cobb J P 1978 Phenomenology of obsessive–compulsive neurosis. British Journal of Psychiatry 132: 233

Stern R S, Marks I M, Mawson D, Luscombe D K 1980 Clomipramine and exposure for obsessive compulsive rituals II: plasma levels, side effects and outcome. British Journal of Psychiatry 136: 161

Surtees P G, Dean C, Ingham J J G, Kreitman N B, Miller P, Sashidharan S P 1983 Psychiatric disorders in women from an Edinburgh community. British Journal of Psychiatry 142: 231

Tarsh M J, Royston C 1985 A follow up study of accident neurosis. British Journal of Psychiatry 146: 18

Teasdale J D 1974 Learning models of obsessional–compulsive disorder. In: Beech H K (ed) Obsessional states. Methuen, London

Thoren P, Asberg M, Cronholm B, Jornestedt L, Traskman L 1980 Clomipramine treatment of obsessive–compulsive disorder: a clinical controlled trial. Archives of General Psychiatry 37: 1281–1285

Tyrer P 1979 Anxiety states. In: Granville-Grossman K (ed) Recent advances in clinical psychiatry 3. Churchill Livingstone, Edinburgh, p 161

Tyrer P 1984 Classification of anxiety. British Journal of Psychiatry 144: 78

Uhlenhuth E H, Balter M B, Millinger G D, Cisin I H, Clinthorne J 1983 Symptom checklist syndromes in the general population: correlations with psychotherapeutic drug use. Archives of General Psychiatry 40: 1167

Valliant G E, Bond M, Valliant O 1986 An empirically validated hierarchy of defence mechanisms. Archives of General Psychiatry 43: 786

Vasquez-Barquero J L 1991 Mental health in primary-care settings. In: Goldberg D, Tantam D (eds) The public health impact of mental disorders, ch 4, p 35

Vasquez-Barquero J L, Monoz P E, Madoz Javrequi V 1981 The interaction between physical and neurotic morbidity in the community. British Journal of Psychiatry 139: 328

Vasquez-Barquero J L, Diez Manrique J F, Pena C, Aldona J, Samaniego Rodriquez C, Mendez Arango J and Mirapeix C 1987 A community mental health survey in Cantabria. A general description of morbidity. Psychological Medicine 17:227

Weissman M M, Myers J K, Harding P S 1978 Psychiatric disorders in a U.S. urban community. American Journal of Psychiatry 135: 459

Weizman A et al 1986 High-affinity imipramine binding and serotonin uptake in platelets of eight adolescent and ten adult obsessive–compulsive patients. American Journal of Psychiatry 143: 335

Wheeler E O, White P D, Reid E W, Cohen M E 1950 Neurocirculatory asthenia. Journal of American Medical Association 142: 878

WHO 1974 Glossary of mental disorders and guide to their classification, 8th revision. World Health Organization, Geneva

Woerner P I, Guze S B 1968 A family and marital study of hysteria. British Journal of Psychiatry 114: 161

Wolff S, Chick J 1980 Schizoid personality in childhood: a controlled follow-up study. Psychological Medicine 10:85

Woodruff R A, Guze S B, Clayton P J 1972 Anxiety neurosis among psychiatric out-patients. Comprehensive Psychiatry 13: 165

23. Eating disorders

C. G. Fairburn

INTRODUCTION

The term eating disorders is generally used to refer to two well-defined psychiatric syndromes, anorexia nervosa and bulimia nervosa. The two are closely related. They share many clinical features, and it is common for people to move from one to the other. Their diagnostic criteria reflect this close relationship.

The ICD-10 and DSM-IIIR diagnostic criteria for anorexia nervosa and bulimia nervosa are essentially the same. They are summarised in Table 23.1. Some refinements are suggested in the proposed scheme for DSM-IV (Wilson & Walsh 1991). In principle, three features are required to make a diagnosis of anorexia nervosa. The first is the presence of certain characteristic overvalued ideas concerning shape and weight. These are often described as the core psychopathology, and they are described in detail below. Their essence is that self-worth is judged largely or solely in terms of shape or weight. The second feature is the active maintenance of a low weight according to population norms: the definition of what constitutes 'low' varies — 15% below the expected weight for the person's age, height and sex is a common figure (or a body mass index (BMI)* below 17.5). The third feature is amenorrhoea (in females not taking an oral contraceptive). One proposal for DSM-IV is that the disorder be divided into two subtypes on the basis of the pattern of eating; a bulimic subtype in which the extreme restraint over eating is interrupted by episodes of uncontrolled overeating (termed 'bulimic episodes' or 'binges'); and a restricting subtype in which restraint over eating is successfully maintained.

Three features are also required to make a diagnosis of bulimia nervosa; first, overvalued ideas concerning shape and weight similar to those found in anorexia nervosa; second, frequent episodes of bulimia; and third, certain extreme behaviour designed to control shape and weight. This behaviour includes strict dieting or fasting, self-induced vomiting, the taking of laxatives or diuretics, and excessive exercising. In clinical practice, and in the proposed DSM-IV scheme, a fourth criterion is added, namely that body weight should not be unduly low. This ruling has the effect of letting the diagnosis of anorexia nervosa 'trump' that of bulimia nervosa. Like anorexia nervosa, bulimia nervosa is divided into two subtypes in the proposed DSM-IV scheme: a purging subtype in which there is either self-induced vomiting or laxative abuse, and a non-purging subtype in which neither of these behaviours is present.

The relationship between the diagnoses of anorexia nervosa and bulimia nervosa is represented schematically in Figure 23.1. The diagnostic status of those people who fall into the central segment of the Venn diagram has been a source of debate. They could be considered to have the bulimic form of anorexia nervosa, bulimia nervosa, or both. As already mentioned, in clinical practice it is usual to restrict the diagnosis of bulimia nervosa to individuals of average or above average weight since those who are underweight require a different treatment approach. If this practice is adopted, individuals in the central segment of the figure are classed as having the bulimic subtype of anorexia nervosa.

In addition to anorexia nervosa and bulimia nervosa, various other eating disorders are encountered in adults. These have not been well characterised. They include disorders resembling anorexia nervosa or bulimia nervosa but not quite meeting their diagnostic criteria, either because one or more features is absent (so called partial syndromes)

---

* The body mass index (or Quetelet's index after a Belgian astronomer) is a convenient way of assessing relative weight without reference to tables of population norms. It is weight in kg/(height in m)^2. The healthy range is 20–25, and underweight may be defined as below 17.5.

Table 23.1   The diagnostic criteria for anorexia nervosa and bulimia nervosa. The ruling that anorexia nervosa 'trumps' bulimia nervosa is adopted

	Anorexia nervosa (restricting subtype)	Anorexia nervosa (bulimic subtype)	Bulimia nervosa
Characteristic extreme concerns about shape and weight	Yes	Yes	Yes
Behaviour designed to control shape and weight	Yes	Yes	Yes
Bulimic episodes	No	Yes	Yes
Low weight according to population norms	Yes	Yes	No
Amenorrhoea	Yes	Yes	Maybe

or because these features are not of sufficient severity (subthreshold disorders), or both. In addition, there are people with disorders quite distinct from anorexia nervosa and bulimia nervosa but with one or two features in common; for example, there are people who vomit when anxious, and people who have difficulty eating or swallowing in public. Both groups are better classed as having forms of anxiety disorder. There is another group of people, who often have severely limited coping resources, who stop eating to bring attention to themselves. Like those with anxiety-related disorders, these individuals do not show the overvalued ideas characteristic of anorexia nervosa and bulimia nervosa. One other group is currently attracting attention, although it has yet to be satisfactorily defined. It consists of people who have recurrent episodes of overeating in the absence of the other core features of bulimia nervosa. This type of

eating disorder is being considered for inclusion in DSM-IV as a new diagnostic category, binge-eating disorder.

The focus of this chapter will be on anorexia nervosa and bulimia nervosa since these are the eating disorders most commonly encountered in psychiatric practice. Binge-eating disorder will be briefly considered as will the changes in eating and weight that accompany certain psychiatric disorders and their treatment.

ANOREXIA NERVOSA

Epidemiology

The study of the incidence and prevalence of anorexia nervosa is complicated by the difficulty deciding on the threshold for what constitutes a 'case' and by problems identifying cases, since many people with anorexia nervosa do not view themselves as having a problem. Estimates of the incidence of the disorder have been derived using case registers (i.e. registers of clinically detected cases) and the figures obtained range from 0.24 to 14.6 per 100 000 of the female population per annum. The majority of studies have found that the incidence has increased in recent decades (Lucas et al 1991), although it is not clear whether this reflects a true increase in incidence or whether it is due to other factors such as the change in the proportion of young women in the population, greater public and professional awareness of the disorder, improved detection and increased likelihood of referral. The proportion of cases that does not come to medical attention is unknown.

Estimates of the prevalence of anorexia nervosa suggest that the disorder is not common. The rate

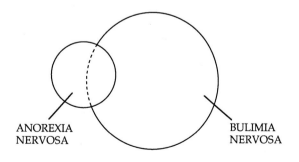

ANOREXIA NERVOSA   BULIMIA NERVOSA

Fig. 23.1   A schematic representation of the relationship between anorexia nervosa and bulimia nervosa.

amongst adolescent girls and young adult women ranges from 0 to 1.1%. There are rather more subthreshold cases and partial syndromes, but their clinical significance is uncertain. In some specific subgroups, for example ballet students, the prevalence appears to be higher. Conversely, the disorder is hardly encountered at all in other groups; for example, it seems to be uncommon in men (less than 10% of cases are male) and it is rare amongst non-whites. The social class distribution seems to be uneven with an overrepresentation of upper socioeconomic groups. Anorexia nervosa is therefore an example of a culture-bound syndrome: it appears to be largely restricted to social groups in which thinness is considered attractive and dieting is widely practised.

Clinical features

The onset of anorexia nervosa is usually in adolescence, although prepubertal cases are encountered and in some people the disorder does not begin until they are in their 20s or 30s. It typically evolves from normal adolescent dieting. At the outset body weight is usually unremarkable, but as the dieting becomes entrenched weight falls significantly and features characteristic of starvation develop. Additional methods of controlling weight or shape may be adopted at any stage. These include intense exercising, self-induced vomiting and the misuse of laxatives. Overvalued ideas concerning shape and weight are not present early on. Despite the low weight and disturbed eating habits, it is often some years before patients come to medical attention. This is largely because they do not view their behaviour as unreasonable.

The psychopathology of anorexia nervosa and bulimia nervosa may be divided into specific and general components: the former consists of features largely peculiar to the eating disorders, whereas the latter comprises features found in other psychiatric conditions. Some of the specific and general features of anorexia nervosa seem to be secondary effects of starvation. The psychopathology of male cases seems to be essentially the same as that of females. (See Andersen (1990) for information on eating disorders in men.)

Specific psychopathology

The 'core psychopathology' of anorexia nervosa and bulimia nervosa comprises a characteristic set of overvalued ideas concerning shape and weight which appears to be of major importance in the maintenance of these disorders. They have been recognised by clinicians of widely different theoretical orientations and have been variously described as a 'morbid fear of fatness', the relentless 'pursuit of thinness', and as a 'weight phobia'. They are not usually present at the outset of the disorder and, even when present, they can be difficult to detect at initial assessment. Sometimes they only become obvious when the patient is advised to eat more and gain weight.

Characteristically, patients with anorexia nervosa and bulimia nervosa evaluate their self-worth largely or solely in terms of their shape and weight: they view fatness and weight gain with fear; they regard thinness and weight loss as desirable; and they place great emphasis upon self-control. Of course, such attitudes are extreme forms of widely held views. Indeed, they are likely to be reinforced by prevailing social values, particularly the current fashion for women to be slim. The presence of these attitudes appears to account for much of the patients' behaviour, particularly the intense interest in appearance and weight. (For a detailed account of the cognitive aspects of anorexia nervosa and bulimia nervosa, see Vitousek & Hollon (1990).)

The dietary restraint of patients with anorexia nervosa is characterised by the selective avoidance of foods regarded as 'fattening', and in some cases by the counting of calories and the setting of a daily calorie limit (usually in the region of 600–1000 kcal). Many patients eat only a limited range of foods. Except in long-standing cases, appetite for food persists, and for this reason the term 'anorexia' is inappropriate. Associated with the food restriction is preoccupation with food and eating. This may account for the characteristic interest in cooking, and the relative frequency with which people with anorexia nervosa choose jobs which involve working with food. More difficult to explain are the episodes of overeating experienced by up to half the patients. These interrupt the attempts to restrict food intake and are a source of much distress. They resemble those encountered in bulimia nervosa and are discussed later in the chapter.

One of the least well understood aspects of anorexia nervosa and bulimia nervosa is the so-called body image disturbance. This appears to include a perceptual component such that all, or parts, of the body are seen as larger than their true size (body shape misperception) and an attitudinal component characterised by an intense dislike of the body or parts of it (body shape disparagement).

General psychopathology

Depressed mood and lability of mood are common features, and in more chronic cases hopelessness and thoughts of suicide may be present. Anxiety symptoms, usually related to situations which involve eating, are also encountered. Outside interests are often reduced and there is usually marked social withdrawal. Obsessional features may be present and frequently these affect eating. Concentration is often impaired, but work performance is usually good, reflecting the influence of perfectionistic standards and a tendency to depend on external criteria to gauge self-worth.

The contribution of starvation

Certain aspects of the psychopathology of anorexia nervosa are probably a direct result of starvation. Many features have been reproduced in experimental studies of starvation, including preoccupation with food and eating, food-related dreams, the consumption of unusual combinations of food and, in a minority, episodes of bulimia. In addition, depressed mood, irritability, obsessional features, impaired concentration, narrowing of interests, social withdrawal, sleep disturbances and a reduction in sexual appetite are also seen. Some of the less common features of anorexia nervosa occasionally develop in starvation, including stealing and hoarding of food and other items. However, it is important to note that the core psychopathology of anorexia nervosa, namely the overvalued ideas concerning shape and weight, does not develop. Instead, these overvalued ideas should be regarded as an independent feature which maintains the starvation.

Physical features of anorexia nervosa

There are many physical abnormalities in anorexia nervosa and their significance has been the focus of much research. There has been particular interest in the possibility that there might be a primary abnormality of hypothalamic function. The strongest argument for such a disturbance rests upon two observations: first, in about 15% of patients, the history suggests that menstruation ceased prior to weight loss; and second, restoration of a healthy weight is not always accompanied by the resumption of regular menstruation. However, it is likely that in both instances the menstrual dysfunction is secondary to abnormalities in eating habits or activity levels since these often precede the onset of weight loss and persist following weight gain. The observation that in bulimia nervosa the menstrual disturbance (if present) generally reverses once healthy eating habits have been established, in the absence of any significant change in weight, supports this view.

Symptoms and signs. Many patients with anorexia nervosa have no physical complaints. However, systematic enquiry often reveals a variety of symptoms, including heightened sensitivity to cold and gastrointestinal complaints such as constipation, fullness after eating, bloating, and vague abdominal pains. Other symptoms include restlessness, lack of energy, low sexual appetite and early morning wakening. In females who are not taking the contraceptive pill, amenorrhoea is by definition present.

On examination some patients are found to be severely emaciated. Unlike those with hypopituitarism, axillary and pubic hair is preserved and there is no breast atrophy. A fine downy lanugo hair is sometimes found on the back, arms and sides of the face. The skin may be dry and rough, and often the hands and feet are cold and blue. There may also be ankle oedema. Blood pressure and pulse are usually low and there may be hypothermia and dehydration. Certain other symptoms and signs are more characteristic of the bulimic subtype of anorexia nervosa and these are described below.

Abnormalities on laboratory investigation. Patients with anorexia nervosa show a wide range of abnormalities on laboratory investigation (see Table 23.2). Most are found in uncomplicated starvation and are reversed by the restoration of a healthy weight and diet. The endocrine changes have attracted most attention, the most striking abnormality being hypogonadotrophic hypogonadism, the effects of which include amenorrhoea and loss of libido. The endocrine changes are thought to be secondary to the disturbed eating habits and weight loss, and in the great majority of cases they reverse with healthy eating and weight gain.

The major medical complications are listed in Table 23.3. Some of these are potentially life-threatening, for example, the electrolyte disturbance may

Table 23.2 Laboratory abnormalities commonly found in anorexia nervosa

Haematological	Endocrine
Leucopenia	Low plasma gonadotrophins
Relative lymphocytosis	Low plasma gonadal steroids
	Elevated plasma growth hormone
Metabolic	Low plasma triiodothyronine
Metabolic alkalosis	Elevated plasma cortisol
Hypokalaemia	
Hypoglycaemia	
Elevated plasma amylase	
Hypercholesterolaemia	
Hypercarotenaemia	

Table 23.3 Principal medical complications of anorexia nervosa

Cardiovascular	*Gastrointestinal*
Bradycardia	Salivary gland enlargement
Hypotension	Delayed gastric emptying
Cardiac arrhythmias	Acute gastric dilatation
Oedema	Superior mesenteric artery syndrome
Cardiac failure	Constipation
	Acute pancreatitis
Neurological	
Seizures	*Metabolic*
	Hypoglycaemia
Endocrine	Dehydration
Amenorrhoea	Tetany
Skeletal	*Other*
Reduced growth	Hypothermia
Osteoporosis and pathological fractures	
Dental	
Erosion of enamel	
Caries	

occasionally lead to epileptic seizures or serious cardiac arrhythmias, and acute gastric dilatation can follow episodes of bulimia or overvigorous attempts at refeeding.

Aetiology

There has been little systematic research on the aetiology of anorexia nervosa, and much of the work has methodological shortcomings. For example, the patient samples are mostly from tertiary referral centres which tend to attract unusual cases, few studies have employed general psychiatric control groups to check that the findings are specific to eating disorders, and often it is unclear whether the variable under investigation is likely to operate as a predisposing, precipitating or maintaining factor. What is not in doubt is that anorexia nervosa results from the interaction of social, psychological and physical factors whose relative contributions differ from individual to individual. There follows a brief account of current views and findings. (For a more detailed discussion on aetiology, see Garfinkel & Garner (1982) and Hsu (1990).)

Predisposing factors

Any account of the aetiology of anorexia nervosa must explain the striking finding that the disorder appears largely confined to a specific social group, namely young white women (Dolan 1991). Epidemiological studies have shown that concerns about being overweight and dieting are especially common in this group.

This may account for the social distribution of the disorder since it is widely accepted that dieting operates as a general vulnerability factor (Hsu 1990). If this is the case, a key question is why do only certain young women who diet go on to develop an eating disorder? To address this question, individual and family factors have to be considered.

A range of vulnerability factors in the individual have been implicated in the aetiology of anorexia nervosa. Amongst the most robust is premorbid weight pathology (25% of patients with anorexia nervosa and 40% of patients with bulimia nervosa have been overweight prior to the onset of the eating disorder). This might well heighten sensitivity about appearance. A more general vulnerability factor is long-standing low self-esteem, often described in this context as a profound sense of ineffectiveness. This is almost ubiquitous and in some cases appears to stem from early adverse experiences such as parental loss or disharmony, or sexual abuse. However, contrary to popular opinion, childhood sexual abuse (present in about a third of patients with eating disorders) seems to be no more common amongst this group than amongst matched patients with other psychiatric disorders. Perfectionism is another characteristic premorbid feature. Clinical observation suggests that it is the combination of low self-esteem and perfectionism that results in these patients being particularly ill-equipped to cope with the developmental demands of adolescence. Under these circumstances dieting becomes personally very significant since it is not only a socially approved behaviour but also powerfully bolsters these individuals' sense of self-control and effectiveness whilst also lessening their concerns about appearance and weight. It is not surprising, therefore, that their dieting and pursuit of weight loss is more extreme and sustained than that of their peers. (For a developmental perspective on the aetiology of eating disorders, see Levine & Smolak (1991).)

Family factors are also relevant to the development of the disorder. It is well established that eating disorders run in families; for example, anorexia nervosa is roughly eight times as common in the female first-degree relatives of anorectic probands as in the general population. The results of twin studies suggest that this vulnerability may in part be genetic in nature (Holland et al 1988). However, if genetic factors do contribute, it is far from clear what is being inherited; for example, it could be a particular physiological or psychological response to dieting such that further dieting is encouraged, or it could be certain personality characteristics.

The most common psychiatric disorders amongst these patients' relatives are not eating disorders; they are affective disorders. The lifetime prevalence of unipolar affective disorder amongst the relatives of anorectic probands is three times that of the general population. Since there appears to be no converse increase in the rate of eating disorders in the relatives of affective disorder probands, the transmissable risk appears to be specific (Strober et al 1990). This observation has parallels, for example in the relationship between alcoholism and depression: these two disorders are frequently associated in individuals, cluster in families, but do not have a common transmitted liability. The mechanism through which a family history of affective disorder increases the risk of developing an eating disorder is not clear. There is also some evidence for an increase in the familial prevalence of substance abuse.

Other family characteristics have been studied (Vandereycken et al 1989). The main findings are that there is an overrepresentation of families from upper socioeconomic groups, maternal age is high (but this is true of several psychiatric disorders), and in some families there is a particular involvement in food, eating, fitness, appearance or weight. The studies of family functioning suggest that interaction is commonly disturbed, but the form of the disturbance varies. No specific abnormalities have been identified, and it has yet to be established whether the disturbances found are a cause or a consequence of the eating disorder.

Precipitating factors

The onset of the eating disorder is often preceded by a significant life event. However, this is by no means invariable and the events themselves have not been adequately studied. In some cases they appear to be specific triggers, as in the case of teasing about appearance or the development of an illness which results in weight loss, but more often they are non-specific in character.

Maintaining factors

In the early stages, as weight is lost, features of starvation develop. Some of these are likely to perpetuate the disorder. For example, the development of depressive symptoms will worsen self-esteem, and the delay in gastric emptying will result in a sensation of fullness even after eating small amounts. The social withdrawal, reduction in outside interests, and possibly also the loss of libido, may also contribute by isolating the person from his or her peers.

External influences also maintain the disorder. Those who have been overweight in the past may well be gratified by the weight loss and complimented on it. There may be secondary effects within the family and these too may be rewarding: many acknowledge in retrospect that dieting and weight loss gave them, sometimes for the first time, a sense of effectiveness and competence. It is partly for this reason that it is so difficult to persuade many of these patients to accept change: relaxing their control over eating and gaining weight have no attractions from their perspective.

Assessment

Relatively few patients with anorexia nervosa refer themselves for treatment: the majority view their behaviour and attitudes as quite reasonable. Often they are persuaded to seek help by concerned relatives or friends and as a consequence attend somewhat reluctantly. The major task of the first interview is therefore to establish common ground between the therapist and the patient. In addition, sufficient information should be obtained to reach a diagnosis and construct an immediate plan of management. In most cases this plan will be to meet the patient again to assess the problem further and decide on the most appropriate form of treatment.

When evaluating these patients six areas need to be assessed. Whenever possible, supplementary information should be obtained from informants, especially the parents, and, if different, the people with whom the patient lives. They can usually provide a detailed picture of the patient's eating habits and social functioning, and they may be able to describe how the disorder developed.

1. The patient's perspective. It is important to

understand the patient's perspective on the problem. The goal is to establish a collaborative working relationship.

2. Attitudes to shape and weight. It is essential to decide whether the core psychopathology of anorexia nervosa and bulimia nervosa is present. Areas to evaluate include the patient's views on shape and weight, the importance attached to appearance, reactions to increases and decreases in weight, and desired shape and weight. The possibility that there may be body image misperception should also be considered.

3. Eating habits. Asking patients to describe a typical day is usually informative. In addition, it is often worthwhile getting them to start monitoring their food intake so that a detailed picture of their day-to-day eating habits may be obtained. The aim is to understand why patients eat in the way that they do. For example, it is important to know if they are attempting to restrict their food intake and, if so, for what reason. They may be setting themselves a daily calorie limit or trying not to eat before a certain time of day. Also of relevance is the range of foods eaten. If patients are actively avoiding eating certain foods, one wants to understand both the reason why and whether they do eat these foods under certain circumstances. Bulimic episodes, for example, are typically composed of foods which are otherwise avoided.

Direct questioning about episodes of bulimia (binge eating) is essential. Such episodes may be defined as discrete bouts of uncontrolled eating in which a genuinely large amount of food is eaten, given the social context. Some patients have so-called subjective bulimic episodes which resemble true bulimic episodes except that the amount of food eaten is not objectively large.

4. Methods of weight control. In every case enquiries should be made about the occurrence and frequency of the various methods of weight control. These include dieting and fasting, vomiting, the taking of laxatives or diuretics, and exercising. Less common methods include the taking of ipecacuanha or amphetamines, and the underuse of insulin in those with diabetes mellitus.

5. General psychopathology. It is especially important to evaluate psychological features of depression. Excluding the presence of a depressive illness can be difficult since anorexia nervosa affects not only body weight, but also concentration, energy, sleep and libido. It is more straightforward, however, to exclude the possibility that a depressive illness is the sole diagnosis since the core psychopathology of anorexia nervosa is not present in depressive disorders.

The evaluation of general psychopathology should also include an assessment of developmental adjustment, personality characteristics with particular emphasis on self-esteem and perfectionistic traits, sexual attitudes and behaviour, and social functioning.

6. Physical state. The physical health of these patients must never be forgotten. Their appearance can be deceptive since many disguise their appearance by wearing loose clothes. A detailed personal and family weight history should be taken and a physical examination which includes weighing is mandatory. The rate of weight loss should be noted. Laboratory tests are not required to make the diagnosis, but it is important to check the electrolytes of patients who are vomiting or taking laxatives or diuretics.

Management

There has been little research on the treatment of anorexia nervosa. Therefore, recommendations about management must necessarily be based on the views of those who specialise in the treatment of the disorder.

There are two aspects to treatment. One is establishing healthy eating habits and restoring a healthy weight, and the second is the reversal of those factors which have been maintaining the disorder. Both are essential. The treatment plan has to be tailored to suit the individual patient and it often involves many different elements. Typically these include education, dietary advice, the use of behavioural and cognitive techniques, and work with the family. The principles of treatment will now be reviewed. (For further information, see Garner & Garfinkel (1985) and Hsu (1990).)

The initial phase of treatment

There are four aspects to the initial phase of treatment.

1. Forming a collaborative therapeutic relationship. This is especially important in patients who are reluctant attenders. Openness, honesty and a direct caring approach are needed.

2. Educating the patient. Patients need to learn about the clinical features of anorexia nervosa, the contribution of starvation to its psychopathology, the factors relevant to its development and maintenance, and the importance of weight gain. They may be recommended certain books; for example, *Anorexia Nervosa* by Palmer (1990) and *Eating Disorders: The*

Facts by Abraham & Llewelyn-Jones (1987). It is obviously essential that therapists themselves are knowledgeable about anorexia nervosa and its treatment. The two best reference books are *Anorexia Nervosa: A Multidimensional Perspective* by Garfinkel & Garner (1982) and *Eating Disorders* by Hsu (1990).

3. Agreeing that there is a need for controlled weight gain. From discussions about the educational material and in particular the contribution of starvation to the patient's present state, it should be possible to establish the need for weight gain. It can be helpful identifying those starvation symptoms the patient finds distressing, for example sensitivity to cold, preoccupation with food and eating, impaired concentration, irritability and depression, since such symptoms are likely to improve with weight restoration. Weight gain can be presented as a planned experiment in which the patient and therapist together explore what changes occur. Therapists must stress that they will ensure that the weight gain will be slow and controlled, and that care will be taken to ensure that the patient does not either lose control over eating or overshoot the target weight range. It should also be acknowledged that the process is difficult, and that it may at times intensify concerns about shape and weight. Throughout it must be emphasised, however, that weight restoration is only one facet of treatment, albeit an essential one: unless it is accomplished, symptoms of starvation will continue to complicate the picture and make other important changes more difficult to achieve.

4. Deciding upon the treatment setting. Most patients with anorexia nervosa may be managed exclusively on an out-patient basis. Some need an initial period of day-patient or in-patient treatment followed by out-patient care. Out-patient treatment is not appropriate if the patient's physical health is a cause for concern, if the weight loss is rapid, or if the patient is depressed and at risk of suicide. Partial or full hospitalisation may also be indicated if no progress is being made with out-patient care or there are no treatment facilities available locally. Occasionally, hospitalisation is needed because the patient's social circumstances are interfering with progress.

Not infrequently, in-patient treatment is indicated, but the patient does not want to be admitted. Under these circumstances, unless immediate hospitalisation is essential, two options are available: either management on a day patient basis or a brief trial of out-patient treatment. If the latter option is chosen, patients should be asked to prove to the therapist that they can gain weight at a reasonable rate (about 1 kg per week). It should be agreed that if they do not succeed, they will be admitted. A few patients refuse admission even though their life is in danger. In such cases compulsory hospitalisation must be seriously considered.

In-patient treatment

Unless the admission is an emergency one because of the patient's poor state of health or the risk of suicide, it should be planned in advance. The patient should visit the ward, meet the staff, and have an opportunity to discuss the treatment programme. In the past elaborate individualised behavioural regimes were used to promote weight gain, but their value is now in doubt. Instead, expert nursing care is the cornerstone of treatment.

Patients should, within a few days of admission, be introduced to the consumption of regular meals and snacks; and, if possible, by the end of 2 weeks these should be of normal quantity and composition, consisting of about 2000 kcal/day. (Nutritional counselling from a dietician can be very helpful at this stage.) A goal should be set of a weight increase of about 1.5 kg a week, with the patient and staff monitoring the weight gain each morning. Average-sized meals and snacks will not be sufficient to achieve this rate of weight gain since between 3000 and 5000 kcal/day are likely to be required. Therefore, in the author's view, this diet should consist of average quantities of a wide range of foods supplemented with high-calorie drinks. This seems preferable to the alternative of encouraging patients to overeat. If a behavioural weight restoration programme is to be used, a simple programme will probably be just as effective as a more complex one. For example, one programme which often works requires patients to gain at least 0.75 kg every 4 days (Fairburn & Cooper 1989). If, with help and support from the staff, they fail to achieve this target, it is agreed in advance that they will spend the following 4 days on bed rest so that eating and exercise levels may be more closely monitored. If, following the bed rest, they achieve the 4 day target, they may then resume full participation in ward activities. If they do not, the period of bed rest is extended.

The issue of what should be the target weight is a controversial one. In principle, it should be a weight at which the patient is eating healthly and not dieting, and one at which normal hormonal functioning is possible. At such a weight, starvation symptoms should no longer be present. A useful rule of thumb is that patients should have a BMI of at least 18, and ideally somewhat higher: this figure should be adjusted upwards or downwards if the patient's premorbid weight was unusually high or low. Patients should understand the reasoning behind the choice of target weight and be encouraged to monitor their weight gain. It is important that the target has a range of about 2.5 kg rather than being a precise figure since it is normal for weight to fluctuate. Once patients enter the target range, the high-calorie drinks should be phased out, leaving them consuming a normal diet sufficient to maintain their weight. It is at this stage that external controls over eating should be gradually withdrawn so that patients can learn to control their own eating. They should be encouraged to shop, cook and eat out with friends and family. Unless considerable effort is put into this maintenance phase, the risk of relapse after discharge is considerable.

Running concurrently with weight restoration should be other forms of therapy. At first, straightforward support is often best, but once the starvation symptoms begin to abate and the patient's psychiatric symptoms have begun to diminish, more focused treatment techniques may be introduced, including cognitive interventions and family therapy.

With an in-patient regime of this type, body weight is usually restored to a healthy range within 2–3 months and the patient is discharged home 2–4 weeks later. The transition from in-patient to out-patient care must be carefully orchestrated, and whenever possible there should be continuity in treatment.

Day-patient treatment

Until recently, there was little interest in the use of day care in the overall management of anorexia nervosa, yet it has some advantages over full hospitalisation. A comprehensive treatment programme can be provided, including the supervision of eating and weight gain, whilst patients remain based in their usual social environment. It might be predicted that day programmes would be associated with less risk of relapse following discharge, but this has yet to be established. (See Piran & Kaplan (1990) for a detailed description of the Toronto day programme.)

Out-patient treatment

This may be the sole form of treatment or it may follow a period of in-patient or day-patient care. There are three main forms of outpatient treatment.

1. Supportive psychotherapy. Patients are encouraged to eat healthily, and, if appropriate, gain weight, whilst at the same time they are assisted in tackling other on-going problems. The approach has never been specified in detail. It has been compared with family therapy in the management of patients who have been discharged from hospital and was found to be as effective, if not superior, except with patients whose disorder began at an early age (onset prior to 19 years) and had not become chronic (history of less than 3 years). In this group, family therapy was superior (Russell et al 1987).

2. Family therapy. This approach may be used as the primary form of treatment, or it may be included as one part of the treatment programme. The latter practice is the one more commonly used. A variety of different forms of family therapy have been advocated (Vandereycken et al 1989); however, their relative merits have yet to be established. Whenever possible, the families of young patients should be involved in their treatment.

3. Cognitive behaviour therapy. Like family therapy, this approach may be used on its own or in conjunction with other forms of treatment. It is probably more suitable for older patients (over 17 years). It aims not only to re-establish healthy eating habits and weight, but also to address the dysfunctional attitudes and styles of thinking. There is particular emphasis on modification of extreme concerns about shape and weight, deficits in self-esteem, perfectionist tendencies, and problems with autonomy and assertiveness (Garner & Bemis 1985). The treatment is usually conducted on an out-patient basis and in most cases takes at least 12 months. It has yet to be satisfactorily evaluated. Many cognitive behavioural procedures may be usefully integrated into any management programme.

The use of drugs and other physical treatments

Drugs have a limited place in the overall management of anorexia nervosa. Short-acting minor tranquillisers may occasionally be used to lessen the anxiety some patients experience prior to eating and, if depressive symptoms persist following weight restoration, antidepressant drugs are indicated. If postprandial fullness is impeding progress, domperidone may be helpful. Tube feeding and intravenous hyperalimentation are rarely indicated. Psychosurgery has been used to treat a small number of intractable cases, but it is doubtful whether it is ever justified.

Occasionally it is appropriate to use drugs to stimulate the resumption of regular menstruation. Most patients whose weight has reached a reasonable level and who are eating healthily restart menstruating within 6 months. If this does not happen, and it seems to merit treatment, referral may be made to an endocrinologist since either clomiphene or luteinising hormone-releasing hormone, or both, are usually effective in inducing menstruation. It is not appropriate to use these drugs with patients who are underweight or who are eating abnormally. Instead, their weight and eating habits need to be addressed.

Self-help groups

Such groups have a definite contribution to make to the management of anorexia nervosa. By providing sufferers and their families with information and guidance, they can help patients enter treatment by suggesting appropriate lines of referral. (In several countries self-help organisations run national information centres which collate and distribute information on sources of help for those with eating disorders.) These groups can also provide support during treatment. Their other important role is to provide long-term support for those who are chronically disabled by the disorder.

The management of the chronic patient

For some patients anorexia nervosa is an intractable disorder. In such cases it is important to adjust one's therapeutic goals (Fairburn & Cooper 1989). However, it is never appropriate to abandon all hopes of change, since recovery, even after many years of unremitting symptoms, does sometimes occur.

Outcome

The course of anorexia nervosa is varied: for some it is a benign self-limiting condition, for others it is an intractable disorder. Little is known about the factors or processes that govern its course or outcome.

The findings of the various medium-term follow-up studies are relatively consistent. First, it is clear that the disorder 'breeds true'. There is no tendency for it to evolve into another psychiatric disorder such as depression. Second, the outcome is remarkably variable. About 20% of patients make a full recovery; about the same proportion remain severely ill; while the remainder show some degree of continuing psychiatric disturbance. Third, whilst a significant number of patients recover in terms of their weight and menstrual function, their overconcern with shape and weight tends to persist and eating habits often remain disturbed. Some patients develop bulimia nervosa. Fourth, psychosocial functioning is often

impaired in those who do not make a full recovery. Fifth, at least two factors appear to predict outcome and these are age at onset and duration of illness at presentation: those with a late age of onset (18 years or later) or a long history fare less well. The outcome in males appears to be essentially the same as that in females.

There have been several studies of the long-term outcome of anorexia nervosa (e.g. Ratnasuriya et al 1991). These indicate that even after many years of illness recovery may take place, although it is uncommon after 12 years. But, just as more patients recover over time, so do more die. Studies with 10–20 year follow-up periods report crude mortality rates between 15 and 20%. These deaths are either a direct result of the illness, often electrolyte imbalance, or due to suicide. It remains to be seen whether modern methods of management will improve the long-term outcome.

BULIMIA NERVOSA

Towards the end of the 1970s reports began to appear concerning a disorder principally characterised by bouts of uncontrolled overeating. People with this disorder closely resembled patients with anorexia nervosa, although there was one major difference: their weight was generally within the normal range. At first, the disorder attracted various names including 'bulimarexia', the 'dietary chaos syndrome', 'bulimia' and 'bulimia nervosa'. The two terms which subsequently gained acceptance were bulimia, the DSM-III term, and bulimia nervosa, the term proposed in a seminal paper by Russell (1979). The latter term is to be preferred for two reasons : first, it avoids the ambiguities that result from using the word 'bulimia' to denote both a behaviour (uncontrolled overeating) and a specific psychiatric syndrome; and second, it emphasises the close links between this disorder and anorexia nervosa. For these reasons bulimia nervosa is now the official term adopted in both ICD-10 and DSM-IIIR.

The diagnostic criteria for bulimia nervosa, and the relationship between this diagnosis and that of anorexia nervosa, have already been discussed.

Epidemiology

There has been considerable interest in the prevalence of bulimia nervosa. Amongst young women in Britain and North America it is generally between 1 and 2% (Fairburn & Beglin 1990). There are many more subthreshold cases and partial syndromes, but their clinical significance is unclear. Male cases are comparatively rare. It is likely that the disorder has become genuinely more common over the past 20 years but there are no satisfactory data on its incidence. What is clear is that in all countries in which anorexia nervosa is found, there has been a dramatic increase in the number of cases of bulimia nervosa: from being regarded as an unusual variant of anorexia nervosa, it is now the most common eating disorder encountered in psychiatric practice. The explanation for this increase is unclear.

Clinical features

The great majority of patients with bulimia nervosa are female. They are on average somewhat older than those with anorexia nervosa, most presenting in their 20s. Many give a history of disturbed eating which stretches back into adolescence and about a third have previously fulfilled diagnostic criteria for anorexia nervosa. Many of the remainder have shown features of anorexia nervosa, but have not met the full criteria. The social class distribution is probably somewhat broader than that of anorexia nervosa. Male cases are rare; they closely resemble female cases although premorbid obesity and homosexuality are possibly more common (Andersen 1990, Carlat & Camargo 1991).

Specific psychopathology

This resembles that found in anorexia nervosa. There are similar overvalued ideas concerning shape and weight and, as one would expect, these are associated with a variety of methods of weight control including intense efforts to diet, self-induced vomiting, the taking of laxatives and diuretics and, in a minority, rigorous exercising. There is also preoccupation with food, eating, shape and weight.

The feature which distinguishes bulimia nervosa from the classic form of anorexia nervosa (i.e. the restricting subtype), apart from body weight, is the profound loss of control over eating. Some patients have as many as ten bulimic episodes a day. Typically, the bouts of overeating are precipitated by unpleasant events or by feeling of depression, anxiety, boredom or loneliness; alternatively, they follow the breaking of rigid and restrictive dietary rules; occasionally they are planned. During these episodes food tends to be eaten rapidly with little attention being paid to its taste or texture and in general it consists of items the patients are attempting to exclude from their diet. Thus, it is usually composed of energy-rich foods which the patient views 'fattening', 'forbidden' or 'dangerous'. Contrary to common opinion, the proportion of

carbohydrate is not high; instead, the distinctive feature is the relatively low proportion of protein (Walsh et al 1992). The popular expression 'carbohydrate craving' is not therefore an appropriate one. The total amount eaten varies greatly, around 3000 kcal per episode being an average figure. The amount of liquid consumed also varies: if self-induced vomiting is to follow, large quantities may be drunk to facilitate regurgitation. The episodes are usually brought to an end by self-induced vomiting, abdominal distension or the exhaustion of food supplies. Afterwards there is often a period of drowsiness and feelings of depression, guilt and self-disgust. Between episodes, the majority of patients do their best to restrict their food intake. A monitoring sheet typical of a patient with bulimia nervosa is shown in Figure 23.2.

In common with anorexia nervosa, most aspects of the psychopathology of bulimia nervosa may be regarded as secondary to the concerns about shape and weight. The episodes of bulimia, however, are difficult to explain along these lines. It would be predicted that fears of weight gain or fatness would lead to constant dieting with success reinforcing further dieting. This is the situation for patients with the restricting form of anorexia nervosa. It would also be predicted that, if for some reason patients fail to adhere to their dietary strictures, they would simply restart dieting as soon as possible afterwards. The clinical features of both bulimia nervosa and the bulimic form of anorexia nervosa are not consistent with either of these predictions. Many patients do not successfully adhere to their dietary regimes, and when they do 'fail' they often react by eating even more. Thus, rather than minimising the 'indiscretion', they tend to magnify it.

Most explanations for the episodes of bulimia assume that they are secondary to the extreme dieting. One postulates a cognitive link between dieting and overeating since the overvalued ideas concerning shape and weight are associated with strict and inflexible dietary rules. Patients report that even minor transgressions are seen as evidence of poor self-control and are followed by the temporary abandonment of control over eating. This view is not incompatible with physiological explanations. For example, it is possible that sustained dieting results in physiological changes that encourage intermittent overeating, perhaps by disrupting satiety. However, something other than a disturbance of satiety must be invoked to account for the composition of bulimic episodes and the extreme restraint between them.

The episodes of bulimia are a source of distress to these patients: they motivate them to seek treatment. They react strongly to the breaking of their dietary

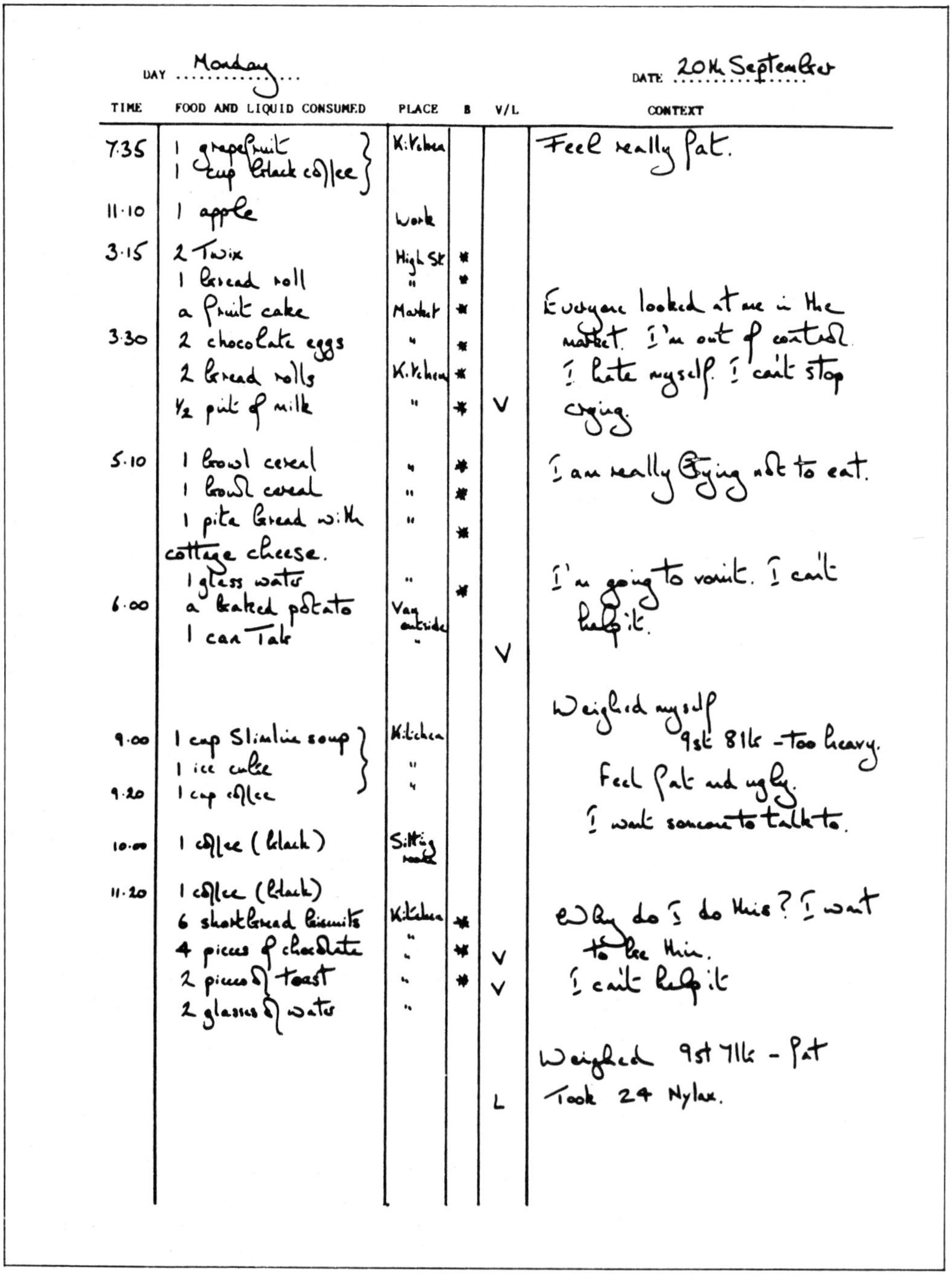

DAY Monday				DATE 20th September	
TIME	FOOD AND LIQUID CONSUMED	PLACE	B	V/L	CONTEXT
7.35	1 grapefruit 1 cup black coffee	Kitchen			Feel really fat.
11.10	1 apple	Work			
3.15	2 Twix	High St	*		
	1 bread roll	"	*		
	a fruit cake	Market	*		Everyone looked at me in the
3.30	2 chocolate eggs	"	*		market. I'm out of control.
	2 bread rolls	Kitchen	*		I hate myself. I can't stop
	½ pint of milk	"	*	V	crying
5.10	1 bowl cereal	"	*		I am really trying not to eat.
	1 bowl cereal	"	*		
	1 pitta bread with	"	*		
	cottage cheese.				
	1 glass water	"	*		I'm going to vomit. I can't
6.00	a baked potato	Van outside			help it.
	1 can Tab	"	*	V	
9.00	1 cup Slimline soup	Kitchen			Weighed myself
	1 ice cube	"			9st 8lb – too heavy.
9.20	1 cup coffee	"			Feel fat and ugly.
					I want someone to talk to.
10.00	1 coffee (black)	Sitting room			
11.20	1 coffee (black)	Kitchen			Why do I do this? I want
	6 shortbread biscuits	"	*		to be thin.
	4 pieces of chocolate	"	**	V	I can't help it
	2 pieces of toast	"	*	V	
	2 glasses of water	"			
					Weighed 9st 7lb – fat
				L	Took 24 Nylax.

Fig. 23.2 A monitoring sheet illustrating the eating habits of a patient with bulimia nervosa. B, bulimic episodes; V/L, vomiting or laxative use; *, episodes of eating viewed by the patient as 'excessive'.

rules, and the resulting possibility of weight gain intensifies their fear of becoming fat. Consequently, they attempt to compensate for these episodes: almost all renew their determination to diet, thereby perhaps increasing their vulnerability to further episodes of overeating, many induce vomiting, some take laxatives or diuretics and a minority rigorously exercise.

Like patients with anorexia nervosa, the 'body image' of patients with bulimia nervosa is disturbed. True body image misperception, as judged clinically, is not common, but body image disparagement is evident in at least a quarter.

General psychopathology

This resembles that found in anorexia nervosa, although these patients have more severe depressive and anxiety symptoms. Personality disorder of the 'borderline' type is present in a small minority, but much more common is severe low self-esteem. Substance abuse is encountered in a small subgroup. In general the anxiety and depressive symptoms appear to be a psychological reaction to the loss of control overeating since they respond to any treatment that reduces the frequency of overeating. However, a minority of subjects appear to have a coexisting depressive disorder since treatment of their eating problem does not lessen their general psychiatric symptoms.

The physical features of bulimia nervosa

Most of the physical features may be directly attributed to the behaviour of these patients, particularly the dieting, overeating, vomiting and laxative use.

Symptoms and signs. The majority of patients have few physical complaints. Those most commonly encountered are irregular or absent menstruation, toothache, vague abdominal pains and weakness and lethargy. On examination, salivary gland enlargement may be present: typically, this involves the parotids and gives the patient's face a chubby appearance. In those who vomit there may be calluses on the dorsum of the hands (Russell's sign) due to the fingers being used to stimulate the gag reflex. Also, there may be significant erosion of the dental enamel of the inner surface of the front teeth. A minority of patients, particularly those who take large quantities of laxatives, have intermittent peripheral or facial oedema.

The body weight of these patients has been the subject of some controversy. Whilst the weight of the majority is unremarkable according to population norms, it has been suggested that they are nevertheless underweight (i.e. below their natural weight). In other words, it is proposed that their natural weight is a high one. This proposal is interesting since it suggests that a tendency to be overweight statistically speaking might be a risk factor for the development of the disorder. Arguments for this view include these patients' reports that they tend to gain weight easily, the data suggesting that they have low energy requirements for weight maintenance (Obarzanek et al 1991), and the presence in some patients of metabolic indices of starvation. Given that energy requirements and resting metabolic rate are to some extent under genetic influence, it is also of note that there is evidence of an increased family history of obesity. However, were this view correct, it would be predicted that successful treatment would result in weight gain, and this is not the case. However, it is possible that a tendency to be overweight may be a risk factor in a proportion of cases.

Abnormalities on laboratory investigation. The abnormality of most clinical importance is the electrolyte disturbance which is encountered in about half those who vomit or take laxatives. Metabolic alkalosis, hypochloraemia and hypokalaemia are the most common disturbances. Usually these abnormalities are of little clinical significance, but they may account for the weakness and tiredness experienced by some. Clinically, serious electrolyte disturbance is occasionally encountered, but rarely does it merit direct treatment; instead, it is generally more appropriate to focus on the treatment of the eating disorder itself, since the normalisation of eating habits will reverse the electrolyte disturbance.

The endocrine status of these patients has not been as extensively studied as in anorexia nervosa. The abnormalities found resemble those in anorexia nervosa, but are not as severe. They are thought to be secondary to the strict dieting (Fichter et al 1990). An exception is the elevated serum amylase level, the pathophysiology of which is not understood.

Aetiology

Since the majority of patients with bulimia nervosa have a history of frank or subthreshold anorexia nervosa, and since the two conditions are so similar, it may be assumed that most factors of relevance to the aetiology of anorexia nervosa will also be relevant to bulimia nervosa. Nevertheless, several factors may specifically increase the risk of developing bulimia nervosa. Already mentioned is a tendency to be overweight. Two others are predispositions to affective disorders and substance abuse: the rate of both disorders appears to be raised in the relatives of these patients. Another factor is the presence of borderline personality traits. However, it is important not to place too much faith in these putative risk factors, since they are derived from studies with many methodological shortcomings, not the least of which is their reliance on clinically detected samples. It must be remembered that most cases of bulimia nervosa are not detected, and the subgroup that tends to be studied may be biased. (For an account of the factors involved in the development of bulimia nervosa, see Striegel-Moore et al (1986).)

Once bulimia nervosa is established, several processes maintain it. These are illustrated in Figure 23.3. First, overconcern with shape and weight drives continued strict dieting. Second, as discussed earlier, this dieting is likely to encourage overeating through both physiological and psychological mechanisms, yet the dieting will also be maintained by the overeating. Third, self-induced vomiting and, to a lesser extent, purgative and diuretic misuse also encourage overeating: faith in their effectiveness undermines attempts not to overeat. Fourth, the episodes of overeating undermine the patients' sense of self-control and their self-esteem, thereby exaggerating feelings of ineffectiveness and intensifying the overconcern with shape and weight.

Assessment

The principles of assessment resemble those for anorexia nervosa. Of particular importance is the evaluation of depressive symptoms since a small subgroup have a coexisting depressive disorder. The 'biological symptoms' of depression are not a useful guide since appetite, weight, energy and gastrointestinal function are all directly affected by the eating disorder. To decide whether there is a depressive disorder, it is usually necessary to see whether the depressive symptoms persist even when the eating problem has improved. Thus, the decision often cannot be made for some weeks.

The physical state of these patients must not be forgotten, especially that of patients who vomit frequently or take laxatives or diuretics. Their electrolyte status must be evaluated, and sometimes monitored.

Treatment

Given that bulimia nervosa has only recently been described, it is remarkable how much has been learned about its treatment. More than 25 controlled trials have been completed and more are in progress. (See Fairburn et al (1992) for an account of the work to date.) Thus, it is possible to base treatment recommendations on research findings.

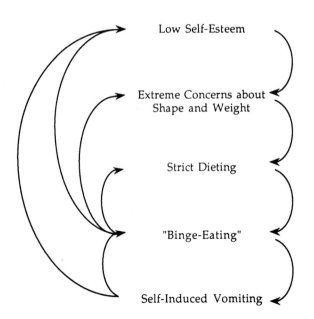

Fig. 23.3 Processes involved in the maintenance of bulimia nervosa.

It is clear from the work on treatment that the great majority of patients may be managed on an out-patient basis. Full or partial hospitalisation is indicated under four unusual circumstances: first, if the patient is too depressed to be managed as an out-patient or there is a risk of suicide; second, if the patient's physical health is a cause for concern; third, if the patient is in the first trimester of pregnancy, since there is evidence that the spontaneous abortion rate may be high; and fourth, if the eating disorder proves refractory to out-patient care. If hospitalisation is indicated it should usually be brief, possibly on a day-patient basis, and regarded as a preliminary to out-patient care.

With regard to out-patient care, the choice lies between treatment with antidepressant drugs and the use of various specific forms of psychotherapy.

Pharmacological treatment studies

Most pharmacological treatment studies have focused on the effects of antidepressant drugs. Other drugs have been studied, including appetite suppressants, opiate antagonists, antiepileptic drugs and lithium. None seems promising and their use is not recommended. In contrast, it is clear that antidepressant drugs have an effect on bulimia nervosa, at least in the short-term. Three groups of findings have emerged. First, these drugs are superior to placebo at reducing many of the features of the disorder. There is a marked reduction in the frequency of overeating and self-induced vomiting and this is accompanied by an enhanced sense of control over eating. At the same time the degree of general psychiatric disturbance lessens substantially. However, the high level of dietary restraint appears not to be affected. The effect of the drugs on these patients' overvalued ideas concerning shape and weight has not been studied. The second group of findings concern the rapidity of the antidepressant drug effect and the dose needed to achieve it. It seems that the time-course resembles that seen in the treatment of depression. It has also been suggested that the dose required is similar, but systematic dose–response studies have yet to be conducted. The third finding is that no consistent predictors of response can be identified. The level of depressive symptoms prior to treatment does not seem to predict outcome.

Maintenance of change following treatment with antidepressant drugs has received remarkably little attention. This is a serious gap in our knowledge since bulimia nervosa tends to run a chronic course. The findings of two recent studies suggest that maintenance is poor, whether or not the patient stays on the drug (see Walsh et al 1991).

Psychological treatment studies

The main focus of psychological treatment studies has been on a form of cognitive behaviour therapy designed specifically for patients with bulimia nervosa. This has been compared with being on a waiting list, antidepressant drug treatment, supportive psychotherapy, focal psychotherapy, a purely behavioural version of the treatment, and exposure with response prevention. With few exceptions, cognitive behaviour therapy has been shown to be superior in its effects. It is at least as effective as antidepressants at reducing the frequency of overeating and vomiting, and it appears to have a much greater effect on the level of dietary restraint. Perhaps because of this, maintenance of change seems good.

Implications for clinical practice

The research on treatment indicates that the best overall approach is the cognitive behavioural one. If clinicians are to use one single form of treatment, this is the one to adopt. Typically, it involves about 20 sessions over 5 months. Detailed manuals have been written describing the treatment (Fairburn & Cooper 1989), and with practice it can be successfully used even without specialist training. All those who see patients with eating disorders should include this form of treatment in their therapeutic armamentarium.

The cognitive behavioural approach is neither necessary nor sufficient for all patients with bulimia nervosa. For some patients it probably constitutes overtreatment. For these patients simpler and briefer therapies are likely to be as effective. For others, cognitive behaviour therapy is not sufficient. There is therefore a need to develop and evaluate treatments for those who do not respond. Combining cognitive behaviour therapy and antidepressant drugs does not seem to be worthwhile, although it is worth trying with patients who have severe unremitting depressive symptoms in case a coexisting depressive disorder is interfering with treatment of the eating disorder.

Outcome

Little is known about the course of bulimia nervosa. Research to date suggests that it is varied. Community-based studies suggest that many cases are transitory and resolve of their own accord. In contrast, clinical experience suggests that the disorder is often long-lasting and resistant to many forms of treatment. Consistent predictors of outcome have yet to be identified. Clearly, bulimia nervosa is a heterogeneous disorder and only those with more enduring forms present for treatment.

BINGE-EATING DISORDER

Serious consideration is being given to the inclusion in DSM-IV of a new category of eating disorder currently termed 'binge-eating disorder' (Wilson & Walsh 1991). The stimulus comes from two sources. First, it has long been recognised that amongst those who seek treatment for obesity there is a subgroup with a distinctive pattern of eating characterised by recurrent episodes of uncontrolled overeating. These individuals are more distressed than those who do not eat in this way, and are thought to respond less well to conventional weight loss programmes. The second stimulus has come from work on the prevalence of bulimia nervosa. This has shown that there is a sizeable group of people who are troubled by repeated episodes of overeating but who do not meet diagnostic criteria for bulimia nervosa (Fairburn & Beglin 1990). Neither this group nor the obese group has been adequately characterised. By bringing them together under the general heading of binge-eating disorder, the hope is that research will be stimulated on their nature and treatment.

At present, little is known about binge-eating disorder; indeed, even the term has yet to be agreed upon. (The lay term is 'compulsive overeating'.) The definition, characteristics and prevalence of the syndrome have still to be defined, and its relationship to other eating disorders specified, particularly the non-purging subtype of bulimia nervosa. Research is also needed on the relationship between this disorder and obesity. Finally, work is needed on treatment; for example, in those patients who are also overweight, it is not clear whether treatment should focus on their weight or eating habits, or both, and, if both, which should be addressed first.

OTHER DISORDERS OF RELEVANCE TO PSYCHIATRIC PRACTICE

Surveys of the eating habits and weight of psychiatric patients indicate that disturbed eating is common and that many in-patients are significantly overweight. Specific eating disorders, in particular bulimia nervosa, sometimes coexist with other psychiatric conditions but often go unrecognised since they are not considered during assessment. With female patients under the age of 40 years, clinicians should be on the alert for problems with eating and weight and consider as a matter of routine the possibility that they might have an eating disorder.

Eating, weight and activity levels are affected in many psychiatric disorders. In mania, weight often falls since energy expenditure is high and some patients are too restless to eat. In social phobias discomfort in company may lead to the avoidance of social eating. In addition, some patients have specific concerns about being seen eating or swallowing; others are afraid of vomiting or choking when eating. Such patients may lose considerable amounts of weight and come to resemble patients with anorexia nervosa, though they may be distinguished since their concerns centre on the act of eating itself rather than on shape or weight. The treatment of such problems is similar in principle to that for phobias (see Ch. 41). There are also patients who stop eating to bring attention to themselves. These do not show the concerns about shape and weight that characterise anorexia nervosa and bulimia nervosa. Most have a personality disorder, and they are best managed along the usual lines (see Ch. 27).

The psychiatric disorder most well known for its effects on appetite, eating, weight and activity level is depression. A reduction in appetite and loss of weight is seen in about half the cases, whereas increased appetite and weight gain occurs in about a third. The explanation for this difference in the pattern of symptoms is not clear: interestingly, it appears to be consistent across episodes (Stunkard et al 1990). Because of the changes in eating and weight, depressive disorders form part of the differential diagnosis of anorexia nervosa and bulimia nervosa. The key distinguishing feature is the core psychopathology of anorexia nervosa and bulimia nervosa which is not present in depression. On occasions, however, depressive disorders coexist with anorexia nervosa or bulimia nervosa.

Various neuropsychiatric disorders affect eating and weight. These include certain types of hypothalamic tumour and the Kleine–Levin syndrome. The disorder of most relevance to psychiatry is dementia. Many demented people lose considerable amounts of weight, especially in the later stages of the illness. The explanation is not clear. In a minority, hyperphagia is seen and it can result in substantial weight gain (Morris et al 1989).

Eating and weight are also affected by certain psychotropic drugs, including neuroleptics, tricyclic antidepressants and lithium carbonate. Usually the result is weight gain, but the mechanisms responsible are unknown. Relevant factors include an increase in food intake accompanied possibly by a change in food choice, decreased activity, and heightened thirst leading to the overconsumption of energy-rich drinks. This weight gain is not a trivial matter since it often interferes with patients' general health and can affect compliance. It is therefore of note that the new selective serotonin re-uptake blocking antidepressants do not produce weight gain; indeed, some even cause weight loss. Such drugs (e.g. fluoxetine) may be of special value when treating overweight patients and those in whom a gain in weight would be a particular problem. Finally, it must not be forgotten that hospitalisation itself may result in weight gain, both by encouraging overeating through the regular provision of large meals and by limiting energy expenditure in the form of exercise.

REFERENCES

Abraham S F, Llewellyn-Jones D 1987 Eating disorders: the facts. Oxford University Press, Oxford

Andersen A E 1990 Males with eating disorders. Brunner/Mazel, New York

Carlat D J, Camargo C A 1991 Review of bulimia nervosa in males. American Journal of Psychiatry 148: 831

Dolan B 1991 Cross-cultural aspects of anorexia nervosa and bulimia: a review. International Journal of Eating Disorders 10: 67

Fairburn C G, Beglin S J 1990 Studies of the epidemiology of bulimia nervosa. American Journal of Psychiatry 147: 401

Fairburn C G, Cooper P J 1989 Eating disorders. In: Hawton K, Salkovskis P, Kirk J, Clark D M (eds) Cognitive behaviour therapy for psychiatric problems: a practical guide. Oxford University Press, Oxford

Fairburn C G, Agras W S, Wilson G T 1992 The research on the treatment of bulimia nervosa: practical and theoretical implications. In: Anderson G H, Kennedy S H (eds) The biology of feast and famine: relevance to eating disorders. Academic Press, New York

Fichter M M, Pirke K M, Pollinger J, Wolfram G, Brunner E 1990 Disturbances in the hypothalamo–pituitary–adrenal and other neuroendocrine axes in bulimia. Biological Psychiatry 27: 1021

Garfinkel P E, Garner D M 1982 Anorexia nervosa: a multidimensional perspective. Brunner/Mazel, New York

Garner D M, Bemis K M 1985 A cognitive-behavioural approach to anorexia nervosa. In: Garner D M, Garfinkel P E (eds) Handbook of psychotherapy for anorexia nervosa and bulimia. Guilford Press, New York

Garner D M, Garfinkel P E 1985 Handbook of psychotherapy for anorexia nervosa and bulimia nervosa. Guilford Press, New York

Holland A J, Sicotte N, Treasure J L 1988 Anorexia nervosa: evidence for a genetic basis. Journal of Psychosomatic Research 32: 561

Hsu L K G 1990 Eating disorders. Guilford Press, New York

Levine M P, Smolak L 1991 Towards a developmental psychopathology of eating disorders — the example of early adolescence. In: Crowther J H, Hobfoll S E, Stephens M A P, Tennenbaum D L (eds) The etiology of bulimia — the individual and family context. Hemisphere, Washington, D C

Lucas A R, Beard C M, O'Fallon W M, Kurland L T 1991 50 year trends in the incidence of anorexia nervosa in Rochester, Minnesota: a population-based study. American Journal of Psychiatry 148: 917

Morris C H, Hope R A, Fairburn C G 1989 Eating habits in dementia: a descriptive study. British Journal of Psychiatry 154: 801

Obarzanek E, Lesem M D, Goldstein D S, Jimerson D C 1991 Reduced resting metabolic rate in patients with bulimia nervosa. Archives of General Psychiatry 48: 456

Palmer J L 1988 Anorexia nervosa. Penguin, London

Piran H, Kaplan A S 1990 A day hospital group treatment program for anorexia nervosa and bulimia nervosa. Brunner/Mazel, New York

Ratnasuriya R H, Eisler I, Szmukler G, Russell G F M 1991 Anorexia nervosa: outcome and prognostic factors after 20 years. British Journal of Psychiatry 158: 495

Russell G F M 1979 Bulimia nervosa: an ominous variant of anorexia nervosa. Psychological Medicine 9: 429

Russell G F M, Szmukler G I, Dare C, Eisler I 1987 An evaluation of family therapy in anorexia nervosa and bulimia nervosa. Archives of General Psychiatry 44: 1047

Striegel-Moore R H, Silberstein L R, Rodin J 1986 Toward an understanding of risk factors for bulimia. American Psychologist 41: 246

Strober M, Lampert C, Morrell W, Burroughs J, Jacobs C 1990 A controlled family study of anorexia nervosa: evidence of familial aggregation and lack of shared transmission with affective disorders. International Journal of Eating Disorders 9: 239

Stunkard A J, Fernstrom M H, Price A, Frank E, Kupfer D 1990 Direction of weight change in recurrent depression. Archives of General Psychiatry 47: 857

Vandereycken W, Kog E, Vanderlinden J 1989 The family approach to eating disorders. PMA, New York

Vitousek K B, Hollon K B 1990 The investigation of schematic content and processing in eating disorders. Cognitive Therapy and Research 14: 191

Walsh B T, Hadigan C M, Devlin M J, Gladis M, Roose S P 1991 Long-term outcome of antidepressant treatment for bulimia nervosa. American Journal of Psychiatry 148: 1206

Walsh B T, Hadigan C M, Kissileff H R, LaChaussee J L 1992 Bulimia nervosa: a syndrome of feast and famine. In: Anderson G H, Kennedy S H (eds) The biology of feast and famine: relevance to eating disorders. Academic Press, New York

Wilson G T, Walsh B T Eating disorders in the DSM-1V. Journal of Abnormal Psychology 100: 362

24. Sleep disorders

C. Shapiro

Sleep complaints are not the most common presenting symptom to a psychiatrist. They are, however, the most ubiquitous symptom in psychiatric patients. There are other reasons for psychiatrists having some understanding of sleep and its disorders: changes in sleep may precipitate psychiatric ill health; many primary sleep disorders are associated with high rates of psychiatric morbidity; sleep disorders may be misidentified as psychiatric illness and vice versa; and a number of drugs used particularly by psychiatrists may alter (and worsen) sleep disorders. Moreover, some of the best biological markers of psychiatric illness come from sleep studies in depression and studies of states of sleep and dreams provide a window to the understanding of psychiatric illness.

For those unfamiliar with current sleep research, this litany may seem to be the overstatement of an enthusiast. In this chapter these statements will be substantiated and five common sleep disorders will be described. For further information see Peter et al (1991), Montplasier & Godbout (1990), Thorpy (1990) and Shapiro & Rathouse (1990).

Sleep and dreams have always been the subject of popular fascination and are frequently depicted in art and described in folk, religious and contemporary literature. In the early part of this century, the interpretation of dreams by Freud expanded the interests of psychiatrists in the subject of sleep and dreams. In the late 1950s the description of rapid eye movement (REM) sleep on electroencephalogram (EEG) criteria by Aserinsky & Kleitman (1953) and Dement & Kleitman (1957) ushered in the current era of sleep research and the development of sleep disorders medicine. At that time, psychiatrists played a leading role, but with the increasing technical complexity of sleep research there has been a shift away from the domain of psychiatry. Although the technical aspects are not particularly esoteric, this hesitancy on the part of psychiatrists to use instrumentation in the study of behaviour and psychiatric illness has many consequences. In the measurement of most psychiatric conditions, rating scales and other psychometric techniques are the dominant modality (Peck & Shapiro 1990) whereas, in the field of sleep and dreams, psychometric instruments are weak and physiological measurements predominate.

Sleep is a normal physiological process. The features of fluctuating physiological activity in REM sleep had been described by many prior to the EEG characterisation. One engaging account is that of MacWilliams, an Aberdonian physiologist, who wrote in 1923:

> disturbed sleep, modified by reflex excitations, dreams, nightmare, etc., sometimes accompanied by extensive rises of blood pressure, increased heart action, changes in respiration, and various reflex effects . . . In addition to the circulation and respiration the disturbances of troubled sleep may extend, in varying degree, over other systems, somatic and visceral, as evidenced by sweating, tremors, vomiting after awaking, etc. It is obvious that such disturbances acting on various functions in different ways may be responsible for important effects in some conditions of disease.

In the newborn infant sleeping 16 hours a day, approximately 8 hours a day is REM sleep, whereas in young adults sleeping 8 hours a day approximately one-fifth of sleep is REM sleep. There is a characteristic architecture to sleep with sleep cycles of 90–100 minutes ending with a REM episode which is typically short (5–10 minutes) early in the night and which progressively lengthens through the night. As a consequence most REM sleep occurs in the last third of the night. In the first two sleep cycles, most 'deep' slow wave sleep (SWS, characterised by large-amplitude slow EEG waves) occurs. During this SWS, approximately 80% of the daily output of human growth hormone (HGH) occurs. SWS is characterised by decreased metabolic rate (Shapiro et al 1984) and REM sleep is characterised by marked autonomic instability and possible dysfunction (Shapiro 1991a).

There are many theories of sleep function. Increasingly, the lay notion that sleep serves a restorative function has gained scientific support (Oswald 1980, Shapiro 1982). There are many theories which emphasised cognitive, memory and psychic aspects associated with REM sleep. In the same way that the observation that enuresis typically occurs in SWS, and therefore cannot be construed as a 'dissociative' experience linked to a 'hysterical neurosis', so all the physiological observations concerning sleep cited above lead to better understanding of behaviour. The growth-retarded child, subject to emotional abuse, may have disrupted sleep, failure of nocturnal HGH release and stunted stature as a consequence. The 'sleepy/lazy' adolescent may be having increased SWS and increased need for restorative sleep; the nocturnally disruptive dementing patient may have a decreased amplitude of circadian rhythm as a result of pineal lesions and there is evidence emerging that exposure to a *Zeitgeber* in the form of bright light may be effective in curtailing nocturnal wandering. The autonomic instability of REM sleep may also be of relevance in triggering the flashback and sleep disruption phenomenon of post-traumatic stress disorder (PTSD).

SLEEP DISRUPTION AND PSYCHIATRIC ILL HEALTH

It is common to recognise a change in sleep pattern in patients with psychiatric illness. Hamilton (1989) has emphasised that one of the most common features of depression is sleep disruption. It is not always appreciated that in 20% of depressed patients with sleep change this is a hypersomnia rather than an insomnia.

The insomnia associated with mania, PTSD, anxiety states, postnatal depression, alcohol dependence and anorexia nervosa can all be perceived as stemming from different psychological and physiological bases. In anorexia, psychological stresses are exacerbated by the disruptive effect of starvation on sleep, the change in metabolism, the altered endocrine state and altered body composition, all of which influence sleep. The disruption of sleep will have the effect of raising metabolic rate and increasing energy requirements. Return of normal sleep architecture may be a useful guide in monitoring recovery.

Several studies have suggested that sleep disruption may cause affective illnesses. Ford & Kamerow (1989) studied close to 8000 subjects on two occasions, 1 year apart, with detailed interviews at each point. Those with either insomnia or hypersomnia were more likely to have a psychiatric illness. Those who developed sleep disruption during the year were more likely to have a psychiatric illness at the end of the year, and conversely in those whose sleep disorder resolved there was a decreased likelihood of having a psychiatric illness at the end of the year. Although these data are correlational, albeit cross-sectional and longitudinal, the authors point to the possibility that 'early recognition and treatment of sleep disturbances can prevent future psychiatric disorders'. Recently, Wilke & Shapiro (1992) have shown that if primiparous woman have part of their labour during what would normally constitute the sleeping period there is a significant increase in postpartum blues. (Interestingly, Coble et al (1991) have shown that REM latency is shorter in the last trimester of pregnancy and postpartum in women with a past history of affective illness than in normal controls.) One occasionally sees patients (such as the articulate 3 month postpartum endocrinologist with financial, domestic and social pressures who said of her insomnia: 'It is making me depressed. It is not that my depression is manifesting as insomnia') who give credence to sleep disruption triggering depression.

Paradoxically, sleep disruption (total or partial) has been shown to elevate mood in people who are depressed. Various studies indicate a 35–70% response rate, with a meta-analysis of 1200 patients from different studies indicating a 60% response level. Unfortunately, the effect is usually brief. Wehr (1990) reviews the subject and gives an interesting historical account of the interest in depriving schizophrenic patients of sleep, linked to psychodynamic ideas of the role of dreams in psychosis in the 1950s. The current interest in sleep deprivation in affective disorders reflects more biological views relating to circadian rhythms and mood. This pendulum has gained some reverse momentum with the observation that many modalities of treatment of depression suppress REM sleep (Shapiro 1991b). The author had a radio mechanic tell him that since his 'breakdown in the early 50s' he had found that if he slept on the couch in the living room he would have a poor sleep and a good mood the next day. If he slept in his bed, he would be aware of somewhat better sleep but worse mood the day following. He spent 30 years trying to balance these needs.

An extension of sleep disruption in elevating mood is the triggering of mania and patients may present with mania after sleep deprivation experiments. For example, a young man with a past history of bipolar illness drove with his brother from Southampton to Edinburgh overnight. The brother described increasing excitement during the drive, starting at 3 a.m. The patient's grandiosity in the car led the brother (who recognised the symptoms) to drive directly to the hospital where the patient had previously been treated. Wehr et al (1987) have described four such cases.

A condition which presents increasingly to psychiatrists is chronic fatigue. There is currently considerable debate about this condition, particularly its relationship with affective disorder and the role of infectious and immunological processes in its aetiology. When referred to as fibromyalgia it is associated with a characteristic sleep EEG profile (Moldofsky 1990). The EEG pattern may be indicative of poor sleep quality which perpetuates the sense of fatigue. In trying to explain this EEG characteristic (an alpha pattern intruding into the sleep EEG) to many patients referred for sleep assessment with chronic fatigue, I have elicited immediate recognition from them by saying that the 'brain waves while you are asleep look as if you are partially awake'. What is not known is whether this 'sleep thumbprint' is a consequence of the condition or if the poor sleep quality indicated by the alpha EEG is a precursor of the chronic fatigue state.

PSYCHIATRIC PRESENTATION OF SLEEP AND SLEEP-RELATED DISORDERS

A number of sleep-related disorders are occasionally mistaken for psychiatric conditions. A small proportion of patients with epilepsy have seizures exclusively during sleep. The mistaken behavioural treatment of nocturnal enuresis when there is a neurological basis for the enuresis is an obvious hazard. Sleep walking is occasionally perceived as a conversion disorder. Exclusive nocturnal asthma was, until relatively recently, frequently misperceived as a hysterical complaint as there were no daytime signs to detect. A complaint of insomnia, particularly in the setting of consultation/ liaison psychiatry, is often misconstrued as depression and a couple of nights of treatment with a hypnotic rather than rushing to commence with antidepressant treatment is a useful strategy. Sleep disruption in general hospital in-patients is poorly documented (Mayou & Hawton 1986).

Recently, Douglass et al (1991) have reported a series of patients with visual and auditory hallucinations treated for schizophrenia with poor response to antipsychotic drugs and apparent excessive sleepiness. Patients with abnormal computerised tomography (CT) scans, EEG abnormalities and a history of alcohol or drug abuse or a relative with affective illness were excluded. All patients fitting these criteria were shown to have HLA blood typing compatible with narcolepsy and, in some, polysomnographic features of narcolepsy. The following quotation of part of a clinical vignette from the paper by Douglass and coworkers emphasises how this type of mistaken diagnosis can be made:

> She had first heard the "voice of God" as a girl. Auditory hallucinations worsened with age and were prominent at night. Recently, at bedtime and associated with waking periods during that night, she had multi-modal hallucinations of being "raped by escaped criminals, hands and feet tied down, and under anaesthesia" (ie, sleep paralysis). She had called the police to complain. During the day, she will experience sexual stimulation by hallucinatory touch and when music played, her hips would be made to rotate. She occasionally had a bad taste in her mouth which she interpreted as being poisoned.

Douglass, who is interested in sleep disorders, had been alerted to this when a 30-year-old 'schizophrenic' woman with a 13 year history of illness had revealed that her father was recently diagnosed as narcoleptic. Even in the 'prepared mind', sleep disorder masquerading as psychiatric illness is not necessarily recognised. Amphetamine is helpful in resolving these patients' hallucinations. Douglass et al emphasise that in some patients cataplectic attacks have been mistaken for catatonia. They estimate that 7% of schizophrenics may be similarly misdiagnosed narcoleptics.

There are few reports of psychiatric concomitants of sleep apnoea but there is an increasing awareness of the cognitive deficits associated with repeated hypoxic episodes (Findley et al 1986). Lee et al (1989) have described a young patient with psychosis based on sleep apnoea with total resolution of the psychosis after tonsillectomy. There are several other reports of psychosis in sleep apnoea patients (Berrettini 1980, Martin & Lefebvre 1981) with resolution of the former with treatment of the latter. Another presentation with psychiatric significance is that of sleep apnoea presenting as pseudodementia (Bradley & Shapiro 1993). When sleep apnoea is first treated there is a dramatic resurgence of REM sleep. As yet, psychiatrists have not used this change in dreaming state as an opportunity to investigate the role of dreaming.

SLEEP STUDIES IN PSYCHIATRY

There are few psychiatric conditions in which an overnight polysomnogram (with or without a daytime multiple sleep latency test) is essential but there are a number of circumstances in which such assessments provide useful additional information. Jacobs et al (1988) studied a consecutive series of insomnia patients attending a specialised clinic in a psychiatric department. The polysomnographic studies contributed to the final diagnosis in 49% of patients. This emphasises that, even with detailed assessment by interviews and psychometric rating scales, assessment of insomnia which has many causes (see below) may still require polysomnography.

There are a number of conditions in which sleep assessment aids in the differential diagnosis. In normal males, REM sleep is invariably associated with a penile erection. This can be construed as part of the autonomic dysfunction alluded to above. It also provides the basis of a test aiding in the separation of psychogenic and organic causes of impotence. If in an overnight study, nocturnal penile tumescence (NPT) studies show repeated erections during REM sleep the patient can be reassured that there is no organic basis for his impotence (Bancroft 1989). Sometimes this reassurance is therapeutic in itself! The converse does not necessarily apply as there may be a failure of NPT in depressed patients (Roose et al 1982). There may also be differences in the physiological substrate of REM-related penile tumescence compared with day-time erectile function. A critical review is given by Meisler & Carey (1990).

Overnight sleep studies may be helpful in the differential diagnosis of myotonia, in which neurological and psychological causes are much debated (Gaudet et al 1991). In this situation, the persistence of muscular tone in affected muscles during REM sleep (during which there is normally a loss of muscle tone) and the absence/suppression of REM sleep have been taken as indications of an organic basis. The converse (i.e. a normal loss of muscle tone in REM sleep) is not evidence of psychogenesis but points in that direction.

Sleep studies in affective disorders

It has been suggested that there is a cluster of changes in the sleep architecture of depressed patients. These changes are: (1) a disruption of sleep continuity and prolongation of sleep latency; (2) a shortening of REM latency (i.e. the time from sleep onset to first appearance of REM sleep); (3) a decrease in SWS; (4) an increase in the SWS proportion in the second sleep cycle compared to the first; and (5) increased REM sleep (particularly in the first third of the night). Recently, the proponents of this theory have suggested that these sleep characteristics are most commonly found in particular subgroups of depressed patients, especially the psychotic, the elderly and those with other (i.e. non-sleep-related) endogenous features (Kupfer & Reynolds 1987). In a meta-analysis of 27 studies comparing drug-free depressed patients with normal controls, Knowles & MacLean (1990) showed that there were robust trends in sleep parameters in

relation to age in both samples and these trends showed a progressively diverging course. There are issues of sensitivity and specificity in using REM latency (the most exhaustively studied sleep feature) as a diagnostic marker for depression. Both Hamilton & Shapiro (1990) and Wehr (1990) have tabulated a dozen conditions in which short REM latency has been reported. Both these reviews list several studies of groups of depressed patients who did not have a short REM latency, e.g. patients with recent-onset depression or depression accompanying medical disorders. In many studies said to have been carried out in drug-free patients the criterion of 'drug-free' was set pragmatically at 2 weeks, but this does not sufficiently preclude the rebound effect of REM suppression following benzodiazepine or tricyclic antidepressant withdrawal. Insufficient attention has been paid to afternoon napping, which is more likely in depressed in-patients and the elderly and may influence results. The sex of the patients may also have a bearing on outcome as Ansseau et al (1985) have shown more variability in REM latency in depressed males than in depressed females. Recently a circannual variation in REM latency in non-depressed patients has been observed, and this may be a further factor to consider (MacFarlane et al 1991). These caveats aside, (1) the observation of greater stability of REM latency in those with a family history of depression (Cartwright et al 1988), (2) the fact that there are now five studies all suggesting that early change in REM latency on starting antidepressant therapy predicts response to treatment, and (3) that persistence of short REM latency at the end of treatment has been shown to predict early relapse (Giles et al 1987) all suggest an integral link between REM sleep architecture and depression. Some of the best evidence that there is a fundamental change in REM sleep in depression comes from studies based on the arecholine REM induction test (RIT) originally described by Gillin et al (1982). They claimed to have identified a trait marker when they found, in both currently depressed and recovered depressed patients, that infusion of a muscarinic agonist, arecholine, would provoke a more rapid onset of subsequent REM periods during sleep. This research has been taken further by Berger et al (1989) who found that 14 out of 16 depressed patients showed early REM onset after pretreatment with a new muscarinic agonist, RS-86, compared with only one of 20 patients with other psychiatric diagnoses.

There are still many issues to be resolved in this area. Early indications point to a lack of alteration in REM latency when psychotherapeutic techniques have been used (Jarrett et al 1988, Buysse et al 1991). Dahl et al (1990) provide tentative evidence in adolescents that suicidal ideation and in-patient status have an influence on REM parameters consistent with the notion of REM sleep abnormality occurring in more severely depressed patients. Kupfer & Ehlers (1989) have argued that there may be two different processes producing a short REM latency. In one type, there is a weakened SWS process, allowing REM sleep to move to an earlier position in the sleep period. This pattern appears to be genetically influenced and strongly age related. In the second type, a stress-related induction of early REM sleep occurs which may be more responsive to treatment with tricyclic antidepressants. If this is correct there is the potential for tailoring treatment to subgroups of depressed patients. The SWS-inducing, REM-suppressing (Shapiro & Driver 1988) and mood-elevating effects of exercise (Cramer et al 1991) may be useful specifically in the first type of depression.

In a recent somewhat skeptical review of REM latency as a diagnostic test for depression, Somoza & Mossman (1990) concluded that it is a 'modestly good discriminator of those mood-disordered patients most likely to require somatic treatments for recovery'. Buysse & Kupfer (1990) review the diagnostic and research role of sleep studies and stress that there are few tests in medicine that are pathognomonic for a disorder. Sleep studies have undoubtedly stimulated considerable research in affective disorders and may have some utility as a diagnostic tool. Their utility is likely to increase with more refined questions (e.g. response to treatment), more features of sleep EEG being utilised, and with pharmacologic challenge tests being incorporated into standard paradigms.

CLASSIFICATION OF SLEEP DISORDERS

It was traditional to classify sleep disorders into those presenting with too little sleep (insomnias), those presenting with hypersomnolence (too much), and those in which 'things went bump in the night' (parasomnias), with a fourth group (circadian disorders) tagged on. The most comprehensive classification, and one which will be made compatible with both ICD-10 and DSM-IV is the International Classification of Sleep Disorders, presented in a 400 page diagnostic and coding manual (American Sleep Disorders Association 1990). Although many of the conditions listed are of limited interest to psychiatrists they should be aware of the structure of the classification, which is shown in Table 24.1. The manual also provides an appendix of differential diagnoses, emphasising that certain conditions may produce either insomnia or

Table 24.1 Outline classification of sleep disorders (American Sleep Disorders Association). The number of specific conditions in each major category are shown in parentheses, followed by three or four examples

1. Dysomnias
   a. Intrinsic sleep disorders (13), e.g. psychophysiological insomnia, narcolepsy, obstructive sleep apnoea, restless legs syndrome.
   b. Extrinsic sleep disorders (14), e.g. inadequate sleep hygiene, insufficient sleep syndrome, nocturnal eating syndrome and alcohol-dependent sleep disorder.
   c. Circadian rhythm disorders (7), e.g. time zone change syndrome, delayed sleep phase syndrome, non-24-hour sleep–wake disorder

2. Parasomnias
   a. Arousal disorders (3), e.g. confusional arousals, sleep walking, sleep terrors
   b. Sleep–wake transition disorders (4), e.g. rhythmic movement disorder, sleep talking, nocturnal leg cramps
   c. Parasomnias usually associated with REM sleep (6), e.g. nightmares, sleep-related painful erections, REM sleep behaviour disorder
   d. Other parasomnias (11), e.g. sleep enuresis, nocturnal paroxysmal dystonia, sudden infant death syndrome

3. Medical/psychiatric sleep disorders
   a. Associated with mental disorders (5), e.g. anxiety disorders, panic disorders, alcoholism
   b. Associated with neurological disorders (7), e.g. dementia, fatal familial insomnia, sleep-related headaches
   c. Associated with other medical disorders (7), e.g. nocturnal cardiac ischaemia, sleep-related asthma, fibrositis syndrome

4. Proposed sleep disorders (11), e.g. sleep hyperhidrosis, menstrual-associated sleep disorder and terrifying hypnogogic hallucinations

hypersomnia, e.g. depression, inadequate sleep hygiene, and obstructive sleep apnoea. As the classification contains almost a dozen 'proposed sleep disorders' in addition to 88 established disorders it is only possible and appropriate here to describe the five disorders which are of greatest interest to psychiatrists.

Narcolepsy

First described in the French literature in 1862 by Caffé and coined by Foot (1866), it is a condition with a classical tetrad of features: hypersomnolence (in 100% of patients); cataplexy (± 90%); sleep paralysis (40%); and hypnogogic hallucinations (± 30%). These four key features run seemingly independent time-courses. At least 50% of patients also suffer from major affective disorders and/or personality problems. The aetiology is unknown. Onset is characteristically in the second decade of life but diagnosis is reputed to be the most delayed of all medical disorders — an average of 9–10 years. Quality of life studies comparing a wide range of different medical conditions suggest that quality of life in narcoleptic patients is worse than in all other groups studied other than quadriplegics.

The sleep attacks these patients experience are usually irresistible and are more frequent in boring situations. For example, patients may say that they have sleep attacks in traffic jams but never if they are speeding. The cataplectic attacks may be dramatic — a women falling to the ground on seeing her sister's wig being lifted off after being entangled by a chandelier, but more often they are partial, for example a sagging of the head, then buckling of the knees and closure of the eyes. They occur especially in the context of strong emotion (mirth, anger or distress) and can be dangerous — so it is important not to tell jokes while swimming, for example. Sleep paralysis is an especially frightening experience and the best treatment is reassurance. Hypnogogic hallucinations are often not described by patients because of a fear of being viewed as 'crazy'. There have been claims that the latter two symptoms may be helped by γ-hydroxybutyrate.

Narcolepsy is associated with an almost pathognomonic polysomnographic feature of direct entry into REM sleep. This observation was first made by Vogel (1960) when studying the dreams of these patients and is now exploited in a diagnostic test. A standard test of sleepiness is the multiple sleep latency test (MSLT) in which a patient is placed in a dark bedroom on five occasions during the day at 2-hourly intervals and given a 20 minute opportunity to attempt to fall asleep. If the patient enters REM sleep on two of the five occasions this is usually taken as diagnostic of narcolepsy. A short sleep onset latency is usually observed and in many patients paradoxically disrupted nocturnal sleep also occurs. For this reason, sedatives are occasionally used in these patients in addition to standard psychostimulants, e.g. methylphenidate and amphetamine. Cataplexy is usually treated with tricyclic antidepressants, such as clomipramine. There are important legal issues in patients with narcolepsy in relation to driving; some can do so safely but others cannot. An opportunity for short sleeps in the workplace or school is a valuable component of treatment. Linking patients with self-help groups is particularly important in this disabling condition.

In the early 1980s, Honda and colleagues described an association between the antigen HLA-DR2 and narcolepsy. It is now recognised that 99% of narcoleptics are HLA-DR2 (and DQw1) positive whereas HLA-DR2 only occurs in 20% of the general population (see Honda & Matsuki 1990). HLA typing is therefore more useful in excluding the diagnosis of narcolepsy in patients with an uncertain clinical history than in confirming the diagnosis. It is thought that, in 80% of patients with a genetic predisposition, a clear precipitating stress can be identified prior to the onset of the disorder. The chance of a first-degree relative having the disorder is increased 40-fold.

The diagnosis is usually not difficult if the appropriate history is taken. There are over three dozen conditions which can cause daytime hypersomnolence, ranging from the insufficient sleep syndrome, specific psychiatric disorders, post-traumatic hypersomnia, circadian disorders and menstrual-associated hypersomnolence. In young men, it is important to enquire about weight fluctuation and heat exposure, as recurrent hypersomnia is a feature of the Kline–Levine syndrome.

Periodic limb movement disorder (PLMD)

This is one of the more frequent but least understood sleep disorders. It is characterised by periodic episodes of repetitive and stereotyped limb movements during sleep. The disorder typically consists of extension of the big toes simultaneous with flexion of the ankle and knee. There is often a partial arousal but most patients are oblivious to having the disorder. The periodicity is related to sleep stage. There are no good epidemiological studies but reports indicate that one-third of individuals aged over 60 years have PLMD and in 10% of insomnia patients PLMD is the cause. The most useful information is usually derived from the bed partner, who may frequently be awakened by being kicked during the night. The number of arousals during sleep does not appear to be clearly related to the level of daytime somnolence, but in patients with 30 or more such movements per hour of sleep, it is common to find complaints of disrupted sleep and daytime fatigue. Treatment with clobazam, clonazepam, selegeline and L-dopa have all been found to be effective. Many PLMD patients present with anxiety and/or depression based on chronic sleep disruption. This condition is also encountered in other sleep disorders (e.g. narcolepsy and obstructive sleep apnoea) and other general medical conditions (e.g. parkinsonism and metabolic disorders, particularly uraemia). It is occasionally a problem in the latter half of pregnancy. PLMD can be induced or aggravated by tricyclic and monoamine oxidase inhibitor (MAOI) antidepressants and by phenothiazines. Withdrawal of benzodiazepines and certain anticonvulsants can also cause a worsening of the condition. The diagnosis is based either on polygraphic studies or on the bed partner's description.

Circadian rhythm disorders

The importance of circadian rhythms is underestimated in many branches of medicine. There are fascinating accounts of one group of premature infants being allowed to have dim light at night and another randomly allocated group being exposed to standard lighting to allow continuous nursing monitoring. The former acquired regular sleep patterns earlier and showed better growth at 1 year (Mann et al 1986). The timing of drug administration has circadian implications for the worsening of symptoms (e.g. the on–off phenomena of parkinsonism) and disease processes influenced by circadian rhythms, e.g. asthma. The effect of a given dose of HGH is greater if it is given at night than if it is administered in the morning. A detailed account of circadian rhythms is given by Moore-Ede et al (1982).

There are interesting claims of increasing psychiatric ill health associated with disruption of biological rhythms (for a review, see Kupfer et al 1988). Jauhar & Weller (1982) found more psychiatric symptomatology in travellers arriving at Heathrow airport from the east or west (i.e. crossing time zones) than in those travelling north and south. Claims of daylight-saving time changes having an impact of psychiatric presentations (Bick & Hannah 1986) have not been substantiated (Shapiro et al 1990).

Up to 25% of the workforce in the Western world is in some form of shift schedule and it is well recognised that the pattern of shifts can have a substantial impact on morbidity (physical and psychological) mortality and also on productivity.

'Jetlag' has been defined as 'consisting of varying degrees of difficulties in initiation or maintaining sleep, excessive sleepiness, decrements in subjective daytime alertness and performance, and somatic symptoms (largely related to gastrointestinal function) following rapid travel across multiple time zones' (American Sleep Disorders Association 1990). There are characteristic polysomnographic features of increased arousals and stage 1 sleep. The disorder is invariably self-limiting but resynchronisation of biological clocks to environmental time can be achieved with benzodiazepines and judicious use of bright light exposure (Czeisler et al 1989). Interestingly, melatonin also can be effective in minimising the impact of jetlag (Arendt et al 1986).

Delayed sleep phase syndrome, in which sleep is regularly delayed in relation to clock time, occurs more in adolescent males than females (10:1 ratio) but is equally distributed in adults and can be a cause of initial insomnia. Treatment by successively delaying sleep each day by a couple of hours until the right phase relationship with environmental time has been achieved is both dramatic and effective.

Parasomnias

Parasomnias have distinctive characteristics but, in some cases, there is considerable overlap. The author has seen an 11-year-old girl who rocked so violently as an infant in her cot (jactatio capitis nocturna) that her mother strapped her down. Ten years later she swung her arm from side to side nightly in her sleep, waking the rest of the household and occasionally sang in her sleep. A behavioural treatment akin to that of the 'pad and buzzer' used in enuretics may be effective in such patients. For the sleep walker, the most important advice is to make sure the sleep environment is safe — bolts on the windows, and requests for ground floor rooms on holidays and business trips. The patient should be taught to recognise that excessive sleepiness, whether as a result of sleep restriction, drugs, alcohol or working shifts, and stress are all likely to exacerbate sleepwalking.

REM sleep behavioural disorder is a condition in which there is an absence of the usual atonia associated with REM sleep and a consequent development of elaborate motor activity associated with dreams. It usually occurs in older men and may occur during the REM rebound associated with alcohol and benzodiazepine withdrawal. Cases induced by tricyclic antidepressants have also been reported. Violence is often a feature. There are no characteristic neuroanatomical or neurophysiological features and treatment consists simply of ensuring safety.

Insomnia

Insomnia is one of the, if not the, most common complaint presenting to general practitioners. A survey of sleep disorders in a representative sample of 1006 households in Los Angeles revealed a 42.5% prevalence of insomnia (Bixler et al 1979). Although use of hypnotic drugs has been declining since the mid-1980s, the consequences of poor management of insomnia can be far-reaching. A study of nearly 27 000 Swedes over a 15 year period (Allgulander & Nasman 1991) indicated that one in three men and one in five women who reported regular hypnotic use had been a psychiatric in-patient at least once during this time.

Although different rates of insomnia have been found in other epidemiological studies (depending largely on the definition of insomnia used), the impact of insomnia on psychiatric health is increasingly well documented. One analysis of the causes of insomnia suggested that, in a broad population, psychiatric disorders accounted for 36% of patients, psychophysiological insomnia for 16%, drugs and alcohol for 12%, PLMD for 12%, and sleep apnoea, pseudoinsomnia, sleep–wake schedule disorder and medical disorders each for 6%. What is not shown in this tabulation is the clear social and personal factors pertinent to insomnia. It is well recognised that at least twice as many females as males seek treatment for insomnia. Grasshoff et al (1990) in a study of 1500 patients in Mannheim showed that the unemployed have the highest rate of sleep disturbance and Kales et al (1976) have suggested that there are characteristic personality patterns in people who complain of insomnia.

An interview with a patient presenting with insomnia should start with the patient's description of his subjective experience and then cover: (1) any objective observations by the patient and spouse/relative; (2) an enquiry into possible general medical and psychiatric causes; (3) details relating to the sleep environment and sleep hygiene; (4) detailed information about drugs, both prescribed and recreational; and (5) specific current stresses. A 2 week sleep diary with annotations regarding caffeine consumption is often helpful in assessing sleep disorders in general and insomnia in particular. The commonest form of insomnia (particularly once other obvious causes are excluded) presenting to a psychiatrist is likely to be psychophysiological insomnia. The diagnostic criteria for this condition serve to describe it and are shown in Table 24.2.

Insomnia is often considered in relation to the timing of sleep difficulty. Initial insomnia is thought of as characteristic of generalised anxiety disorders and terminal insomnia as characteristic of depression. This is correct, but more depressed patients have 'initial' rather than terminal insomnia.

Awakening during the sleep period is seen in a number of medical conditions in which pain is a feature and in the elderly. Treatment of the primary cause is the best treatment.

There is considerable evidence that most insomniacs overestimate the amount of time it takes them to fall asleep and underestimate the disruption during their sleep (Carscadon et al 1976). A number of studies have shown that sleep duration and conti-

Table 24.2 Diagnostic criteria for psychophysiological insomnia

1. A complaint of insomnia combined with a complaint of decreased functioning during wakefulness

2. Indications of learned sleep-preventing associations are found:
   a. Trying too hard to sleep, suggested by an inability to fall asleep when desired, but ease of falling asleep during other relatively monotonous pursuits, such as watching television or reading
   b. Conditioned arousal to bedroom or sleep-related activities, indicated by sleeping poorly at home, but sleeping better away from the home or when not carrying out bedtime routines

3. Evidence for increased somatised tension, e.g. agitation, muscle tension, increased vasoconstriction

4. Polysomnographic monitoring demonstrates:
   a. An increased sleep latency
   b. Reduced sleep efficiency
   c. An increased number and duration of awakenings

5. No evidence of other medical or psychiatric disorders that would account for the sleep disturbance

6. Other sleep disorders can coexist with the insomnia, e.g. inadequate sleep hygiene, obstructive sleep apnoea syndrome, etc.

nuity may be no different in well-matched good and poor sleepers (Adam et al 1986). These authors have, however, shown that poor sleepers have higher core body temperatures during the night. Reliance on sleep quantity (whether subjective or by polygraphic measurement) as an indicator of insomnia is no longer tenable. There are a variety of qualitative changes that may occur during sleep which influence the sense of 'being restored' afterwards. If any of a variety of pathophysiological changes to normal sleep process occurs it may be expected that sleep will be perceived as poor and insomnia may be the presenting complaint. In alcoholics, there is suppression of normal HGH release during SWS. This dissociation may be responsible for the subjective sleep complaints that are so common in alcohol dependence. Other possible 'qualititative' changes include: raised body temperature during sleep; increased metabolism (and greater oxygen consumption) during sleep; failure of normal nocturnal prolactin release; an alpha EEG pattern during sleep, for whatever reason; and circadian dysrhythmia. These features are not assessed in routine clinical situations at present. A patient's complaint of poor sleep should therefore not be dismissed. The limit of what is available in terms of medical investigation should be both exploited and recognised. Pragmatic palliative treatment should be employed. Short-term use of hypnotic medication should not always be avoided. This does not obviate the need for treating the provoking problem where a cause can be estab-

lished, instruction in sleep hygiene, and providing some training in relaxation techniques if appropriate. The latter two objectives can be cost-effectively achieved in a group setting.

REFERENCES

Adam K, Tomeny M, Oswald I 1986 Physiological and psychological differences between good and poor sleepers. Journal of Psychiatric Research 20: 301–316

Allgulander C, Nasman P 1991 Regular hypnotic drug treatment in a sample of 32,679 Swedes: association with somatic and mental health, inpatient psychiatric diagnoses and suicide, derived with automated record-linkage. Journal of the American Psychosomatic Society 53: 101–108

American Sleep Disorders Association 1990 The international classification of sleep disorders: diagnostic and coding manual. American Sleep Disorders Association

Ansseau M, Kupfer D J, Reynolds 3rd C F, Coble P A 1985 "Paradoxical" shortening of REM latency on first recording night in major depressive disorder: clinical and polysomnographic correlates. Biological Psychiatry 20: 135–145

Arendt J, Aldhous M, Marks V 1986 Alleviation of jetlag by melatonin: preliminary results of controlled double blind trial. British Medical Journal 292: 1170

Aserinsky E, Kleitman W 1953 Regularly occurring periods of eye motility and concomitant phenomena during sleep. Science 118: 273–274

Bancroft J 1989 Human sexuality and its problems. Churchill Livingstone, Edinburgh, pp 432–439

Berger M, Riemann C, Hochli D, Spiegel R 1989 The cholinergic rapid eye movement sleep induction test with RS-86: state or trait marker of depression? Archives of General Psychiatry 46: 421–428

Berrettini W H 1980 Paranoid psychosis and sleep apnea syndrome. American Journal of Psychiatry 137: 493–494

Bick P A, Hannah A L 1986 The effect of daylight saving time on the incidence of psychiatric presentations. Royal College of Psychiatrists Annual Meeting, University of Southampton, (Abstract), p 5

Bixler E, Kales A, Soldatos C R, Kales J D, Healey S 1979 Prevalence of sleep disorders in the Los Angeles metropolitan area. American Journal of Psychiatry 136: 10

Bradley T D, Shapiro C M 1993 "Lesson of the week": CPAP for the treatment of unusual cases of sleep apnea. In press

Buysse D J, Kupfer D J 1990 Diagnostic and research applications of electoencephalographic sleep studies in depression: conceptual and methodological issues. Journal of Nervous and Mental Disease 178: 405–414

Buysse D J, Kupfer D J, Frank E, Monk T H 1991 Longitudinal sleep studies in depressed patients treated with psychotherapy. Sleep Research 20: 173

Caffé C 1862 Maladie du sommeil. Journal des Connaisances Médicales et Pharmaceutiques 29: 323

Carskadon M A, Dement W C, Mitler M M, Guilleminault C, Zarcone V P, Spiegel R 1976 Self reports versus sleep laboratory findings in 122 drug-free subjects with complaints of chronic insomnia. American Journal of Psychiatry 133: 12

Cartwright R D, Stephenson K, Kravitz H, Eastman C 1988 REM latency stability and family history of depression. Sleep Research 17: 119

Coble P A, Reynolds 3rd C F, Kupfer D J, Houck P, Day N L, Scher M S 1991 REM latency in childbearing women with and without a history of affective disorder. Sleep Research 20: 176

Cramer S R, Nieman D C, Lee J W 1991 The effects of moderate exercise training on psychological well-being and mood state in women. Journal of Psychosomatic Research 35: 437–449

Czeisler C A, Kronauer R E, Allan J S et al 1989 Bright light induction of strong (type O) resetting of the human circadian pacemaker. Science 244: 1328–1333

Dahl R E, Puig-Antich J, Ryan N D et al 1990 EEG sleep in adolescents with major depression: the role of suicidality and inpatient status. Journal of Affective Disorders 19: 63–75

Dement W C, Kleitman N 1957 The relationship of eye movements during sleep to dream activity: an objective method for the study of dreaming. Journal of Experimental Psychology 53: 339–346

Douglass A B, Hays P, Pazderka F, Russell J M 1991 Florid refractory schizophrenias that turn out to be treatable variants of HLA-associated narcolepsy. Journal of Nervous and Mental Disease 179: 12–17

Findley L J, Barth J T, Powers D C, Wilhoit S C, Boyd D G, Suratt P M 1986 Cognitive impairment in patients with obstructive sleep apnea and associated hypoxemia. Chest 90: 686–690

Foot A 1866 Narcolepsy (sudden periodical sleep seizures). Dublin Journal of Medical Science 82: 165

Ford D E, Kamerow D B 1989 Epidemiologic study of sleep disturbances and psychiatric disorders: an opportunity for prevention? Journal of the American Medical Association 262: 1479–1484

Freud S 1900 The interpretation of dreams. Translated by Strachey J. Hogarth Press, London

Gaudet L, Chow E, Greben D, MacFarlane J G, Shapiro C M 1991 Sleep studies in three cases of dystonia. Sleep Research 20: 375

Giles D E, Roffwarg H P, Rush A J 1987 Reduced rapid eye movement latency: a predictor of recurrence in depression. Neuropsychopharmacology 1: 33–39

Gillin J C, Sitaram N, Mendelson W B 1982 Acetylcholine, sleep and depression. Human Neurobiology 1: 211–219

Grasshoff U, Hohage F, Schramm E, Wendt G, Weyerer S, Berger M 1990 Insomnia and professional status. In: Horne J (ed) Sleep '90. Pontenagel Press, Bochum, pp 214–216

Hamilton M 1989 Frequency of symptoms in melancholia (depressive illness). British Journal of Psychiatry 154: 201–206

Hamilton M, Shapiro C M 1990 Depression. In: Peck D F, Shapiro C M (eds) Measuring human problems. Wiley, Chichester, pp 25–65

Honda Y, Matsuki K 1990 Genetic aspects of narcolepsy. In: Thorpy M J (ed) Handbook of sleep disorders. Marcel Dekker, New York, pp 217–234

Jacobs E A, Reynolds 3rd C F, Kupfer D J, Lovin P A, Ehrenpreis A B 1988 The role of polysomnography in the differential diagnosis of chronic insomnia. American Journal of Psychiatry 145: 346–349

Jarrett D B, Miewald J M, Kupfer D J 1988 Acute changes in sleep-related hormone secretion of depressed patients following oral imipramine. Biological Psychiatry 24: 541–554

Jauhar P, Weller M P I 1982 Psychiatric morbidity and time zone changes: a study of patients from Heathrow airport. British Journal of Psychiatry 140: 231–235

Kales A, Caldwell A B, Preston T, Healey S, Kales J D 1976 Personality patterns in insomnia: theoretical implications. Archives of General Psychiatry 33: 1128–1124

Knowles J B, MacLean A W 1990 Age-related changes in sleep in depressed and healthy subjects, a meta-analysis. American College of Neuropsychopharmacology 3: 251–259

Kupfer D J, Ehlers C L 1989 Two roads to rapid eye movement latency. Archives of General Psychiatry 46: 945–948

Kupfer D J, Reynolds 3rd C F 1987 Sleep research in affective illness: state of the art circa 1987. Sleep 10: 199–215

Kupfer D J, Monk T H, Barchas J D (eds) 1988 Biological rhythms and mental disorders. Guildford Press, New York

Lee S, Chiu H F K, Chen C 1989 Psychosis in sleep apnoea. Australian and New Zealand Journal of Psychiatry 23: 571–573

MacFarlane J, Shahal B, Moldofsky H, Shapiro C 1991 Circannual variation in abbreviated REM onset latency. Abstracts of the 150th Annual Meeting of the Royal College of Psychiatrics, Brighton, July 1991

MacWilliam J A 1923 Some applications of physiology to medicine: blood pressure and heart action in sleep and dreams: their relation to haemorrhages, angina and sudden death. British Medical Journal ii: 1196–1200

Mann N P, Haddow R, Stokes L, Goodley S, Rutter N 1986 Effects of night and day on preterm infants in a newborn nursery: randomised trial. British Medical Journal 293: 1265–1267

Martin P R, Lefebvre A M 1981 Surgical treatment of sleep-apnea-associated psychosis. Canadian Medical Association Journal 124: 978–980

Mayou R, Hawton K 1986 Psychiatric disorder in the general hospital. British Journal of Psychiatry 149: 172–190

Meisler A W, Carey M P 1990 A critical reevaluation of nocturnal penile tumescence monitoring in the diagnosis of erectile dysfunction. Journal of Nervous and Mental Disease 178: 78–89

Moldofsky H 1990 The contribution of sleep–wake physiology to fibromyalgia. In: Friction J R, Awad E (eds) Advances in pain research and therapy, vol. 17. Raven Press, New York, pp 227–240

Montplaisir J, Godbout R 1990 Sleep and biological rhythms: basic mechanisms and application to psychiatry. Oxford University Press, New York

Moore-Ede M C, Sulzman F M, Fuller C A 1982 The clocks that time us: physiology of the circadian timing system. Harvard University Press, Massachusetts

Oswald I 1980 Sleep as a restorative process: human clues. Progress in Brain Research 50: 279–287

Peck D F, Shapiro C M 1990 Measuring human problems: a practical guide. Wiley, Chichester

Peter J H, Penzel T, Podszus T, von Wichert P 1991 Sleep and Health Risk. Springer-Verlag, Berlin

Roose S P, Glassman A H, Walsh B T, Cullen K 1982 Reversible loss of nocturnal penile tumescence during depression: a preliminary report. Neuropsychobiology 8: 284–288

Shapiro C M 1982 Energy expenditure and restorative sleep. Biological Psychology 15: 229–239

Shapiro C M 1991a Health risks associated with autonomic nervous system malfunction. In: Peter J H, Penzel T, Podszus T, von Wichert P (eds) Sleep and health risk. Springer-Verlag, Berlin, pp 124–136

Shapiro C M 1991b The role of REM sleep in psychiatric disorder. In: Idzikowski C, Cowen P J (eds) Serotonin, sleep and mental disorder. Wrightson Biomedical, pp 251–262

Shapiro C M, Driver H 1988 Sommeil et ses implications militaires. In: Rouseel B, Jouvet M (eds) Proceedings of the 27th DRG Seminar, Laboratoire de Medecine Experimentale, Université Claude Bernard, Lyon, France. Stress and sleep. NATO colloqium. Plenum Press, New York, pp 133–146

Shapiro C M, Rathouse K 1990 Sleep disorders. In: Peck D F, Shapiro C M (eds) Measuring human problems: a practical guide. Wiley, Chichester, pp 375–398

Shapiro C M, Goll C C, Cohen G, Oswald I 1984 Heat production during sleep. Journal of Applied Physiology 56: 671–677

Shapiro C M, Blake F, Fossey E, Adams B 1990 Daylight saving time in psychiatric illness. Journal of Affective Disorders 19: 177–181

Somoza E, Mossman D 1990 Optimizing REM latency as a diagnostic test for depression using receiver operating characteristic analysis and information theory. Biological Psychiatry 27: 990–1006

Thorpy M J (ed) 1990 Handbook of sleep disorders. Marcel Dekker, New York

Vogel G 1960 Studies in psychophysiology of dreams III. The dream of narcolepsy. Archives of General Psychiatry 3: 421–428

Wehr T A 1990 Effects of wakefulness and sleep on depression and mania. In: Montplaisir J, Godbout R (eds) Sleep and biological rhythms: basic mechanisms and applications to psychiatry. Oxford University Press, New York, pp 42–86

Wehr T A, Sack D A, Rosenthal N E 1987 Sleep reduction as a final common pathway in the genesis of mania. American Journal of Psychiatry 144: 201–204

Wilke G, Shapiro C M 1992 Sleep loss and postnatal blues and depression. Journal of Psychosomatic Research (in press)

25. Sexual disorders

J. Bancroft

INTRODUCTION

For the majority of people, the most important relationship in their adult lives is sexual. Many experience problems within such relationships. The general quality or enjoyment of the sexual relationship may be impaired or, more specifically, the physiological responses necessary for satisfactory sex, such as erection or orgasm, may fail. These responses are not only susceptible to psychological influences, but can also be affected by a host of physical and pathological processes as well as by drugs and alcohol. Sex is, par excellence, a psychosomatic process and the understanding of the possible interactions between psychological and physical mechanisms is of fundamental importance. The majority of sexual problems that present for help arise within heterosexual relationships, but other types of sexual difficulty also need to be considered. Homosexuals not only have their share of sexual difficulties but also suffer the consequences of being stigmatised. Some seek help to establish heterosexual relationships. Other people have sexual preferences which are incompatible with stable relationships of either a hetero- or a homosexual kind, sado-masochism and fetishism being examples. Occasionally people with such preferences seek professional help. Problems of gender identity are also important, with transsexualism, the most extreme form, presenting particular difficulties. Some forms of sexual activity (e.g. sexual assault, sexual abuse of children, or exhibitionism) are illegal and help may be sought to avoid prosecution or, in those who have already been convicted, to prevent further conflict with the law.

Since the last edition of this book there have been some dramatic changes in this clinical field. Three principal factors have been responsible:

1. Acquired immune deficiency syndrome (AIDS) and the epidemic of human immunodeficiency virus (HIV) infection; this has resulted in some major reappraisals of sexuality, the need for sex education and for sex research and much public debate. So far the impact on patterns of sexual behaviour has been most marked within the homosexual community. As yet there is little evidence of changed behaviour amongst heterosexuals.

2. A dramatic increase in awareness of sexual abuse of children. Not only are many more children being identified as victims of sexual abuse, much of it within the family, but many adults, mainly women, are now revealing their earlier experiences of sexual abuse. The full significance of this extraordinary change is far from clear at this time, and this issue has become surrounded with confusion and controversy.

3. The medicalisation of male sexuality; this has mainly resulted from a major increase in the involvement of the medical profession, in particular surgeons, in the management of erectile dysfunction. Whereas previously erectile problems were generally considered to be psychogenic in the large majority of cases, with psychological methods the mainstay of treatment, the situation has now reversed in that many believe physical disease to be responsible in the majority of cases, and physical methods of treatment, such as intracavernosal injection of drugs or surgical implantation of penile prostheses are now widely used. This is also a controversial area, with the pendulum swinging in the mind–body dualism of medical thought.

Each of these three areas of change and controversy will be considered more closely in this chapter.

HETEROSEXUAL RELATIONSHIPS

Incidence of problems

It is virtually impossible to establish the true prevalence of sexual difficulties in the general population. There are many ways in which a sexual relationship can be problematic; many such problems reflect transient difficulties in the general relationship. Many couples are relatively disinterested in the sexual dimension of their relationship. Apart from the problem of obtaining representative samples for enquiry, answers to sensitive questions concerning sex will vary considerably in their validity (Bancroft 1989, Clement 1990).

In an American study of 100 apparently normal couples, a fifth of the women and a third of the men were sexually dissatisfied, and the proportions reporting some specific sexual dysfunction were even higher (Frank et al 1978). Kinsey et al (1948) reported the incidence of complete erectile impotence in men, revealing a marked age factor with 0.8% at the age of 30, 6.7% at the age of 50 and 55% by the age of 74 years. Approximately 35% of their male subjects experienced occasional erectile failure (Gebhard & Johnson 1979). A number of studies, whilst unrepresentative in their samples, produced similar figures, suggesting that the prevalence of erectile dysfunction is in the region of 7–8% (Bancroft 1992). It undoubtedly increases with age, reflecting the variety of physical processes that accompany ageing.

In a substantial and representative Dutch study, 26% of men and 43% of women reported some problems with sexual enjoyment and arousal, with a further 9% of women expressing actual sexual aversion. A total of 12% of men and 33% of women had difficulty or dissatisfaction with orgasm, with a further 5% of women being anorgasmic (Frenken 1976). Other studies have reported orgasmic inability in women ranging from 4% (Garde & Lunde 1980) to 15% (Hunt 1974). Obviously the severity and importance of these problems vary. Garde & Lunde (1980) interviewed a representative sample of 40-year-old Danish women: 35% reported having sexual problems of some kind, with 15% describing too little motivation, 7% 'derived nothing from intercourse' whilst 6% 'felt it to be an obligation'. Of these women, 11% would have welcomed advice whilst 5% said they wanted 'sexological treatment'. The proportion who would actually seek such help would no doubt be smaller.

When we turn to the people who do seek professional help, of what do they complain? A consecutive series of 1110 patients presenting at sexual problem clinics in Edinburgh was described by Warner et al (1987). The presenting problems for the men and for the women are shown in Table 25.1. This shows a striking sex difference: a substantial majority of the men present with complaints about their physiological function — erectile or ejaculatory problems; a comparable majority of the women complain about lack of desire or enjoyment, with much less attention to physiological factors. Tiefer (1991) has criticised the diagnostic schema in DSM-IV for sexual dysfunctions, pointing out that diagnosis is based on a very genitally oriented, physiological response concept of sexual interaction. This tallies with how men conceptualise their difficulties, but, according to Tiefer, works to the disadvantage of women. It is certainly true that, whereas diagnostic categories are defined in terms of the 'sexual response cycle' (i.e. desire, arousal and orgasm, according to the ideas of Masters & Johnson (1970) and Kaplan (1974)), much of the sex therapy is concerned with poor communication, feelings of emotional insecurity or problems in coping with sexual intimacy. In general, such problems are articulated much more clearly by women than by men. (ICD-10 differs from DSM-IV in paying more attention to 'satisfaction and enjoyment' in the sexual relationship.)

There are some obvious reasons for this sex difference: absence of erection or inability to control ejaculation has a much more limiting effect on sexual activity than impaired vaginal response or orgasmic difficulty in the woman. But this nevertheless underlines an important difference in the attitudes of men and women to their sexual relationships. As yet, no method of classifying sexual problems satisfactorily takes into account the complex interplay of subjective experience and physiological response.

Sexual problems present in a variety of clinical settings. In an Edinburgh study of a family planning clinic population, 75% of 1000 consecutive women attenders completed a questionnaire. Of these women, 12% said that they had a sexual problem (Dickerson et al, unpublished study). Studies of gynaecological clinics (Levine & Yost 1976, Frenken & Van Tol 1987), psychiatric clinics (Swan & Wilson 1979), sexually transmitted disease clinics (Catalan et al 1981) and general practice clinics (Golombok et al 1984) reveal a substantial proportion with some sexual problem. It is not always clear whether this is linked to the clinical problems, though in some cases the association is very striking. Thus, up to 50% of male diabetics have problems with erections (McCulloch et al 1980), though diabetic women appear to be relatively immune (Tyrer et al 1983). However, in a study of 1180 males attending a general medical out-patient clinic no less than 34% were found to have some form of sexual dysfunction (Slag et al 1983). Patients with spinal injuries, multiple sclerosis, hypertension, epilepsy, colostomies or ileostomies, mastectomies and those on renal dialysis all appear to have more than their fair share of sexual difficulties. It is nevertheless often difficult to distinguish between direct effects of the disease process on sexual physiology, psychological reactions to the disability, and the sexual side-effects of drug treatment, reminding us once again of the complex psychosomatic nature of sexuality (Bancroft 1989).

The psychosomatic circle

The psychosomatic nature of human sexuality is represented schematically in Figure 25.1. Cognitive factors and the sensory input from touch influence the neurophysiological substrate in the limbic system and the spinal centres of the cord. This in turn is responsible for the general bodily changes that follow. Awareness of these bodily changes completes the circle and can either be exciting or anxiety-provoking. At each point of the system, both excitatory and inhibitory mechanisms are operating. The system can 'reverberate' either positively, with mounting excitement and eventual orgasm, or negatively with inhibition of genital response.

It is possible to identify factors that can interfere at particular points of the circle, e.g. with peripheral control of genital response, or the integrity of spinal centres. But to understand the effects of such a factor on the sexuality of the individual, one has to consider its impact on the whole system rather than just at the point of action. Thus, slight physiological impairment of erectile capacity in one man may cause little psychological reaction in either him or his partner, and hence remain of negligible significance. In another case, when the man or his partner attaches particular importance to erectile performance, similar

Table 25.1 Principal problems of men and women presenting at a sexual problem service in Edinburgh. (Problems of those presenting as couples, both with problems of equal importance, are not included)

Male problems	Percentage presenting	Female problems	Percentage presenting
Low sexual interest	7	Low sexual interest	35
Lack of enjoyment	1	Lack of enjoyment	12
Other orgasmic problems	5	Orgasmic dysfunction	7
Dyspareunia	1	Dyspareunia	11
Erectile failure	50	Vaginismus	13
Premature ejaculation	13	Sexual aversion	3
Problems relating to homosexuality	3		
Transsexualism	4	Problems relating	
		to homosexuality	0.2
Sexual deviance	2	Transsexualism	2
Sexual offences	3	Miscellaneous	15
Miscellaneous	12		
	100		100
	(n = 533)		(n = 577)

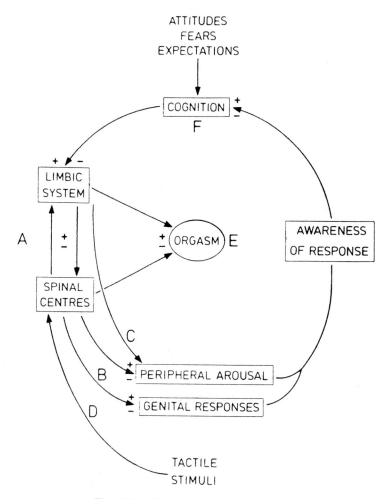

Fig. 25.1   The psychosomatic cycle of sex.

impairment may lead to a markedly adverse reaction and escalating difficulty to the point of complete erectile failure. Similarly, due to such psychological reverberation in the system, the problem may continue long after the precipitating factor has ceased to operate, e.g. a transient drug effect may lead to persisting problems after the drug is withdrawn. Let us, in summarising the principal aetiological factors, consider each point of this circle in turn.

Central mechanisms

The limbic system and the spinal centres represent the 'black box' of our sexuality; we know very little about their workings. Hormones may play an important part at this level. The role of reproductive hormones in the sexuality of men is becoming increasingly clear.

Androgens are necessary for normal levels of sexual interest and for ejaculation. Their effects on erectile function are more complex. Erections occurring during sleep (nocturnal penile tumescence or NPT) are androgen-dependent, whereas those in response to erotic stimuli in the waking state are not. This raises the possibility that the part of the limbic system responsible for sleep erections is linked in some way to the neurophysiological substrate for sexual interest or appetite, and that both are dependent on androgens (Bancroft 1988). Drugs may exert sexual side-effects by affecting this part of the system, as may generalised metabolic disturbances and some cases of depressive illness. The role of hormones in female sexuality is much less clear; women appear to vary considerably in their behavioural sensitivity to hormones (Bancroft 1989).

Functional disturbance of the limbic system or spinal cord may affect sexual function, though it is difficult to predict what effect will be produced by a particular lesion. There is a common association between temporal lobe and other types of epilepsy and low sexual interest, at least in men. In many such cases this may result from a lowering of plasma free testosterone induced by anticonvulsant medication (Toone et al 1983).

Genital responses

In both men and women, genital responses rely predominantly on vasocongestion. The peripheral blood vessels and the nerves controlling them may be directly affected by disease. Factors affecting the function of the pelvic floor muscles may also be relevant, particularly in women.

One of the consequences of the 'medicalisation' of male sexual dysfunction, and the involvement of surgeons, mentioned earlier, has been an intensive period of investigation of the pathophysiology of erection. The current view is that penile erection depends not only on a dilatation of the penile arteries and hence increased arterial flow into the penis but, possibly more important, also on the relaxation of the smooth muscle which is present in abundance in the specialised tissues of the corpora cavernosa, forming the walls of the sponge-like sinusoidal spaces. This relaxation allows the filling and distension of these spaces and the passive compression of the venous drainage between them. This reduction of venous outflow results in the build up of pressure within the corpora close to systolic pressure. Providing the 'hydraulic' integrity of this system is intact, this high pressure, augmented by periodic contractions of the striped muscles enveloping the corpora, produces the rigidity of erection required for effective vaginal entry (Bancroft 1989). Physical causes of erectile failure include insufficient arterial supply due to narrowing or obstruction of the penile or pelvic arteries, damage to the nerve supply that controls these various vascular and smooth muscle responses, and failure of the erectile tissue, for reasons which are not yet well understood, to occlude venous drainage during the development of erection, leading to so-called 'venous incompetence'.

The precise neurotransmitter mechanisms involved in this highly sophisticated example of biological engineering are not yet understood. However, a variety of drugs, which share in common the capacity to relax smooth muscle, have been found effective in producing erection when injected into the corpora cavernosa. Examples of such drugs are papaverine, phentolamine and prostaglandin E_1. These now form the basis of diagnostic tests of various kinds, either by simply establishing the capacity for erection (and hence reducing the likelihood of a primarily arterial cause), or aiding in other techniques for assessing blood flow into and venous drainage out of the penis (see Buvat et al (1990) for an authoritative review of these diagnostic methods). Such injections are also being used as a method of treatment, and will be considered below.

The role of drugs in the iatrogenic causation of erectile failure remains uncertain. Whereas direct pharmacological interference with ejaculation is well established with drugs such as adrenergic blockers, direct interference with the vascular mechanisms leading to erection is less certain. Indirect effects also have to be considered, e.g. via action on the central nervous system or, in the case of hypotensive agents and diuretics, by lowering blood pressure and hence blood flow in restricted vessels. (For a comprehensive review of drug effects on sexuality, see Rosen (1991).)

In women, pain during intercourse is particularly important. It is commonly caused by vaginal infections or deep pelvic pathology, but may also result from an inadequately lubricated vagina. As this lubrication is normally a response to sexual stimulation, a vicious circle readily becomes established, when anticipation of pain further inhibits lubrication. Oestrogen deficiency in the postmenopausal or lactating woman may also cause vaginal dryness and soreness. It is unusual to find women with impaired vaginal response resulting from nerve damage.

Some women have a particular tendency to react to local pain, or its anticipation, with marked spasm of the pelvic floor muscles. This, if persistent, results in vaginismus, making sexual intercourse painful or impossible. The reason for this tendency to spasm is usually not clear.

Orgasm is a neurophysiological mystery. Though the physiological basis is probably similar in males and females, an important difference in the male is the association with seminal emission. The combination of emission and the rhythmic muscle contraction that accompanies orgasm results in ejaculation. If, for any reason, emission occurs without orgasm, there is no pumping, ejaculatory effect. This may occur with high levels of anxiety and is common amongst men with severe premature ejaculation. Interference with the nerve supply or pharmacological block may result in orgasm without emission, the so-called 'dry run orgasm'. Occasionally, neural disturbance, as in diabetes, may lead to other alterations of ejaculatory function, sometimes resulting in retrograde ejaculation into the bladder (Fairburn et al 1982). Premature ejaculation is very common in young men, but most acquire control as they gain experience. The reasons why some fail to do so are not clear, but any factor that causes the man to be anxious during sexual activity — and anticipation of inadequate ejaculatory control can have that effect — will make the acquisition of control more difficult. In women, the effect of anxiety on orgasm is strikingly different to that in men, usually resulting in a delay. Thus, women typically have to learn to let go of control in order to experience satisfactory orgasm whilst men have to acquire it.

Psychological factors and associated emotional states

It is widely believed that anxiety has a disruptive effect on sexual response. Anger or resentment is also commonly implicated as a cause of sexual difficulty. 'Performance anxiety' or the spectator role, becoming too concerned about how one is responding and not enough about what one is feeling, has also been emphasised as an important factor leading to sexual dysfunction (Masters & Johnson 1970).

Recently, a series of well-controlled laboratory-based studies have investigated the relevance of such emotional states to sexual response in the male (see the review by Cranston-Cuebas & Barlow 1990). These have demonstrated that:

1. Experimental induction of anxiety often facilitates sexual response, though this is more likely to occur in men who are not already experiencing sexual difficulties.

2. Performance demand, induced in the experimental situation again distinguishes 'functional' from 'dysfunctional' men, apparently facilitating response in the former and hindering it in the latter.

3. Heightened arousal, induced by whatever means, appears to accentuate the typical pattern. Thus, in functional men who tend to focus on erotic cues in the experimental setting, this focus is enhanced and the sexual response facilitated. Dysfunctional men, who characteristically focus on non-erotic cues in sexual situations are even more likely to do so. In other words, the arousal increases the response, erotic in the functional group, non-erotic in the dysfunctionals.

4. Distraction (i.e. being asked to listen to a non-erotic cue whilst attending to an erotic stimulus) substantially reduces the erotic response in functional men. In dysfunctional men, it makes either little difference or even increases the response. The assumed explanation for this difference is that the dysfunctional men are already attending to non-erotic cues, which may be even more countererotic than the distracting cue.

5. When asked to report on their level of genital response to erotic stimuli, functional men tend to report accurately or to over-report their response; dysfunctional men tend to underreport.

Thus, we find functional and dysfunctional men reacting to these emotional states and cognitive processes differently. But we do not know whether that difference is a cause of the dysfunction, representing some characteristic that *precedes* the dysfunction, or is a consequence of dysfunction, so that once men regard themselves as dysfunctional, for whatever reason, they react differently, possibly accentuating the problem in the process. It remains possible that whilst cognitive mechanisms of the kind studied by Barlow and his colleagues play a part in sexual dysfunction, they are insufficient as an explanation. Other mechanisms, of a more neuro-physiological kind, involving direct inhibition of sexual responses, may be involved, although we can only speculate on this point.

Apart from this experimental approach to studying the cognitive and affective mechanisms involved, we can also consider, in a more descriptive way, the types of psychological problem that are commonly associated with sexual difficulties. It is important to remember, however, that demonstrating an association is not the same thing as showing causation. The mediating mechanisms remain obscure. Nevertheless, these common psychological issues form much of the subject matter of psychological methods of treatment. The therapist aims to identify these issues in each case, to 'work through' them in some sense, and hopes to see behavioural change without necessarily understanding how the change comes about. We will consider the principles the therapist follows later; let us first consider briefly the common problems.

There are many reasons for feeling anxious or angry in a sexual context. Some of them are best understood in developmental terms — result of earlier experiences which precede the current sexual relationship. Others reflect the ongoing difficulties in the current sexual relationship. They can be considered under the following headings.

1. Misunderstandings and ignorance. The most important are misleading standards of 'normality' which generate anxiety and guilt if they are not attained. 'Normal' frequency of intercourse, the 'normality' of simultaneous orgasm and female orgasm from vaginal stimulation alone are common examples.

2. Negative feeling about sex. As a result of earlier learning, sex may be viewed as wrong or sexual pleasure as immoral in some way. Sexual pleasure is sometimes confined to 'bad' or at least illicit relationships, making it difficult to enjoy sex in a good, loving relationship. Sexual arousal may threaten the person's need for self-control. This may reflect a general tendency to keep control, as in many obsessional personalities, or more specifically a fear of what will happen during sexual abandonment. Sex may be feared as painful or dangerous. For women, in particular, this can become a self-fulfilling prophecy because the resulting muscle spasm can cause pain when intercourse is attempted. The fear of pregnancy is the most rational fear associated with sex and has probably succeeded in spoiling more sexual relationships than any other single factor. But in spite of modern methods of fertility control, there are still some women (and occasionally men) who feel that sex unassociated with the possibility of pregnancy is wrong. Fear of venereal disease is adaptive in many situations, but occasionally, in the form of a phobia, it becomes an obstacle to any satisfactory sexual relationship.

With many of these fears and misunderstandings we have to ask why they persist in spite of experience or information to the contrary. As with most neurotic (i.e. maladaptive) fears, two explanations have to be considered. First, there may be a 'neurotic disposition' which is associated in an ill-understood way with inappropriate learning of anxiety responses. Secondly, the fear may continue because of 'secondary gain'. Thus, the avoidance of intercourse because of 'irrational fears' may serve the purpose of avoiding the mature adult sexual role that intercourse symbolises. In such cases, the sexual problem is a manifestation of a more general personality problem.

3. Low self-esteem. This may be specifically related to body image or be more general, as with a person who is depressed. In either case, sexual enjoyment is likely to be impaired. A man who is experiencing failure in his job feels less effective, less 'potent' as a man, and this can adversely affect him sexually. When women feel unattractive or 'unfeminine', for whatever reason, they often find they are less able to enjoy sex. Although low self-esteem, when a manifestation of depression, can have these direct psychological effects, there are probably other ways, as yet not understood, in which depressive illness affects sexual interest and response.

4. Relationship problems. Resentment and insecurity in the sexual relationship are two emotions which cause particular havoc. There are many causes for such emotions, but some are sufficiently common to deserve special mention, for example different expectations of marriage. Attitudes to the woman's role in marriage are undoubtedly changing. There are an increasing number of women who now resent what is traditionally expected of them, often with good reason. It is not unusual to find couples who enjoyed sex before marriage but experienced a decline in the one or two years after marriage. Beforehand, sex was not taken for granted and could be used by the woman to 'express her love'. After marriage, she is 'contracted to provide it'. In a similar way, many men after marriage feel under pressure to perform sexually.

Many young wives now feel considerable conflict between their role as housewife and mother and their role as an independent career woman. Caring for preschool children is especially stressful and may be compounded by the woman's loss of her previous work role and the social isolation that often ensues. Two people entering marriage usually have a lot of 'personal growth' still to work through. At different times, each person will go through an individual crisis, putting strains on the marital relationship. How a couple deals with these various problems depends not only on the circumstances of the 'here and now' but also earlier experiences, in particular what they have learnt from their parents about close intimate relationships and communicating strong feelings.

5. Unsuitable circumstances. It is easy to overlook the importance of unsuitable circumstances such as lack of privacy or warmth. Also affecting those who are overworked is lack of appropriate time. Trying to squeeze one's sex life into a few minutes between an exhausting day and badly needed sleep is not the way to maintain a good sexual relationship. The often dramatic improvement in sexual interest and enjoyment that is experienced on holiday is testament to the negative effects of day-to-day pressures.

The effects of earlier sexual abuse or assault

In recent years there has been an extraordinary increase in the number of women (and to a lesser extent men) reporting sexual abuse during their childhood, often within an incestuous relationship. One must assume that only recently has it become acceptable and credible to reveal such earlier experiences. Sex therapists are currently struggling with the realisation that for many years they must have been working with many clients who were concealing past histories of this kind. At the same time there is a danger, in the present climate, of attributing too many current problems to such early experiences. In many respects, sex therapists seem to have retreated into a thoughtful phase, attempting to adapt their therapeutic principles to take this new awareness into account and to achieve an appropriate sense of balance between the importance of current and early experiences. This reappraisal is, of course, more problematic for therapists with behavioural rather than psychodynamic backgrounds.

With childhood sexual abuse the sense of betrayal, anger and guilt that result are important causes of later sexual difficulty. Problems that result can be expressed either as difficulty or reluctance to participate or enjoy sexual activity, or a tendency to engage in relatively casual sexual encounters with little emotional commitment but a somewhat compulsive need to be sexually active. Such women often take risks both in relation to pregnancy and sexually transmitted disease. (For a review, see Wyatt (1991).)

Following sexual assault during adulthood, the consequences are less complex and more readily understood. Reactions can often be considered as examples of post-traumatic stress disorder. Also, there is often a sense of loss that requires to be resolved, e.g. loss of one's identity as a sexual person, loss of trust and loss of feelings of emotional safety. Depression is a common sequel. Sexual problems, whilst common, are variable in type. (For a review, see Becker (1991).) One of the main challenges facing the sex therapist is whether to deal with these unresolved issues in individual or couple therapy.

Clinical management

When a sexual problem presents at the clinic, decisions need to be made: first, whether any physical assessment and investigation is required and, secondly, whether simple advice or counselling is appropriate, whether more systematic sex therapy is indicated, or whether physical methods of treatment should be considered. The criteria for seeking physical investigations cannot be briefly stated and are outside the scope of this chapter (see Bancroft 1989, Buvat et al 1990) but the occurrence of pain clearly requires assessment. Recent loss of sexual interest in the absence of obvious psychological explanation is also an indication. Most cases of erectile dysfunction need systematic assessment and a simple scheme to follow has been provided elsewhere (Bancroft & Wu 1985).

In most cases, the objective of counselling or psychological treatment is the establishment of optimal psychological conditions for the couple to respond sexually. The reduction of performance anxiety or 'fear of failure', increase in feelings of emotional security, and the resolution of chronic resentment in the sexual relationship are of paramount importance. The therapist helps to achieve these objectives principally by setting limits (e.g. a temporary ban on intercourse), by facilitating communication, and helping in the expression and consequent resolution of resentment. Such an approach, combined with education about sexual function, constitutes the essence of modern sex therapy for couples. In some cases, when the basic problems are more intractably rooted in the individual's personality, long-term individual psychotherapy may be indicated.

The physical aspects, however, must not be neglected. Unfortunately there are few physical causes of sexual difficulty which are both common and treatable. Vaginal infections and the sexual side-effects of drugs are probably the most important examples. But it is nevertheless necessary to ensure that physical factors are dealt with properly when they occur. Even in cases where irreversible physical pathology is involved, counselling has an important role to play, with two principal objectives: to establish the optimum psychological conditions to permit the couple to make the best of their sexual relationship within the limits imposed by the physical impairment; and, in the light of any such change, to help the couple decide whether other non-psychological forms of treatment, such as surgery, are indicated and acceptable to them. Recent developments, such as the use of intracavernosal injections for erectile failure, will be considered below. But in most respects they do not achieve 'cure' of the problem but rather 'a way round it'. As stressed earlier, many of the difficulties that arise stem from psychological reactions to the physical impairment rather than the physical disease itself. In other cases, the physical condition is *only* important because of the psychological reactions to it. Reactions to colostomies and mastectomies and the fear of heart attacks in people with ischaemic heart disease are important examples. In all such cases, the basic counselling approach is similar but an understanding of the medical implications is necessary, either to assess how much impairment can be attributed to the physical lesion or to appreciate the emotional impact of the physical condition. For these various reasons, it is necessary to have medical expertise available in any clinical service for sexual problems, even though most of the counselling can be satisfactorily provided by non-medical therapists.

The aims of simple counselling, which have been described more fully by Annon (1974), are as follows:

1. To provide limited information about sexual response, in particular to counteract false or misleading expectations.

2. To make specific suggestions about approaches to lovemaking that might be useful (e.g. direct clitoral stimulation, agreeing on limits, trying different positions, etc.).

3. To give permission and reassurance. Permission is usually implicit in the suggestions made, but is often of crucial importance. Suggestions to use masturbation techniques, for example, may effectively counter the patient's previous belief that masturbation is wrong.

4. To facilitate communication. Talking with a couple about sex often provides a model of communication and a vocabulary which makes it easier for them to discuss the issues between themselves.

The main requirement of the counsellor in these circumstances is therefore comfort in talking about sexual matters combined with a reasonable knowledge and understanding of the varieties of human sexual response. Such counselling is largely based on common sense and need only occupy one or two half-hour sessions. It can therefore be provided by a wide range of health professionals who do not have to regard themselves as experts in sex therapy. It is particularly useful at those points in the health care service where ordinary sexual problems are likely to be identified, e.g. family planning clinics, postnatal clinics, vasectomy counselling, sexually transmitted disease clinics, and medical clinics dealing with patients after coronaries or other acute medical episodes. If simple counselling is ineffective, or the problem obviously complex enough to require more specialist management, sex therapy may be indicated.

Principles of sex therapy

The principles of sex therapy are basically those of behavioural psychotherapy in general, i.e. a combination of 'doing' and 'understanding', getting patients to try things and helping them to understand the difficulties that they have in carrying them out. There are three main components of such treatment: behavioural, educational and psychotherapeutic. They are combined in the following framework, which also provides the structure of each treatment session:

1. Set appropriate behavioural assignments ('homework'; the behavioural component)
2. Examine the patient's attempts to carry out these assignments
3. As a result, identify those obstacles (attitudes, fears or other feelings) that underlie the difficulties encountered
4. Help the patient to modify or reduce those obstacles so that the behaviour can be carried out successfully (the educational and psychotherapeutic components)
5. Set the next behavioural assignments

The particular strength of this combination is that the setting of relevant target behaviours is a rapidly effective way of uncovering the crucial inter- or intrapersonal problems that underlie the sexual difficulty. Such an approach is a combination of behavioural change and discovery. The therapist can reasonably assume that relevant material will emerge during the course of treatment. It is therefore not necessary to elicit all the information during the initial assessment. This means that there need be no delay in getting the couple or individual patient actively involved and started on a behavioural programme, provided that appropriate assignments suggest themselves. Let us consider the three components of treatment in more detail.

The behavioural component

This is best described for the treatment of couples when very similar assignments can be given initially whatever the nature of the couple's problem. These early assignments concern the couple's method of communication during lovemaking, both verbally and physically, and their ability to protect and assert themselves to make each other feel secure. The 'sensate focus' stages of Masters & Johnson (1970) are particularly effective for this purpose. The couple are asked to accept limits to their lovemaking, i.e. no direct genital or breast contact or any attempts at intercourse. They are encouraged to take time to touch one another anywhere except the genital areas. Initially the objective of the 'toucher' is to find ways of enjoying touching; the person being touched simply has to protect him- or herself against anything that is unpleasant. At a later stage, the 'toucher' aims to give pleasure as well, and relies on communication from the partner about what or where is enjoyable to the touch. Eventually genital touching is incorporated, following the same principles. These assignments rapidly reveal problems of resentment, feeling of insecurity or lack of trust in the couple (e.g. can the partner be trusted to keep to the limits?) as well as negative feelings about taking the initiative or experiencing pleasure without first giving pleasure.

Once the couple can manage a particular behavioural assignment without difficulty and with emotional comfort, they move on to the next stage. Behavioural progress is often halted for some time whilst crucial inter- or intrapersonal conflicts are resolved. As treatment proceeds, behavioural tasks become more tailormade for the couple, and specific techniques dealing with premature ejaculation, vaginismus or other special dysfunctions may be incorporated into the programme. Often the most important issues are dealt with before genital touching is attempted. In other cases, the main problems are revealed at the genital stage, when fears of sexual arousal or loss of control and 'performance anxiety' are commonly encountered.

The educational component

Overcoming ignorance and countering false expectations about what is 'normal' or socially acceptable is as important in this context as in the simple counselling approach. A didactic teaching session about normal male and female anatomy and sexual physiology is usually included before the behavioural programme reaches the stage of genital touching. The couple's attention is focused on those aspects of anatomy and physiology which are especially relevant to their problems, e.g. the pelvic floor muscles for the woman with vaginismus or normal ejaculatory physiology for the premature ejaculator. Physical examination, when it is carried out, provides a further opportunity for education.

The psychotherapeutic component

The setting of appropriate behavioural tasks may be all that is required of the therapist for improvement to occur. But, in the majority of cases, difficulties in carrying out the behavioural assignments will occur sooner or later and the psychotherapeutic skills of the therapist then become important. This is the aspect of therapy which is most difficult and which has been least well defined in the literature. This aspect can only be dealt with briefly in this chapter but a much more thorough description of this and other aspects of sex therapy can be found in Bancroft (1989). The principal psychotherapeutic objectives of the therapist are: (1) to facilitate understanding of why the couple or individual has difficulty with specific behaviours;

(2) to make explicit the couple's commitment to specific changes; (3) to use 'reality confrontation' in which the patient's inconsistencies between attitudes and behaviour or between beliefs and factual evidence are brought out into the open; (4) to facilitate the expression of affect; (5) to use an understanding of the relevant background problems to plan further behavioural assignments appropriately.

Efficacy of sex therapy

Assessing the value of a psychological treatment for sexual problems in a relationship is far from straightforward. Attempts to do so have been confounded by a tendency to categorise cases according to the specific type of physiological dysfunction (e.g. erectile dysfunction, orgasmic dysfunction), whereas the goals of sex therapy involve much broader dimensions of the relationship than physiological response. Thus, we are faced with a fundamental problem: how does one define success with such treatment? There is also the problem of long-term effects. Relationships are dynamic, and continue to be influenced by a variety of factors over time. Thus, major improvement in a sexual relationship following sex therapy may be obscured by newly developed pressures which create tensions between the couple. Nevertheless, the objectives of sex therapy, in a long-term sense, are to help the couple to learn new and better ways of dealing with their relationship issues when they arise, not simply to reverse current symptoms.

Long-term follow-up has proved difficult. Perhaps couples who have been successfully helped by sex therapy prefer to forget that stage of their lives some years later. Because of these various qualifications, it is only possible, in a short space, to give a crude guide to the efficacy of sex therapy. More detailed analyses of outcome can be found in Arentewicz & Schmidt (1983) and other studies are reviewed in Bancroft (1989). Approximately 50–70% of couples who undergo a reasonable course of sex therapy report substantial benefits. The most consistently good results are for vaginismus, and the worst for low sexual desire. For other types of dysfunction the outcome is very variable, reflecting the varied relationship problems that accompany the dysfunction, as well as the often imponderable contribution of physical factors. Most follow-up studies have been limited by high attrition rates. Hawton et al (1986) were more successful than most in this respect. Of 140 couples treated 1–6 years previously, 75% were contacted (at least one partner). Of these, 75% had experienced a continuation or recurrence of the original problem, though in a third this did not cause concern. Almost a half of them were able to deal effectively with the recurrences, often by adopting strategies learnt during therapy. Thirteen per cent of the original group had separated.

Hawton & Catalan (1986) reported a prospective study of prognostic factors in sex therapy. They found that the quality of the non-sexual relationship, motivation for treatment, particularly in the male partner, and progress by the third treatment session all had prognostic significance. More studies of this kind are required.

Individual therapy

The treatment described above is designed primarily for couples, though the basic principles are equally well applied to individuals. A proportion of patients presenting with heterosexual problems have no current sex partner, or have partners who will not participate or whom the patient does not want to involve. Individual therapy is appropriate, providing that goals of therapy can be chosen which are relevant to that individual alone and not dependent on another particular person. If these individual goals are achieved, and as a consequence the patient becomes more confident and comfortable with his or her sexuality, then positive consequences in sexual relationships may well follow. Quite often the individual problem fits well into the approach outlined above for the couple. If the patient is inhibited about sex, uncomfortable about his or her body and genitals, uneasy about sexual arousal or orgasm, or generally unable to enjoy sexual feelings in a relaxed fashion, then similar behavioural assignments can be followed as for the couple. Individual sensate focus can be used with initial limits on genital touching. In the course of this, relevant attitudes are likely to be revealed. Eventual ability to masturbate to orgasm and feel comfortable and enjoy the experience may be an important step forward for that person. For individuals who have been victims of sexual assault or abuse, either as a child or adult, helping them 'work through' their anger and deal appropriately with their guilt is often necessary before behavioural progress can be made. Various specific techniques can be added to the individual's sensate focus programme, just as they are in couple therapy. Thus the 'stop–start' or 'squeeze' techniques for premature ejaculation can be used if the man tends to ejaculate quickly during masturbation as well as with a partner. Women with vaginismus can use graded vaginal dilation first with fingers and subsequently with glass or plastic dilators. Men with erectile impotence can sometimes be helped individually if their performance anxiety has affected their ability to obtain erections during masturbation as well as with their partner (see Bancroft (1989) for further details).

Group therapy

The use of group therapy for sexual dysfunction increased noticeably during the early 1980s, but there has been a noticeable decline in this respect over the last few years (Leiblum & Rosen 1989). Usually the group approach involved the same basic principles as described for couple and individual therapy, but applied in a group setting. The advantages of the group are several. The relationship between patient and therapist is less crucial. The group tends to be cohesive, reducing the likelihood of drop-outs from treatment; there is a loyalty to the group or, alternatively, a fear of loss of face that keeps them going. The group may well have shared objectives. Explanations, interpretations and 'permission-giving' that come from the group, may have more impact than those coming from a therapist. Progress of individual members acts as encouragement for others, whereas individuals experiencing setbacks may get support from the group. There are practical advantages in the economic use of the therapist's time and in provision of educational material (e.g. films). However, there are also disadvantages. Many people are reluctant to join a group, fearing exposure and loss of confidentiality. Many issues of sex therapy are simply too complex to be dealt with in this format. At the present time, the main interest in groups is for helping the victims and perpetrators of sexual abuse or assault.

Drug treatment

The last few years have seen a dramatic increase in interest in pharmacological methods of treatment, and there is much on-going research. The main impact has been the use of drugs injected into the corpora cavernosa of the penis to produce an erection lasting usually for 1–2 hours. Papaverine and prostaglandin E_1, both smooth muscle relaxants, are the two most widely used for this purpose. Although such use is mainly for diagnosis, repeated self-injections are being used as a form of treatment (Brindley 1986, Virag et al 1991), and are sometimes irresponsibly marketed by private clinics as 'a cure for impotence'. Obviously this route of administration is not generally acceptable, the reliance on such injections is regarded by many as an 'artificial' form of sexual response, and repeated use may lead to fibrosis within the penis. They are welcomed by a proportion of couples, however, particularly those with intractable physical causation such as diabetes or multiple sclerosis. The combination of pharmacologically induced erections with psychological methods of treatment offers interesting possibilities that are only just being explored (e.g. see Kaplan 1990).

The search for a centrally acting drug that will enhance both sexual desire and genital response is gathering pace. Recent attempts to introduce a new dopamine agonist for this purpose have foundered because of the substantial D_2 side-effects. Several studies have evaluated yohimbine, an α_2 antagonist as a treatment for erectile dysfunction, usually with results which are inconclusive but suggestive of modest benefits (e.g. see Reid et al, 1987, Riley et al 1989). The author has had promising (uncontrolled) clinical results with yohimbine in men with psychogenic erectile dysfunction, particularly when erections occur but are poorly maintained. He advises 5 mg three or four times daily on 2 or 3 days a week. Studies with a new, pharmacologically superior α_2 antagonist are currently in progress.

Anxiety-reducing drugs have not been shown to be effective in dealing with the various forms of sexual anxiety. The use of hormones such as testosterone is clearly indicated in male hypogonadism. It may also be beneficial in eugonadal men complaining of loss of sexual interest, though in such cases counselling is probably also required (O'Carrol & Bancroft 1984).

The role of hormones in the treatment of female sexual dysfunction is much less clear, apart from the use of oestrogens to counter vaginal dryness in postmenopausal women. Some women may benefit from androgens but such effects are very unpredictable and more evidence will be required before clear clinical guidelines emerge (Bancroft 1989).

Other forms of treatment

Surgical techniques are being widely used for erectile dysfunction, particularly of the irreversible 'organic' variety. The commonest method is the surgical implantation of a silastic prosthesis into the penis, giving a semipermanent erection. Inflatable devices are also available but are technically and surgically much more complex. Re-operation is commonly required (Kabalin & Kessler 1989). Adequate follow-up of such cases has been sparse, but most couples do appear to benefit, although commonly the main

benefit is to the man's self-esteem rather than the partner' sexual fulfilment (Tiefer at al 1988).

Vascular surgery to correct vascular occlusion or 'leaks' continues to be explored but as yet the results are very unconvincing. There are no real indications for surgical treatment for sexual dysfunction in women, except in those rare cases where an anatomical abnormality is contributing to the problem (e.g. hymeneal strands).

The use of external vacuum devices for erectile dysfunction has increased substantially in the past few years. A recent study showed these to be more acceptable than self-injection (Turner et al 1991)

HOMOSEXUAL RELATIONSHIPS

It is not known how many people in our society are predominantly homosexual. Figures given by Kinsey and his colleagues (1948) are probably overestimates because of the inclusion of subgroups (e.g. criminals) with unusually high prevalence. Gagnon & Simon (1973) re-analysed the Kinsey data, concentrating on a more representative group of 2900 young men, of whom 30% had been involved in a homosexual experience in which one or other person had attained orgasm. The large majority of these experiences had occurred in adolescence and more than half before the age of 15 years. This left about 3% with extensive homosexual as well as heterosexual histories beyond adolescence and 3% with exclusive homosexual histories. A similar reanalysis of the women showed that only 6% (as compared with 30% of the men) had undergone at least one homosexual experience; only 2% had any significant amount of homosexual experience and less than 1% were exclusively homosexual. Other large-scale (but unrepresentative) studies of American men have reported about 1% exclusive homosexuality and 1–3% bisexuality (Hunt 1974, Pietropinto & Simenauer 1977).

A proportion of homosexuals seek professional help; in many cases, the problems are no different to those experienced by heterosexuals but others are mainly suffering the consequences of belonging to a stigmatised minority. Some homosexuals seek help because they want to be heterosexual, which raises complex ethical issues (Bancroft 1991a). Finally, homosexuals seek help for problems in their homosexual relationships. Are these relationships more vulnerable than those of the heterosexual world or are their problems any different? The almost universal nature of the stigma attached to homosexuality is not easy to explain. Legal proscription of homosexuality exists in most Western societies, though the situation is changing in many countries. The law was changed in England in 1967. In Scotland, all forms of male homosexuality remain illegal although prosecution is unlikely unless privacy is not maintained or the age of consent is breached. In most countries the law does not specifically concern itself with female homosexuality. Even in those countries where the law has changed, legal discrimination persists in various forms. The age of consent tends to be higher (i.e. 21 years) for homosexual than heterosexual relationships (i.e. 16 years). Men may solicit women but they may not solicit other men. 'Privacy' is defined in a much more restrictive sense for homosexual than for heterosexual acts. The penalties are more severe than for equivalent heterosexual offences. Any form of homosexuality is illegal for members of the armed forces or merchant navy. Admitting to being homosexual in orientation is grounds for dismissal from the services. A recent consideration of this issue by a parliamentary committee has resulted in no change.

Are homosexuals more susceptible to psychological problems? The best evidence comes from early large-scale studies by Weinberg & Williams (1974) and Bell & Weinberg (1978) from the Kinsey Institute. They found a higher incidence of loneliness, lower self-acceptance, and more depression and suicidal ideas in male and female homosexuals than in heterosexual controls. This was reflected not only in a higher incidence of seeking professional help but also of previous suicidal attempts. It is nevertheless important to stress that these problems were confined to a minority of the homosexuals and most were well adapted and happy. Also, there have been substantial changes in the lifestyles of gay men and social attitudes to homosexuality since those studies were carried out. At the time of writing, homosexual men are under a new and very substantial threat, that of HIV infection and AIDS. Apart from the fact that in urban centres where AIDS is common, few homosexual men have escaped the bereavement of a close friend or lover, many gay men are faced with the very uncertain prospect of developing the disease from previous contacts, others are reluctant to get tested for HIV, fearing the results, and yet others are currently healthy but living in the knowledge that they are HIV-positive and will develop AIDS at some very uncertain time in the future. The stress of such a situation cannot be overestimated. But, apart from the effects of AIDS, any tendency for homosexual men and women to be more at risk for psychological problems probably results in large part from the social stigmatisation they experience.

McWhirter & Mattison (1984), following an in-depth study of 156 long-term male relationships, suggested five developmental stages for male homosexual relationships: (1) blending (year 1); (2) nesting (years 2–3); (3) maintaining (years 4–5); (4) building (years 6–10); (5) releasing (years 11–20).

Bell & Weinberg (1978) used factor analysis to arrive at a typology of homosexual relationships. They described: the 'close coupled' pair, similar to the happily married and faithful heterosexual couple; the 'open couple' in which a reasonably stable relationship is maintained with a fair amount of 'extramarital' sexuality; 'functionals' were not in stable relationships but enjoyed a wide variety of partners; 'dysfunctionals', conforming to the stereotype of the 'unhappy homosexual', had recurring problems in their sexual relationships, often involving sexual dysfunction or discomfort with their homosexual identity; and 'asexuals' with low sexual interest were inclined to lead a solitary existence. The proportions of males and females in each category in their study is shown in Table 25.2. Apart from the greater number of lesbians in the close coupled category, there is also evidence that the male homosexuals found the 'open couple' and 'functional' lifestyles easier to cope with than did the lesbians. This study was carried out prior to the 1970s, during which decade there were substantial changes in the behaviour of gay men.

Both of the above studies were carried out prior to the AIDS epidemic. The impact of HIV and AIDS, which is now being intensively studied in the gay community, has no doubt changed the pattern even further. Many homosexual men have adopted 'safer' sexual lifestyles, and it remains to be seen whether there will be a fundamental change in the 'openness' of male homosexuality.

Table 25.2   Typology of homosexuality (Bell & Weinberg 1978)

	Percentage males (n = 686)	Percentage females (n = 293)
Close coupled	10	28
Open coupled	18	17
Functional	15	10
Dysfunctional	12	5
Asexual	16	11
Unclassifiable	29	28
	100	100

Origins of sexual preferences

During normal sexual development, the three main components of our sexuality — sexual responsiveness, the formation and maintenance of emotional dyadic relationships, and 'gender identity' — become integrated into mature adult sexual relationships. Through childhood, these three components remain relatively detached from one another. Around puberty, we normally start to incorporate our sexual responsiveness into our relationships with other people as our sexual preferences become organised. There are a wide variety of factors which may push us away from, or pull us towards, a particular type of relationship; and it is difficult to escape the conclusion that social learning plays an important part in determining our sexual preference. But is there a 'preparedness to learn' either homosexual or heterosexual preferences and, if so, does this result from earlier learning, for example during infancy, or is it determined by innate characteristics? It is a striking fact that, whereas homosexual behaviour is commonplace amongst non-human primates and other mammals, exclusive homosexual preference appears to be a uniquely human phenomenon, and one which probably varies in incidence from one type of society to another. This would suggest that, whereas biological factors may influence whether homosexual activity occurs, the establishment of an exclusive homosexual orientation is probably a result of social learning (Bancroft 1989). Genetic studies of twins show a substantially higher concordance for homosexuality amongst monozygotic than dizygotic pairs (Heston & Shields 1968), and there is evidence of increased incidence of homosexuality amongst the close relatives of homosexuals (Pillard et al 1982), but this may simply mean that genetic similarity increases the likelihood of responding to environmental influences in a *similar* rather than a *particular* way. In both males and females, attempts to find endocrine differences between homosexual and heterosexual adults have been inconclusive. The possibility that hypothalamic activity of male homosexuals shows female characteristics, resulting from early hormonal influences on brain organisation, has been proposed by Dorner (1979) but more recent evidence has laid this hypothesis to rest (Gooren 1990). More recently, attempts to find a biological difference between homosexual and heterosexual men have focused on structural differences in the hypothalamus. Thus, Swaab & Hofman (1990) have reported from post mortem evidence that the suprachiasmatic nuclei of homosexual men are larger than those of heterosexuals. The significance of this preliminary finding is exceedingly questionable at this juncture.

There is, however, convincing evidence that endocrine mechanisms operating prenatally can influence gender role behaviour in childhood and later life in both humans and animals (Money & Ehrhardt 1972). It is therefore possible that biological factors may *indirectly* affect later sexual preferences by their direct effects on gender role and identity development. There is now a consistent body of evidence, both from prospective studies of children with gender non-conformity and retrospective studies of adults, that a substantial proportion of adult homosexuals have shown gender nonconformity during childhood (for a review, see Bancroft 1989). This may be an important influence leading to later development of homosexual preferences, though, once again, it is clearly not a *necessary* factor.

Let us consider the ways in which gender identity might affect development of sexual preferences, interacting in complex and varied ways with other social factors. In this respect, we need to consider not only gender identity of the cross-gender type (e.g. a boy feeling or behaving in a feminine way) but also the lack of confidence in one's assigned gender that may stem from an absent or emasculating father, an overprotective mother, a physical disability or genital abnormalities during development. Any of these features in a boy could have the following effects:

1. Make him unattractive to the opposite sex or undermine his self-confidence in relating to girls, so that attempts at heterosexual contact are likely to be unrewarding or even punishing
2. Make him attractive to other males who seek 'unmasculine' partners
3. Lead him to escape from the competitiveness of the male world to the homosexual world where there are different criteria for gender success (Hooker 1967)

In a comparable way, we can consider the consequences of sexual anxiety or guilt, particularly in relation to the opposite sex. Such negative feelings may be learnt during childhood, a result of incestuous feelings or experiences, or the consequences of a sexually repressive environment in the home. Such anxiety may act as a 'push' factor away from heterosexual relationships. For those who have had problems in their dyadic relationships, particularly lacking a secure relationship with one or other parent, sexual relations with others may offer them an alternative. Thus, if a boy has never had a good relationship with his father, a close relationship with another male may hold special appeal.

Such explanations are unlikely to account for more than a proportion of adults with homosexual orientation. Various factors may therefore increase the likelihood of homosexual and reduce the likelihood of heterosexual interaction. The histories of many individuals simply suggest the relatively early onset of sexual attraction to the same sex. But probably the most crucial additional influence, in determining whether an individual ends up with a homosexual or heterosexual identity, is the socially derived meaning given to homosexuality in any particular culture. If, as in some primitive societies, homosexual interaction is accepted as a normal aspect of sexual behaviour and development (Herdt 1981) then such behaviour is perfectly compatible with the establishment of heterosexual relationships, permitting the expression of a 'bisexual potential'. But in other societies, such as our own, adolescents are strongly encouraged to see themselves as *either* heterosexual *or* homosexual, so that evidence of a capacity for homosexual attraction and enjoyment precludes the possibility of a heterosexual identity. This is the 'social polarisation' effect. One implication of such a view is that sexual orientation, once established, is immutable. There is, however, increasing evidence that many women and, to a lesser extent, men change or modify their sexual preferences at different stages of their lives (Blumstein & Schwartz 1976). There is an increasing tendency to view homosexuality less in terms of 'identity' of the individual, and more in terms of 'relationships' between people (Peplau & Cochran 1990). With the inevitable impact of HIV on sexuality in general, it is difficult to predict how our concepts of sexual orientation will change and evolve over the next decade.

Helping the homosexual

Problems with existing sexual relationships

Sexual or interpersonal difficulties in homosexual couples can be approached in the same way as with heterosexual couples, using couple, individual or group therapy. Masters & Johnson (1979) reported good results in treating sexual dysfunction in homosexual pairs using their usual couple therapy approach.

The consequences of stigmatisation

Here the person needs the type of counselling used for members of any stigmatised minority group, helping to distinguish between intra- and interpersonal conflicts, attributing guilt in an appropriate way and learning to manage one's identity in public.

Dissatisfaction with the homosexual role

A desire for a heterosexual lifestyle or some of its accompaniments, such as children, may lead the homosexual to seek treatment. Twenty years ago such a request was not unusual; now it is relatively uncommon, although with the social reaction to the AIDS epidemic, we may see it once again increase in frequency. Twenty years ago someone with such a request would probably have been offered treatment aimed at suppressing his homosexual feelings, either by drugs or psychological methods such as aversion therapy. It is now regarded as not only more acceptable ethically, but also more efficacious to help such people explore alternatives to homosexuality; in other words, to add to their behavioural repertoire. Even help of that kind remains ethically controversial, though most therapists would feel that an individual should be allowed, and hence be helped, to explore heterosexual relationships if he or she really wants to. (See Bancroft (1991a) for a fuller discussion of the ethical aspect.) Masters & Johnson (1979) reported relatively good results with homosexuals who came to them with a potential heterosexual partner prepared to cooperate in couple therapy of the kind described earlier in the chapter. Obviously an important first step had already been taken in finding a partner willing to cooperate in treatment. Those seeking such help are seldom in that position. There are a variety of other ways, mainly based on simple common-sense counselling about heterosexual skills and relationships, which can be used with an individual lacking a suitable partner (see Bancroft (1989)). However, the first task of the counsellor is to ensure that he is not simply colluding with social pressures to conform, but rather acting to allow the individual more freedom of choice. And, realistically, the proportion of men or women with clearly established homosexual identities who will change significantly as a result of such interventions is probably small.

OTHER SEXUAL PREFERENCES

Fetishism and sado-masochism are two types of sexual preference which, whilst relatively common in some degree, are only seldom presented as problems. They carry less obvious social stigma because they can often be concealed behind an apparently normal heterosexual or homosexual front; but they often conflict with stable sexual relationships, and most often help is requested because of the strain that is imposed on such relationships.

Fetishism

The word 'fetish', which from its Portuguese origins implies an artistically created artifact, also conveys a special symbolism or 'magical' meaning — the love token or erotic icon. Sexual fetishes, however, vary from a particular physical attribute or body part to a truly inanimate sexual symbol. As the fetishist becomes more preoccupied with his fetish, so his sexual partner becomes less relevant and, in extreme cases, redundant. Hence the fetish serves to weaken the sexual relationship. There are three principal types of sexual fetish to consider: (1) a part of the body; (2) an inanimate extension of the body, e.g. an article of clothing; and (3) a source of specific tactile stimulation (e.g. a specific texture). The use of women's clothes as a fetish overlaps with transvestism and will be further considered below. Fetish objects often reflect current fashions. Rubber, leather and shiny black plastic are common fetish textures nowadays. In Kraft Ebbing's time in the late 19th century, furs, velvets and silks were the popular textures.

It seems likely that fetishism results from a specific conditioning of sexual response to particular stimuli. Penile erection is a peculiarly conditionable response (Rachman & Hodgson 1968, Bancroft 1974) and the probable lack of any comparable conditionable sexual response in women may account for the apparent rarity of fetishism amongst females. A simple conditioning model is not sufficient, however. Other factors must operate to maintain the response and it remains a mystery why such specific learning occurs in these cases. Does it reflect a peculiarity of learning in certain individuals or does it indicate problems in those people when trying to incorporate sexual responses into their dyadic relationships, resulting in isolation of their sexuality? If conditioning occurs at an early age, before any mature concept of sexuality has developed, are bizarre associations more likely to develop? It is certainly tempting to assume that the fetish object has some significance beyond that of a randomly conditioned stimulus. Occasionally, bizarre fetishes are found in association with a neurological abnormality such as temporal lobe epilepsy. In such cases, the stimulus could well be more randomly conditioned as a result of a neurophysiological disturbance of learning.

Sado-masochism

Although the terms sadism and masochism are often used loosely to cover any situation in which an individual gains a reward from either hurting or dominating another person, or being hurt or dominated, the terms are properly used when the rewards involved are clearly sexual. The sadist plays the active role in the infliction of pain, psychological humiliation or ritualised dominance; the masochist, the passive role. Submission is commonly manifested in 'bondage', i.e. being tied up or constrained so that you are unable to protect yourself and at the mercy of your assailant. Whereas fetishism is distinctly rare amongst women, sado-masochism is by no means unusual, although the more serious use of sado-masochistic sexual activity is rarely found amongst women (Spengler 1977). It is, however, much more common for both men and women to be aroused by the fantasy of such activities than the reality. Moderate pain inflicted as an expression of sexual excitement in the form of the 'love bite' is by no means unusual; this phenomenon is also widespread amongst other species. But, for the most part, sado-masochism remains difficult to understand. It is perhaps best seen as a ritualised form of sexual stimulation in which the need for dominance, the psychological significance of passivity, the sexualisation of anger and the arousing effect of pain interact.

SEXUAL OFFENDERS

The most important categories of sexual offence are sexual assault and rape, and the sexual abuse of children and minors. Rape offenders seldom present for professional help, even though in some instances a definite sexual preference for coercive sexual behaviour develops (Abel et al 1980). Furthermore, the courts are relatively unlikely to ask for a psychiatric report on a rapist. With sexual abuse of children, however, psychiatric help is frequently sought, either as part of the legal process or in order to avoid it, and for this reason we will focus mainly on this form of sexual offence. This difference, however, reflects an interesting aspect of social attitudes that sees sexual abuse of children as more 'pathological' than the sexual assault and rape of adults. The significance of this, and in particular the extent to which social attitudes and expectations about male sexual behaviour may foster rape in our society, has been discussed more fully elsewhere (Bancroft 1991b). The consequences of rape for the woman may well require psychiatric help (see above).

Sexual abuse of children

With the recent dramatic increase in the extent to which adults reveal their childhood experiences of being sexually abused, the prevalence of this form of child abuse becomes an issue of some importance. There is no good reason to believe that there has been a substantial increase in such abuse, but certainly we are hearing more about it.

The various prevalence studies leave us with a bewildering range of reported prevalence rates, ranging from 6 to 62% of females and 3 to 31% of males with such experiences (Peters et al 1986). It is difficult to make sense of such disparate rates, although methods of sampling, survey techniques and, in particular, what is regarded as sexual abuse obviously account for a fair amount of the variance. Earlier researchers, such as Kinsey, did not assume that a sexual experience involving a child and an adult was *necessarily* harmful to the child. Hence neutral terms were used, and Kinsey et al (1953) reported that 24% of women had described a 'prepubertal sexual experience with a postpubertal male'. Workers in the child sexual abuse field eschew such neutral terminology. Harmful consequences, even if not obvious or immediate, are assumed, and hence all such behaviour, including genital exhibition or verbal communications about sex, is regarded as 'abuse', or in some cases as 'assault' (e.g. see Katz & Mazur 1979). Children with such experiences are labelled as 'victims'. There is no doubt that most cases of sexual exploitation of children by adults are harmful to the child, often to a devastating extent. However, to assume that harm invariably follows any such childhood experience, regardless of its nature, its participants or its consequences, is not only likely to confound 'prevalence rates' of 'abuse' and contribute to the variance in reported figures but, more important, may also contribute to a potentially pathogenic situation for the children involved. This has become a highly contentious area. Wyatt (1991), one of the principal workers in the field, has described the 'schism' between the 'sexual abuse' workers who are struggling to tackle what they see as a frightening and widespread problem, and the more traditional 'sex researchers' who are sceptical about some of the assumptions and assertions.

The problems of evaluating prevalence rates from surveys of adults pale into insignificance besides the difficulties of evaluating the evidence from young children where sexual abuse is suspected. This problem is not only crucial for the child, but has an important bearing on societal reactions to child sexual abuse. In general, sexual contact between adults and children is an exceedingly emotive topic. Any adult involved in such behaviour is committing an offence and no category of offence is so strongly reviled by the general public. The strength of this societal reaction, and the consequences to the alleged perpetrator, are not always just; civil liberties may be endangered. Yet there also seems to be a reluctance to accept that child sexual abuse, particularly when occurring within the family, is anything other than a rare aberration perpetrated by evil or sick individuals. Evidence that such behaviour might be widespread is unacceptable to our society; it threatens too strongly our notion of the sanctity of the family.

Masson (1984) presented his controversial historical analysis of the evolution of Freud's ideas about sexual abuse, and his conversion from believing such abuse to be a common cause of neurosis, to regarding accounts of such abuse as 'wish-fulfilling fantasies'. In his book he describes the frequency with which physical and sexual abuse of children was reported in the French medical literature of the mid-to-late 19th century. He also describes a further literature developing the idea that 'children lie' about such incidents. The implication is that, for a while, evidence of common and often horrific sexual abuse of children by their parents was publicised, at least in the medical literature. Then came a phase of 'denial', which appears to have continued until recently. Recent well-publicised episodes, such as the Cleveland affair and (at the time of writing still under enquiry) the Orkney ritual sexual abuse case, have shown how quickly public opinion can turn against those who report child sexual abuse as common within the family. At the same time, it is difficult to avoid questioning the approach taken by the professional agencies in some of these cases. Is there any middle ground between believing that children 'never lie' about such matters and regarding their reports as examples of fantasy? Is there a danger that, if it appears to be too common, intrafamilial sexual abuse will be swept under the carpet, as appeared to happen in the late 19th century?

In the meantime, health professionals continue to struggle to help appropriately in such cases, both with the children and the families, and with adults who are revealing their childhood experiences. Sexual offences considered by the courts are twice as likely to involve girls as boys, possibly because boys are less likely to report the incidents. The major change has been in awareness of intrafamilial child sexual abuse. The taboo against incest appears to be weaker than was assumed to be the case. The explanations for such abuse are not yet well formulated. The concept of the paedophile, the adult, almost always male, who has a sexual preference for a prepubertal or peripubertal child, is most often useful in explaining cases of extrafamilial sexual abuse. Paedophiles are mainly attracted to girls in the 8–11-year-old age group, or boys of 11–15 years old, the ages when childhood sexuality is probably most noticeable. Many paedophiles have problems establishing satisfactory adult relationships (Mohr et al 1964) and may be attracted to children because they are less threatening. In some cases, there is evidence of a fixation of sexual development at a stage of childhood sexual experimentation; the individual who enjoyed such encounters as a child and who is unable to progress for one reason or another into a more mature sexual relationship continues to harbour fantasies of those early positive experiences which form the basis of his adult sexual thoughts and interest. However, there is now increasing evidence that many paedophiliacs may have been sexually abused by adults themselves when children. This raises the question of whether their later behaviour as the abuser is best understood in non-sexual terms (e.g. the need to exercise control rather than be controlled).

In the intrafamilial cases involving children close to puberty, the sexuality of the behaviour is often fairly apparent, the 'pathology' lying mainly in the irresponsibility and preparedness to exploit the adult–child relationship. With sexual abuse of very young children, the motivation is usually more difficult, and one wonders to what extent this is a variant of physical abuse, motivated by hostility, need to control, or pleasure in inflicting pain or humiliation.

The effects on the children do depend on the nature of the relationship with the perpetrator. When this occurs within the family, the threat to the family and the enormous responsibility that this places on the child is probably as harmful as the specifically sexual consequences. Summit (1983) has described the 'child sexual abuse accommodation syndrome' which 'allows for the immediate survival of the child within the family but which tends to isolate the child from eventual acceptance, credibility or empathy within the larger society'. There are five components to this syndrome (1) *secrecy*, the need to keep quiet about the abuse for fear of the consequences of revealing it; (2) *helplessness*, the difficulty, in view of the need for secrecy, for the child to avoid further abuse; (3) *entrapment and accommodation*, the development of various maladaptive behaviour patterns which have a destructive effect on personality development; (4) *delayed and unconvincing disclosure*, usually at times of conflict with the family, resulting in rejection of the child's story and a further damaging sense of being 'unbelieved'; (5) *retraction*, the threat of disintegration of the family, following disclosure, leading to retraction of the child's story, resulting in further 'invalidation' of the child.

The effects of sexual abuse on the sexuality of the child have been described by Friedrich (1988). They depend on the age of the child, the frequency of the abuse, as well as the relationship with the abuser. Abused children may masturbate excessively, show inappropriate sexual knowledge, become preoccupied with sexual thoughts and pursue sexual games with other children. The effects on the sexuality of adulthood were considered earlier in this chapter.

Indecent exposure and exhibitionism

Exhibitionism or 'indecent exposure' is one of the more common forms of sexual offence, and offenders are quite often referred for psychiatric help. It is also a very difficult behaviour to understand. As with many other forms of sexual offence, it is difficult to distinguish between sexual and non-sexual determinants. In certain circumstances, genital display does have a simple sexual significance. It is the most common form of sexual interaction amongst children and may precede sexuality between adults. But, with the exception of exposure by the mentally handicapped, most of these offences are not apparently aimed at establishing further sexual contact with the 'victim'. The theme of mastery and insult is much more noticeable, suggesting that genital display is being used as an expression of hostility. Such display is common amongst many species of primates, especially the males. But, as with sexual assault, the picture is complicated by the 'sexualisation' of the behaviour that is evident in a proportion of cases. Some exhibitionists are sexually aroused at the thought of exposing and use fantasies of exposing whilst masturbating. It is in these cases that the exhibitionist behaviour is most likely to be persistent. In other cases, the impulse to expose is a more occasional event, occurring against a background of otherwise fairly normal sexual preferences. Other consequences of indecent exposure have to be taken into consideration in understanding its possible determinants. Not only is the offender likely to be punished, but his wife and family will feel humiliated. In many cases one is struck by the apparent need of the exhibitionist to provoke these reactions and one wonders then whether the behaviour would be as likely to occur if it were not regarded as an offence. Certainly, for the vast majority of exhibitionists, their behaviour should be seen as harmless, although unseemly and often transiently unpleasant or frightening for the 'victim'. A large number of women must have witnessed such acts. Gittleson et al (1978) found that 44% of a group of nurses had had this experience, usually in their early teens. Exhibitionism varies in a number of aspects.

The age of the victim. A minority of exhibitionists expose persistently to prepubertal girls and in some of them this may lead eventually to more direct sexual contact with children (Rooth 1973). The commonest age of victim is at or around puberty.

The nature of the act. Sometimes the exposure is clearly sexual, associated with an erect penis and sexual excitement. Masturbation usually occurs either during the exposure or shortly after. In other cases, the penis is flaccid and there is no obvious sexual arousal. The reaction of the female is important and an exhibitionist may go on exposing until he produces a desired response. Rooth (1971) describes a typical ideal exposure as:

one of dominance and mastery. The exhibitionist, usually timid and unassertive with women, suddenly challenges one with his penis, briefly occupies her full attention and conjures up in her some powerful emotions such as fear and disgust, or sexual curiosity and arousal...he experiences a moment of intense involvement in a situation in which he is in control. The reaction that he most dislikes is indifference.

The frequency of exposing behaviour. An important distinction, as already mentioned, is between the person who only has occasional urges to expose, often at times of crisis or emotional distress, and those for whom the idea of exposing is always sexually stimulating.

Risk taking. Some exhibitionists are careful to avoid being caught or recognised. Others seem to behave in a way that ensures that they are caught, e.g. exposing from their car, so that their registration number leads to their arrest.

Exhibitionists are unremarkable in their intelligence or social class, though there is some evidence that they are 'underachievers'. Rooth (1971) describes them as 'immature' and suggests that they commonly have dominant, overprotective mothers and passive and ineffectual fathers; they marry women who take over this maternal role, and they have relatively stable marriages of the mother/son type. These must be regarded as clinical impressions, but marital sexual problems are undoubtedly common amongst them.

Management of sexual offenders

In the current climate of concern about child sexual abuse and sexual assault, much attention is being given to methods of intervention with the victim. Much less attention has been given to helping the offender, both to avoid further offences and to establish a more acceptable sexual lifestyle. This in part reflects the difficulty of the task. In particular, it reflects our uncertainty and ignorance about why people behave in this way. Unfortunately, it is a minority of such individuals whose behaviour can be understood simply in sexual terms, and more often other factors about need for control, emotional insecurity or feelings of inadequacy are pre-eminent. In the last few years there has been an increase in attempts to help such individuals, mainly in the USA. It is too early to judge whether real progress is being made. In this country there is widespread pessimism about helping the individual with conventional methods. Appropriate group or special institutional methods possibly offer the best prospects, but await validation.

In general, the legal process is effective; the large majority of sexual offenders are deterred by their first conviction and are not seen again. But those who re-offend usually present formidable problems. Drugs are sometimes useful for reducing sexual interest and hence lessening the likelihood of sexual offence behaviour. Although oestrogens were used in the past for this purpose, they have now largely given way to the following: cyproterone acetate, an antiandrogen; benperidol, a butyrophenone; or medroxyprogesterone acetate, a progestagen that has some antiandrogenic effects. None of these drugs is free from side-effects and they should be used with proper supervision, as their effects are difficult to predict in a particular case (Bancroft 1989). They also raise some crucial ethical issues. Although they can be used in the context of a normal doctor–patient relationship and with fully informed consent on the part of the patient, they have frequently been used as a condition of treatment imposed by a court, or as part of a process of early release or parole from prison. In such cases it is difficult, if not impossible, to ensure adequate or proper consent and the use of the drug should then be seen as a form of 'social control' rather than medical treatment. This then requires suitable legal scrutiny to ensure that such treatment is not abused (Bancroft 1991a).

TRANSVESTISM AND TRANSSEXUALISM

Gender identity problems, particularly those involving transvestism and transsexualism, deserve separate consideration, not only because of their complexity and interest, but also because of the specialised and demanding treatment involved.

Cross-dressing (i.e. dressing in the clothes of the opposite sex) is one factor that these various forms of behaviour have in common. Four categories of cross-dresser can be described, each emphasising one particular aspect of the phenomenon.

The fetishistic transvestite. This is a man (probably never a woman) who wears female clothes as fetish objects. The clothes are sexually arousing and, usually, wearing them leads to masturbation. Cross dressing in this case is a sexual act.

The transsexual. A male or female who believes himself or herself to be a woman or man, or has a strong desire to be accepted as such in spite of his or her anatomy. In this case, cross-dressing is part of the process of expressing one's preferred gender. Both the male and female transsexual are likely to seek medical help to alter their bodies to be consistent with their psychological gender (sex reassignment).

The 'double role transvestite'. Usually a male who spends part of his life as a normal heterosexual male and part of his life dressing and 'passing' as a woman. Cross-dressing is usually similar to that of the transsexual but there is no desire to change sex permanently.

The homosexual transvestite. A man or woman who is sexually attracted to members of the same sex and who cross-dresses, but with less intention of being considered of the opposite sex. This cross-dressing is not necessarily sexual and often takes the form of caricature rather than serious impersonation.

These four examples demonstrate the three principal dimensions of the cross-dressing experience: the fetish component; the cross-gender identity and role; and sexual orientation. Most of the variety of cross-dressing behaviour can be accounted for by inter-action of these three dimensions. There is very little that can be said about the determinants of these behaviours, which remain in most respects mysterious (Green 1974). The most important condition is transsexualism, because of the major and often devastating impact that this has on the individual's life. In males, childhood transsexualism is rare and the majority of such boys followed into early adulthood have so far shown homosexual rather than transsexual identities (Green 1985, Zuger 1978). It remains possible that some of them will eventually adopt the 'transsexual position' and this is one possible route to adult transsexualism. Many others start off with a fetishistic transvestite pattern which, over a period of time, becomes more transsexual, the cross-dressing

losing its sexual effects. It is as though the repeated fetishistic cross-dressing undermines or produces conflict with the masculine gender identity, leading in some cases to adoption of a female identity as a solution (Bancroft 1972). In other cases, this process appears to stop, at least for a relatively long time, at the 'double role transvestite' stage.

In some cases where homosexual attraction is present, but a homosexual identity unacceptable, the transsexual role allows the same attraction to continue whilst maintaining a heterosexual identity. In many cases, the strength of the transvestite or the transsexual urge varies with the success or failure of the individual's ordinary sexual relationships. Thus, a resurgence of these feelings often follows a breakdown in a sexual relationship or marriage rather than precedes it.

In females, transsexualism is less common. The fetishistic dimension is not relevant to the female. In the author's experience, the avoidance of homosexuality is more striking as a causative factor in female transsexuals. They are also more likely than the male transsexual to be involved in a relatively stable sexual relationship. The role of the partner is therefore more relevant. Often the partner's own sexual or gender identity needs are best met by having a transsexual partner, and sometimes the partner may put pressure on the transsexual to seek sex reassignment because of her own need to avoid a homosexual identity.

Management

Management of transsexualism presents one of the most demanding challenges in clinical sexology, requiring the collaboration of behavioural, endocrinological and surgical specialists working as a team. Though surgical aspects are complex, it is the psychological management that is most time-consuming. It is unlikely that a transsexual will seek help to reduce or eliminate his transsexual feelings. As indicated above, the transsexual urge does wax and wane and there may be relatively prolonged periods of remission. This in itself makes evaluation of any treatment procedure difficult. Occasionally people have claimed 'cures' of transsexualism, but they are usually based on short periods of follow-up and may be no more than a period of remission expedited by treatment. Usually the transsexual wants help with sex reassignment, most tangibly in the forms of hormone therapy, facial hair electrolysis and surgery to reassign genitalia or remove or augment breasts. The use of such measures remains controversial. But a number of responsible clinicians have worked long enough and cautiously enough in this field to conclude that, with careful selection, at least a proportion of transsexuals will benefit from such reassignment.

In a recent review of the follow-up literature of sex reassignment surgery, Green & Fleming (1990) concluded that the preoperative factors indicating a favourable outcome include: (1) a reasonable degree of psychological stability, with no history of psychosis; (2) successful adaptation in the desired role for at least a year, with physical appearance and behaviour convincing; (3) sufficient understanding of the limitations and consequences of surgery; and (4) preoperative psychotherapy in the context of a gender identity programme.

Hormone therapy and facial electrolysis may be introduced at an earlier stage than surgery, but the decision to use surgery should only be made once it has become evident that the individual has the psychological and physical attributes, i.e. outward appearance, to adapt successfully. Hormone therapy involves oestrogens (possibly combined with progestagens) for the male to female, and androgens for the female to male. Oestrogens will probably induce breast growth, redistribution of body fat along more feminine lines, some change in skin texture and some slowing of facial and body hair growth. The extent of these effects is difficult to predict.

Oestrogens may also suppress sexual interest and response, which may or may not be acceptable to the patient. Androgens will increase muscle bulk, deepen the voice and increase body and facial hair growth. Clitoral enlargement is to be expected, often accompanied by an increase in sexual interest and response. Acne may be a problem.

Surgical reassignment for the male transsexual involves removal of testes and the corpus spongiosum of the penis, preserving scrotal and penile skin to shape the labia and vaginal barrel, and with some methods, deploying the corpora cavernosa on either side to provide an erectile base for the labia. Usually some additional skin graft is required to obtain a satisfactory vaginal barrel. Surgical breast augmentation is often required.

The female has fewer options from surgical treatment. Hysterectomy and oophorectomy are usually involved. Mastectomy is often important, as concealment of breasts can be difficult or uncomfortable as well as limiting. Surgical creation of a penis remains surgically difficult, though some progress is being made. The principal problem is in ensuring satisfactory passage of urine through the surgically created urethra, without urinary fistulae developing. Once these technical problems are solved, there may be possibilities for erection, at least of artificial kind.

REFERENCES

Abel G G, Becker J V, Skinner L J 1980 Aggressive behaviour and sex. Psychiatric Clinics of North America 3: 133

Annon 1974 The behavioural treatment of sexual problems. In: Brief therapy. Enabling Systems, Honolulu

Arentewicz G, Schmidt G 1983 The treatment of sexual disorders. Basic Books, New York

Bancroft J 1972 The relationship between gender identity and sexual behaviour: some clinical aspects. In: Ounsted C, Taylor D C (eds) Gender differences: their origins and significance. Churchill Livingstone, Edinburgh

Bancroft H 1974 Deviant sexual behaviour: modification and assessment. Clarendon Press, Oxford

Bancroft J 1988 Reproductive hormones and male sexual function. In: Sitsen J M A (ed) Handbook of sexology, vol 6. Pharmacology of sexual function. Elsevier, Amsterdam

Bancroft J 1989 Human sexuality and its problems, 2nd edn. Churchill Livingstone, Edinburgh

Bancroft J 1991a Ethical aspects of sexuality and sex therapy. In: Bloch S, Chodoff P (eds) Psychiatric ethics. 2nd edn. Oxford University Press, Oxford

Bancroft J 1991b The sexuality of sexual offending: the social dimension. Criminal Behaviour and Mental Health 1: 181–192

Bancroft J 1992 Impotence in perspective. In: Gregoire A, Pryor J (eds) Impotence: an integrated approach to clinical practice. In press

Bancroft J, Wu F C 1985 Clinical algorithms; erectile impotence. British Medical Journal 290: 1566

Becker J V, Kaplan M S 1991 Rape victims: issues, theories and treatments. Annual review of sex research 2: 267–292

Bell A P, Weinberg M S 1978 Homosexualities. A study of diversity among men and women. Mitchell Beazley, London

Blumstein P W, Schwartz P 1976 Bisexuality in women. Archives of Sexual Behavior 5: 171

Brindley G S 1986 Maintenance treatment of erectile impotence by cavernosal unstriated muscle relaxant injections. British Journal of Psychiatry 14: 210

Buvat J, Buvat-Herbaut M, Lemaire A, Marcolin G, Quittelier E 1990 Recent developments in the clinical assessment and diagnosis of erectile dysfunction. Annual Review of Sex Research 1: 265–308

Catalan J, Bradley M, Gallway J, Hawton K 1981 Sexual dysfunction and psychiatric morbidity in patients attending a clinic for sexually transmitted diseases. British Journal of Psychiatry 138: 292

Clement U 1990 Surveys of heterosexual behavior. Annual Review of Sex Research 1: 75–92

Cranston-Cuebas M A, Barlow D H 1990 Cognitive and affective contributions to sexual functioning. Annual Review of Sex Research 1: 119–162

Dörner G 1979 Hormones and sexual differentiation of the brain. In: Porter R, Whelan J (eds) Sex, hormones and behaviour. Ciba Foundation symposium 62. Excerpta Medica, Amsterdam

Fairburn C G, Wu F C W, McCulloch D K et al 1982 The clinical features of diabetic impotence: a preliminary study. British Journal of Psychiatry 140: 447

Frank E, Anderson C, Rubinstein D 1978 Frequency of sexual dysfunction in 'normal' couples. New England Journal of Medicine 299: 111

Frenken J 1976 Afkeer van seksualiteit. Van Loghum Slaterus, Deventer (English summary, p 219)

Frenken J, Van Tol P 1987 Sexual problems in gynecological practice. Journal of Psychosomatic Obstetrics and Gynaecology 6: 143–155

Friedrich W N 1988 Behavior problems in sexually abused children. In: Wyatt G E, Powell G J (eds) The lasting effects of child sexual abuse. Sage, Newbury Park, CA, pp 171–191

Gagnon J, Simon W 1973 Sexual conduct: the social sources of human sexuality. Aldine, Chicago

Garde K, Lunde I 1980 Female sexual behavior. A study in a random sample of 40 year old women. Maturitas 2: 255

Gebhard P H, Johnson A B 1979 The Kinsey data: marginal tabulations of the 1938–1963 interviews conducted by the Institute for Sex Research. Saunders, Philadelphia

Gittleson N L, Eacott S E, Mehta B M 1978 Victims of indecent exposure. British Journal of Psychiatry 132: 61

Golombok S, Rust J, Pickard C 1984 Sexual problems encountered in general practice. British Journal of Sexual Medicine. 11: 210–212

Gooren L 1990 Biomedical theories of sexual orientation: a critical examination. In: McWhirter D P, Sanders S A, Reinisch J M (eds) Homosexuality/heterosexuality. Concepts of sexual orientation. 2nd Kinsey Symposium. Oxford University Press, New York.

Green R 1974 Sexual identity conflict in children and adults. Duckworth, London

Green R 1985 Gender identity in childhood and later sexual orientation: follow up of 78 males. American Journal of Psychiatry 142: 339–341

Green R, Fleming D T 1990 Transsexual surgery follow-up: status in the 1990's. Annual Review of Sex Research 1: 163–174

Hawton K, Catalan J 1986 Prognostic factors in sex therapy. Behaviour Research and Therapy 24: 377

Hawton K, Catalan J, Martin P, Fagg J 1986 Long term outcome of sex therapy. Behaviour Research and Therapy 24: 665–675

Herdt G H 1981 Guardians of the flutes: idioms of masculinity. McGraw-Hill, New York

Heston L L, Shields J 1968 Homosexuality in twins: a family study and a register study. Archives of General Psychiatry 18: 149

Hooker E 1967 The homosexual community. In: Gagnon J H, Simon W (eds) Sexual deviance. Harper & Row, New York

Hunt M 1974 Sexual behavior in the 1970s. Playboy Press, Chicago

Kabalin J N, Kessler R 1989 Penile prosthesis surgery: review of 10 year experience and examination of re-operations. Urology 33: 17–19

Kaplan H S 1974 The new sex therapy. Brunner/Mazel, New York

Kaplan H S 1990 The combined use of sex therapy and intrapenile injections in the treatment of impotence. Journal of Sex and Marital Therapy 16: 195–207

Katz S, Mazur M A 1979 Understanding rape victims; a synthesis of research findings. Wiley, New York

Kinsey A S, Pomeroy W B, Martin C R 1948 Sexual behaviour in the human male. Saunders, Philadelphia

Kinsey A S, Pomeroy W B, Martin C R, Gebhard P H 1953 Sexual behaviour in the human male. Saunders, Philadelphia

Leiblum S R, Rosen R C 1989 Principles and practice of sex therapy. 2nd edn. Guilford, New York

Levine S B, Yost M A 1976 Frequency of sexual dysfunction in a general gynaecological clinic: an epidemiological approach. Archives of Sexual Behavior 5: 229

McCulloch D K, Campbell I W, Wu F C, Prescott R J, Clarke B F 1980 The prevalence of diabetic impotence. Diabetologia 18: 279

McWhirter D P, Mattison A M 1984 The male couple. How relationships develop. Prentice Hall, New Jersey

Masson J M 1984 The assault on truth. Freud's suppression of the seduction theory. Farrar, Strauus & Giroux, New York

Masters W H, Johnson V E 1970 Human sexual inadequacy. Churchill, London

Masters W H, Johnson V E 1979 Homosexuality in perspective. Little Brown, Boston

Mohr J W, Turner R E, Jerry M B 1964 Paedophilia and exhibitionism. University of Toronto Press, Toronto

Money J, Ehrhardt A A 1972 Man and woman, boy and girl: differentiation and dimorphism of gender identity from conception to maturity. Johns Hopkins University Press, Baltimore

O'Carroll R, Bancroft J 1984 Testosterone therapy for low sexual interest and erectile dysfunction in men: a controlled study. British Journal of Psychiatry 145: 146

Peplau L A, Cochran S D 1990 A relationship perspective on homosexuality. In: McWhirter D P, Sanders S A, Reinisch J M (eds) Homosexuality/heterosexuality. Concepts of sexual orientation. 2nd Kinsey symposium. Oxford University Press, New York.

Peters S, Wyatt G, Finkelhor D 1986 Prevalence. In: Finkelhor D et al (eds) Sourcebook on child sexual abuse. Sage, Beverly Hills, CA, pp 15–59

Pietropinto A, Simenauer J 1977 Beyond the male myth: a nationwide survey. Times Books, New York

Pillard R C, Poumadere J, Carretta R A 1982 A family study of sexual orientation. Archives of Sexual Behavior 11: 511

Rachman S. Hodgson R 1968 Experimentally induced 'sexual fetishism': replication and development. Psychological Record 18: 25

Reid K, Surridge D H C, Morales A et al 1987 Double-blind trial of yohimbine in the treatment of psychogenic impotence. Lancet ii: 421–423

Riley A J, Goodman R E, Kellett J M, Orr R 1989 Double blind trial of yohimbine hydrochloride in the treatment of erection inadequacy. Sexual and Marital Therapy 4: 17–26

Rooth F G 1971 Indecent exposure and exhibitionism. British Journal of Hospital Medicine April: 521

Rooth F G 1973 Exhibitionism, sexual violence and paedophilia. British Journal of Psychiatry 122: 705

Rosen R C 1991 Alcohol and drug effects on sexual response: experimental and clinical studies. Annual Review of Sex Research 2: 119–180

Slag M F, Morley J E, Elson M K et al 1983 Impotence in medical clinic outpatients. Journal of the American Medical Association 249: 1736

Spengler A 1977 Manifest sado-masochism of males: results of an empirical study. Archives of Sexual Behavior 6: 441

Summit R C 1983 The child sexual abuse accommodation syndrome. Child Abuse and Neglect 7: 177–193

Swaab D F, Hofman M A 1990 An enlarged suprachiasmatic nucleus in homosexual men. Brain Research 537: 141–148

Swan M, Wilson L J 1979 Sexual and marital problems in a psychiatric out-patient population. British Journal of Psychiatry 135: 310

Tiefer L 1991 Historical, scientific, clinical and feminist criticisms of "the sexual response cycle" model. Annual Review of Sex Research 2: 1–24

Tiefer L, Pedersen B, Melman A 1988 Psychosocial follow-up of penile prosthesis implant patients and partners. Journal of Sex and Marital Therapy 14: 184–201

Toone B K, Wheeler M, Nanjee N, Fenwick P, Grant R 1983 Sex hormones, sexual activity and plasma anticonvulsant levels in male epileptics. Journal of Neurology, Neurosurgery and Psychiatry 46: 824

Turner L A, Althof S E, Levine S B, Bodner D R, Kursh E D, Resnick M I 1991 A comparison of the effectiveness of two treatments for erectile dysfunction: self-injection therapy versus external vacuum devices. Paper at Annual Meeting, International Academy of Sex Research, Barrie, Ontario

Tyrer G, Steele J M, Ewing D J, Bancroft J, Warner P, Clarke B F 1983 Sexual response in diabetic women. Diabetologia 24: 166

Virag R, Shoukry K, Floresco J, Nollet F, Greco E 1991 Intracavernous self-injection of vasoactive drugs in the treatment of impotence: 8-year experience with 615 cases. Journal of Urology 145: 287–293

Warner P, Bancroft J and members of the Edinburgh Human Sexuality Group 1987 A regional service for sexual problems: a 3-year study. Sexual and Marital Therapy 2: 115–126

Weinberg M S, Williams C J 1974 Male homosexuals: their problems and adaptation. Oxford University Press, New York

Wyatt G E 1991 Child sexual abuse and its effects on sexual functioning. Annual Review of Sex Research 2: 249–266

Zuger B 1978 Effeminate behavior present in boys from childhood: 10 additional years of follow up. Comprehensive Psychiatry 19: 363–369

26. Psychiatric disorders of childbirth

J. L. Cox

INTRODUCTION AND HISTORICAL CONSIDERATIONS

Since the 5th century BC physicians have given particular attention to the psychiatric disorders that follow childbirth. Hippocrates described puerperal psychoses and speculated that they might have a physiological cause such as milk diverted from the breast to the brain. During the Middle Ages, witchcraft beliefs were more widely prevalent and some witches were believed to kill and eat small babies (see Cohn 1975). It was not until the mid 19th century that reliable clinical observations were again made, by two French psychiatrists: Marcé and Esquirol.

In 1858 Marcé, who was working in the mental hospital at Ivry-sur-Seine, described a series of 310 women with a mental illness associated with childbirth and observed a clinical syndrome different from that found at other times. He noted that delirium and lability of mood were common and that the illness often started on the fourth or fifth postpartum day (*nouvelles accouchées*). Hamilton, (1962), in a comprehensive review of these early French studies, has helped to re-establish their historical importance:

> to a remarkable degree he (Marcé) was able to describe the varieties, nuances and details of puerperal mental illness. He noted many ways in which cases which occur after childbirth differ from ordinary mental illness. He believed that the observed psychological phenomena were closely related to changes in the pelvic organs.

Twenty years earlier, Esquirol had made another highly pertinent observation: 'large numbers of mild to moderate cases' of puerperal mental illness were cared for at home and 'never recorded'. Esquirol also pointed out that studies restricted to women admitted to hospital could be particularly misleading. However, despite this caveat, most subsequent observations have been descriptions of women with a psychosis that required in-patient treatment and only in the last 25 years have prospective surveys of non-hospitalised women been carried out.

PSYCHOLOGICAL AND SOCIAL CONSIDERATIONS

In a useful monograph on postnatal depression, Breen (1975) drew a distinction between childbirth as a 'hurdle' which must be overcome and as a 'process' which is continuous and results in irreversible physical or psychological changes. Breen preferred this latter analogy, and likened pregnancy to puberty — regarding it as a 'biosocial event' that may necessitate a reassessment of personal relationships as well as an acceptance of a new biological role. A child-bearing woman may, for example, have to renegotiate her relationship with her husband and her mother, as well as establish an entirely new bond with her baby.

Psychoanalysts have also made a distinctive and clinically relevant contribution to the understanding of the parturient woman. The intense identification that may occur between mother and baby as well as with her own mother has been described by Deutch (1947). If the relationship with her own mother is hostile this may interfere with her ability to be a good mother herself and the conflict may then be projected on to the baby. Mothers who were themselves deprived of adequate maternal affection in childhood may become envious of the baby who demands the attention that they never had themselves. Some support for these theories is provided by Nilsson & Almgren (1970), who showed that a postpartum psychiatric disorder was more likely to occur in women who had a poor relationship with their mother or were uncertain of their female identity. In a prospective study in Edinburgh the absence of a mother through earlier death was found to increase the likelihood of severe emotional disturbance immediately after delivery (Cox et al 1982) and several women said that they now felt closer to their mother and could understand more fully what she had experienced during childbirth.

From a sociological perspective the fact that most child-bearing women are more closely scrutinised by the medical profession than at almost any other time in their lives is of much interest. Nevertheless, the 'under-utilisers' have been investigated by McKinlay (1970) and shown to come from lower social classes and to have a greater risk of both obstetric and psychological complications. Milio (1975) has even suggested that this under-utilisation occurs because maternity services are middle-class institutions primarily organised for middle-class women, and that working-class women are therefore alienated. The sick role of the pregnant women is also emphasised by the increased medicalisation of child-bearing, with the result that many mothers regard themselves as patients and pregnancy as a sickness.

Postpartum taboos

Many societies have definite rules governing how a mother should behave in the weeks that follow childbirth. In Jamaica, for example, a period of ritual seclusion follows childbirth which is particularly intense for the first nine nights, and Kitzinger (1982) described this as similar to the seclusion that follows bereavement. This is followed by a secondary, but less restricted, seclusion for a further 13 nights, when the mother remains at home with her baby and is looked after by her own mother. In India, among the lower Hindu castes, a postpartum woman is regarded as impure for 40 days and during this time she and her child should not come out of confinement. In a gypsy community, Okley (1975) reports that childbirth is polluting, and to prevent contamination cooking is carried out by other women, or by older children. Among Punjabi women living in Britain the length of the confinement after childbirth varies, and depends on whether other women in the household can help, as well as on economic considerations (Homans 1982). In China the postpartum period is referred to as 'doing the month', when extra attention is given to the mother by her family, as well as by her wider social network (Pillsbury 1978).

Postnatal rituals, however, are also found in contemporary Western societies. There is, for example, a similar 6 week period after birth, when special observations of the mother are carried out, that is enshrined in present-day obstetric practice. The postnatal clinic usually takes place at 6 weeks and is customarily regarded as a signal that full domestic and marital responsibilities should be resumed. Because of present-day ambiguity about social norms postpartum and the usefulness of such obstetric postnatal 'rituals', there is a lack of clarity for the mother about when to return to work and about the extent of her husband's involvement with child-care. It is these ambiguities which provide some limited support for the hypothesis that the lack of these 'rites of incorporation' are related to the aetiology of postnatal depression.

DISORDERS OF PREGNANCY

Though psychiatric disorder is most severe in the puerperium, it can also occur during pregnancy. One in five married mothers attending an antenatal clinic in London was regarded as having a psychiatric disorder of some kind by Kumar & Robson (1984). Much lower rates (5%) were found in Edinburgh (Cox et al 1982), though symptoms of anxiety were common in unmarried women from working-class backgrounds. Clearly, the proportion of women with a psychiatric disorder will be considerably influenced by the criteria used and the sample investigated. Furthermore, the distinction between neurosis and appropriate, or even facilitatory, anxiety during pregnancy is often hard to make. Nevertheless, comparisons of psychiatric morbidity in pregnant women and in non-child-bearing controls show a higher frequency of psychiatric symptoms in the former (Robin, 1962, Cox 1979). These symptoms are not usually regarded as requiring treatment and psychiatric referral is unusual. A policy of 'wait and see' is more commonly implemented, so that the psychiatric disturbance may become submerged in the physiological symptoms that precede childbirth. A further difficulty in determining the frequency of psychiatric disturbance in pregnancy is the emotional lability characteristic of the last trimester and also the limitations of anxiety or depression questionnaires which have not been adequately validated for use with child-bearing women.

When a mother is known to have had a previous bipolar or schizophrenic illness more detailed observation is indicated and careful consideration has to be given to the need for continuing with prophylactic medication. During the first trimester it is usually wise to avoid all psychotropic drugs; a counselling approach that acknowledges a mother's fears of childbirth and allows expression of negative attitudes is often beneficial, as are attempts to alleviate socioeconomic hardships.

DISORDERS OF THE PUERPERIUM

The relationship between childbirth and psychiatric disorder in the puerperium is complex. There are several possibilities:

1. That childbirth is itself a sufficient and specific physiological or psychological stress and is therefore immediately causal
2. That those women most vulnerable to a puerperal psychiatric illness include those with specific difficulties concerning sexual activity, mothering and reproduction (Tetlow 1955) or with a strong genetic predisposition
3. That the puerperium increases vulnerability to other life events such as bereavement, loss of job, marriage or divorce.

Psychiatric disorders of the puerperium will be discussed under the following conventional headings:

1. Puerperal neuroses
2. Puerperal psychoses
3. Transitory mood disturbances.

Puerperal neuroses

Postnatal depression is not only the most frequent but also the most disabling neurotic disorder at this time. Within 6 weeks of childbirth 10–15% of mothers may become seriously depressed (Pitt 1968, Paykel et al 1980, Cox et al 1982, Kumar & Robson 1984, Watson et al 1984) and if untreated this illness may last for 6 months or more and cause considerable family disruption.

In our Edinburgh study, for example, 13 of the 103 women interviewed had a depressive illness in the puerperium, and a further 17 had milder depressive episodes (which nonetheless lasted for 4 weeks in all but two). Of those mothers with severe depression at least half remained depressed for a year and most had not received any sustained psychiatric treatment. It is therefore a considerable public health problem that general practitioners and other primary care workers diagnose postnatal depression so infrequently despite being in regular contact with the mother, and that so little information about this disorder is available (see Cox 1986). This apparent neglect may be explained by the following factors:

1. An assumption that all mood disturbances in the puerperium are 'just postnatal blues', i.e. they are not only common but are also transitory and therefore of no clinical importance.
2. Transfer from hospital to home may occur at or about the time when the illness begins and so the likelihood of an accurate diagnosis being made is diminished.
3. The health visitor, the general practitioner and the family may be more concerned with the physical health and developmental milestones of the baby than with the mood of the mother.
4. Limited psychiatric training of general practitioners, midwives and health visitors may delay the diagnosis.
5. The mothers may not report their depressed mood to their general practitioner, because they do not recognise their distress as illness or because they fear that their guilt and inadequacy will be reinforced.

The early identification of postnatal depression is therefore difficult and is not facilitated by the absence of useful antenatal predictors, other than a hereditary predisposition or a previous psychiatric history. The illness often develops unexpectedly or 'out of the blue' and for this reason may cause additional family distress. No association was found in any of three prospective studies between postnatal depression and parity, or with being unmarried. Furthermore, women were not likely to become depressed if they had had an assisted delivery, were older or from a lower social class. The only predictive finding in our study, which replicated that of Pitt (1968), was that women observed to be emotionally unstable in the first week after delivery were more at risk of developing a depressive illness subsequently.

Clinical features

A mother with postnatal depression usually exhibits several of the following symptoms, which are often disguised as loneliness or worry about a physical illness:

1. Excessive anxiety about her baby's health that cannot be diminished by reassurance.
2. Self-blame: the mother believes that she cannot live up to her own expectations of a 'good mother', nor is she as competent as her own mother. She may also compare herself unfavourably with others in the neighbourhood and even remain at home to avoid their criticism.
3. Sleep difficulty due to mood disturbance is a commonly reported symptom but may be masked by the disruption of night feeds or by a noisy hospital routine.
4. A depressed mood is not itself a common complaint though tears and other depressive behaviour can frequently be observed. The mother may recognise, however, that she is not her normal self, and her husband may also have noticed this change and have urged her to obtain medical help.
5. Suicidal thoughts or a fear of harming the baby.
6. Irritability and loss of libido leading to deterioration in the marital relationship.

7. Worry at her rejection of the baby and a reluctance to feed or handle it.

8. A fear that the baby may not be hers, or could be seriously deformed in some way.

Treatment

The diagnosis is made by taking a psychiatric history with particular reference to the symptoms described, and by careful observation of the mental state. The diagnosis may by missed, however, if clinical attention is diverted to the physical well-being of the baby or if the mother has a physical illness or a postpartum complication such as an infected episiotomy or breast abscess. Other difficulties of assessment may be caused if an inappropriate emphasis is given to psychodynamic aspects of assessment, although this model can be useful in management.

The diagnosis must be established as quickly as possible so that treatment, which may include counselling and antidepressant drugs, can be commenced. Breast-feeding is not contraindicated if antidepressants are prescribed, but should be discontinued if treatment with lithium carbonate is maintained. Some depressed mothers are best advised to change to bottle-feeding to enable them to get adequate sleep and also to allow the husband or others to help more with the care of baby. The mother can usually be reassured that the prognosis is good but that it may be several months before she is fully back to her normal self. Some mothers are glad to talk about their hateful feelings towards themselves or their baby and are greatly relieved when they are not criticised. Confirmation of this clinical observation has recently been obtained in a controlled intervention study of counselling. In this study it was shown that depressed mothers who were given non-directive counselling by a health visitor recovered more fully than a control group of depressed mothers who had routine treatment; 18 (69%) of the 26 depressed mothers in the counselled group recovered, compared with only nine (38%) of the 24 in the control sample (Holden et al 1989). The results of this study therefore suggest that providing training for health visitors or other primary care workers in these simple counselling skills would be beneficial. Women who do not improve with counselling alone may require treatment with antidepressants as well as a more complex psychotherapy such as cognitive therapy. Occasionally the depression is maintained by having to cope with severe behavioural disturbance in an older child; in this circumstance collaboration with a child psychiatrist may be very valuable.

As treatment may be started early in the puerperium, midwives must be familiar with the symptoms of the illness, the likely prognosis and also the side-effects of medications. Premature discharge home of a depressed mother should be avoided and the indications for admission to a psychiatric unit carefully considered. Women who do not improve with anti-depressant medication and those who have fleeting delusions are best admitted to a mother and baby in-patient unit, or to a day unit with a nursery; the latter facility is particularly useful when close to the mother's home and if the nursery can accommodate an older child as well as babies.

Prevention

Primary prevention would be assisted by better education of the health professionals involved; the teaching requirement for midwives on these topics at present is only 2 hours, although a course of 26 hours is necessary to cover the field adequately. Prophylactic medication, such as antidepressants, lithium or phenothiazines, should be considered in women who are at high risk of developing a puerperal mental illness.

Secondary prevention, i.e. early detection, may be carried out by closely following up mothers with severe postnatal blues as they are known to have a greater likelihood of becoming depressed later on. In addition, a brief self-report scale, such as the ten-item Edinburgh Postnatal Depression Scale (Cox et al 1987) can be used to screen for depressive illness, and has been shown to be acceptable to mothers as well as to primary care workers when used at a postnatal (Murray & Carothers 1990) or child welfare clinic, or at home.

A raised incidence of depression postpartum has been found in several prospective studies and Pitt (1968) estimated a seven-fold increase in the onset of psychiatric disorder in the puerperium. Edinburgh data suggest that the increased risk is substantially less, and not more than four-fold. The specificity of postnatal depression was questioned by Cooper et al (1988) who found a similar prevalence to that reported in non-puerperal women. Likewise, O'Hara et al (1990) in a prospective controlled study in the USA found no difference between puerperal women and their controls in the prevalence of depression at 9 weeks postpartum, although there was a greater frequency of depression in puerperal women at 3 and 6 weeks. In a recent controlled study of 232 women in Stoke-on-Trent a three-fold increase in the risk of a depression commencing within 5 weeks of childbirth compared with controls was found, though the prevalence of depression at 6 months was similar in both groups (Cox et al 1991b). Thus, the birth event, because of either biological or psychological changes, may initiate depression which may last as long as a year; the closer the onset of such depression to childbirth, the greater the likelihood that biological (neuroendocrine) factors are important in aetiology.

Other neurotic disorders

Phobias, anxiety states and obsessive–compulsive disorders may also occur and interfere markedly with child-care. A mother with a germ phobia, for example, may have great difficulty washing nappies and become upset if her baby does not develop a precise routine. Another mother with an anxiety state may be so worried that her baby might stop breathing at night that she responds to every sound and so generates separation anxiety. Agoraphobia can be especially disabling in the puerperium, as such mothers may avoid public transport because they fear their baby may cry and so attract the critical attention of other passengers.

Puerperal psychoses

Problems of classification

The major mental illnesses that follow childbirth can generally be diagnosed using familiar criteria for affective, schizophrenic and organic psychoses. They are relatively rare and occur following 0.2% of live births. Such women are generally admitted to a psychiatric hospital; manic illnesses, because of their greater disruption, are more likely to be admitted earlier in the puerperium than depressions.

Although there is no separate category of puerperal psychosis in ICD-10 or in DSM-IIIR, certain symptoms such as confusion, perplexity and lability of mood are persistently reported in the absence of a definite physical cause (Brockington et al 1979). Furthermore, as the management of puerperal psychosis presents particular difficulties which do not occur with other psychoses, the absence of puerperal psychoses from ICD-10 and DSM-IIIR, although consistent with the principle that diagnostic categories are based on symptoms, impedes research and hinders the improvement of clinical facilities. However, the specificity of the diagnosis of puerperal psychosis remains in doubt and the lack of evidence for hormonal differences between psychotic and non-

psychotic mothers, or between mothers with and without more minor mood disturbances postpartum, suggests that if hormonal changes are important aetiological factors, the mechanism is more likely to depend on differences in receptor sensitivity to the hormonal milieu than to the hormonal levels themselves. Furthermore, the controlled follow-up by Platz & Kendell (1988) of matched groups of women with puerperal psychoses and similar illnesses unrelated to childbirth found no significant differences in the subsequent psychiatric morbidity of the two, or in the morbidity of their first-degree relatives.

However, the increased likelihood of admission postpartum is not in doubt. Thus, Kendell et al (1987), using linked data from separate obstetric and psychiatric case registers, have confirmed the finding of earlier studies that there is a substantial increase in the likelihood of a mother being admitted to a psychiatric unit within 90 days of parturition, a risk of 2.2 per 1000 births (see Fig. 26.1). In the first 30 days after childbirth they found nearly seven times as many admissions as the average monthly rate before pregnancy (68 versus 10); and for primiparae the risk of being admitted with psychosis within this 30 day period was no less than 35 times higher than before pregnancy. This dramatic rise in the admission rate postpartum suggests either that powerful biological factors are involved or that the parapartum weeks are exceptionally stressful, and that such stress greatly exceeds other stressful events such as the loss of a job or bereavement.

Their finding that being unmarried, having a first baby, perinatal death and delivery by caesarean section were associated with an increased risk of psychiatric admission does, however, give support to those who believe that psychological stresses make a substantial contribution to this high psychiatric morbidity postpartum.

Although little definite can be said about the relative frequency of different syndromes in the puerperium from studies of women who have been admitted to specialised mother and baby units, or which rely on retrospective case note data, it is nevertheless clear that depressive and manic presentations are much commoner than schizophrenic or organic ones. However, not all women who are admitted to hospital have psychotic illnesses. In Edinburgh a quarter were admitted because of minor depressive disorders or with a diagnosis of personality disorder (Dean & Kendell 1981). Mothers with a previous history of manic–depressive illness or with a previous puerperal psychosis have a very high risk (one in three or one in five) of an affective disorder after

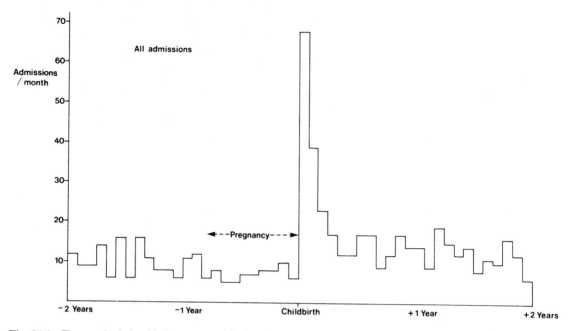

Fig. 26.1 Temporal relationship between psychiatric admission and childbirth (derived from a series of 54 087 births in Edinburgh from 1970–1981).

childbirth. Kumar and his colleagues have recently shown that when these high-risk women do relapse after childbirth the onset of psychotic symptoms is preceded (on the fourth day postpartum) by evidence of increased sensitivity of dopamine receptors in the hypothalamus (Wieck et al 1991).

Clinical presentation

The following symptoms are of particular importance in establishing the diagnosis of a psychosis in the puerperium:

1. Severe insomnia and early morning waking
2. Lability of mood, sudden tearfulness or inappropriate laughter
3. Persistent perplexity, disorientation or depersonalisation
4. Unusual behaviour, such as restlessness, excitement or sullen withdrawal
5. Unexpected rejection of the baby or a conviction that the baby is deformed or dead
6. Paranoid ideas that may involve hospital staff or close family relations
7. Suicidal or infanticidal threats
8. Excessive guilt, depression or anxiety.

The initial mood disturbance may be difficult to distinguish in the first instance from the 'postnatal blues'. Such mothers are therefore best kept in the postnatal ward for further observation or, if they are discharged, must be visited at home by the general practitioner, community midwife or community psychiatric nurse to ensure that a psychosis has not developed.

The decision whether or not to admit the mother to a psychiatric hospital is therefore difficult and, if in doubt, as when a mother has a borderline psychotic illness, admission should usually be arranged even if this may temporarily disrupt the mother–baby relationship, or be contrary to the wishes of the relatives. The risk if a major illness is not diagnosed, or is only partially treated at home, is considerable and may include a serious attempt to harm the baby or commit suicide. Fortunately, this latter event is less likely to occur during pregnancy or in the first postnatal year than at other times and motherhood may therefore be protective (Appleby 1991).

These considerations also influence whether or not the baby should be admitted with the mother. The advantages of doing so include maintaining the physical proximity of mother and baby, which may allow breast-feeding to continue, and the mother is also helped to retain her confidence in her own ability to care for her baby. However, some mothers are too disturbed and unpredictable to be entrusted with any child-care tasks and others have infanticidal thoughts; in these circumstances there may have to be a delay before admitting the baby. Other considerations include the presence of other psychotic patients in the ward who might pose a threat to the baby, as well as the possible disruption of a ward milieu by the baby's demands. If the baby is admitted, its administrative status in the hospital must be clarified, adequate nursing facilities provided, and good liaison maintained with midwives and nursery nurses. A separate room properly equipped as a nursery is usually essential. These facilities are best provided in a mother and baby unit, but some babies can be managed on general admission wards, provided the above factors are carefully considered. It is always desirable to observe the mother and baby together for at least a week prior to discharge, so that it is clearly established that she is now able to cope with her infant.

The management of puerperal psychoses involves a careful explanation to the patient and her family as to why she needs to be in hospital. The husband is frequently alarmed and puzzled by his wife's behaviour, and so needs considerable reassurance. As she recovers from her illness the mother should be encouraged to look after the baby, and may be helped by a structured behavioural programme. Electroconvulsive therapy (ECT) is particularly effective in the treatment of puerperal psychoses even if the symptomatology is not typically that of a depressive illness. Phenothiazines and lithium are useful in the treatment of mania but control of lithium therapy can be difficult immediately after delivery. Any coexisting physical illnesses such as pelvic sepsis or breast abscess require joint management with the obstetrician. The postnatal examination should not be overlooked because the patient is in a psychiatric unit, and advice about future contraception should be given.

The prognosis for the acute illness is usually good, but the risk of recurrence following a subsequent pregnancy is very high — of the order of one in five. Careful observation of the mother after discharge is also necessary because unexpected relapse may occur; close liaison with the general practitioner, health visitor and community psychiatric nurse is therefore vital.

Transitory mood disturbances of the first postpartum week ('postnatal blues')

At least 50% of mothers (Pitt 1973) experience unfamiliar episodes of crying, irritability, depression and emotional lability in the 10 days after childbirth, a syndrome often referred to as 'postnatal blues'. Such mood disturbances, though familiar to midwives, may cause considerable distress to both the mother and her relatives. The tearfulness seems unwarranted by the circumstances and the customary belief that the days following childbirth are a time for pleasure and celebration. The midwife may regard the postnatal blues as fleeting and trivial — an assessment that has had some support in the past by psychiatrists. However, recent research has shown that severe postnatal blues may be linked to more serious psychiatric disorders, so they should arouse the concern of clinicians as well as the interest of the researcher. An obstetrician or psychiatrist, for example, is often confronted by a tearful and depressed mother who wants to go home and has then to decide whether this mood disturbance is indeed transient, or denotes the onset of a major psychiatric disorder. It may be wise to keep such women in hospital for a further period of observation although the mother herself may think she would be better at home.

The cause of postnatal blues is unknown but associations have been found with increased levels of urinary cyclic adenosine monophosphate (CAMP) and also with reduced plasma levels of free tryptophan. No associations, however, have been found so far with changes in the levels of oestrogen or progesterone in the puerperium (Gelder 1978), although evidence of modification of platelet adrenoreceptor activity by oestrogens may be a clue to the way in which sex hormones mediate their effect on central brain synapses. There is evidence that depression and mood instability are maximal on the fifth postpartum day and that women with higher neuroticism scores are more likely to experience 'the blues' (Kendell et al 1981, 1984), although why this should be so is unknown. This study also revealed that one-third of women with severe postnatal blues developed a depressive illness later in the puerperium, which suggests that the aetiology of the two phenomena may be linked. O'Hara et al (1991) report an association between the blues and the depressed component of the premenstrual syndrome, a finding which suggests that both disorders share a common neuroendocrine distur-bance, or are linked to the underlying personality. The Maternity Blues Questionnaire (Kennerley & Gath 1989), which has satisfactory validity and is sensitive to daily mood changes, may assist further research into the nature of these transitory mood disturbances.

POSTNATAL DEPRESSION AND CHILD DEVELOPMENT

The possible relationship between severe mood disturbance in the puerperium, when mother–child bonding occurs, and subsequent child development is of much interest. The temperamental characteristics of the child may be established at this time so that any disruption of normal maternal bonding by mental illness may have a lasting effect. Several studies reviewed by Murray & Stein (1989) have shown that a depressed woman is more unresponsive to her infant's cries, and usually more withdrawn, overintrusive or hostile. It is possible that the infant's way of relating to others may be influenced by this early relationship to a depressed mother. Thus, Cogill et al (1986) found adverse long-term effects of postnatal depression on the later behaviour and cognition of the child. Stein et al (1991) investigated the 19-month-old infants of women who had experienced an earlier postnatal depression and compared them with infants of the same age of non-puerperally depressed mothers. They found that women who had been depressed played less with their children and that the children behaved in a more negative way towards them; although such associations could be explained by an adverse marital relationship, the personality of the father, or by the baby's temperament. It nevertheless is likely that the sequence of mother–baby interactions, which is an important part of mothering behaviour, will be interrupted if the mother is unresponsive because of depression, or if she overcompensates for her low self-esteem by intruding into the baby's physical or psychological 'space' (see Stern 1977). The positive reinforcement by the baby of the mother's mothering behaviour is also a crucial determinant of mother–child interaction, and could influence the duration of depression; a baby who looks 'ugly' or does not conform to the stereotype of a 'good baby' might impair the mother's self-esteem.

Psychotropic drugs, if taken during the first trimester of pregnancy, increase the risk of congenital malformation and should be avoided. Lithium increases the risk of congenital cardiac abnormalities and the likelihood of conception should therefore be considered before embarking on long-term lithium therapy in a young woman. Dietary sodium restrictions during pregnancy can also influence lithium control.

Alcoholism or bouts of heavy drinking during pregnancy are associated with a risk of the baby developing the fetal alcohol syndrome, a disorder characterised by growth deficiency, microcephaly, shortened palpebral fissures and mental handicap (Clarren & Smith 1978; see also Ch. 4).

PUERPERAL PSYCHIATRIC DISORDER IN DEVELOPING COUNTRIES

It is possible that the puerperal psychiatric disorders described above are much the same in both industrial and developing countries, although the management may differ depending on the availability of medical resources as well as on local cultural beliefs about childbirth. The organic and schizophrenic puerperal illnesses, though rare in the UK, are nevertheless more common than affective psychoses in some developing countries (Ebie 1972, Swift 1972). In a prospective community study of non-psychotic postnatal depression in Uganda, 10% of the 180 women interviewed had a depressive illness after childbirth (Cox 1983), although these women were more likely to seek help from a traditional healer than from a doctor.

It is commonly assumed in Britain that postnatal depression may be caused by confinement in hospital rather than at home, or by changes in the role of women. However, the finding that many rural Ugandan women became depressed in the puerperium, and that depression was not more likely to follow a hospital delivery or more likely to occur in co-wives, suggests that biological factors should also be considered. Guilt or self-blame were unusual in the Africans; the depressed Scots, on the other hand, constantly worried about their failure to meet their own standards or those of their neighbours.

SUMMARY AND CONCLUSIONS

The puerperium is undoubtedly a time when a woman has an increased risk of developing a psychiatric disorder. The relative frequencies of these disorders, their possible interrelationships and the psychiatrist's role in management are illustrated in Table 26.1. Both clinical and research evidence indicate that a spectrum of disorders may exist, from mild emotionality at one extreme to florid psychosis at the other. It is possible that a physiological trigger, which may result from a reduction of hormone levels in the puerperium, may increase the risk that a mother will have an emotional disturbance at this time. It is likely, however, that the actual mood experienced may be determined by the immediate environment and by the mother's own personal memories or other recent stressful life events. The picture puzzle of these postpartum psychiatric disorders therefore still persists and may only be fully solved when aetiological research has included a full understanding of social factors — such as consulting behaviour and the meaning of the childbirth event — as well as physiological causes. Childbirth is not a

Table 26.1 Spectrum of mood disturbances in the puerperium

	Postnatal blues	Puerperal neuroses	Puerperal psychoses
Frequency	50%	15% (13% depression)	0.2% Affective psychoses common; schizophrenic and organic psychoses rare
Peak time of onset	4–5 days after childbirth	2–4 weeks after childbirth	1–3 weeks after childbirth
Duration	Usually 2–3 days	4–6 weeks if treated; up to 1 year if not	6–12 weeks
	Severe 'blues' may ⟶	Postnatal depression ⟶	Affective psychosis
Profession of first contact	Midwife (hospital); obstetrician	Midwife (community); health visitor; general practitioner	Midwife; health visitor; general practitioner; psychiatrist (rarely)
Psychiatric referral	Virtually never	Unusual	Common — especially if marked behaviour disturbance
Possible treatments	Nil; but observation if severe	Counselling; antidepressants	Admit to mother and baby unit; neuroleptics; antidepressants; ECT; lithium; counselling and advice about further pregnancy

straightforward single life event and may best be considered as a cascade of life events; some, such as the birth itself, are initiated by physiological changes whilst others, such as the new social role of the mother, are determined by sociocultural variables.

The contribution of the psychiatrist is not confined to the treatment of these disorders since the role of educator is also of paramount importance. Health visitors, social workers, community psychiatric nurses and general practitioners, for example, are the key primary care workers and they need training in the recognition and treatment of puerperal mental illnesses. However, the psychiatrist must first develop clinical competence by seeing obstetric referrals for this teaching to be effective. The main task is then to alert other professionals to the importance of psychiatric knowledge about the management of postnatal mental illness and, in this indirect way, to enable the mother's distress to be relieved, and the negative impact of mental illness at this time on the family to be diminished. The need for health authorities to purchase a postnatal mental illness service led by a consultant psychiatrist has been argued by Oates (1988), who emphasised the distinctive clinical skills necessary. The contribution of this service to the long-term prevention of psychiatric disorder in the mother and her family needs to be more fully evaluated.

REFERENCES

Appleby L 1991 Suicide during pregnancy and in the first postnatal year. British Medical Journal 302: 137–140

Breen D 1975 The birth of a first child. Tavistock, London

Brockington I F, Schofield E M, Donnelly P, Hyde C 1979 In: Sandler M (ed) Mental illness in pregnancy and the puerperium. Oxford University Press, Oxford

Clarren S K, Smith D W 1978 The fetal alcohol syndrome. New England Journal of Medicine 298: 1063–1067

Cogill S R, Caplan H L, Alexandra H, Robson K M, Kumar R 1986 Impact of maternal postnatal depression on cognitive development of young children. British Medical Journal 292: 1165–1167

Cohn M 1975 Europe's inner demons. Chatto-Heinemann, Sussex University Press

Cooper P J, Campbell E A, Day A, Kennerley H, Bond A 1988 Non-psychotic psychiatric disorder after childbirth: a prospective study of prevalence, incidence, course and nature. British Journal of Psychiatry 152: 799–806

Cox J L 1979 Psychiatric morbidity and pregnancy: a controlled study of 263 semi-rural Ugandan women. British Journal of Psychiatry 134: 401–405

Cox J L 1983 Postnatal depression: a comparison of Scottish and African women. Social Psychiatry 18: 25–28

Cox J L 1986 Postnatal depression: a guide for health professionals. Churchill Livingstone, Edinburgh

Cox J L, Connor Y, Kendell R E 1982 Prospective study of the psychiatric disorders of childbirth by personal interview. British Journal of Psychiatry 140: 111–117

Cox J L, Holden J M, Sagovsky R 1987 Detection of postnatal depression: development of the Edinburgh postnatal depression scale. British Journal of Psychiatry 150: 782–786

Cox J L, Murray D M, Chapman G 1992 A controlled study of the onset, duration and prevalence of postnatal depression. British Journal of Psychiatry, accepted for publication.

Dean C, Kendell R E 1981 The symptomatology of puerperal illnesses. British Journal of Psychiatry 139: 128–133

Deutch H 1947 The psychology of women, vol 2. Motherhood. Research Books, London

Ebie J C 1972 Psychiatric illness in the puerperium among Nigerians. Tropical Geographical Medicine 24: 253–256

Gelder M 1978 Hormones and post partum depression. In: Sandler M (ed) Mental illness in pregnancy and the puerperium. Oxford University Press, Oxford

Hamilton J A 1962 Post-partum psychiatric problems. Mosby, St Louis

Holden J, Sagovsky R, Cox J L 1989 Counselling in a general practice setting: a controlled study of health visitor intervention in the treatment of postnatal depression. British Medical Journal 298: 223–226

Homans H 1982 Pregnancy and birth as rites of passage. In: MacCormack C P (ed) Ethnography of fertility and birth. Academic Press, London

Kendell R E, McGuire R J, Connor Y, Cox J L 1981 Mood changes in the first three weeks after childbirth. Journal of Affective Disorders 3: 317–326

Kendell R E, MacKenzie W E, West C, McGuire R J, Cox J L 1984 Day-to-day mood changes after childbirth: further data. British Journal of Psychiatry 145: 620–625

Kendell R E, Chalmers L, Platz C 1987 The epidemiology of puerperal psychoses. British Journal of Psychiatry 150: 662–673

Kennerley H, Gath D 1989 Maternity blues, I. Detection and measurement by questionnaire. British Journal of Psychiatry 155: 356–362

Kitzinger S 1982 The social context of birth: some comparisons between childbirth in Jamaica and Britain. In: MacCormack C P (ed) Ethnography of fertility and birth. Academic Press, London

Kumar R, Robson K M 1984 A prospective study of emotional disorders in childbearing women. British Journal of Psychiatry 144: 35–47

McKinlay J B 1970 The new late comers for antenatal care. British Journal of Preventive and Social Medicine 24: 52

Milio N 1975 Values, social class and community health services. In: Cox C, Mead A (eds) A sociology of medical practice. Collier-MacMillian, London

Murray L, Carothers A D 1990 Validation of the Edinburgh postnatal depression scale on a community sample. British Journal of Psychiatry 157: 288–290

Murray L, Stein A 1989 The effects of postnatal depression on the infant. In: Oates M R (ed) Psychological aspects of obstetrics and gynaecology, vol 3, Baillière Tindall, London

Nilsson A, Almgren P E 1970 Paranatal emotional adjustment: a prospective investigation of 165 women. Acta Psychiatrica Scandinavica suppl 220

Oates M 1988 The development of an integrated community-orientated service for severe postnatal mental illness. In: Kumar R, Brockington I F (eds) Motherhood and mental illness, vol 2, Wright, London

O'Hara M W, Zekoski E M, Philipps L H, & Wright E J 1990 A controlled prospective study of postpartum mood disorders: comparison of childbearing and non-childbearing women. Journal of Abnormal Psychology 99: 3–15

O'Hara M W, Schlechte J A, Lewis D A, Wright E J 1991 Prospective study of postpartum blues: biologic and psychosocial factors. Archives of General Psychiatry 48: 801–806

Okley J M 1975 The traveller-gypsies. Cambridge University Press, Cambridge

Paykel E S, Emms E M, Fletcher J, Rassaby E S 1980 Life events and social support in puerperal depression. British Journal of Psychiatry 114: 339–346

Pillsbury B L K 1978 "Doing the month": confinement and convalescence of Chinese women after childbirth. Social Sciences and Medicine 12: 11–22

Pitt B 1968 Atypical depression following childbirth. British Journal of Psychiatry 114: 1325–1335

Pitt B 1973 Maternity blues. British Journal of Psychiatry 128: 431–435

Platz C L, Kendell R E 1988 Matched control follow-up and family study of puerperal psychoses. British Journal of Psychiatry 153: 90–94

Robin A A 1962 Psychological changes of normal parturition. Psychiatric Quarterly 35: 129–150

Stein A, Gath D H, Bacher J, Bond A, Cooper P J 1991 The relationship between postnatal depression and mother–child interaction. British Journal of Psychiatry 158: 46–52

Stern D 1977 The joint relationship: infant and mother. Fontana, London

Swift C R 1972 Psychosis during the puerperium among Tanzanians. East African Medical Journal 49: 651–657

Tetlow C 1955 Psychoses of childbearing. Journal of Mental Science 101: 629–639

Watson J P, Elliott S A, Rugg A J, Brough D I 1984 Psychiatric disorder in pregnancy and the first post-natal year. British Journal of Psychiatry 144: 453–462

Wieck A, Kumar R, Hirst A D, Marks M N, Campbell I C, Checkley S A 1991 Increased sensitivity of dopamine receptors and recurrence of affective psychosis after childbirth. British Medical Journal 303: 613–616

Wrate R M Rooney A C, Thomas P F, Cox J L 1985 Postnatal depression and child development: a three year follow-up study. British Journal of Psychiatry 146: 622–627

27. Personality disorders

C. P. L. Freeman

INTRODUCTION

There is a new optimism and renewed activity in the study of personality disorder. In the last edition of this textbook this introduction was critical and pessimistic. I advocated the temporary suspension or permanent abandonment of the use of personality disorder labels within psychiatry. I still believe that for clinical use this is not an unreasonable course. But simply ignoring personality disorder labels will not cause them to go away. There is no doubt that, despite all its shortcomings, the introduction of Axis 2 in DSM-III has provided a great stimulus for research in this area. One may not go as far as Millon (1984) who stated that "the long drought is over and a revival of the rich heritage of the forties and fifties is underway". Nevertheless much effort has been put into personality disorder research in the last five years and most authorities agree that the way forward is through a separate axis such as Axis 2 and more careful operational definitions of different personality disorder labels. However, it is the author's impression that in American psychiatry the term Axis 2 is already becoming a judgemental, pessimistic and value-laden term. Patients are described as being 'a bit Axis 2-ey' or being 'very Axis 2 laden'.

The reader will have to accept that in discussing personality disorders we move into an area where science and systematic enquiry have so far been of limited help and that some of the personality types to be described represent little more than the personal opinions of eminent psychiatrists. If a diagnostic label tells you little about the patient, communicates nothing of certainty to a colleague and predicts little about the past, present or future of the individuals so labelled, it is doubtful if it is worth using. If in addition it stigmatises the patient, makes him less likely to receive adequate treatment, or is used as a reason for not offering treatment at all, then it can be positively harmful.

Whereas psychologists have contributed a great deal to the concept of personality and personality types in both normal and ill individuals, psychiatrists have not studied their concepts of personality disorder with anything like the same thoroughness.

The pattern of traits and behaviour that make up an individual's personality are unique and it is perhaps not surprising that it proves difficult or impossible to subdivide individuals into discrete personality disorder categories. There are no reliable ways of dividing individuals into those of 'normal' personality and those of 'abnormal' personality. Welner et al (1974) showed that it was not always clear why patients initially received diagnoses of personality disorder, except that they had a significantly higher frequency of impulsive and manipulative behaviour, temper tantrums, suicide attempts and severe marital discord than a control in-patient population.

Although a comprehensive discussion of normal personality is beyond the scope of this chapter some reference must be made to it here. Mention is also made of those theories and personality measures which have been used extensively on patient as well as non-patient populations. The biological basis of personality and personality development are covered in Chapters 4 and 5.

NORMAL PERSONALITY

Definition

There are as many definitions of personality as there are psychologists and psychiatrists who have written about the subject. It is a concept which probably causes much less trouble to the layman than to the professional. Personality as it is commonly understood is what makes one individual different from another, so in its simplest sense personality can be defined as 'the characteristic patterns of behaviour and modes of thinking that determine a person's adjustment to the environment'. A complete description of an individual's personality might include factors such as intellectual abilities, attitudes, beliefs, moral values, emotional reactivity and motives acquired in the process of growing up.

Most definitions of normal personality include some or all of the following features:

1. Present since adolescence
2. Stable over time despite fluctuations in mood
3. Manifest in different environments
4. Recognisable to friends and acquaintances.

Classification of normal personality

In order to have some understanding of the way abnormal personalities have been described a brief account is given of the main approaches to the description of normal personality. Five models of personality,

1. The type model
2. The trait model
3. The psychodynamic model
4. The social learning theory/situational model
5. The interactionist model

will be briefly discussed. They are not mutually exclusive and the trait model which has been most used in psychiatric research is discussed more fully.

The type approach

This is the oldest approach and still the one that is used most commonly by psychiatrists in describing abnormal personality. Type theories usually group people into discreet categories and try to explain behaviour on the basis of a few types. Although such type theories are appealing because they provide a simple way of looking at a problem, personality is probably too complex for such an approach. Most individuals do not conform to extreme types but fall somewhere in the middle. The earliest of such theories attempted to classify individuals on the basis of body build (Kretschmer 1925, Sheldon 1954). Short, plump individuals (endomorphs) were said to be sociable, relaxed and even-tempered. Tall, thin individuals (ectomorphs) were described as restrained, self-conscious and fond of solitude. Heavy set, muscular individuals (mesomorphs) were characterised by being upright, sturdy and fond of physical activity. Sheldon also described three types of temperament which corresponded with these body builds: viscerotonics who, he said, 'sucked hard at the

breast of mother earth' and loved physical proximity with others; cerebrotonics linked with ectomorphs; and somatotonics linked with mesomorphs. All subsequent attempts to link specific personality characteristics with body build have shown very low correlations and therefore these classifications are clinically useless. Nevertheless, there is no doubt that a person's physique and physical appearance do have some effect on the personality, primarily because of the limits it may impose on the individual's abilities and the reactions it evokes from others.

The Swiss psychoanalyst Carl Jung coined the terms introvert and extrovert to describe two basic types of personality (Jung 1928). Jung recognised, however, that these two types were extremes and that 'normal man had a balance of both attributes'. He also acknowledged that classification according to introversion and extroversion was not the only method possible but he did feel that it had great practical significance. Perhaps the most widely accepted by the general public, but least valid, of type approaches are the 12 signs of the zodiac and the personal attributes which are said to be associated with them.

The trait approach

The assumption of such theories is that there are universal traits present to differing degrees in all people and which influence behaviour in the same ways in different situations and at different times, so that trait measures can be used predictively. In fact this assumption is fallacious. Traits are inferred from behaviour and the direction of causality cannot be reversed so that the trait is used to explain behaviour. If we observe that an individual behaves in an uncontrolled and impulsive way in a number of different situations, it might be reasonable to characterise him along a trait which measured control versus lack of control. However, we could not use the presence of that trait to explain his uncontrolled behaviour. The trait approach has been particularly popular in psychology because a number of apparently valid objective personality tests have been derived from it.

Personality traits are therefore frequently used as independent variables in psychiatric research.

16 Personality Factor Questionnaire (16PF). Raymond Cattell, a British psychologist working in the USA, has over a 30 year period developed a trait description of personality (Cattell & Butcher 1968). Although Cattell prefers the term factor to trait the two are synonymous. Sixteen personality factors were obtained by factor analysis of a large number of ratings and each factor was assigned two names, one for a high score, the other for a low. Twelve factors were obtained from factor analysis of ratings of one person by another and four from self-ratings. These were combined to form the 16PF, which is a 100-question yes/no test. By plotting an individual's test scores a characteristic personality profile is derived. Examples of the pairs of factors are 'tense' versus 'relaxed', 'controlled' versus 'uncontrolled' 'venturesome' versus 'timid' and 'happy-go-lucky' versus 'serious'.

Eysenck's dimension of personality. There are close parallels between the work of Eysenck and Cattell, though Eysenck is probably better known in Britain. His research has been carried out from an explicitly stated basis of learning theory; it has been publicised in popular scientific writings and has been more closely associated with the problems of psychiatry than Cattell's. It has also often been presented along with a systematic attack on psychoanalysis and dynamic psychology in general. Eysenck's description of personality by reference to orthogonal dimensions is attractive because it is simple, but it does not have the descriptive power of Cattell's multivariate approach.

Eysenck's personality system is made up of four dimensions, viz:

Extroversion–introversion
Neuroticism–stability
Psychoticism–stability
Intelligence.

A succession of personality inventories have been produced to measure such traits. The Maudsley Personality Inventory (MPI) was the first. This was superceded by the Eysenck Personality Inventory (EPI) and, more recently, by the Eysenck Personality Questionnaire (EPQ), which contains items for measuring psychoticism and also a lie scale. A huge amount of experimental work has been generated by this approach to personality and Eysenck himself has tried to link his theory with a very wide range of human behaviour. He has applied his measures not just to normal and abnormal personality but to mental illness as well, indicating that using his dimensional scheme each patient can be measured for his degree of neuroticism, introversion and psychoticism. Criminals and psychopathic patients are said to be characterised by high extroversion and high neuroticism: obsessional and anxiety state patients by high neuroticism and high introversion.

The Minnesota Multiphasic Personality Inventory (MMPI). The MMPI (Hathaway & McKinley 1951) is not based on any particular personality theory but was designed to lessen the conflict between a psychiatrist's conception of abnormal personality and that of other professional workers dealing with abnormality amongst more normal persons. Thus, the inventory is couched in clinical terms with scales which measure such traits as depression, hypochondriasis, hysteria and paranoia. It is a lengthy inventory of 550 statements about attitudes, emotional reactions, physical and psychological symptoms and past experiences to which the subject answers 'true', 'false' or 'cannot say'. The test does not assume any specific personality traits but was constructed in an empirical fashion. The designers gave hundreds of test questions to groups of individuals who differed on particular criteria, and then selected questions which discriminated between the various groups. Although it was originally designed to identify people with serious personality disorders, the MMPI has also been widely used in studying normal populations.

Narrow band theories. These differ from more comprehensive theories of personality in that they restrict their analysis to one particular area of behaviour. In one sense such narrow band theories are not really theories of personality at all, because they cover very limited aspects of human behaviour. Nevertheless, they provide a different and interesting approach and recently have been increasingly used in research on psychiatric patients.

A good example is the internal–external *locus of control* approach of Rotter (1966). Rotter maintained that people could be classified along a continuum, with individuals at the internal end viewing their behaviour and what happens to them as directly under their personal control. At the external end are people who view their behaviour as influenced by events that are completely out of their control and due to such factors as chance, powerful figures in authority and fate. Thus, individuals at the internal end will feel confident that they can bring about changes in their life and environment and that these will be due to their own efforts, whereas those at the external end will feel comparatively powerless to produce change. There are similarities between this approach and that of Seligman and his analysis of depression in terms of learned helplessness.

Other examples of narrow band theories are the 'need for achievement trait' of McClelland et al (1953) and the 'sensation seeking scale' (SSS) of Zuckerman et al (1964). Type A 'coronary-prone behaviour' is also a narrow band concept (see below).

The psychodynamic model

The psychoanalytic approach differs considerably from others in that unconscious motives, rather than traits or situations, are said to direct behaviour. Freud believed that the id was largely instinctual and inherited and closely linked to biological processes. Freud's theory is based almost entirely on the study of emotionally disturbed people who came to him for treatment and it may not be an accurate or appropriate description of the normal, healthy personality. It is also difficult to test in that widely differing and even opposing behaviours may be attributed to the same unconscious conflict. For example, aggressiveness may result in punitive or abusive behaviour, or by the mental mechanism of reaction formation may result in over-concern and protectiveness. Nevertheless, Freud's model of personality consisting of the id, ego and superego, with characteristic phases of development and defence mechanisms, has had a profound influence on psychiatry and on society in general. There have been many modifications and reappraisals of the psychoanalytic approach to personality. Adler, Horney, Fromm and Sullivan all stressed that the unconscious and the id were less powerful than Freud had thought. They felt that personality was shaped more by the individual's life experience than by instincts. They stressed that people were more rational in their decision making and planning than Freud had supposed and their behaviour less governed by instinctual drives.

Carl Rogers (1951) 'self-theory' is another psychodynamic approach to personality. The central tenet of Rogers' theory is that the individual's view of himself, his self-concept, determines his view of the world and his behaviour. Someone with a strong sense of self views the world quite differently from someone whose self-concept is weak. The self consists of all the cognitions, perceptions and ideas that relate to 'I' or 'me' and the individual evaluates every experience in relation to this self-concept. The most important aspect of personality is the congruence between the individual's view of himself and reality and his view of himself as compared with his ideal self. The greater the congruence of these three elements, the happier and more satisfied the individual. Maslow (1967) has taken Rogers' theory further and developed the concept of *self-actualisation*. Although the concept of self-actualisation is never clearly defined it appears that both Rogers and Maslow believe that the basic force motivating human behaviour is a drive towards fulfilment of potential within the limits of heredity.

Maslow studied a group of eminent historical figures and from them developed a list of the characteristics of self-actualisers and of behaviours leading to a state of self-actualisation.

The situationist approach (social learning theory/situational model)

This model looks at the environment for important factors that might determine the behaviour of individuals. Personality differences result from differences in learning experiences. People behave consistently only insofar as the settings they encounter and the roles they are expected to play remain stable. Thus, the type and intensity of external stimulation are seen as the most powerful determinants of behaviour. For example, if subject A scored much higher on the submissiveness factor on the 16PF than subject B, a trait theorist would predict that, in most situations, subject A would behave more submissively than subject B. The social learning theorist would expect that subject B had learnt to be more submissive than subject A in certain situations and that the rank order of subjects A and B would depend not on the strength of a particular trait but on the meaning of the situation as perceived by subjects A and B. A brief but comprehensive review of both the situationist and trait theories is provided by Powell (1986).

The most consistent and vehement proponent of the situationist approach has been Mischel (1968, 1981). He states that 'with the possible exception of intelligence, highly generalised behavioural consistencies have not been demonstrated, and the concept of personality traits as broad dispositions is thus untenable'. Mischel points out that there is a low correlation between personality dimensions derived from questionnaires and observed behaviours. Correlations between questionnaires are high but behavioural responses in a range of different situations correlate poorly with them. Mischel therefore concludes that the predictive power of personality traits is not great. He also points out the circularity of the trait argument. If a person consistently acts in an obsessional, pedantic way, then we rate them high on a trait of obsessionality and this might be a reasonable description of their behaviour. It does not make sense, however, to turn the argument round and say that this individual's obsessional behaviour is accounted for by their high score on an obsessional trait. The trait does not cause the behaviour, it is merely a description of the behaviour.

Powerful evidence for the situationist theory came from the work of Haney et al (1973). A group of students were selected in such a way that none of them had any known antisocial tendencies. A mock prison was set up, some students being randomly allocated to being guards and others to being prisoners. After a few days the guards started to display antisocial behaviour and brutality towards the prisoners. This behaviour was completely different to their 'normal' behaviour and was clearly dependent on the situation. Mischel also points out that there is a human tendency to simplify characters and that we tend to ignore the many inconsistencies in behaviour that we observe and concentrate on the aspects which are consistent with our assumptions. In other words, we all have stereotypes of personalities: people we regard as typically introverted or gregarious. These individuals do not have all the characteristics of a category but, so long as they have one or two and exhibit them in certain situations, we readily assign them to the category concerned.

The interactionist model

In many ways this model reflects the obvious common-sense view that neither the person nor the setting in which he finds himself determines the behaviour in isolation. Behaviour is modified as a result of a continuous feedback between the individual and the situations he encounters. The interactionist model pays heed to the individual in terms of his intelligence, cognitive processes and motivation and to the situation in terms of the psychological meaning that it has for the individual. It does not deny the existence of traits or their importance. As a simple example an individual who is highly anxious may in one setting talk excessively and appear agitated and in another talk minimally and appear withdrawn. The level of anxiety may be the same but the behaviour as determined by the situation is quite different. A good review of the interactionist approach is provided by Magnusson & Endler (1977). So far this approach has had little impact on psychiatry whilst being much debated within psychology.

Consistency of personality

One of the basic assumptions that is made in most definitions of personality and of personality disorder is that behaviour which is determined by personality rather than by illness is consistent over time and from situation to situation. Unfortunately, research has failed to show as much personality consistency as most theorists would lead us to believe.

Longitudinal studies of individuals have shown some consistency of personality traits. Block (1971)

reported a group of 100 subjects followed over a 25 year period. They had been rated twice at school and then again 20 years later in their mid-30s. Over the 20 year period from senior high school to their mid-30s only 29% of items showed a significant positive correlation. The highest correlations for males were between 0.5 and 0.6 and for females between 0.4 and 0.5 (Block's study can, of course, be criticised on the grounds that, at the time of his first two ratings, the personalities of his subjects could hardly be said to be fully formed). Evidence for personality consistency across different situations is even less impressive. Studies of traits such as honesty, self-control, dependency and aggression have usually found low correlations between measures of the trait in one situation and measures in another, for example, comparing aggressive behaviour at home with aggressive behaviour at work. Similarly, attempts to equate responses on personality tests with behaviour in real life have been disappointing. Correlations between independent measures of behaviour and measures derived from personality tests are typically low.

Whether this is because the traits are described too broadly or because some individuals are consistent in their inconsistency is not known. Social psychiatrists point to behaviour being 'situation-specific' rather than 'trait-specific'. In other words, a person behaves in a certain way because of the particular situation in which he finds himself. Of course, many qualities of the individual do remain constant. Physical appearance, gestures and way of speaking tend not to change and, to the extent that these are included in a personality description, there is some consistency.

Studies which have looked at general traits such as anxiety or hostility have found that individual differences in the strength of a trait account for little of the variability of behaviour. What appears to matter most is the interaction of the differences in individuals with the differences in situations. In other words, it is not very useful to talk about general traits such as hostility or anxiety without considering the situation in which they may be exhibited. The importance of this in helping people with personality disorders is that one's efforts may be much more fruitfully directed towards finding situations in which the individual behaves less deviantly than in trying to change personality with psychotherapy.

DEFINITIONS OF ABNORMAL PERSONALITY

Personality disorder is not a subject addressed directly by personality theorists. The terms personality disorder or abnormal personality imply a judgement that certain traits or features of the personality are 'good' or 'bad'. Wherever possible, personality theorists avoid making such judgements. Powell (1986) points out that the meaning of the term 'personality' in 'personality disorder' bears little if any relationship to that in 'personality theory'. For personality theorists, personality disorders are a secondary phenomenon. What a psychiatrist calls personality disorder is really a behaviour disorder and such problem behaviours may be exhibited by more than one personality group with different mechanisms pertaining to each. For example, isolated, friendless, asocial behaviour may be the result of extreme anxiety about interacting with others and therefore related to introversion. However, it could just as easily be related to psychopathy and due to total disregard for others and their needs and wishes. Powell has suggested a three-part description to replace the standard single-label approach. This would consist of (1) a single score on an appropriate psychometric test assessing the personality trait creating most difficulty; (2) a statement which describes the specific behaviours that are causing problems; and (3) a description of the social context and the situations in which the personality problems exhibit themselves. Whilst this approach has much merit there is little evidence at present that psychiatrists are prepared to give up single diagnostic labels describing personality. Such an approach could, however, be used to help to persuade trainees to justify and describe the personality labels they use.

The World Health Organization (WHO 1978) defines abnormal personality in ICD-9 as:

> deeply ingrained maladaptive patterns of behaviour generally recognisable by the time of adolescence or earlier and continuing throughout most of adult life, although often becoming less obvious in middle or old age. The personality is abnormal either in the balance of its components, their quality and expression or in its total aspect. Because of this deviation or psychopathy the patient suffers or others have to suffer and there is an adverse effect on the individual or on society.

The ICD-9 classification allowed more than one diagnosis to be made so that an illness and personality disorder label could both be given to a patient if required, e.g. obsessional neurosis and anankastic personality, or schizophrenia and schizoid personality. No guidance was given on how to distinguish personality disorder from neurosis or from normal personality. In essence what ICD-9 represented as far as personality disorder was concerned was a consensus view of what labels were thought appropriate, based on a meeting of eminent psychiatrists from all over the world held in Tokyo in 1971.

DSM-III classification of personality disorder

DSM-III (APA 1980) distinguishes between personality traits and personality disorders. Personality traits are defined as enduring patterns of perceiving, relating to, and thinking about the environment and oneself, and are exhibited in a wide range of important social and personal contexts. Personality disorders are defined as personality traits which have become inflexible and maladaptive and cause either significant impairment in social or occupational functioning or subjective distress. They are recognisable by adolescence or earlier and persist throughout most of adult life, though often becoming less obvious in middle or old age. Personality disorder diagnoses are made on a separate axis, Axis II, from those of psychiatric illness. It is therefore possible to make a diagnosis of psychiatric illness or personality disorder alone, or to make both diagnoses in the same patient. It is also possible to indicate a premorbid personality disorder. For example, illness diagnosis on Axis I = schizophrenia, paranoid, chronic. Personality diagnosis on Axis II = schizoid personality disorder. The clinician is not restricted to a single specific personality disorder diagnosis; if the patient meets the criteria for more than one, multiple categories can be used. Table 27.1 shows the DSM-III classification.

One distinctive feature of DSM-III is the hierarchical organisation of its typology. There are three loosely defined clusters. The first of these incorporates schizoid, schizotypal and paranoid personality disorders and as a group these are odd and eccentric individuals (Cluster A). A second cluster is composed of histrionic, antisocial, borderline and

Table 27.1 Types of personality disorder recognised in DSM-IIIR

301.00	Paranoid
301.20	Schizoid
301.22	Schizotypal
301.50	Histrionic
301.81	Narcissistic
301.70	Antisocial
301.83	Borderline
301.82	Avoidant
301.60	Dependent
301.40	Obsessive–compulsive
301.84	Passive–aggressive
301.90	Personality disorder not otherwise specified (sadistic personality disorder, self-defeating personality disorder)

narcissistic types, which often appear dramatic, emotional and erratic (Cluster B). The third cluster, described as anxious or fearful, includes the avoidant, dependent, passive–aggressive and compulsive personalities (Cluster C). It has been suggested that the first cluster is related to Eysenck's psychoticism scale, the second to extroversion and the third to the introversion and neuroticism dimensions.

In a study looking at the diagnostic overlap and internal consistency of DSM-III criteria, Pfohl et al (1986) found that 54% of patients with at least one DSM-III personality diagnosis met criteria for more than one personality disorder. Two-thirds of borderline personality disorder patients met criteria for histrionic personality disorder and two-thirds of histrionic patients met criteria for borderline personality. There was also marked overlap between borderline and narcissistic personality disorders. Paranoid and schizoid personality disorders were both rare. Passive aggressive disorder occurred so frequently in patients with other personality disorders and so rarely in the absence of other personality disorders that the need for this diagnosis as a separate entity was called in question by the authors.

Abnormal personality and ICD-10

The changes in the classification of personality disorder that have appeared in ICD-10 are listed in Table 27.2. The terms paranoid, schizoid, impulsive, obsessional, histrionic and dependent have all remained and the term sociopathic personality disorder has replaced antisocial personality disorder. Two new categories have been introduced. The first is *personality traits of psychiatric significance* (character accentuation). This is an important innovation. It implies a level of personality function less disturbed than that required for a personality disorder but still of psychiatric significance. Clinically this will allow the noting of personality traits such as obsessionality or schizoidness, which are important in the understanding of a clinical problem, but which do not warrant the label of personality disorder.

The second innovation is the concept of *enduring personality change* (not attributable to gross brain damage or disease). This refers to the personality changes that can occur after a catastrophic experience, after prolonged stress such a imprisonment or torture or in the aftermath of a psychiatric illness. The latter includes changes that may occur after affective disorders but not the changes of process schizophrenia.

THE EPIDEMIOLOGY OF PERSONALITY DISORDER

This section concentrates on the relatively few studies that have looked at the prevalence of personality disorder in the community. There are a large number of studies, usually with very small sample sizes, that have looked at the prevalence of personality disorder in association with psychiatric conditions or in special populations. From this latter group it is almost impossible to draw any conclusions because the samples are drawn from such highly selected populations. Table 27.3 summarises the main studies that have been carried out.

Essen-Moller's study in Sweden is one of the first. This was conducted by personal interview of a sample of 2550 subjects. The prevalence figures must be treated with great caution as no precise definitions of personality disorder were given nor were the borders between personality disorder and illness clearly drawn.

The Epidemiologic Catchment Area (ECA) study found low rates of personality disorder as diagnosed by the Diagnostic Interview Schedule (DIS) with lifetime prevalences of 2.1% for men and 3.3% for women, and no abnormal personalities were found in the female population over the age of 45 years. The highest rates for both sexes were between the ages of 24 and 44 years. The findings from a number of different studies carried out on the ECA project can be summarised as follows. Personality disorder decreases with increasing age, is consistently higher in men than in women and shows no racial differences. There are tendencies to find higher rates in urban rather than rural areas and in those who have had shorter periods of education.

Drake & Vaillant (1985) studied 369 middle-aged inner-city men, on whom data had been collected 33 years before, at around the age of 14 years. Of these, 23% were judged to have a DSM-III personality disorder. The study found that men with personality disorder in the community were severely impaired and that their impairment was more than just a judgement of middle class morality or psychiatry. Such men felt subjective dysphoria and had difficulty in finding satisfaction in loving and working. The study confirmed the long-term dysfunction of individuals with personality disorder, even when the personality disorder was not of the antisocial type. It also clearly supported the view that the problems in question began in childhood and adolescence. Boys who later developed personality disorder showed clear evidence of adaptive difficulties by the age of 14 years. They

Table 27.2   Comparison of current classification of personality disorder

ICD-10 description	DSM-IIIR description	Cluster
Paranoid — excessive sensitivity, suspiciousness, preoccupation with conspirational explanation of events, with a persistent tendency to self-reference	*Paranoid* — interpretation of people's actions as deliberately demeaning or threatening	*Cluster A* Odd/eccentric
Schizoid — emotional coldness, detachment, lack of interest in other people, eccentricity, and introspection and fantasy	*Schizoid* — indifference to relationships and restricted range of emotional experience and expression	
No equivalent	*Schizotypal* — deficit in interpersonal relations with pecularities of ideation, appearance and behaviour	
Histrionic — self dramatisation, shallow mood, egocentricity and craving for excitement, with persistent manipulative behaviour	*Histrionic* — excessive emotion and attention-seeking	*Cluster B* Flamboyant/dramatic
Dyssocial — callous unconcern for others, with irresponsibility, irritability and aggression, and incapacity to maintain enduring relationships	*Antisocial* — evidence of repeated conduct disorder before the age of 15 years	
No equivalent	*Narcissistic* — pervasive grandiosity, lack of empathy, and hypersensitivity to the evaluation of others	
Impulsive — inability to control anger, to plan ahead, or to think before acts, with unpredictable mood and quarrelsome behaviour *Borderline* — unclear self-image, involvement in intense and unstable relationships	*Borderline* — pervasive instability of mood, and self-image	
Anankastic — indecisiveness, doubt, excessive caution, pedantry, rigidity and need to plan in immaculate detail	*Obsessive–compulsive* — pervasive perfectionism and inflexibility	*Cluster C* Fearful/anxious
Dependent — failure to take responsibility for actions, with subordination of personal needs to those of others, excessive dependence, with need for constant reassurance and feelings of helplessness when a close relationship ends	*Dependent* — persistent dependent and submissive behaviour	
Anxious — persistent tension, self-consciousness, exaggeration of risks and dangers, hypersensitivity to rejection, and restricted lifestyle because of insecurity	*Avoidant* — pervasive social discomfort, fear of negative evaluation and timidity	
	Passive–aggressive — pervasive passive resistance to demands for adequate social and occupational performance	

Table 27.3 Personality disorder in the community

Study	Site	Measure	Results	
Essen-Moller (1956)	Sweden	—	29% males 19% females	Personality disorder
Srole (1962)	Manhattan, USA	MMPI	10% probable	Personality disorder
Leighton (1963)	Stirling Co, USA	Personal interview	11% men 5% women	Sociopathy
			7% men 6% women	Personality disorder
Epidemiologic Catchment Area (ECA) study Various (1984)	USA	Diagnostic Interview Schedule (DIS)	6% prevalence 0.8–2.1% men 0.3–0.5% women	
Drake & Valliant (1985)	USA	DIS (men only)	23% DSM-III	Personality disorder
Casey (1986)	Nottingham, UK	Personality Assessment Schedule (PAS)	7% personality difficulties 7% personality disorder 4% severe personality disorder	

were behind their peers in developing skills, in age-appropriate tasks, had poor intellectual endowments, poor physical health and emotional problems. These impairments were not due solely to low social class or lack of educational opportunity.

Men with personality disorders had chronically unsuccessful work histories and impaired interpersonal relationships. Almost one-third had never married and marriages that did occur were unstable. Despite their poor psychological functioning these men were unlikely to have become psychiatric patients. Eighty per cent had never received psychiatric attention and only 10% had had more than 12 out-patient contacts. Being a psychiatric patient did not seem to be dependent on the severity of the personality disorder or the degree of poor social functioning. Some features of this study are summarised in Table 27.4.

Casey & Tyrer's study (1986) is one of the few on a UK population. They used the Personality Assessment Schedule (PAS), which in its original form generated categories similar to ICD-9. However, this has now been revised to produce grades of severity from personality difficulty to gross personality disorder. In total, 82% of their sample showed no personality abnormality (90% in women, 74% in men).

The same authors have carried out a similar study looking at conspicuous psychiatric morbidity in urban general practice. In that study the general practitioner made personality disorder the primary diagnosis in 8.9% of the sample and the psychiatrist in 6.4%.

When the subjects were then interviewed with a structured research interview a third were shown to have personality disorder in addition to their psychiatric presentation. This and a similar study in rural practice (Casey 1985) are interesting in that they failed to uphold the view that hysterical and asthenic personality disorder are particularly associated with being a woman.

In summary, then, the prevalence of personality disorder in a general population has been demonstrated to be as low as 2.1% and as high as 18%. In patients presenting to a general practitioner with obvious psychological symptoms about 7% will have personality disorder as the primary diagnosis and about one-third will have personality disorder complicating their psychiatric presentation.

SOME IMPORTANT CONTRIBUTIONS

Schneider's psychopathic personalities

Schneider defined abnormal personality as a variation upon an accepted yet broadly conceived range of average personality. The variation may be expressed as an excess or deficiency of certain personal qualities and whether this is judged 'good' or 'bad' is immaterial to the issue. The saint and the poet are equally as abnormal as the criminal. All three of them fall outside the range of average personality as we conceive it so that all persons of note may be classed as 'abnormal personalities'. He thus saw abnormal personalities as being very numerous, but within that

Table 27.4 Comparison of middle-aged men with and without DSM-III personality disorder (a community study)

	Men with personality disorder (n = 86) (%)	Men without personality disorder (n = 283) (%)
Poor mental health	79	14
Received psychiatric attention	20	—
Unemployed for more than 4 years	42	9
Adult social class IV or V	79	36
Never married	29	3
Takes no responsibility for children	41	6
Absence of friends	40	7
Poor social competence	58	10

Modified from Drake & Valliant (1985)

large group were two subgroups, both of which he labelled as psychopathic personality. These were defined as 'abnormal personalities who either suffer personally because of their own abnormality or make the community suffer because of it' (Schneider 1950).

Schneider did not use the term neurosis at all and it is clear that most of what we now regard as neurosis and personality disorder would be included in Schneider's psychopathic personalities. It is also clear that Schneider did not include all criminals or delinquents in his concept, and the idea that the individual himself had to be suffering from his behaviour seems crucial. Schneider warns against using the term psychopathic or abnormal personality too freely and recommends that a lively portrait drawn as simply as possible is probably the best way of describing individuals. He also warned against the use of sub-categories of psychopathic personality and felt they had little scientific value, but that they could be of some service in everyday clinical practice. He described the following subtypes:

Hyperthymic psychopaths
Depressive psychopaths
Insecure psychopaths
  (sensitives and anankasts)
Explosive psychopaths
Affectionless psychopaths
Weak-willed psychopaths
Fanatic psychopaths
Attention-seeking psychopaths
Labile psychopaths
Asthenic psychopaths.

Although in his book *Psychopathic Personalities* (1950) Schneider describes each of these types in some detail, there is much overlap between the descriptions.

Behaviours such as nervousness, anxiety and attention-seeking seems to be common to several types. His category of affectionless psychopathy probably comes closest to the modern use of the term, which is synonymous with antisocial behaviour.

Schneider believed that abnormal personalities were essentially determined by innate constitution and that personality development consisted of an unfolding of inborn characteristics. He did not think that external factors played an important part in the development of abnormal personality and assumed that the main aetiological factor was a genetic one.

Schneider disliked systematic typologies and preferred what he called unsystematic typologies. He felt that, with the former, clinical facts are ignored in order to prevent the system of classification breaking down. He regarded his own terms for different sorts of psychopath as descriptions and not diagnoses, and on most occasions in the clinical setting he would go no further than a diagnosis of psychopathy: 'Individual personality is rich and complex so that any one characteristic is scarcely likely to represent the whole person. In actual practice therefore these type descriptions are not very useful'.

Peter Tyrer and the Nottingham group

Over the past decade Peter Tyrer and his colleagues from Nottingham have been responsible for most, if not all, the important research on personality disorder emanating from the UK. Much of this work is summarised in their recent book (Tyrer 1988). In the late 1970s they developed the PAS (see later), and in the 1980s carried out studies on the classification of personality disorder, the reliability and validity of its diagnosis, the prevalence in the general UK

Table 27.5 Suggested division between mature and immature personality disorder

Mature personality disorders			Immature personality disorders		
ICD-10	DSM-IIIR	PAS	ICD-10	DSM-IIIR	PAS
Anankastic	Obsessive-compulsive	Asthenic	Dyssocial	Borderline	Sociopathic
		Anankastic	Impulsive	Antisocial	Sensitive-aggressive
		Hypochondriacal	Histrionic	Narcissistic	Explosive (impulsive)
		Anxious Dysthymic	Dependent Anxious	Histrionic Passive-aggressive	Histrionic Avoidant
Paranoid	Schizotypal				
Schizoid	Schizoid	Schizoid			Passive-dependent
	Paranoid	Paranoid			

From Tyrer (1988).
PAS, Personality Assessment Schedule.

population and the prevalence in a variety of psychiatric conditions. Tyrer has also resurrected the idea of mature versus immature personality disorders. These are summarised in Table 27.5. As is suggested by the terms, immature personality disorders tend to change with age, whereas mature ones remain stable over time. Immature personality disorders have earlier onset, with abnormal features being evident from childhood. The mature disorders only become apparent in late adolescence and then remain stable, often into old age. The approach of the Nottingham group, which has ploughed a lonely furrow in personality disorder research in the UK, provides an interesting contrast to a recent book edited by Oldham (1991) which typifies the current American approach to personality disorders within psychiatry. There is much preoccupation with DSM-IIIR labels, with adding new types of personality disorder and with studies on comorbidity.

The work of Graham Foulds

The relationship of personality disorder to psychiatric illness

The usual distinction drawn between illness and personality disorder is that the former is characterised by symptoms which are qualitatively different from anything expected in health, and that the onset of illness represents a definite change in the individual's level of functioning. In contrast, personality disorder is enduring and described in terms of traits and attitudes which sustain the normal continuity of the personality. Such a separation is too simple and does not do justice to the complexity of the relationships

between personality, personality disorder, personal distress, symptoms and illness. The most comprehensive account of the problem is by Foulds (1976). Unfortunately, Foulds' terminology is a little confusing, but he does provide a clear discussion of the various relationships involved. He uses the term 'personality deviance' to refer to those with abnormal personality and only uses the term 'personality disorder' when such deviance has led to breakdown or to formal restraint. Similarly, 'personal symptomatology' refers to all those with recognised psychiatric symptoms whether or not they have resulted in personal breakdown. The five possible types of relationship are summarised in Figure 27.1.

Model 1

In this model the two arenas of personality disorder and illness are mutually exclusive and each individual must be a member of one of these classes only, or of neither. This is the method that until recently was assumed by the ICD.

Model 2

Here, all those with illness fall within the personality disorder class, but not all those with personality disorder are ill. This is the model that Foulds himself originally proposed in his hierarchical model of psychiatric disorders. At its simplest this implies that all individuals who develop a psychiatric illness have an underlying personality disorder. On clinical grounds it is clear that this model is wrong and that individuals of quite normal personality can, given

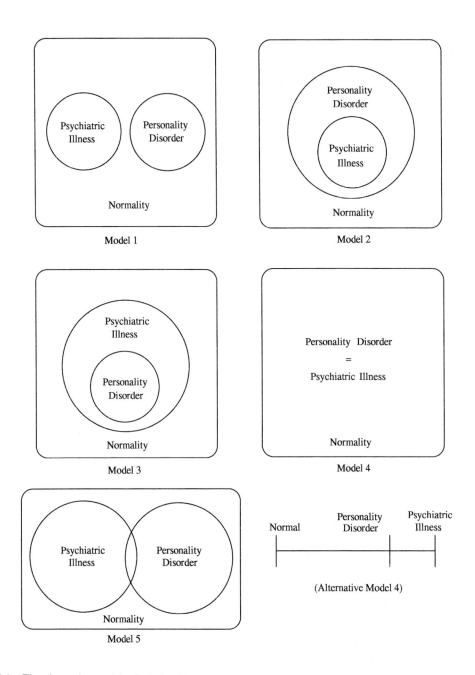

Fig. 27.1 Five alternative models of relationship between personality disorder and psychiatric illness (modified from Foulds 1976).

sufficient stress, develop psychiatric disorders. The fact that some psychiatrists operate using this model and believe it to be true is probably due to the frequency with which personality disorder and illness occur together, and to their failure routinely to reassess personality on recovery from illness after having made a personality disorder diagnosis when the individual was ill.

Model 3

All those with personality disorder fall within the illness class. Although a great many individuals with personality disorder do have symptoms there is no evidence that they all do so. This model is therefore the least convincing.

Model 4

In this model no distinction is made between personality traits and symptoms, at least as far as neurotic disorders are concerned. Personality disorder and neurotic illness are seen as part of a single dimension differing only in severity. This is the view of Schneider and also the view expressed by Slater & Roth (1969). In other words, neurotic symptoms are seen as manifestations of a given type of personality and constitution, and behaviour such as seeking relief in alcohol, outbursts of temper, lying and thieving or acts of cruelty are seen in the same light.

Model 5

In this model, personality disorder and illness exist separately, but with a large area of overlap, so that there is a group of people who at any given time are both personality disordered and have symptoms of illness. Foulds favoured model 5 and then went on to consider three levels of personality disorganisation and three levels of illness, all of which were interrelated, giving a total of nine possible categories (see Fig. 27.2);

Personality categories:
1. Normal personality
2. Discordant personality
3. Personality disorder

Illness categories:
1. Personally healthy
2. Personal symptomatology
3. Personal illness

The term personally disturbed, or personal systomatology, is used to describe individuals who have symptoms and suffer but cope and are not receiving treatment. Foulds gives examples of his nine classes, which are perhaps useful to repeat here:

1. *Personally healthy, normal personality.* A person with no symptoms whose traits and attitudes are reasonably congruent with his self-concept and the concept others have of him and who does not unduly alarm society.

2. *Personally healthy, discordant personality.* A man with no symptoms who worries about his aggressiveness but manages to sublimate it sufficiently to keep out of trouble.

3. *Personally healthy, personality disorder.* A sadist with no symptoms who commits a murder. This is the classical but rarely seen cold, callous psychopath unacquainted with guilt.

4. *Personally disturbed, normal personality.* A man who bears with his obsessional ruminations and otherwise utilises his compulsive, meticulous creativity.

5. *Personally disturbed, discordant personality.* A man who copes with periods of depression — perhaps by heavy, but not addictive drinking — whose irresponsibility and abnormal egocentricity are coped with by his wife.

6. *Personally disturbed, personality disorder.* A man who copes with some phobic symptoms by avoidance but is constantly in trouble for ill-treating his wife after drinking bouts.

7. *Personally ill, normal personality.* A man of normal personality who has a series of stressful experiences and develops an acute anxiety state.

8. *Personally ill, discordant personality.* A man with strong submissive, dependent needs whose wife has always helped him to cope who develops a depressive state after her death.

9. *Personally ill, personality disorder.* An aggressive psychopath, who commits a crime and wanders off in a fugue.

Tyrer et al (1983) he found that most patients with neuroses do not have personality disorder but a significant minority do. There was a tendency for passive–dependent personalities to be linked with anxiety neurosis, anankastic personalities with obsessional neurosis and both anankastic and passive–dependent personalities with phobic disorders. Of neurotic patients, 60% had no personality disorder diagnosis at all, and of all neurotic disorders the highest prevalence of personality disorder occurred in obsessional states.

STANDARDISED CLINICAL ASSESSMENTS OF PERSONALITY

Interview instruments

An important contribution is the recent work of Tyrer & Alexander (1979), who have developed a structured interview, the Personality Assessment Schedule

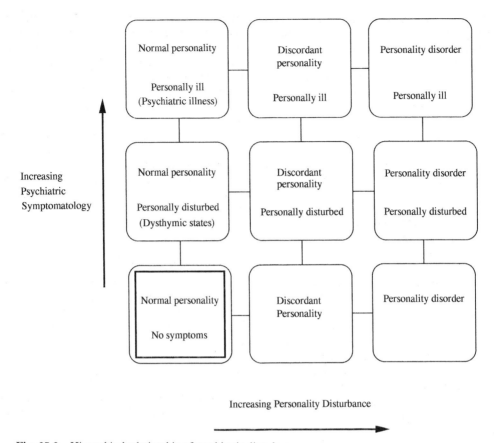

Fig. 27.2   Hierarchical relationship of psychiatric disorders.

(PAS), for the rating of personality disorder. The schedule allows for the rating of 24 personality variables in three ways — by personal observation of the subject, by interview with the subject and by interview with an informant. Personality assessments are only made if a relative or close friend who has known the patient for 10 years is available for interview and if the rater has seen the patient at least three times, one of which is at a time when the patient has no formal psychiatric disorder.

In their own studies Tyrer & Alexander found that the difference between normal and abnormal personality was a matter of degree rather than of qualitative difference. Factor analysis of ratings from a combined group of subjects with and without personality disorder showed that the underlying structure of the factors that accounted for most of the variance was the same in both groups. A cluster analysis of patient ratings produced anankastic,

sociopathic, schizoid and non-personality disordered clusters. This resulted in 63% of those who were personality disordered falling into the sociopathic or passive–dependent groups. This work provides a fresh approach to the assessment of personality disorder by the use of a standardised clinical interview similar in style to the Present State Examination (PSE) and by the routine and systematic interviewing of an informant.

A similar approach has been reported by Mann et al (1981). Their interview, the Standard Assessment of Personality (SAP), has the virtue of being brief, taking only about 10 minutes to administer to a close informant. However, the authors assumed that discreet personality types existed and then devised questions and prompts to elicit them. They added two further categories to those found by Tyrer & Alexander. The term 'anxious' describes individuals with lifelong anxiety or anxiety proneness (trait anxiety), and 'self-conscious personalities' are those who are unduly sensitive and readily upset, but without the coldness or crankiness associated with schizoid personality or the suspiciousness of paranoid personality. So far only small-scale studies have been carried out and certain personality types have not appeared frequently enough for any conclusions to be drawn about them. Because of the assumptions that these authors start with, it is unlikely that they will shed any new light on the understanding of abnormal personality, but the approach may be useful as an assessment technique in everyday clinical practice.

Stangl et al (1985) have produced a structured interview for the DSM-III personality disorders (SIDP). The SIDP takes between 60 and 90 minutes to administer and there is a further 30 minute interview with an informant. There are 160 questions, grouped under 16 sections such as self-esteem, level of social interaction and dependency. The interview, of course, cannot add to the validity of DSM-III categories themselves as it is specifically designed to elicit them. However, in a preliminary study, inter-rater reliability reached 0.70 or higher for histrionic, borderline and dependent personality subtypes.

The structured clinical interview for DSM-III personality disorders (SCID-II) is a 120-item semistructured interview (Spitzer et al 1985). It is designed only to be used by a skilled clinician and covers all the DSM-III personality disorders. It is designed for a relatively rapid assessment of personality disorder and has been widely used to assess the presence of Axis II disorders in the presence of Axis I diagnoses.

The Personality Disorder Examination (PDE) covers all DSM-IIIR personality disorders (Loranger et al 1985). It is longer, having 328 items and takes at least $1\frac{1}{2}$ hours to administer.

Two other instruments, the Schedule for Affective Disorders and Schizophrenia (SADS) (Spitzer et al 1978) and the National Institute of Mental Health Diagnostic Interview Schedule (NIMH-DIS) (Robbins et al 1979) include diagnostic criteria for antisocial personality disorder but not for other types.

Self-report measures

Two self-report measures are said to generate personality disorder diagnoses. The Personality Diagnostic Questionnaire (PDQ) (Hyler et al 1983) is a 152-item self-administered forced-choice questionnaire which covers all 11 DSM-III Axis II personality disorders. It takes about 30 minutes for the patient to complete. This instrument markedly overdiagnoses personality disorders: in one recent large UK study, some patients with bulimia nervosa met diagnostic criteria for all 11 personality disorders at the same time (M. Tattersall, personal communication). The Millon Clinical Multi-axial Inventory (MCMI) is a computer-scored 175-item self-report instrument which takes about 20 minutes. It can also be scored by hand (Millon 1982). Millon's concept of personality disorders divides them into two clusters, which he calls basic personality patterns and pathological personality disorders. The latter includes borderline, schizotypal and paranoid disorders. The MCMI is out of step with other instruments in that it also has scales which measure some DSM-III Axis I diagnoses.

SPECIFIC PERSONALITY LABELS

What follows is an account of the main personality disorder labels currently used in psychiatry. Most space is given to antisocial personality disorder because it is the only one which has been widely studied in a reasonably systematic way.

Histrionic personality disorder

Chodoff & Lyons (1958) found that the following traits were associated with the concept of the hysterical personality:

1. Egoism, vanity, egocentricity, self-indulgence
2. Exhibitionism, dramatisation, lying
3. Unbridled display of affect, excitability, inconsistency
4. Emotional shallowness
5. Lascivious sexualisation of non-sexual functions
6. Sexual frigidity and sexual immaturity.

It is interesting that nearly all such personality disorder descriptions are judgemental of the individual concerned and rarely include any positive features. The above description has been criticised as simply a man's stereotyped view of femininity, typically a male psychiatrist's view of female patients that he finds difficult or threatening. This type of personality disorder is certainly diagnosed much more frequently in females.

Such individuals are described as lively, dramatic, flirtatious and always drawing attention to themselves. They tend to over-react to situations and express their emotions intensely. Personal relationships are said to be shallow and lacking in genuineness, and such people are often described as manipulative and demanding.

Relationship with hysterical syndromes

Ljungberg (1957) found that no one particular type of personality disorder was associated with hysterical syndromes. Slavney & McHugh (1974) found no evidence of hysterical signs and symptoms in his group of hysterical personality disorders. Similar conclusions were reached by Ziegler & Imboden (1962), who concluded that the 'hysterical personality pattern was not a pre-requisite for the occurrence of conversion symptoms'. They felt that the concept covered such a scattered constellation of traits that in no way could it be considered a discrete diagnostic entity. They suggested that if anything was central to the concept it was the tendency to role playing and to acting out parts in life in an unconvincing and exaggerated manner. This concept is similar to the one originallly described by Jaspers, who suggested that hysterical personalities seemed to wish to appear both to themselves and to others as more than they really were.

Slavaney & McHugh (1974) compared a group of in-patients with a diagnosis of hysterical personality as defined by DSM-II with a group of mixed in-patient controls. Index patients were found to be typically young women, hospitalised after suicide attempts or with symptoms of depression. They were often the product of an unhappy early environment, had made previous suicide attempts and, if married, their marriages were generally unhappy. They were generally described as being 'dramatic' and treatment usually involved several months in hospital. However, there were no differences in family history of mental illness, parental separation, neurotic symptoms in childhood, attitude towards sex, marital status, history of abdominal surgery or unexplained illnesses, or in abuse of alcohol or drugs. The feature which most clearly distinguished the index group from controls was the high frequency of depressive symptoms. These tended not to be treated with antidepressants; instead, the symptoms were seen as expressions of emotional instability and self-dramatisation. Lazare & Klerman (1968) found a similar relationship between personality and symptoms when they examined hysterical features in depressed women. It is possible, then, that at least in some cases applying the label of hysterical personality disorder prevents a certain sort of female patient receiving adequate treatment for her depressive symptoms.

Changing the name from hysterical to histrionic, as in DSM-III, does not really solve anything. Until the identification of the hysterical personality is more reliable and valid it must remain a suspect term; and

theories which claim to explain why such behaviour is exhibited by patients or studies which show that such behaviour runs in families, must be treated with caution.

Obsessional personality disorder (compulsive, anankastic)

There is no clear-cut boundary between obsessional personality traits and obsessional symptoms in terms of the individual's behaviour. Consider the case of two middle-aged housewives who both report extreme concern with cleanliness and order. One spends a lot of time cleaning and tidying her home and is extremely proud of this. She is in no way distressed by her obsession with cleanliness and order, nor are her family. The second spends an equal amount of time in cleaning and tidying but is distressed by her obsession and unable to resist it. It interferes with her everyday life and her family are equally distressed by her obsessional concern and behaviour. Although their behaviour is virtually identical the former would probably be labelled obsessional personality and the latter obsessional neurosis. Distinction between personality and illness thus depends on the individual's or other people's view of the behaviour. If the traits and attitudes seem egosyntonic the behaviour is labelled 'personality'; if the behaviour causes distress it tends to be labelled 'illness'.

The traits usually included in any description of obsessional personality are excessive cleanliness, orderliness, pedantry, conscientiousness, uncertainty, inconclusive ways of thinking and acting and a fondness for collecting things, including money. The picture is of an exceedingly systematic, methodical and thorough person, who likes a well-ordered life, is consistent, punctual and meticulous in his use of words, dislikes half-done tasks, finds interruptions irksome, and pays much attention to detail. Such personality features are, of course, advantageous in many walks of life.

The relationship between obsessional personality traits and obsessional neurosis is not as clear as is often thought. Black (1974) collated the results of a number of studies which had looked at obsessional personality traits in obsessional patients before illness developed. By no means all obsessional patients showed such traits, their absence being noted in between 16 and 36% of cases. In one study that had the advantage of a control group (Kringlen 1965), 53% of the non-obsessional neurotic controls showed moderate or marked obsessional personality traits, indicating that the personality–illness relationship is less than specific and that personality is only one factor associated with the development of an obsessional illness.

More recent studies have shown little or no association between obsessional personality disorder and clinical obsessive–compulsive disorder. Surprisingly, higher rates of other personality disorders were found.

The psychoanalytic concept of the 'anal character, the triad of obstinacy, parsimony and orderliness' has found little support from psychometric observations and there is little evidence that obsessionality is particularly linked with a tendency to disagree or with meanness. A number of studies have, however, found a relationship between measures of neuroticism, introversion, extroversion and obsessionality, with obsessionality being highly correlated with both introversion and neuroticism.

Borderline personality disorder

Over the last 15 years an enormous literature has appeared about the 'borderline syndrome', and the concept of borderline personality disorder has achieved nosological recognition in DSM-III. Because there is little agreement about what the term means it is difficult to give a succinct description of features which are said to typify a borderline patient. Features such as impulsivity, unpredictability and unstable and intense interpersonal relationships are said to be characteristic. Inappropriate, sudden, intense outbursts of anger, and loss of temper leading to suicidal gestures, self-mutilation, accidents or fights may occur. Shifts of mood from normal to depression, anxiety or irritability frequently occur, though they are usually brief. There may be chronic feelings of emptiness or boredom with intolerance of being left alone, so that such individuals will often strive always to be in company. Another central feature is said to be confused or uncertain identity, manifested by uncertainty about the individual's goals in life, moral and social values, and loyalties to friends and family. For some the term borderline refers to the border between psychosis and normality and arose from psychoanalytic treatment. Other terms that have been used to describe borderline patients are borderline state, psychotic character, pseudoneurotic schizophrenia, borderline psychosis and schizotypal personality disorder.

Kroll et al (1982) compared DSM-III criteria with those of Gunderson & Kolb (1978) and those of Spitzer et al (1979). Concordance in case selection between the various diagnostic criteria was no greater than chance. The authors comment that the concept is already in danger of over-use, in that practically all non-schizophrenic, non-affective disorder and non-classically neurotic patients will be seen to fall somewhere within the concept of borderline disorder. In other words, it will become a non-discriminatory synonym for personality disorder. The term is not in widespread use in the UK and is hardly used at all by general psychiatrists. Such caution seems entirely justified given the vagueness of the concept.

The most comprehensive review so far published is by the Danish psychiatrist Aarkrog (1981). She describes all the main uses of the term in the literature to date. She concludes that, as used at present, it is no more specific than a term such as psychosis, though it is clear from her own work that she does feel there is a role for the term if it is defined along the lines described by Gunderson & Kolb (1978).

Kroll and his colleagues (1982) examined a group of UK psychiatric patients using the Diagnostic Interview for Borderlines (DIB). Patients identified as borderline personality had all been labelled as personality disordered using the ICD-9 classification with labels such as explosive, hysterical, inadequate or immature. A substantial proportion of patients had concomitant mood disorders with a diagnosis of neurotic depression on ICD-9 or depressive disorder on DSM-III. This raises the possibility that both the DIB and ICD-9 personality diagnoses were being used to describe depressed patients who were responding to their subjectively unpleasant dysthymia with hysterical and self-destructive behaviours. In other words, their personality characteristics were being exaggerated by their depressive illness and it remains unknown how they would have appeared when well.

Akiskal et al (1985) have shown that non-schizotypal borderline patients had shortened REM latencies indistinguishable from a group of patients with primary affective disorders, but clearly different from normal controls and a group of non-borderline personality disorders. They suggested that there may be a group of patients with both affective disorder and borderline personality disorder in whom the frequently recurring affective illness may have prevented optimum ego development, leading to chronic personality maladjustment, and that the borderline rubric was nosologically heterogenous and unwieldy. A similar conclusion was reached by Pope et al (1983), who were unable to distinguish borderline personality disorder as defined by DSM-III from either histrionic or antisocial personality disorder on phenomenology, family history, treatment response of 4–7 years follow-up data.

The interrelationships of the various elements of the borderline concept are illustrated in Fig. 27.3, and the main features of borderline personality as described by Gunderson and by DSM-III are compared in Table 27.6.

Relationship of borderline and schizotypal personality disorder to schizophrenia

There is now evidence from several sources that individuals with borderline personality disorder do not have first-degree relatives with a higher than usual prevalence of schizophrenia whereas there is an association between chronic schizophrenia and relatives with schizotypal personality. Brief psychotic-like episodes occur in both borderline and schizotypal personality disorder and do not by themselves help in discriminating the phenotypic variation of schizophrenia that the schizotypal category is intended to identify.

Gunderson et al (1983) have suggested that the following features characterise the personality-disordered relatives of schizophrenics most clearly, and that these should form the core of schizotypal personality disorder: social isolation and anxiety; suspicious superficial and distant interpersonal relationships; odd, eccentric, 'off-putting' appearance and behaviour; frequent somatic problems; detached and flattened affect; and serious social dysfunction at school and work. They also argue that magical thinking, illusions and odd speech should be removed from the DSM-III criteria for the disorder. McGlashan (1983), reporting the Chestnut Lodge follow-up study, confirmed the lack of association between schizophrenia and borderline personality and suggested that the latter may be more closely related to affective disorder.

Schizotypal personality

DSM-III includes two categories of borderline conditions: the schizotypal personality disorder and the borderline personality disorder. The former is derived partly from research studies on the concept of pseudoneurotic schizophrenia and from the American–Danish adoption studies of schizophrenia in which the term borderline schizophrenia was used to describe individuals with certain characteristic features who were the first-degree relatives of schizophrenic patients.

A number of rating scales exist for eliciting schizotypal features such as those of Meehl (1984), Spitzer & Endicott (1979) and Baron (1981). Spitzer

Table 27.6 The borderline concept: a comparison of DSM-III and Gunderson & Singer's (1975) criteria

---

Main features according to DSM-III
1. Instability in a variety of areas
2. Interpersonal relationships are often intense and unstable with marked shifts in attitude
3. Impulsivity and self-damaging behaviour
4. Interpersonal behaviour characterised by:
   Idealization
   Devaluation
   Manipulation
5. Inappropriate intense anger — 'temper tantrums'
6. Identity disturbance:
   Self-image
   Gender identity
   Long-term goals
   Career choice
7. Affective instability
8. Intolerance of being alone
9. Chronic feelings of emptiness and boredom

Main features according to Gunderson & Singer criteria
1. Presence of intense affect (usually hostile or depressed)
2. History of impulsive behaviour
3. Social adaptiveness/good level of achievement
4. Brief psychotic experiences characterised by being:
   a. Stress related
   b. Reversible
   c. Transient
   d. Ego alien
   e. Unsystematic
5. Intrapsychic phenomena characterised by:
   Fabulizing
   Confabulatory
   Combinatory thinking
6. Interpersonal relationships either:
   Superficial and transient or
   Intense and clinging

---

has argued strongly for the separation of schizotypal from schizoid personality disorder and borderline personality disorder on the basis that brief losses of reality testing and psychotic-like experiences mainly occur in schizotypal patients. However, George & Soloff (1986) when examining a cohort of borderline patients, found that nearly all of the cohort exhibited such phenomena and that it was difficult to separate borderline and schizotypal patients using such criteria. Other features such as social isolation and oddness of speech may be more discriminating. To meet DSM-III schizotypal criteria the individual must not meet DSM-III criteria for schizophrenia, but must have four of the following symptoms:

1. Magical thinking, e.g. superstitiousness, belief in clairvoyance, telepathy, etc.
2. Ideas of reference
3. Social isolation

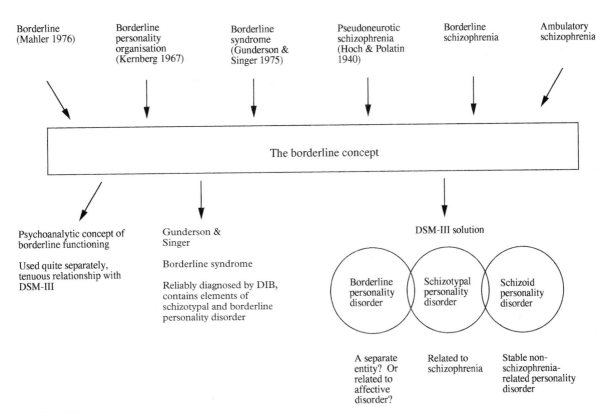

Fig. 27.3   The borderline concept.

4. Recurrent illusions, such as sensing the presence of a force or person not actually present
5. Odd speech — this has to be speech that is digressive, vague, over-elaborate, circumstantial or metaphorical, but without definite incoherence or looseness of associations
6. Inadequate rapport in face-to-face interaction
7. Suspiciousness or paranoid ideation
8. Undue social anxiety or hypersensitivity to real or imagined criticism.

Schizotypal personality is differentiated from schizoid personality because the latter has no oddities of behaviour, thinking, perception or speech.

In a series of papers from the Danish Adoption Study, Kendler et al (1981) have shown that schizotypal individuals do have genetic links with chronic schizophrenia and that these are not found in individuals with schizoid personality or borderline personality disorder. The first long-term follow-up of patients with schizotypal personality disorder comes from the Chestnut Lodge study (McGlashan 1983).

Although on small numbers, this study extended over a period of 33 years and showed that, in terms of outcome, schizotypal patients were closer to schizophrenic patients than to those with borderline personality disorder. Where patients met criteria both for schizotypal and borderline personality their outcome was more like that of a pure borderline group.

Schizoid personality disorder

Individuals with this condition are characterised by having little or no desire for social involvement. They prefer to be solitary and have few if any close friends. They pursue solitary interests and appear reserved and withdrawn to others. They are often said to have 'no sense of humour' or to be 'dull'. The stereotype of such individuals is of tall, asthenic build, gawky appearance, ill-fitting, unfashionable clothes and poor social skills. They may also appear to be self-absorbed or absent-minded.

The original description by Kretschmer (1936), who thought he had clearly identified a characteristic premorbid personality for schizophrenia, did not refer to the same traits. He described schizoid individuals as suspicious, over-sensitive, reckless, callous, paranoid, shy and delicate. There is still no clear consensus as to whether either type of schizoid personality disorder precedes schizophrenia, or whether, in those cases where schizophrenia does develop, the so-called schizoid personality disorder simply represents a prodromal phase of the disorder in individuals who do not at that stage meet diagnostic criteria for schizophrenia but have odd speech which is digressive, vague and circumstantial, ideas of reference, magical thinking, paranoid ideas and social isolation. Such individuals are categorised by DSM-III as schizotypal (see above). Follow-up studies of schizoid personality from childhood and adolescence suggest that it is a stable and persistent personality organisation.

Narcissistic personality disorder

Like borderline personality this type of disorder owes its origin to psychoanalytic ideas and has also been included as a category in DSM-III. Two authors, Kernberg (1967) and Kohut (1968), have largely been responsible for popularising the concept, and Akhtar & Thomson (1982) have provided a good review. The main features of this type of personality are as follows: a grandiose sense of self-importance or uniqueness; and a preoccupation with fantasies of unlimited success, power, brilliance, beauty or ideal love. Some authors stress the lack of warmth, empathy and concern for others that such individuals exhibit, others the intolerance of failure, the marked feelings of rage, shame and humiliation in response to criticism. Yet others stress the chronic feelings of boredom or emptiness such individuals suffer. Kohut goes as far as to say that the diagnosis can only be made on the basis of the spontaneous transference that develops during analysis and not on the basis of any overt symptomatology or behaviour.

Narcissistic personality disorder appears to share many features with borderline disorders, not the least being a general disagreement about what the label means. In narcissistic disorder the self is said to be more cohesive and less likely to disintegrate into quasipsychotic states under stress than in the borderline state in which psychotic episodes are common. Those concerned are also more likely to achieve success at work and socially, and to exhibit less self-destructive behaviour than borderline patients. Narcissistic personality disorders are distinguished from hysterical personality disorders by

retention of the capacity for warmth, empathy and love for others in the latter. The boundary between narcissistic personality and antisocial personality is blurred. Promiscuity and manipulative and antisocial behaviour are said to occur in both, but in narcissistic personality disorder such behaviour is episodic and there is not the complete disregard for social standards that occurs in antisocial personality. Also the individual's work record is usually good.

Relatively few patients have been studied and the disorder has rarely been described outside psychoanalytic practice. There is also little information on what sort of early life experience predisposes an individual to this personality structure. It seems that the term would rarely fit British psychiatric patients although one certainly meets people in professional life who possess the characteristics described. One might expect that the very nature of the individuals' view of themselves would draw them towards an intensive and special therapy like psychoanalysis.

Antisocial personality disorder

The terms psychopathy, psychopathic personality disorder, sociopathy and antisocial personality are synonyms for a recurrent pattern of antisocial, delinquent or criminal behaviour that begins in childhood or in early adolescence and is manifested by disturbances in many areas of life such as family relations, schooling, military service, and marriage. Of all these terms psychopathy is the most misleading, though still the most commonly used in the UK. This is because many authors have used the term psychopathic personality disorder in its German sense to cover the whole range of abnormal personality.

Historical background: evolution of the concept

In 1801 Philip Pinel described *manie sans délire*. These were individuals who showed impulsive, senseless acts of violence amounting to murderous fury but whose intellectual functions of perception, judgement, memory and imagination were all intact. Some of the cases that Pinel described might now be regarded as explosive forms of antisocial personality. In 1812 the American physician Benjamin Rush described 'derangement of the moral faculties', by which he meant individuals with sound reason and good intellect with innate or lifelong irresponsibility, and without shame, being unaffected by the consequence their behaviour had on others. In 1835 the Bristol physician J. C. Prichard introduced the term *moral insanity*, indicating that the primary deficiency appeared not to be in intellect but in the individual's moral qualitites:

> There are many people suffering from a form of mental derangement in whom the moral and active principles of the mind are strongly perverted or depraved, the power of self government is lost or greatly impaired and the individual is found incapable, not of talking or reasoning on any subject proposed to him, but of conducting himself with decency and propriety in the business of life.

The Edinburgh psychiatrist Thomas Clouston thought that many of Prichard's descriptions were probably of manic illness but did agree that there were individuals who seemed to be incapable of knowing right from wrong and that for such individuals the term *moral idiot* or *moral insanity* should be used. It is important to appreciate that the 19th century meaning of moral probably referred more to emotional or affective responses, in contrast to cognitive ones, rather than to any ethical sense of right or wrong. These early writers saw such states as being constitutional, and probably inherited.

The next series of developments confused rather than clarified the picture. The Frenchman Morel proposed that a degenerative process was responsible for the behaviour of such individuals and that this process was inherited, increasing in severity in successive generations. Confusion arose because at around the same period it was increasingly being realised that some individuals had lifelong mental handicap (moral idiocy), and some authors saw the two concepts as linked. For instance, Magnan (1893) in Paris subscribed to Morel's concept of doomed hereditary descent and thought that progression could occur from mania in the first generation to idiocy or imbecility in the fourth. Magnan described *héréditaries dégénérés*, who were idiots, imbeciles and the feeble-minded, and *dégénérés supérieurs,* who were of average or superior intellect but who had moral defects.

The first use of the term psychopathic was by Koch in 1891. He defined his *psychopathic inferiorities* as 'all mental irregularities whether congenital or acquired which influence a man in his personal life and cause him, even in the most favourable cases, to seem not fully in possession of normal mental capacity, though even in the bad case the irregularities do not amount to mental disorder.' Within this group he included both behavioural and symptomatic conditions and much of what we would today call neurosis. Koch stressed that there was a physical basis to such conditions, though he admitted this could not be demonstrated anatomically or chemically. Gradually the term inferiority was dropped and for the next 30

years psychopathy was a relatively neutral term implying that a person's disposition or temperament deviated appreciably form the average.

Both Henry Maudsley and Emil Kraepelin subscribed to the degenerative view, though the later editions of Kraepelin's textbook show that he became unhappy with this view and finally adopted the term psychopathic personality. Kraepelin regarded psychopathies partly as undeveloped psychoses and partly as constitutional abnormalities of personality. He divided them into seven subgroups: excitable, unstable, impulsive, eccentric, liars and swindlers, antisocial, and quarrelsome.

In 1939 Henderson described three broad groupings of psychopaths:

1. Predominantly aggressive
2. Predominantly inadequate
3. Predominantly creative.

His concepts of aggressive and inadequate types have survived but not his creative category. By the latter he meant intensely individualistic people who carve out a way for themselves in life, irrespective of the people and obstacles which get in their path. Such people may have great qualities of leadership and drive and yet an unevenness in their personality which makes them markedly different from others. He gave Joan of Arc, Napoleon and Lawrence of Arabia as examples who gained their objectives by knowing that they were right rather than by methodical planning.

In more recent times one of the most influential reviews and persuasive descriptions has been that of Cleckley (1966) in his book *The Mask of Sanity*. Cleckley used the term sociopathy and regarded it as synonymous with antisocial personality. He described a group of individuals with average or superior intelligence, an absence of irrationality and other symptoms of psychosis, who have no sense of responsibility, a disregard for the truth and no sense of shame. They indulge in antisocial behaviour with no regret and seem unable to learn from experience. They have poverty of affect and an apparent lack of genuine insight. They show little response to special consideration and kindness and also have unrestrained and unconventional sex lives. The age of onset of these characteristics is no later than 20 years. This description of a cold, callous, abnormally aggressive and irresponsible individual, unable to make enduring friendships and not profiting from experience, has become the stereotype of modern psychopathic or antisocial personality. Many of the features described are incorporated in the ICD description of personality disorder with predominantly sociopathic or asocial manifestations. However, despite its popularity it is not a very reliable description. Psychopaths are not the only individuals who fail to profit by experience, many of them do learn coping skills remarkably well, especially in institutions, and many do form enduring relationships. Scott (1960) reviewed all the major definitions of psychopathy and concluded that they all contained four common themes:

1. An exclusion of psychotic illness or subnormality
2. The disorder is persistent from an early age
3. Behaviour is described as abnormally aggressive or inadequate, seriously irresponsible, asocial or antisocial
4. Society is impelled to deal with such individuals.

Psychopathic disorder was given official recognition in the Mental Health Act 1959 (HMSO 1959) and defined as 'a persistent disorder or disability of the mind (whether or not including subnormality of intelligence) which results in abnormally aggressive or seriously irresponsible conduct on the part of the patient, and requires or is susceptible to treatment'. (No such definition was included in the Scottish Act.) A similar definition has been retained in the English Mental Health Act 1983 but, again, omitted from the Mental Health Act (Scotland) 1984 (see Ch. 33).

Because the term psychopathic personality was used inconsistently, sometimes to refer to the whole spectrum of deviant personalities and at other times to refer only to antisocial or aggressive psychopaths, DSM-I (APA 1953) adopted the term sociopathic personality disturbance. However, sociopathy and psychopathy continued to be used interchangeably and in subsequent editions of the DSM the term antisocial personality was introduced in a further attempt to reduce confusion.

Gunn (1978) has suggested that the term psychopathic should be abandoned altogether. His studies showed a high prevalence of neurotic symptoms in offenders labelled as psychopathic and he suggested that such individuals may be responding to neurotic stresses and anxiety by exhibiting antisocial behaviour rather than possessing a discrete cluster of neurotic symptoms. He therefore suggested that such individuals should be included with the neuroses as 'neurotic state (antisocial type)'.

Clinical picture

Much of what follows must be treated cautiously. It is frequently not possible to tell from the literature exactly what kind of individuals are being described in a given study. Although many individuals with antisocial personality are criminals, not all criminals are psychopaths; but in many studies the terms criminality and antisocial personality have been used interchangeably. Some authors (e.g Guze et al 1969) also regard trouble with the police as a formal requirement for a diagnosis of antisocial personality.

The precursors of antisocial personality appear in childhood or early adolescence. At least two studies have shown that a proportion of children suffering from the 'hyperactive child syndrome' of restlessness, short attention span and unresponsiveness to discipline go on to develop antisocial behaviour. There is usually a history of difficult behaviour at school, including truancy, suspension from class and lack of response to ordinary disciplinary measures. Similarly, the subject's work record is usually poor and characterised by frequent changes of job, leaving jobs without warning and persistent absenteeism.

Sexual experience begins earlier than in other adolescents and is likely to be characterised by promiscuity in both sexes. Marriage tends to occur early, and to be stormy and shortlived, ending in separation or divorce. Both Cloninger & Guze (1973) and Guze et al (1970) have shown that women with antisocial personalities tend to marry men of the same type and that women may involve themselves with a succession of such men.

A criminal record is frequently obtained. No one particular type of crime is characteristic, but offences tend to be impulsive or poorly planned. Reporting of psychiatric symptoms is usual when such individuals come into contact with doctors. Typical neurotic symptoms of anxiety and depression are common, as are alcohol and drug abuse. Guze et al (1971) also found that conversion symptoms were common and a number of studies have found that adolescent girls identified as antisocial or delinquent tend to produce multiple symptomatology (somatization disorder or Briquet's syndrome) as adults.

Antisocial behaviour begins in childhood or adolescence and one should be cautious about making the diagnosis if when taking a history no evidence of antisocial behaviour can be found before the age of 20 years. Some milder degrees of this personality type tend to settle down in the late 20s or early 30s, but in the majority the antisocial behaviour continues. The concept of the maturing or burnt-out antisocial personality is a misleading one. Although such individuals do tend to exhibit less overt antisocial behaviour during their 30s and 40s this improvement does not extend to their interpersonal relationships or to their drug or alcohol abuse, and many such people continue to cause havoc amongst their families well into middle age.

A large number of studies support the clinical impression that psychopaths as a group have at least average global intelligence. Some investigations have shown that psychopaths consistently score higher on performance tasks that verbal IQ tests. Others have shown that psychopaths have a capacity to think more divergently, suggesting that they have a capacity to see things in novel and unusual ways, unhampered by ordinary constraints. Intelligence has been measured mainly in groups of individuals whose antisocial behaviour is so persistent or so poorly planned that they are sent to prison or psychiatric hospitals. If, as seems reasonable, such people are less intelligent than those who avoid being caught we must conclude that the total population of psychopaths is on average more intelligent than the general population.

Follow-up studies of psychopathy

Robbins (1978) followed up a group of children originally referred to a child guidance clinic to a mean age of 43 years. She has also followed up a group of young black males to a mean age of 33 years. She concludes that antisocial behaviour or personality does seem to be a real syndrome, at least as far as American males are concerned. The syndrome rarely occurs in the absence of serious antisocial behaviour in childhood. She found that 50% of her highly antisocial adults had shown moderate to high antisocial behaviour as children. There was no one particular type of childhood behaviour that predicted adult behaviour, nor were there any particular family variables. The best predictor from childhood was wide-ranging and varied antisocial behaviour; in other words, the child who has been involved in multiple different antisocial activities is more likely to persist in antisocial behaviour into adulthood. She also found that only about 40% of antisocial children become antisocial adults. Surprisingly, social class was not an important predictor of severe antisocial behaviour, though it may make some contribution to lesser degrees of such behaviour. The importance of Robbins' work cannot be underestimated. There are no other long-term studies which are so well documented, and unlike many other authors she used relatively hard measures of antisocial personality such as truancy, alcohol and drug abuse, school drop-out, arrests, vagrancy and financial problems, rather than less tangible features such as guilt and lack of remorse.

Electroencephalogram (EEG) studies in psychopathy

The typical finding is of generalised, widespread slow (theta) wave activity occurring in between 31 and 58% of psychopaths, with some studies showing that extremely aggressive and dangerous psychopaths are likely to have a higher prevalence of EEG abnormalities than those who are more passive.

A second type of abnormality is the 'positive spike' phenomenon. This term refers to bursts of activity, positive in polarity, at 6–8 and 14–16 Hz recorded over the temporal lobe. Kurland et al (1963) found that between 40 and 45% of highly impulsive and aggressive psychopaths had such positive spikes compared with a prevalence in the general population of 10–12%. Some authors, such as Schwade & Geiger (1965) have associated this EEG pattern with sudden outbursts of aggressive or destructive behaviour precipitated by trivial or innocuous stimuli, uncoordinated behaviour during the 'attack' and no expression of guilt, remorse or anxiety afterwards.

A third abnormality also located in the temporal lobes was reported by Hill (1952). He found that about 14% of severely aggressive psychopaths had abnormal slow wave activity which was not widespread but localised in the temporal lobes. This abnormality was found in only 2% of normal controls and 4.8% of schizophrenic patients.

These EEG abnormalities have led to two theories of psychopathic behaviour. The fact that the EEG activity of psychopaths bears some resemblance to that of children has led investigators to propose that psychopathic behaviour reflects cortical immaturity. If this is so it might be expected to lessen with age. Though the evidence for this is contradictory, Gibbens et al (1955) found that psychopaths with EEG abnormalities had a better prognosis than those with normal EEGs and postulated that the former outgrew their cortical immaturity. The second theory is that the EEG abnormality represents some underlying minimal brain damage. Hare (1970) has suggested that specific EEG abnormalities reflect dysfunction in the temporal lobe and possibly in the limbic system. He links this with the finding that the limbic system appears to play an important role in the regulation of fear-motivated behaviour. In particular, the ability to inhibit a response in order to avoid punishment (passive avoidance learning) may be under limbic control. However, only a minority of psychopaths have definite evidence of minimal brain damage and many individuals with minimal brain damage do not show psychopathic behaviour. Therefore, the most that can be said is that perhaps there is an interaction between cortical immaturity or minimal brain damage or both and early experience and environment.

Finally, psychopaths have been found to have a slower rate of cortical recovery as measured by cortical-evoked potentials. The latter are probably a measure of cortical excitability and, if so, the psychopath's slow recovery rate would indicate lowered cortical arousal. This would support a large number of studies which have examined autonomic measures of arousal in psychopaths, and also those theories which suggest that psychopaths are chronically under-aroused and that much of their behaviour is sensation-seeking and motivated by a desire to increase arousal.

Lykken (1957) and Schacter & Lantane (1964) showed that in tasks of avoidance learning antisocial personalities did not learn to avoid electric shocks as quickly as normal or neurotic individuals, but that when given intravenous adrenalin their learning curve changed to normal. These findings led to the hypothesis that psychopathic individuals may have been born with a relative autonomic underactivity. The attractiveness of this theory was that it helped to explain the psychopath's characteristic excitement-seeking behaviour and failure to respond to the normal dangers or deterrents that cause most people to refrain from antisocial acts. Despite its attractiveness these theories should be viewed with caution. Lykken studied institutionalised psychopathic patients and did not control for this. It may also be that such personalities view experimenters and experiments differently from normals, treating them in a more flippant and playful way.

Family studies

It is well established that antisocial behaviour runs in families and that antisocial individuals tend to come from families characterised by social disturbance, disruption, and alcohol dependence and other alcohol problems. Guze studied a series of American female criminals, half of whom were diagnosed as sociopathic, and found that one-half of their first-degree male relatives were alcoholic and one-third sociopathic (Cloninger & Guze 1973). Despite the biased and distorted reviews by Eysenck (1973, 1977), attempts to show a genetic basis for antisocial behaviour have been less convincing. Twin studies have tended to focus on antisocial behaviour, delinquency and criminality without distinguishing between them. Concordance rates in monozygotic twins have nearly always been higher than in dizygotic twins for such behaviour, but the differences are much smaller than for other psychiatric disorders in which a genetic basis is suspected. The best study, which was based on the Danish twin register, found the lowest concordance rate: 36% in monozygotic twins and 12% in dizygotic twins (Christianson 1970). Earlier studies, such as those by Lange & Legras which showed huge differences in monozygotic and dizygotic concordance rates, can be almost entirely discounted because of methodological deficiencies. Nor is it justified to group all twin studies carried out over a 40 year period together and come up with an average figure. There are, however, a series of adoption studies carried out by Cadoret et al in Iowa (1975, 1978) and by Crowe (1972, 1974) which have shown that, when the children of criminals or those with antisocial personality have been adopted early in life by non-relatives, they are more likely to reveal antisocial and criminal behaviour as adults than control children whose biological parents were not criminals or antisocial personalities. There would thus appear to be some genetic predisposition in some cases of antisocial behaviour, but how much of the total variance can be accounted for in genetic terms has yet to be established.

TYPE A CORONARY-PRONE BEHAVIOUR

In the 1950s two Californian cardiologists, Meyer Friedman and Ray Rosenman, produced the concept of type A coronary-prone behaviour. Generalising from their clinical impressions of patients who had suffered myocardial infarction they identified a constellation of behaviours that included sustained aggression, ambition, competitiveness, and a chronic sense of time urgency. Other features were a sense of impatience, being constantly alert and committed to vocational goals. The contrasting, more relaxed individuals who did not display these features were labelled type B. Type A is generally regarded as a behaviour pattern or response style, rather than as a fixed personality trait or attribute. Type A characteristics tend not to be present all the time, but only emerge when the individual is confronted by an appropriate challenge. Type A behaviour appears to be more prevalent in those who have received higher education and who are in jobs of administrative responsibility. It may be a response style exhibited mainly in Western urban cultures. It seems to be seen less commonly in American blacks, in rural settings and in western Europe when compared to the USA.

There is, however, considerable evidence from American studies relating type A behaviour with ischaemic heart disease. In a follow-up study lasting over 8.5 years of 3000 employed middle-aged Californian men (Rosenman et al 1975), the age-corrected risk of myocardial infarction amongst type A individuals (approximately half the total group) was twice that of type B individuals. Even after reliable predictors of ischaemia such as high arterial pressure and serum cholesterol were allowed for, there was still a link between type A behaviour and cardiac disease.

It has been suggested that type A individuals respond with heightened neuroendocrine and sympathetic nervous system changes when confronted by psychological challenges, and there is evidence that they have greater increases in adrenaline in response to stress than type B subjects.

Attempts have been made to modify type A behaviour (Friedman 1982). Several hundred post-myocardial infarction patients were randomly assigned to type A modification or to cardiological counselling groups. Follow-up assessments show that type A behaviour had indeed been modified and that the rate of non-fatal reinfarction in the group who had received type A modification was half that of the cardiological counselling sample.

It may well be that type A behaviour does not prove to be a robust factor and that its relationship to myocardial disease is only present in middle-aged Californian executives. Nevertheless, this 'narrow band approach' of linking specific traits or response styles to particular physical or psychiatric illnesses may prove useful in other areas. Comprehensive reviews are provided by Steptoe (1981, 1985).

MANAGEMENT OF PERSONALITY DISORDERS

When thinking about the management of these conditions it is best to keep a number of principles in mind and it may well be that it is the general structure of a management plan that is more important than any specific aspect of treatment. The principles can be listed as follows:

1. Progress will be slow; do not look for sudden change but enduring change over longer periods of time. Change in deeply ingrained patterns of behaviour is involved and it is not surprising that it is slow, if it happens at all.

2. Make sure that all Axis I disorders are given specific treatments; for example, those for depressive episodes, social anxiety, panic attacks, can be effective without change in the underlying personality structure. Patients with personality disorders often have these aspects overlooked and the Axis I disorder is seen as further evidence of their disturbed personality functioning.

3. Think about the *situation* as well as the person. For many individuals management is more appropriately aimed at helping the individual change their life circumstances so that these are less discordant with their personality. This may not be easy but is often easier than effecting underlying personality change.

4. Do not raise expectations of treatment that you cannot meet. The sacred 50 minute 'hour', once a week, so beloved of psychotherapists, is often quite inappropriate for such patients. It may be much more appropriate to see such individuals for half an hour every month or 6 weeks over a number of years rather than intensively over a number of weeks, only to find that no change occurs in such a short period of time. If brief or focal psychotherapies are being used, the aims of such treatment should be clearly spelt out so that the patient is aware that this course of treatment is about learning a specific skill or dealing with a particular aspect of their functioning rather than helping them change their functioning completely.

5. Be aware that it is change in the individual's functioning in the real world which you are attempting to effect, not just change in the therapeutic situation. The fact that someone functions well in a highly structured therapeutic community or whilst their dependency needs are being met in an individual psychotherapy relationship may give no indication as to how they may function in other settings.

6. Most psychiatric training schemes have 6 month rotations. Such patients do badly, being passed from trainee to trainee, and yet trainees clearly need experience of being involved in the management of such disorders. It may be better during training years to take on only one or two such patients and stick with them through different rotational placements.

Certain specific treatments have been advocated for personality disorders and these are summarised in Table 27.7.

CONCLUSIONS

1. The publication of DSM-III and its Axis II for personality disorders has proved to be a great boost to personality disorder research. DSM-III is far from perfect but represents a first attempt to define personality disorders operationally using a categorical approach.

2. The development of standardised assessments of personality which are reasonably reliable is a major advance. To some extent these represent the equivalents for personality disorder of the Present

Table 27.7   Summary of treatment used for personality disorder

Type of treatment	Personality disorder categories			
	Antisocial	Dependent	Inhibited	Withdrawn
Group psychotherapy	Widely used, of unproven worth	Not adequately evaluated	Not adequately evaluated	Unhelpful
Individual psychotherapy	May be effective in borderline and explosive group	May be effective but 'transference cures' common	May be effective	Useful in some patients but not adequately evaluated
Behaviour therapy	Anger control and social skills training of some value	Assertiveness training probably effective	Social skills training may be effective	Social skills training of proven value
Cognitive-behaviour therapy	May be effective. Now being widely advocated but so far little definite evidence		No evidence	No evidence
Drug treatment	Established efficacy of antipsychotic drugs in short-term treatment. Possible efficacy of lithium in aggressive individuals	Tricyclic antidepressants may be useful if mood disturbance prominent	As for dependent group	Unhelpful
Serotonin re-uptake blockers, SSRIs	May be effective across a wide range of personality disorders. Have been evaluated in 'borderline' and 'impulsive' disorders			

State Examination (PSE) and the Schedule for Affective Disorders and Schizophrenia (SADS). As discussed earlier in the chapter, they are available for DSM-III and ICD-9 categories and for borderline and schizotypal personality disorders.

3. Recent research has shown that certain personality disorder categories, such as schizotypal, anankastic and schizoid may be valid categories. They can, to some extent, be reliably separated from other personality disorder types and follow-up studies have shown stability over time. Others, such as the narcissistic, avoidant and hysterical types, overlap considerably with each other and may need to be redefined before they can be useful working concepts.

4. The research findings on borderline personality disorder are contradictory, though there is a tendency for the borderline concept as defined by Gunderson & Singer to be more reliable and valid.

5. The introduction in ICD-10 of 'personality traits of psychiatric significance' and 'enduring personality change' are useful additions and will hopefully allow personality factors to be taken into account more readily when making clinical assessments.

RECOMMENDATIONS

1. DSM-III and the ICD-10 definitions need to be more tightly and operationally defined. At present, there are marked variations in the length, detail and vagueness of the categories. For example, the DSM-III criteria for antisocial personality run to almost two pages, whereas those for dependent personality are covered in seven lines. The same or very similar traits are described differently in different personality disorder descriptions, e.g. lacking closer friendships, socially isolated, and socially withdrawn are used in schizoid, schizotypal and avoidant personality disorders, respectively.

2. Personality disorder descriptions should be based much more on specific behaviours, specific events and objective historical details, and less on

criteria that cannot be readily identified. For example, antisocial personality disorder includes recklessness as a criterion and goes on to define this by 'as indicated by driving while intoxicated or recurrent speeding' and failure to honour financial obligations is qualified by 'as indicated by repeated defaulting on debts, failure to provide child support, failure to support other dependants on a regular basis'. In contrast, avoidant personality includes 'desire for affection and acceptance' as one criterion with no mention of how this is to be recognised. The bald statement as written would appear to be a normal human attribute and not part of any personality disorder. Similarly, criteria in histrionic personality such as being 'vain and demanding' or 'over-reaction to minor events' need to be defined and qualified before they can be reliably used.

3. Consideration should be given to the use of a prototypical approach to personality disorder classification rather than a categorical one. This implies that personality disorder descriptions should be seen as prototypes of typical cases rather than categories which have discreet or overlapping boundaries. The implication clinically would be that instead of saying that an individual had a schizoid personality disorder, one would describe such a patient as having some features of schizoid prototype and these features would then be specified. An individual patient could be described as having clusters of features derived from more than one personality disorder prototype. This approach has the advantage that, clinically, the shorthand labels can be used without implying that an individual has all the features of that category, and atypical cases can more easily be dealt with. A fuller description of this approach is given by Livesley (1985). It is also possible that measures could be devised describing how much individuals differ from such given prototypes.

4. Personality disorder diagnoses should be used sparingly. As mentioned earlier, the majority of neurotic patients do not have a concomitant personality disorder. Diagnoses should not be based solely on patients' behaviour when ill or when observed in in-patient settings. Corroborative evidence must be sought from a reliable informant and from the patient's behaviour before illness or after recovery.

5. Clinicians should familiarise themselves with the standardised assessments of personality now available and incorporate elements of these into their routine mental state examination. At present, 'previous personality' usually merits only one or two questions in the typical psychiatric history and personality disorder diagnoses are often made on very scant and unreliable evidence.

6. Given the resources available in a National Health Service setting, the management of personality disorder should concentrate on helping individuals find a role and a situation in which they can live with less dissonance and conflict, rather than on attempting to change long-standing and deeply ingrained personality patterns, in other words concentrating on situations and situation-specific behaviours rather than attempting to alter traits themselves.

REFERENCES

Aakrog T 1981 The borderline concept in childhood, adolescence and adulthood. Acta Psychiatrica Scandinavaica suppl 293

Akhtar S, Thomson A J 1982 Overview: narcissistic personality disorder. American Journal of Psychiatry 139: 12

Akiskal H S, Yerevanian B I, Davis G C, King D, Lemmi H 1985 The nosologic status of borderline personality, clinical and polysommographic study. American Journal of Psychiatry 142: 192

APA 1953 Diagnostic and statistical manual. Mental disorders, 1st edn. American Psychiatric Association, Washington, DC

APA 1980 Diagnostic and statistical manual. Mental disorders, 3rd edn. American Psychiatric Association, Washington, DC

Baron M 1981 A diagnostic interview for schizotypal features. Psychiatry Research 4: 213

Black A 1974 The natural history of obsessional neurosis. In: Beech H R (ed) Obsessional states. Methuen, London, p 19

Cadoret R J, Cunningham L, Loftus R, Edwards J 1975 Studies of adoptees from psychiatrically disturbed biological parents. Journal of Paediatrics 87: 301

Cattell P B, Butcher H J 1968 The prediction of achievement and creativity. Bobbs-Merrill, London, p 53

Chodoff P, Lyons H 1958 Hysteria: the hysterical personality and "hysterical" conversion. American Journal of Psychiatry 114: 734

Christianson K O 1970 Crime in a Danish twin population. Acta Genetica Medica Gemellei 19: 323

Cleckley H 1966 The mask of sanity: an attempt to clarify some issues about the so-called psychopathic personality. C V Mosby, St Louis

Cloninger C R, Guze S B 1970 Psychiatric illness and female criminality: the risk of sociopathy and hysteria in the antisocial woman. American Journal of Psychiatry 127: 303

Cloninger C R, Guze S B 1973 Psychiatric illness in the families of female criminals: a study of 288 first degree relatives. British Journal of Psychiatry 122: 697

Crowe R R 1972 The adopted offspring of women criminal

offenders. Archives of General Psychiatry 27: 600

Crowe R R 1974 An adoption study of antisocial personality. Archives of General Psychiatry 31: 785

Drake R E, Vaillant G E 1985 A validity study of Axis II of DSM-III. American Journal of Psychiatry 142: 553

Eysenck H J 1973 The inequality of man. Maurice Temple Smith, London

Eysenck H J 1977 Crime and personality. Granada Paladin, St Albans

Foulds G A 1976 The hierarchical nature of personal illness. Academic Press, London, p 31

George A, Soloff PH 1986 Schizotypal symptoms in patients with borderline personality disorder. American Journal of Psychiatry 143: 212

Gunderson J G, Kolb J E 1978 Discriminating features of borderline patients. American Journal of Psychiatry 135: 792

Gunderson J G, Siever L J, Spaulding E 1983 The search for a schizotype. Archives of General Psychiatry 40: 15

Gunn J, Robertson G 1976 Psychopathic personality: a conceptual problem. Psychological Medicine 6: 631

Guze S B, Goodwin D W, Crane J B 1969 Criminality and psychiatric disorders. Archives of General Psychiatry 20: 583

Guze S B, Goodwin D W, Crane J B 1970 A psychiatric study of the wives of convicted felons: an example of assortative mating. American Journal of Psychiatry 126: 1773

Guze S B, Woodruff R A, Clayton P J 1971 A study of conversion symptoms in psychiatric out-patients. American Journal of Psychiatry 128: 643

Hare R D 1970 Psychopathy: theory and research. John Wiley New York

Henderson D 1939 Psychopathic States. W W Norton, New York

Hill D 1952 EEG in episodic psychiatric and psychopathic behaviour: a classification of the data. Encephalography and Clinical Neurophysiology 4: 419

HMSO 1959 Mental Health Act 1959 Her Majesty's Stationery Office, London

Hyler S, Reider R, Spitzer R et al 1983 Personality diagnostic questionnaire (PDQ) New York: New York State Psychiatric Institute

Jung C G 1928 Contributions to analytical psychology. Routledge & Kegan Paul, London, p 295

Kendler K S, Gruenberg A H, Straus J S 1981 An independent analysis of the Copenhagen samples of the Danish adoption study of schizophrenia. II. The relationship between schizotypal personality disorder and schizophrenia. Archives of General Psychiatry 38: 982

Kernberg O F 1967 Borderline personality organization. Journal of the American Psychoanalytic Association 15: 641

Koch J L A 1891 Die Psychopathischen minderwestigkeiten. Maier, Ravensberg

Kohut H 1968 The psychoanalytic treatment of narcissistic personality disorder. Psychoanalytic Study of the Child 23: 86

Kretschmer E 1936 Physique and character, 2nd edn (revised Miller). Routledge & Kegan Paul, London

Kringlen E 1965 Obsessional neurotics: a long term follow-up. British Journal of Psychiatry 111: 709

Kroll J, Casey K, Sines L, Roth M 1982 Are there borderlines in Britain: a cross validation of US findings. Archives of General Psychiatry 39: 60

Kurland H D, Yeager C T, Arthur R J 1963 Psychophysiological aspects of severe behaviour disorders. Archives of General Psychiatry 8: 599

Lazare A, Klerman G L 1968 Hysteria and depression: the frequency and significance of hysterical personality features in hospitalized depressed women. American Journal of Psychiatry 124: 48

Lion J R 1981 Personality disorders: diagnosis and management (revised for DSM-III). Williams & Wilkins, Baltimore

Livesley J W 1985 The classification of personality disorders. Canadian Journal of Psychiatry 30: 353

Ljungberg L 1957 Hysteria: a clinical, prognostic and genetic study. Acta Psychiatrica et Neurologica Scandinavica suppl 112

Lykken D T 1957 A study of anxiety in the sociopathic personality. Journal of Abnormal and Social Psychology 55: 5

McClelland D C, Atkinson J W, Clarke R A, Lowell E L 1953 The achievement motive. Appleton-Century-Crofts, New York

McCord W, McCord J 1964 The psychopath. Van Nostrand, New York.

McGlashan T H 1980 Schizotypal personality disorder: Chestnut Lodge follow-up study. Archives of General Psychiatry 43: 329

McGlashan T H 1983 The borderline syndrome II. Is it a variant of schizophrenia or affective disorder: Archives of General Psychiatry 40: 1319

Magnan V 1893 Lecons cliniques sur les maladies mentales. Bataille, Paris.

Magnusson D, Endler, N S 1977 Personality at the crossroads. John Wiley New York

Mann A H, Jenkins R, Cutting J C, Cowen P J 1981 The development and use of a standardised assessment of abnormal personality. Psychological Medicine 11: 839

Maslow A H 1967 Self-actualization and beyond. In Bugental J F T (ed) Challenges of humanistic psychology. McGraw-Hill, New York, p 396

Meehl P E 1984 Manual for use with checklist for schizotypic signs. Minneapolis, Psychiatric Research Unit, University of Minnesota Medical School

Millon T 1981 Disorder of personality DSM-III Axis II. John Wiley New York

Millon T 1982 Millon clinical multiaxial inventory (2nd edition) Minneapolis MN: Interpretive Scoring Systems

Millon T 1984 On the renaissance of personality assessment and personality theory. Journal of Personality Assessment 48: 450

Mischel W 1977 The interaction of person and situation in Magnusson D, Endler N S (eds) Personality at the crossroads: current issues in interactional psychology. Lawrence Erlbaum, Hillsdale, New Jersey.

Mischel W, Peake P K 1982 Beyond deja vu in the search for cross-situational consistency. Psychological Review 89: 730

Morel B A 1839 Traite des degenerescences physiques, intellectuelles et morales de l'espere humaine. J B Baillière, Paris

Oldham JM 1991 Personality disorders: new perspectives on diagnostic validity. American Psychiatric Press, Washington, DC

Peck D, Whitlow D 1975 Approaches to personality theory. Methuen, London

Pfohl B, Stangl D, Zimmerman M 1982 The structured interview for DSM-III personality disorders (SID-P). University of Iowa Hospitals and Clinics, Iowa

Pfohl B, Coryell W, Zimmerman M, Stangl D 1986 DSM-III personality disorders: diagnostic overlap and internal consistency of individual DSM-III criteria. Comprehensive Psychiatry 27: 21

Pinel P 1801 Traite medico-philosophique sur l'alienation mentale, ou la manie. Richard Caille et Ravier, Paris

Pope H G, Jonas J M, Hudson J I, Cohen B M, Gunderson J G 1983 The validity of DSM-III borderline personality disorder. Archives of General Psychiatry 40: 23

Powell G E 1986 Personality. In: McGuffin P, Shanks MF, Hodgson RJ (eds) Scientific principles of psychopathology. Grune & Stratton, London

Pritchard J C 1835 A treatise on insanity and other disorders affecting the mind. Sherwood, Gilbert & Piper, London

Robbins L N 1978 Study of childhood predictors of adult antisocial behaviour: replication from longitudinal studies. Psychological Medicine 8: 611

Rogers C R 1951 Client-centered therapy. Houghton Mifflin, Boston

Rogers C R 1977 Carl Rogers on personal power. Delacorte, New York

Rosenman R H, Brand R J, Jenkins C D et al 1975 Journal of the American Medical Association 233: 872

Rotter J B 1966 Generalized expectancies for internal versus external central reinforcement. Psychological Monographs 80, No 1

Rush B 1812 Medical enquiries and observations upon the diseases of the mind. Philadelphia

Schacter S, Lantane B 1964 Crime cognition and the autonomic nervous system. In: Levine D (ed) Nebraska symposium on motivation. University of Nebraska Press, Nebraska

Schneider K 1950 Psychopathic personalities. Translation of 9th edn by Hamilton M 1958. Cassell, London

Schwade E D, Geiger S E 1965 Abnormal electroencephalographic findings in severe behaviour disorders. Diseases of the Nervous System 17: 307

Scott P 1960 The treatment of psychopaths. British Medical Journal i: 1641

Sheldon W H 1954 Atlas of men: a guide for somatotyping the adult male at all ages. Harper Row, New York

Slater E, Roth M 1969 Clinical Psychiatry, 3rd end. Ballière, Tindall & Cassell, London

Slavaney P R, McHugh P R 1974 The hysterical personality: a controlled study. Archives of General Psychiatry 30: 325

Spitzer R L, Endicott J 1979 Justification for separating schizotypal and borderline personality disorders. Schizophrenia Bulletin 5: 95

Spitzer R L, Endicott J, Gibbon H 1979 Crossing the border into borderline personality and borderline schizophrenia. Archives of General Psychiatry 36: 17

Spitzer RL, Williams JB et al 1985 Structured clinical interview for DSM-III personality disorders (SCID-II). Biometrics Research Department, New York State Psychiatric Institute, New York

Stangl D, Pfohl B, Zimmerman M, Bowers W, Correnthal C 1985 A structured interview for DSM-III personality disorders. Archives of General Psychiatry 42: 591

Steptoe A 1981 Type A coronary-prone behaviour. In: Psychological factors in cardiovascular disorder. Academic Press, London

Steptoe A 1985 Type A coronary-prone behaviour. British Journal of Hospital Medicine 24: 257

Tyrer P, Alexander J 1979 Classification of personality disorder. British Journal of Psychiatry 135: 163

Tyrer P, Casey P, Gall J 1983 Relationship between neurosis and personality disorder. British Journal of Psychiatry 142: 404

Tyrer P 1988 Personality disorders: diagnosis, management and course. Butterworth/Wright, London

WHO 1978 Ninth revision of the international classification of diseases. World Health Organization, Geneva

Ziegler F J, Imboden J B 1962 Contemporary conversion reactions: a conceptual model. Archives of General Psychiatry 6: 279

28. Mental retardation

A. K. Zealley

CHANGING PERCEPTIONS OF MENTAL RETARDATION

Someone who cannot manage an everyday task with ordinary ease may need some extra explanation, or a different demonstration, or repeated practice. It is this that suggests that much of the help which intellectually limited people need lies at the hand of teachers, with both a capital and a small 't'. For the great majority, perhaps 95%, of people who have drawn the 'short straw' in the matter of innate intellectual ability there is force in the view that medicine is no more relevant than it is for the average person.

Since the early 19th century, and roughly coincidental with urban industrialisation, there have been three phases in how the 'mental retardation problem' has been seen. These successive perceptions have been more or less shared both by the professional people involved and by the informed man in the street.

Initially, mental retardation was seen as a threat, once its visibility became more obvious with the move away from the land. Fuelled by eugenecist views in the later 19th and early 20th centuries, it was feared that 'moral defectives' would damage the quality of the racial stock.

Second came the 'medicalisation' of mental retardation, after World War I. Unfortunately, the medical ethos of the time was centred on finding cures, rather than on working out the best care. Institutions were the order of the day. 'Control' by means of sedation was usual. Together with persisting confusion between psychiatric illness and mental retardation, there developed an assumption — shortly before World War II — that it was for medicine to take the lead role with regard to these matters.

With the 1950s came the third phase. This is still current and developing, predicated on the view that what mentally retarded people need is help to achieve as satisfactory and normal a life as possible. Concepts such as 'normalisation', 'integration' and 'community care' gathered pace in the 1970s. There was perhaps too much emphasis on the *location* of the care that was to be provided, rather than on its extent and nature; indeed, this is still the case in some circles.

It is now axiomatic that help for a person who is mentally retarded needs to be tailored to his personal needs and circumstances, and to those of his family. Coupled with this is the recognition that the person himself may well have preferences, and that these must enter the equation too. To give effect to this sort of philosophy of care provision there needs to be ongoing collaboration between all the several strands — health service, education, housing, social services, employment services and the voluntary sector.

The difficult matter of ensuring adequate quality of the various services taken up by a mentally retarded person is of course magnified by a dispersed care philosophy. Yet the monitoring of quality is a necessary element. An indisputable problem in leavening up quality is of course finance. It is clear that for most of this century the problems faced by those with intellectual limitations have been understood by senior officialdom. Thus, it has to be concluded that the insufficiency of many services they need has been a function of deficient political will, relative to other calls on the public purse.

Changes in attitudes to the mentally retarded cannot be ordained from on high. And it must be acknowledged that those who have worked over the years in hospitals for these people have had their own personal interests at heart, as well as those of their charges. These interests have certainly retarded the pace of change in what services are provided and where. At the same time it must be said that failure to carry such staff along with the thinking of senior planners, by dint of insufficient communication, consultation and support, has in part been responsible for whatever reactionary attitudes and obstructive tactics have been evident.

In essence, it must be remembered that there are three aspects to the problems of someone who is mentally retarded:

1. The *impairment* itself; for example, brain injury as a result of prenatal or perinatal trauma or infection
2. The *disability* which results; for example, inability to read or to perform arithmetic so as to be able to handle money
3. The *social handicap* in which the disability results; for example, resultant problems with regard to occupational, leisure or personal relationship possibilities.

While there is indeed scope for medical advances in respect of *impairment* prevention, or at least mitigation, help for the *disability* and the *social handicap* is likely to be at the hands of professionals and others in the fields of education and of social provision. Psychiatrists in the field of mental retardation have an important role in stimulating coordinated service planning and delivery.

The prevailing national policy of returning residents of hospitals for the mentally retarded to the community at large now commands widespread medical support. But with two important caveats:

1. The living arrangements to which these people are discharged from hospital must ensure an enhanced quality of life, not the opposite.
2. There is a small minority of mentally retarded people for whom care in *any* location is going to demand many skilled contributions, including those from the medical profession and those in professions allied to medicine. Whether that mix of care contributions is provided under the aegis of the health service or of another organisation matters less than that it is recognised to be needed by this small proportion of retarded people. Moreover, it will be costly, if it is to be adequate.

Man has relied on his problem-solving ability to achieve his current state of dominance in the world. *Homo sapiens* has been able to adapt to a wide range of environments. The individual with limited intelligence is at a disadvantage in problem-solving and adjustment to new or complex situations.

It is clear from everyday experience that although intelligence facilitates adaptation, it is by no means the only factor. Emotional stability, age, physical health and, in some situations, strength, enhance the capacity to adapt. In a different way factors such as social class, wealth, skin colour and education will operate to frustrate or support an individual's coping mechanisms. From the start it is essential to realise that while limited intelligence is a sine qua non of mental retardation, many other individual and social influences determine whether an individual's limited intellectual capacity necessarily proves a real disability.

There have been many attempts to define mental retardation but the definitions are relative because they are so closely tied to social and cultural factors.

The definition which appears in ICD-9 is as follows: 'A condition of arrested or incomplete development of mind which is especially characterised by subnormality of intelligence'.

The formulation used in the Mental Deficiency Act (1927) has been widely used. It is similar to that in the ICD, but with an important age factor added: 'A condition of arrested or incomplete development of mind existing before the age of 18 whether resulting from inherent causes or induced by disease or injury'.

It can rightly be said that the use of so precise a cut-off as 18 years of age is arbitrary. A person who becomes mentally retarded as a result of a head injury, or of encephalitis, when he is 15 years old would meet this age criterion for mental retardation; if he is 19 years old at the time of the injury or illness, he would not — and indeed may be considered by some to suffer from one of the variants of 'presenile dementia'.

Essentially, the concept of mental retardation implies that the person concerned has been affected by the condition for most of his life. He has not previously enjoyed normal intellectual ability and all that goes with it, and then suffered its reduction.

In recent years, the term employed to refer to people with this sort of disadvantage has changed several times. This has usually been because the existing term had acquired pejorative connotations in the eyes of many in the field, though not necessarily of those so identified. While 'mental deficiency' and 'mental subnormality' are terms now seldom used, 'mental handicap' still has currency as it is the official UK term used by Health Departments.

But certain psychiatric illnesses may result in a variety of 'mental' handicaps, unrelated to intelligence. The term mental handicap is therefore not ideal. While 'people with learning difficulties/disabilities' also has currency, it is both long-winded and emphasises just one — albeit key — characteristic.

The World Health Organization (WHO) now employs the term mental retardation, including it in the draft of ICD-10. It is also the term used by the American Psychiatric Association in DSM-IIIR. The term will therefore be used in this chapter.

In the USA, reputedly the spiritual home of the intelligence test, the criterion of intelligence has been widely employed in deciding whether a subject was suffering from mental retardation. Clarke (1965) has critically reviewed the shortcomings of the IQ (intelligence quotient) as the criterion for diagnosing mental retardation: (1) the IQ and social competence are not perfectly related; (2) the IQ is not constant, i.e. there are test–retest differences; (3) the same IQ as measured by different tests may not mean the same thing. But she did point out that a considerable degree of intellectual subnormality as measured on reputable and appropriate IQ tests should be a sine qua non of classification as a mental defective. Despite its limitations, it was used recently to determine on a sliding slide the charge to be levied at a residential establishment for the mentally retarded. The lower the IQ, the higher the charge (Campaign for Mentally Handicapped People 1983).

The criterion of educability has formed an important theme in the development of provisions for the retarded. This is essentially an administrative problem: children in ordinary classes who could not profit from this education posed problems for themselves, their teachers and their classmates. The creation of special classes integrated into ordinary schools, as well as special schools themselves, have taken place to meet this need.

The criterion of social competence has been one much favoured in the UK (see Craft 1979). But social competence is only relative to the norms operating in that society at that particular time; this creates problems when society is changing at an accelerating rate or when, as now, the level of unemployment makes employability an unreliable criterion.

LEGISLATION

The important UK Acts were those of 1904, 1927, 1959 (1960 in Scotland) and 1983 (1984 in Scotland). The English Act of 1959 abolished the categories of idiot, imbecile and feeble-minded and replaced them with the categories of subnormality, severe subnormality and psychopathy. In the sense that the earlier terms—idiot, imbecile and so on—were opprobrious the 1959 English Act with its degrees of subnormality represented an advance, but in many ways the Mental Health (Scotland) Act 1960 was more consistent; it had only two general categories—mental illness and mental deficiency—and did not attempt to delineate degrees of handicap. This Act also introduced informal admission (as did the English Act), which did much to accelerate the opening of the doors of hospitals for the mentally retarded e.g. for holiday admissions and for brief admissions precipitated by a crisis in the family.

The UK Mental Health Acts (1983 in England and Wales, 1984 in Scotland) use the term mental disorder, and define it as meaning mental illness or mental handicap however caused or manifested (but excluding promiscuity or other immoral conduct, sexual deviancy, and dependence on alcohol or drugs). The Acts do not define mental illness or mental handicap but they do define two other terms, mental impairment and severe mental impairment. The former is defined thus: 'a state of arrested or incomplete development of mind not amounting to severe mental impairment which includes significant impairment of intelligence and social functioning and is associated with abnormally aggressive or seriously irresponsible conduct on the part of the person concerned.' The definition of severe mental impairment is similar, with the substitution of 'severe' for 'significant'.

Most mentally retarded people are to be regarded as suffering from arrested or incomplete development of mind, so far as their legal position is concerned; and while there will typically be associated impairment of intellectual and social functioning, only a minority will show abnormally aggressive or seriously irresponsible conduct. Only a minority of mentally retarded people are therefore liable to compulsory admission to hospital under the auspices of these Acts.

INTELLIGENCE

Intelligence tests seek to measure a person's capacity for intelligent behaviour in solving problems in relation to other people of a similar age. A child is thus compared with the norm for his age. It is assumed that intelligence grows in this way to the age of roughly 14 years. Although experience and emotional maturity augment an adult's capacity for problem-solving, it seems that there is rarely much growth in pure intelligence beyond adolescence. Different tests measure differing facets of intelligence such as verbal, nonverbal or social intelligence. Some believe that there is an underlying trait or number of traits which constitute pure intelligence which is independent of previous educational experience. In practice, it has proved impossible to divorce intelligence tests from all cultural and educational bias.

Most tests have been devised to contrast the performance of the child with that of a standardised example of his peers. Thus, a 6-year-old who solves the problems appropriate for a 6-year-old is said to have a mental age of 6 years. If the 6-year-old solves the problems of an 8-year-old, then he has a mental age of 8 years. The ratio of mental to chronological age gives us a measure of the child's relative intelligence, and in this respect the mentally retarded child will always function at a mental age well below his chronological age. The IQ is arrived at by the formula

$$\frac{\text{mental age}}{\text{chronological age}} \times 100.$$

Detailed discussion of intelligence testing is found in Vernon (1960).

It is wrong to place too great reliance on a single score or a single test; and it is only when several different assessments carried out over a period of time consistently show that a child is falling behind his peers that retardation should be diagnosed. The child's co-operation, emotional upsets, physical illness, emotional or social deprivation all influence the quality of the test results. Intelligence tests are of some value in predicting a child's final level of intellectual capacity but even for the normal child, their validity declines as the duration of the prediction grows (Clarke & Clarke 1965). The rate at which the retarded or brain-damaged child's intelligence grows has not yet been fully determined and it is quite possible that unexpected changes in the rate of intellectual growth may be observed in certain cases.

Most intelligence tests are designed for use with children of school age. Some psychologists have endeavoured to assess babies and measure their developmental quotient in a way analogous to the IQ.

Gesell, for instance, has devised a scale which studies four aspects of behaviour: (1) social behaviour; (2) language; (3) hand–eye coordination; (4) bodily coordination (Gesell & Armatruda 1941).

Intelligence tests have been devised on the assumption that intelligence is normally distributed in the population. The normal (Gaussian) distribution is shown in Figure 28.1. It is generally assumed in this country that those who have an IQ below 70 are of sub-normal intelligence (their intelligence level lies more than two standard deviations below the mean for the population). It has often been shown that there are more people of very low intelligence than can be explained by this normal distribution alone. This important group is represented by the shaded area of the diagram.

This excess of severely and moderately retarded individuals has been termed the pathological group in contrast to the subcultural group, most of whom are only mildly mentally retarded. This latter group is normal in all respects except that, for a mixture of genetic and environmental reasons to be discussed later, it is less well endowed intellectually than the majority of the population. It is balanced at the other end of the distribution by a group of highly intelligent individuals who are abnormally well endowed. No corresponding group counterbalances the pathological group because no disease provokes an excess of intelligence.

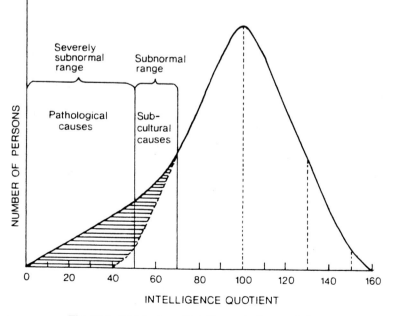

Fig. 28.1 Distribution of intelligence in the population

The term pathological is chosen because the retardation in these cases is caused by various disease processes arising in individual genes or chromosomes or from damage before, during or after birth. The means by which the pathology arises will be discussed later in the chapter, but it is important at this stage to recognise that most members of this group have characteristics which make special demands on services that are different from the subculturally retarded. Many have physical handicaps in addition to their retardation. Whereas those mildly affected will often have dull parents, the pathological/severely retarded patient may come from any social background and have parents of below, average or superior intelligence. In a survey of a mental retardation hospital population, Penrose classified patients by the father's occupation and showed that it was uncommon for parents in professional or managerial occupations to have mildly retarded offspring; but they were just as likely to have severely retarded children as parents from any other social class (Penrose 1972).

DIAGNOSIS OF MENTAL RETARDATION

Considering the social and economic importance of the problem, the means whereby mental retardation is first ascertained are surprisingly haphazard. The route from first suspicion that a child may be of subnormal intelligence to the provision of appropriate services is still not clearly signposted in this country; and luck and determination on the part of the parents, teacher or family doctor play a larger part than they should in the journey. In a number of cases mental retardation may be suspected or predicted at birth or shortly after. In these cases the problem is usually severe and associated with other physical defects such as hydrocephaly, brain injury at birth or microcephaly. It may be associated with recognisable characteristics as in mongolism, or the infant may suffer damage that is known to carry a high risk of irreversible brain damage, as in cases where prolonged hypoxia is followed by recovery due to heroic measures to resuscitate. The paediatrician and paediatric neurologist will keep a record of those children whom he considers at risk of being mentally retarded and should liaise closely with the specialised services for the retarded from the start.

More commonly, retardation is not suspected at first, but the parents come to notice that their child lags behind his siblings or other children in reaching such milestones as sitting up, walking and talking. At this stage the parents commonly seek guidance from their family doctor. Most textbooks on child development contain charts which plot the progress of the average child as he advances through infancy (Gesell & Armatruda 1941). Parents or doctor will often consult charts and compare the child's progress with that of the statistical norm. If the young child appears to be consistently taking twice as long to reach the common milestones as other children, the family doctor is justified in considering mental retardation as a possible diagnosis. At this stage he will often seek specialist help in excluding other possible reasons for the retarded development.

When unrecognised, sensory defects such as deafness or poor vision may handicap a child's learning capacity. Nutritional deficiencies or chronic illness may cause a child to lag in reaching the normal milestones. Bowlby (1965) has shown that emotional deprivation can give rise to apparent retardation. Every child requires emotional and sensory stimulation to achieve his maximum potential.

The diagnosis of mental retardation can only be made after careful and repeated assessment. Parents are naturally worried about the attainments of their offspring and the family doctor is understandably tempted to reassure them even when his experience tells him that this may not be justified. If he has reasonable grounds for suspecting disability, it is better to enlist help at an early stage than to reinforce parental denial until a further crisis occurs.

The parents' anxiety may cloud their perception of these milestones, with the result that a certain amount of wishful thinking enters into their account of dates at which a child first walked or talked. Conversely, parents with high expectations may overlook a child's accomplishments. In other cases obvious signs of retardation are ignored, not out of any lack of attention but because people are liable to deny what they do not wish to see.

In milder cases the child may enter school before his retardation becomes apparent. Faced with the demands of the education system, it becomes clear sooner or later that the child cannot keep pace with his contemporaries, or routine intelligence testing may reveal a low IQ. Often the child will become frustrated when he cannot meet the various demands made of him. Behaviour problems of various kinds may thus draw attention to a previously unnoticed intellectual retardation. School and health services should also look out for other causes of the child's slowness. A search should be made for specific learning difficulties such as dyslexia, impaired hearing or vision, autism or physical illness.

It is very uncommon for significant degrees of mental retardation to escape recognition at some stage during childhood. There are many mildly retarded individuals who make no particular demand on specialised services during their childhood. Some of these may return to special notice later when they are exposed to particular social crises such as loss of parents, illness or arrest. In such circumstances the retardation may be recognised once more as a reason for the difficulties the individual experiences in coping with new and stressful circumstances.

Once mental retardation is suspected, a detailed history should be taken. The family and social background may reveal a family history of retardation and some estimate of the parents' intelligence may be gleaned from their own school and occupation record. A careful account of the pregnancy and delivery may provide clues to potentially damaging influences such as drugs, infections or birth injury. The child's development should be carefully traced past various milestones. The examiner should be concerned about social as well as physical accomplishments. A detailed account of the child's capacity to cope with formal learning should be obtained. Particular note should be made of discrepancies in performance as this may point to specific learning defects or emotional difficulties. Having taken a history from the child and his parents, psychological assessment is usually the next step. The child should be physically examined with special reference to the nervous system. Ideally the diagnosis should be arrived at by a team of specialists working closely with the parents and the referring family doctor, social worker and teacher. The importance of providing such joint assessment services must be emphasised.

It is important that assessment using criteria of intelligence tests and social competence does not place the patient in a category from which he cannot move at a later stage. Assessment must be a continuous process throughout the individual's development. It should not be concerned primarily with individual test results, but with the constellation of strengths and weaknesses. Psychologists such as Mittler (1970) now make it clear that a careful analysis of an individual's motor, perceptual and psycholinguistic skills is important. The work of the Clarkes, summarised in Clarke & Clarke (1965), shows that performance at the time of initial assessment may be transformed to a much higher level of function with suitable training.

PREVALENCE OF MENTAL RETARDATION

To ask what is the prevalence of mental retardation in a country raises so many imponderables that the answer in any general sense appears irrelevant. When it is asked of a specific community with a definite purpose

in mind, the question becomes extremely pertinent.

Mentally retarded people will only be ascertained if they have come to the notice of health, social or educational agencies. The extent to which this occurs will depend, on the one hand, on the adequacy and number of these agencies and the prevailing social attitudes towards retardation and, on the other, on the extent to which their retardation proves a real handicap. As discussed previously, the more complex a society becomes, the greater stress it places on the mental resources of the handicapped individual. These social and psychological variables have greatest influence on the *apparent* prevalence of *mild* degrees of retardation. Those who are very severely retarded would be recognised as being in need of special care and protection in any society. Even amongst this severely retarded group, several different agencies cater for their needs. Therefore, any attempt to count their numbers must involve all these agencies.

Some centres have devised registers in which the names of all mentally retarded people are recorded irrespective of the agency which made the first contact. Computerised case registers of this kind are valuable both for research and planning.

It may be predicted that more than 2% of a population will have an intelligence level which is more than two standard deviations below the mean—corresponding to an IQ of less than 70. The figure of 2% is much higher than most prevalence studies have revealed, though the figure would include the large number of people of limited intelligence who never come to the attention of any specialist agency for the mentally retarded. Study of this latter group would be fruitful in obtaining an understanding of the ways in which such people achieve a successful adaptation in society.

The size of this 'unascertained' group is of more than theoretical importance. At times of social stress produced by high unemployment or growing industrialisation, this group's latent handicap becomes significant and they may require support from the state. It may be that this decompensation could be avoided if they were provided with better services at the outset. They might well benefit from a prolonged education which took into account their slower rate of development and learning.

Table 28.1 reminds one that there are three mildly retarded people for every person with a more severe degree of retardation.

The close correlation between overcrowding, poverty, irregular unskilled employment and educational backwardness has been strikingly demonstrated in a survey of 17 000 British schoolchildren (Davie et al 1972).

Table 28.1 Main clinical features of the different degrees of mental retardation

Profound	Severe	Moderate	Mild
	sometimes called severe mental retardation		
IQ 20	IQ 35	IQ 50	IQ 70
0.05% of population	0.5% of population		1.5% of population
Less than 1% of cases	5% of cases	20% of cases	75% of cases
Usually need extensive or total help with daily living	Many need much help with daily living, though able to wash and usually to be predominantly continent; often physically disabled, (including epilepsy, especially younger patients); locomotor problems include ataxia, spasticity, athetosis	Often capable of substantial autonomy in daily living, with some supervision	Often not ascertained as retarded and may only need help if problems in living arise; overrepresented among clients of housing departments
Normally only able to communicate minimally	Capable of only limited communication, often not by means of speech	Normally able to communicate adequately, to follow their own leisure interests, and to do simple household jobs	Often marry and may hold a routine job
Often some organic brain pathology			Organic brain pathology uncommon

Some surveys have been based on intelligence test findings alone; such a survey of Scottish schoolchildren revealed that approximately 1.5% were of subnormal intelligence. Dahlberg (1937) reported that 3% of Swedish schoolboys were in need of special education by reason of retardation. In view of the limitations of simple intelligence tests discussed earlier, these findings can only act as rough guidelines. It would, however, be interesting to trace the subsequent progress of those schoolchildren who were found to be subnormal in a survey of this kind, but made no use of any special services.

Of more value are a number of field surveys which have combined intelligence test scores with other social or educational criteria. The classic study of this kind was conducted by Lewis (1929). Three urban and three rural areas of England and Wales were selected for intensive study. The teachers of each school in the area were asked to nominate the 15% of each age group whom they considered most backward. This group was given an intelligence test and those who scored the lowest marks were individually tested and examined. Lewis also examined all children who had any kind of neurological disturbance.

Other children who did not attend school were contacted through local mental retardation services, health visitors, district nurses and family doctors. To obtain data on adults in the selected areas, Lewis obtained information from those social work, local authority, medical and voluntary agencies which might deal with or know of retarded people. He then tried to contact and assess those adults who had been so identified. The survey was thus an enormous task for one man to undertake before the advent of computers.

This survey revealed that slightly less than 1% of the population was mentally retarded. He found a higher incidence in rural than in urban areas. He also observed that for each severely retarded person, there were four moderately and 15 mildly retarded individuals. This observation has been confirmed in subsequent studies. Finally, Lewis noticed that the incidence of retardation varied greatly with age.

He showed that the prevalence of retardation rises with age until the late teens and thereafter declines. This presumably reflects the process of ascertainment whereby increasing numbers of mentally retarded people are revealed by the educational system as its demands extend, and—amongst the more severely retarded—as the capacity for parents to cope with a growing retarded child declines.

In reviewing similar findings from other countries, Gruneberg (1964) felt that this apparent resorption of retarded people back into the community after adolescence was the most remarkable observation to come from these field studies. He concludes: 'Either these individuals are continuing to be extremely handicapped in later life and are unknown because the services they need are unavailable, or they have stopped being retarded in any real sense at all and do not need any special protection, help or services.' This important question remains unanswered, though it is likely that many of these people are simply lost from official view once schooldays are past.

There have been several more recent field studies of the prevalence of retardation in this country, for instance Goodman & Tizard (1962), Kushlick (1964), Scally & Mackay (1964) and Innes et al (1968). While these show considerable variation in the prevalence of mild degrees of retardation, they find that the prevalence of moderate and severe mental retardation is remarkably constant at approximately 3.7 per 1000 population. As anticipated, those who are severely handicapped come to attention irrespective of the cultural setting and services available, while the mildly affected cases are sensitive to these variables.

It seems that mental retardation of all degrees is marginally more common in males. Penrose (1972) has claimed that this would be explained on the grounds that male intelligence is more widely distributed about the mean than female. It is also probable that mentally retarded males are more likely to utilise services than females who can often be maintained at home for a longer period with less social distress than men.

Lewis (1929), Kushlick (1964) and Goodman & Tizard (1962) have all found retardation to be more prevalent in rural areas. It has been suggested that there is a drift of the more able to the towns whereas the retarded remain in their rural communities. In contrast to these findings, more recent studies in north-east Scotland have found a higher prevalence of retardation of all severities in the city of Aberdeen than in the surrounding countryside (Innes et al 1968). The true position may possibly be changing.

Following a painstaking study of the Aberdeen population, Birch et al (1970) were able to trace the highest prevalence of retardation to a particular section of the urban community. It has long been known that the frequency of mental retardation is highest amongst children of parents in social class V. Birch found that the highest prevalence of mild subnormality was to be found in a subgroup within this class. He identified

this subculture as being of manifest low status with 'minimal education, poverty, family disorganisation and unwillingness or inability to plan the major economic and marital aspects of their lives'. This study has helped to focus on a social group at risk with a high prevalence of subcultural retardation.

Some forms of mental retardation are easily identified and this has allowed a very accurate description of their prevalence. Down's syndrome, for instance, occurs once in 660 live births (that is, 1.5 per 1000 live births). Approximately 8.5% of the retarded population have this condition. The prevalence in a hospital population is higher—about 10%. The prevalence of some metabolic disorders is now known with accuracy as routine screening tests become available.

Surveys of the kind described above have a number of important uses. They may help the epidemiologist obtain clues concerning the causation of retardation. The best known example of this kind of use was the observation that Down's syndrome was much more common amongst the children of elderly mothers. The incidence varies from one in 1050 births when the mother is a teenager, to one in 50 when she is aged 45 years. This observation was a crucial step in the chain of discovery which led to the chromosomal defect responsible for Down's syndrome being found to occur in the ageing maternal germ cells.

AETIOLOGICAL FACTORS IN MENTAL RETARDATION

Referring back to Figure 28.1, there are clearly two different but overlapping varieties of mental retardation:

1. The subcultural group in which polygenic inheritance of low normal or borderline intelligence is compounded by the factors of social and educational deprivation
2. The pathological group in which genetic, chromosomal, infective, toxic or traumatic factors have led to the condition.

In addition, there is a third group of subjects suffering from childhood psychoses ranging from childhood autism to brain-damaged children exhibiting autistic features.

SUBCULTURAL MENTAL RETARDATION

The concept of subcultural retardation appears to have been introduced by E. O. Lewis (1933). He classified cases of mental retardation into pathological and subcultural types, the latter showing no recognised pathogenesis but representing an extreme variant of the normal distribution of mental endowment. Stein & Susser (1962) recognised two types of mental retardation: those with presumptive brain damage and those who appear to be without brain damage. The first type is distributed evenly between the different social classes, whereas the second is found only amongst families in social class V. They argued that this second type is a 'cultural' syndrome of mental retardation; it accounted for 75% of all the educationally subnormal.

It has, however, been shown that there is a slight excess liability for severe mental retardation to arise in social class V than in other social classes. This may be a function of poorer take-up of preventive and other health and related services in social class V.

Hospital surveys have produced some contradictory results. Berg & Kirman (1959) found evidence of aetiological (i.e. pathological) factors in 36.5% of cases, probable aetiological factors in 32.5% and none at all in 31%. This last group probably included a large proportion of subcultural cases.

It has been calculated that 20 per 1000 of the American population have an IQ of more than two standard deviations below the mean, i.e. an IQ less than 70 (Stevens & Heber 1964). But most authorities accept for planning purposes an administrative prevalence (that is, the number of subjects who will need services) of 3 per 1000. It is this gap between the administrative prevalence and the postulated prevalence of IQ less than 70 which makes an explanation based simply on polygenic inheritance unacceptable as a working hypothesis.

Sociologically oriented studies such as that sponsored by the National Children's Bureau (Wedge & Prosser 1973) emphasise the relationship between social disadvantage and mental retardation. But social disadvantage is often compounded by the parents' social incompetence, in turn related to the low IQ of so many parents of children with subcultural mental retardation. American studies have suggested that the mother's IQ was the single most important predictor of mental retardation in the children of slum families in Milwaukee. They noted that not all slum families produced children needing special education. It seemed to be the combination of living in the slum and having a mother of IQ less than 80 that determined the need. While mothers with IQ less than 80 comprised less than half the total group of mothers, they accounted for almost 80% of children with IQ less than 80.

With the foregoing in mind, this provisional definition of subcultural retardation is suggested: 'Subcultural retardation is a limitation of intelligence based partly on polygenic inheritance but compounded by severe social and educational disadvantage so that the majority of these subjects require services (educational, social work or medical) on this account at some stage in their lives.'

Subcultural retardation: research findings

A Scottish study (Blackie et al 1975) revealed that mild retardation clustered in social classes IV and V while severe cases were the mode in classes I and II. 'Accepting attitudes' toward the handicapped child and a negative attitude toward family planning were characteristic of social classes IV and V. Language development occurred much earlier in social classes I and II (compared with classes IV and V) although the majority of the children were more severely handicapped. Multiple incidence (i.e. more than one mentally retarded child in the same family) was correlated with mild handicap in the index case and also with social classes IV and V.

In Aberdeen, Birch et al (1970) surveyed all mentally retarded children aged 8–10 years and collected data about their families. They showed that within classes IV and V there were certain family conditions associated with a greater risk of mental retardation in the children: five children or more, substandard housing, person to room ratio of two or more, family disorganisation (as shown by debt, rent arrears, etc.) and poverty. Birch and his colleagues found that all their multiple-incidence families were in social classes IV and V. They also found that for mildly retarded subjects the percentage of their siblings who were mentally retarded was 12 times that of the comparison population (i.e. control children from social classes IV and V).

In short, Birch et al showed that it is not so much classes IV and V but a problem subgroup of families within these social classes who contribute disproportionately to the 'pool' of mentally retarded subjects.

Heber & Garber (1971) reported that the IQ of children of mothers with IQ below 80 showed a progressive decline with age. The authors go on to state that the excess prevalence of mental retardation appears to relate to retarded parents living in the slum area rather than the slum itself. They started an educational programme for 20 families from this slum area with mothers with IQ less than 80 and the youngest child less than 6 months old. On randomised allocation a further 20 families received standard welfare care. Four years later, the IQ of the experimental group had risen to a mean of 122, while that of the control group was 96. Even this latter figure is perhaps better than expected and suggests that the control children were benefiting from being involved in the study.

Strategies for intervention

While Wedge & Prosser (1973) have suggested that disadvantaged families require better housing, Heber & Garber (1971) have concentrated on identifying families at risk and then introducing preschool education for the child and further education for the mother. Their results seem to indicate that this massive 'injection' of education is effective but the financial implications are considerable.

PATHOLOGICAL MENTAL RETARDATION

Table 28.2 sets out some non-genetic conditions associated with mental retardation, relating them to the stage of development at which the pathological factor operates.

Infections and intoxications

Syphilis

In times past, syphilis was an important cause of many pathological changes in the nervous system of the developing fetus. Mental retardation was a common accompaniment. Today, it is very rare for a child to be born with congenital syphilis in Western cultures, partly because of routine screening.

Rubella (German measles)

This disorder, particularly when it infects a mother during the first trimester of pregnancy, is still an important determinant of a wide variety of abnormalities in the child (Dudgeon 1967, Cooper et al 1969). Cardiac anomalies, deafness, cataracts as well as mental handicap (Chess et al 1971) are all found in a proportion of such children, the term 'rubella syndrome' having been coined for infants thus affected.

The incidence is greatest when the infection occurs at the very start of pregnancy. Because infection with rubella virus may be subclinical and pass unnoticed, there is a case for testing all teenage schoolgirls to ascertain the small proportion who have not acquired natural immunity by their teen years. Girls at risk can then be offered active immunisation against the disorder. In this way termination of pregnancy may be avoided, a situation particularly distressing if there has been some problem of fertility in the couple concerned.

Other infections

Other infections affecting the fetus include toxoplasmosis, influenza, and cytomegalic inclusion body disease. The exact manner in which these infections cause mental retardation is still being evaluated.

Table 28.2   Some non-genetic conditions associated with mental retardation

Antenatal	Perinatal	Postnatal/childhood
Maternal infection: Cytomegalovirus Rubella Syphilis Toxoplasmosis	**Prematurity:** Predisposing to cerebral palsy **Physical injury to baby during labour with/without:** Birth asphyxia/hypoxia Intraventricular haemorrhage	**Infections:** Encephalitis Meningitis
Endocrine disorders: Hypothyroidism/cretinism Hypoparathyroidism		**Injury:** Accidents 'Non-accidental injury'
Maternal intoxication: Alcohol Lead Mercury Drugs, e.g. thiouracil		**Metabolic:** Hyperbilirubinaemia (Rhesus incompatibility ± prematurity) Hypoglycaemia
Maternal illness during pregnancy: Antepartum haemorrhage Toxaemia		**Status epilepticus:**
Maternal physical damage: Hypoxia Injury		**Toxic:** Lead poisoning

Bacterial meningitis has long been recognised as liable to result in subsequent mental retardation. Overall it remains unclear just how important infections are as a cause of mental retardation, but the subject demands and is getting a good deal of attention. The possible development of a safe vaccine to reduce the incidence of mental retardation due to cytomegalovirus is an important priority.

Environmental and related factors

Further environmental factors that may cause damage to the brain around the time of birth include bilirubin encephalopathy (*kernicterus*). The disorder is now preventable by exchange transfusion techniques, and is usually due to rhesus incompatibility between the fetus and the mother. It may however also result from other sorts of blood incompatibilities. In other instances, this sort of encephalopathy may be associated with prematurity or with neonatal sepsis.

The encephalomyelitis that may occur following vaccination or triple vaccine is the commonest type of encephalitis occurring in Britain. These disorders are associated with a high mortality, and mental retardation may occur in those that survive. Other sorts of encephalitis—such as that following measles and mumps—are not as common. Encephalopathy may also be associated with lead or carbon monoxide poisoning, the former becoming less common now with the reduction in the amount of lead-based paint in use for house decorations or manufacture of painted toys.

Brain damage may occur in relation to childbirth due to obstetrical difficulties. The types of lesion that are common include tears in the meninges with damage to blood vessels and brain tissue. Such bleeding naturally causes cerebral damage, and subsequent retardation—both intellectual and physical—can clearly be expected. Improvements in obstetrical skills are lessening the incidence of such damage; but at the same time children are now being prevented from dying at birth by improved intensive care. In this way—the outcome of pyrrhic therapeutic victories—the number of children who are destined to spend their lives as residents in facilities for the mentally retarded is being constantly replenished. Cerebral palsy (i.e. congenital spastic paralysis, congenital diplegia, etc.) includes a range of chronic non-progressive disorders of motor function (Ingram 1966). The aetiology of cerebral palsy includes any of a wide variety of antenatal, perinatal and postnatal factors, with prematurity perhaps the most important. It is common to divide the syndromes of cerebral palsy into different clinical groups according to the particular clinical presentation. The work of Ingram in this field is outstanding and the reader is referred to published work by this author for more detailed expositions. Regarding the intelligence of patients with cerebral palsy, it must be remembered that perhaps as many as 50% of patients may be of normal or above normal intelligence. The intelligence of those with the extrapyramidal type of palsy tends to be higher than that of the spastic group while, understandably, patients who suffer from spastic tetraplegia are usually the most mentally retarded.

Hydrocephalus

A number of conditions that are characterised by increase in the volume of the cerebrospinal fluid are brought together under the general heading of hydrocephalus. The disorder results in enlargement of the cerebral ventricles and of the head. Causation includes a developmental malformation of uncertain origin; rarely it may be due to stenosis of the aqueduct, and sometimes to failure of development of the foramina of Luschka and Magendie in the roof of the fourth ventricle. Such anomalies are often associated with spina bifida and meningomyelocele.

Hydrocephalus may not be noted until the infant is perhaps 3 months old. Then there occurs rapid enlargement of the head circumference, with increased tension of the fontanelle, and widening of the cranial sutures. Untreated, the pressure caused by the dilatation of the lateral ventricles causes cortical atrophy and there is frequently a rapid decline in physical and mental development. Sometimes the disorder may arrest spontaneously and only a mild degree of handicap is the outcome. Operative procedures may be attempted to provide a shunt—incorporating a valve such as the Holter valve—by means of a polythene tube between the cerebral ventricles and the right side of the heart. However, it is often the case than even apparently successful surgical results may be associated with serious mental retardation so that the 'success' of the procedure cannot be regarded as unqualified. Revision operations are often required, due to valve malfunction or other blockage of the shunt.

GENETIC DEFECTS LIABLE TO BE ASSOCIATED WITH MENTAL HANDICAP

There is an account of the genetics of psychiatric disorders in Chapter 12. Table 28.3 lists certain of

Table 28.3 Examples of genetic conditions associated with mental retardation

Pathoplastic genes							Abnormal chromosomes
Gross brain disease	Metabolic disorders affecting						
	Amino acids	Carbohydrates	Lipids	Mucopolysaccharides	Purines	Urea cycle	
Tuberose sclerosis	Hartnup disease	galactosaemia	Gaucher's syndrome	Hunter's syndrome	Lesch–Nyhan syndrome	aminosuccinicaciduria	Down's syndrome
Neurofibromatosis	homocystinuria		Niemann–Pick's disease	Hurler's syndrome		citrullinuria	Fragile X syndrome
	phenylketonuria (PKU)		Tay–Sachs disease	Morquio's syndrome Sanfillipo's syndrome			Klinefelter's syndrome
							Triple-X syndrome
							Turner's syndrome
							Cri du chat syndrome

the many genetic disorders associated with mental retardation, some of which are outlined below.

Chromosomal abnormalities

The normal number of human chromosomes is 46, comprising 22 pairs, and two X chromosomes in females and an X and a Y chromosome in males. The autosomal (i.e. non-sex) chromosomes are of very different size and characteristics, and are clearly distinguished. Until recently it was only possible to group them into seven principal groups. Trisomy is the name given to the existence of an additional chromosome over and above the usual pair. Trisomy may be of the autosomal or of the sex chromosomes. If a chromosome fails to separate correctly during a meiotic division preceding ovum or sperm formation, there may be a resultant aneuploidy. This is the commonest sort of chromosomal abnormality. While this may affect all cells, sometimes mosaicism may occur, so that a mixture of normal and aneuploid cells exist. In other instances there may be apparent damage to two chromosomes, so that translocation of parts of the affected chromosomes can occur. There then follows a joining up of the broken chromosomal portions in an abnormal way—hence the term 'translocation'.

It is likely that about 5% of all fetuses have chromosomal abnormalities; and that about 90% of these abort. Of live newborn infants, 0.5% have such abnormalities, of which one-third affect sex chromosomes and two-thirds affect autosomal chromosomes. Certain abnormalities of chromosome karyotype are associated with mental retardation and the more common of these will now be described.

Abnormalities of autosomal chromosomes

Down's syndrome (mongolism; trisomy 21). The first detailed description of this disorder is attributed to the English physician Langdon Down in 1866. There are many theories as to the aetiology of the disorder, and it is recognised that there are a number of different types. It is known that maternal age has an influence on the incidence of the disorder. Further, it is probable that increased paternal age and also X-ray radiation may sometimes be implicated. Among patients with an IQ less than 50, one-third have Down's syndrome. Indeed, few Down's syndrome patients have an IQ greater than 50. One in 660 live births is a Down's syndrome baby, though the incidence at 20 years of age is only about one in 2000. For mothers aged 45 years and over, the incidence is one in 50 (Ratcliffe et al 1970).

Patients with Down's syndrome usually have trisomy of chromosome 21. It may be complete, there being three of chromosome 21 in every cell, instead of the usual pair. Mothers of such patients have a normal chromosomal pattern; and these cases account for 95% of Down's syndrome patients. In about 4% of cases of Down's syndrome, it is a result of translocation. Here, fusion occurs at a certain stage of fetal development between a chromosome in group D (as is chromosome 21) and genetic material from another chromosome. In translocation cases, unaffected parents and siblings may be found possessing the translocation chromosome: these carriers have only 45 chromosomes, while the patient has 46 and may manifest all or few features of Down's syndrome. In about 1% of cases, the patient has a mosaic pattern—only a proportion of cells have trisomy, the rest of the body's cells having a normal chromosome constitution.

Numerous stigmata characterise the disorder, including oblique palpebral fissures, small flattened skull, high cheek bones, tongue apparently too big for the mouth, broad hands with stubby fingers, a single transverse palmar crease, and incurved little fingers. Often the tongue is fissured, height is less than average, ears are small and rounded and a squint is common. Brushfield spots may be seen on the iris. There are frequently abnormalities in the dermatoglyphs, as described by Penrose & Smith (1966). While hand, finger and foot prints are of course unique to every individual, chromosomal abnormalities affect the formation of dermal ridges and patterns; in mosaics, the extent of the mosaicism parallels the extent of the dermatoglyphic abnormality (Penrose 1963, Loesch 1974).

The feet are commonly short and broad, with a large cleft between the first and second toes. There is usually poor development of male external genitals and cryptorchidism is frequent. Pubic hair is usually straight. About 50% of cases have congenital cardiac pathology. Death due to this used to be common, particularly in the early years of life, but owing to cardiac surgery this is no longer so in developed countries. Mental retardation is a prominent feature of the syndrome, most patients being moderately or severely retarded. While it is commonly reported that these patients are cheerful and fond of rhythmic movements and dancing, and characterised by relatively easy and cooperative management at home, this is not always the case in those who survive to late adolescence and adult life. By this stage, they may manifest a variety of behavioural difficulties that may make formalised care necessary.

Senile plaques in the brain occur early, apparently a feature of genetic programming. Cognitive deterioration is usual from middle age onwards, and hypothyroidism quite commonly develops. Using auditory event-related potential studies, it has been shown that all those Down's syndrome patients showing signs of dementia on clinical psychological testing also show a marked increase in P300 latency. This starts to be evident around 37 years of age, whereas in control subjects (both normal volunteers and people with fragile X syndrome) the feature did not start to appear until 17 years later, around 54 years of age (Blackwood et al 1988).

An infant born with Down's syndrome may nowadays be expected to have a lifespan extending well into late middle age. In Western society those with serious congenital heart defects will often be successfully operated on; and there are now more adults with the syndrome than children—a position not yet reached in many developing countries (Fryers 1986). It is, however, of interest to note that female patients with Down's syndrome living in institutions appear to have a higher mortality rate than those living outside. This is not the case with male patients (Dupont et al 1986). Whereas there used to be considerably higher mortality rates in all age groups 50 years ago compared to the general population, the difference now has been shown to be relatively small. Indeed, in relation to congenital heart disease, a large-scale study in Scotland revealed no difference in mortality between Down's syndrome children with such disease and those without it (Murdoch 1985). This is assumed to be due to improved drug treatment, diet and general care. An important implication is that future services for the mentally retarded must take account of an ageing population (Carter & Jancar 1983).

Trisomy 13 (Patau's syndrome). This disorder, affecting only one in 7600 live births, was first described by Patau et al (1960), and is characterised by numerous abnormalities, including cleft palate and lip, polydactyly, sloping forehead, low-set ears, and cardiac and ophthalmic defects. Almost all die by the age of 3 years; half die within a month of birth. Like Down's syndrome and trisomy 18 (see below), trisomy 13 is associated with greater maternal age.

Trisomy 18 (Edward's syndrome). This syndrome occurs in one in 3500 live births, and appears to be rather more common in females than males. The infant is characterised by a prominent occiput, cardiac abnormalities, a small chin, low-set ears, and quite severe mental retardation. As is the case with other chromosomal abnormalities, there are dermatoglyphic anomalies. Half the cases survive more than 2 months, very few a matter of years.

The cat-cry syndrome (cri du chat). In this disorder, affecting only one in 50 000 live births, there is absence of part of chromosome 5. Lejeune et al reported the chromosomal abnormality in 1963. The mental defect is severe in these cases and microcephaly is usual, along with facial abnormalities. A distinctive cat-like cry, high-pitched and wailing, is typical. The patient may survive to adulthood.

Abnormalities of the sex chromosomes

These disorders are usually typified by a lesser degree of mental retardation, and there may even be normal or above average intelligence. Many deviations of the normal sex chromosome pattern for men and women have been described, some of which are very rare.

Fragile X syndrome (Martin–Bell–Renpenning syndrome). Thirty years ago (Renpenning et al 1962) a syndrome was reported which was observed to run in families as an apparently X-linked form of mental retardation: the observation was a sequel to an earlier report (Martin & Bell 1943) of a pedigree of mental retardation showing sex linkage. Male offspring of possible female carriers were at risk and no special clinical features of the syndrome were noted. Somewhat later, a liability to large, floppy ears, prognathism and macro-orchidism was added to the clinical description, together with serious impairment of speech: these features were not, however, found in all cases. In more recent years it has been noted that a fragile site at band q27–28 on the X chromosome is strongly associated with X-linked mental retardation in males. This fragility is revealed when, for example, blood lymphocytes are cultured in a medium deficient in folic acid.

Fragile X syndrome has been found in 9.2 per 10 000 of the general male population (Herbst & Miller 1980). It has been estimated that between 2 and 20% of mentally retarded males have this disorder undiagnosed, and it is the second commonest known cause of mental retardation in males.

In a cytogenetic survey of a mentally retarded school-age population with special reference to fragile sites, Webb et al (1987) found that fragile X syndrome was second only to Down's syndrome as a cytogenetic entity contributing to mental retardation among school-age children.

The identification of affected individuals is most important, since the risk of hereditary mental retardation in other family members can then be determined, permitting genetic counselling. Ultimately it ought thereby to be possible to prevent this common form of mental retardation, the severity of which is usually moderate, though all degrees are seen (Neilsen 1983). Recent studies suggest reduced intellectual functioning in about a third of female carriers as well, with a liability to have poor muscle tone, hyper-extensibility of joints, prominent ears and elongated faces (Chudley et al 1983, Madison et al 1986). Among male cases a higher level of cognitive functioning has been shown in the performance area (e.g. copying designs, completing puzzles) than in the verbal and memory areas. Speech tends to be higher pitched than in normal males, and hypernasality is common.

Fragile X has also been found in normal males (Daker et al 1981) and it has been transmitted through a male, through two generations (Webb et al 1981). Prenatal diagnosis of fragile X syndrome has now been shown to be feasible (Jenkins et al 1981, Shapiro et al 1982). It has been suggested that the fragility of the fragile X chromosome might possibly be remediable— both in vitro and in vivo—by use of substances such as folic acid (Lejeune 1982). If validated, this suggestion could open promising therapeutic doors in the prevention of mental retardation. (See Davies 1989, Hirst et al 1992.)

Klinefelter's syndrome. In this syndrome, male patients have atrophy of the testes which is evident at puberty, and there may be signs of feminisation such as gynaecomastia. It occurs in one in 1400 (0.7 per 1000) live births. The commonest karyotype is XXY, but a variety of others have been described as well as certain mosaic patterns. More than half of the cases have a female-type chromatin characteristic in cells, showing one or more Barr bodies. The degree of mental retardation is very variable, and some cases are of normal or above average intelligence. Probably because of the sexual abnormality, some patients may become behaviourally abnormal in adolescence. Diabetes mellitus is rather common, but in other respects health is usually good.

Turner's syndrome (XO). This disorder, affecting one in 3300 (0.3 per 1000) live births, is associated with absence of Barr bodies in cells (i.e. chromatin-negative). There is usually deletion of the Y chromosome, with only a single X chromosome remaining. Bodily these patients are female, but there is failure to develop normal secondary sex characteristics. Mental retardation is not usual, though it may occur. Webbing of the neck, dwarfism, and other deformities may be found, including cubitus valgus. Kidney and cardiac defects are common, a third of cases having coarctation of the aorta. Treatment with oestrogens by way of substitution may be attempted.

The XYY syndrome. A small number of patients with this chromosomal pattern was reported by Jacobs et al (1965). An association between this sex chromosome anomaly and aggressive or criminal behaviour was originally suspected, but now appears of doubtful significance. It affects one in 1400 (0.7 per 1000) live births. Patients are usually over 1.9 m tall, but have no other special physical characteristics. Mental retardation is not invariable, but many subjects have been identified in hospitals for the retarded.

The XXX syndrome. This so-called 'superfemale' disorder affects one in 1600 (0.6 per 1000) live births. It is compatible with normal mental and physical status, though a proportion of such women are mentally retarded and have underdeveloped sexual characteristics.

Aberrant single genes associated with mental retardation

Nearly 10% of patients with severe mental retardation are found to have some abnormality—dominant or recessive—either of a particular autosome or of sex chromosome constitution.

Autosomal dominant disorders

There is a group of abnormalities in which a single dominant gene of variable expression and penetrance is responsible. The disorders are rare, though one of them—tuberous sclerosis—accounts for almost 1% of the population of mental retardation hospitals.

Tuberous sclerosis. The incidence of this disorder is between one in 20 000 and one in 40 000 live births. There are skin lesions that include a so-called 'butterfly rash' over the face, often beginning in the crease between the nose and the cheeks. The rash usually begins in the preschool years, and essentially consists of hyperplastic vascular and connective tissue. Macules also develop over the trunk. Epilepsy is usual. One-third of cases are not mentally retarded, but patients with numerous physical abnormalities usually are.

Tumours may be found in other parts of the body also, including the heart, kidneys, liver and also the retinae. *Café-au-lait* areas may be seen in the skin. Death is due to such complications as heart failure and pneumonia, though life expectancy is variable according to the severity of pathological features. There is no specific treatment.

Sturge–Weber syndrome (encephalofacial angiomatosis). This disorder is not thought to be hereditary and relatives are not affected. There is classically a facial naevus, usually in the distribution of the fifth cranial nerve. Coupled with this there is angiomatous malformation within the skull; this commonly becomes calcified and therefore evident on radiography. Glaucoma may result from a capillary haemangioma affecting the anterior chamber of the eye. Half the patients are mentally retarded and epilepsy affects the majority.

Neurofibromatosis (von Recklinghausen's disease). The genetic abnormality here is of autosomal dominant type. Incidence is as high as one in 3000 live births. Clinically, there are pigmented patches distributed over much of the skin, mostly corresponding to the distribution of the subcutaneous nerves. These patches increase during childhood and adolescence. Skin tumours may arise, which are polyp in nature and sometimes very numerous. Intracranial tumours may also develop, including neurofibromas of the cranial nerves, especially the acoustic nerve: they are prone to sarcomatous change.

Only about one-third of these patients are mentally retarded, and this is not usually severe. The prognosis is chiefly governed by the development or otherwise of malignant change in the lesions. Treatment can only be symptomatic.

Autosomal recessive disorders

So far as mental retardation is concerned, these disorders are represented by syndromes associated with *metabolic* disorders. There are a large number of metabolic abnormalities which may be associated with varying degrees of intellectual defect. It should be stressed at the outset that the presence of a particular abnormality does not imply the probability of any particular degree of intellectual impairment. Further, a great many of these disorders which have been delineated in recent years are very rare and only a few cases have been reported in the literature.

It is convenient to describe the metabolic abnormalities in groups, according to the nature of the metabolic abnormality. For example, there are the disturbances of protein metabolism (hereditary aminoacidurias), disturbances of carbohydrate metabolism, the mucopolysaccharidoses, disturbances of lipid metabolism, and a group of disorders, all of which are rare, that are not so much metabolic as anatomical abnormalities inherited as Mendelian dominants. This last group comprises the phakomatoses. A fuller account of the genetic aspect of these conditions may be found in Chapter 12.

Disorders of protein metabolism: hereditary aminoacidurias

It may be said that, where the genetics of these disorders have been thoroughly clarified, they are almost always recessive in type. These inborn errors of metabolism are mostly very rare, and only one will be described.

Phenylketonuria. This metabolic disorder was first discovered in 1934 by Folling, and it has been studied extensively. It accounts for over 1% of institutionalised mentally retarded people, being exceeded in frequency—among those who are mentally retarded where the aetiology is known—only by mongolism and fragile X syndrome (Berg 1959, Penrose 1963, Kolb 1968). Incidence is about one in 14 000 live births, ranging between one in 5 000 and one in 20 000 in different parts of the UK (0.2 to 0.05 per 1 000).

Basically the metabolic defect consists of an inability to convert an essential amino acid—phenylalanine—to tyrosine on account of the relevant enzyme, phenylalanine hydroxylase, being inactive or absent. A screening test is applied to all newborn babies in Britain, either the Guthrie (microbiological) test or a biochemical phenylalanine determination on capillary blood. The affected patient is commonly severely handicapped, though on occasion the degree of defect is much less than this. However, it has been found that, if it is possible to use a diet low in phenylalanine for feeding the baby, mental retardation can be avoided (Koch et al 1963). It is essential that such a diet should be instituted while the child is still only weeks or at the most a few months old, otherwise mental retardation is bound to be the consequence of the cerebral damage that occurs. The blood level of phenylalanine has to be kept below 10 mg per 100 ml during the first year of life, and it is still uncertain how long the dietary restriction has to be enforced in order to avoid mental retardation. Children with phenylketonuria whose special diet was stopped at the age of 6 years failed to show increases in mean IQ, reading and spelling ability, whereas those who continued the diet up to the age of 10 years improved on these measures (Fishler et al 1989). All the phenylketonuric children studied scored more poorly on tests of visual perception and on visual–motor skills. The authors concluded that it was prudent to continue the diet throughout the teens, given the stresses of school years for these people.

In an interesting case study, Harper and Reid (1987) found that a restricted protein/high-energy diet resulted in significant improvement in the behaviour disorder of a severely mentally retarded adult woman in her 50s who suffered from phenylketonuria.

It must also be remembered that a minimum of phenylalanine is essential in the diet.

Disorders of carbohydrate metabolism

Again, many different types of these disorders have been reported, though only a few cases are to be found among the residents of facilities for the mentally retarded.

In common with the majority of metabolic abnormalities that are liable to be associated with mental retardation, these disorders are mostly of relatively recent discovery, principally over the past 25 years.

Galactosaemia. This disorder is inherited as an autosomal recessive abnormality. Incidence is about one in 30 000 live births in the UK, less common elsewhere: it is thus decidedly rare. Galactose accumulates in the blood owing to failure to convert it to glucose on account of an enzyme defect. The relevant enzyme is absent from the liver and red blood cells.

Like phenylketonuria, galactosaemia gives some hope for prevention of serious mental retardation in persons born with the relevant metabolic abnormality. Exclusion of galactose from the diet, provided this is done early, is reported as preventing all clinical manifestations of the disease, including the physical failure to thrive as well as the mental retardation. It seems probable that in due course—perhaps around the age of 5 or 6 years—the child may be able to ingest galactose without risk, at least in limited quantities, as a result of the development of alternative pathways for its metabolism.

Mucopolysaccharidoses

Gargoylism (Hurler's disease). This disorder is usually due to an autosomal recessive gene, though sex-linked recessive transmission has been reported in male subjects. The metabolic abnormality causes an accumulation of a mucopolysaccharide and glycolipids in the brain and other organs. Clinically, the subject has a large head, corneal clouding, thickened long bones, hepatosplenomegaly and kyphosis: there is a progressive though often slow deterioration that starts in early infancy. Death usually occurs prior to adolescence. The disease got its name from the typical facial appearance.

Other mucopolysaccharidoses. These include the more benign Hunter's syndrome, in which the mental retardation may be mild, corneal clouding is absent, and survival into adulthood common.

Disorders of fat metabolism (lipidoses)

Here, lipid is deposited in cells of the nervous system with resultant physical and mental abnormalities. Two such diseases will be mentioned.

Cerebromacular degeneration (amaurotic family idiocy). In the infantile and juvenile forms of this disease there appears to be an autosomal recessive genetic abnormality, but in the adult type—where the onset may be in the later teens or 20s—the genetics are less certain. The infantile form is also known as Tay–Sachs disease. It is commonest in Jews, and this distinguishes it from other types of cerebromacular degenerations which are found in all races. The incidence of Tay–Sachs disease among American Jews is one in 6000. Lipids accumulate throughout the central nervous system, including the ganglion cells of the retina. It is this latter feature which causes the progressive blindness. The disorder usually manifests itself in the earlier months of life, when the child appears listless and weak, with slow mental development. Spasticity is common, and the characteristic 'cherry-red spot' is to be seen at the macula of the retinae. The disorder is invariably progressive, and death has usually occurred before the age of four years.

In the juvenile type of the disorder, the clinical picture may not present itself until the child is of school age. Visual difficulties may then present, and the disorder may thereafter progressively impair both physical and mental development, with ataxia, fits and blindness. Death is usual before the age of 20 years. No specific treatment is available for the cerebromacular degenerations.

Niemann–Pick disease. Transmitted as an autosomal recessive abnormality, this too is a disorder which occurs especially in Jews: between a third and a half of cases are Jewish. There is abnormal storage of sphingomyelin. A number of forms of the disease have been described. On account of this abnormality, brain functioning is affected. It may manifest itself at any time from early infancy to young school years. There are both physical and mental abnormalities, with hepatic and splenic enlargement causing abdominal prominence, anaemia, and occasionally a similar 'cherry-red spot' at the macula to that seen in the cerebromacular degenerations. The deterioration in mental functioning is commonly accompanied by epilepsy.

A third type of disorder, considered to be related to the lipidoses, is that group known as the progressive leucodystrophies. They comprise many syndromes in which the white matter of the brain degenerates in a diffuse, symmetrical fashion. Onset may occur at any time from infancy onwards. The mode of inheritance is autosomal recessive, except in certain types of the disorder where a sex-linked recessive gene is responsible. The leucodystrophies invariably have a bad prognosis, as no treatment is available. Progressive mental and physical deterioration, commonly with ataxia, blindness, deafness and fits, is the sort of pattern followed. Death is usual before 2 years of age.

X-linked disorders

There are several X-linked disorders associated with mental retardation. Recent interest here has centred on the X-linked type of mental handicap where there is a fragile site at the end of the long arm of the X chromosome.

X-linked recessive inheritance is typified by males only being affected, with transmission through healthy female carriers. Any female children of an affected male are all carriers.

Besides fragile X syndrome, other X-linked mental handicap disorders include the Lesch–Nyhan syndrome (hyperuricaemia with choreoathetosis), due to deficiency of the enzyme hypoxanthineguanine, phosphoribosyltransferase (HGPRT). Self-mutilation is common, as are torsion spasms, typically of the neck muscles. Custom-made mouthguards and gloves are valuable in minimising self-injurious behaviour (Wurtele et al 1984).

The association of haemoglobin H (HbH) disease with mental retardation was first reported in 1981 (Weatherall et al 1981). A further entity has now been defined—the α-thalassaemia/mental retardation (ATR-X) syndrome. Where there is deletion involving the α-globin gene complex on chromosome 16p, HbH disease may be associated with mild to moderate mental retardation. But where there is non-deletion, a (usually) mild form of HbH disease may be associated with severe mental retardation. This is characterised by microcephaly and short stature, hypertelorism, convulsions, mid-face hypoplasia, and genital abnormalities.

All the non-deletion patients are chromosomal males. It therefore seems probable that a mutation on the X chromosome is responsible, with sex-linked recessive inheritance. This illustrates a further instance of the X chromosome comprising the locus of a mental retardation syndrome (Donnai et al 1991).

Epilepsy and mental retardation

A liability to epileptic seizures adds a substantial burden to that already carried by the parents of a mentally retarded child. Epilepsy is one of the commonest added disabilities in these people, and is especially likely in those with more severe degrees of mental retardation. In the latter cases, fits represent an indicant of the same neurological disorder which underlies the mental retardation.

While epilepsy only affects about 0.6% of all school-children, 3–6% of children whose IQ lies between 50 and 70 have a persisting tendency to fits. Where IQ is less than 50, 44% of patients have been found to have one or more seizures by the age of 22 years (Richardson et al 1981). Mentally retarded males were found to be four times as likely to have fits as females. A recent study from Scandinavia on a random sample of over 300 mentally retarded adults showed that 18% had had epilepsy at some time, and that 8% had had a fit in the past year (Lund 1985a). Of equal significance was the finding that, among those patients who had had a fit in the past year, it was possible to establish a Present State Examination psychiatric diagnosis in over 50% compared to 26% in those without seizures. The combination of epilepsy and psychiatric disorder in the mentally retarded often appears to reflect underlying brain pathology in the form of widespread cortical and subcortical damage, with psychiatric disorders dominated by behaviour problems.

Neuroleptic drugs do not precipitate seizures in mentally retarded patients who have no history of fits when low to moderate drug dosages are used. But in those with a history of epilepsy who are either receiving inadequate anticonvulsant medication, or whose fits are poorly controlled despite adequate anti-convulsant levels, the frequency of fits is liable to increase. It is possible that thioridazine is less epileptogenic than other phenothiazines (James 1986). Improvement in the overall wellbeing of these patients when carefully planned reductions are made in the number of anticonvulsant drugs prescribed has been demonstrated (Fischbacher 1982, 1985).

The experience of persistent or severe epilepsy, especially if from an early age, is liable to be associated with deterioration in intellectual function. It is possible that this may be related not so much to high seizure frequency as to the result of long-term anticonvulsant treatment (Corbett & Trimble 1983).

Psychiatric disorder and mental retardation

It is in the context of those mentally retarded people who are also psychiatrically ill that psychiatric competence finds a particular relevance. The matter is increasingly important now, given the climate that urges community care on a wide scale for mentally retarded people. The doctrine of 'care in the community' is liable to be insisted upon in a wholesale fashion, yet the coincidence of severe mental retardation and significant psychiatric or behaviour disorder results in instances in which it is plain that round-the-clock medical and nursing care is necessary (Reid 1985).

Prompt and accurate diagnosis of coincidental psychiatric illness is thus vital, especially in view of the scope for effective treatment measure, which in turn may enable care to continue being provided in as domestic an environment as possible.

Table 28.4 outlines some of the ways in which the clinical presentation of psychiatric illness may be modified by coexistent mental retardation.

About 27% of a random sample of 302 adult mentally retarded patients were found to be suffering from a psychiatric disorder. Nearly 11% were behaviour disorders, while a range of other diagnoses accounted for the rest. Interestingly, there were no instances of

Table 28.4 Some observations on the presentation of psychiatric disorders in mentally retarded people

Schizophrenia	Difficult to ascertain; disruption of thought processes in light of their underdevelopment; normal fantasy in the mentally retarded may be misinterpreted as evidence of psychosis; altered (especially strange) behaviour; poverty of thought; motor mannerisms of schizophrenia are similar to those of severe mental retardation
Manic–depressive disorder	Change in overall level of activity, $\uparrow$ or $\downarrow$; excitability; may be attempts to injure self (or others) often ineffectually; changed appearance, sleep and eating patterns; mood variability
Neurosis	Usually precipitated by environmental circumstances; conversion symptoms, phobias are common; distress following losses including actual or presumed bereavement
Personality disorder	Liable to be diagnosed where patient's environment is apparently inimicable to him; self-perceptions of the mentally retarded as someone who has 'failed'/disappointed his parents/family may be aetiological
Organic psychiatric disorder	With increased life expectancy, enhanced risk of Alzheimer dementia in Down's syndrome is now more evident; in severe retardation, brain injury may be both its cause and also the cause of associated psychiatric disorder/symptoms; epilepsy common, with its own clinical concomitants, e.g. hyperkinesis; aggression and self-harm are associated with the brain injury of Lesch–Nyhan syndrome and of inadequately managed phenylketonuria
Behaviour disorder	Repeated purposeless activities, self-injury including head banging; rocking; excess emotionality
Sexual disorder	Usually manifests as a relative lack of sexual discreteness

alcohol or drug abuse (Lund 1985b). The rate of significant psychiatric disorder in people in hospitals for the mentally retarded was reported as two to three times greater than in those attending training centres (Ballinger & Reid 1977). Importantly, they point out that even relatively minor 'behavioural quirks' and psychiatric symptoms may cause problems for those who are dependent on others.

Several factors predispose mentally retarded people to psychiatric illness, including the frequent existence of brain damage and the personal and social consequences of being retarded. The subject is clearly described by Reid (1982, 1983), who stresses the contemporary psychiatrist's role in an area of disability management in which far more distinct professional contributions can be made than was the case a few decades ago. One worrying result of the widespread dispersal of mentally retarded people into the community from institutional care has recently been identified in Denmark. A rapid rise in the number of psychiatric retarded subjects admitted to psychiatric illness hospitals has occurred. It is pointed out that the diagnosis of psychiatric illness in these patients is complicated by the coincidental mental retardation, with divergent clinical pictures in many cases. The need for medical and other staff knowledgeable about retardation is clear, and is particularly necessary when factors such as associated sensory deficits, epilepsy and cerebral palsy are present.

Because hospitals for the mentally retarded now look after an increasing concentration of the severely disabled, they are unsuitable for the temporary admission of less disabled people with a psychiatric disorder. Equally, an ordinary psychiatric illness hospital is ill-equipped to cope sensitively with the latter cases (Lund 1985c).

Bearing in mind the descriptions outlined in Table 28.4, it is of interest that Fraser et al (1986) found that behaviour disturbances were not usually expressions of psychiatric disturbances. They found that clinical features were usually reliably diagnosed at psychiatric interview, though they also found and accepted that the communicativeness of an interviewee limited the detection of depression in the mentally retarded.

CHILDHOOD PSYCHOSIS

Introduction

The term childhood psychosis is used here in a special sense; it excludes childhood schizophrenia or late-onset psychosis (Kolvin 1971) and also manic-depressive illness in childhood. It refers to those children with the condition Wing has called early childhood autism

(Wing 1966); and those other children who are thought to be brain damaged but also show some or many of the features of the autistic child.

Phenomenology of early childhood autism

Wing (1966) describes symptoms under the headings of auditory perceptual problems, disorders of speech; visual perceptual problems, motor behaviour, odd and repetitive behaviour, abnormalities of mood and 'autistic behaviour'.

Here it is proposed to group the phenomena into five main categories: autistic behaviour, auditory and visual perceptual problems, motor phenomena, obsessive and ritualistic behaviour and disorders of speech.

Autistic behaviour

Whereas early authors (Kanner & Eisenberg 1955) had suggested that autistic aloneness and failure to form relationships were the central or primary disorder and the other symptoms were in a sense derivative, it is now clear (Rutter 1966) that the autism may improve substantially in later childhood and adolescence while the other symptoms remain unchanged. It is therefore proposed that 'autism' is a central symptom but one which is not related causally to other symptoms, except possibly some of the motor phenomena. The features which comprise autism are these: as a baby the child did not respond to his mother's voice or hold out his arms to be lifted up; later on he seemed aloof, would turn his head away when talked to, seemed indifferent to the presence of others, would not play with other children, and failed to make or maintain eye contact.

Auditory and visual perceptual disorders

There seems to be increasing agreement that some type of auditory imperception is a feature of autistic children. Often they are, or have been considered to be, deaf because they make no reaction to loud noises; on the other hand, they can usually detect the traditional rustle of a sweet-paper and enjoy music, many being able to sing even when they cannot talk. It does seem as if there is a specific difficulty in decoding auditory information, especially speech.

In the visual modality, these children seem to find it difficult to 'separate figure from ground'. They use peripheral as opposed to central vision and can identify moving objects better than stationary ones. An object may be identified by moving it up and down in front of the eyes; parents often develop the habit of waving their arms when approaching the child so that he will recognise them.

Motor phenomena

Overactivity or hyperkinesis is very common between ages three and five; it is often replaced in adolescence with apathy and hypokinesis (Rutter et al 1967). Special movements such as flapping wrists, flicking fingers, jumping up and down and whole-body spinning are characteristic. Many have a peculiar tiptoe gait which mimics that seen in congenital equinovarus deformities. Finger movements on the edge of the visual field are common in these children, as in the partially blind. Secondary self-stimulation such as rocking, head banging, self-biting and scratching are common though not diagnostic. However, in a hospital population it is clear that self-injury is much commoner amongst psychotic patients than among other subgroups, e.g. Down's syndrome.

Obsessive and ritualistic behaviour

Kanner described an obsessive desire for the maintenance of sameness. One autistic boy, aged 20 years, was moved to another ward and caused much concern by repeatedly running away from his new ward and returning to the old one. Collecting objects such as bits of plastic, pieces of paper or cotton reels are common features. Sometimes one object, a piece of cloth, a toy or a piece of string with knots in it, are retained as 'special' objects. Often the piece of string or cloth is used in flicking rituals. Sometimes obsessive rigidity leads to an insistence on exactly the same eating utensils placed in exactly the same manner on the table, or to complex food fads. One man aged 50 years ate only crisps, bread, cheese and milk for 30 years. For the crisps he had a special ritual: he tipped them into his left jacket pocket where he proceeded to crush them and then ate the fragments with great enjoyment.

Disorders of speech

Speech often starts at about 2 years of age and is then lost; other children never begin to speak. In some cases speech begins late, perhaps at age 5 or 6 years, and progresses slowly. Lenneberg et al (1964) have shown that in Down's syndrome there is a delay in all stages, i.e. babbling, echolalia, single words, phrases and so on. This is not the case in autism: when the child begins to speak, he reveals a fairly advanced phrase level of language. Also there are specific peculiarities about the speech of autistic children: echolalia, pronominal reversal, use of personalised neologisms and a preference for 'no' rather than 'yes'.

Echolalia is characteristic; the last words of what is said to the child are repeated, often with the same tone and inflection. Sometimes this repetitive speech is delayed from the actual time of hearing but the original speaker's tone and inflection are retained. One patient endlessly repeated the admonitions of the charge nurse: 'Jocky mustn't be a bad boy, he mustn't pull down the curtains, Jocky must be a good boy', and so on. Further information on childhood autism may be found in Chapter 29.

Autism with fragile X chromosome marker

An association of the fragile X chromosome with autism has been reported (Gillberg et al 1986). In a series of ten boys with both conditions, features not inherent in the diagnosis of autism were seen: epilepsy, brainstem dysfunction and a range of psychiatric symptoms. The authors suggest that up to 20% of autistic boys may have the fragile X chromosome abnormality as one important background factor, possibly of major aetiological significance. Other studies have raised the possibility that all fragile X boys may be liable to exhibit autistic features.

Brain-damaged children with autistic features

This forms the larger group and presents the major problem in management in the context of the hospital for the mentally retarded. Goldfarb (1961) found that he could subdivide his 'schizophrenic' (his term) children into organic and non-organic groups. Rutter's follow-up study (Rutter et al 1967) showed how many of these children later developed epilepsy or other evidence of brain damage or dysfunction.

In essence these children go through a protracted period of hyperkinesis. They are mentally retarded and they also show some or many of the features of autism: most commonly they show body spinning, finger flicking, obsessional rituals and attachments to objects. Many show gaze avoidance and a tendency to take the adult by the hand to whatever object they want. Language, which may or may not have started well, falls further and further behind the age expectation. Self-injurious behaviour is characteristic and makes this group of children most difficult to manage. In late adolescence and early adult life the hyperactivity is often replaced by apathy.

It is possible that some of these children represent cases of Rett's syndrome, first described in Germany in the 1960s, and reported again recently by Hagberg

et al (1983) and by others. Hagberg described a progressive syndrome of autism, dementia, ataxia and loss of purposeful hand movement, exclusively in girls. The series was drawn from three European countries, and revealed normal development up to between seven and 18 months. Developmental stagnation then occurred, and was followed by rapid deterioration of higher brain functions within a further 18 months. There then followed a period of apparent stability lasting through decades, with additional insidious neurological abnormalities supervening. The restriction to girls suggests a dominant mutation on one X chromosome, with male hemizygous conceptuses being non-viable.

OUTLINE OF SERVICES FOR THE MENTALLY RETARDED

The majority of subnormal children and adults live at home and make few demands on any specialised services. Even amongst the severely retarded, Kushlick showed that 80% of children and nearly 50% of severely retarded adults were cared for at home (Kushlick 1966).

It is essential to bear in mind that the *family* remains the principal source of support for the mentally retarded. In providing services the contemporary view is that this should be assisted and enhanced, avoiding concentration on residential care. Having said that, it must equally be emphasised that 'care in the community' is in danger of becoming a fashionable shibboleth, a cry taken up all round because of a swing of the pendulum against institutional care. There is no doubt that many mentally retarded people who now live in hospitals are quite capable of living in ordinary houses in ordinary communities. Often the fact that they are not doing so is a function of formerly overt, and nowadays somewhat covert, prejudice on the part both of the relevant local authorities and of the public at large. Such prejudice is quite as prevalent among well-educated sections of society as among the least sophisticated; indeed, the latter appear to assimilate their mentally handicapped citizens more equably than the middle classes.

But the impact of a seriously mentally retarded person on the rest of the family must not be underestimated. Quite heroic measures and adaptations are often made in the home, where life may come to pivot almost totally around the handicapped person. Tensions may arise among his siblings, who perceive—rightly or wrongly—positive discrimination in his favour, not just in respect of his obvious disabilities but in everything. Because the parents may not both judge the position in the same way, marital strife may slowly foment and family disintegration is by no means rare, leaving a train of unfulfilled aspirations around the perplexed key figure (Gath 1977).

Obviously, serious family discord is not inevitable in such circumstances. Many families seem to be happily welded together around their retarded member (Gath 1973). But the concept of 'the greatest happiness of the greatest number' must be kept in mind when decisions are being made about where a retarded person should live. If he could articulate his wishes clearly, he too—like most people—might prefer to live with others who see the world from his angle.

It is easier to help a mentally retarded person to settle into life in a group home while he is still relatively young than when parental death forces the issue once he is middle-aged. One is, of course, assuming a residential setting of domestic scale, whatever administrative background it may have—hostel, sheltered housing, group home, and so on.

This caveat concerning community care is mentioned simply to remind the reader that such care is not without its own penalties. For many mentally retarded people, the community at large can be an unsympathetic place. This may be so despite the support provided by social work and community nursing professionals. The risk of simply translating institutional ghettos into council estate mini-ghettos is real; and the potential for undetected exploitation is greater in the latter context.

Clearly the mentally retarded and their families have as much right as any others to health and social services, and should be treated as 'normally' as possible. For example, there is usually no reason why a mentally retarded person who has pneumonia and requires admission to hospital should not be treated in an ordinary ward; and yet it is not uncommon for such patients to be treated in a special ward for the psychiatrically disturbed sick.

Assessment of need

There is an urgent need for properly organised assessment of any child as soon as retardation is suspected. Some areas are moving toward the provision of assessment centres as suggested in *Better Services for the Mentally Handicapped* (Department of Health and Social Security 1971). Some centres will be organised by education or social work departments while others have been centred on paediatric or mental retardation hospitals and clinics. It is probably less important under whose auspices assessment is organised than that it should occur. There are advantages in experimenting with different organisational frameworks for assessment

centres as long as the impact of each is carefully evaluated. There is, however, no doubt that the professional representation at the time of assessment should be broad and that assessment should start early in the child's life and be a recurrent process.

The assessment team should include social worker, educational psychologist, teacher, paediatrician and a medical specialist in mental retardation, along with the family doctor and the parents of the individual child. This nuclear team should have access to other related specialist services such as paediatric neurology, speech therapy, physiotherapy, genetics and orthopaedic surgery.

Mittler (1970) has stressed the importance of thorough assessment of the individual child, not only by routine intelligence tests but with detailed assessment of particular facets of learning over a long period of time, so that each child is the subject of a unique remedial programme. By focusing on specific disabilities, a plan of action can be devised for the individual child and the parents' help enlisted in carrying out some of the remedial education. Parents often welcome opportunities to participate in this. It is generally agreed that the earlier a remedial programme is started the better the prospect of the child making optimal use of his capabilities. By involving the parents in the teaching programme, planned education can start immediately after assessment, however sparse the resources may be. Parents often complain that they received least support when the infant was newly diagnosed as mentally retarded and yet found this the most agonising stage to cope with.

The assessment period therefore presents an ideal opportunity for the social worker and often the family doctor to encourage the parents to discuss their feelings and fears about their retarded child. In those uncommon situations where gross abnormality is apparent at birth, outright rejection is not uncommon and urgent help is required. Contrary to what is often believed, rejection is rare once the parents have come to know the child and then to realise he is abnormal. By then they may have had some months or years of living and caring for him and building up expectations for his future.

For the parents at this stage to have to revise these ambitions provokes mixed feelings—grief that these hopes are lost; anger that this should have happened to them or that they had been wrongly reassured in the past; denial that the child is backward; anxiety about future children they may have and the effect of this child on his siblings; and often guilt and recrimination as they search for antecedents in their lives that could have caused this. These and other conflicting emotions coexist and it is clearly a time when the family needs a chance to talk about and adjust to the crisis. The initial assessment affords the social worker an opportunity of initiating a relationship which will be developed in later interviews. The social worker will have to work in close liaison with others involved in the child's care to avoid conflicting opinions being given which would add to the parents' anxieties.

In addition to the educational and social needs of the child, the degree of any physical handicap should be ascertained. The paediatrician clearly has a central role in diagnosis and assessment. It is important that appropriate speech therapy and physiotherapy are started as early as possible for the dysarthric or spastic child.

During the assessment period a plan of action should evolve from discussion between the specialists concerned and the family. Possible need for future day or residential care can be considered. Parents should be invited to visit future residential facilities that may be anticipated for their child, so that entrance at a later age will be to familiar surroundings and a staff with whom parents and child have already established some relationship. Joint assessment from the earliest stage helps to avoid tangled communications and hopefully keep the parents as active participants in the care of their child.

It has been proposed that responsibility for ensuring assessment and service provision for the mentally retarded should lie with the health service up until school age; with the education authorities throughout school years; and with local authority social work departments thereafter. At all times there is obviously a need for close and integrated working by all types of staff.

In 1979, the Jay Report into mental handicap nursing and care was published (HMSO 1979). Nearly half the members of the committee were social workers who—like Mrs Peggy Jay who chaired the committee—felt that all mentally retarded people would be happy living in the community. The report disregarded the important minority who are either very severely disabled, often physically as well as mentally, or prone to major behavioural disorder or concomitant mental illness. There is, however, no doubt that the report correctly stressed the need for improved resources for the care of the mentally retarded whether in the community or in hospital.

Social work

As has been noted, the majority of subnormal children and adults live in their own homes. Amongst the more severely handicapped, parents often complain of the isolation they feel during the early years before their child enters school or a day centre. During this period the family can be helped by their general practitioner or health visitor. The local authority social worker and, in some areas, voluntary associations for the mentally retarded should help the family discuss the anxieties and problems which arise. Recently there has been considerable extension of social work activity with mentally retarded people and their families. In some parts of the UK, specialist social workers are now deployed by local authorities expressly to work with the mentally retarded. This move away from the 1970s trend towards the generic social worker, 'jack of all trades', is to be welcomed. Some area social work teams have organised regular group discussions amongst parents with mentally retarded children with considerable benefit. Practical difficulties at home may be relieved by the provision of home helps, home laundry services for the incontinent, and in some areas local voluntary associations have organised babysitter services. In most areas it is possible for the social worker to arrange short-term admission of a severely disabled child while parents have a brief holiday. This is one circumstance in which it may be reasonable for such 'relief admission' to be to a hospital: purely social holidays in hospital for less disabled people can seldom now be justified.

Education

All mentally retarded children should receive a planned education from as early an age as possible. Education authorities in England are now accepting responsibility for educating all young people, however severe the disability. Ample evidence now exists of the beneficial effect of early stimulation on the development of young children. Parents of handicapped youngsters have an important role in this, but need guidance in the application of the best techniques. Valuable groundplans were outlined in the report on special educational needs (Warnock Report: Department of Education and Science 1978); and Mittler (1972) has emphasised the part that parents can play in early language programmes. Some areas are developing toy 'libraries' for the retarded. Here parents may select and try out toys appropriate for their children. Many firms are taking an interest in designing appropriate toys.

There is no reason why the majority of mentally retarded children should not attend play groups and nursery schools alongside normal children. Young children are very tolerant of handicap in others, and the victimisation and ridicule which parents fear rarely if every occurs until an older age. Some voluntary associations have provided their own play groups for pre-school retarded children. The need for improved nursery school provision, particularly in socially deprived areas, is now well recognised. Even those severely retarded children who have hitherto been referred either to hospital or to local authority junior training or special care centres have become the concern of education authorities. There are disappointingly few teachers skilled and interested in educating the severely retarded at present. It is hoped that this situation will change as appropriate training programmes develop. For the present the optimum role for the teacher of the severely retarded may be that of consultant to the nurses and assistants who currently work with these children.

Day centres

For those who for mental or physical reasons are too handicapped to attend a special school, education authorities should provide day care centres. In some areas this service has been augmented by more medically orientated day hospitals (Craft et al 1971) where intensive nursing and medical care can be given. The orientation will differ slightly between those that originate from the health services and those that are organised by the social services, but in either case there must be close liaison between the two services within the centre. As mentioned above, an individually designed education programme should be available to each child attending a day centre.

Speech therapy and physiotherapy are an essential part of the treatment programme in most centres. The children should receive as wide a range of stimulation as possible using carefully chosen play, music, painting and similar techniques.

It is now clear that the education and training of the mentally retarded should continue long past the conventional school-leaving age (Clarke & Clarke 1969). The transition from junior to senior day or occupation centre should therefore not imply the end of a continuing learning programme for the individual. Local authorities have a statutory duty to provide both day care centres through education departments, and training centres through social work departments. It is important that they should be centrally situated in their community with easy access by public transport. The assessment procedures outlined earlier should be repeated at intervals as the individual gets older.

The adult mentally retarded person should be encouraged to attain as great a degree of independence as his disability will allow. Some adolescents benefit from a period away from home, living in a hostel to assist them in the transition from dependence on parents to a more independent way of life (Baranyay 1971). Industrial rehabilitation units and training centres cater for all people who require to learn or retrain for a new trade and a number of retarded individuals are accepted on these courses. The disablement resettlement officer advises the individual on his suitability for such training. Sometimes he will be able to use his knowledge of local job opportunities to find a suitable niche. A similar service is available for mentally retarded people. When talking of community care it is important to recognise that it is often extremely difficult to obtain employment for the mentally retarded and that some kind of special sheltered employment is often the only available option. The more severely retarded may only be able to cope with the simplest forms of occupation. Local authorities provide senior occupation centres which should continue the social education of the adult along lines similar to those initiated at the day centre or special care centre. The focus is on learning to be self-sufficient, e.g. by coping with housework, cooking and shopping.

Some of those who attend day centres live in special hostels but the majority come from their own homes. Loss of parents or long periods of hospitalisation may make it impossible for the handicapped person to remain at home. This need not necessarily mean that the individual must return to residential care since many are able to live in supervised lodgings with selected landladies (Craft et al 1971). It must be remembered that only about half of all moderately or severely mentally retarded people live in hospital, while the majority with mild disability live outside hospital.

Residential care

As stated earlier, recent years have seen a shift away from residential towards community care. In the past, admission to hospital was most often undertaken on a long-term basis and subnormality institutions were isolated, self-supporting communities. Despite the advantage of home care described above, there remains an important place for residential arrangements, whether in hostels or hospital, and whether on a short- or long-term basis.

Patterns of care have been influenced by experiments such as that conducted at Brooklands between 1958 and 1960. Two groups of 16 carefully matched severely retarded children aged between 4 and 10 years were studied. At the start they were all in-patients in a large mental retardation hospital. One group was then moved to a large house where the children were then organised into two family groups with their own house-mothers. Their daily programme was organised on a nursery school pattern. Toilet and washing breaks were taken at appropriate times and took only a short time, in contrast to the prolonged ritual which these procedures become in some hospitals when a 'block' of children are toileted at a time. After 2 years the Brooklands children were reassessed and contrasted with the group who stayed in hospital. Although there remained no difference between the groups in non-verbal IQ, the verbal and social intelligence of the Brooklands children increased at more than twice the rate of the control group (Tizard 1966).

Tizard and coworkers made a further study of the different styles of care to be found in five hospitals, eight local authority hostels and three voluntary homes all caring for severely retarded children (King et al 1971). They found that the hostels and homes were significantly more child oriented than hospitals, allowing more contact between staff and children, and greater continuity of care. It was shown that these advantages were for the most part independent of staff:child ratios. Their findings do not criticise the individual nurses but the social organisation of the hospital as an institution.

Hostels

Hostels located in ordinary residential areas should be the most frequently used form of residential accommodation. Ideally they should be small with not more than 12 residents and situated near to schools or sheltered workshops. The hostel should be as home-like as possible and cater for short and long stay. Most now favour a hostel which mixes age groups, sexes and degrees of disability. This facilitates a home-like constellation of interdependence, where the older or more competent gain self-esteem by having responsibility both for organising their home and caring for the more disabled who are in turn stimulated to attain their potential.

Usually hostels are staffed by a warden or house-parents who help to stimulate social learning and independence. Baranyay (1971) has shown the value of their role in hostels for severely retarded adolescents. It is a difficult task, often undertaken by people with a social work background (with or without formal training) or by psychiatrically trained nurses. For all but the most severely handicapped the hostel will be a stage in the person's progress towards independence. A further step in this direction is entry into a group home where a small group of about six retarded individuals live together and support each other. Initially they will require regular visits from the social worker or community nurse, but later may become essentially self-supporting.

Sweden has been in the forefront of countries which advocate small group homes for the retarded. They stress the importance of 'normalisation'—the advantage of living with a small group in which personal relationships can flourish. 'A normal home-like environment enables the mentally handicapped person to learn simply by living. The home must always be the starting point to which modifications are made to meet particular needs' (Grunewald 1971).

In Britain, those characteristics of group homes and their potential occupants which are conducive to successful operation have been studied by Malin (1983) in Sheffield. Such homes have not been without their critics, not least concerning their liability to try and fit the residents' requirements to the home's style, rather than the other way round. While the best hospital living arrangements may readily beat indifferent community living with regard to quality of life, there is little doubt that well-devised and managed community care for the great majority of mentally retarded people will be preferable. Two further factors must also be remembered: first, the majority of mentally retarded people already live in the community, with their families; and second, the best sort of domestic-scale community living is likely to be more costly to run than the institutions which were once regarded as such a social advance by earlier generations. With regard to that small but important minority of mentally retarded people who are more severely disabled, multiply disabled or psychiatrically disordered (or some combination of all three), it has been emphasised elsewhere that there remains and will remain a need for the sort of medical, nursing and paramedical care that can only sensibly be provided in a hospital albeit small scale.

Hospital care

It is commonly stated that most of the current residents in hospitals for the mentally retarded could live in the community. This assumes an improved service for patients at home and in hostels which is only now beginning to materialise. The current task for the staff of hospitals for the mentally retarded must be to accelerate the change in their own attitude towards their role, and break down the stultifying effect of institutionalisation pari passu with preparing increasing numbers of patients for a return to the community.

Valuable advice on caring for mentally retarded people in hospital has been forthcoming from the National Development Group for the Mentally Handicapped

(1978), a body set up in 1975 to advise ministers on the development of policy. Perhaps significantly, this particular publication resulted from a request to the Group by the Secretary of State to advise on improvement of services *within existing resources*. The same group had published a pamphlet the previous year (1977) on day services for the mentally retarded, a matter of particular importance to families still providing a home for the patient.

Like the National Development Group, which has now been disbanded, the Development Team for the Mentally Handicapped is independent of government. It was established in 1975 to advise local health and social service authorities on the planning of services for the mentally retarded and their families. While hospitals must not work in isolation from local authority services, many have developed their own network of community supports to aid in rehabilitation. Some hospitals provide hostels, group homes and clubs of their own. Community nurses and hospital-based psychiatric social workers visit and encourage patients who are making their first steps back to a normal life in the community at large.

A 'health service' type of residential provision of some sort is almost certainly needed by that small minority of profoundly mentally retarded young people whose disabilities are extensive. Minns et al (1989) described the formidable task of designing alternatives to current hospital provision for patients such as this whom they surveyed. These patients had a mean chronological age of 10.8 years, but their developmental age for such matters as posture, manipulation, vision and communication was about 4 months. All of them were tetraplegic and doubly incontinent: they could not walk, talk, change position, self-feed, dress or bath; over three-quarters were liable to epileptic fits, and a great many were blind and/or cortically deaf. Staff caring for such gravely damaged people have a task which is a non-stop, 24 hour one.

Alongside changes in the patient's environment, there have been changes in outlook towards treatment from a rather nihilistic custodial approach to a planned 'treatment' programme. The word 'treatment' in its narrowly medical sense is not, of course, in most cases appropriate for techniques which owe more to psychology and education than they do to medicine. Nonetheless, they are at present largely implemented by nurses and doctors. The aim in this form of treatment is to ensure that the patient achieves his maximum potential. A plan should be devised for each patient based on the assessment process described earlier. Temporary hospital admission to learn a particular skill or overcome a particular anxiety may be part of such a

programme. Gunzberg (1968) has emphasised that patients need to acquire simple social skills that will enable them to cope in society. In this way patients who cannot read learn to recognise important notices such as 'Exit', 'Push', 'No Entry', 'Ladies', 'Gents' and so on. They work at learning how to cross the road, use the telephone, cope with money, fill in simple forms and acquire similar skills which help them to fit into contemporary society.

Operant conditioning techniques can be devised to treat individual behaviour problems or reinforce desired behaviour. Here, the giving of rewards must be closely linked in time with the desired response and takes the form of extra affection, food, toys or similar 'bonuses'. Nurses and parents can both learn to use these techniques (Larsen & Bricker 1968).

Psychiatric and behaviour disturbance in mentally retarded people has been carefully investigated, revealing the technical difficulties of identifying the determinants of problematical conduct (Leudar et al 1984, Fraser et al 1986). In view of the practical importance of behaviour problems in these patients, improved means of detecting and treating depressive and neurotic disorders in such populations are likely to facilitate the move to care in the community for the majority of mentally handicapped people.

Occupation and art therapy have more than a diversional function for the retarded. In this setting manual skills are developed, and the retarded patient's repertoire of achievement is enhanced by producing objects of his own making. Most hospitals provide industrial therapy units which simulate ordinary work conditions and can provide both sheltered employment for some and rehabilitation for others. It is important that both these functions are recognised and that a patient's skill in completing contract work does not necessarily mean he continues to do the same task endlessly, but is given the chance of learning new and more complex skills. The contemporary unemployment problem in the UK discriminates against people with few specific skills to offer. While the mentally retarded are substantially represented in this group, many employers have learned that such individuals are often strong and single-minded and get real satisfaction from doing jobs that would be tiresomely repetitive and boring to others.

Physiotherapy and speech therapy are both essential aspects of treatment for those patients who suffer from such associated features as spasticity or speech disorders. Drug treatment has only a limited role. Tranquillisers of the phenothiazine group may be of value in reducing acute behaviour disturbance and hyperactivity, but are not normally recommended in the longer term. Other tranquillisers and antidepressants have indications similar to those in general psychiatry. Care should be taken in treating the retarded epileptic to ensure that he is not unduly sedated, as diminished fits may be achieved only at the cost of such lethargy that no learning is possible. There has lately been much interest in the place of drugs in the treatment and care of mentally retarded people. It is often alleged that learning performance may be reduced by drugs, and that the useful effect of reinforcement contingencies may be interfered with. However, other studies fail to support such views, and at present what is needed is a better understanding of advantageous subject-treatment combinations, with high vigilance for adverse effects (Aman & Singh 1986).

Each clinical team should organise and review the programme for its own patients by holding weekly meetings at which all members of the team—nurses, physiotherapist, doctor, social worker, psychologist, and occupational therapist—may discuss their individual contributions to the total programme. The hospital must not operate in isolation from other services described earlier and its own staff will be involved in domiciliary work and consultation in day centres and local authority hostels.

The education department now takes responsibility for hospital schools and educating those severely retarded children who had previously been excluded from the hospital school. In an experimental school in Cambridge even the most severely physically disabled attend in ordinary school hours under the care of skilled teachers, and return to their ward at the end of the day.

PERSONAL RELATIONSHIPS, SEX AND MARRIAGE

Mentally retarded people used to be considered either uninterested in close personal relationships that could lead to marriage, or to be ill-equipped to sustain any such social convention, if so inclined. Indeed, the early years of this century heard dire predictions of the results of any failure to inhibit the 'disproportionate reproduction of the mentally unfit', with grave consequences for the national 'gene pool' (Craft 1979). In fact, even today mentally retarded couples raise relatively few children; and many recognise the heavy responsibilities implicit in parenthood and choose to avoid it. But such people need the same knowledge about fertility and its control as non-retarded people; and will need it to be presented in a style, and at a pace, commensurate with their ability to grasp what is taught (Craft & Craft 1978). Their entitlement to such advice,

and to a sexual life at all, has been conceded only quite lately: caregivers have traditionally sought to suppress manifestations of sexuality in their charges. If living in hospitals, these patients may have had little experience of normal family affections and their display. They may thus be at an added disadvantage when embarking on marriage themselves, with little awareness of the 'elastic' necessary to keep a marital show on the road. For this and doubtless other reasons, divorce or permanent separation is as common amongst mentally retarded married couples as in others. In the 1960s about a third of such couples were known to local children's departments or officers of the National Society for the Prevention of Cruelty to Children (NSPCC) because of cruelty or neglect, especially when there were more than two children in the family.

Today, few hospitals for the mentally retarded have accommodation for married couples. But there is increasing awareness of the need to make sex education a part of training experience, for both in-patients and the much greater number in the community at large. Staff familiar with helping mentally retarded people are crucial for this, and this is so for genetic counselling personnel too. Contraception is now more practicable than ever before, and advice as to choice of method must be readily accessible. Though not a prerequisite for discharge from hospital (as it is in some parts of the USA), sterilisation is one option commonly adopted by non-disabled people today; and along with 'the pill', intrauterine devices and so forth, can be discussed with a mentally retarded woman to ensure she only becomes pregnant by choice. Contemporary cautions about sexual activity and human immunodeficiency virus (HIV) infection apply as much to people who are mentally retarded as they do to everyone else.

Hostels and other forms of supported accommodation will increasingly include married quarters for these patients; and of course many can sustain a normal house or flat tenancy, given reasonable support. In large measure, the mutual support which such a couple may afford can be a decidedly cost-effective arrangement, as well as having other more obvious personal advantages.

PREVENTION OF MENTAL RETARDATION

The WHO (1985) has set down performance targets for the prevention of conditions causing serious limitation of intellectual development. The setting of practicable targets in this field is difficult but necessary to help gauge progress.

Low birth weight children who are brought up in deprived circumstances are most likely to attain only poor intellectual competence. Improved obstetric and neonatal care has caused a substantial drop in early deaths among low birth weight babies. Despite predictions to the contrary, this has occurred without a serious increase in the number of damaged survivors (Powell et al 1986).

The total of *impaired* low birth weight survivors appears to be remaining constant. Thus, the incidence of impairment in these small babies is falling. It is disappointing that, in the UK, the number of low birth weight babies as a proportion of all birth weights has remained constant in recent years: 7% in 1977, 7.2% in 1981, 7.1% in 1984. This is roughly double the Swedish figure. These 'light for dates' babies are not distributed evenly in all parts of the UK, nor in all parts of any particular locality. They are more often found in areas of social disadvantage, though the relationship between environmental and biological factors is complex.

Antenatal screening

In the majority of cases of Down's syndrome, the disorder is due to the random occurrence of a chromosome abnormality which is more likely to occur at greater maternal ages: it is 20 times more likely at 40 than at 20 years of age. About a quarter of the 1000 babies with Down's syndrome born in 1980 in the UK were to mothers aged over 35 years. Amniocentesis can often provide a positive diagnosis at around 18–20 weeks, which is a late stage for many couples to contemplate therapeutic termination. Chorionic villus sampling (CVS) enables a diagnosis to be made at about the eighth week of gestation, though the safety and efficiency of the technique are still under scrutiny. If CVS proves a sound technique, it will be necessary to ensure that women at risk come to antenatal care earlier than occurs at present.

The possibility of a simple Down's syndrome screen for all pregnant women has been raised by Cuckle & Wald (1984). They found that unusually low levels of α-fetoprotein (AFP) in maternal blood are associated with Down's syndrome. AFP level is already checked in connection with neural tube defect (NTD) screening, which has probably been an important factor in the declining incidence of NTD during the last 10 years. Where a high serum AFP level is found, diagnostic ultrasound can detect, for example, open spina bifida and anencephaly with considerable accuracy. Preventive screening for fragile X syndrome has been proposed (Leading article 1986, 1987). Prospective screening of newly diagnosed children with idiopathic mental retardation irrespective of sex, together with

their relatives, is now considered basic good clinical practice.

Fragile X syndrome is second only to Down's syndrome as a cause of mental retardation. About one in 544 schoolgirls in an English city were recently found to be carrying the fragile X mutation, with a one in two risk that any son of theirs would be mentally retarded and a one in six risk for any daughter. It may shortly be necessary to give serious thought to the vast task of retrospective screening of all mentally retarded children and young adults, together with relevant relatives. The scope for substantially reducing the prevalence of this type of mental retardation would appear great.

Stages of prevention of mental retardation

Four stages at which measures can be taken to prevent or limit the extent of mental retardation may be defined. These are shown below with a summary indication of the procedures or considerations relevant at each (Taylor 1986).

Preconceptual

- Rubella immunisation
- Genetic counselling
- Health promotion for potential mothers—including advice about diet, smoking, alcohol use
- Medical care of diabetics contemplating pregnancy
- Availability of contraception and family planning advice, to avoid unwanted pregnancies.

Prenatal

- Identification of 'at risk' groups, and genetic counselling
- AFP level
- Rubella screening
- Syphilis screening
- Maternal age
- Rhesus incompatibility check
- Fetal cell screening for genetic/chromosome abnormalities
- Diagnostic ultrasound
    Diagnosis of growth retardation
    Microcephalus
    Hydrocephalus
    Neural tube defects
    Multiple births
    Placental abnormalities
- Improved antenatal care services, with special reference to factors conducive to low birth weight babies, including outreach care at local clinics.

Perinatal/neonatal

- Improved obstetric and neonatal care (with the aim of reducing hypoxia, hypoglycaemia and trauma)
- Neonatal screening/treatment for hypothyroidism, phenylketonuria
- Prompt surgical treatment for hydrocephaly
- Use of anti-D immunoglobulin in mothers at risk of future rhesus incompatibility.

Postnatal

- Improved uptake of immunisations (e.g. measles) to reduce incidence of encephalitis/meningitis
- Prevention of further damage of impaired children, e.g. expert control of epilepsy, physiotherapy for the non-ambulant
- Prevention of circumstances conducive to child abuse, to road traffic accidents, to home accidents.

REFERENCES

Aman M G, Singh N N 1986 A critical appraisal of recent drug research in mental retardation: the Coldwater studies. Journal of Mental Deficiency Research 30: 203–216

Ballinger B R, Reid A H 1977 Psychiatric disorder in an adult training centre and a hospital for the mentally handicapped. Psychological Medicine 7: 525–528

Baranyay E P 1971 The mentally handicapped adolescent. Pergamon Press, London

Berg J M 1959 Discussion on the aetiology of mental defect. Proceedings of the Royal Society of Medicine 52: 789–791

Berg J M, Kirman D H 1959 Some aetiological problems in mental deficiency. British Medical Journal ii: 848–852

Birch H G, Richardson S A, Baird S, Horobin G, Illsley R 1970 Mental subnormality in the community. Williams & Wilkins, Baltimore

Blackie J, Forrest A D, Witcher G 1975 Subcultural mental handicap. British Journal of Psychiatry 127: 535–539

Blackwood D H R, St Clair D M, Muir W J, Oliver C J, Dickens P 1988 The development of Alzheimer's disease in Down's syndrome assessed by auditory event-related potentials. Journal of Mental Deficiency Research 32: 439–453

Bowlby J 1965 Child care and the growth of love. Penguin Books, Harmondsworth

Campaign for Mentally Handicapped People 1983 Newsletter 34 (Autumn). Campaign for Mentally Handicapped People, London

Carter G, Jancar J 1983 Mortality in the mentally handicapped: a 50 year survey at the Stoke Park Group of Hospitals (1930–1980). Journal of Mental Deficiency Research 27: 143–156

Chess S, Korn S J, Fernandez P B 1971 Psychiatric disorders of children with congenital rubella. Butterworths, London

Chudley A E, Knoll J, Gerrard J W, Shepel L, McGahey J, Anderson J 1983 Fragile (X)-linked mental retardation. I: Relationship between age and intelligence and the frequency of expression of fragile (XXq28). American Journal of Medical Genetics 14: 699

Clarke A M 1965 In: Clarke A M, Clarke A D B (eds) Mental deficiency: the changing outlook, 2nd edn. Methuen, London

Clarke A M, Clarke A D B 1969 Recent advances in the study of subnormality. National Association for Mental Health, London

Cooper L Z, Fedun B A, Matters B A, Krigman S 1969 Maternal rubella and the risk to the foetus. In: Proceedings of the International Symposium on Rubella Vaccines. Karger, Basel

Corbett J A, Trimble M R 1983 Epilepsy and anticonvulsant medication. In: Rutter M (ed) Developmental neuropsychiatry. Guildford Press, New York

Craft M 1979 Tredgold's mental retardation, 12th edn. Baillière Tindall, London

Craft M, Craft A 1978 Sex and the mentally handicapped. Routledge & Kegan Paul, London

Craft M, Freeman H, Lockwood H, Wilkins R 1971 Day hospital care for the mentally subnormal. British Journal of Psychiatry 119: 287–294

Cuckle H S, Wald N J 1984 Maternal serum alpha-fetoprotein measurement: a screening test for Down's syndrome. Lancet: 926–929

Dahlberg P 1937 On the frequency of mental deficiency. Upsala Lakreforenings Fordhandinav 5: 439

Daker M G, Chidiac P, Fear C N, Berry A C 1981 Fragile X in a normal male: a cautionary tale. Lancet i: 780

Davie R, Butler N, Goldstein H 1972 From birth to seven. Longman, London

Davies K E (ed) 1989 The fragile X syndrome. Oxford University Press, Oxford

Department of Education and Science 1978 Special educational needs: report of committee of enquiry into the education of handicapped children and young people. (Warnock report.) Cmnd 7212. Her Majesty's Stationery Office, London

Department of Health and Social Security 1971 Better services for the mentally handicapped. Her Majesty's Stationery Office, London

Donnai D, Clayton-Smith J, Gibbons R J, Higgs D R 1991 The non-deletion α-thalassaemia/mental retardation syndrome: further support for X linkage. Journal of Medical Genetics 28: 742–745

Dudgeon J A 1967 Maternal rubella and its effect on the foetus. Archives of Diseases in Childhood 42: 110–125

Dupont A, Voeth M, Videbech P 1986 Mortality and life expectancy of Down's syndrome in Denmark. Journal of Mental Deficiency Research 30: 111–120

Fischbacher E 1982 Effect of reduction of anticonvulsants on wellbeing. British Medical Journal 285: 423–424

Fischbacher E 1985 Mental handicap and epilepsy: are we still overtreating? In: Wood C (ed) Epilepsy and mental handicap. Royal Society of Medicine, London

Fishler K, Azen C G, Friedman E G, Koch R 1989 School achievement in treated PKU children. Journal of Mental Deficiency Research 33: 493–498

Fraser W I, Leudar I, Gray J, Campbell I 1986 Psychiatric and behaviour disturbance in mental handicap. Journal of Mental Deficiency Research 30: 49–57

Fryers T 1986 Survival in Down's syndrome. Journal of Mental Deficiency Research 30: 101

Gath A 1973 The school-age siblings of mongol children. British Journal of Psychiatry 123: 161–167

Gath A 1977 The impact of an abnormal child upon the parents. British Journal of Psychiatry 130: 405–410

Gesell A, Armatruda C 1941 Developmental diagnosis. Hoeber, New York

Gillberg C, Persson E, Wahlstrom J 1986 The autism-fragile-X syndrome (AFRAX): a population-based study of 10 boys. Journal of Mental Deficiency Research 30: 27–39

Goldfarb W 1961 Childhood schizophrenia. Harvard University Press, Cambridge, MA

Goodman N, Tizard J 1962 Prevalence of imbecility and idiocy amongst children. British Medical Journal i: 216–219

Gruneberg H 1964 Epidemiology in mental retardation. Stevens H A (ed) University of Chicago Press, Chicago

Grunewald K 1971 The needs of the mentally handicapped and their satisfaction through different patterns of care. Bolton Symposium, CEH, London

Gunzberg H 1968 Social competence and mental handicap. Baillière, Tindall & Cox, London

Hagberg B, Aicardi J, Dias K, Ramos O 1983 A progressive syndrome of autism, dementia, ataxia, and loss of purposeful hand use in girls: Rett's syndrome: report of 35 cases. Annals of Neurology 14: 471

Harper M, Reid A H 1987 Use of a restricted protein diet in the treatment of behaviour disorder in a severely mentally retarded adult female phenylketonuric patient. Journal of Mental Deficiency Research 31: 209–212

Heber R, Garber H 1971 An experiment in the prevention of cultural-familial mental retardation. In: Primrose D A (ed) Proceedings of the 2nd Congress of the International Association for the Scientific Study of Mental Deficiency. Swets & Zeitlinger, Amsterdam

Herbst D S, Miller J R 1980 Non-specific X-linked mental retardation. II: The frequency in British Columbia. American Journal of Medical Genetics 7: 461–469

Hermelin B, O'Connor N 1970 Psychological experiments with autistic children. Pergamon Press, London

Hirst M C, Suthers G K, Davies K E 1992 X-linked mental retardation: the fragile X syndrome. Hospital Update 18: 736–742

HMSO 1979 Report of the committee of enquiry in to mental handicap nursing care 1979. Chair, Peggy Jay. Cmnd 7468-I & 7468-II. Her Majesty's Stationery Office, London

Ingram T T S 1966 The neurology of cerebral palsy. Archives of Diseases in Childhood 41: 337–357

Innes G, Kidd C, Ross H S 1968 Mental subnormality in north east Scotland. British Journal of Psychiatry 114: 35–41

Jacobs P A, Brunton M, Melville M M 1965 Aggressive behaviour mental subnormality and the XYY male. Nature 208: 1351–1352

James D H 1986 Neuroleptics and epilepsy in mentally handicapped patients. Journal of Mental Deficiency Research 30: 185–189

Jenkins E C, Brown W T, Duncan C J et al 1981 Feasibility of fragile X chromosome prenatal diagnosis demonstrated. Lancet ii: 1292

Kanner L, Eisenberg L 1955 Notes on the follow-up studies of autistic children. In: Koch P H, Zubin J (eds) Psychopathology of childhood. Grune & Stratton, New York

King R D, Raynes N V, Tizard J 1971 Patterns of residential care. Routledge & Kegan Paul, London

Koch R, Acosta P, Ragsdale N, Donnell G N 1963 Nutrition in the treatment of phenylketonuria. Journal of the American Dietetic Association 43: 212–215

Kolb L C 1968 Noyes' modern clinical psychiatry, 7th edn. Saunders, Philadelphia

Kushlick A 1964 The prevalence of recognised subnormality of IQ under 50 among children in the south of England. Proceedings of the International Congress of Scientific Study of Mental Retardation 2: 550

Kushlick A 1966 Social problems of the mentally subnormal. Social Psychiatry 1: 73–82

Langdon Down J 1866 Observations on an ethnic classification of idiots. Clinical Lectures and Reports of the London Hospital 3: 259–262

Larsen L A, Bricker W A 1968 A manual for parents and teachers of severely and moderately retarded children. Institute on Mental Retardation. Papers and Reports V: No 22

Leading article 1986 Preventive screening for fragile X syndrome. Lancet ii: 1191

Leading article 1987 Fragile X syndrome: an important preventable cause of mental handicap. British Medical Journal 295: 564

Lejeune J 1982 Is the fragile X syndrome amenable to treatment? Lancet i: 273–274

Lejeune J, Lafourcade J, Berger R et al 1963 Trois cases de deletion partielle du bras court d'un chromosome 5. Comptes Rendus Hebdomadaires des Séances de l'Académie des Sciences (Paris) 257: 3098–3102

Lenneberg E H, Nichols I A, Rosenberger E F 1964 Language development. In: McRich D, Weinstein E A (eds) Mongolism in disorders of communication. Williams & Wilkins, Baltimore

Leudar I, Fraser W I, Jeeves M A 1984 Behavioural disturbance in mental handicap: typology and longitudinal trends. Psychological Medicine 14: 923–935

Lewis E O 1929 Report of the mental deficiency commission 1925–1927. His Majesty's Stationery Office, London

Lewis E O 1933 Types of mental deficiency and their social significance. Journal of Mental Science 79: 298–304

Loesch D 1974 Dermatoglyphic characteristics of 21 trisomy mosaicism in relation to the fully developed syndrome and normality. Journal of Mental Deficiency Research 18: 209–269

Lund J 1985a Epilepsy and psychiatric disorder in the mentally retarded adult. Acta Psychiatrica Scandinavica 72: 557–562

Lund J 1985b The prevalence of psychiatric morbidity in mentally retarded adults. Acta Psychiatrica Scandinavica 72: 563–570

Lund J 1985c Mentally retarded admitted to psychiatric hospitals in Denmark. Acta Psychiatrica Scandinavica 72: 202–205

Madison L S, George C, Moeschler J B 1986 Cognitive functioning in the fragile-X syndrome: a study of intellectual, memory and communication skills. Journal of Mental Deficiency Research 30: 129

Malin N 1983 Group homes for mentally handicapped people. Her Majesty's Stationery Office, London

Martin J P, Bell J 1943 A pedigree of mental defect showing sex-linkage. Journal of Neurology 6: 154–157

Menkes J H, Hurst P L, Craig J M 1954 A new syndrome: progressive familial infantile cerebral dysfunction associated with an unusual urinary substance. Paediatrics 14: 462–467

Minns R A, Wong B, Brown J K, Fraser W I 1989 Neuro-developmental study of profoundly handicapped children in hospital care. Journal of Mental Deficiency Research 33: 439–454

Mittler P 1970 Psychological assessment of mental and physical handicap, Methuen, London

Mittler P 1972 Education of the mentally handicapped. British Journal of Hospital Medicine 8: 155–158

Murdoch J C 1985 Congenital heart disease as a significant factor in the morbidity of children with Down's syndrome. Journal of Mental Deficiency Research 29: 147–151

National Development Group for the Mentally Handicapped 1977 Day services for mentally handicapped adults. Pamphlet No 5. Her Majesty's Stationery Office, London

National Development Group for the Mentally Handicapped 1978 Helping mentally handicapped people in hospital. Her Majesty's Stationery Office, London

Neilsen K B 1983 Diagnosis of the fragile-X syndrome (Martin Bell syndrome). Clinical findings in 27 males with the fragile site at Xq28. Journal of Mental Deficiency Research 27: 211–226

Patau K, Smith D W, Therman E, Inhorn S L, Wagner H P 1960 Multiple congenital anomaly caused by an extra autosome. Lancet i: 790–793

Penrose L S 1963a The biology of mental defect, 3rd edn. Sidgwick & Jackson, London

Penrose L S 1963b Finger-prints, palms and chromosomes. Nature 197: 933–938

Penrose L S 1972 The biology of mental defect. Sidgwick & Jackson, London

Penrose L S, Smith G F 1966 Down's anomaly. Churchill, London

Powell T G, Pharoah P O D, Cooke R W I 1986 Survival and morbidity in a geographically defined population of low birthweight infants. Lancet: 539–543

Ratcliffe S G, Stewart A L, Melville M M, Jacobs P A 1970 Chromosome studies on 3500 newborn male infants. Lancet ii: 121–122

Reid A H 1982 The psychiatry of mental handicap. Blackwell Scientific, London

Reid A H 1983 Psychiatry of mental handicap: a review. Journal of the Royal Society of Medicine 76: 587

Reid A H 1985 Psychiatry and mental handicap. In: Craft M, Bicknell J, Hollins S (eds) Mental handicap: a multi-disciplinary approach. Baillière Tindall, London

Renpenning H, Gerrard J W, Zaleski W A, Tabata T 1962 Familial sex-linked mental retardation. Canadian Medical Association Journal 87: 954–956

Richardson S A, Koller H, Katz M, McLaren J 1981 A functional classification of seizures and its distribution in a mentally retarded population. American Journal of Mental Deficiency 85: 457–466

Rutter M 1966 In: Wing J K (ed) Early childhood autism. Pergamon Press, London

Rutter M, Greenfeld D, Lockyer L 1967 A 5–15 year follow-up study of infantile psychosis II. Social and behavioural outcome. British Journal of Psychology 113: 1183–1199

Scally B G, Mackay D N 1964 Mental subnormality and its prevalence in Ireland. Acta Psychiatrica Scandinavica 40: 203–211

Shapiro L R, Wilmot P L, Brenholz P et al 1982 Prenatal diagnosis of fragile X chromosome. Lancet i: 99–100

Stein Z, Susser M 1962 Families of dull children. Journal of Mental Science 166: 1296–1310

Stevens H A, Heber R 1964 Mental retardation: a review of research. University of Chicago Press, Chicago

Taylor J 1986 Mental handicap; partnership in the community? OHE paper No 83 Office of Health Economics/MENCAP/The Mental Health Foundation/Centre for Health Economics, York

Tizard J 1966 Care and treatment of subnormal children in residential institutions. Association for Special Education

Vernon P E 1960 Intelligence and attainment tests. University of London Press, London

Wada Y, Taka K, Minagawa A, Yoshida T, Morikawa T, Okamura T 1963 Idiopathic hypervalinemia: probably a new entity of inborn error of valine metabolism. Tohoku Journal of Experimental Medicine 81: 46

Weatherall D J, Higgs D R, Bunch C et al 1981 Hemoglobin H disease and mental retardation—a new syndrome or a remarkable coincidence? New England Journal of Medicine 305: 607–612

Webb G C, Rogers J G, Pitt D B, Halliday J, Theobald T 1981 Transmission of fragile (X) (q27) site from a male. Lancet ii: 1231–1232

Webb T P, Thake A I, Bundey S E, Todd J 1987 A cytogenetic survey of a mentally retarded school-age population with special reference to fragile sites. Journal of Mental Deficiency Research 31: 61–71

Wedge P, Prosser H 1973 Born to fail? Arrow Books/National Children's Bureau, London

WHO 1985 Targets for health for all. World Health Organization, Copenhagen

Wing J K 1966 Early childhood autism. Pergamon Press, London

Wurtele S K, King A C, Drabman R S 1984 Treatment package to reduce SIB in a Lesch–Nyhan patient. Journal of Mental Deficiency Research 28: 227–234

29. Psychiatric disorders of childhood

P. Hoare

INTRODUCTION

Child psychiatry is concerned with the assessment and treatment of children's emotional and behavioural problems. These are very common with prevalence rates of 10–20% in several community studies (Richman et al 1982, Rutter et al 1970a, Shepherd et al 1971). The Isle of Wight (IoW) study (Rutter et al 1970a) showed that less than one in ten disturbed children were seen by specialist psychiatric services, with the majority looked after by general practitioners, paediatricians, community health doctors and other professionals working with children such as teachers and residential care staff. Clearly, familiarity with the range and management of children's emotional and behavioural problems is essential for all doctors involved in the care of children.

For the psychiatrist in training, knowledge of child development and experience in child psychiatry are important for several reasons. First, it demonstrates that childhood experiences are influential in the development of the adult personality. Second, it provides an explanation for the continuity or discontinuity of psychopathology between childhood and adult life. Third, it shows the ways in which parental psychiatric illness can adversely affect the child's development. This can happen directly through effects on the parent–child relationship or indirectly through the child's exposure to deviant parental role models. Fourth, it provides the basis to evaluate the significance of childhood experience in the development of adult psychopathology. Finally, it gives the trainee the competence to assess families and their functioning.

Psychological disturbance in childhood is most usefully defined as an abnormality in at least one of three areas — emotions, behaviour or relationships. However, unlike most other branches of medicine, it is *not* helpful to regard these abnormalities as strictly defined disease entities with a precise aetiology, treatment or prognosis. Rather, it is preferable to regard them as deviations or departures from the norm which are distressing to the child or to those involved with his upbringing. Although child psychiatric disorders do not conform to the strict medical mode of illness, this does not mean that they are trivial or unimportant. Some disorders such as autism or conduct disorder have major implications for the child's development and adjustment in adult life.

In childhood, the distinction between disturbance and normality is often imprecise or arbitrary. Isolated symptoms are common and not pathological. For example, many children will occasionally feel sad, unhappy or have temper tantrums. This does not mean that the child is disturbed, as disturbance is determined by the number, frequency, severity and duration of symptoms rather than by the form of the symptomatology. In addition, disturbed children rarely have unequivocally pathological symptoms such as hallucinations or delusions. In clinical practice, it is often more important to establish why the child is the focus for concern rather than adopt the more narrow perspective of whether the child is disturbed or not.

Another distinctive feature of childhood psychiatric disturbance is that several factors rather than one usually contribute to the development of disturbance. This makes their assessment and treatment more difficult, so that an essential prerequisite for successful treatment is the correct evaluation of the relative contribution of the different aetiological factors.

Aetiological factors are usually categorised into two groups, constitutional and environmental. The former include hereditary factors, intelligence and temperament. The three major environmental influences are the family, schooling and the community. Another factor, physical illness or disability, if present, can have a profound effect on the child's development and on his vulnerability to disturbance.

Three other considerations are of general importance in understanding children's behaviour: the situation-specific nature of behaviour, the impact of

649

current stressful life circumstances and the role of the family. Several studies (Rutter et al 1970a, Shepherd et al 1971) have shown that children's behaviour varies markedly in different situations. For instance, a child may be a major problem at school but not at home, or vice versa. Consequently, there may well be an apparent discrepancy between the account of the child's behaviour from the parents and that from the teachers. The most likely explanation for this discrepancy is that the child does indeed behave differently, as the demands and expectations on the child vary in the two situations. It is therefore essential to obtain several independent accounts of the child's behaviour wherever possible in order to obtain an accurate and realistic assessment of the problem. The situation-specific nature of the behaviour also has implications for treatment. It is important to explain to parents and teachers the reasons for the discrepancy, thereby reducing the chances of misunderstanding.

Children are immature and developing individuals. Childhood is also a period of life characterised by change and the necessity for adaptation. Consequently it is not surprising that symptoms of disturbance may arise at times of stress when the demands upon the child are too great. Recent research (Goodyer et al 1985, Goodyer 1990) has shown that stressful life events are associated with an increased psychiatric morbidity among children, findings similar to those reported for adults (Brown & Harris 1978). Some stresses such as the birth of a sibling or starting school are, of course, normal and usually uneventful, whereas others such as marital break-up or life-threatening illness are serious with long-term implications for the child's well-being.

The child may cope successfully with these stresses, which as a result enhance the child's self-esteem and confidence. Alternatively, the child may be overwhelmed, responding with the development of symptomatic behaviour. The latter may involve regressive behaviour (behaving in a more immature, dependent fashion), or be more clearly maladaptive, for instance aggression, excessive anxiety or withdrawal. A crucial feature of assessment is the identification of the stressful factors that may be contributing to the problem, as this will influence treatment strategies and also the prognosis.

The family is a most powerful force for the promotion of health as well as for the production of disturbance in the child's life. Assessment of parenting qualities, the marital relationship and the quality of family interaction are essential components of child psychiatric practice. It is a frequent observation that it

is the parents who are disturbed and not the child. One consequence of this observation is that in many cases the focus of treatment is likely to be the parents or the whole family rather than the referred child. Indeed in many instances, the main emphasis of treatment may be the promotion of normal healthy family interaction as much as in the specific treatment of the child's disturbed behaviour.

Finally, many disturbed children do not complain openly about their distress nor admit to problems. It is usually their parents or other adults involved with their care who bring the child to the attention of professionals. Disturbed children also frequently manifest their distress or unhappiness indirectly through the development of symptoms such as abdominal pain, aggression or withdrawal. Direct questioning of the child on first acquaintance is unlikely to reveal the true extent of the child's feelings and his degree of distress. Sensitive observation during the interview and the use of indirect approaches such as play therapy techniques are necessary to elicit a more accurate view of the child's feelings. This is only likely to be successful once a relationship of trust has been established between the child and the therapist.

NORMAL AND ABNORMAL PSYCHOLOGICAL DEVELOPMENT

Children are not small adults, but developing individuals. A child aged 2 years is very different from a teenager, whereas a 25-year-old may not differ much from someone 10 years older. During childhood, the child undergoes a remarkable transformation from a helpless, dependent infant to an independent, self-sufficient individual with his own views and outlook, capable of embarking on a career and living separately from his family.

Knowledge of the *mechanisms*, *processes* and *sequences* underlying these events is necessary in order to understand the nature of psychological disturbance in childhood. This knowledge is conveniently divided into three components: developmental theories, personality development and developmental psychopathology. The first two have been discussed in Chapter 5, so it may be advisable to consult that chapter when reading this section. The third aspect, developmental psychopathology, is discussed below.

Developmental psychopathology

This lengthy phrase describes the two most important dimensions involved in the evaluation of a child's behaviour: firstly, the developmental (is the behaviour age-appropriate?) and secondly, the psychopathological (is the behaviour abnormal?). The developmental aspect is illustrated by separation anxiety. This is a normal reaction in children between the ages of 9 months and 4 years, but the same response in a 6-year-old would be abnormal.

Childhood psychopathology is most usefully classified under three main headings: abnormalities of behaviour, emotions and social relationships. Many behavioural problems can be conceptualised as a deficit in or an excess of a particular skill or behaviour. For instance, a child with encorpresis or enuresis can be regarded as showing a deficit in toileting skills. Similarly, the aggressive child can be seen as displaying excessively belligerent or oppositional behaviour at an inappropriate time. This conceptualisation also has implications for treatment strategies, as the latter often use behavioural techniques in order to increase or decrease the frequency of certain behaviours.

Anxiety is central to the understanding of emotional disturbance. It has physical manifestations such as palpitations or dry mouth as well as psychological components such as fear or apprehension. Exposure to anxiety is a normal, indeed essential, part of a child's experience. It arises in many situations: in respond to external threat; in new or strange situations; and in response to the operation of conscience. Anna Freud (1936) developed the concept of *defence mechanism(s)* to explain the processes whereby individuals cope with excessive anxiety. These responses are entirely healthy and appropriate in many situations. They only become maladaptive when used excessively or exclusively, thereby preventing the individual from learning to cope with a normal degree of anxiety.

The common defence mechanisms are *denial, rationalisation, regression* and *displacement.*

Denial is an inability or reluctance to accept the psychological impact of a potentially stressful event or situation. For example, a child denies stealing even though it is obvious to everyone that he is responsible. This is because open admission of the theft would produce such a loss of self-esteem and induce such a sense of guilt that it becomes intolerable.

Rationalisation is a strategy to excuse or minimise the psychological consequences of an event. For example, the child who fails to gain selection to the school team may say to his friend 'I don't really like football anyway, so I'm not bothered about playing for the team'.

Regression is the recurrence of developmentally immature behaviour, often at times of stress. For example, many children have a recurrence of enuresis at the start of primary school.

Displacement is the transfer of hostile or aggressive feelings from their original target to another person, usually less important, for instance getting angry with a sibling rather than with an adult.

Social relationships are often impaired in disturbed children. This may be the primary failure in some instances such as autism but more commonly it is a secondary phenomenon. Children with neurotic or conduct disorders are usually socially isolated and unpopular with their peer group as they exclude themselves or are excluded as a result of their deviant behaviour. In addition, the behaviour usually brings them into conflict with parents or other adults such as teachers.

GENERAL FEATURES OF PSYCHIATRIC DISTURBANCE

Diagnostic classification

As discussed earlier, psychiatric disorders rarely have a single cause. The usual pattern is for several factors to be involved, with a broad distinction into constitutional and environmental factors. One consequence of this multiple causation is that it is inappropriate to devise a diagnostic classification on the basis of aetiology, as the relative contribution of each factor is often unclear. Diagnostic practice is therefore descriptive or phenomenological, with three main categories of abnormality: disorders of *emotions, behaviour* and *relationships.*

Definition of disturbance

A commonly used definition of disturbance is 'an abnormality of emotions, behaviour or relationships, which is sufficiently severe and persistent to handicap the child in his social or personal functioning and/or to cause distress to the child, his parents or to people in the community'.

Another feature of contemporary diagnostic practice in child psychiatry is the adoption of a multiaxial framework to describe the various abnormalities or disabilities that frequently coexist. This is a further recognition of the multifactorial nature of disturbance in childhood. The two commonest systems are the ICD and DSM-IIIR (see Ch. 14 and Table 29.1). The two systems have similar underlying principles with an emphasis on a clinical-descriptive approach to diagnosis and the categorisation of disorder along five

Table 29.1   The ICD-10 and DSM-IIIR classificatory systems

	DSM-IIIR	ICD-10
Axis 1	Clinical syndrome	Clinical syndrome
Axis 2	Mental retardation, pervasive developmental disorder and specific developmental disorders	Disorders of psychological development
Axis 3	Physical disorders or conditions	Intellectual retardation
Axis 4	Severity of current psychosocial stressors	Medical illness
Axis 5	Highest level of adaptive functioning in past year	Abnormal psychosocial conditions

separate dimensions with the child having a position on each dimension, even when there is no abnormality. ICD-10 uses diagnostic guidelines and DSM-IIIR operationally defined criteria to provide the basis for diagnosis. An important difference between ICD-10 and DSM-IIIR is that the latter allows for more than one diagnosis on the clinical syndrome axis, whereas ICD-10 prefers a single diagnosis, an approach more widely used.

DSM-IIIR shows important changes compared with its predecessors. Childhood autism has been reclassified in a new category called pervasive developmental disorders. This is now included on Axis 2 along with mental retardation. Earlier versions of the DSM had classified childhood autism in the category of childhood psychosis. The term 'psychosis' is not strictly correct when applied to childhood autism, as psychosis implies a period of normal development, which is usually not present in autism. 'Pervasive developmental disorder' is probably a more satisfactory term as it emphasises the developmental aspect. The choice of 'pervasive' is more problematic, as although the autistic behaviour occurs in most situations, the disorder does not affect all aspects of development. For example, some cognitive attainments such as memory may be normal or even superior.

ICD-10 is also radically different from ICD-9 (see Table 29.1). There is a new category or axis called 'disorders of psychological development', as well as a reorganisation of the axis concerned with childhood psychiatric disorders, now known as 'behavioral and emotional disorders with onset usually occurring in childhood or adolescence' (F9). ICD-10 still adopts the convention that disorders occurring in childhood which fulfill the criteria for other syndromes, for example schizophrenia or affective disorder, should be classified with these disorders rather than being included in the specific childhood category (F9).

Disorders of psychological development are divided into three main categories, specific developmental disorders of speech and language, specific developmental disorders of scholastic skills and the pervasive developmental disorders. The latter include childhood autism, Rett's syndrome and Asperger's syndrome (see below).

The following list, excluding the separately classified pervasive developmental disorders, describes the main psychiatric syndromes of childhood in ICD-10:

1. Conduct disorders (F91)
2. Emotional disorders (F93)
3. Mixed disorders of conduct and emotions (F92)
4. Hyperkinetic disorders (F90)
5. Disorders of social functioning (F94)
6. Tic disorders (F95)
7. Other behavioural and emotional disorders (F98)
8. Unspecified mental disorder (F99).

Conduct disorders are characterised by serious repetitive and persistent antisocial behaviour such as aggression or stealing. The disorder often involves damage to or destruction of property and is unresponsive to normal sanctions. Conduct disorder is frequently associated with adverse psychosocial conditions, including unsatisfactory family relationships and failure at school.

The main feature of emotional disorder is a disturbance of affect or mood, often arising in response to stress. This group includes separation anxiety, phobic and social anxiety subcategories. The group shares many features of neurotic disorders in adult life. Many disturbed children show a mixture of emotional and behavioural symptoms, so that a mixed category is clinically useful.

Hyperkinetic disorders cover a range of disorders characterised by overactivity, distractibility, impulsivity, aggression and short attention span. Large differences in the prevalence of this syndrome have been reported between the USA and the UK (see section on overactivity and hyperactivity). This is probably a reflection of different diagnostic practices in the two countries, as many children diagnosed as hyperkinetic in the USA would be diagnosed as conduct disordered in the UK.

Disorders of social functioning include elective mutism and attachment disorders. Tic disorders range in severity from simple tics to the disabling Gilles de la Tourette syndrome. The final residual category, other behavioural and emotional disorders, contains the important clinical syndromes of encopresis and enuresis.

Epidemiology of disturbance

Epidemiological research has been an important research interest in the UK for the past 25 years. It has provided accurate information about the frequency and distribution of disturbance throughout childhood and adolescence (Rutter et al 1970a), the differences between urban and rural areas (Rutter et al 1975), and the effects of illness and handicap on vulnerability to disturbance (Rutter et al 1970b) as well as providing clues about the relative importance of various aetiological factors (Rutter et al 1975).

Most studies have shown prevalence rates of between 10 and 20%, depending on the criteria for deviance. The first and most influential study was the IoW study carried out by Rutter and his colleagues (1970a). Using strict definitions of disorder, they found rates of approximately 7% among 10–11-year-old children. Follow-up of these children into adolescence indicated a prevalence rate of around 7%, with more than 40% of the children with conduct disorder continuing with major problems. Disorders arising for the first time during adolescence were more adult-like in presentation, with a preponderance in girls. Over 80% of the disorders were in the emotional, conduct or mixed categories. Emotional disorders were more common among girls, with anxiety as the commonest type. By contrast, conduct disorders, and to an important extent mixed disorder, were more common among boys with an association with specific reading retardation. A comparative study of 10-year-olds living in London (Rutter et al 1975) showed a rate of disturbance over twice that on the IoW study. This study also showed that the difference in prevalence rate was entirely accounted for by the increased frequency of predisposing factors among children and their families in London compared with those on the IoW study. These factors were family discord, parental psychiatric disorder, social disadvantage and inferior quality of schooling.

The IoW study (Rutter et al 1970b) also showed that children with chronic illness or handicap had much higher rates of disturbance than healthy children. For instance, children with neurological disease, such as epilepsy or cerebral palsy, had a rate over five times that of the general population, while children with other illnesses such as asthma and diabetes were twice as likely to be disturbed as healthy children.

Studies of pre-school children, most notably by Richman et al (1975), have found that about 20% of children have significant behavioural problems, with 7% classified as severe. Follow-up studies (Richman et al 1982) indicated that about 60% of the problems persisted, most commonly among overactive boys of low ability. An important association was found between language delay and disturbed behaviour. Finally, problems were more likely to continue when there was marital discord, maternal psychiatric ill-health and psychosocial disadvantage such as poor housing and large family size.

ASSESSMENT PROCEDURES

Assessment is more time-consuming in child psychiatry than in other branches of psychiatry. It has three components: history taking and examination; psychological assessment; and information about the child and family from other professionals.

History taking and examination

This has many similarities to traditional methods, though with important modifications. Interview skills are essential to the elucidation, understanding and treatment of emotional and behavioural problems in children. Training in interview skills should be an important part of medical undergraduate and postgraduate training. Recent research (Maguire & Rutter 1976) has revealed the lack of skills among doctors in training and also how these skills can be improved.

Points of general importance include: clarification of the nature of the problem and the reason for referral; obtaining adequate factual information; eliciting emotional responses and attitudes to past events and observing behaviour during the interview; establishing the trust and confidence of the child and family; and providing the parents with a summary of problems and a provisional treatment plan at end of the initial interview.

There are no absolute rules about interviewing;

indeed, flexibility is essential. However, the following guidelines are useful:

1. The interview room should be large enough to seat the family comfortably and also to allow the children to use play material in a relaxed manner
2. Avoid having a desk between the interviewer and the family; for instance, put the desk against the wall of the interview room
3. Do not spend the interview writing notes but rather encourage eye-to-eye contact, taking the minimum notes necessary.
4. Play material must be suitable for a wide age range and include crayons and paper, jigsaws, simple games, books (provides rough estimate of reading ability), doll's house, play telephones and miniature domestic and zoo animals
5. The play material should be gradually introduced as appropriate and not left around in a haphazard manner
6. Interview parents and young children together
7. Older children and adolescents like to be seen separately from their parents at some point during the interview
8. Older children and adolescents are able to talk about problems openly once trust has been established
9. Too direct questions usually elicit denial from the child so that open-ended questions are much more preferable.

The interview should provide information about the following (bold type indicates essential facts):

1. **Presenting problem(s): frequency; severity; onset; course; exacerbating/ameliorating factors; effect on family; help given so far**
2. Other problems or complaints:
   a. General health: eating; sleeping; elimination; physical complaints; fits or faints
   b. Interests, activities and hobbies
   c. **Relationship with parents and sibs**
   d. Relationship with other children; special friends
   e. Mood: happy, sad, anxious
   f. Level of activity, attention span and concentration
   g. Antisocial behaviour
   h. **Schooling: attainments; attendance; friendships; relationship with teachers**
   i. Sexual knowledge, interests and behaviour (when relevant)
3. Family structure:
   a. **Parents: ages; occupations; current physical and psychiatric state**; previous physical and psychiatric history
   b. Sibs: ages, problems
   c. Home circumstances
4. Family function:
   a. **Quality of parenting: mutual support and help; level of communication and ability to resolve problems**
   b. **Parent–child relationship: warmth, affection and acceptance; level of criticism, hostility and rejection**
   c. Sibs' relationship
   d. Pattern of family relationships
5. Personal history:
   a. Pregnancy and delivery
   b. Early mother–child relationship: postpartum depression; early feeding patterns
   c. Temperamental characteristics: easy or difficult; irregular, restless baby or toddler
   d. Developmental milestones
   e. **Past illnesses and injuries: hospitalisation**
   f. Separations greater than 1 week
   g. Previous schooling
6. **Observation of child's behaviour and emotional state**
   a. **Appearance: nutritional state; signs of neglect or injury**
   b. **Activity level: involuntary movements; concentration**
   c. **Mood: expressions or signs of sadness, misery, anxiety**
   d. **Reaction to and relationship with the doctor: eye contact; spontaneous talk; inhibition and disinhibition**
   e. **Relationship with parents: affection/resentment; ease of separation**
   f. Habits and mannerisms
   g. Presence of delusions, hallucinations, thought disorder
7. Observation of family relationships:
   a. Patterns of interaction
   b. Clarity of boundaries between parents and child
   c. Communication
   d. Emotional atmosphere of family: mutual warmth/tension; criticisms
8. Physical examination:
   A. Screening neurological examination:
      a. Note any facial asymmetry
      b. Eye movements: ask child to follow a moving finger and observe eye movement for jerkiness, incoordination
      c. Finger–thumb apposition: ask child to press the tip of each finger against the thumb in

rapid succession and observe for
clumsiness, weakness
  d. Copying pattern: drawing a man
  e. Observe grip and dexterity in drawing
  f. Observe visual competence when drawing
  g. Jumping up and down on the spot
  h. Hopping
  i. Hearing: capacity of child to repeat
     numbers whispered 2 m behind him
B. **Further medical examination (if relevant)**

Formulation

At completion of the assessment, the clinician should
be able to make a formulation. This is a succinct
summary of the important features of the individual
case. The formulation consists of the following: statement of main problems; diagnosis and differential
diagnosis; relative contribution of constitutional and
environmental factors to the aetiology; probably short-
term and long-term outcome; further information
required (including special investigations); initial
treatment plan. The formulation should be included
in the casenotes, thereby providing the clinician with a
record of his views at referral.

Psychological assessment

Psychological assessment, carried out by a child
psychologist, is an invaluable and integral part of the
overall assessment of a child's problems in many
situations. It can provide information about three
aspects of development: general intelligence, educational attainments and special skills. Assessment is
usually based on the administration of standardised
assessment procedures. These tests are norm referenced or criterion referenced. The former compares
the child's ability with other children of the same age,
whereas the latter is on a pass/fail basis, for instance
whether he can tie his shoelaces. Ideally, the test items
should have good discriminatory value (distinguish
between children of different ability), predictability
(give similar results when repeated) and validity
(agreement with other independent evidence, be
compatible with existing theoretical models and have
predictive value). An important aspect of the assessment is that the tasks are carried out in a standardised
fashion, thereby increasing their reliability and validity.

Developmental assessment in infancy and early childhood

The commonly used tests are the Bayley Scales of
Infant Development (Bayley 1969), Griffiths Mental

Development Scale (Griffiths 1954) and the Denver
Developmental Screening Test (Frankenberg et al
1975).

Intellectual assessment of school-age children

The most popular test is the Wechsler Intelligence
Scale for Children — revised form (WISC-R)
(Wechsler 1974). This covers an age range from 6 to
14 years. There are 12 subtests measuring different
aspects of the child's ability. Commonly, the tests are
divided into 'verbal' and 'performance' categories
yielding a 'verbal IQ' and a 'performance IQ'. The
'verbal' subtests commonly used are *information
comprehension, arithmetic, similarities* and *vocabulary,*
whilst the 'performance' subtests are *picture completion,
picture arrangement, block design, object assembly* and
coding. Each subtest has a mean score of 10 so that
combining these 10 tests gives a 'full scale' IQ of 100
with a standard deviation of 15. The 'normal'
distribution of the test scores means that it is possible
to state that 66% of children will be within the IQ
range 85–115, 95% within the IQ range 70–130 and
99% within the IQ range 55–145. Other tests used
include the Stanford–Binet (Form L–M) (Thorndike
1973) and the British Ability scales (BAS) (Elliott et
al 1983).

Tests of educational attainment

There are two commonly used reading tests, the
Schonell Graded Word Reading Test (Schonell &
Schonell 1950) and the Neale Analysis of Reading
Ability (Neale 1958). The latter is more comprehensive but takes longer to administer. It provides
information about speed, accuracy and comprehension of reading. The scores are transformed into
reading ages of so many years and months, for
instance 6 years 11 months. Other attainment tests
include the Schonell Graded Spelling Test (Schonell
& Schonell 1950). There is no satisfactory standardised test of mathematical skills, although appropriate
subtests scores of the WISC-R and the BAS can be
used as a guide to mathematical ability.

Specific skills

The Reynell Development Language Scale (Reynell
1969), the Bender Motor Gestalt Test and the
Vineland Social Maturity Scales are examples of tests
to assess the child's acquisition of particular abilities
and skills. These are often helpful with some specific
problems.

Limitations of assessment

Caution should always be exercised in the interpretation of test results. It is wrong to attribute undue significance to a single result, most often done with the IQ score. Many factors influence test results, including fatigue, motivation, poor testing conditions and the use of inappropriate tests. The results should be evaluated in the context of the overall assessment and the report from the child psychologist. A great deal of harm, upset and distress may result when a child is incorrectly classified, or labelled as too able or too dull on the basis of an unreliable psychological assessment.

Additional information

A distinctive feature of child psychiatry practice is the importance attached to obtaining independent evidence about the child's behaviour. This is for two reasons: firstly, a child's behaviour varies from one situation to another, so that it is helpful to have information about the child's behaviour in several contexts; secondly, parental accounts of the child's behaviour are likely to be distorted in many cases, as it is the parents who may be disturbed rather than the child. Consequently, an important part of assessment is to obtain reports from other professionals involved with the family such as schools, health visitors or general practitioners. Another common practice is the use of questionnaires to supplement information provided by referrers and other more formal reports. Several questionnaires (Rutter et al 1970a, Richman et al 1982, Achenbach & Edelbrock 1983) have been devised to assess different age ranges and have satisfactory psychometric properties. The most commonly used questionnaires for school-age children in the UK are the Rutter Parents' and Teachers' Scales, also known as Rutter A and Rutter B, respectively. These scales have established reliability and validity as well as classifying children into neurotic or emotional, conduct or antisocial and mixed categories.

DISORDERS IN PRESCHOOL CHILDREN

Except for rare but severe disorders such as childhood autism, psychiatric disorders in this age group are mostly departures or delays from normality rather than psychiatric illness as such. Moreover, the child's behaviour and development are so influenced by the immediate surroundings that it is often the environment which is responsible for the problems rather than the child. Most of these problems are treated by general practitioners and paediatricians, with only a minority being referred for specialist advice.

Aetiology

Four factors contribute to these problems in varying degrees in the individual child: temperamental factors; physical illness or handicap; family psychopathology; social disadvantage. The New York Longitudinal Study (Thomas et al 1968) showed clearly that children with certain temperamental characteristics, the so-called 'difficult child' and the 'slow to warm up child', were more likely to develop problems. Similarly, physical illness or handicap can directly or indirectly retard developmental progress as well as increase parental anxiety, both of which increase the likelihood of behavioural disturbance. Parental psychiatric illness, marital disharmony and poor parenting skills are instances where disturbances in the parents adversely affect the child's behaviour. Several authors (Brown & Harris 1978, Richman 1977) have shown high rates of depression among mothers with pre-school children. Social disadvantages such as poor housing or inadequate recreational facilities also increase the risk of disturbance among preschool children (Richman 1977).

Frequency of problems

Table 29.2 shows the prevalence of common problems among 3- and 4-year-olds in the general population (Richman & Lansdown 1988).

Problems are mainly about eating, sleeping and elimination, with a marked decrease in wetting and soiling over a 1 year period. Affective symptoms such as unhappiness and also relationship problems are infrequent but, when they arise, they are probably of some significance. Community studies (Richman et al 1975) indicate that 20% of children are regarded by their mothers as having problems, with 7% rated as severe.

Common problems

This section discusses those problems that are particularly characteristic of the pre-school period, whilst others such as soiling that also occur in older children are discussed in a later part of the chapter.

Temper tantrums

These usually arise when the child is thwarted, angry or has been hurt. They can occur in isolation or as

Table 29.2   Problem behaviours among 3- and 4-year-olds

	3-year-olds (%)	4-year-olds (%)
Poor appetite	19	20
Faddy eater	15	24
Difficulty settling at night	16	15
Waking at night	14	12
Overactive and restless	17	13
Poor concentration	9	6
Difficult to control	11	10
Temper	5	6
Unhappy mood	4	7
Worries	4	10
Fears	10	12
Poor relationships with siblings	10	15
Poor relationships with peers	4	6
Regular day wetting	26	8
Regular night wetting	33	19
Regular soiling	16	3

From Richman & Lansdown (1988).

part of a wider problem. They comprise a variety of behaviours, including screaming and crying, often resulting in collapse to the floor with banging of the feet. The child can be aggressive towards other people around him, but rarely injures himself. Most tantrums 'burn themselves out' so that specific intervention is not necessary. If it is, then the following points are useful: if necessary, restrain from behind by folding arms around child's body; minimise any additional attention to the child and only respond and praise when behaviour is back to normal.

Eating disorders

These range in severity from a minor problem such as the finicky child to the severe disabling problem of non-organic failure to thrive (NOFTT) (see also the section on child abuse). Minor problems will usually respond to patient and attentive listening to the parents' concerns, counselling and specific advice. Two specific syndromes, NOFTT and deprivation dwarfism, have been recognised. They usually present to, and are managed by, paediatricians.

Non-organic failure to thrive (NOFTT). This usually manifests itself in the first year of life as persistent failure to gain weight. The child is below the third percentile for weight with additional evidence of developmental and cognitive delay. Examination and investigation reveal no cause for the failure to gain weight. The infant is irritable, lethargic and apathetic. The most striking feature is the poor mother–child relationship manifest by the critical and rejecting attitude of the mother towards the infant's feeding. This often occurs in the context of more widespread emotional and social deprivation with individual characteristics in the child such as adverse temperamental factors and aversion to feeding also making a contribution. The clinical picture varies widely, with the more severe proving extremely intractable (Skuse 1985).

Admission to hospital (to ensure the child's safety and to assess the mother–child relationship) is frequently necessary. Extensive support and counselling is the mainstay of treatment, though in many situations this is not successful. Alternative care arrangements for the child, including foster care and ultimately adoption, may be required in the most severe cases.

Deprivation dwarfism. This syndrome, first described by Powell et al in 1967, occurs in the toddler and older child. It usually presents as idiopathic short stature. It shares many features of NOFTT, including developmental and cognitive delay, behaviour problems and abnormal eating habits. The latter include food searching, scavenging, hoarding and gorging. These are clearly evident when the child is observed at home or when admitted to hospital for investigation. The family circumstances are similar to those in NOFFT with a poor mother–child relationship and social/emotional deprivation. Long-standing modification of the family interaction patterns is often difficult to achieve and sustain so that placement of the child in a new family may be the most sensible and realistic option.

Pica. The ingestion of inedible material such as dirt or rubbish, termed pica, is a normal transitory phenomenon during the toddler period. Persistent ingestion is found amongst mentally retarded, psychotic and socially deprived children. Lead poisoning is a possible but uncommon danger from pica.

Sleep problems

These are common, with up to 20% of 2-year-olds waking at least five times per week (Richman 1981, Eaton-Evans & Dugdale 1988). The two most frequent problems are reluctance to settle at night and persistent waking up during the night. Several factors contribute to the problem, including adverse temperamental characteristics in the child, perinatal problems and maternal anxiety. It is also important to distinguish between those responsible for the onset of the problem and those maintaining it. Medications such as trimeprazine and promethazine are frequently prescribed but usually ineffective. Their only genuine indication is to provide a brief respite for the parents as well as ensuring that the child has an uninterrupted night's sleep. The most successful management is a behavioural strategy (see treatment section). Douglas & Richman (1984) provide a useful summary of these techniques. Other sleep problems in older children are discussed in the miscellaneous section.

Psychiatric aspects of child abuse

Originally, the term 'child abuse' was restricted to the 'battered baby syndrome' (Kempe & Kempe 1978), but it has now been extended to include *physical abuse, emotional abuse, sexual abuse* and *neglect*. Recent enquiries and controversies, particularly the Cleveland affair (Department of Health and Social Security 1988), have highlighted the importance of this topic for all doctors involved in the care of children (i.e. general practitioners, paediatricians, school doctors and child psychiatrists). The main professional responsibility for child protection lies with social workers though other professions are frequently involved at various stages.

This section will concentrate on the psychiatric aspects relating to infants and younger children, as Chapter 30 discusses the adolescent issues. It is also important to remember that the different aspects of child abuse are frequently present in the same child and family and that many comments about the detection, management and treatment apply equally well to all aspects of child abuse. Several books (Kempe & Kempe 1978, Jones 1982, Porter 1984, Bentovim et al 1988) provide useful accounts of current practice.

Physical abuse (non-accidental injury) (for a general review see Mrazek & Mrazek 1985)

Diagnostic awareness and suspicion are the key elements in the detection and recognition of physical abuse. The common characteristics of abused children and their families are summarised below, although the most important factor to recognise is that child abuse can occur in all sections of society:

Vulnerability factors in the abused child:
- Product of unwanted pregnancy
- Unwanted child in family
- Low birth weight
- Separation from mother in neonatal period
- Mental or physical handicap
- Habitually restless, sleepless or incessantly crying
- Physically unattractive.

High risk factors among the parent(s):
- Single parent
- Young
- Abused themselves as children
- Low self-esteem
- Unrealistic expectations of the child and his development
- Inconsistent or punishment-oriented discipline
- Adverse social circumstances
- Low income or unemployment
- Social isolation
- Current stress such as housing crisis, domestic friction, exhaustion or ill health
- Large family.

Management. Three separate stages can be identified in the investigation of suspected child abuse: first, detection and disclosure; second, child protection and legal considerations; third, therapeutic and practical support for the child and family in the immediate and long-term. These stages usually follow one another in a sequential manner.

Stage 1 involves the social work department and frequently general practitioners and/or paediatricians. Stage 2 is the convening of a case conference to obtain a comprehensive assessment of the child's needs and the initiation of statutory measures of care to ensure the protection of the child. This stage is also concerned with decisions about pursuing criminal proceedings against the perpetrator of the abuse, who is usually one of the child's carers. Stage 3 is the institution of a therapeutic plan to remedy the psychological sequelae of the abuse for the child and also to improve the quality of parenting. The latter includes practical help to lessen the burden of child-care as well as specific advice/counselling on parenting skills.

The child psychiatrist can make a useful contribution in two ways: firstly, to act as an outside consultant to other professionals and agencies working with the family on various aspects of detection, management and treatment; secondly, to provide individual and family therapy for the child, the parents or the family in particular instances depending upon the assessment.

In addition to its immediate effects, child abuse may have medium-term and long-term sequelae. Many abused children continue to be exposed to emotional abuse and neglect throughout their childhood so that they often show symptoms of disturbance such as unhappiness, wariness, inability to trust others, low self-esteem and poor peer relationships. This child-hood experience in turn predisposes abused children to become abusing parents as adults (Kempe & Kempe 1978).

Emotional abuse

This term has been introduced to describe the severe impairment of social and emotional development resulting from repeated and persistent criticism, lack of affection, rejection, verbal abuse and other similar behaviour shown by the parent(s) to the child over a long period of time. Affected children display a variety of symptoms, including low self-esteem, limited capacity for enjoyment, severe aggression and impulsive behaviour as well as more specific syndromes such as NOFTT and deprivation dwarfism. Diagnosis is made through observation and interview of the parent(s) and child, separately and together. Parents rarely have any overt psychiatric disorder, though personality disturbance and a history of parental childhood deprivation is common. Management involves similar principles to those outlined for stage 3 of physical abuse.

Sexual abuse (for detailed discussion see Ousten 1990)

This became a topic of major public and paediatric concern in the late 1980s (Department of Health and Social Security 1988). A commonly used definition is as follows: 'the involvement of dependent children and adolescents in sexual activities they do not truly comprehend, to which they are unable to give informed consent, or which violate social taboos of family roles'.

Fundamental to child sexual abuse is the misuse of adult power. The range of activities includes fondling, masturbation, rape and buggery. The term also covers some activities not involving physical contact such as posing for pornographic photographs or films. The abuser is frequently known to the child and is often a member of the family (incest).

The presentation of the sexual abuse varies widely depending on the nature of the abuse and on the relationship between the abused child and the perpetrator. Open disclosure/accusation is more likely when the offender is outside the family, whereas physical symptoms involving the anogenital region and/or emotional or behavioural disturbance are commoner when a family member is responsbile. As with physical abuse, diagnostic awareness and suspicion are the key elements in the detection and recognition of the abuse.

Investigation (see Bentovim et al 1988). Sensitivity and tact are clearly essential when conducting the examination and interview of the child during the initial investigation. Separate detailed questioning and interviewing of the parents are also necessary.

Management (see Bentovim et al 1988). The same principles apply in sexual abuse as in physical abuse. The role of the child psychiatry team is more directly relevant in sexual abuse, as interviewing skills, psychotherapeutic expertise and the use of specialised equipment (anatomically accurate dolls) are often necessary at the detection and also the treatment stages of management. Detailed accounts of this work, including the use of the anatomical dolls, are described in the book by the Great Ormond Street Child Sex Abuse Team (Bentovim et al 1988). The establishment of specialised assessment teams in every locality is another important recommendation of the Cleveland enquiry (Department of Health and Social Security 1988).

Neglect

This varies markedly, ranging from relative inadequacy and incompetence in providing safety, shelter, love and security for the child to severe failure in the provision of basic essentials, often combined with emotional and social deprivation. Though more difficult to quantify than physical or sexual abuse, the condition is certainly more common, at least in its milder forms, than these other two forms of abuse. Additionally, it may be more long-lasting with potentially more serious consequences for the child's development. It is often noticed and reported by relatives, neighbours, health visitors and teachers. Adverse social circumstances and poor parenting are usually found with the necessity for alternative family placement for the child the most suitable solution in the long term in many cases.

Munchausen's syndrome by proxy (Meadow 1982)

This remarkable variant of physical abuse often occurs against the same background of parental psychopathology and social disadvantage as in other forms of abuse. The essential feature of this syndrome is the fabrication of physical illness in the child by the parent(s), usually the mother. Common examples include factitious recurrent bleeding and unstable control of diabetes or epilepsy. Extensive investigation and admission to hospital are carried out with fruitless results. It is only when the possibility of parental abuse is recognised that the explanation becomes apparent.

Management. As soon as the diagnosis is established, the parents should be confronted. The main priority is the protection of the child, including where necessary removal of the child from the family home. The immediate and longer-term aims of treatment are similar to that for child abuse as the underlying psychopathology and social circumstances are similar. The role of the child psychiatrist is usually confined in most cases to offering counselling for the parents and/or family therapy when indicated.

CHILDHOOD AUTISM (PERVASIVE DEVELOPMENTAL DISORDER), SCHIZOPHRENIA AND RELATED SYNDROMES

These conditions were previously combined under the general term 'childhood psychosis', as they are severe and disabling, with clear-cut abnormalities. However, autistic children do not experience hallucinations or delusions, the characteristics of psychosis, and, moreover, have had the abnormalities from early infancy. For these reasons, it seems more sensible to separate childhood autism from other psychotic conditions in childhood and to include the condition under the new category 'pervasive developmental disorder'.

Childhood autism (pervasive developmental disorder)

Kanner's (1943) original description of 11 children with 'an extreme autistic aloneness' has not been bettered, with its astute observation of 'an inability to relate in an ordinary way to people and to situations' and 'an anxiously obsessive desire for the maintenance of sameness'. Subsequently, opinions have fluctuated about the diagnosis, aetiology and treatment. Most authorities now agree that three features are essential to the diagnosis: a general and profound failure to develop social relationships; language retardation; and ritualistic and compulsive behaviour. Additionally, these abnormalities should be manifest before 30 months.

Prevalence

Community surveys (Lotter 1966, Wing & Gould 1979) have found prevalence rates of two per 10 000 increasing to 20 per 10 000 when individuals with severe mental retardation and some autistic features are included. Boys are affected three times as often as girls.

Clinical features

Impaired social relationships. Parental recollections of infancy often reveal that as an infant the child was slow to smile, unresponsive and passive with a dislike of physical contact and affection. Contemporary social deficits include failure to use eye-to-eye gaze and facial expression for social interaction, rarely seeking others for comfort or affection, rarely initiating interaction with others, a lack of empathy and of cooperative play. The children are aloof and indifferent to other people.

Language abnormalities. Language acquisition is delayed and deviant and about 50% of autistic children never develop language. When present, language abnormalities are many and varied, including immediate and delayed echolalia (repetition of spoken word(s) or phrase(s)), poor comprehension and use of gesture, pronominal reversal (use of 'you' when 'I' is meant) and abnormalities in intonation, rhythm and pitch.

Ritualistic and compulsive behaviour. Common abnormalities are rigid and restricted patterns of play, intense attachments to unusual objects such as stones, unusual preoccupations and interests (timetables, bus routes) to the exclusion of other pursuits with a marked resistance to any change in the environment or daily routine. Tantrums and explosive outbursts often occur when any change is attempted.

Other features. Autistic children often exhibit a variety of stereotypies, including rocking, finger twirling, spinning and tip-toe walking. They are often overactive with a short attention span. Seventy per cent of autistic children are in the retarded range of intelligence and only 5% have an IQ above 100. Occasionally, some have remarkable abilities in isolated areas, for instance computation, music and rote memory. Twenty-five per cent will develop epilepsy during adolescence, though not usually severe.

Association with other conditions. Autistic behaviour occurs in some patients with a diverse group of conditions, including rubella, phenylketonuria, tuberose sclerosis, neurolipoidoses, and infantile spasms (Rutter 1985). More recently, Rett's syndrome, with its marked autistic features, has been described (Hagberg et al 1983, Kerr & Stephenson 1985). This condition, which has only been observed in girls, has the following features: a period of normal development with subsequent loss of cognitive and motor skills, acquired microcephaly and hand stereotypies. The condition usually manifests itself around 5 years of age.

Aetiology

Most people favour a primary cognitive deficiency with an organic basis for the following reasons: neurological abnormalities are common; the association with epilepsy and various neurological syndromes; the increased rate of perinatal complications; and the higher concordance among monozygotic compared with dizygotic twins (Rutter & Schopler 1988). Application of new investigative techniques such as computerised tomography (CT), magnetic resonance imaging (MRI) and positron emission tomography (PET) have not revealed any consistent abnormality, though increased brain serotonin levels have been reported. The relationship between autism and the fragile X syndrome is also unclear, as the different rates in the various studies may be a reflection of the degree of mental handicap rather than of aetiological significance. A most interesting psychological perspective on the autistic deficit has been provided by the series of experiments described by Hobson (1986). Hobson concluded that the primary deficit in autism is a lack of empathy, namely, the inability to perceive and interpret emotional cues.

Treatment

Explaining the significance of the diagnosis is a vital first step in helping parents to accept the presence of handicap with a consequent lessening of parental guilt about aetiology. Counselling and advice are likely to be necessary throughout childhood. Rutter (1985) suggested that treatment aims should have four components: the promotion of normal development; the reduction of rigidity and stereotypies; the removal of maladaptive behaviour; and the alleviation of family stress. Behavioural methods, including operant conditioning and shaping (see behavioural treatment section), are the most likely way to achieve some success with the first three aims, whilst counselling is important for the fourth. Special schooling, where the child's special social and educational needs are recognised, is very beneficial, sometimes on a residential basis. Drugs do not have an important role in management.

Outcome

Many individuals with autism are unable to live independently, with only 15% looking after and supporting themselves (Lockyer & Rutter 1969). Many are placed in institutions for the mentally handicapped, though national policy now favours community care. Autistic children with an IQ of 70 or more receiving proper education and coming from middle-class families do comparatively well. In most individuals, there is some improvement in social relationships, though many are still handicapped. Parents often find it helpful to join the National Society for Autistic Children.

Schizoid personality/Asperger's syndrome

Child psychiatrists are reluctant to diagnose personality disorder, as this diagnosis implies that the condition is unlikely to change, a situation somewhat in conflict with the notion that the child is a developing individual. Recently, however, Wolff & Chick (1980) and also Wing (1981) have described a small number of children with very distinctive but uncommon personality characteristics. Wolff & Chick use the term schizoid for these children, whereas Wing prefers the term Asperger's syndrome (Asperger 1944). These children are described as distant, aloof and lacking in empathy. Other features include obstinate and aggressive outbursts when under pressure to conform, often at school, along with undue rigidity, sensitivity to criticism and unusual interests to the exclusion of everything else. In some ways they show features of childhood autism, but in a minor degree. Adult adjustment is variable, with many finding employment, though with an increased risk of anxiety and depressive reactions and obsessional disorders.

Schizophrenia (see also Chs 18 and 30)

This is a rare disease during childhood. Even during adolescence it has a frequency of less than three per 10 000. Symptomatology consists of delusions, hallucinations, distortions of thinking and of movement, most commonly catatonia. It can present acutely with bizarre behaviour or insidiously with gradual withdrawal and failing schoolwork. There is good evidence of a genetic component, with approximately 10% of relatives having the disease. Diagnostically, it often can be difficult to distinguish from a major mood disturbance such as manic–depressive psychosis.

Treatment

This must be comprehensive, including treatment with neuroleptics such as chlorpromazine or haloperidol, and individual and family therapy, as well as help with education. Favourable prognostic factors include high intelligence, acute onset, precipitating factors and a normal premorbid personality.

Other related syndromes

Disintegrative disorder (Corbett et al 1977, Rutter 1985).

This term refers to a group of conditions characterised by normal development until around 4 years of age followed by profound regression and behavioural disintegration, loss of language and other skills, impairment of social relationships and the development of stereotypies. It can follow a minor illness or more definite neurological disease such as measles encephalitis. The prognosis is poor due to the underlying degenerative pathology in many cases.

Delirium-like conditions

Conditions with impairment of consciousness, hallucinations and illusions are common among children with acute infections. Rarely, a non-infective agent, for instance acute intermittent porphyria, is responsible.

EMOTIONAL DISORDERS

The primary abnormality is a disturbance of mood or affect with similar symptomatology and classification to neurotic disorders in adults. Traditionally, these disorders are further divided into phobic, anxiety, obsessional, depressive and hysterical states, though many children show a mixture of symptoms so that allocation to a single category is not possible. ICD-10 and DSM-IIIR have modified this classification with the inclusion of new categories such as separation anxiety disorder and social sensitivity disorder. They have also replaced hysteria with dissociative (conversion) disorders as somatisation disorder. The IoW study (Rutter et al 1970a) found a prevalence rate of 2.5% for emotional disorders with a female preponderance. Prognosis is generally favourable as many problems arise in response to an acute stress and resolve once the stressful effects lessen.

Anxiety states

Clinical features

This is the commonest type of emotional disorder. Anxiety has physical and psychological components, the former referring to palpitations and dry mouth, the latter to the subjective sense of fear and apprehension. Somatic symptoms, particularly abdominal pain, are common. Again, many symptoms may represent the persistence and exaggeration of normal developmental fears and range in severity from an acute panic attack to a chronic anxiety state over several months. Predisposing factors include temperamental characteristics, overinvolved and overconcerned parents and the 'special child syndrome'. The latter refers to children who are treated in an overprotected manner by their parents. This may arise in several ways, for instance the child is much wanted, or previous ill health during pregnancy or infancy with consequent 'anxious' attachment between the child and its parents. In turn, this 'anxious' attachment leads the parents inadvertently to reinforce normal fears and anxieties.

Treatment

Several approaches, including individual, behavioural and family therapy, are used, often in combination depending upon the assessment and formulation. Anxiolytic drugs do not have a major role except in certain situations and for a specified period.

Phobic states

Clinical features

Phobias are common and normal among children. For instance, toddlers are fearful of strangers, whereas adolescents are anxious about their appearance or weight. Pathological fears often develop from ordinary fears that are exacerbated by parental and/or social reinforcement. A phobia is defined as a special form of fear for specific objects or situations, for instance dogs or heights, which are not dangerous in reality. Its characteristics are that it is irrational, beyond voluntary control and leads to avoidance of the feared situation. This avoidance behaviour is the main reason the fear is maladaptive, as it leads to increasing restriction and limitation of the child's activities.

Treatment

A behavioural approach using graded exposure to the feared situation is the most commonly used treatment. The rationale of this approach is that continued exposure to the feared stimulus reduces the anxiety associated with the stimulus, thereby decreasing avoidance behaviour. The success of this method often depends on the ability of the therapist to devise a treatment programme that combines gradual exposure without inducing too much anxiety. Occasionally, anxiolytic drugs are used in conjunction with this behavioural approach.

School refusal (Hersov & Berg 1980)

This term, also known as school phobia, refers to the child's irrational fear of going to school. It is also known as the masquerade syndrome (Waller & Eisenberg 1980) as it can present in a variety of disguises, including abdominal pain, headaches and viral infection. The child is reluctant to leave home in the morning to attend school (in contrast to the truant who leaves home but does not arrive at school). It occurs most commonly at the commencement of schooling, change of school or the beginning of secondary school.

Most cases can be understood in terms of the following three mechanisms, often in combination: first, separation anxiety, the child and/or the parent being fearful of separation, of which school is the cause; second, a specific phobia of some aspect of school attendance, such as travelling to school or mixing with other children, or some part of the school routine, for instance certain subjects, gym or assembly; third, a more general psychiatric disturbance such as depression or low self-esteem. The latter is more frequent among adolescents. Typically, most school refusers have good academic attainments and are conformist at school but oppositional at home. School refusal can present acutely or insidiously, often becoming a chronic problem in adolescence.

Treatment

The initial essential step is to recognise the condition, that is, to avoid unnecessary and extensive investigations for minor somatic symptoms or advising prolonged convalescence following minor illness. For recent-onset cases, early return to school with firm support for the parents and liaison with the school is the most successful approach. For more intractable cases, extensive work with the child and parents, along with a graded return to school is advisable. A specific behavioural programme for the phobic elements may be necessary as well as the use of anxiolytic drugs in some instances. The chronic problem often requires a concerted approach, sometimes involving a period of assessment and treatment at a child psychiatric inpatient unit. Many clinicians also use family therapy to tackle the major relationship problems that exist in many cases.

Outcome

Two-thirds usually return to school regularly, whilst the remainder, usually adolescents from disturbed families, only achieve erratic attendance at best. Follow-up studies into adult life have found that approximately one-third continue with neurotic symptoms and social impairment (Hersov & Berg 1980).

Depression (see Kazdin 1990 & Ch. 30)

There is an important distinction between sadness and unhappiness on the one hand and depressive disorder on the other. Transitory mood swings are a normal phenomenon, affecting many children, particularly adolescents. Moreover, sadness and unhappiness are features found in several other psychiatric disorders, including chronic anxiety and conduct disorders. By contrast, depressive disorder is characterised by a sustained lowered mood, anhedonia (inability to derive pleasure from life), low self-esteem, suicidal ideas and disturbances of eating and sleeping.

Until recently, it was thought that this syndrome did not occur in prepubertal children, except perhaps following certain illnesses such as infectious mononucleosis. However, the development of reliable interview schedules and questionnaires (Rutter 1988) has changed this view so that it is recognised that depressive illness does occur, though uncommonly (prevalence less than 1%). Bipolar or manic–depressive illness is even more infrequent (Antony & Scott 1960).

Assessment

A comprehensive assessment involving individual and family interview(s) is essential as well as information from the school. The interview with the child has particular importance as it can involve the disclosure of suicidal ideas and also provide the child with the opportunity to unburden himself as well as establishing a trusting relationship with the therapist. The assessment of suicidal risk is important (see Ch. 30). Detailed enquiry should be made about current stresses, particularly life events involving threat and loss of self-esteem and about recent illnesses, particularly viral infections.

Treatment

Tricyclic antidepressants (imipramine or amitriptyline) are successful for some children with definite depressive disorder, though side-effects are common and occasionally disabling. Individual and family therapy are used in most cases. Attempts should be made wherever possible to ameliorate any contributory stressful factors. Recently, some clinicians have also attempted to use cognitive behavioural approaches in older children and adolescents.

Outcome

Approximately two-thirds will respond to treatment with the remainder continuing to show symptoms or to be vulnerable to further episodes.

Obsessive–compulsive disorder

Definition

An obsession is a recurrent, intrusive thought that the individual recognises is irrational but cannot ignore. A compulsion or ritual is the behaviour(s) accompanying these ideas, the aim of which is to reduce the associated anxiety (see Fig. 29.1).

Clinical features

Most children display obsessional behaviours at some time, for instance avoiding cracks on paving stones or walking under ladders. These have no clinical significance. It is only when the behaviour interferes with ordinary activities that it amounts to illness. Common obsessional rituals are hand washing and dressing.

Obsessional thoughts often have a foreboding quality, for instance that 'something could happen' to a parent or sibling, that he might die or get run over. The rituals, though maladaptive, are maintained because they produce temporary reduction in anxiety. Commonly, the child involves other members of the family in the performance of rituals so that he assumes a controlling role within the family.

The illness is rare (community prevalence 0.3%) but commoner among older children and adolescents with an acute or gradual onset. In addition to anxiety symptoms, many children exhibit depressive features.

Treatment

Behavioural methods, particularly response prevention, are often successful in eliminating the obsessive–compulsive behaviour. Response prevention consists of training the child to become aware of the cues that trigger the symptom and then using distraction techniques to make the performance of the ritual impossible. Medication, usually clomipramine, is helpful sometimes for anxiety and depressive symptoms. Involvement of other members of the family, whether specifically in family therapy or to assist the child in the elimination of rituals, is necessary. Some cases require in-patient admission.

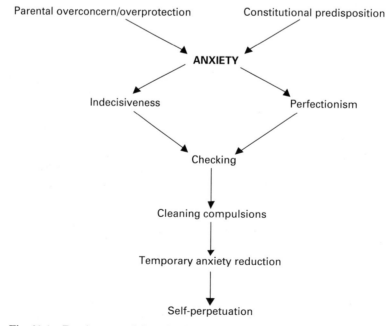

Fig. 29.1 Development of obsessional symptoms.

Outcome

Two-thirds do well, with the remainder continuing to have problems, usually in a fluctuating fashion.

Hysteria or somatisation disorder

Somatisation disorder is a new category in DSM-III and ICD-10, for a reasonably well-defined group of disorders previously classified as hysterical. The primary feature of somatisation disorder is the development of multiple somatic symptoms without any pathological basis in response to some form of stress. As the term hysteria continues to be used in clinical practice, this section discusses the two groups separately in the recognition that they show many similarities.

Hysteria

Clinical features. These comprise conversion and dissociative states, both of which are rare in childhood (Goodyer 1981). Conversion disorder refers to the development of physical symptoms, usually of the special senses or limbs, without any pathological basis in the presence of identifiable stress and/or affective disturbance. The emotional conflict is said to be 'converted' into physical symptoms which are less threatening to the individual than the underlying psychological conflict. A dissociative state is the restriction or limitation of consciousness due to psychological causes; examples include amnesia and fugue.

It is dangerous to diagnose the condition solely by the exclusion of organic disease as follow-up studies have found that a substantial minority subsequently develop definite organic illness, most notably amblyopia (Caplan 1970). Misdiagnosis is most likely when physical signs are absent and coincidental emotional upset is present (Rivinus et al 1975). There should always be positive psychological reasons to explain the development of the symptoms. Common reasons include major life events or stresses for the child, a similar illness among other family members/peers or underlying depressive disorder.

Minor degrees of these disorders are extremely common and frequently occur as a transitory phenomenon during the course of many illnesses. A more general term 'abnormal illness behaviour' has been coined to describe the situation when the individual persists with and exaggerates symptoms following from an illness, akin to the physician's phrase 'functional overlay'.

Treatment. Successful treatment depends on recognition that the symptoms are 'real' for the child, and that psychic pain is as distressing as physical pain. Anger and confrontation are unhelpful. A firm sympathetic approach with little attention to the symptom per se as well as avoiding rewarding the symptom is probably best. Allow the child to give up his symptoms with a good grace, perhaps by providing him with some face-saving reason for improvement. Identify and treat any affective disturbance. The outcome is good for the individual episode, though other psychological problems may persist.

Somatisation disorder (see Lask & Fosson 1989)

Clinical features and management. Many children complain of somatic symptoms which do not have a pathological basis. Common symptoms are abdominal pain, headaches and limb pains with a prevalence rate of approximately 10% (Apley & MacKeith 1968, Faull & Nicol 1986). This condition is usually managed by general practitioners, though it sometimes results in referral for specialist opinion. Persistent unexplained somatic symptoms are commonly a reflection of underlying anxiety or a response to stressful events.

Management involves the minimum necessary investigation to exclude any pathology, the identification of stressful circumstances and a sensitive explanation of the basis for the symptoms. Prevention of restrictions and active encouragement of normal activities are essential. Occasionally, specialist referral for psychiatric help is necessary to treat the underlying psychopathology.

CONDUCT DISORDERS (see Robins 1991)

Clinical features

This is usually defined as persistent antisocial or socially disapproved of behaviour that often involves damage to property and is unresponsive to normal sanctions. The IoW study (Rutter et al 1970a) found a prevalence rate of 4% when the mixed disorder category was included with a marked male predominance (at least 3:1). There is no absolute criterion for deviance as social and cultural values determine the seriousness or importance that is attached to antisocial behaviour. Common symptoms include temper tantrums, oppositional behaviour, overactivity, irritability, aggression, stealing, lying, truancy, bullying and wandering away from home/school.

Delinquency (see Ch. 30). This is a legal term referring to a young person who has committed a criminal offence. It is common among older children and adolescents. Stealing, vandalism, arson and fire-setting are common forms of delinquency (male:female, 10:1).

Traditionally, a distinction has been made between socialised and unsocialised behaviour disorder. The former describes behaviour that is in accord with peer group values but contrary to those of society, for instance antisocial gang behaviour such as stealing and vandalism. Unsocialised antisocial behaviour implies more disturbed behaviour as it is often done as a solitary activity against a background of parental rejection or neglect and poor peer relationships. Learning difficulties, especially specific reading retardation, occur more commonly among children with conduct disorders. This is a further reason why school is unpopular and a source of discouragement for these children. Additionally, many children with conduct disorder have affective symptoms such as anxiety or unhappiness, as well as low self-esteem and poor peer relationships. When these symptoms are prominent, it is often appropriate to classify the disorder as mixed, implying both emotional and behavioural symptomatology.

Aetiology

Four factors — the *family*, the *peer group*, the *neighbourhood* and *constitutional* — make some contribution in most cases, but the family is usually the most important. Families of children with conduct disorder are characterised by a lack of affection and rejection, marital disharmony, inconsistent and ineffective discipline and parental violence and aggression. The families are often large, which aggravates the problems of supervision and care. Constitutional factors present in some cases include low intelligence and learning difficulties along with adverse temperamental features such as overactivity and impulsiveness. Oppositional peer group values are an important feature in older children and adolescents. Many children with conduct disorder live in areas of urban deprivation with poor schooling. The intractable and chronic nature of these problems is a major reason for the continuation of conduct disorder into adolescence and adult life.

Treatment

Help for the family, by counselling for the parents or by family therapy, is often used. A behavioural approach for some symptoms such as aggression and oppositionality is often successful. Educational support through remedial teaching or the provision of special education can be important in some cases. For many families, however, the role of psychiatric services is limited to practical support, for instance with rehousing in order to alleviate social disadvantage, the most important but mundane contribution.

Prognosis

Two-thirds of individuals continue to show problems into adult life. Bad prognostic features are many and varied symptoms, problems at home and in the community along with anti-authority and aggressive attitudes (Robins 1991).

DISORDERS OF ELIMINATION

Enuresis

This term refers to the involuntary passage of urine in the absence of physical abnormality after the age of 5 years. It may be nocturnal and/or diurnal. Bed-wetting continuously, though not usually every night, since birth is termed primary enuresis. When there has been a 6 month period of dry beds at some stage, recurrence of bed-wetting is termed secondary or onset enuresis. Diurnal enuresis is much less common than nocturnal, but more common among girls and among children who are psychiatrically disturbed. Depending upon definition, approximately 10% of 5-year-olds, 5% of 10-year-olds and 1% of 15-year-olds have nocturnal enuresis. Most of them are not psychiatrically ill, though a substantial minority, approximately 25%, do have signs of psychiatric disturbance.

Aetiology

A combination of individual factors such as positive family history (approximately 70%), low intelligence, psychiatric disturbance and small bladder capacity along with environmental factors such as recent stressful life events, large family size and social disadvantage, are present in many cases.

Treatment

It is important to exclude a physical basis for the enuresis by history, physical examination and, if necessary, investigation of the renal tract. Assuming no physical pathology, the most important initial step is to minimise the handicap, that is, to point out to the parents the very favourable natural outcome of the condition, and to relabel the child's enuresis as immaturity rather than laziness or wilfulness. A star chart (the accurate recording of enuresis plus positive reinforcement for dry nights) provides an accurate baseline as well as a successful treatment in its own right. A buzzer or bell-and-pad is successful with older co-operative children. The success of this approach is probably because the child becomes more aware of the sensation of a full bladder, along with the encouragement he receives from parents for dry nights. The new models of the buzzer are extremely compact and do not require a pad placed between the sheets, thereby increasing patient compliance considerably. It is useful to combine a buzzer with a star chart. Tricyclic antidepressants, such as imipramine 25–50 mg nocte, are very effective at stopping enuresis, though the enuresis tends to return when they are stopped. Many paediatricians believe it is wrong to prescribe potentially lethal drugs for a benign condition such as enuresis, as accidental or intentional overdose of the prescribed tricyclics, often by other siblings, can occur.

Encopresis and soiling

Most children are continent of faeces and clean by their fourth birthday. Encopresis is the inappropriate passage of formed faeces, usually on to underclothes, in the absence of physical pathology after 4 years of age. Soiling, the passage of semisolid faeces, is often used synonymously with encopresis. Symptoms vary widely in severity, ranging from slight staining of underclothes to encopresis with the smearing of faeces

on to walls. Encopresis is uncommon, with a community prevalence among 8-year-olds of 1.8% for boys and 0.7% for girls. Psychiatric disturbance is common among children with encopresis. Enuresis may also be present.

Clinical features

Figure 29.2 shows a convenient way to classify encopresis with a broad distinction between children who retain faeces with eventual overflow incontinence and those who deposit faeces inappropriately on a regular basis. Some children have never achieved continence, a situation called continuous or primary encopresis, whilst others have had periods of cleanliness followed by relapse, so-called discontinuous or secondary encopresis. Figure 29.2 also lists the common different patterns of interaction between encopretic children and their parents. For instance, children with retentive encopresis have usually been subjected to coercive and obsessional toilet training practices, and the encopresis is seen as a reaction, often of anger and aggression, towards this practice. Similarly, many children with continuous non-retentive encopresis come from disorganised chaotic families where regular training and toileting are not the norm. Encopresis can also arise in some children as a response to a stressful situation. Finally, encopresis can reflect a poor parent–child relationship, often long-standing and usually associated with other aspects of psychiatric disturbance. The clinical picture is often, however, not clear-cut with several different elements making some contribution. There may also be a previous history of constipation or occasionally of anal fissure.

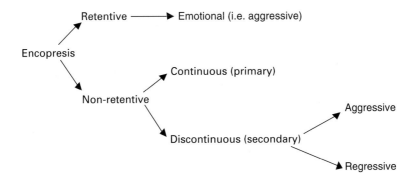

Fig. 29.2   Classification of encopresis. Emotional — obsessive, coercive toilet training practices; continuous — inadequate and disadvantaged families with poor training; aggressive — reflection of poor parent–child relationship; regressive — responsive to itress.

Treatment

A physical aetiology such as Hirschsprung's disease must be excluded before commencement of psychological treatment. The assessment must include an account of previous treatments and, most importantly, the current attitude of the parents and the child to the problem. Treatment has two aims: the promotion of a normal bowel habit; and the improvement of the parent–child relationship. Initially, bowel washouts and/or microenemata may be necessary to clear out the bowel. Judicious use of bowel smooth muscle stimulants (Senokot), stool softeners (Dioctyl) and bulk agents (lactulose) is helpful for the child with retention. Suppositories may also be useful from time to time. These treatments must be combined with parental and child education about the dietary importance of fibre. The psychological component includes behavioural (star chart) and individual psychotherapy to gain the cooperation and trust of the child, along with parental counselling or family therapy in order to modify attitudes and hostile interactions between the child and his parents.

Prognosis

It usually resolves by adolescence, though other problems may persist. Occasional reports of persistence into adult life have been published (Fraser & Taylor 1986).

OVERACTIVITY AND HYPERACTIVITY SYNDROMES (Taylor 1986)

The terms overactivity, hyperactivity, attention deficit disorder and hyperkinetic syndrome are often used synonymously so it is important to define their usage in each instance.

Overactivity and/or hyperactivity

These terms refer to excessive motor activity and restlessness which are present in some but not all situations. About one-third of children are described by their parents as overactive and 5–20% of schoolchildren are so described by teachers. The overactivity ranges in severity from normal childish exuberance to the severe and disabling hyperkinetic syndrome. Numerous studies, reviewed by Taylor (1986), have shown a ten-fold difference in prevalence between the USA and the UK (USA ten per 1000 children, UK one per 1000). The most likely explanation for this difference is probably terminology rather than a true difference in prevalence. British psychiatrists tend to limit the term hyperkinesis to the small number of children with the hyperkinetic syndrome with the remainder classified as conduct disorder (since many conduct-disordered children have overactivity as an important feature of their disturbance).

A convenient way to classify overactivity is as follows:

1. The upper end of the normal activity range
2. A major symptom of the rare hyperkinetic disorder
3. A feature of many children with conduct disorder
4. A reflection of developmental delay or immaturity by itself, or in association with general intellectual retardation
5. A feature of childhood autism or psychosis
6. An uncommon reaction to high anxiety or tension
7. A response to some drugs, for instance barbiturates or benzodiazepines

Attention deficit disorder

This is a term mainly used in North America to describe a large group of children (approximately 5–10% of the population) whose principal abnormalities are a short attention span and distractibility. The children are overactive in some situations, aggressive and have learning difficulties. The primary abnormality of the disorder is said to be a defect in attention and vigilance processing within the brain. A major weakness of this explanation is, however, the absence of convincing experimental evidence in support. Another disadvantage of this terminology is that it could include some children who are inattentive for other reasons, for instance daydreaming or excessive anxiety. DSM-IIIR has recognised the difficulties with this diagnostic category so that the disorder is now just one of four categories for children with disruptive overactive behaviour.

Hyperkinetic syndrome

In the UK this category is restricted to the small number of children (less than 0.1%) who have severe pervasive hyperactivity (i.e. present in all situations), are restless, distractible and have a short attention span. Hyperkinetic children are reckless and impulsive, prone to accidents, and find themselves in trouble because of unthinking breaches of rules rather than because of deliberate defiance. They are socially disinhibited, showing a lack of caution or reserve with adults. Behaviour can be aggressive at times with marked mood swings. Other associated features are a male predominance (at least 3:1), low intelligence, learning difficulties and often some signs of neurological impairment. The hyperactivity is at its peak between the ages of 3 and 8 years.

Aetiology

Originally, the hyperkinetic syndrome was regarded as the prototype for syndromes attributable to 'minimal brain damage' (Strauss & Lehtinen 1947). This theory proposed that minor abnormalities or anomalies of brain structure and function produced a stereotyped clinical picture characterised by hyperkinesis. This was said to mimic to a lesser degree the well-known effects of definite brain damage. Unfortunately, the theory was extended in such a way that the reasoning became tautological, for instance certain behaviours were said to be pathognomonic of brain damage. Many writers, including Bax & MacKeith (1963), have exposed the conceptual flaws of this theory so that it has now been largely discredited.

Many studies, reviewed by Taylor 1986, have shown that several factors, both genetic and environmental, contribute to the development of the syndrome. Two other theories have recently attracted increasing attention, the role of food additives and that of lead intoxication.

Feingold (1975) maintained that hyperactivity was an allergic response by the child to certain food additives, commonly tartrazine. He therefore proposed a diet which excluded these substances. His subsequent findings appeared to show beneficial results. However, evidence for the general efficacy of these exclusion diets, other than as a placebo response, is unconvincing, though recently Egger et al (1985), using a sophisticated methodological design, showed that children with severe hyperactivity and mental retardation did respond. It is, however, unclear whether these results would apply to the majority of children with the hyperkinetic syndrome.

Whilst the toxic properties of lead are not in doubt, the relationship between lead intoxication and behaviour, particularly hyperactivity, is still unresolved. A recent study (Thomson et al 1989) of 501 Edinburgh children found a dose–response relationship between high blood levels of lead and abnormal hyperactivity scores on the Rutter Scale questionnaire. This study supported earlier reports that high blood lead levels can produce behaviour and cognitive disorders in some children (Needleman et al 1979). The main uncertainty is still the strength and clinical importance of the statistically significant findings found in the various studies.

Treatment

Medication, usually with stimulant drugs such as methylphenidate (up to 0.3 mg/kg·day) can be very valuable for children with severe hyperkinetic syndrome, but it should be restricted to this small group of children and not prescribed for every hyperactive child. Most importantly, drug treatment should be combined with behavioural approaches. Side-effects of methylphenidate include loss of appetite, insomnia, reduced growth rate and labile moods. Drug 'holidays', whereby the drug is stopped for periods of time are very useful, not only to minimise side-effects but also to show whether medication is still necessary. Behavioural techniques, parental counselling and the alteration and manipulation of the child's environment, particularly at school, to reduce and minimise distraction are the main components of treatment programmes in most cases. As discussed earlier, the general role of exclusion diets is still 'not proven'.

Outcome

Hyperactivity and attention deficits lessen considerably by adolescence, though other major problems such as learning difficulties and behaviour problems persist. A substantial minority continue to have problems in adult life, mainly of an antisocial nature.

MISCELLANEOUS DISORDERS

Developmental disorders

Language disorders (see Campbell & McIntosh 1992)

Delayed speech is a frequent source of parental concern as well as a common reason for specialist paediatric referral. All children without meaningful words by 18 months should be investigated thoroughly. The commonest cause of significant speech delay is mental retardation. The following list shows the important causes:

1. Intellectual retardation
2. Deafness
3. Specific speech/language disorder
4. Social deprivation
5. Childhood autism.

Specific language disorder is a delay in the acquisition of speech and language compared with other aspects of development (Bishop 1987). It is usually divided into receptive and expressive types, implying a disorder in the understanding of language or in the production of speech, respectively. Expressive disorder (prevalence five per 1000) is twice as common in boys as in girls, whereas the rarer receptive disorder (prevalence one per 10 000) has an equal sex prevalence. Children with language disorder are more vulnerable to disturbance, mainly because of the anxiety and embarrassment caused by the disorder (Cantwell & Baker 1985). Richman et al (1982) found that approximately 25% of 3-year-olds with specific language delay had behavioural problems.

Stuttering or stammering. This is an abnormality of speech rhythm consisting of hesitations and repetitions at the beginning of syllables and words. It is a normal, though transitory phenomenon, occurring around 3–4 years of age. When it persists (as it does in approximately 3% of the general population), this is often due to inadvertent parental overconcern leading to further anxiety and low self-esteem.

Elective mutism. This is not strictly a language disorder, as the main problem is the child's refusal to talk in certain situations, most commonly at school, rather than an inability to speak. Mild forms of the disorder are common but transitory, usually at the commencement of schooling, while the severe form has a prevalence of one per 1000 (Kolvin & Fundudis 1981). Other features include a previous history of speech delay, excessively shy but stubborn temperament and parental overprotectiveness.

A combination of behavioural and family therapy techniques to promote communication and the use of speech is most commonly used, though some cases require in-patient assessment. Prognosis is good for approximately 50%, with failure to improve by the age of 10 years a poor prognostic sign.

Reading difficulties

Though mainly of educational concern, the child psychiatrist may get involved because of the associated behavioural or emotional problems. Two main types are recognised: first, *general reading backwardness* when the retardation is a reflection of generalised intellectual delay; second, *specific reading retardation* when the attainment in reading is significantly below the expected level when age and general intelligence are taken into account. The problem is usually 'significant' when the delay is at least 2 years.

Dyslexia. This is a concept similar to that of specific reading retardation, implying a neuropsychological substrate for the specific reading difficulties. The use of this term is contentious, so that the more neutral expression, specific reading retardation, is preferred by many clinical psychologists.

The aetiology is multifactorial, involving genetic, social, perceptual and language deficits. A noteworthy feature is the strong association between specific reading retardation and conduct disorder with the behaviour problem probably arising secondary to the frustration and disillusionment associated with the reading difficulty. Treatment involves detailed assessment of the precise nature of the problem by a clinical or educational psychologist, followed by an individualised remedial programme carried out by a specialised teacher in collaboration with the psychologist. Help with the behavioural problem is also necessary in order to prevent more serious problems arising during adolescence.

Other developmental disorders

Two other scholastic disorders, *specific arithmetic disorder* and *specific spelling disorder*, and *specific motor disorder* (also known as the clumsy child syndrome or developmental dyspraxia) have been described.

The two scholastic disorders relate to specific difficulties with arithmetic and spelling. Their aetiology, prevalence and prognosis are not well delineated, though it is assumed that they have many similarities to specific reading retardation. Treatment involves the same general principles as for reading disorder.

Specific motor disorder (Gordon & MacKinlay 1986, Henderson 1987, Campbell & McIntosh 1992,) is characterised by a serious impairment in the development of motor coordination involving fine and gross motor skills. Common features are an awkward gait and poor skills in dressing, drawing and constructional tasks. Neurological assessment reveals neurodevelopmental immaturities such as choreiform movements, 'soft' neurological signs and abnormal reflexes. By definition, there is no diagnosable neurological disorder. Treatment involves a coordinated physiotherapy and remedial educational programme. Psychiatric support may be necessary for the attendant emotional and behavioural problems.

Habit disorders

Tics

These are rapid, involuntary, repetitive muscular movements, usually involving the face and neck, for instance blinks, grimaces and throat clearing. Simple tics occur as a transitory phenomenon in about 10% of the population with boys outnumbering girls three to one and with a mean age of onset around 7 years. They range in severity from simple tics involving the head and neck to complex tics extending to the limbs and trunk and finally to the Gilles de la Tourette syndrome (Gilles de la Tourette 1885). The latter comprises complex tics accompanied by coprolalia (uttering obscene words and phrases) and echolalia (the repetition of sounds or words). Like stammering, tics are worse at times of stress and may be exacerbated by undue parental concern. The differential diagnosis of tics in childhood is principally from chorea where the movements are less co-ordinated and predictable, not stereotypic in form and cannot be suppressed. Other features of tics are a positive family history and a previous history of neurodevelopmental delay. Many tics resolve spontaneously, but those that persist can be extremely disabling and difficult to treat.

Treatment. Several approaches are used singly or in combination, depending on assessment. Medication is effective but should be reserved for severe cases. Haloperidol (0.5–1.5 mg b.d.) is the drug of choice for the Tourette syndrome. If unsuccessful, alternative drugs are pimozide and clonidine. Many children with simple tics respond to explanation and reassurance along with advice for the parents. Individual and/or family therapy may be indicated when anxiety and tension are clearly making important contributions to the problem. Behaviour therapy in the form of relaxation and/or massed practice can also be helpful.

Prognosis. Simple tics have a good outcome with complete remission, whereas in the Tourette syndrome the condition fluctuates in a chronic manner, with 50% continuing with symptoms even into adult life.

Finger or thumb sucking and nail biting

These are extremely common and usually of no pathological significance. Excessive finger/thumb sucking can lead to deformity of teeth and fingers. Occasionally, they are signs of more a serious disturbance which itself requires treatment.

Rocking and head banging

Many normal and otherwise healthy toddlers indulge in these habits when they are in their cot, causing much anxiety and distress to their parents who are also embarrassed by neighbours' complaints about the noise. Most children spontaneously cease these habits by around their fourth birthday so that reassurance and support for the parents is usually effective.

More serious self-injurious behaviour occurs among some severely retarded children, some blind children and children with the Lesch–Nyhan syndrome.

Masturbation

This usually attracts attention and concern when it happens excessively. Most infants and toddlers engage in and enjoy touching their genitalia. During middle childhood, this appears less common and/or the child is more discrete. At adolescence, masturbation is probably universal among boys, though less common among girls. Excessive masturbation requires investigation and help. Causes include: local skin irritation, particularly among infants; sexual abuse among older children; and emotional deprivation where the masturbation represents an attempt by the child to obtain some pleasure from an otherwise unloving environment. Some mentally retarded adolescents cause much embarrassment to their parents by masturbating in public. Clear guidelines for the parents about what is acceptable and what is not (i.e. masturbation in private is allowable) are the best way to help, along with encouragement for the parents to enforce these rules.

Sleep disorders (see section pre-school children)

Night terrors

The usual pattern is for the child to wake up in a frightened, even terrified state, not to respond when spoken to, nor appear to see objects or people. Instead, he appears to be hallucinating, talking to and looking at people/things not actually present. The child may also be difficult to comfort, with the period of disturbed behaviour and altered consciousness lasting up to 15 minutes, occasionally longer. Eventually, the behaviour settles, with or without comfort, and the child goes back to sleep, awakening in the morning with no recollection of the episode. The latter point is invaluable in helping to allay parental anxiety about the episodes. Night terrors arise from stage 4 or deep sleep. The peak incidence is between 4 and 7 years, falling to 1–3% in older children. It is also helpful to identify and ameliorate any identifiable stresses that may occasionally contribute the problem. Recently, a new behavioural approach based on waking the child 15 minutes prior to the expected time of the night terror has been reported with apparent success (Lask 1988).

Nightmares

These are frightening or unpleasant dreams, occurring during REM (rapid eye movement) sleep. The child may or may not wake up but there will be a clear recollection of the dream if he does wake up and also in the morning. There is no period of altered consciousness or inaccessibility as in night terrors. Again, daytime anxieties and/or frightening television programmes in the evening may be contributory factors.

Sleep-walking (somnambulism)

The child, usually aged between 8 and 14 years, calmly arises from his bed with a blank facial expression, does not respond to attempts at communication and can only be awoken with difficulty. The child is in a state of altered consciousness at the deep level of sleep (stages 3 or 4). Any contributory anxiety should be treated as well as giving the parents some advice about the safety and protection of the child during these episodes.

Eating disorders (see pre-school section and Ch. 30)

Obesity

This is a common problem affecting around 10% of children, depending on the definition. Psychological problems may be responsible for the onset of the obesity and/or may arise secondary to the obesity. The role of the psychiatrist or psychologist is to identify and treat these problems and, more importantly, to enlist the cooperation of the child and family in adherence to a dietary regime. Other treatment components include a behavioural programme to modify eating patterns, for instance making the child more aware of the cues associated with excessive eating. A major problem with treatment programmes is that they may not modify eating habits sufficiently to ensure that weight loss is maintained when the programme is finished.

Anorexia nervosa

This condition, defined as a morbid fear of being fat, accompanied by behaviour designed to produce weight loss, does occur in prepubertal children, both girls and boys, though much less frequently than among adolescents. Bulimia, defined as periodic bouts of 'binge eating' or the consumption of high-calorific food over a brief period often followed by self-induced vomiting, rarely occurs in children. The

main features of these conditions are discussed in Chapters 23 and 30.

PSYCHOLOGICAL EFFECTS OF ILLNESS AND HANDICAP

Approximately 15% of children have some form of chronic illness or handicap. The IoW study (Rutter et al 1970b) showed clearly that this group of children had a high rate of disturbance, namely, a rate of 33% for children with chronic illness involving the central nervous system and 12% for children with other chronic illnesses, compared with 7% in the general population. The IoW study also showed that children with chronic illness or handicap had the same range of disorders as other disturbed children, thereby implying that the mechanisms involved in this increased morbidity are probably indirect and non-specific.

Illness or handicap imposes psychological stress on the child and family not only at the time of diagnosis but also in the long term. Although these effects may be considered separately in some of the following sections, the two processes clearly interact with each other.

Effects on the child

Three aspects are important: the acquisition of skills and of outside interests; the development of self-concept; and the development of adaptive coping behaviour. Many illnesses or handicaps inevitably limit and restrict the child's ability or opportunity to acquire everyday skills and to develop interests and hobbies. For example, the child with cerebral palsy is by definition motor handicapped. Other examples are the dietary restrictions of diabetes, the exercise limitations of asthma and the avoidance by epileptic children of activities such as cycling or swimming. Additionally, educational problems are common among this group of children for a variety of reasons, including increased absence from school, specific learning difficulties, especially among children with epilepsy, and low expectations of parents and teachers.

Illness and handicap can adversely affect the child's self-concept in several ways through its effects on the child's body image, self-esteem and his ideas about the causation of the disability. Many children have a distorted view of their body, believing the handicap to be very prominent or disfiguring. These ideas can often be reinforced by comments from parents and peers. Self-esteem can also be impaired by a faulty cognitive assessment of the situation and a pessimistic and despondent response to that evaluation. This leads the child to have low self-esteem with a gloomy view about his illness and about his prospects for the future. This is particularly likely and also potentially very disabling among older children and adolescents. The other factor influencing the child's self-concept is his explanation for the cause of his disability. Young children below the age of 6 years often regard their disability as a punishment for some misdemeanour, whilst during middle childhood the child commonly thinks he has 'caught' the illness from someone or something. It is only from around 10 years onwards that adult ideas of causation begin to appear.

Successful adaptation to a disability depends on the acquisition of a range of coping behaviours and defence mechanisms to lessen anxieties to an acceptable level. Effective coping strategies include rationing the amount of stress into containable amounts, obtaining information from several sources, rehearsing the possible outcomes of treatment and assessing the situation from several viewpoints. Parents, nursing staff and paediatricians have an important role in promoting this repertoire of skills among children with disability. Additionally, the use of defence mechanisms such as denial, rationalisation or displacement can be helpful for the child during the initial stages of adjustment to the illness or disability.

Effects on the parents

The parents can respond in various ways in the short term (see later section) and also in the long term. Most parents eventually achieve some degree of adaptation, though for a minority maladaptive behaviour patterns emerge and are prominent. The common reaction is overprotection whereby the parent is unable to allow the child to experience the normal disappointments and upsets of childhood, so that the child leads a 'cotton wool' existence. Less frequently, the parent(s) may be rejecting and indifferent to the child because the child's disability is so damaging to their self-esteem, or because the disability has exacerbated an already precarious parent–child relationship. Overprotection and rejection are sometimes combined together in the parental reaction to the child's disability.

The parents may also find it difficult to provide appropriate discipline and control through fears that such control may aggravate the child's illness. For example, parents of children with epilepsy may think that thwarting the child's wishes may induce an epileptic fit.

Finally, the stress of coping with the child's illness may exacerbate parental marital disharmony, though in a minority it may paradoxically unite them as they face the adversity together.

Effect on siblings

This can manifest itself in several ways: the oldest sibling may be given excessive responsibility such as looking after the handicapped sibling; the sibs may lose friendships because they are reluctant to bring their friends home in case their handicapped sibling is an embarrassment; finally, the sibling's own developmental needs may be neglected with consequent resentment and frustration.

Breaking bad news to parents

This distressing but inevitable aspect of paediatrics comes in various guises, for instance the birth of a child with Down's syndrome or with cystic fibrosis. Unfortunately, most undergraduate and postgraduate training includes very little teaching about this important subject. Though the details vary for each case, the following general principles are important:

1. Information should be given by the most senior and experienced doctor involved with the child's care
2. Both parents must be seen together if at all possible as this reduces misinformation and allows the parents to be mutually supportive from the outset
3. Allow adequate time for the interview (not 10 minutes at the end of a ward round)
4. Privacy is essential, not only as a matter of courtesy but also because it allows parents to express emotions more freely
5. Begin the interview by asking the parents to tell you what they know about the problems
6. Tell parents frankly and honestly in simple and non-technical language the nature of the problem, explaining the reasons for the investigations and the basis for the diagnosis
7. Encourage the parents to ask questions (by asking open-ended questions)
8. Emphasise the positive as well as the negative aspects of the diagnosis, for instance the child will be able to have physiotherapy and special equipment, will be able to go to school and will receive effective control for pain
9. Facilitate the expression of emotions by the parents, namely, respond sympathetically and sensitively to the parent(s)' distress and crying

10. Make a definite offer of a further appointment to talk things over again
11. Many parents find it helpful to continue the discussion with a nurse or social worker after the interview

The importance of these guidelines has been confirmed in a recent study by Wooley et al (1989). This retrospective study involved interviewing the parents of 70 children who had life-threatening illnesses. The parents greatly appreciated the opportunity to discuss the implications of the illness at an open, sympathetic, direct and uninterrupted interview at the time of diagnosis. They disliked evasive or unsympathetic brief interviews. The degree of satisfaction or dissatisfaction was not influenced by the current psychiatric morbidity of the parents, though the measures used were not particularly sensitive.

Reactions to hospitalisation

Admission to hospital is a common experience during childhood, with approximately 25% admitted by the age of 4 years. For most children, this is a short admission for a brief treatable illness, whilst a minority (approximately 4%) remain in hospital for at least a month. While most parents and their children cope successfully with the admission, some, particularly those with repeated admissions for minor illnesses, show evidence of disturbance which may have been the reason why the child was admitted in the first place (Quinton & Rutter 1976).

Admission to hospital can have adverse effects in the short term as well as the long term. The contributory factors can be grouped under three headings: the child and family; the nature of the illness; and the attitudes and practices of the hospital and its staff. Important factors within the child and family include the age and temperament of the child, previous experience of hospital, previous parent–child relationship and current family circumstances. Children between the ages of 1 and 4 years are particularly stressed by separation from familiar figures. Similarly, children with adverse temperamental characteristics, such as poor adaptability and irregularity of habits, are more vulnerable. If the child had a favourable experience when in hospital previously, this will ease the stress of any subsequent admission. If the parent–child relationship was poor prior to admission, hospitalisation is likely to exacerbate this problem because of the additional stress. Adverse family circumstances, for instance financial, may also be aggravated by admission.

The nature of the illness, particularly the associated pain and the necessity for painful procedures, influences the child's response. Again, an emergency admission is likely to be more stressful than an elective procedure.

The attitudes of the staff and hospital practices can minimise the distress of the child. Helpful and favourable aspects include good rooming-in facilities, adequate preparation for painful or unpleasant procedures, nursing and medical staff trained to minimise distress and to offer comfort when required. The ward should be organised so that parents and sibs are encouraged to visit, as well as ensuring the ready availability of playleaders and teachers. Medical and nursing staff should also have access to social work resources as well as to psychological and psychiatric services. Finally, liaison between the medical and psychiatric teams and the establishment of a staff support group to enable staff to discuss their own anxieties about working in a stressful environment are likely to be beneficial.

MISCELLANEOUS TOPICS

Stillbirth and neonatal death (Forrest et al 1981, 1982, Bourne & Lewis 1991)

Parental responses vary considerably, though most couples are profoundly shocked initially, followed by a bereavement response to the loss of the child. Hospital staff should be sensitive and responsive to the parents' feelings and wishes. The issue of a certificate of stillbirth or a death certificate and the funeral arrangements are extremely distressing for the parents. Mourning is facilitated by the parents seeing and holding their dead child, as well as having a photograph to remember the child. The results of investigations, including the post mortem examination, should be communicated to the parents to allay their anxiety and to advise about future pregnancies.

Oglethorpe (1989), reviewing subsequent parenting after perinatal bereavement, argues cogently for the importance of these principles as well as suggesting ways to minimise the risk of the 'replacement child syndrome' for future pregnancies.

Sudden infant death syndrome (SIDS)

This has become the commonest cause of death for infants aged between 1 month and 1 year. The sudden and unexpected nature of the event produces profound shock, disbelief and numbness, followed by a bereavement response. Mourning may continue for several months. The family doctor and health visitor usually have important roles during this time. Skilled counselling is essential, as most parents feel responsible for the child's death and are overcritical of themselves in consequence. The provision of home monitoring facilities requires careful consideration and discussion as false alarms are frequent, thereby increasing parental tension and anxiety.

Care of the dying child

Parents usually undergo two periods of grief response, firstly at the time of diagnosis ('initial phase') and then at the approach of death ('terminal phase'). These phases have the features of a grief response, namely, shock and numbness, denial, development of somatic symptoms and/or affective features such as anger, anxiety or depression, followed by some degree of acceptance. Most concern is often expressed about what to tell the child. This is obviously influenced by the child's age and intelligence. Generally speaking, current hospital practice is to facilitate discussion with the child about his illness and its implications. Parental wishes should, however, be respected, whilst indicating to the parents the advantages of openness. Consequently, there are no absolute rules but rather that a sensitive and flexible approach is likely to be beneficial. Recent research (Wooley et al 1991) has emphasised the value of a 'key worker' in helping the child and family make a more satisfactory adjustment to the implications of the disease and its likely outcome.

Suicide and deliberate self-harm

These problems are uncommon among preadolescent children. Chapters 30 and 32 discuss the relevant aspects of the problem as applied to children and adolescents.

TREATMENT METHODS

Several factors are usually responsible for the development of disturbance, so it is unlikely that one treatment method will resolve the problem. All treatment approaches also rely upon common elements that are not only necessary but also essential for a successful outcome. These elements include active cooperation between the therapist and the child and family, agreement between them about the aims of treatment, and a mutual trust to enable these aims to be achieved. Again, the relative efficacy of different

treatments is not clearly established so that the choice of treatment is often a reflection of the therapist's training and experience rather than a policy commanding general agreement. Careful analysis of the following elements is therefore necessary in order to devise an effective treatment programme:

1. Individual:
   a. Physical illness or handicap
   b. Intellectual ability
   c. Type of symptomatology
2. Family:
   a. Developmental stage (for instance a family with pre-school children or one with adolescents)
   b. Psychiatric health of parents
   c. Marital relationship
   d. Parenting qualities
   e. Communication patterns within the family
   f. Ability to resolve conflicts
   g. Support network, for instance availability of extended family
3. School:
   a. Scholastic attainments
   b. Child's and parents' attitudes to the authority of the school
   c. Peer relationships
4. Community
   a. Quality of peer relationships and of role models
   b. Neighbourhood and community resources.

The formulation of the problem along these four dimensions determines the suitability and likely success of treatment.

The three main types of treatment available are *drug treatment*, the *psychotherapies* and *liaison* or *consultation work*. The latter refers to the common practice whereby the child psychiatrist or a member of the psychiatric team does not have direct contact with the referred child, but rather helps those involved with the child to understand and modify the child's behaviour. Psychotherapies are treatments that use a variety of psychological techniques to ameliorate disturbance. They include individual therapy, behaviour therapy, family therapy and group therapy as well as counselling and advice for parents.

Drug treatment

This does not have a major treatment role in child psychiatry. A recent review (Campbell & Spencer 1988) commented sadly on the absence of empirical data to provide an adequate basis for the use of psychotropic drugs in child psychiatry. Consequently, drugs should only be used to treat specific symptoms and only for a defined period of time. They are more likely to produce symptomatic relief than to cure. Table 29.3 summarises the important indications and side-effects of various drugs used in child psychiatry.

Psychotherapies

These are the commonest treatment approach in contemporary child psychiatric practice.

Individual psychotherapy (Wolff 1986)

Though there are several theoretical orientations, including psychoanalytic (Freud 1946) and Rogerian (Reisman 1973), the therapist has the same therapeutic tasks in each. These are: to develop a trusting, non-judgemental relationship with the child; to enable the child to express his feelings and thoughts; to understand the meaning of the child's symptoms, including his behaviour during the therapeutic session; and finally to provide the child with some understanding and explanation for his behaviour. The indications for individual psychotherapy are not clearly established, though usually it is given to children with a neurotic or reactive disorder rather than those with a constitutionally based disorder. For younger children the medium for communication is play, such as sand-play or drawing, whilst for older children verbal exchange and discussion are possible.

Behavioural psychotherapy (McAuley & McAuley 1977)

This approach is based upon the application of the findings of experimental psychology, particularly learning theory, to a wide range of problems such as enuresis, encopresis, tantrums and aggression. Its characteristics are as follows:

1. Define problem(s) objectively with reference to the antecedents, the behaviour itself and the consequences (the 'ABC' approach)
2. Emphasis on current behaviour rather than on past events
3. Set up hypotheses to account for the behaviour
4. Pretreatment baseline to determine the frequency and severity of the problem
5. Devise a behavioural programme on an individual basis to test the hypothesis
6. Evaluate the outcome of treatment programmes
7. Tackle one problem at a time.

As with other psychotherapies, success depends on the establishment of a trusting relationship with the patient and the close supervision of the treatment programme, together with the involvement of teachers and parents in many cases.

Cognitive–behaviour therapy (see Chs 30 and 40 and Braswell & Kendall 1988)

The application of cognitive techniques to the treatment of disturbed adolescents and older children has been one of the most recent developments in treatment (Braswell & Kendall 1988). The same principles and strategies, with appropriate modification, have been applied to a wide range of problems. Difficulties in its application include the ability of children to verbalise their cognitions, the

Table 29.3 Drug treatment in child psychiatry

Drug	Usage	Comment
Anxiolytics (e.g. diazepam)	Anxiety/phobic conditions	Short-term adjunct to behavioural treatment
Phenothiazines (e.g. chlorpromazine)	Schizophrenia/hyperkinetic syndrome	Extrapyramidal side-effects common
Butyrophenones (e.g. haloperidol)	Complex tics/Tourette syndrome	Extrapyramidal side-effects common
Tricyclic antidepressants (e.g. imipramine/amitriptyline)	Enuresis Depression	High relapse rate Not very effective in children
Stimulants (e.g. methylphenidate)	Hyperkinetic syndrome	Effective short term, but long-term side-effects (growth, sleep, appetite)
Hypnotics (e.g. trimeprazine/promethazine)	Persistent sleep disorders in pre-school children	Only short-term

stability of their beliefs and the assignment of age-appropriate 'homework' tasks. Despite these limitations, there is little doubt that this approach is likely to be used increasingly in the future.

Family therapy (Barker 1986; see also Chs 30 and 40)

This is an extremely popular treatment approach at present. The rationale underlying family therapy is that the child's disturbed behaviour is symptomatic of the disturbance within the family as a group.

There are many different theoretical approaches and techniques (see Barker 1986), but all usually involve interviewing the whole family on each occasion for about an hour. Most family work is short-term, lasting about 6 months, with approximately monthly sessions. The emphasis is on current behaviour, verbal and non-verbal, observed during the session rather than on past events. The main aim is to improve communication within the family so that dysfunctional patterns of behaviour are replaced by more healthy and adaptive behaviour.

The evidence for the effectiveness of family therapy is convincing (Gurman et al 1986), though its comparative efficacy and range of application is less clear.

Group therapy (see Ch. 30)

Older children and adolescents often benefit from group therapy when the aim is to improve interpersonal relationships, particularly with the peer group, using a variety of theoretical models (for instance psychodynamic and social skills).

Supportive psychotherapy and counselling

The former is frequently used for the child with chronic illness or handicap; the focus may be either the child or the parents. It is especially beneficial at the time of diagnosis and also in the longer term when the implications of the disability become more evident. Parental counselling is also used to help the parents understand their child's behaviour problems, the factors that may have led to them and those that are responsible for their continuation, along with an emphasis on the parent–child relationship and the improvement of parenting skills. Counselling may therefore help parents to devise and implement a behavioural programme to modify the child's behaviour as well as to promote normal development.

Liaison and consultation psychiatry (Mrazek 1985)

This is a collaborative approach between the child psychiatry team and the professionals directly involved with the child, for instance hospital staff, teachers and residential care staff, in order to help them to understand the child's disturbed behaviour, and their own possible contribution to the problem and to suggest ways to improve the situation. Although the child psychiatrist may see the referred child in the first instance, subsequent contact is usually with the staff rather than with the child. This approach can also include the establishment and supervision of a staff support group whose aim is to look at the attitudes and emotional responses of the staff towards the behaviour shown by the children under their care.

REFERENCES

Achenbach T M, Edelbrock C S 1983 Manual for Child Behaviour Checklist and Revised Behaviour Profile. Achenbach, Burlington, VT

Anthony E J, Scott P D 1960 Manic–depressive psychosis in childhood. Journal of Child Psychology and Psychiatry 1: 53–72

Apley J, MacKeith R 1968 The child and his symptoms. Blackwell, Oxford

Asperger H 1944 Die 'Autistischen Psychopathien' im Kindesalter. Archive für Psychiatrie und Nervenkrankheiten 117: 76–136

Barker P 1986 Basic family therapy, 2nd edn. Collins, London

Bax M, MacKeith R (eds) 1963 Minimal cerebral dysfunction. Clinics in developmental medicine 10. SIMP/Heinemann, London

Bayley N 1969 Bayley scales of infant development: birth to two years. Psychological Corporation, New York

Bentovim A, Elton A, Hildebrand J, Tranter M, Vizard E 1988 Child sexual abuse within the family: assessment and treatment. Wright, Bristol

Bishop D 1987 The causes of specific developmental language disorder ("developmental dysphasia"). Journal of Child Psychology and Psychiatry 28: 1–8

Bourne S, Lewis E 1991 Perinatal bereavement. British Medical Journal 302: 1167–1168

Braswell L, Kendall P 1988 Cognitive–behavioral methods with children. In Dobson K (ed) Handbook of cognitive–behavioral therapies. Guilford Press, New York

Brown G W, Harris T 1978 Social origins of depression: a study of psychiatric disorder in women. Tavistock, London

Campbell A, McIntosh N (eds) 1992 Forfar and Arneil's textbook of paediatrics, 4th edn. Churchill Livingstone, Edinburgh

Campbell M, Spencer E 1988 Psychopharmacology in child and adolescent psychiatry: a review of the past five years. Journal of the American Academy of Child and Adolescent Psychiatry 27: 269–279.

Cantwell D, Baker L 1985 Psychiatric and learning disorders in children with speech and language disorders: a descriptive analysis. Advances in Learning and Behaviour Disabilities 4: 29–47

Caplan H L 1970 Hysterical 'conversion' symptoms in childhood. MPhil dissertation, University of London

Corbett J A, Harris R, Taylor E, Trimble M 1977 Progressive disintegrative psychosis of childhood. Journal of Child Psychology and Psychiatry 18: 211–219

Department of Health and Social Security 1988 Report of Inquiry into Child Abuse in Cleveland 1987, Cm 413. Her Majesty's Stationery Office, London

Douglas J, Richman M 1984 My child won't sleep. Penguin, Harmondsworth

Eaton-Evans J, Dugdale A E 1988 Sleep patterns of infants in the first year of life. Archives of Disease in Childhood 63: 647–649

Egger J, Carter C, Graham P, Gumley D, Soothil J F 1985 A controlled trial of oligoantigenic treatment in the hyperkinetic syndrome. Lancet i: 540–545

Elliott C, Murray D J, Pearson L 1983 The British Abilities Scales (new edition). National Foundation for Educational Research/Nelson, Windsor

Faull C, Nicol R 1986 Abdominal pain in six year olds: an epidemiological study in a new town. Journal of Child Psychology and Psychiatry 27: 251–261

Feingold B F 1975 Hyperkinesis and learning difficulties linked to artificial food flavors and colors. American Journal of Nursing 75: 797–803

Forrest G, Claridge R S, Baum D 1981 Practical management of perinatal death. British Medical Journal 281: 31–32

Forrest G, Standish E, Baum D 1982 Support after perinatal death: a study of support and counselling after perinatal death. British Medical Journal 285: 1475–1478

Frankenberg W K, Dodds J B, Fandal A W, Kazuk E, Cohrs M 1975 Denver Screening Test. Ladoca Project and Publishing Foundation, Denver

Fraser A M, Taylor D C 1986 Childhood encopresis extended into adult life. British Journal of Psychiatry 149: 370–371

Freud A 1936 The ego and the mechanisms of defence. Hogarth Press, London

Freud A 1946 The psychological treatment of children. Imago, London

Gilles de la Tourette G 1885 Étude sur une affection nerveuse caractérisée de l'incoordination motrice accompagné d'echolalie et de copralalie. Reprinted in Archives of Neurology 9: 158–200

Goodyer I 1981 Hysterical conversion reactions in childhood. Journal of Child Psychology and Psychiatry 22: 179–188

Goodyer I 1990 Life experiences, development and childhood psychopathology. Wiley, Chichester

Goodyer I, Kolvin I, Gatzanis S 1985 Recent undesirable life events and psychiatric disorder in childhood. British Journal of Psychiatry 147: 517–523

Gordon N, MacKinlay I 1986 Motor learning difficulties: 'clumsy' children. In: Gordon N, MacKinlay I (eds) Children with neurodevelopmental disorders, book 1. Neurologically handicapped children: treatment and management. Blackwell, Oxford

Griffiths R 1954 The abilities of babies. McGraw Hill, New York

Gurman A, Kniskern D, Pinsof W 1986 Research on the process and outcome of marital and family therapy. In: Garfield S, Bergin A (eds) Handbook of psychotherapy and behaviour change. Wiley, New York

Hagberg B, Aicardi J, Dias K, Ramos O 1983 A progressive syndrome of autism, dementia, ataxia and loss of purposeful hand use in girls: Rett's syndrome. Archives of Neurology 14: 471–479

Henderson S 1987 The assessment of 'clumsy' children: old and new approaches. Journal of Child Psychology and Psychiatry 28: 511–527

Hersov L, Berg I (eds) 1980 Out of school. Wiley, Chichester

Hobson P 1986 The autistic child's appraisal of expressions of emotions: an experimental investigation. Journal of Child Psychology and Psychiatry 27: 321–342

Jones D M (ed) 1982 Understanding child abuse. Hodder & Stoughton, Sevenoaks

Kanner L 1943 Autistic disturbances of affective contact. The Nervous Child 2: 217–250

Kazdin A 1990 Childhood depression. Journal of Child Psychology and Psychiatry 31: 121–160

Kempe R, Kempe C H 1978 Child abuse. Fontana, London

Kerr A M, Stephenson J 1985 Rett's syndrome in the West of Scotland. British Medical Journal 291: 579–582

Kolvin I, Fundudis T 1981 Elective mute children: psychological development and background factors. Journal of Child Psychology and Psychiatry 22: 219–232

Lask B 1988 Novel and non-toxic treatment for night terrors. British Medical Journal 297: 592

Lask B, Fosson A 1989 Childhood illness: the psychosomatic approach. Wiley, Chichester

Lockyer L, Rutter M 1969 A five to fifteen year follow-up study of infantile psychosis. III. Psychological aspects. British Journal of Psychiatry 115: 865–882

Lotter V 1966 Epidemiology of autistic conditions in young children. I. Prevalence. Social Psychiatry 1: 1241–1247

McAuley R, McAuley P 1977 Child behavioural problems. An empirical approach to management. MacMillan, London

Maguire G P, Rutter D R 1976 History taking for medical students: I. Deficiencies in performance. Lancet ii: 556–558

Meadow R 1982 Munchausen syndrome by proxy. Archives of Disease in Childhood 57: 92–98

Mrazek D 1985 Child psychiatric consultation and liaison to paediatrics. In: Rutter M, Hersov L (eds) Child and adolescent psychiatry: modern approaches, 2nd edn. Blackwell, Oxford

Mrazek D, Mrazek P 1985 Child maltreatment. In: Rutter M, Hersov L (eds) Child and adolescent psychiatry: modern approaches, 2nd edn. Blackwell, Oxford

Neale M D 1958 Neale Analysis of Reading Ability manual. MacMillan, London

Needleman H, Gunnoe C, Leviton A et al 1979 Deficits in psychologic and classroom performance of children with elevated dentine lead levels. New England Journal of Medicine 300: 689–695

Oglethorpe R 1989 Parenting after perinatal bereavement — a review of the literature. Journal of Reproductive and Infant Psychology 7: 227–244

Ousten J (ed) 1990 The consequences of child sexual abuse. Occasional papers 3. Association of Child Psychology & Psychiatry, London

Porter R (ed) 1984 Child sexual abuse within the family. Tavistock, London

Powell G, Brazel J, Blizzard R 1967 Emotional deprivation and growth retardation simulating idiopathic hypopituitarism. I Clinical evaluation of the syndrome. New England Journal of Medicine 276: 1271–1278

Quinton D, Rutter M 1976 Early hospital admission and later disturbances of behaviour: an attempted replication of Douglas's findings. Developmental Medicine and Child Neurology 18: 447–459

Reisman J M 1973 Principles of psychotherapy with children, 2nd edn. Wiley, New York

Reynell J 1969 Reynell Developmental Language Scales. National Foundation for Educational Research, Windsor

Richman N 1977 Behavioural problems in pre-school children, family and social factors. British Journal of Psychiatry 131: 523–527

Richman N 1981 A community survey of characteristics of one-to-two-year-olds with sleep disruptions. Journal of the American Academy of Child Psychiatry 20: 281–291

Richman N, Lansdown R 1988 Problems of pre-school children. Wiley, Chichester

Richman N, Stevenson J, Graham P 1975 Prevalence of behaviour problems in three-year-old children: an epidemiological study in a London borough. Journal of Child Psychology and Psychiatry 16: 277–287

Richman N, Stevenson E J, Graham P 1982 Pre-school to school: a behavioural study. Academic Press, London

Rivinus T, Jamison D, Graham P 1975 Childhood organic neurological disease presenting as psychiatric disorder Archives of Disease in Childhood 50: 115–119

Robins L 1991 Conduct disorder. Journal of Child Psychology and Psychiatry 32: 193–212

Rutter M 1985 Infantile autism and other pervasive developmental disorders. In: Rutter M, Hersov L (eds) Child and adolescent psychiatry: modern approaches, 2nd edn. Blackwell, Oxford

Rutter M 1988 Depressive disorders. In: Rutter M, Tuma A M, Lann I S (eds) Assessment and diagnosis in child psychopathology. Fulton, London

Rutter M, Schopler E 1988 Autism and pervasive developmental disorders. In: Rutter M, Tuma A M, Lann I S (eds) Assessment and diagnosis in child psychopathology. Fulton, London

Rutter M, Tizard J, Whitmore K 1970a Education, health and behaviour. Longmans, London

Rutter M, Graham P, Yule W 1970b A neuropsychiatric study of childhood. Clinics in developmental medicine 35/36, SIMP/Heinemann, London

Rutter M, Yule B, Quinton D, Rowlands O, Yule W, Berger M 1975 Attainment and adjustment in two geographical areas: III. Some factors accounting for area differences. British Journal of Psychiatry 126: 520–533

Schonell F J, Schonell F F 1950 Diagnostic and attainment testing. Oliver & Boyd, Edinburgh

Shepherd M, Oppenheim A N, Mitchell S 1971 Childhood behaviour and mental health. University of London Press, London

Skuse D 1985 Non-organic failure to thrive: a reappraisal. Archives of Disease in Childhood 60: 173–178

Strauss A, Lehtinen L 1947 Psychopathology and education in the brain injured child. Grune & Stratton, New York.

Taylor E (ed) 1986 The overactive child. SIMP/Blackwell, Oxford

Thomas A, Chess S, Birch H 1968 Temperament and behaviour disorders in childhood. New York University Press, New York

Thomson G, Raals G, Hepburn W, Hunter R, Fulton M, Laxen D 1989 Blood-lead levels and children's behaviour — results from the Edinburgh lead study. Journal of Child Psychology and Psychiatry 30: 515–528

Thorndike R L 1973 Stanford Binet Intelligence Scale, Form L-M, 1972 Norms tables. Houghton Mifflin, Boston

Waller D, Eisenberg L 1980 School refusal in childhood — a psychiatric–paediatric perspective. In: Hersov L, Berg I (eds) Out of school. Wiley, Chichester

Wechsler D 1974 Manual for the Wechsler Intelligence Scale for Children — revised. Psychological Corporation, New York

Wing L 1981 Asperger's syndrome: a clinical account. Psychological Medicine 11: 115–129

Wing L, Gould J 1979 Severe impairments of social interaction and associated abnormalities in children: epidemiology and classification. Journal of Autism and Developmental Disorders 9: 11–30

Wolff S 1986 Child psychotherapy. In: Bloch S (ed) Introduction to the psychotherapies, 2nd edn. Oxford University Press, Oxford

Wolff S, Chick J 1980 Schizoid personality in childhood: a controlled follow-up study. Psychological Medicine 10: 85–100

Wooley H, Stein A, Forrest G, Baum D 1989 Imparting the diagnosis of life threatening illness in children. British Medical Journal 298: 1623–1626

Wooley H, Stein A, Forrest G, Baum D 1991 Cornerstone care for families of children with life-threatening illnesses. Developmental Medicine and Child Neurology 33: 216–224

30. Psychiatric disorders of adolescence

W. Parry-Jones

INTRODUCTION

Adolescent psychiatry has a close natural alliance with both child and adult psychiatry, with overlap in aetiology, assessment and treatment. However, clinical work is uniquely different, due to the effects of the maturational stage of adolescence, which is widely regarded as a time of turmoil, unhappiness, rebellion and antisocial behaviour. While many adolescents experience personal suffering and misery, emotional and behavioural disturbance is not a prerequisite. However, misbehaviour, alienation and apparent unhappiness is a continuing source of concern. Inevitably, the adolescent psychiatrist deals with a wide range of young people whose mental state and behaviour are considered abnormal or unacceptable. The term 'adolescent disturbance' is used to cover this spectrum of conditions. Involvement with family members is almost inevitable and skills in interviewing parents and conducting family interventions are intrinsic. There is a need to collaborate closely with other services and agencies, and the clearest definition of the adolescent psychiatrist's central role and responsibilities is required. If interdisciplinary work is to be effective, psychiatrists have to be confident about the nature of their contribution and able to convey this to colleagues. Only a small proportion of adolescent disturbance calls for active psychiatric intervention, especially if this is viewed in orthodox clinical terms. However, distinctive psychiatric skills are significant in consultation with other disciplines.

Specialisation in adolescent psychiatry has a brief history (Parry-Jones 1984, 1993). During the second half of the 19th century, childhood mental disorders began to be described, recognising psychological and organic factors. Puberty became regarded increasingly as a physiological cause of mental disturbance, and pubescent or adolescent insanity was referred to frequently. Adolescents were admitted routinely to asylums, receiving no special age-related care until the late 1940s, when the first adolescent units opened. Exclusively adolescent in-patient services developed rapidly, on a regional basis, in the late 1960s, in response to concern about the welfare of adolescents in adult mental hospital wards. Subsequently, there has been remarkable growth of adolescent services and hospital treatment of serious adolescent psychiatric disorder is usually in age-appropriate surroundings. Nevertheless, significant deficiencies remain, reflecting the tendency for health services to be slower in providing for adolescents than for children or adults. Psychiatric services are variable and incomplete, especially for acute disturbance, emergencies, rehabilitation and long-term care. Particular shortcomings include limited provisions for older adolescents, the mentally retarded, aggressive conduct-disordered teenagers and drug abusers. Accessibility of services, especially in-patient units, is often unsatisfactory and overlap with adult services is inadequate and unplanned. Joint planning and coordination of services delivered by mental health, education and social services and voluntary organisations can be limited (Health Advisory Service 1986).

As adolescent psychiatry is relatively new, there is considerable variation in thinking about optimal ways of understanding and managing disturbance; and selecting the most effective approach, for personal practice and wider service organisation, is difficult. It is necessary to remember that adolescent psychiatry is a medical specialty and its proper boundaries and functions fall conventionally within a medical remit. The clinical psychiatric model, emphasising individual disorder and treatment, has many advantages. Traditional reliance on detailed diagnostic assessment enables both psychiatric and non-psychiatric problems to be identified, intervention planned systematically, with clarification of the contributions of psychiatrists and associated professionals. Although popular in many adolescent services, a single theoretical and treatment model restricts the range of disorders treated. In view of the variable, incomplete nature of current adolescent services and the diversity of presenting problems, an eclectic approach is advocated. Continuities between adolescent psychiatry and the child and adult fields mean that the adolescent psychiatrist should be a generalist theoretically and practically.

SCOPE OF ADOLESCENT PSYCHIATRY

Concept and definition of adolescence

Although the physical and psychological characteristics of adolescence have been described for centuries, its current format emerged in the late 19th century, influenced by social, cultural and economic factors (Parry-Jones 1993). It carried new age-related expectations and problems, generated by lengthening compulsory education, delayed assumption of adult responsibilities and associated dependence on parents. By the end of the 19th century, adolescence was a popular focus of study and phase-specific forms of psychiatric disorder were well-established.

In Western society, there is no satisfactory definition of adolescence, which is regarded usually as extending from the onset of puberty to attainment of physical maturity and adult status. Broadly, it covers the age range of 12–20 years, incorporating early (12–15 years), mid (14–16 years) and late adolescence (17–20+ years). In many parts of the world, however, adolescence is not clearly designated, with children introduced early to adult social and economic responsibilities, and little transition between childhood and adulthood.

Adolescent development

Adolescent disturbance comprises specific psychiatric disorders and reactions to developmental and situational stresses. It is necessary to consider the interrelationship between these components and take the broadest view of aetiology. Effective understanding of adolescent disturbance, identification of psychopathology and its management, require thorough familiarity with phenomena of normal adolescence, information about the lives of adolescents and their families and appreciation of internal and external stressors. A fundamental clinical task is disentangling essentially normal, age-appropriate behaviour from psychopathology.

Adolescence is characterised by rapid biological and psychological changes, intensive readjustment to family, school, work and social life, coupled with unrelenting preparation for adulthood. Clinically, the concept of adolescence as a period demanding completion of a sequence of phase-specific tasks is valuable, creating a frame of reference for assessment and treatment. Particularly significant for psychiatric treatment are cognitive changes, with acquisition of capacity for abstract thought. The theme of normal development pervades adolescent psychiatry, but it is not discussed separately in this chapter, since it is covered comprehensively elsewhere (Bancroft & Reinisch 1990, Coleman & Hendry 1990, Lewis & Volkmar 1990). Instead, emphasis is placed on clinical aspects of adolescent and family development when they have relevance to aetiology, diagnosis, treatment and prognosis. Particular attention is given to the clinical significance of maturational stress.

Psychiatric disorder in adolescence

No psychiatric disorders are unique to adolescence. Disorders include conditions commencing in infancy and childhood (see Ch. 29) and those arising initially in adolescence, with symptoms resembling those in adulthood. In this chapter, emphasis is placed on distinctive features of adolescent presentations and disorders prominent at this time. During early adolescence, therefore, the main manifestations are of childhood disorders, in conjunction with those beginning to appear, eg. anorexia nervosa, substance abuse and stress-related disorders accompanying biological and social change. By late adolescence, conditions such as schizophrenia begin to emerge. Common manifestations of adolescent disturbance take the form of emotional upset, delinquent or antisocial behaviour, conflict with parents, change in friendship patterns, alienation, school difficulties, eating problems, substance abuse and sexual problems. No single theory provides a sound rationale for assessment, classification and intervention in dealing with such presentations. The most satisfactory model is all-encompassing, involving interaction of biological, psychological and social factors, in the aetiology and maintenance of problems.

Difficulties related to the process of adolescent development may arise variously. For example, on entering puberty, children with pre-existing medical, psychiatric, developmental or temperamental difficulties may experience particular problems. There may be issues relating to the timing of puberty, or problems generated by physical, cognitive, emotional, social, psychosexual and moral maturation. Developmental changes have the capacity of being either stressful or supportive. Wide variation in age of onset and rate of growth spurt, for example, and impact of both early and late development, may have positive or negative effects. In boys, delayed maturation can generate inferiority feelings and, in girls, early menarche may be experienced negatively, or positively — signifying maturity.

At all stages, adolescence is influenced by facilitating or obstructive family influences and, in assessment and treatment, this interactionary process needs consideration. For example, concurrence of adolescence with parental mid-life changes frequently impairs parental function. Conflict between adolescents and parents is rarely long-standing and, generally, parental influence remains significant throughout adolescence. Nevertheless, adolescent challenge to parental standards and attainments can pose a major threat, destabilising family homeostasis. Essentially similar processes occur in recombined, reconstituted and nuclear families.

Estimation of prevalence and incidence of adolescent psychiatric disorder is still limited, especially in specific populations, such as those with mental retardation or developmental disabilities. Variation in prevalence rates relates to differences in sampling methods, case definition criteria and assessment procedures (Costello 1989, Brandenburg et al 1990). Nevertheless, findings suggest that at least 12% of children and adolescents have clinically identifiable psychiatric disorders.

CLINICAL ASSESSMENT

Adolescents are unlikely to acknowledge problems, finding it difficult to request help. Self-referral is infrequent and, generally, referral is initiated by others, presenting problems often reflecting contravention of parental expectations or social rules and requirements. Preparation for the initial interview, by the general practitioner or other referrer, is especially important in clarifying reasons for help. However, the psychiatrist is wise to assume limited preliminary preparation, until the position is clarified at first interview. The obtrusiveness of adolescent disturbance, its arousal of anxiety in others, and the adolescent's sense of urgency about resolving difficulties, generate the need for rapid clinical response. Prompt consultation and planned emergency provisions are essential.

Assessment should be broad based and the following sequence provides a framework for the initial meeting: (1) joint interview with the adolescent and parents, clarifying reasons for referral, the psychiatrist's role and plans for the session, establishing the history of presenting problems, the adolescent's personal history, including developmental and medical aspects, and the family history; (2) interview with the adolescent; (3) physical examination; (4) interview with parent(s); (5) assembly of additional information from school or other sources, with appropriate consent.

Initial professional contact, including correspondence and telephone calls, is particularly important. Attention needs to be given to the reception of the young person and parents and to stage management of the first interview. Joint meetings assist alliance building, by clarifying the purpose and structure of the interviews, while facilitating preliminary observations about the adolescent's mental state, parental attitudes and interactive features. Predictable feelings and attitudes of the parents need consideration, with a sensitive response to their predicament. Disappointment about the adolescent's progress, and anger, recrimination and guilt about past events, is to be anticipated. There may be ambivalence about consultation and its connotations of parenting failure, with annoyance and relief at the prospect of intervention. Clinic refusers are frequent and steps need to be taken routinely to minimise non-attendance. Success is likely to be related to adequate preparation of adolescents and parents by the referrer. If serious opposition to attendance is anticipated, a home visit may be indicated.

Particular attention has to centre on establishing trust and confidence, especially in youngsters who are withdrawn, uncommunicative, angry, sulky or fearful of being thought 'mad'. Adolescents quickly detect phoneyness and resist an 'open up, trust me, all will be well' approach. Content of early interviews should be as unambiguous as possible, with clear evidence that the consulting room is neutral and the intention is to be unbiased, without attributing blame or undermining adolescent values and convictions. The most constructive approach is to regard assessment and treatment as a collaborative process, each step being explained and discussed, in intelligible terms, with oral consent being sufficient in most situations. Face-to-face interviews can be daunting and imaginative use has to be made of strategies for reducing tension and confrontation.

Legal and ethical issues need to be given thorough consideration, especially where there are no clear guidelines. Confidentiality is of central importance, with clarification of the extent to which revelations will remain private. Boundaries of personal and public thoughts and feelings in families need to be reflected explicitly in the stage management of interviews. Reassurance about confidentiality has to be tempered by reality, indicating that, under some circumstances, information may have to be conveyed to others. In contacts with schools or employers, written consent is preferable. Adolescents under 16 years of age, with sufficient understanding of the proposals, may consent to examination. The consent of an over 16-year-old is sufficient in itself and separate permission from parent or guardian is unnecessary. Imposition of intervention without consent occurs only when emergency action is needed, because of threatened or actual life-endangering behaviour, due to major disturbance of thinking or perception. It is conventional under such circumstances, with young people under 16 years, to accept authority of parents or guardians. In the absence of such consent, or with young people over 16 years, appropriate compulsory powers provided by mental health legislation should be utilised.

Mental state examination

Despite the greater degree of informality and flexibility necessary with adolescents, mental state examination needs to be conducted systematically, using the framework employed with other age groups. Recording of the examination should include reference to physical appearance, behaviour and manner of relating, speech, mood, thinking, perception, orientation, attention and concentration, memory and insight.

Physical examination

The physical health of adolescent patients must not be overlooked, particularly since the decline of school health screening programmes. Physical examination represents an important medical contribution in multi-disciplinary work. While examination is undertaken routinely on adolescent in-patients, it is not always deemed necessary for out-patients. Fears about complicating the therapist's role are misplaced and examination can establish credible evidence of interest in the patient. Even if the yield of abnormalities is small, examination provides opportunity to discuss physical changes of adolescence more openly, facilitating revelation of personal health worries. Specific indications for examination include known or suspected physical illness or anomalies, self-concern about illness and evidence of precocious, or delayed, puberty. If the family believes the adolescent's illness is due to physical causes, it is wise to undertake detailed examination. Routine use of growth charts is recommended, with rating of pubertal stages.

Special investigations

The differential diagnosis may necessitate special medical and psychological investigations, which need to be selected carefully and completed swiftly, with appropriate explanation to the adolescent and parents. This would apply if there was disturbance of growth, weight loss or the possibility of seizure disorder. It is becoming increasingly possible to use organ imaging techniques, but these are mainly research tools. New techniques for visualising chromosomes have increased interest in the genetics of psychiatric disorders. Referral questions for investigation by a child psychologist must be explicit, in relation, for example, to the requirement for testing intellectual capacity and educational attainment, or neuropsychological screening (see Ch. 29).

Interviewing parents and siblings

Information from parents about the adolescent, their personal histories, their marriage, the nuclear and extended family, home background and friends is essential in assessment. Problems of parents, especially single or adoptive, quality of parenting and the nature of adolescent–parent interaction require exploration. Attention needs to be paid to the family's developmental stage and capacity to cope with the adolescent's challenge. Reasons for interviewing or involving siblings should be clear. Such action requires the consent of the adolescent, parents and the siblings themselves, and the usual rules of confidentiality apply. This lays the foundation for extending assessment to include joint meetings with part, or whole, family groups. Throughout, the psychiatrist has responsibility to provide feedback to parents about the adolescent's disorder and progress.

Assembling additional information

Diagnosis is unlikely to be reliable without sampling behaviour and mental state in settings outside the consulting room. School visits can be helpful in evaluating day-to-day social and academic functioning, providing an effective index of degree of disturbance and enhancing understanding of relationships with peers and adults. Elective home visits extend the scope of assessment and treatment, e.g. assessing housebound adolescents or undertaking specific therapeutic tasks, such as setting up response prevention programmes or modelling management of anorectic patients in family meals, as part of treatment relocation from clinic to home. Home visiting is intrusive and expensive in time and money, requiring well thought out reasons and objectives for cost effectiveness.

Standardised interviews and rating scales

Clinicians and researchers have access to an increasing range of diagnostic tools (Orvaschel 1985, Gutterman et al 1987), usually comprising separate parent and adolescent versions. Highly structured interviews include the Diagnostic Interview for Children and Adolescents (DICA) (Herjanic & Campbell 1977) and the Diagnostic Interview Schedule for Children (DISC)

(Costello et al 1984). Widely used semistructured interviews include the Kiddie Schedule for Affective Disorders and Schizophrenia (K-SADS) (Endicott & Spitzer 1978), the Child Assessment Schedule (CAS) (Hodges et al 1982) and the Interview Schedule for Children (ISC) (Kovacs 1985). Behaviour rating scales covering a range of psychopathology are the Behaviour Problem Checklist for Children and Teachers (Quay 1983), the Conners Parent and Teachers Questionnaires (Conners & Barkley 1985) and the Achenbach Parent and Teacher Questionnaires (Achenbach & Edelbrock 1983). There are several self-report inventories and scales for use with adolescents.

DIAGNOSIS AND CLASSIFICATION

The diagnostic process need not differ from that employed in other age groups, consideration being given to the clinical history, mental state, life circumstances and associated family, educational, work, social and legal problems. There may be reluctance to diagnose psychiatric disorder in adolescents from fears of adverse effects of medical labelling, reflecting some misapprehension of the meaning and application of the diagnostic process. Diagnosis is popularly viewed as especially difficult and unreliable, since adolescent disorders are regarded as atypical versions of more clearly defined adult forms. This is not necessarily the case, although adolescent presentations are often complex and not immediately part of recognisable nosological entities. Rather than transposing adult diagnoses, it is more constructive to accept that typical adolescent presentations occur, with characteristics shaped by pathoplastic effects of maturation. In view of possible clinical ambiguity in adolescent disturbance, diagnostic precision is vital, in improving communication, understanding causation, treatment planning and prognostic evaluation. The non-hierarchical diagnostic approach, implicit in DSM-IIIR, has revealed that many adolescents display psychopathology fulfilling criteria for several disorders, e.g. depression associated with conduct disorder, eating disorders, substance abuse and anxiety. The concept of co-morbidity has been introduced also in ICD-10, but it remains unclear whether it represents discrete, but related, disorders or an artefact of classification.

A formulation is useful in all cases and the following framework is commended: (1) essential features; (2) differential diagnosis; (3) aetiology, identifying predisposing, precipitating, perpetuating and protective factors; (4) management and treatment plan, including investigations needed; (5) prognosis. Although prognosis in adolescent disorders is influenced by maturational processes and associated disturbances, it relates principally to the nature and course of disorder and its susceptibility to existing treatments. Prognostic pointers need serious consideration and overoptimism about outcome, because adolescence is transient, is misplaced. Without attention to prognosis, decisions about intervention risk over-reacting too urgently or underestimating the seriousness of the problem, because the adolescent will 'grow out of it'.

CLINICAL SYNDROMES

Follow-up studies of pre-school and older children indicate that a significant proportion of early onset disorders persist into adolescence and beyond (see Ch. 29). These include autism, conduct disorder, psychoses and some developmental disorders. In autistic children, for example, there may be maturational gain in adolescence but, generally, there is behavioural deterioration and an increasing risk of seizures. Similarly, a high proportion of hyperactive children remain disabled in adolescence and adulthood (Thorley 1988).

Neurotic, stress-related and somatoform disorders

Concepts of emotional disorder and neurosis

Although all adult neurotic disorders occur in adolescence, generalised anxiety, with regressive symptoms, is the common presentation. Phobic, hysterical or obsessive–compulsive features may present transiently, preceding clinical pictures with more enduring features. More clearly defined disorders of late adolescence merge with those typical of adulthood. It is important, however, to recognise poorly differentiated, early adolescent emotional disorder, although outcome is generally good. In ICD-10, the concept of 'developmental appropriateness' is used to distinguish between such emotional disorders, with childhood or early adolescent onset, and neurotic disorders.

Anxiety disorders

The commonest presentation is that of the over-anxious teenager, showing excessive, non-specific worrying and fearful behaviour, unnecessary concern about the future, excessive demands for reassurance, inability to relax, preoccupation with past behaviour, and somatic complaints. Separation anxiety can arise suddenly, with unrealistic worries about harm occurring to an attached person or fears of non-return. Commonly, such anxieties are associated with reluctance or refusal to go to school. Some anxious youngsters display persistent and excessive shrinking from contact with strangers, interfering with social functioning and peer relationships. Phobic anxiety, particularly social phobias and agoraphobia, may originate in adolescence. Although true school phobia may be manifested, it is not necessarily a feature of school refusal (Berg 1991). Specific fears can present acutely as panic attacks.

Crucial to management is clarification of the pattern and causation of symptoms. It may be sufficient to identify the problem and support existing coping methods. With serious symptoms, a more systematic approach relieving distress and disability involves behavioural techniques, e.g. relaxation training and desensitisation. Anxiety management training is useful in the treatment of panic attacks. Although brief use of benzodiazepines may be beneficial, caution is needed because of risks of dependence.

Obsessive–compulsive disorder (OCD)

OCD generally begins in adolescence or young adulthood, sometimes in mid-childhood. Onset is usually gradual, with no special premorbid personality. The clinical picture is essentially the same as in adults (Rapoport 1989). Odd behaviours are usually the first features, with obsessional ideas becoming evident on enquiry. Ruminations and rituals are likely to be recognised by the adolescent as alien and senseless. Obsessional slowness may be present and, commonly, a phobic component. The disorder can be seriously handicapping, interfering with social activities, relationships, education and work. Involvement of family members in rituals can lead to distress and, sometimes, to control over the household. OCD can be associated with anxiety and depression, and adolescents with anorexia nervosa and Tourette's syndrome have high rates of obsessional symptoms.

OCD occurs in 0.2% of child and adolescent outpatients (Hollingsworth et al 1980) and up to 1.0% of in-patients. Diagnosis is missed easily and frequency of the disorder, especially milder forms, may be much higher. The connection between OCD and compulsive behaviour in normal children and adolescents is unclear and learning theories provide inadequate theoretical explanation. Genetic and family factors have been implicated and the strongest case for a physical basis concerns altered serotonin function.

Diagnostically, the absence of another psychiatric disorder is critical, because obsessional symptoms occur more widely than the disorder and can be associated with other clinical features. Internal resistance is not a diagnostic requirement (Allsopp & Verduyn 1989).

Where there are bizarre ideas and behaviours, schizophrenia may be suggested and morbid rumination may indicate depression. Separation from Tourette's syndrome and primary phobic disorders can be difficult.

Treatment needs to consider the relative severity of obsessional thoughts, compulsions and family disruption. Psychotherapeutic techniques are a common component in establishing therapeutic relationships and in family work (Bolton et al 1983). Reports of behavioural methods with adolescents mainly refer to single case studies (Green 1980). Principal treatment components comprise in vivo exposure, modelling and response prevention, preferably self-imposed and monitored, habituation training and thought stopping, although adolescents find these techniques difficult. Responses of family members can perpetuate disorder and counselling and support of parents and siblings, with frequent feedback, are required, in addition to strategies for using the parents in treatment. The most important drug is clomipramine hydrochloride (Flament et al 1985) and increasing experience is being obtained with fluoxetine and fluvoxamine (Riddle et al 1990).

Follow-up suggests a chronic, but variable, course associated with episodic remissions. There is strong continuity from childhood to adulthood, that for obsessive–compulsive symptoms being stronger than for the disorder itself (Zietlin 1986).

Reaction to severe stress and adjustment disorders

Stresses accompanying maturational changes of adolescence can provoke healthy, transient, adjustment reactions, associated with prominent emotional and behavioural manifestations, such as irritability, depression and temper outbursts. Provided symptoms are not persistent and there is no significant disturbance of daily functioning, it is unnecessary to categorise such states as psychiatric disorders.

Acute stress reaction

Exceptional physical or mental stress, such as produced by natural catastrophe, assault or multiple bereavement, can lead to transient disorders, usually subsiding within hours or days.

Post-traumatic stress disorder (PTSD)

The essential feature is the development of characteristic symptoms in response to a distressing event, outside the range of usual human experience and likely to cause pervasive distress in almost anyone. Increased reporting of traumatic experiences provides greater opportunity for the study, in juveniles, of the effects of personal injury and abuse and consequences of witnessing fearful scenes. Characteristic symptoms of PTSD comprise: persistent re-experiencing of the traumatic event; persistent avoidance of stimuli associated with the event or numbing of general responsiveness; and manifestations of increased arousal, sleep difficulties, impaired concentration, exaggerated startle response, irritability and anger outbursts. Anxiety and depressive symptoms are common and may warrant separate diagnosis. Diagnosis is not made if the disturbance lasts less than 1 month (Eth & Pynoos 1985, Lyons 1987, Yule & Williams 1990, Terr 1991).

Adult diagnostic criteria have been applied, but influence of developmental stage generates differences. Adolescents often present in a depressed, moody state. Manifestations of guilt are more salient than in younger children, together with a tendency to alternate between compliant withdrawal and aggressiveness.

Not all adverse reactions to major traumatic events meet PTSD criteria and consideration needs to be given to other diagnoses, including adjustment disorder, anxiety and depression; exacerbation of pre-existing conditions and co-morbidity occurs commonly. PTSD is increasingly important in compensation litigation. There are no entirely satisfactory screening and diagnostic instruments and it is best to use a variety of measures of anxiety, fears and depression, additional to the Impact of Event Scale (Horowitz et al 1979) and the PTSD Reaction Index (Pynoos & Eth 1986).

Adjustment disorders

These are mild, transient conditions, without antecedent psychiatric disorder, related closely in time and content to recognisable stresses, within the range of common experience. They are generally reversible, lasting only a few months. Death of a close friend or relative is an important precipitant and is likely to be a potential risk factor for subsequent psychopathology. Individual adolescent vulnerability plays a major part in shaping manifestations. This diagnosis has been misused as a non-stigmatising label for responses to a wide range of normal and abnormal stressors.

Treatment

Objectives involve removal of the stressor, provision of physical safety and care, early psychiatric intervention and family contact. Individual treatment should be directed primarily towards supporting the adolescent's

coping strengths. There is growing evidence of the benefits of crisis intervention and counselling to ameliorate acute trauma and minimise risks of subsequent disorder. Intervention is required within 24 hours if possible, before maladaptive responses become established.

In treating adolescents with PTSD, the essential component is re-exposure to traumatic cues, in a structured, supportive fashion, with attempts to enhance coping strategies for dealing with intrusive phenomena. Generally, there is scope to work with parents and possibly whole families. Long-term treatment may involve group work, intensive individual psychotherapy and psychotropic medication. Despite the potential for chronic disabling symptoms, difficulty in establishing therapeutic alliance with PTSD sufferers is common.

Dissociative (conversion) disorders

Disorder may be construed variously, by reference to conversion and dissociation, individual response to intolerable predicaments and abnormal illness behaviour. The latter seems most pertinent in the management of young people, providing a more credible and pragmatic explanation for adolescents than reliance on the concept of unconscious motivation. There is limited literature relating to adolescent hysterical states (Dubowitz & Hersov 1976). Clinical features include motor disorders, such as limb paralysis, aphonia and fits resembling epileptic seizures. Such presentations need to be taken seriously and responded to promptly, with thorough physical examination and investigation. Careful differential diagnosis is crucial, to eliminate the possibility of physical disease.

Effective treatment is likely to involve combined use of dynamic and behavioural psychotherapy (Brooksbank 1984). Exploratory psychotherapy may progress to an examination of the psychological meaning of the illness, but is unlikely to be helpful in adolescents who are poorly motivated or of low intelligence. If successful, firm prediction of recovery and continuing support may be sufficient. Various retraining techniques may be employed, often calling for considerable ingenuity, e.g. biofeedback confirming return of motor function in limb paralysis.

Hypochondriacal disorder

Although some adolescents are health conscious, preoccupation with fear of disease, persisting despite medical reassurance, in the absence of physical disorder, is an uncommon feature of adolescent emotional disorders, but may occur in anxiety or depression. In young people preoccupied with health worries, there should be appropriate physical examination and investigation. Underlying emotional difficulties need to be understood and it is often useful to interpret symptoms in terms of the avoidance of difficulties.

Neurasthenia

Occasionally, adolescents present with complaints of mental or physical fatigue and weakness, in the absence of anxiety or depression, commonly following physical illnesses such as influenza or glandular fever. The aetiology, diagnosis and treatment of myalgic encephalomyelitis present problems in view of the viral, toxic, environmental or psychological causes implicated. Whatever the causation, prolonged fatigue symptoms can generate psychological problems for the adolescent and the family. These provide a legitimate treatment focus, without disputing the origins of the disorder. Conflicting advice about the need for rest results in uncertainty in coping with fatigue symptoms.

Depersonalisation and derealisation

Both occur within the range of normal adolescent experience, under conditions of fatigue, excitement or stress and may feature in acute anxiety, panic disorder, phobic and depressive states. Very rarely, depersonalisation occurs as an enduring syndrome, beginning in adolescence. Anxiety management techniques or psychotropic drugs are likely to be most effective, especially when symptoms are secondary to other disorders.

Conduct disorder

Conduct disorder is characterised by persistent dyssocial, aggressive or defiant behaviour, representing serious violation of age-appropriate social expectations. Such behaviour may arise initially in adolescence or continue from childhood and needs to be viewed in the context of the adolescent's life history, as well as current factors. Its significance is often difficult to assess, since unreasonable behaviour and poor impulse control is likely during adolescence, and adult complaints may reflect a low tolerance threshold. Transient manifestations and occasional minor forms of public disorder must be distinguished from persistent, pervasive symptoms constituting conduct disorder. Problems are more serious than in mischievous, rebellious behaviour, in which basic rights of others are not violated. Conduct disorder is not the equivalent of juvenile delinquency and cannot be equated with antisocial behaviour as part

of adjustment reactions or personality disorder. Types of behaviour forming the basis of the diagnosis include repeated lying, stealing, severe destructiveness, fire-setting, excessive fighting and bullying, cruelty to persons or animals, truancy, running away, severe temper tantrums, defiant provocative behaviour and persistent disobedience. In classification, the socialised–unsocialised distinction is retained because of the prognostic importance of problems in peer relations and integration. The condition can overlap with emotional disorders and several mixed categories are listed in ICD-10, e.g. depressive conduct disorder.

There is limited evidence about prevalence because of difficulties in case definition and the changing nature of conduct disturbance during development. Conduct disorder in adolescents needs to be taken seriously, in terms of the wide range of emotional, social and relationship problems that can ensue, although not all youngsters displaying antisocial behaviour continue to do so in adult life (Robins 1978, 1991). Influential aetiological theories focus on the sociological bases of antisocial behaviour, a view supported by high rates of such behaviour in inner-city areas, characterised by social disorganisation and family instability. Parental psychopathology has been implicated, but precise causal connections are difficult to establish. Other factors include neurological impairment and underlying psychotic features. Since multiple influences contribute to the presentation of conduct disturbance, diagnostic assessment needs to be comprehensive, incorporating a detailed medical history and neurological examination.

Types of conduct disorder

Deliberate fire-setting is a particularly dramatic and dangerous form. Most perpetrators are boys who have experienced abnormal family life, and it is usually symptomatic of wider conduct disturbance (Jacobson 1985a, b). It is crucial to assess the degree of dangerousness and differentiate between high- and low-risk fire-setters. Recidivists are likely to have high levels of curiosity about fire, involvement in fire-related activities, greater antisocial behaviour and may reveal overt revenge fantasies and sexual excitement. Residential assessment and treatment requires constant vigilance to minimise the risks. *Runaways* present complex management problems, especially when leading alienated urban lifestyles. Generally, they have a background of social alienation and parental estrangement, and share common motivations in their flight from situational stresses. Repetitive running away, associated with serious personal risk, may be a suicidal equivalent. Runaways are likely to express loneliness, fear and resentment, but are difficult to engage in consistent treatment (Tomb 1991). Victims of *bullying* are more likely to be encountered by the psychiatrist than the perpetrators, but it is important to consider characteristics of both groups (Lowenstein 1978). Distinction has to be made between bullying by a small number of individuals and mobbing, involving a large group of the victim's peers (Hill 1989). *Stealing* may occur with or without confrontation of the victim, the latter being characteristic of mugging, purse snatching and armed robbery. Persistent *truancy* is usually associated with educational backwardness, family disadvantage and delinquency. There is little evidence about effectiveness of clinical treatment (Berg 1985). Law-breaking behaviour is widespread among young people but, when it leads to conviction, the term *juvenile delinquency* is applicable (Rutter & Giller 1983).

The new category of *family-based conduct disorder* in ICD-10 requires that there be no significant disturbance or abnormalities of social relationships outside the family. Types of behaviours likely to be involved include persistent negativistic, hostile, defiant, provocative, destructive behaviour, violence against family members and fire-setting within the home. It is unclear whether situation-specific emphasis facilitates prognosis. Adolescent disturbance is often characterised by conflict with parents or substitute care givers, with complaints about the adolescent's anger, defiance or unmanageability. Family disputes may be attributed to adolescent demands for independence, parental disapproval and disappointment with the adolescent's behaviour and developing personality and over-reaction to the teenage lifestyle. Angry outbursts and temper tantrums, however, occur frequently in adolescents coping with biological changes and mounting academic and family responsibilities, and may be age-appropriate, despite parental complaints of its obtrusiveness. Parent-adolescent alienation does not necessarily lead to psychiatric disorder, although there may be complete breakdown of communication and trust. 'Dropping out' from activities desired by parents, truancy, recurrent staying out late or absconding may occur. Complete parental estrangement, withdrawal from the peer group and loss of career orientation generally appear in late adolescence, following depression, severely disturbed family relationships and wider social, economic and cultural influences. Unemployment prospects heighten alienation from work, with reluctance to strive for employment, poor punctuality and unwillingness to conform to employers' requirements. Prolonged unemployment can lead to depression and the stigma of not belonging to any workforce.

Treatment

Management and treatment need to match specific medical, family, psychodynamic or environmental vulnerabilities. Various attempts have been made to encourage pro-social behaviour, using the peer group, parents and residential communities. No specific medication is indicated, although short-term empirical use of neuroleptics is justifiable in aggressive or hyperactive youngsters. With multiple intervention strategies, and the complexity of measuring effectiveness, it is difficult to comment usefully on outcome (Kazdin 1987).

Personality disorders

From infancy, temperamental and personality qualities become increasingly identifiable, e.g. degree of dependence, sociability, and frustration tolerance. Personality is formed by genetic factors and the influence of physical and psychological experience. Reciprocal responses between child, parents and others, and the effects of life events are crucial. The question of personality dysfunction hardly arises in infancy and childhood but, by adulthood, abnormal personalities are identifiable and distinguishable from psychiatric disorder. In adolescence, scope for diagnostic uncertainty is considerable. By the age of 20 years, emotionally healthy people have completed the bulk of their maturation, but this may be delayed or impeded by disrupted childhood and poor parenting. Not all juveniles with problems in personality development exhibit personality disorders as adults, but some abnormalities are overtly persistent, even by early adolescence. There is a popular view, not necessarily in the adolescent's best interest, that it is improper to diagnose personality disorder while the young personality is being formed. Without recognition of early prognostic indicators to long-term personality difficulties, pace and form of therapeutic intervention may be inappropriate. Nevertheless, it is difficult to define and categorise unequivocally personality disorders in this age group, and measurement is problematic. The nature of the deficit needs to be focused on, and distinction made between, personality variation and personality disorder (Wolff 1984). The relationship between temperament, normal personality variation, personality accentuation and personality disorder is unclear and is probably not a simple continuum (Rutter 1987).

Types of personality disorder

Current classification of personality disorder is inadequate for adolescence since, at this stage, forms of disorder have not crystallised. Although features suggesting paranoid, cyclothymic, histrionic or antisocial personality disorder occur, manifestations commonly encountered include poor socialisation and communication, low self-esteem, frustration tolerance and impulse control, and tension discharge outbursts. Coping capacity with negative life events is often critical. Origins of difficulties are obscure, little being known, for example, about development of negative self-concepts. Children with abnormal social development and 'schizoid' features, which may be reflected in their antisocial behaviour, are identified inadequately (Wolff & Cull 1986).

Borderline personality is a controversial concept in British psychiatry, whose trend goes against diagnostic ambiguity (Aarkrog 1981). The DSM-IIIR definition refers to 'instability in a variety of areas, including inter-personal behaviour, mood and self-image'. For those under 18 years of age, the imprecise term 'identity disorder' is often employed. Features include poor anxiety tolerance, fears of being alone or close to others, educational deterioration, substance abuse, chaotic interpersonal relationships, disorders of eating and sexual behaviour and defiant oppositional acts. Causation is speculative, involving possible genetic, constitutional and developmental factors. Compared with antisocial personality disorder and dysthymic disorder, borderline personality is more likely to be associated with exposure to chronically disturbed caretakers, prolonged separation, abuse and neglect (Zanarini 1989).

Assessment and diagnosis

Diagnostically, evidence is required, from adolescence or earlier, of enduring, maladaptive behaviour patterns covering a wide range of activities, causing subjective discomfort, abnormal responses and recognisable difficulties in relationships and coping with age-appropriate expectations. Assessment requires detailed history taking, with corroboration from schools and other sources.

A range of interview schedules, involving subjects and informants, is available (Tyrer 1988), but minimal use has been undertaken with adolescents. Significant co-morbidity can exist, e.g. with depressive disorder, although caution has to be exercised because clinical depression can influence personality assessment during acute episodes.

Treatment

Intervention is discouraged by diagnostic ambivalence, connotations of poor prognosis, few guidelines concerning techniques, doubts about treatment effectiveness and lack of outcome research. Treatment is rendered difficult by problems relating, and gaining access, to young people. Realistic therapeutic objectives require recognition of the potentially life-long nature of problems, their complex aetiology and the unlikelihood of complete resolution. Strategies are essentially psychotherapeutic, involving subjects individually or in groups, the family and other contextual factors, such as the school peer group. Sometimes, it may be feasible to consider ways of reversing processes that perpetuate and consolidate disorders. Individual psychotherapy in borderline disorders requires considerable experience and the capacity to set clear objectives and firm limits (Egan 1986). Social skills and cognitive behavioural techniques may facilitate development of self-control and ability to 'stop and think before one acts' (Kendall & Braswell 1985).

Psychoactive substance abuse

In most adolescent populations, drug and alcohol use is a serious social concern and a major public health problem. Alcohol and drugs are overused with no evidence of abating and, in many parts of the world, adolescents grow up in an environment where substance abuse is commonplace. Abuse is increasing in all age groups and contributes significantly to adolescent morbidity and mortality. Precise prevalence rates are difficult to achieve, particularly since drug use patterns change rapidly, e.g. expanding use of 'crack' cocaine in the USA. First drug and alcohol experiences occur earlier, and are perceived, like cigarette smoking, as 'grown-up' habits, providing a vehicle for challenge. Peer group pressures, family influences, easy access, media glamorisation, and natural curiosity make refusal difficult, and adolescents are expected to experiment. The decision whether or not to do so can now be regarded as a developmental problem.

Drugs and alcohol provide psychological relief from newly experienced emotional turmoil, yet experimentation is dangerous and dependency unpredictable. Addictive behaviours are maintained by powerful motivation, and interventions need to be highly effective. Concern about drugs like marijuana is justified clinically, but alcohol abuse is more prevalent, its effects are cumulative, possibly more chronic. Principal medical complications of drug misuse involve trauma, intentional and accidental overdosage, withdrawal effects and hazards of parenteral use, including human immune deficiency virus (HIV) infection. The main psychiatric consequences are depression, suicidal ideation, attempted suicide and drug-induced psychosis. Accidents, homicides and suicides have strong correlation with drug and alcohol abuse.

Alcohol

Young people are drinking more often, earlier and have established a greater than average increase in such indicators of alcohol-related harm as drunkenness offences and road accident deaths. Regular drinkers fall commonly into the 17–21-year-old age group. Among younger adolescents, frequency of regular drinking increases rapidly with age.

There is no single theory why alcohol misuse begins (Hawker 1978). Pressures to conform with peer group habits are high and alcohol features prominently in entertainments and recreation, with rapid growth in purchasing outlets. At least one half of young drinkers are likely to have had their first drink at home and parental models are crucial. Young people whose parents make significant use of alcohol, drugs and tobacco are more likely to use these themselves and to have psychiatric and social difficulties. There is evidence also that children from households where alcohol is forbidden can be at risk. Many who start drinking outside the home, in school, parks, clubs and in the company of peers, emerge as the heaviest drinkers and have problems in parental relationships and hostility towards authority.

Personality problems and emotional disturbance are major contributory factors. Many young people regard alcohol as an escape from loneliness and stress, and shy youngsters find it assists social mixing. There may be feelings of parental rejection or indifference, lack of peer acceptance, emotional isolation and low self-esteem. Increasing alcohol intake may be a clue to suicide risk. Substance abuse to ward off reality during this stage may compromise seriously further ability to make adequate adjustment to an increasingly complex society and to deal with daily problems and frustrations.

Hawker (1978) showed that, in most young people, alcohol caused no problems for themselves or others, although some displayed socially disruptive behaviour under its influence. Four per cent of boys and 3% of girls drank because they liked getting drunk and 10% reported episodic amnesia. Frequent drinkers got drunk relatively more often than infrequent drinkers and experienced greater hangover symptoms. In the long-term, critical milestones are age at first drinking, daily regular drinking and age of experiencing amnesia.

Management follows that used with adults. Cognitive strategies are useful in strengthening abstinence, e.g. by self-definition as a non-drinker and viewing other drinkers negatively. Avoidance of high-risk situations and engagement in alternative activities is important. Effective prevention requires changes in the law relating to drinking and driving offences, drunkenness and licensing, and increased tax on alcohol. Scope for health education is considerable, despite the dilemma concerning total abstention or safe limits, the objectives should include moderation, drinking only in appropriate circumstances, social disapproval of drunkenness and greater acceptance of abstention.

Cannabis

Cannabis is widely used among older adolescents. Only a minority develop dependence and intermittent use does not appear to be adverse, although acute psychoses can be precipitated.

Stimulants

Frequently abused stimulant drugs include cocaine, amphetamines, methylphenidate, phenmetrazine, diethylpropion and ephedrine. Acute paranoid psychotic states, resembling schizophrenia, can occur following chronic use. Rapid rise in cocaine use is of special concern. It is a short-acting stimulant, generating powerful dependence, which can be swallowed, injected or inhaled, especially in the form of 'crack'. The latter can produce acute respiratory failure and bronchial spasm.

Hallucinogens

This group includes lysergic acid diethylamide (LSD), psilocybin ('magic mushrooms'), mescaline and phencyclidine (PCP or 'angel dust'). Enduring affective and psychotic disorders can occur, sometimes with 'flashbacks'. In small dosage, PCP induces drunkenness; higher levels produce excitement, aggressiveness and hallucinations.

Opiates

This group includes heroin, morphine, codeine and synthetic opiates, which can be swallowed, smoked, inhaled or injected. Tolerance develops rapidly, resulting in increasing dosage. Serious adverse effects include constipation, nausea, vomiting, respiratory depression and coma.

Depressants

Commonly abused drugs include benzodiazepines, barbiturates and a variety of other hypnotics and sedative psychotropic drugs. Use reduces anxiety, inducing a feeling of freedom from tension and aggression.

Caffeine

There is widespread consumption of caffeine in soft drinks, coffee, tea, cocoa and 'over-the-counter' medications. Effects of caffeinism include restlessness, insomnia, flushing, diuresis, muscle twitching, gastrointestinal disturbance, rambling speech, tachycardia or cardiac arrhythmia. Reduced intake can produce withdrawal symptoms, e.g. irritability, lethargy and headaches, but rapid discontinuation is usually possible.

Inhalants

Despite considerable preventive efforts, there is little evidence of reduction in the use of, or mortality from, the deliberate inhaling of solvents, gases and other volatile substances (Watson 1986, Cooke et al 1988, Ashton 1990). Solvents implicated have been toluene and acetone, included in glues, typewriting correction fluids and aerosols. Use has also been made of petrol, paint stripper and butane gas. Currently, 3.5–10% of adolescents have experimented with solvents and 0.5–1.0% of secondary school pupils are abusers (Ramsey et al 1989).

Occasional abusers form the largest group and experimental misuse is usually transient in youngsters with various personality problems. Habitual abusers are chiefly boys aged 13–15 years, with high rates associated with single parents, paternal alcoholism, unemployment, large families and low socioeconomic status. Masterton (1979) differentiated between socially determined abuse, the product of the subculture and social disorganisation, and psychologically determined abuse, responding to individual underlying disorder.

Inhalation produces excitement, disinhibition, delusions and perceptual disturbance and aggressive, risk-taking behaviour. Large dosage causes increasing drowsiness, convulsions and coma. Death results from accidents, suicide, or respiratory depression, due to inhalation of vomit, vagal inhibition and cardiac arrhythmia. Despite concern about brain damage, misuse of volatile solvents, as commonly practised by secondary school pupils, is unlikely to result in neurological or neuropsychological impairment (Chadwick et al 1989). Nevertheless, annual deaths in Britain have increased to over 100 (Ramsey et al 1989).

Assessment and diagnosis of drug abuse

Accurate identification of drug-related problems is critical in the differential diagnosis and management of adolescent disturbance. The presence and extent of abuse is difficult to establish, as such problems are likely to be denied strongly, necessitating highly specific questioning. There is a danger of misinterpreting events as essentially 'normal' adolescent disturbance. Parents and professionals may overlook substance abuse or deny its connection with emotional, social and behavioural problems. Ultimately, crises such as law-breaking, running away or school expulsion may precipitate treatment (Williams et al 1989). Warning signs include unusual mood lability and 'personality changes'. Impaired school performance occurs commonly, with absenteeism and truancy. There may be evidence of uncharacteristic delinquency, alienation from 'straight' friends, and deteriorating family relationships. Physical changes, e.g. in eating and sleeping routines, may be noticeable. Full physical examination is required, confirming or excluding the presence of intoxication or withdrawal, clarifying routes of drug administration and identifying medical consequences. Urinary drug screening should be undertaken, with, if appropriate, more extensive testing, e.g. for HIV and hepatitis B antigen.

Treatment of drug abuse

Treatment should commence in the least restrictive programme. Initially, short-term abstinence needs to be assured and, for individuals who evade confrontation and need a restricted environment, hospitalisation is required, although suitable facilities are scarce. During this period, adolescents can begin to examine the impact of abuse and acknowledge need for treatment. The next step is assessment of problems involved in the maintenance of abstinence. Out-patient treatment is the preferred option, despite compliance problems. It calls for experienced staff, a range of individual, group and family treatments, school liaison and a climate of free expression and spontaneous action (Friedman & Glickman 1986). Reduction of high-risk behaviour among intravenous drug users is crucial. Long-term aftercare is essential to maintain behaviours learned in treatment, and recovery requires consistent family involvement. Major efforts have been made at preventive education starting in the preadolescent period. Effectiveness is reduced by the high-dependency effects and cash returns to dealers, which are powerful reinforcers.

Sexual disorders, offences and problems

Disorders of gender identity and sexual preference

Gender identity refers to the sense of belonging to one sex and awareness of being male or female. It is learned at an early stage and needs to be distinguished from sex role identity, concerning the consistency with male or female behaviour of a particular culture, which develops later in childhood or early adolescence (Douvan 1979). There is no reliable information about the prevalence or incidence of adolescent gender identity disorders. Problems include: transsexualism; cross-gender identification, without acknowledged homosexual orientation or a desire to change sex; and established homosexual behaviour or orientation (Zucker & Green 1991).

Various treatments have been employed, including behaviour therapy, individual psychotherapy, family therapy and parent counselling (Zucker 1990), but prospects of successful outcome are limited and difficulties arise in setting therapeutic objectives. While it may be possible to achieve agreement about short-term goals, e.g. reducing social difficulties, longer-term goals, e.g. changing sexual orientation, are problematic. Parents concerned whether effeminate behaviour in boys might forecast homosexuality will be reluctant to accept plans for adaptation to homosexual orientation (Green 1987).

Sexual offences

Indecent exposure, like other adolescent sexual problems, generally reflects clumsy, immature attempts to achieve sexual gratification and recognition. Cases of voyeurism and the touching or fondling of strangers may be similarly explicable. Prevalence of sexual abuse and assault of, or by, adolescents remains unclear because of under-reporting. Offences include rape, incest, paedophilia, sexual killing and involvement in pornography and prostitution.

In assessment and management of sexually abused adolescents, the principles outlined in Chapter 29 apply. Rigorous care has to be taken, in cases of alleged abuse, to counteract the tendency to reach conclusions which cannot be substantiated. Despite the requirement to report juveniles suspected of being at risk, and the over-riding necessity for protection, difficult decisions may arise with older adolescents having a history of sexual abuse by a family member, who are no longer at risk, because of potential loss of therapeutic alliance.

Teenage parenthood

Sexual maturity is occurring earlier and births and abortions in teenage girls are increasing. For example, in Britain in 1969, there were 6.8 births per 1000 among 16-year-olds, but the rate had risen to 8.7 by 1986 (Frater 1986). There is no evidence of specific psychopathology leading to schoolgirl pregnancy or substantial evidence of positive intent (Shaffer et al 1978, Black 1986). Runaways are particularly vulnerable to the risks of prostitution and pregnancy. Few physical disadvantages accompany teenage child-bearing, provided antenatal care is adequate. Educationally, however, girls are seriously disadvantaged, employment difficulties are likely and teenage marriage lacks stability. There are fewer teenage fathers, because many teenage pregnancies are fathered by men aged over 20 years, some of whom fail to acknowledge paternity. Generally, teenage fathers are affected less adversely than mothers. Neonatal mortality is higher, and there is evidence that children of teenage parents have higher rates of cognitive deficits and psychosocial problems.

Eating disorders

Problems with eating, body weight and shape are increasingly referred to adolescent psychiatrists. Anorexia nervosa may arise in prepubertal children (Fosson et al 1987), but occurs typically in mid- or late adolescence. Bulimia nervosa is increasingly common among adolescents. Obesity is rarely the main referral reason, despite high prevalence and effects on self-esteem and peer relationships. Rumination disorder and pica occur rarely in isolation, other than in mentally retarded adolescents, but may feature in anorexia nervosa or bulimia nervosa.

Anorexia nervosa

Girls predominate, especially during late adolescence, accounting for 90–95% of cases. Prevalence rates of 0.5–1.0% have been recorded and evidence advanced of increasing incidence. Diagnosis and management resembles that in adults.

Complex sociocultural aetiological factors need to be related to underlying psychobiological and maturational processes. Adolescence in girls is accompanied by increased deposition of adipose tissue and consequent feelings of fatness may predispose to dieting. Abstinence has a powerful manipulative effect in family relationships and, at a time of age-appropriate turmoil, the sense of personal control from relentless dieting appeals to some adolescents. Persistent self-induced weight loss may become a maladaptive way of coping with maturational changes, associated with fears about adult sexuality and autonomy. Since teenage slimming is widespread, it is difficult to distinguish psychopathology from transient age-appropriate behaviour. The extent to which an overwhelming fear of fatness exists is the most useful index of serious disorder. If dieting fails to maintain desired weight, there may be complete breakdown of control with binging, and self-induced vomiting or purging may become incorporated in weight control.

Family interaction and issues concerning autonomy and emancipation usually feature prominently in treatment. Family therapy is most effective in young patients with illnesses of short duration, but less beneficial with older adolescents (Russell et al 1987). Depending upon the severity of weight loss and its medical consequences, treatment may need to begin in hospital and progress to out-patient care. Some programmes avoid explicit emphasis on weight restoration, focusing on personal and interpersonal issues and normalisation of eating and related behaviours. While these may be appropriate with adults, structured weight-oriented programmes are often required with younger patients and weight restoration alone may succeed.

Weight gain is a complex, prolonged process, complicated by ambivalence towards treatment and change. Weight gain programmes require dietary counselling and psychoeducational, behavioural, cognitive and psychotherapeutic strategies, e.g. concerned with problems of meal completion, manipulative conduct, and conformity to social functions of eating. Parental or family involvement is often crucial. There should be planned progression from minimal responsibility to full control of food intake and weight management. There is no consensus about frequency of weighing or whether patients should be informed about exact weight. Target weight needs to be seen as appropriate, reflecting the uniqueness of individual physique and set weight, so that power struggles between therapist and patient diminish and treatment goals are understandable. Detailed consideration needs to be given to the most effective method of calculating target weight, matching it to the patient's age, sex, height, maturational stage, eating attitudes, shape, weight gain, physical and nutritional knowledge. Using several methods to corroborate the chosen target is most helpful. In postmenarchic girls, non-negotiable, long-term target weights, concerned largely with menstrual onset, are likely to achieve the greatest compliance (Parry-Jones 1991).

Bulimia nervosa

This disorder has a prevalence of approximately 1.0% in adolescents (Fairburn & Beglin 1990). Anorexia nervosa may have occurred previously, but body weight, although a focus of concern, is usually normal. It is a chronic, often secretive, disorder, requiring prolonged treatment, especially in patients with concomitant psychopathology. Its management resembles that for anorexia nervosa. Hospitalisation is only required when binging, vomiting and purging are out of control, if there is a major weight loss or if there are serious medical complications.

Obesity

Obesity, usually defined as the body weight being 20% above normal, affects 20–30% of young people (Parry-Jones 1988). Causation is multifactorial, including physiological predisposition, family eating patterns and overeating in response to anxiety, depression, disturbed relationships and maturational stress. In addition to medical complications and increased vulnerability to other eating pathology, obesity generates personal and family problems. Teasing and bullying by peers leads to self-consciousness and isolation. Family tensions may be generated by maintaining reducing diets. Treatment outcome is discouraging, lost weight being regained rapidly without consistent family support and strong motivation. Cognitive and behavioural methods, involving the family and, if possible, the school peer group are most successful.

Mood disorders

Depression

Presentation of adolescent depression is often complex and, initially, not clearly part of the 'adult' entity. Several characteristic patterns are distinguishable, e.g. lowering of mood is more influenced by environment and is less fixed, reflecting typical adolescent mood fluctuation. Continuities with childhood and adult disorder, however, should not be overlooked (Parry-Jones 1989). Although depressive behaviour may be displayed from early childhood, capacity to articulate feelings of lowered mood only emerges with adolescent cognitive maturity. Nevertheless, adolescents are often unwilling to talk spontaneously about deeper feelings and, rather than lowered mood, may refer, more ambiguously, to a sense of emptiness or absence of feelings. Research on depression in young people has expanded (Rutter et al 1986, Goodyer 1992). Systematic interview schedules have been developed and the similarity between adolescent and adult depression has been confirmed (Strober et al 1981), although puberty has modifying effects on psychological markers of depression (Puig-Antich 1986).

Prevalence. Data on prevalence of adolescent depressive disorders in non-clinic populations are inadequate, although there is more information about the frequency of depressive symptoms. Kashani et al (1987) reported a prevalence of 4.7% for major depression and 3.3% for dysthymic disorder, significantly higher than rates for preadolescents. Rutter et al (1976) revealed a 1 year prevalence of affective disorder of 1.4 per 1000 in 10–11-year-olds and a three-fold increase in the rate from preadolescence to adolescence. A sharp rise in depressive feelings during pubescence was also demonstrated. During adolescence, the sex ratio changes progressively, girls outnumbering boys by up to 4:1. Some studies suggest that about 25% of adolescent psychiatric patients suffer from clinical depression.

Mild depressive episode. Coping with pubertal changes, separating from the family, developing intimate relationships and preparing for work may produce an unhappy, demoralised state. Relinquishment of childhood gratifications has to be mourned, the ending of school years can be unsettling, and a new awareness of the problems facing humanity increases the emotional burden. Usually, such maturational tasks are achieved comfortably, with only transient mood lowering and little interference with everyday functioning. Some adolescents experience persistent sadness, hopelessness and apathy, which interferes with performance and leads to personal suffering. Although usually mild, there may be expressions of self-denigration, and feelings of loneliness and hopelessness may precipitate suicidal ideas. Fears of failure may be prominent, such as not becoming an effective adult, or making a successful sexual relationship. In the background, there are likely to be behavioural problems, and difficulties with school, family and peers.

Depressive episodes may follow bereavement or personal setbacks and disappointments, such as breaking up a close relationship or academic failure, with loss of an important hope or ambition. Problems in the adolescent's social life at home, school or in the peer group may be precipitants, the intensity of depression depending on the degree of loss and susceptibility to the implications of reversal. Personality features predisposing to depression may be recognised during adolescence and depressive cognitions can commence in late childhood. Adolescents who habitually adopt these ways of thinking and lack self-esteem are more likely to become depressed when faced with reversals. Processes interacting with cognitive development to produce low self-esteem and negative self-evaluation are ill-understood and the significance of these apparent vulnerability factors is uncertain.

Lowered mood may not always be conspicuous or described spontaneously, although characteristic depressive symptoms are confirmed on detailed inquiry. For such presentations, the unsatisfactory term 'masked depression' has been used (Carlson & Cantwell 1980). While this is not a separate diagnostic entity, retaining the term in adolescent practice emphasises that depression can go unrecognised. Presentations concealing depression can take the form of restless boredom, persistent search for new activities, fatigue, bodily preoccupations and physical symptoms. Alternatively, there may be uncharacteristic antisocial and risk-taking behaviour, promiscuity or drug abuse. There may be association between depression and both substance abuse and conduct disorder (Marriage et al 1986, Kovacs et al 1988).

Moderate and severe depressive episodes. Serious depressive episodes are rare before puberty, increasing in mid- and late adolescence to adult levels. Developmental processes accounting for this change are ill-understood (Rutter 1986). Clinical features are essentially the same as in adulthood, comprising single or recurrent episodes of depression, with or without psychotic symptoms, and depression alternating with mania or hypomania. As in adults, moderate–severe depression has prominent somatic symptoms, but retardation may not be as salient. Compared with depression, largely understandable in reactive terms, there is likely to be less mood changeability. A family history of affective disorder is often present.

Recognition of the first episodes of bipolar disorder is difficult, especially in younger adolescents, until a cyclical pattern emerges. Instead, attempts tend to be made to construe symptoms in terms of personal and interpersonal difficulties. In differential diagnosis, affective disturbance in early schizophrenia has to be considered. Although little is known about the course of adolescent depressive disorders and prediction of relapse is difficult, adolescent depression can be a chronic, recurring and debilitating disorder, persisting into adulthood.

Diagnostic assessment. The central task is disentangling depressive disorder from age-appropriate reactions. Consideration needs to be given to evidence of change in behaviour and mental state, the extent to which these are in keeping with age and development, and the frequency, persistence and pervasiveness of abnormalities. Physical examination is essential because depressive symptoms can follow physical diseases. Measures suitable for use with adolescents include the Hamilton Rating Scale for Depression, the Birleson Depression Inventory and the Children's Depression Rating Scale.

Treatment. Most depressed teenagers are manageable at home, only a small proportion requiring hospitalisation for intensive assessment and treatment. It is important not to over-react to minor, stage-related mood changes, when what is needed is reassurance of parents or other significant adults. Intervention in 'understandable' depression ranges from direct practical help in resolving personal, situational and relationship problems, to individual psychotherapy, systematically planned to develop a more assertive and confident outlook. When there is a chronically negative self-view it may be difficult to shift the focus onto assets and achievements, away from losses, regrets and inadequacies. Cognitive therapy can be effective (McAdam 1986), because it is problem-oriented, concerned with current experiences and discourages dependency and regression. The burden borne by the parents and siblings can be considerable. Parents may feel responsible for the adolescent's state and unsure how to deal with mood disturbance in a young person who is cut-off and unaffected by reassurance. However, elaborate family involvement is not appropriate in all cases, especially with older adolescents.

There are few well-controlled studies of antidepressants in adolescents and limited evidence of efficacy. Clinical experience, however, suggests that medication may be beneficial for the small number of patients with biological or psychotic symptoms. A tricyclic antidepressant is advocated, and should be administered in maximum dosage for several weeks before concluding it is ineffective. Failure to respond, or inability to tolerate tricyclics, indicates use of an alternative, such as fluoxetine. Caution is needed not to undermine attempts to cope constructively with painful feelings by resorting to medication. Lithium carbonate is as effective in adolescent manic–depressive disorder as in adults (Youngerman & Canino 1978) and, following several major affective episodes, it is appropriate for long-term prophylactic treatment, although compliance may be poor. Minor tranquillisers and hypnotics are best avoided. Electroconvulsive therapy (ECT) may be indicated in severe, protracted depression resistant to other treatments.

Manic episodes

Despite doubts about the occurrence of mania in children, its adolescent presentation, as manic episodes or part of bipolar disorder, is well established, with prevalence of 0.6–1.0% in mid- and late adolescence (Carlson & Kashani 1988). Hypomania and mania in adolescents is similar to that in adults, although difficulties may arise in identifying the first episode (Carlson 1990). Differential diagnosis includes substance abuse and schizophrenia. Hospitalisation is usually necessary in severe mania to ensure patient safety. Treatment of the acute condition is by neuroleptic medication or lithium carbonate, although the latter is best used prophylactically.

Suicide and suicidal behaviour

Suicide is very rare before puberty, but the incidence rises rapidly and it becomes the third leading cause of death for adolescents, following accidents and homicides (Hawton 1986). Male suicides outnumber females at all ages and in all cultures, and rates have been increasing in males. This pattern is reversed in attempted suicide, although female rates appear to be declining. Methods vary widely, according to country and culture, with drug overdose, hanging, jumping from heights, car exhaust fumes and shooting being most frequent. Self-poisoning is the commonest form of parasuicide, the usual agents being analgesics and psychotropic drugs. There is likely to be a background of broken homes, disturbed relationships with parents and family history of suicidal behaviour. Precipitants include multiple losses or changes, such as fears of failure, recent quarrels, break-up with a boy- or girlfriend, trouble with teachers or school work, or social embarrassment. Few adolescents who attempt suicide have psychiatric disorder and serious suicidal intent is often low. Instead, there may be a range of motives, such as relief from intolerable stress, retaliation or manipulation. Suicide of a friend or relative, or media coverage of the death of a cult figure, may be influential. Suicide pacts are infrequent.

Assessment

Serious attention should be given to subtle or blatant verbal warnings referring to dying or suicide, and behavioural warnings, such as suicide notes or isolating behaviour. Key risk factors are male sex, previous self-destructive behaviour, persistent depression, suicide plans, family history of depression or suicide, isolation and alienation from family, friends or other social support systems and selection of a violent method, carried out in isolation with little likelihood of interruption. When depression is associated with conduct disorder, impulsivity, drug and alcohol abuse the risk may be higher.

Management

Not all young persons are assessed psychiatrically, although this is recommended practice. Examination in hospital, at the crisis point, is most effective, and delayed appointments are often unsuccessful. Difficulty in engagement is common, often due to negative family attitudes. Some psychiatrists hospitalise all suicidal adolescents, irrespective of risk, but a discriminating approach is preferable, provided immediate out-patient treatment is available. In addition to treating depression, attention needs to be given to developing more effective coping behaviour. Ten per cent of adolescents who attempt suicide repeat within a year (Hawton et al 1982). Repeaters have higher rates of drug and alcohol abuse, associated psychiatric disturbance, long-term problems, poor peer relationships, early parental loss and are likely to live away from home.

Self-mutilation

Self-injuring activities include cutting, scratching, cigarette burns, tattooing, bruising, biting and inserting needles (Raine 1982). Additional to its occurrence in schizophrenia and mental retardation, it arises typically in teenage girls displaying personality problems with impulsive–aggressive behaviour, poor relationships and low self-esteem, often in association with eating disorders, appearing to relieve intolerable tension or relationship impasse. A sequence can be identified, involving build-up of tension, anticipatory excitement at the prospect of injury, feelings of detachment on self-injury, discharge of tension and calmness, even sleep, before experiencing shame and guilt.

Self-mutilation is notoriously difficult to treat. The least possible response should be made that is compatible with essential first-aid. Psychiatric treatment addresses the underlying emotional and personality problems, although this may be complicated by poor verbal communication. Intervention should involve a search for more adaptive strategies for alleviating tension and achieving gratification, e.g. relaxation techniques.

Schizophrenia and schizotypal disorders

There is no unique adolescent psychosis and the view that adolescent 'turmoil' represents a 'normal psychosis' is outdated (Rutter et al 1976). Adolescent disorders need to be seen in the context of all psychoses occurring in children and adults, and adult diagnostic criteria are applicable. Adolescence has a pathoplastic influence, giving disorders staged characteristics and colouring the content of symptoms (Parry-Jones 1992). Schizophrenia is rare in childhood, but incidence increases at puberty, and the usual age of onset is 15–45 years. In the initial clinical picture, first-rank symptoms may be fleeting, difficult to elicit or absent (Garralda 1985). The common presentation is the acute syndrome, with falling off in social and academic performance, mood disturbance, incoherent speech, bizarre actions, hallucinations, delusions and preoccupation with inner thoughts.

Differential diagnosis

Careful syndromal diagnosis is essential, but it is characteristic of adolescent psychoses that precise diagnosis may be difficult, and lengthy observation and assessment necessary. Adolescents with severely disturbed emotional and personality development are hard to understand and may appear incoherent, but few develop psychotic disorders. Diagnostic problems arise if there are affective features, insidious personality deterioration or clouding of consciousness. Distinguishing between first episodes of schizophrenia and mania is particularly difficult, but this should encourage rigorous diagnostic endeavours, avoiding unqualified use of the term 'adolescent psychosis'. Not uncommonly, apparently affective disorders emerge as schizophrenia. Paranoid states, without typical schizophrenic features, are unusual. Acute transient psychotic disorders, attributable to stressful experiences occur, but distinction from schizophrenia is uncertain. Possible organic causes of psychosis, e.g. toxic confusional and drug-induced states and rare neurodegenerative conditions, need investigation. Early signs of subacute sclerosing panencephalitis may resemble schizophrenia, until progressive dementia with myoclonus and epilepsy supervenes. Seizure disorder, especially with temporal lobe involvement, can be associated with schizophrenia-like psychosis, and anticonvulsants can produce psychotic states.

Treatment

Treatment is concerned with a wider range of problems and handicaps than the psychotic process and intervention has to be tailored pragmatically to symptoms and needs. The overall aim is out-patient or day hospital care, but hospitalisation is commonly necessary. Management of a few schizophrenic adolescents in a general-purpose, multidisciplinary unit may generate problems (Parry-Jones 1992), due to differing staff attitudes towards the concept of psychosis, fears about diagnostic 'labelling', disagreement about the patient's capacity to control psychotic behaviour and ambivalence about antipsychotic drugs.

Individual intervention centres on straightforward

communication about the disorder and routine maturational, social and educational problems. It should be supportive and non-confrontational, and stressful group therapy is inappropriate. Family work aims at providing candid information and support, reducing high expressed emotion, encouraging realistic expectations, acceptance of relapses and long-term disabilities.

Neuroleptic treatment is the mainstay in acute and chronic schizophrenia and allied disorders, with depot preparations for maintenance when there is unreliability with oral medication. There is scope for behaviour modification, particularly reducing withdrawn, socially unacceptable behaviour. Appropriate educational provisions, especially residential, are hard to find, and there may be difficulties in obtaining employment. Facilities for rehabilitation and long-term care of teenagers with chronic schizophrenia are unsatisfactory, and overlap with adult services is often inadequate and unplanned. Even after vigorous treatment, adolescents with schizophrenia are likely to display a fluctuating course, with progression to a chronic stage, characterised by negative symptoms. Favourable prognostic pointers include acute onset associated with stress, affective features, higher intelligence and good premorbid personality. Generally, the younger the onset, the worse the prognosis (Kydd & Werry 1982).

Sleep disorders

In addition to sleep disturbance associated with psychiatric disorder, such as depression and PTSD, adolescents may suffer from other conditions which have received little attention (Stores 1990). Many adolescents have difficulty sleeping regularly through the night and have an increased need for daytime sleep (Price et al 1978, Carskadon & Dement 1987). Normal daytime somnolence has to be distinguished from narcolepsy and hypersomnolence occurring in the Kleine–Levin syndrome. Sleepwalking and night terrors may start in early adolescence, but are usually out-grown. Terrifying dreams or nightmares may be precipitated by frightening experiences occurring during acute stress and anxiety.

Tic disorders

Tics in adolescents are usually short lived and recovery takes place without treatment. Sometimes symptoms persist for a longer period, although recovery usually occurs within a few years. Tourette's syndrome usually begins in adolescence, characterised by motor and vocal tics, coprolalia, echolalia, sleep disturbance, learning difficulties and behaviour disorder. Associa-

tion with OCD has been established. Tics need to be distinguished from other movement disturbances and neurological disorders, such as Huntington's chorea.

In the treatment of Tourette's syndrome emphasis needs to be given to supporting the adolescent and family and enabling normal daily life and schooling to proceed. Haloperidol is an established treatment, but other drugs have been used, including pimozide, clonidine and fluoxetine (Cohen et al 1988).

Organic disorders

Assessment and differential diagnosis of suspected organic psychiatric disorder in adolescents, e.g. disorders associated with head injury, intracranial infections, cerebral tumours, endocrine and metabolic disorders, does not differ from that for adults. Detailed physical examination and neuropsychiatric assessment is essential, with selective use of special investigations.

Dementing disorders occur rarely in childhood and adolescence. Huntington's chorea can arise, although generally commencing after the age of 25 years. Neurological signs, especially choreiform movements, usually precede psychiatric symptoms, including depressive and schizophrenia-like features, culminating in progressive intellectual impairment. Other causes of dementia include the lipoidoses, leucodystrophies, hepatolenticular degeneration and subacute sclerosing panencephalitis. Although the pace of deterioration varies, the outcome is fatal or results in profound intellectual impairment. Occurrence after a period of normal function heightens the distress of parents and siblings, emphasising the need for family support during relentless deterioration. The opportunity for individual work is variable, but there may be scope for medication, e.g. neuroleptics in Huntington's chorea.

Psychiatric disorders associated with chronic physical illness

Adjustment problems can arise in long-term illnesses such as epilepsy, diabetes mellitus, asthma, ulcerative colitis, rheumatoid arthritis, cystic fibrosis, muscular disorders and physical deformities. However, chronic illness is not necessarily associated with psychological disturbance (Kellerman et al 1980, Zeltzer et al 1980). Responses may be more critical in life-threatening diseases, such as leukaemia, which can interrupt normal maturation, prolong dependence and interfere with peer group activities. Treatment refusal may occur as part of an autonomy struggle with parents and staff. The psychiatrist's role involves individual work and provision of explanation and support to parents and staff. Participation in groups of adolescents with similar disorders provides peer support, facilitating adaptation to disability and treatment compliance.

Epilepsy

Accurate diagnosis is essential before any form of psychiatric treatment is undertaken. Social management of epilepsy is particularly important in adolescent onset. Adolescents resent being stigmatised and overprotected and their need for control may lead to refusal of medication. Consideration needs to be given to the effects of anticonvulsants, injuries sustained during seizures and attitudes of family, peers, school staff and employers. Parents require help in reducing anxiety and over-protection, while adolescents need support and guidance in anticipating, reasonably confidently, a fairly normal life. Special psychiatric aspects concern emotional disturbance in temporal lobe disorders and schizophrenia-like psychoses.

Acne

Acne can be associated with intense anxiety, shame, depression and despair, aggravated by inappropriate self-treatment. Sufferers may fail to receive adequate treatment, if the condition is dismissed as a passing teenage problem. Topical treatment, usually with benzoyl peroxide, is generally employed before using antibiotics or isotretinoin.

Cancer

Increased chances of long-term survival have rapidly changed the pattern of presenting psychological problems in adolescents (Koocher et al 1980). These vary with the type of cancer, sites affected, course and forms of treatment. Feelings of inferiority and difference from peers occur. Painful diagnostic and therapeutic procedures, like biopsies and bone marrow aspirations, and concern about disfigurement and residual cosmetic defects following surgery, cause anxiety. Problematic side-effects of treatment commonly arise from cytotoxic chemotherapy and radiotherapy. Consequences of repeated hospitalisation and treatment include interruption of ordinary peer relations, school absences and boredom and stress in hospital. Worry about uncertain outcome is less problematic than for the parents.

Psychiatric input involves mental state assessment and identification of adjustment difficulties, with treatment emphasis on normalisation and psychosocial rehabilitation. Most worries and conflicts are resolvable by ventilation of feelings and brief, focused help, fostering the adolescent's coping skills and self-help capacity. Specific treatment techniques, e.g. relaxation training and systematic desensitisation, are indicated with depression, procedure-related pain and anxiety and school difficulties. Reaction to adverse cosmetic effects of treatment and persistent maladaptive thinking may necessitate prolonged psychotherapy. The psychiatrist is well placed to work with parents and siblings, and in supporting and training specialist staff, especially those involved in terminal care.

Surgical treatment

Teenagers should receive personal preparation for surgery to reduce preoperative anxiety and distress and aid postoperative adjustment and recovery. Management of postoperative pain is an appropriate area for psychiatric input.

Sensory handicaps

Early onset deafness interferes with language and speech development, and deaf children and adolescents have increased rates of emotional and behavioural disorders (Freeman et al 1975). Undetected partial deafness should be considered in academic underachievement. In assessment and management, principal issues are overcoming communication difficulties and understanding practical, day-to-day problems. Rates of psychological problems in visually impaired children and adolescents are also higher than in the general population (Freeman 1977), with 45% showing disorder.

HIV infection and acquired immune deficiency syndrome (AIDS)

There is limited information about HIV seroprevalence rates among adolescents, but approximately 1% of all AIDS cases are adolescent and numbers are increasing rapidly (Hein 1989). Adults suffering from AIDS were often exposed to the virus as teenagers and many adolescents, particularly runaways and gay males, are exposed to HIV infection by risky sexual behaviour and drug abuse. Young male prostitutes are particularly vulnerable. Increasingly, adolescents are concerned about AIDS because relatives, friends or cult figures are infected. Although most teenagers are likely to know that the disease is transmitted by sexual intercourse and re-used needles, there may be misconceptions and ignorance. Knowledge about safer sex practices, e.g. abstinence, reduced number of sexual partners and encounters and condom use, is likely to be limited, HIV-infected haemophiliac adolescents, and their distressed parents, present particularly difficult management problems.

Neuropsychiatric features include possible early subacute encephalitis and the AIDS dementia complex (ADC). In adolescents, this may present with impaired attention, concentration and memory and frontal lobe dysfunction. The infected teenager is susceptible to a wide range of intercurrent infections. The psychiatrist's role in HIV spectrum disease, becoming clarified with increasing clinical experience (Krener & Miller 1989), requires full integration into the multidisciplinary team, with specialised knowledge of the chronic illness (Krener 1991).

EFFECTS OF GENERAL HOSPITALISATION

Despite recommendations for specialised medical adolescent in-patient services (British Paediatric Association 1985), there has been limited development of such resources in Britain. Generally, adolescents requiring hospital treatment are managed in paediatric or adult wards. While technical care may be of a high order, adolescents may encounter problems in both settings in relation to privacy, age-appropriate freedom, involvement in decision-making and consent, and understanding and communication by staff lacking specific familiarity with maturational needs (Gillies & Parry-Jones 1992).

MENTAL RETARDATION

Incidence of psychiatric disorders and disturbed behaviour in mentally retarded adolescents is higher than in the general population (Rutter et al 1970, Corbett 1985). Diagnostic interviewing needs to be flexible, taking into account effects of limited cognitive capacity on communication and understanding, and direct observation of behaviour is required. Difficulties assimilating information, experimenting socially and conforming to peer group behaviour, with lack of expressive ability, can leave mentally retarded teenagers isolated and socially rejected. Although disorders resemble those in non-retarded adolescents, there may be diagnostic difficulties, e.g. identifying schizophrenia in the presence of severe retardation. A wide range of disturbed behaviour occurs. Violent, aggressive, self-stimulating and self-injurious behaviour is a major concern and constitutes the most frequent reason for pharmacological control. The overriding treatment emphasis is on acceptance and integration in the community and improvement in living skills.

TREATMENT

General principles

Treatment is usually multimodal and flexibility and versatility are crucial. An eclectic approach permits a range of techniques, adapting intervention to individual needs. Psychiatric intervention is necessary only within a small section of the spectrum of adolescent disturbance, and input at the point of service delivery frequently requires joint work with other services and agencies. Collaboration is enhanced by familiarity with their functions, resources and practice, and reduction of interprofessional tensions is facilitated by acknowledging the distinctive competences and central role responsibilities of each discipline (Parry-Jones 1986).

Referral reasons are often more concerned with not knowing what to do than with intrinsic disorders. However, clear courses of therapeutic action are rarely available and the risk–benefit ratio of intervention should be considered against likely outcome without treatment. The necessity and timing of psychiatric treatment is controversial, because of difficulties distinguishing healthy behaviour from disorder, but residual ambiguity does not negate intervention. Decisions are essential concerning design and implementation of interventions, treatment adherence, progress monitoring, and termination. Non-adherence to treatment can be a major challenge, and engaging commitment is facilitated by focusing on clearly relevant issues and actions to produce change. Unnecessary prolongation of out-patient contact risks increased dependency and invalidism and, generally, it is best to withdraw with further progress still to be made.

Therapeutic relationship

Development of trust depends on the therapist's honesty, evenhandedness and respect for confidentiality. Being 'tough', expressing negative views or criticism will not necessarily jeopardise good relationships. Difficult decisions, threats of absconding, dropping out of treatment or acting out are best countered by openness and directness. Future appointments need to be clear, with full expectation that they will be kept. Dropout rates and prematurely terminated treatment are not necessarily higher than with adults. Alleged proclivity to drop out of psychotherapy can often be explained in terms of the therapist's emotional response to unilateral termination and failure to acknowledge adolescent attempts at independence (Suzuki 1989). Follow-up of some non-attenders, especially suicide attempters, is essential.

Location of treatment

Most adolescents are manageable as out-patients, but home visiting is an important service component. Some treatments need to be home based, e.g. response prevention programmes for OCD. Despite careful definition of selection criteria, in-patient admission has to fulfil diverse purposes (Steinberg 1982). Twenty-four hour observation and assessment is crucial, especially if there is a safety requirement. Residential treatment facilitates initiation and monitoring of intensive techniques which would be impracticable on an out-patient basis. Limited development of day care has been achieved.

Main therapeutic approaches

A wide therapeutic perspective avoids factionalism, resolving the dichotomy between physical and psychodynamic approaches. Rigorous attention should be paid to evidence of evaluative research. Although psychological methods predominate, consideration needs to be given to the combined or sequential use of psychotherapy and pharmacotherapy.

Managing emergencies

Prompt response is necessary since disturbed behaviour can be obtrusive and deemed uncontainable in the home, school, or neighbourhood. Certain circumstances necessitate urgent intervention, including risk of serious self-harm, acute alcohol or drug intoxication, aggressive and violent behaviour, absconding and homelessness (Steinberg 1989). Clinical emergencies may be precipitated by acute psychotic episodes, severe mood disturbances and acute stress reactions.

The priority is ensuring the safety of the adolescent and others. General or psychiatric hospitalisation, or an alternative place of safety, may be indicated. Time-limited crisis intervention should be provided following emergencies. Adolescents and families are more amenable to therapeutic intervention following unexpected hospitalisation, violence, attempted suicide or family breakdown. Crisis intervention utilises rapid assessment and focused, flexible, short-term strategies.

Ethical issues

Rigorous confidentiality needs to be maintained. Clarification of authority for intervention is important, since few adolescents seek help themselves. Whenever possible, the adolescent's full agreement should be obtained. At the age of 16 years, the young person's consent becomes paramount. Under that age, unless there is clear evidence of sufficient understanding of what is proposed, parental consent is decisive, although problems can arise when an adolescent aged under 16 years opposes intervention. Parental agreement is desirable with young people of any age, but alternative authority may be derived from a Care Order, the Mental Health Act 1983 or the Mental Health (Scotland) Act 1984. Consent has to be based on detailed explanation of what treatment entails. Special issues arise in family therapy, for example: involvement of family members, not registered as patients, in a way amounting to personal treatment; the use of personally disturbing procedures; and failure to provide adequate explanation of strategies and a range of treatment options. Meticulous clarification of the reasons for intervention and definition of the participative basis of family members is essential.

Transfer to adult services

Transfer to adult services should be planned carefully, with attention to the timing, allowing opportunity for the patient, relatives and staff to adjust to the transition. Limited resources in some adolescent units necessitate temporary admission of violent or self-destructive patients to adult wards. Such transfers are usually urgent and well-established links with adult services forestall difficulties.

Psychological and social treatments

Professional relationships with patients and families

Intervention involves staff of different disciplines and experience and psychotherapies need to be eclectic and flexible. Many problems arising in everyday work complicate staff–patient relationships. Staff may experience anxiety, ambivalence, irritation and anger in handling disturbed adolescents, and establishing emotional empathy may be difficult. Constructive use of dependency problems is often avoided by staff, who are trained to steer clear of becoming 'over-involved' (Ryder & Parry-Jones 1982). Particular problems may arise between parents and staff, especially young, inexperienced workers, who may appear to blame or depreciate the parents, and flaunt easy relationships with previously uncommunicative or oppositional teenagers. Staff need opportunities to acknowledge difficulties, with skilled support and supervision, which should avoid being over-elaborate and time-consuming.

Individual work

The level at which individual work is pitched requires careful planning. The best received approach is likely to be brief, focused intervention, with short-term goals concerned with problem-solving and developing and maintaining a sense of control. This recognizes that, for many adolescents, talking about intimate feelings is an unaccustomed task, whereas 'action-oriented' techniques are more acceptable. Treatment of silent, non-productive adolescents poses a serious challenge.

Insight-oriented psychotherapy requires consideration of the teenager's capacity to verbalise thoughts and feelings and think conceptually. Evans (1982) has given an account of adolescent psychiatric practice from a predominantly psychoanalytic viewpoint, but some psychotherapists doubt the treatability of certain adolescent disorders, favouring other supportive and educational techniques to avoid unforeseen failures or aggravation. Transference issues can present problems, especially in multidisciplinary residential settings. Integrating different forms of psychotherapy makes treatment more specific to problems and development, e.g. individual psychodynamic and behavioural methods in eating disorders or behavioural and family techniques in OCD. Current adolescent psychotherapy lacks empirical demonstration of efficacy, tending to display an expectation that benefits can be taken on trust (Parry-Jones 1990a).

Limit setting and control

Limit setting is important in staff-adolescent relationships and the need for clear boundaries requires therapeutic use of authority in management (Bruggen 1979). Deficient authority, evident in the lives of many adolescents, occurs symptomatically, for example, in school non-attendance and limit-testing antisocial behaviour. As part of a phase of treatment, assertion of authority, for example, enables re-establishment of a school routine or regaining healthy weight.

Younger staff may experience difficulties in being authoritative, fearful of jeopardising good relationships built on an easy going, 'equal footing' basis. In residential units, adolescents are likely to regard the staff as more restrictive and less tolerant than the staff views itself. Parents need to see staff use of authority as complementing, not usurping, their control.

Small group work

Group work is used frequently, especially as an adjunct to therapeutic community participation. Despite popularity, it poses special problems for the therapist and there is little information about outcome, indications and contraindications or selection criteria. Emphasis on action, rather than introspection, encourages structured activities, such as role play. Once alliance is established, attachments and differences can emerge and individuals share common experiences and practice growing up in a supportive environment. Indiscriminate inclusion of patients in open groups has limited clinical justification. Group therapy may benefit youngsters who are difficult to engage individually, with interpersonal problems or showing withdrawal and isolation, and the chronically physically ill.

Therapeutic communities

It is questionable how far the ethos of the adult therapeutic community is transferable to adolescent work, requiring control and leadership, but the principles have found application in many residential training and therapeutic institutions (e.g. see Rose 1990). Evaluation is difficult, but the method appears most beneficial for long-stay, homogeneous populations. However, this restricts the diversity of patient intake and pace of treatment necessary for effective general-purpose units.

Behavioural and cognitive therapies

There is considerable scope for behaviour therapy in disorders, such as obsessional states and single phobias, either alone or with other treatments (Werry & Wollersheim 1989). Reported use of cognitive therapy with adolescents is limited, although experience suggests its usefulness in depression, anxiety and panic. Use of self-monitoring and behavioural assignments appeals to young patients. Self-instructional training can be used with adolescents with deficits in self-control, who are impulsive, attention disordered, disobedient and aggressive (Kendall & Braswell 1985).

Anxiety management training

Anxiety management combines relaxation training, symptom explanation and techniques for controlling intrusive anxious thoughts. The latter is achieved by distraction or by repeating reassurance to neutralise their content.

Social skills training

Approaches involving instruction, role play, modelling and feedback are particularly appropriate and successful with adolescents. Despite considerable face value appeal, evidence about long-term effectiveness remains limited, with few evaluative studies (Hansen et al 1989).

Self-management

Many adolescent treatment procedures are adaptable for self-management, making them more acceptable and enjoyable, enhancing a sense of personal responsibility. It applies particularly to behavioural approaches, such as self-directed response prevention in OCD (Brigham 1989).

Creative and experiential therapies

Therapeutic use of art ranges from opportunities for recreation and disinhibition, to psychotherapy (Merry 1986). Using role play to clarify feelings and behaviour, or rehearse new responses, is constructive. Psychodrama is generally a group activity and, like sculpting and role play, requires experienced leadership (Wynn 1986). Various exercises and activities are used for enhancing the sense of belonging within groups, promotion of responsibility, trust and self-esteem. Long-term benefits, however, are unproven.

Parental and family work

Intervention with parents or families needs planning in the light of the overall diagnostic formulation, since elaborate family involvement is not always appropriate. Time allocated to the adolescent, the parents, or the whole, or part, family group requires careful balancing. Most adolescents accept family interviews as an appropriate medium for issues impinging on all family members. This permits separate sessions with the adolescent and parents, preserving privacy of personal disclosures. The form of conjoint intervention should match the stage reached in the adolescent–parent relationship, acknowledging changing balance of responsibility and independence. With all adolescents, it is appropriate to emphasise responsibility for their own thoughts, feelings and actions. Despite expectation of increasing acceptance of adult responsibilities, the inevitable ambiguity of this transitional stage generates adjustment difficulties for both parties.

Intervention with parents

Parents play a key part in supporting treatment and as agents of change. Intervention with parents has to be differentiated from family therapy, parent education and marital therapy. This approach emphasises the appropriate and adaptive development of parenting and the modification of attitudes and responses to the adolescent's behaviour, especially where they perpetuate dysfunction.

Parental willingness and capacity to form a treatment alliance needs evaluation. Knowledge of individual and marital histories clarifies the relationship between parenting styles and the parents' personal and developmental difficulties. Intervention objectives need to be agreed, with an explicit focus on parenting, not individual psychopathology. Parental attitudes towards adolescence require exploration. It may be viewed negatively, as a period to be endured until the young person is old enough to pursue adult life. At a personal level, earlier painful feelings and unresolved conflicts may be aroused. At the interpersonal level, implications of adolescent detachment for the marital relationship may be problematic and counselling may be indicated. Regarding the adolescent's capacity for emancipation, there may be separation-inducing perceptions and expectations, conveying confidence in the ability to grow and become independent, or separation-inhibiting perceptions, conveying lack of confidence (Stierlin et al 1971).

Exercise of parental authority and control may be the principal therapeutic focus in parent–adolescent conflict and estrangement. Some degree of challenge and confrontation is appropriate to adolescent maturation and need not be seen as a personal assault by parents, especially at a time of reappraisal in their own lives. A positive view of adolescence, as a creative force in the family, is encouraging and parental morale and successful coping has to be fostered. Individual or couple therapy should be arranged formally, or referral made to other services.

Family therapy

The most commonly used forms are psychodynamic methods, structural or strategic family therapy, behavioural methods and various eclectic approaches, which represent typical practice in adolescent psychiatry (Bruggen & Davies 1977; Will & Wrate 1985, Barker 1986). A problem-oriented method, with pragmatic objectives, benefits from greater flexibility and is particularly suitable in issues regularly precipitating family conflict. Identifying reciprocal changes and planning their implementation provides a model for family negotiation and communication. There are insufficient scientific grounds for an exclusively family-oriented approach applied indiscriminately. Evidence is weak for causal links between observable family interaction and presenting adolescent psychopathology, and there has been limited evaluation of family therapy. Adolescent disorder is rarely best understood in terms of family psychopathology, although family factors can precipitate, exacerbate or maintain problems in predisposed individuals. Particular indications include issues specific to adoption and divorce. In its selection, therefore, there has to be full awareness of positive and negative aspects (Walrond-Skinner 1978).

Physical treatments

Psychopharmacology in adolescence

There is limited information about the use and response to psychotropic drugs (Campbell et al 1985). Licensing restrictions, applying to marketing of psychotropic drugs for children, are unclear regarding adolescents, but use has been limited on ideological grounds and from fear of side-effects. There is scope for the judicious use of some drugs, avoiding polypharmacy (Jackson 1985).

Consent and compliance

Oral or written consent should be obtained, based on information about the respective risks and benefits with, and without, medication. To promote compliance, adolescents need active engagement and information about expected changes and monitoring.

Psychotropic medication

Anxiolytics, sedatives and hypnotics. Although safe and effective for brief administration, prolonged use of benzodiazepines produces adverse effects. There is no place for the use of barbiturates and it is rarely necessary to prescribe hypnotics. Beta–blockers are indicated in the short-term treatment of anxiety with prominent autonomic symptoms.

Anticholinergics and antihistamines. There is no evidence that these drugs warrant a place in adolescent treatment, apart from the use of anticholinergic drugs in treating acute dystonic and parkinsonian effects of antipsychotic drugs.

Antidepressants. The current view, based largely on uncontrolled studies, is that antidepressants are less effective in adolescent than in adult depression (Ryan 1990). There is evidence, for example, that despite a wide range of plasma levels, imipramine is not an effective antidepressant in adolescent major depression (Ryan et al 1986). With careful identification of target symptoms, however, medication may prove useful. Relatively little is known about adolescent response to antidepressants and suggested usage relies on adult data. Imipramine and amitriptyline remain standard antidepressants, but fluoxetine and fluvoxamine have fewer side-effects. The latter are reported to be effective in OCD. Dietary precautions with monoamine oxidase inhibitors make them unsuitable for adolescents. Baseline measurements of blood pressure and pulse rate should be recorded before administration, with an electrocardiogram if there are cardiac concerns, and serum levels should be monitored.

Psychostimulants. Dextroamphetamine and methylphenidate hydrochloride are used in the treatment of hyperactivity in children, but there have been fewer studies of their effects in adolescence. In the latter, there is risk of abuse and dependence, and the possibility of reduction in growth velocity (Biederman 1988).

Neuroleptics. There is no contraindication to the full use of the phenothiazines and butyrophenones in psychotic states, the guidelines being those applicable to adults. Side-effects, particularly acute dystonic reactions, tardive and withdrawal dyskinesia and neuroleptic malignant syndrome are the main concern. Use of neuroleptics for behaviour problems and aggressiveness remains controversial and is to be discouraged or applied selectively.

Lithium. It is wholly appropriate to consider the use of lithium treatment for bipolar disorder (Youngerman & Canino 1978, Steinberg 1980), with close cooperation between doctor, patient and family ensuring compliance. Treatment may produce hypothyroidism, but current lower lithium doses and serum levels generate fewer side-effects.

Anticonvulsants. Additional to seizure control, anticonvulsants have been employed in treatment of behaviour disorders. Carbamazepine is most widely used, but its benefit in hyperactivity, aggression and impulsivity awaits assessment.

Electroconvulsive therapy

There have been few studies of the use of ECT in adolescents. It is rarely indicated, except in severe, prolonged major depression or uncontrolled mania (Bertagnoli & Borchardt 1990).

RESIDENTIAL TREATMENT AND CARE

Psychiatric in-patient hospital treatment

The optimal role of in-patient units has remained controversial, because of the potential diversity of admission policies and therapeutic regimes. The Health Advisory Service (1986) clarified the nature of the required residential service, emphasising the benefits of general-purpose units. Clinical practice in such units is demanding and stressful, the organisation of interdisciplinary work is complex, and maintenance of a stable therapeutic ethos requires perceptive management (Steinberg 1986). Future planning needs to consider the wide range of poorly delineated demands relating to the care of disturbed adolescents, and current lack of uniformity in the organisation of residential services, causing gaps and unplanned overlap (Parry-Jones 1990b).

Reasons for referral and selection criteria

Reasons for referral reflect differing views about the function of hospitalisation and admission policies of individual units. The latter may be unclear because units are small, highly selective, operate outside mainstream psychiatry and have infrequent use by general practitioners, adult psychiatrists and paediatricians. The varied needs of hospital referrals include educational appraisal, care, control and provision of a safe place, diagnostic assessment, treatment and further work with involved adults (Steinberg 1982). These relate to identifiable psychiatric disorder and unmanageable behaviour, of which the latter is not necessarily within the scope of the psychiatric service, whose principal resource is 24 hour medical and nursing care.

Operational policies vary widely in relation to treatment and length of stay. Hospitalisation cannot provide the definitive treatment and, wherever possible, intervention should be focused on the changes necessary for short stay. All patients should be assessed prior to admission and intervention decisions related to the definite, or possible, presence of individual psychiatric disorder unequivocally requiring 24 hour nursing and medical care. Highly selective admission policies, in short-stay, general-purpose units, with inadequate staffing and secure facilities, have limited provision for severely disturbed adolescents. Local authority resources for 'difficult to place' patients, have been diminishing and demand for places in youth treatment centres exceeds availability.

Therapeutic objectives and outcome

Hospitalisation should be undertaken with great discrimination, so that the therapeutic objectives are clearly defined. Most in-patient units operate a general-purpose approach, with diverse, individually planned treatments, in an institutional setting providing a therapeutic living experience. Attempts to simplify the situation, by adopting single-treatment approaches, e.g. the therapeutic community, or by limiting disorders treated, can have serious implications where one unit serves a large population. Sometimes, attention is directed at problems necessitating admission or one focal problem (Harper 1989). The short-term treatment model is employed increasingly (Khan 1990).

The duration of stay is influenced by the severity and treatment resistance of disorders, non-clinical factors, e.g. deficiency of alternative placements and by different ideological approaches to hospitalisation. If the objective is to make a diagnosis, control symptoms and review treatment, short admission is appropriate. Lengthy admission is inevitable, however, if substantial psychodynamic and personality changes are sought.

Adolescent in-patient care carries the added burden of promoting normal development, although this does not necessarily militate against hospitalisation designed primarily for symptom control. While brief hospitalisation is advocated, there is a group of highly resistant, disturbed adolescents requiring lengthy in-patient care. Despite disadvantages created by a small number of long-stay patients in a short-stay unit, this arrangement may be inevitable, in the absence of more appropriate accommodation.

There have been several outcome studies (Ainsworth 1984, Turner et al 1986) and consumer surveys (Wells et al 1978, Pyne et al 1986), although research and evaluation represent a relatively minor concern compared with the demands of clinical work, consultation and administration. This is of major significance in adolescent psychiatry, since well-validated knowledge remains small, aetiological models controversial and treatment largely empirical. Further, while scope for cost–benefit evaluation of mental health care is extensive, its application in adolescent psychiatry has been negligible.

REFERENCES

Aarkrog T 1981 The borderline concept in childhood, adolescence and adulthood: borderline adolescents in psychiatric treatment and five years later. Acta Psychiatrica Scandinavica suppl 293, 64: 1–300

Achenbach T M, Edelbrock C S 1983 Manual for the Child

Behaviour Checklist and Revised Child Behaviour Profile. University of Vermont, Burlington, VT

Ainsworth P 1984 The first 100 admissions to a regional general purpose adolescent unit. Journal of Adolescence 7: 337–348

Allsopp M, Verduyn C 1989 A follow-up of adolescents with obsessive–compulsive disorder. British Journal of Psychiatry 154: 829–834

Ashton C H 1990 Solvent abuse. British Medical Journal 300: 135–136

Bancroft J, Reinisch J M 1990 Adolescence and puberty. Oxford University Press, Oxford

Barker P 1986 Basic family therapy. Blackwell Scientific, Oxford

Berg I 1985 The management of truancy. Journal of Child Psychology and Psychiatry 26: 325–331

Berg I 1991 School avoidance, school phobia, and truancy. In: Lewis M (ed) Child and adolescent psychiatry. A comprehensive text book. Williams & Wilkins, Baltimore, pp 1092–1098

Bertagnoli M W, Borchadt C M 1990 A review of ECT for children and adolescents. Journal of the American Academy of Child and Adolescent Psychiatry 29: 302–307

Biederman J 1988 Pharmacologic treatment of adolescents with affective disorders and attention deficit disorder. Pharmacological Bulletin 24: 81–87

Black D 1986 Schoolgirl mothers. British Medical Journal 293: 1047

Bolton D, Collins S, Steinberg D 1983 The treatment of obsessive–compulsive disorders in adolescence: a report of 15 cases. British Journal of Psychiatry 142: 456–466

Brandenburg N A, Friedman R M Silver S E 1990 The epidemiology of childhood psychiatric disorders: prevalence findings from recent studies. Journal of the American Academy of Child and Adolescent Psychiatry 29: 76–83

Brigham T A 1989 Self-management for adolescents: a skills training programme. Guilford Press, Hove

British Paediatric Association 1985 Report of the working party on the needs and care of adolescents. British Paediatric Association, London

Brooksbank D 1984 Management of conversion reaction in five adolescent girls. Journal of Adolescence 7: 359–376

Bruggen P 1979 Authority in work with young adolescents: a personal review. Journal of Adolescence 2: 345–354

Bruggen P, Davies G 1977 Family therapy in adolescent psychiatry. British Journal of Psychiatry 131: 433–447

Campbell M, Green W H, Deutsch S I 1985 Child and adolescent psychopharmacology. Sage, London

Carskadon M A, Dement W C 1987 Sleepiness in the normal adolescent. In: Guilleminault C (ed) Sleep and its disorders in children. Raven Press, New York, pp 53–66

Carlson G A 1990 Child and adolescent mania — diagnostic considerations. Journal of Child Psychology and Psychiatry 31: 331–341

Carlson G A, Cantwell D P 1980 Unmasking masked depression in children and adolescents. American Journal of Psychiatry 137: 445–449

Carlson G A, Kashani J H 1988 Manic symptoms in a non-referral adolescent population. Journal of Affective Disorders 15: 219–226

Chadwick O, Anderson R, Bland M, Ramsay J 1989 Neuropsychological consequences of volatile substance abuse: a population based study of secondary school pupils. British Medical Journal 298: 1679–1684

Cohen D J, Brunn R D, Leckman J F (eds) 1988 Tourette's syndrome and tic disorders. Wiley, New York

Coleman J C, Hendry L 1990 The nature of adolescence, 2nd edn. Routledge, London

Conners C K, Barkley R A 1985 Rating scales and checklists for child psychopharmacology. Psychopharmacology Bulletin 21: 809–815

Cooke B R B, Evans D A, Farrow S C 1988 Solvent misuse in secondary school children — a prevalence study. Community Medicine 10: 8–13

Corbett J 1985 Mental retardation: psychiatric aspects. In: Rutter M, Hersov L (eds) Child and adolescent psychiatry: modern approaches. Blackwell Scientific, Oxford, pp 661–678

Costello E J 1989 Developments in child psychiatric epidemiology. Journal of the American Academy of Child and Adolescent Psychiatry 28: 836–841

Costello E J, Edelbrock C, Dulcan M K et al 1984 Development and testing of the NIMH Diagnostic Interview Schedule for Children in a clinic population. Final report. Centre for Epidemiologic Studies, National Institute of Mental Health, Rockville, M D

Douvan E 1979 Sex role learning. In: Coleman J C (ed) The school years. Methuen, London

Dubowitz V, Hersov L 1976 Management of children with non-organic (hysterical) disorders of motor function. Developmental Medicine and Child Neurology 18: 358–368

Egan J 1986 Etiology and treatment of borderline personality disorder in adolescents. Hospital and Community Psychiatry 37: 613–618

Endicott J, Spitzer R L 1978 A diagnostic interview: the Schedule for Affective Disorders and Schizophrenia. Archives of General Psychiatry 35: 837–844

Eth S, Pynoos R (eds) 1985 Post-traumatic stress disorder in children. American Psychiatric Press, Washington, DC

Evans J 1982 Adolescent and preadolescent psychiatry. Academic Press, London

Fairburn C G, Beglin S J 1990 Studies of the epidemiology of bulimia nervosa. American Journal of Psychiatry 147: 401–408

Flament M, Rapoport J, Berg C J, Sceery W, Kilts C, Mellstrom B, Linnoila M 1985 Clomipramine treatment of childhood obsessive–compulsive disorder. A double-blind controlled study. Archives of General Psychiatry 42: 977–983

Fosson A, Knibbs J, Bryant-Waugh R, Lask B 1987 Early onset anorexia nervosa. Archives of Disease in Childhood 62: 114–118

Frater A 1986 Teenage pregnancy in under sixteens 1969–1984, England and Wales. Brook Advisory Centres Education and Publications Unit, Birmingham

Freeman R D 1977 Psychiatric aspects of sensory disorders and intervention. In: Graham P J (ed) Epidemiological approaches in child psychiatry. Academic Press, London, pp 275–304

Freeman R, Malkin S, Hastings J 1975 Psychosocial problems of deaf children and their families: a comparative study. American Annals of Deafness 120: 391–405

Friedman A S, Glickman N W 1986 Program characteristics for successful treatment of adolescent drug abuse. Journal of Nervous and Mental Disorders 174: 669–679

Garralda M E 1985 Characteristics of the psychoses of late onset in children and adolescents (a comparative study of hallucinating children). Journal of Adolescence 8: 195–207

Gillies M, Parry-Jones W Ll 1992 Suitability of the paediatric setting for hospitalised adolescents. Archives of Disease in Childhood (in press)

Goodyer I M 1992 Depression in childhood and adolescence. In: Paykel E S (ed) Handbook of affective disorders, 2nd edn. Churchill Livingstone, Edinburgh, pp 585–600

Green D 1980 A behavioural approach to the treatment of obsessional rituals: an adolescent case study. Journal of Adolescence 3: 297–306

Green R 1987 The "sissy boy syndrome" and the development of homosexuality. Yale University Press, New Haven, C T

Gutterman E M, O'Brien J D, Young J G 1987 Structured diagnostic interviews for children and adolescents: current status and future directions. Journal of the American Academy of Child and Adolescent Psychiatry 26: 621–630

Hansen D J, Watson-Perczel M, Christopher J C 1989 Clinical issues in social-skills training with adolescents. Clinical Psychology Review 9: 363–391

Harper G 1989 Focal inpatient treatment planning. Journal of the American Academy of Child and Adolescent Psychiatry 28: 31–37

Hawker A 1978 Adolescents and alcohol. Edsall, London

Hawton K 1986 Suicide and attempted suicide among children and adolescents. Sage, London

Hawton K, O'Grady J, Osborn M, Cole D 1982 Adolescents who take overdoses: their characteristics, problems and contacts with helping agencies. British Journal of Psychiatry 140: 118–123

Health Advisory Service 1986 Bridges over troubled waters. Her Majesty's Stationery Office, London

Hein K 1989 AIDS in adolescence: a response to the challenge. Journal of Adolescent Health Care 10: 510–536

Herjanic B, Campbell W 1977 Differentiating psychiatrically disturbed children on the basis of a structured interview. Journal of Abnormal Child Psychology 5: 127–134

Hill P 1989 Adolescent psychiatry. Churchill Livingstone, Edinburgh, pp 286–287

Hodges K, McKnew D, Cytryn L, Stern L, Kline J 1982 The Child Assessment Schedule (CAS) diagnostic interview: a report on reliability and validity. Journal of the American Academy of Child Psychiatry 21: 468–473

Hollingsworth C E, Tanguay P E, Grossman L, Pabst P 1980 Long-term outcome of obsessive–compulsive disorders in childhood. Journal of the American Academy of Child Psychiatry 19: 134–144

Horowitz M J, Wilner N, Alvarez W 1979 Impact of event scale: a measure of subjective stress. Psychosomatic Medicine 41: 209–218

Jacobson R 1985a Child firesetters: a clinical investigation. Journal of Child Psychology and Psychiatry 26: 759–768

Jacobson R 1985b The subclassification of child firesetters. Journal of Child Psychology and Psychiatry 26: 769–775

Jackson A H 1985 Teaching pediatric psychopharmacology: an interdisciplinary model. Journal of the American Academy of Child Psychiatry 24: 103–108

Kashani J H, Carlson G A, Beck N C 1987 Depression, depressive, symptoms, and depressed mood among a community sample of adolescents. American Journal of Psychiatry 144: 931–934

Kazdin A E 1987 Conduct disorders in childhood and adolescence. Sage, California

Kellerman J, Zeltzer L, Ellenberg L, Dash J, Rigler D 1980 Psychological effects of illness in adolescence. I. Anxiety, self-esteem, and perception of control. Journal of Pediatrics 97: 126–131

Kendall P C, Braswell L 1985 Cognitive-behavioural therapy for impulsive children. Guilford Press, New York

Khan A U 1990 Short-term psychiatric hospitalisation of adolescents. Year Book Medical, Chicago

Koocher G P, O'Malley J E, Gogan J L, Foster D J 1980 Psychological adjustment among pediatric cancer survivors. Journal of Child Psychology and Psychiatry 21: 163–173

Kovacs M 1985 The Interview Schedule for Children (ISC) Psychopharmacological Bulletin 21: 991–994

Kovacs M, Paulanskas S, Gatsonis C, Richards, C 1988 Depressive disorders in childhood III. A longitudinal study of comorbidity with and risk for conduct disorders. Journal of Affective Disorders 15: 205–217

Krener P G, Miller F B 1989 Psychiatric response to HIV spectrum disease in children and adolescents. Journal of the American Academy of Child and Adolescent Psychiatry 28: 596–605

Krener PG 1991 HIV-spectrum disease. In: Lewis M (ed) Child and adolescent psychiatry. A comprehensive textbook. Williams & Wilkins, Baltimore, pp 994–1004

Kydd R R, Werry J S 1982 Schizophrenia in children under sixteen years. Journal of Autism and Developmental Disorders 12: 343–357

Lewis M, Volkmar F R (eds) 1990 Clinical aspects of child and adolescent development, 3rd edition. Lea & Febiger, Philadelphia

Lowenstein L F 1978 The bullied and the non-bullied child. Bulletin of the British Psychological Society 31: 316–318

Lyons J A 1987 Post-traumatic stress disorder in children and adolescents. A review of the literature. Journal of Developmental and Behavioural Pediatrics 18: 349–356

McAdam E 1986 Cognitive behaviour therapy and its application with adolescents. Journal of Adolescence 9: 1–15

Marriage K, Fine S, Moretti M, Haley G 1986 Relationship between depression and conduct disorder in children and adolescents. Journal of the American Academy of Child Psychiatry 25: 687–691

Masterton G 1979 The management of solvent abuse. Journal of Adolescence 2: 65–75

Merry J 1986 Art in the education of the disturbed adolescent. In: Steinberg D (ed) The adolescent unit. Wiley, Chichester, pp 43–51

Orvaschel H 1985 Psychiatric interviews suitable for research with children and adolescents. Psychopharmacology Bulletin 21: 737–746

Parry-Jones W Ll 1984 Adolescent psychiatry in Britain: a personal view of its development and present position. Bulletin of the Royal College of Psychiatrists 8: 230–233

Parry-Jones W Ll 1986 Multidisciplinary teamwork: help or hindrance? In: Steinberg D (ed) The adolescent unit. Wiley, Chichester, pp 193–200

Parry-Jones W Ll 1988 Obesity in children and adolescents. In: Burrows GD, Beumont PJV, Casper R C (eds) Handbook of eating disorders, part 2. Obesity. Elsevier, Amsterdam, pp 207–219

Parry-Jones W Ll 1989 Depression in adolescence. In: Herbst K, Paykel E (eds) Depression: an integrative approach. Heinemann, Oxford, pp 111–123

Parry-Jones W Ll 1990a Psychotherapy with adolescents. Current Opinion in Psychiatry 3: 346–350

Parry-Jones W Ll 1990b Adolescent psychiatric services: development and expansion. In: Hendriks J H, Black M (eds) Child and adolescent psychiatry: into the 1990s.

Occasional paper OP8. Royal College of Psychiatrists, London, pp 83–89

Parry-Jones W L1 1991 Target weight in children and adolescents with anorexia nervosa. Acta Paediatrica Scandinavica suppl 373: 82–90

Parry-Jones W L1 1992 Adolescent psychoses: treatment and service provision. Archives of Disease in Childhood 66: 1459–1462

Parry-Jones W L1 1993 History of child and adolescent psychiatry. In: Rutter M, Hersov L, Taylor E (eds) Child and adolescent psychiatry, modern approaches, 3rd edn. Blackwell Scientific, Oxford (in press)

Price VA, Coates T J, Thoresen C E 1978 Prevalence and correlates of poor sleep among adolescents. American Journal of Diseases of Children 132: 583–586

Puig-Antich J 1986 Psychobiological markers: effects of age and puberty. In: Rutter M, Izard C E, Read P B (eds) Depression in young people: developmental and clinical perspectives. Guilford Press, New York, pp 341–381

Pyne N, Morrison R, Ainsworth P 1986 A consumer survey of an adolescent unit. Journal of Adolescence 9: 63–72

Pynoos R S, Eth S 1986 Witness to violence: the child interview. Journal of the American Academy of Child Psychiatry 25: 306–319

Quay H C 1983 A dimensional approach to behavior disorder: the Revised Behavior Problem Checklist. School Psychology Review 12: 244–249

Raine W J B 1982 Self mutilation. Journal of Adolescence 5: 1–13

Rapoport J L 1989 Obsessive–compulsive disorder in children and adolescents. American Psychiatric Press, New York

Ramsey J, Anderson H R, Bloor, K, Flanagan R J 1989 An introduction to the practice, prevalence and chemical toxicology of volatile substance abuse. Human Toxicology 8: 261–269

Riddle M A, Hardin M T, King R et al 1990 Fluoxetine treatment of children and adolescents with Tourette's and obsessive compulsive disorders: preliminary clinical experience. Journal of the American Academy of Child and Adolescent Psychiatry 29: 45–48

Robins L N 1978 Sturdy childhood predictors of adult antisocial behaviour replications from longitudinal studies. Psychological Medicine 8: 611–622

Robins L N 1991 Conduct disorder. Journal of Child Psychology and Psychiatry 32: 193–212

Rose M 1990 Healing hurt minds: the Peper Harow experience. Tavistock/Routledge, London

Russell G F M, Szmukler G I, Dare C, Eisler I 1987 An evaluation of family therapy in anorexia nervosa and bulimia nervosa. Archives of General Psychiatry 44: 1047–1056

Rutter M 1986 The developmental psychopathology of depression: issues and perspectives. In: Rutter M, Izard C E, Read P B (eds) Depression in young people: developmental and clinical perspectives. Guilford Press, New York, pp 3–30

Rutter M 1987 Temperament, personality and personality disorder. British Journal of Psychiatry 150: 443–458

Rutter M 1989 Annotation: child psychiatric disorders in ICD-10. Journal of Child Psychology and Psychiatry 30: 499–513

Rutter M, Giller H 1983 Juvenile delinquency: trends and perspectives. Guilford Press, New York

Rutter M, Tizard J, Whitmore K 1970 Education, health and behaviour. Longman, London

Rutter M, Graham P, Chadwick O, Yule W 1976 Adolescent turmoil: fact or fiction. Journal of Child Psychology and Psychiatry 17: 35–56

Rutter M, Izard C E, Read P B (eds) 1986 Depression in young people: developmental and clinical perspectives. Guilford Press, New York

Ryan N D 1990 Heterocyclic antidepressants in children and adolescents. Journal of Child and Adolescent Psychopharmacology 1: 21–31

Ryan N D, Puig-Antich J, Cooper T B, Rabinovich H, Ambrosini P, Davies J, King J, Torres D, Fried J 1986 Imipramine in adolescent major depression: plasma level and clinical response. Acta Psychiatrica Scandinavica 73: 275–288

Ryder R, Parry-Jones W L1 1982 Fears of dependence and its value in working with adolescents. Journal of Adolescence 5: 71–78

Shaffer D, Pettigrew A, Wolkind S, Zajicek, E 1978 Psychiatric aspects of pregnancy in schoolgirls: a review. Psychological Medicine 8: 119–130

Steinberg D 1980 The use of lithium carbonate in adolescence. Journal of Child Psychology and Psychiatry 21: 263–271

Steinberg D 1982 Treatment, training, care or control? The functions of adolescent units. British Journal of Psychiatry 141: 306–309

Steinberg D (ed) 1986 The adolescent unit: work and teamwork in adolescent psychiatry. Wiley, Chichester

Steinberg D 1989 Management of crises and emergencies. In: Hsu L K G, Hersen M (eds) Recent developments in adolescent psychiatry. Wiley, New York, pp 87–114

Stierlin H, Levi L D, Savard R J 1971 Parental perceptions of separating children. Family Process 10: 411–427

Stores G 1990 Sleep disorders in children. British Medical Journal 301: 351–352

Strober M, Green J, Carlson G 1981 Phenomenology and subtypes of major depressive disorder in adolescence. Journal of Affective Disorders 3: 281–290

Suzuki R 1989 Adolescents' dropout from individual psychotherapy — is it time? Journal of Adolescence 12: 197–205

Terr L 1991 Childhood traumas: an outline and overview. American Journal of Psychiatry 148: 10–20

Thorley G 1988 Adolescent outcome for hyperactive children. Archives of Disease in Childhood 63: 1181–1183

Tomb D A 1991 The runaway adolescent. In: Lewis M (ed) Child and adolescent psychiatry. A comprehensive textbook. Williams & Wilkins, Baltimore, pp 1066–1071

Turner T H, Dessetor D R, Bates R E 1986 The early outcome of admission to an adolescent unit: a report on 100 cases. Journal of Adolescence 9: 367–382

Tyrer P J 1988 Personality disorders: diagnosis, management and course. Wright, Bristol

Walrond-Skinner S 1978 Indications and contraindications for the use of family therapy. Journal of Child Psychology and Psychiatry 19: 57–62

Watson J M 1986 Solvent abuse: the adolescent epidemic? Croom Helm, London

Wells P G, Morris A, Jones R M, Allen D J 1978 An adolescent unit assessed: a consumer survey. British Journal of Psychiatry 132: 300–308

Werry J S, Wollersheim J P 1989 Behavior therapy with

children and adolescents: a twenty-year overview. Journal of the American Academy of Child and Adolescent Psychiatry 28: 1–18

Will D, Wrate R M 1985 Integrated family therapy. A problem-centred psychodynamic approach. Tavistock, London

Williams R A, Feibelman N D, Moulder C 1989 Events precipitating hospital treatment of adolescent drug abusers. Journal of the American Academy of Child and Adolescent Psychiatry 28: 70–73

Wolff S 1984 The concept of personality disorder in childhood. Journal of Child Psychology and Psychiatry 25: 5–13

Wolff S, Cull A 1986 "Schizoid" personality and antisocial conduct: a retrospective case note study. Psychological Medicine 16: 677–687

Wynn B 1986 Creative therapy. In: Steinberg D (ed) The adolescent unit. Wiley, Chichester, pp 73–82

Youngerman J, Canino I 1978 Lithium carbonate use in children and adolescents. Archives of General Psychiatry 35: 216–224

Yule W, Williams R M 1990 Post-traumatic stress reactions in children. Journal of Traumatic Stress 3: 279–295

Zanarini M C 1989 Childhood experiences of borderline patients. Comprehensive Psychiatry 30: 18–25

Zeltzer L, Kellerman J, Ellenberg L, Dash J, Rigler D 1980 Psychological effects of illness in adolescence. II. Impact of illness in adolescents — crucial issues and coping styles. Journal of Pediatrics 97: 132–138

Zietlin H 1986 The natural history of psychiatric disorders in children. Oxford University Press, Oxford

Zucker K J 1990 Treatment of gender identity disorders in children. In: Blanchard R, Steiner B W (eds) Clinical management of gender identity disorders in children and adults. American Psychiatric Press, Washington, DC, pp 1–23

Zucker K J, Green R 1991 Gender identity disorders. In: Lewis M (ed) Child and adolescent psychiatry. A comprehensive textbook. Williams & Wilkins, Baltimore, pp 604–613

31. Old age psychiatry

A. Jacques

INTRODUCTION

In Britain 15.8% of the population was aged over 65 years in 1991. The male-to-female ratio falls steadily from 1:1.2 in the 65–69 year age band to 1:3.0 at over 85 years (patients will therefore generally be referred to as female). Table 31.1 shows how the elderly population has expanded during the present century. The very elderly group, the 'old-old', will continue to expand for several further decades, whilst the 'young-old' population has already peaked. In other developed countries the pattern is similar, and in developing countries an even more rapid population explosion will occur later (WHO 1986).

Only 5% of the total elderly population of Britain lives in institutional care. Altogether, perhaps 15% of the elderly have a serious psychiatric problem, so psychiatric illness is a community problem. On the other hand, about 65% of psychiatric hospital residents in Britain are aged over 65 years, and this figure may increase in the future.

Despite its growing importance, old age psychiatry is still an underdeveloped specialty. Some services are still plagued by long waiting lists, inadequate staffing levels and poor morale. Colleagues still sometimes see old age psychiatry as a 'dustbin' or 'warehouse' subject, and the pessimism and carelessness of 'ageism' or 'gerontophobia' can occasionally infest even the most enthusiastic services. Nevertheless, considerable progress has been made in transforming a 'back-ward' non-specialty to a subject of major clinical, teaching and research interest.

HISTORY

The idea that elderly psychiatric patients might need separate attention first arose in the late 1940s. The gradual increase in older age groups (due to better housing, nutrition and social conditions during their childhood in the late 19th century) led to an increase in the elderly population of the long-stay wards of mental hospitals. Most of these patients were presumed to be suffering from 'senile dementia', but inevitably some had other, reversible conditions. Roth's (1955) simple demonstration that five diagnostic groups of elderly patients (senile dementia, arteriosclerotic dementia, delirium, depression and late paraphrenia) had different prognoses for discharge and survival showed the importance of accurate diagnosis. *Psychogeriatric assessment wards* for the elderly (Robinson 1975) began to be set up in the 1950s in a few hospitals and the idea gradually spread.

In the 1960s, problems of waiting lists for long-term care and assessment wards, and of 'misplacement' of dementing patients in medical wards (Kidd 1962) preoccupied psychiatrists. One solution was the development of *day hospitals* as an alternative to admission. Unfortunately it has not been proven that day hospitals either avoid or delay admission (Greene & Timbury 1979, Eagles & Gilleard 1984).

The 1970s was a decade of plans for coping with the population explosion of elderly people. (Department of Health and Social Security 1972,

Table 31.1 Population trends and projections for the United Kingdom 1901–2011

Year	Population (millions)		
	65–74 years	75–84 years	> 85 years
1901	1.29	0.47	0.06
1931	2.46	0.84	0.11
1951	3.69	1.55	0.22
1971	4.71	2.12	0.47
1991	5.03	3.12	0.89
2001	4.79	3.23	1.17
2011	5.18	3.15	1.32
Age change 1901–2011(%)	+300	+570	+2050
Age change 1991–2001(%)	–4.5	–3.6	+23

Adapted from the Central Statistical Office (1991).

Scottish Home and Health Department 1979). The concepts of *relief admission* (to relieve carers in a crisis) and *respite admission* (regular, preplanned breaks from caring) were introduced and, together with specialist *EMI (elderly mentally infirm) homes* for dementia sufferers in some areas (de Zoysa & Blessed 1984), began to show that continued increases in long-stay hospital provision might not be necessary.

In the 1980s the burgeoning of private sector *nursing* and *residential homes*, some specialising in dementia, has meant that in many areas unsatisfactory accommodation in old asylums has been closed down. Increased interest in *community care* led to patchy development of sitter services, day care and attempts at multiagency care planning. It is as yet unclear to what extent good community care can replace institutional care for dementia (Challis & Davies 1986). It is hoped, possibly over-optimistically, that the 1990s will be the decade when community care ideas are put into effective practice (Department of Health/Department of Social Security 1989).

Paralleling this slow evolution of services has been an equally slow growth of old age psychiatry as a specialty. The first consultants with a special interest in the field were appointed in the 1950s, a special section of the College of Psychiatrists was founded in the 1970s and in 1989 subspecialty status was granted.

THE OLD AGE PSYCHIATRY SERVICE

Catchment area

Most old age psychiatrists believe that a defined catchment area for a service is not only desirable but essential. Care is provided locally for patients and relatives who may find travel difficult, 'boundary disputes' between services are unlikely and some attempt at planning the use of scarce resources is possible. There are inevitable inequalities between areas that are rich and poor in resources, or between active, optimistic teams and passive, pessimistic teams, though such differences may lessen with better education and audit. However, the catchment principle has stood the test of time, and now fits uneasily with concepts of 'purchaser–provider' relationships, and 'cross-boundary flow' (Department of Health 1989).

Age limit policy

Clear, carefully negotiated age policies on presenile dementia and on functional disorders are vital for good relationships between old age psychiatry and other specialties. Most old age services do not take referrals for diagnosis of presenile dementia, but provide day, respite or long-term care to selected cases. Very young dementia sufferers do not fit easily with their elderly counterparts, and the boundaries between presenile dementia proper, and head injury, Korsakov's syndrome and other disorders are vague, so it is wise to be selective. Many services have an older cut-off age, perhaps of 70 or 75 years, for functional disorders, placing the emphasis on careful physical assessment as well as psychiatric treatment.

A comprehensive approach

In the few areas which offer pure dementia services, staff recruitment and morale may pose problems. Debates about *segregation or integration* of dementia sufferers have been prolonged. Old long-stay hospital wards were often examples of segregation at its worst, suffering from 'back-ward' mentality, distant from relatives and familiar territory, and rarely visited by outsiders. Meacher's broadside (1972) against some specialist EMI homes was an early plea for integration of dementia sufferers with the non-demented elderly. Rabins (1986) has emphasised the merits of 'segregated' dementia services, which can provide a separate environment where staff build up special skills and patients feel safe from the frequently stigmatising attitudes of their fit contemporaries. Wilkin et al (1985) concluded that there may be a 'right mix' for any institution. Residential homes which had over about 30% of dementing residents appeared less successful than those with lower percentages.

In old age psychiatry services, similar conflicts of interest between 'organic' and 'functional' patients are found. About half of most services' referrals are for organic disorders, though they require much more than half of the resources.

Multidisciplinary teamwork

The multiple problems of elderly patients require multiple assessment and treatment skills. Psychiatric expertise should be backed up by readily available advice from geriatric medical colleagues and access to other specialist medical services. The multidisciplinary team of doctors, clinical psychologist, community psychiatric nurses, hospital nurses, occupational therapist, physiotherapist, social worker and pharmacist should regularly attend patient reviews in respite and long-stay care as well as in the more attractive day hospital and assessment wards. Good access to speech therapy and to dietetic, chiropody and dental services are essential.

The practice of inviting relevant outsiders to multidisciplinary discussions on particular patients is becoming more widespread. Such 'network meetings' may involve the patient herself if she is able to participate, relatives, other friends or neighbours, home help, voluntary sector staff, area team social workers, general practitioner, primary care nurses, solicitor, police and clergy.

A range of services

Domiciliary assessment

Most referrals come from general practitioners, and consultants customarily see patients in their own homes. This not only provides better information on the social circumstances of the patient, her practical abilities and family relationships, but it avoids the disturbing or artificial effect of out-patient clinics, and usually starts the psychiatrist on a better footing with the patient. It often allows useful contact with relatives, though lack of privacy to interview the patient on sensitive topics, or the interference of a 'helpful' relative can lessen the value of the visit. Domiciliary assessment helps avoid hasty decisions and unnecessary admission. In some areas other members of the multi-disciplinary team contribute to domiciliary assessment and in a few areas the multi-agency approach of the 'dementia team' is used.

Out-patient clinics

Only some services run out-patient clinics. These help to overcome the few limitations of domiciliary visiting. More privacy can be accorded to patient or informants. Physical examination and investigations can be carried out and a geriatric opinion obtained.

Open-access clinics, called *memory clinics* (Philpott & Levy 1987), have been started in a few centres, usually as part of research projects. A multi-disciplinary group involving perhaps a psychiatrist, clinical psychologist, community psychiatric nurse (CPN) and social worker can investigate complaints of memory problems from the general public, concerned families or professionals. Such a system may overcome the reluctance of general practitioners to refer patients with possible early dementia, allows differential diagnosis which would otherwise be neglected and gives some reassurance to the 'worried well'.

Day hospital

Day hospitals now exist in most areas. In some, mainly rural, districts facilities are shared with geriatric medicine or other services. The trend in recent years has been away from 'granny sitting' for patients with milder dementia. This role is being increasingly taken over by local day centres, run by social services or voluntary organisations, thus allowing day hospitals to concentrate on their diagnostic, assessment, treatment and rehabilitative functions, and to offer long-term intensive support to those who need nursing care.

Flexibility in day care is essential if the actual needs of patients and carers are to be met. For carers in employment, for example, a 5-day day hospital may mean that they know where their relative is while they are working, but gives them no respite from caring when they are at home. In many areas, evening or weekend day care is now being offered, whilst 'night hospital' has been developed in one or two places.

Day hospital care can help effectively in the management of affective disorders and psychosis in the community. For dementia, it has been shown to be highly acceptable to carers (Gilleard et al 1984b) and it may be that, if sufficiently intensive and flexible, it can prevent admission to hospital.

Assessment beds

Dementing patients should be assessed in a separate ward from the 'functional' group, though there are of course some patients with both types of disorder and some who need considerable assessment before it is clear which category of bed is most suitable, so flexibility is required. Since domiciliary and day hospital assessment have become the norm, and as respite care has reduced the load of crisis admissions to short-stay wards, the need for assessment beds for dementia is lessening. Only a few patients need in-patient diagnosis. Some can benefit from in-patient treatment of specific behaviour problems. However, assessment beds are still often used for what are essentially 'relief' admissions, with no clear assessment purpose. If that function can be transferred to the respite facility, and if patients waiting for longer-term care do not wait for transfer for long periods, then the need for dementia assessment beds proper is perhaps as low as 0.3 per 1000 of the population over 65 years of age.

Respite beds

Respite for carers is of course an essential function of much day centre and day hospital care. Live-in respite care is most suited for dementing patients who live with their carers. A few patients are confused or develop minor infections as a result of the move, so respite care is unsuitable for patients who live alone. Very few patients fail to return home, and a clear contract between the hospital and relatives avoids unplanned 'ditching' of patients.

A choice of respite services is now available in most areas, ranging from holidays for groups of couples arranged by the Alzheimer Society, through fostering breaks with specially trained families, residential or nursing home care, to geriatric and psychiatric hospital care for those who need nursing. The system is most helpful if admissions come at regular intervals, planned with the relatives so that each comes *before* the stress of caring becomes too great, rather than giving relief *after* a crisis. In severe cases this may mean that the patient spends half (or even more) of her time in hospital and half at home with day hospital support.

Because hospital respite care has developed rapidly without central planning it has of necessity been fitted into available spaces. The beds may be in either assessment or long-stay wards, and neither is entirely satisfactory. It would be much better to have specially designated and designed small wards for respite care, roughly 0.8 beds per 1000 of the population over 65 years of age. A recent innovation is the *dementia resource centre*, a small local unit providing support, day care and respite care in one place.

Continuing care

The need for long-term hospital care for those with functional disorders is very small. Residential homes are able to cater for most who cannot return home after admission, with the exception of the few psychotic or chronically depressed patients who make no response to drug treatments or have intractable side-effects. These sorry patients fit equally badly into a ward of young disturbed patients as into a ward of dementia sufferers.

There is still a place for continuing hospital care for dementia. Nursing and residential homes are unlikely, unless highly specialised, to be able to tolerate disruptive residents (Capewell et al 1986). Better training and greater numbers of staff, regular support by consultants, CPNs and other psychiatric team members, judicious drug treatments, and the promise of admission if a difficult situation does not improve, should enable such patients to survive longer in non-hospital care. Some services even offer 'respite care' for homes. A small number of hospital beds, and certainly less than the old norms of 3/1000 elderly for England and

Wales (Department of Health and Social Security 1972) or 5/1000 for Scotland (Scottish Home and Health Department 1979), should suffice, depending on local conditions.

Liaison psychiatry

A third of referrals to most services are from geriatricians and general physicians. High rates of psychiatric disorder have been demonstrated in geriatric patients (Bergmann & Eastham 1974, Copeland et al 1975). The value of a separate old age psychiatry liaison service has been shown by Scott et al (1988). The special diagnostic and treatment skills of the old age psychiatrist and special knowledge of local services allow patients to be more effectively treated in the medical wards, enable better discharge planning and help avoid unwise disposal or unnecessary long-term care. Organic disorders comprise 60% of referrals. In a good liaison service, which makes itself readily available, most referrals will be for diagnosis and advice, rather than for transfer.

Liaison geriatric medicine

The chances of finding physical illness among a psychogeriatric population are very high, and in many cases this illness will contribute to the psychiatric disorder, or interfere with treatment or rehabilitation. Readily available advice from a geriatric physician in the out-patient clinic, day hospital and wards can be very helpful, and can minimise the transfer of patients between the services.

Joint activities

To overcome the problems of overlap between psychiatric and geriatric services (RCPsych 1979), and to help each other with difficult patients, some centres have developed the concept of joint working (Arie & Dunn 1973, Pitt & Silver 1980). Part of the service is managed together by the two specialties, as in a joint assessment ward, joint day hospital or joint long-stay care. The patients involved will be both physically and mentally disabled, or require further assessment to determine which service should become responsible. The logical consequence is a 'department of care of the elderly' in which all facilities are shared.

Links with community services

Old age psychiatrists are very aware that their patients do not depend on the efforts of the psychiatric service alone if they are to be maintained in the community. A wide network of caring agencies and professions is also involved (Table 31.2). Home helps are rightly said to be the backbone of community care. In their different ways the primary care nurses also contribute greatly, though they have traditionally concentrated their efforts on the physically disabled. Some enthusiastic health visitors contribute greatly to care planning, which is also the particular interest of social workers and will become their special responsibility in 1993. Social services departments provide day care, respite care and other services. Workers in a growing number of voluntary organisations offer advice, support, counselling, and sitter services, day care or other respite services. Some housing associations have recently been developing extra-care housing for dementia sufferers. A growing private sector is providing not only residential and nursing home care, but is now expanding into the delivery of home support services. This expansion has been greatly encouraged by the community care legislation which is due to take effect in 1993 (Department of Health/Department of Social Security 1989) with its emphasis on a 'mixed economy of care'.

In the last decade these organisations have shown great initiative in developing alternative forms of care for elderly people with psychiatric disorders. An effective old age service spends much of its efforts on liaising with agencies who share the care of patients living in the community, and on supporting them, whether in care planning, training and support of staff, project development, or just by paying them a regular visit. Two particular models of cooperation have been developed.

1. The mental health liaison meeting for the elderly

Representatives of the various agencies covering a particular community meet regularly, usually monthly, and discuss those patients with mental disorders who are of mutual interest to at least two of them. Such meetings help in care planning, avoid overlaps or gaps in care, and are mutually supportive and educative. Patients may be referred between the services. The meetings also develop a political role. Gaps in service provision become obvious and ideas about how to fill these gaps can be pursued. The liaison group is an efficient, effective and remarkably cheap method of organising care in the community.

2. The community dementia team

A dementia team (Lodge & McReynolds 1985) is also a multiagency group, and is formed by representatives of the relevant bodies, usually by secondment or special appointment. After local consultation and advertisement, it provides an open-access point for people in the community who are worried about dementia in themselves, their relatives or those they care for professionally (cf. the 'memory clinic' concept, but here the emphasis is on care planning rather than diagnosis). Inevitably most referrals come from professionals, but informal referral of patients who would otherwise fail to come to the attention of mainstream services is encouraged. A particular member of the team, who may come from any of the agencies involved, is selected to make an initial assessment and may become the 'key worker' for that patient and family over the succeeding months or years, introducing the patient to the services she needs, and

Table 31.2 Community services for elderly people with psychiatric disorders

Service	Potential providers
Informal support and supervision	Family, friends, neighbours, shopkeepers, police, clubs, church groups, 'granny sitting' circles
Home help	Social services Private
Sitting services, day or night	Voluntary agencies Private, including nursing agencies A few hospitals and social services departments
Meals on wheels	Social services Voluntary agencies
Aids, adaptations and safety	District nurses Occupational therapists (community or hospital based) Housing departments Gas and electricity companies
Incontinence care	District nurses and health visitors, some specialist incontinence nurses Laundry services (social services or community health)
Day care	Social services Voluntary agencies Some private
Respite care	Informal carers Social services Voluntary agencies Private
Planning and coordination of care — the 'key worker'	Informal carers Community psychiatric nurses Health visitors General practitioners Social workers

providing continuing support. The team's role over-laps with that of the primary care team, and in areas where the primary care team takes an active interest in organising community care it is probably superfluous.

Links with residential and nursing homes

Between 30 and 80% of residents in Part III homes are likely to suffer from dementia (Ineichin 1990) and perhaps 40% suffer from significant depressive symptoms (Mann et al 1984). Links between the old age psychiatry service and residential or nursing homes may be informal or formal. The consultant may regularly visit homes within his catchment area to review known patients' progress and give informal support to staff. CPNs may provide a regular advice and support service, particularly where hospital patients are discharged to the homes. Formal training sessions by doctor, CPN or clinical psychologist, and formal liaison groups, are found in a few areas. Some psychiatrists are on the admission panels for local authority, voluntary organisation or private homes.

Partnership with carers

Carers' groups have always been part of normal day hospital practice. Now Alzheimer society, social work and other community-based carers groups are commonplace. Carers form an essential part of the treatment team in dementia, having much information to provide about the patient, and wishing to be involved in decisions which are made throughout the illness. In day and respite care the psychiatric team is truly 'sharing care' with relatives and needs to recognise this.

Community bias

Attention in old age psychiatry is moving away from the problems of seemingly endless waiting lists for long-stay care to the opportunities of community care coupled with, if anything, short contact with hospital. This trend is welcomed by almost all patients and most families. Indeed, long-term care of patients with dementia is more and more being seen as the responsibility of extra-care housing, residential and nursing homes, which may give patients a better living environment than hospital, and sometimes also better care. Psychiatric services which are less involved in providing long-stay care can concentrate their efforts on specialist advice and treatment.

INTERVIEW METHODS

Interviewing the patient

Interviewing elderly psychiatric patients requires special skills.

Normal changes of ageing

In response to the almost universal slowing of all mental processes the interviewer must slow his pace, and learn patience. Elderly people tend to be more cautious in their responses to questions, so the interviewer may need to be more encouraging than for a younger patient, and use more multiple-choice or forced-choice questions. A tendency to greater intro-spection makes some elderly people more reticent about personal problems than is the norm for younger generations. A 'transference' effect may add to this. Inevitably, the interviewer is considerably younger than the patient, and may be treated as an inexperienced person, who needs to be protected from unpleasant reality.

In addition, *'counter-transference'* attitudes may interfere with the interviewer's willingness to ask personal questions of someone who could be their grandparent. Some doctors seem to believe that elderly people have inevitably led sheltered lives. They therefore avoid important questions about alcohol or sexual behaviour. Even worse is the still prevalent tendency to infantilise elderly people. This can have strange effects on interviewers, who fail to explain the interview process, 'speak down' to the patient, assume that she lacks understanding, general knowledge or wisdom, ignore her right to make or be involved in decisions, or speak to her relatives as if they were her parents. Some elderly people prefer a formal approach to interviewing. On the other hand, many become less inhibited than younger adults are about touch, probably because it has less obvious sexual connotations. Not only a shake of the hand, but holding the hand and other reassuring bodily contact is often both acceptable and helpful.

Elderly people of the present generation sometimes have surprisingly fatalistic, ageist *attitudes towards ill-ness*. This affects not only patients themselves but also their families and even professional carers, who may treat quite serious symptoms as evidence of 'just old age', fail to report them, or underplay their significance. Persistence may be required to elicit the full clinical picture.

Difficulty with or *dislike of change* is also common. This may be a real biological aspect of ageing or may be culturally determined. Introducing new concepts or new activities can lead to considerable resistance, most obvious when the doctor is recommending a course of action or therapy. Considerable time and gradual persuasion may be necessary to get the patient to consider even quite simple changes. Major changes such as accepting a home help for the first time or leaving home may be met in the first instance by total resistance.

Disabilities

Disabilities, often unconnected with the patient's psychiatric disorder, may interfere with the interviewing process. *Impairment of hearing* is the commonest, and, if not recognised, can easily lead to misdiagnosis of mental impairment. Access to a voice amplifier or communicator is essential. In severe cases it is necessary to write questions or use behavioural evidence of the mental state. *Visual impairment* brings difficulties with certain tests. Like deafness it may not be mentioned by a proud or self-conscious patient, and so is misconstrued. Patients who are *physically ill,* fatigued or in discomfort may not concentrate, so questioning will have to be simple, repetitive and carefully explained. *Parkinsonism* leads to mumbled speech which hinders interviewing, and can tempt the interviewer to diagnose depression or dementia.

Mental impairment

Impaired comprehension means that the interviewer has to explain carefully the rationale, content and duration of the interview. These explanations will have to be repeated several times for patients who show poor concentration, forgetfulness or suspiciousness. Difficulty with attention span, receptive dysphasia, poor vocabulary and grammar, impaired comprehension and abstract thinking all mean that questions or instructions should use simple words and simple one-clause sentences, dealing with only one item at a time, avoiding abstractions. It is not unusual for a patient to recall only the beginning (primacy effect) or the end (recency) of a long sentence. And retention of an instruction to be carried out in the future ('future memory') is likely to be impossible. Since attention and concentration are often impaired it is usually necessary to intersperse short periods of questioning with informal chat. A patient whose impairment of simple mental tasks is being revealed will need the reassurance of a spell of interesting reminiscence before new embarrassment is caused. Patients with expressive dysphasia may need assistance from the interviewer who guesses what words she is trying to say, or with prompt cards. Considerable skill and inventiveness is required to interview a patient who has no idea that the interviewer is a doctor, has severe receptive dysphasia or has no insight into her condition. Skill is also required in dealing with the defensive patient who has developed the ability to side-track interviewers into repetitive reminiscence to cover amnesia.

Interviewing informants

In general psychiatry it is usual for the patient to be able to give enough information about their history to allow accurate diagnosis. This is much less true in old age psychiatry. In organic disorders, interviewing the patient can *never* give a reliable or comprehensive history. Even at very early stages of dementia, sufferers fail to time-code information properly, so that vital questions about the natural history of the illness cannot be answered. However, the patient's history should not be ignored. Her attitude to her illness is important in assessing insight, working out treatment strategy and predicting compliance. And she may have more knowledge of some details than even her close relatives have. Furthermore, some patients do not have any available informant, or their informants themselves may have dementia or other disabilities.

It is important, even in severe dementia, to ask the patient's permission before seeing the relative. Relatives (and professionals) often need to be reminded that they are not legally in charge of the patient, even though they may feel or act in loco parentis. The doctor must also remind himself that he is the patient's *advocate* as well as trying to help the relatives. He may have to balance the distress and clearly expressed demand for help of an exhausted relative against uncomprehending or incoherent resistance from the patient.

The relatives' history itself may be inaccurate, either because they wish to emphasise their need for help, or because they wish to carry on caring without outside intrusion. Clarifying questions are very important, to pin down the exact time when a symptom started, or how often it has been obvious. These details are most important in diagnosis and in assessing what action is needed.

A useful procedure with informants for a patient who may have dementia is:

1. Explain the purpose, structure and timing of this interview, and of the interview with the patient.
2. Obtain the general history of the mental decline and enough information to indicate that the

impairment is *global*. Pin down *timing* as accurately as possible and clarify whether the process has been acute, gradual or irregular.

3. Details of relevant past history, personality, abilities and medical history will provide a *baseline* which is essential to diagnosis, and gives some currently relevant information.

4. Using a *problem check-list*, such as Table 31.5 or that of Gilleard (1984), list the problems experienced by the relatives, patient and others. There may be as many as 15–20 dementia-related problems for one patient. Clarify the seriousness, circumstances, timing, frequency, consequences and variations of each problem separately and record any treatment or management strategies which have been tried. Review the problem list with the relative and ask them if any other significant problems have been missed out. This essential part of the interview enables the relative to feel that all their concerns have been covered, yet the whole process has been quick and effective.

5. Ask about current supports, make a *timetable* of regular visitors or outings during the week and establish how long the patient can be left alone. This locates gaps and overlaps in care and support.

MENTAL STATE EXAMINATION

Much of the mental state examination is, as in younger patients, composed of information gathered during history-taking, by observation of the patient's behaviour and responses to questions. Organic mental testing is central to much of the work of the old age psychiatrist, and there is little evidence that any psychological test or test battery can give better information for diagnosis than a properly conducted mental state examination. A few points are worth stressing:

1. The principles of interviewing elderly people, particularly about explanation, pace, breaks from questions and simplicity of communication apply equally to mental testing.

2. No individual item tests only one function. For example, to ask 'What day is it today?' can lead to information about receptive dysphasia, general comprehension, immediate memory, recent memory, motivation and affect, expressive ability, hearing and sight as well as telling how oriented the person is. The serial 7 test may reveal dyscalculia or dysphasia as well as poor concentration. Very non-specific tests such as clock-drawing (Shulman et al 1986) can be invaluable.

3. Impairments can interact. A patient who has significant receptive dysphasia will be unable to participate in other mental tests which involve spoken questions or commands; this must not be taken to mean that she is impaired in these respects. Poor attention or low mood may interfere with all testing.

4. Although some standard questions are useful, imagination and flexibility are also essential. For example, questions about general knowledge, remote memory and new learning must all be varied according to the individual's premorbid intelligence, education, interests and experience. And, as information emerges, the doctor may need to employ additional tests to explore, say, parietal lobe function or dysphasia.

5. A patient's performance may vary from time to time. Mood, motivation, fatigue, time of day, and her attitude to the particular examiner may all make the difference between good and bad performance in tests. The doctor should never assume that what she has presented to him is how she always is. Mental state examination gives a tiny snapshot of her whole mental condition. Indeed, variations in presentation at different times provide useful information for both diagnosis and functional assessment.

6. The mental state examination is carried out for diagnostic purposes or to monitor progress. It is not an assessment of the practical needs of the patient. That is a separate exercise.

FURTHER INVESTIGATIONS

Rating scales

Intellectual rating scales, such as Hodkinson's Abbreviated Mental Test (1973), the information–orientation section of the Clifton Assessment Procedure for the Elderly (CAPE) (Pattie & Gilleard 1976) or the Mini-Mental State Examination (MMSE) (Folstein et al 1975), provide a general rating of mental impairment which can be used to assess severity or chart progress or decline. They are not diagnostic, though they are widely used as screening tests. They do not substitute for a thorough mental state examination, for they do not provide enough evidence to demonstrate the global impairment of delirium or dementia.

Ratings of behaviour using scales such as the Crichton Behaviour Rating Scale (Robinson 1975), and the behaviour section of the CAPE, are in regular use. Again these are not in any way diagnostic, and many of the items they test could relate to a variety of illnesses or disabilities. They do, however, give some estimate of severity of general impairment, after diagnosis has been carried out, and can be used to chart changes, or predict the level of care needed by the patient (Pattie & Gilleard 1976).

Standard depressive rating scales are not very appropriate to old age psychiatry, since questions about biological symptoms will not clearly distinguish depressive from physical illness.

Research interview schedules

Two major instruments were introduced in Britain in the 1980s, the Geriatric Mental State Schedule of Copeland et al (1986), which links with the AGECAT computerised diagnostic program, and the Cambridge Diagnostic Examination (CAMDEX) of Roth et al (1986), both covering the major diagnoses of old age psychiatry. These are making epidemiological surveys more reliable and valid, and providing a common language for researchers. They are not for routine use, but can be useful in examining difficult cases.

Psychological testing

The role of the clinical psychologist in mental state assessment in the elderly has expanded and contracted at different times over recent decades. Most claims that particular psychological tests (Kendrick 1987) can distinguish early dementia from normal ageing, or distinguish pseudodementia from true dementia, have failed to convince, largely because they have been validated on pure samples of classical cases, rather than samples from the grey areas. Nevertheless, psychological testing can be an extremely useful adjunct to examination, providing more detail about particular impairments, and adding weight for or against a particular diagnosis. The subject has been reviewed in Chapter 5 of Woods & Britton (1985).

Activities of daily living

The psychological abilities examined in mental state or psychological testing represent only a sample of brain activity that may be affected by brain damage. Behaviour rating scales give some evidence of other impairments, but the most practically useful evidence comes from assessment of the 'activities of daily living'. This is the special province of the occupational therapist, and is best carried out on a visit to the patient's own home, rather than in an artificial 'ADL suite'. Improved performance under scrutiny, performance anxiety, variations with mood, motivation, time of day and the relationship with the therapist must be taken into consideration when interpreting the results.

Table 31.3 Routine screening tests and the differential diagnosis of dementia

Test	Diagnosis
Full blood count	Alcohol dementia
Vitamin B_{12} and folate	Vitamin B_{12} and folate deficiency
Urea and electrolytes	Metabolic disorders
Calcium and phosphate	Parathyroid disorder
Syphilis serology	General paralysis of the insane (GPI)
Human immunodeficiency virus (HIV) testing where appropriate	Acquired immune deficiency syndrome (AIDS) dementia
Chest radiography	Secondary tumour
Computerised tomography (CT), magnetic resonance imaging (MRI) or single-photon emission CT (SPECT) scan where appropriate	Vascular dementias Normal pressure hydrocephalus Tumour

Blood tests and X-rays

Screening of the elderly in the community has generally brought little success in case-finding, but screening of groups of elderly people at special risk of physical illness has been much more productive. Elderly patients with any major psychiatric diagnosis are such a group. The list in Table 31.3, plus ward urine testing and bacteriology, are a useful minimum.

Special tests

The electroencephalogram (EEG) still has some place in old age psychiatry, but mainly in the diagnosis of possible fits. There were hopes that measuring auditory and visual evoked potentials could help in diagnosis, but, like almost every other special test, they lack sufficient specificity and sensitivity where they are needed, that is, in distinguishing mild dementia from normal ageing, and depression from dementia. The same criticism applies to the dexamethasone suppression test.

Computerised tomography (CT), magnetic resonance imaging and single-photon emission CT (SPECT) scanning are variably available. Again they are not perfect diagnostic tools, and, being relatively expensive, and in the case of SPECT invasive, are not in routine use. The sense of this practice is emphasised by the fact that probably 95% of dementias in old age are of the commoner types. A scan should be ordered when there are unusual clinical features or course, specific reasons to suspect a space-occupying lesion, subdural haemorrhage or hydrocephalus, or a particularly difficult differential diagnosis. The value of MRI in showing white matter and vascular lesions, and the possibility that SPECT can distinguish specific features of dementia of Alzheimer type (DAT) at early stages suggest that use of these tests will increase. When specific treatments for DAT or vascular dementias are available, diagnosis at the earliest possible stage will be essential.

THERAPIES

Psychotherapy

Most older neurotic patients do not suit or show interest in explorative psychotherapy, and therapists tend to agree that brief, problem-solving therapy related to current life difficulties is more likely to be relevant and effective. In effect, a counselling approach is often best. Possibly the biggest problem encountered is the resistance of some older people to change (Brink 1979).

The psychodynamic issues that are relevant to older people differ from those which preoccupy young adults. Coming to terms with the losses of old age and with decreasing independence and increasing dependence is often central. This is particularly difficult for active, independent personalities who have never anticipated such changes. Coming to terms with the past is also likely to be relevant, typical issues being regrets, renunciation of hopes, forgiveness or lack of forgiveness of perceived wrongs, and putting past preoccupations into perspective (Butler 1963). Although for many people reminiscence is an entirely enjoyable experience, some achieve that enjoyment by idealisation and denial, and others fail to find happiness in their recollections or are entrenched in bitterness. Erikson's (1963) counterpoint of 'ego integrity' versus 'despair' is relevant here.

Changed relationships and power structures in the family and among friends may cause both external and internal conflicts. Previously held expectations of old age may cause a variety of problems. Many had expected that they would be surrounded by a family who have instead moved away physically or emotionally; many looked forward to activities which they are kept from by disability or illness. Most are unprepared for the fact that old age can last for a very long time (average expectation of life at the age of 65 years is now 13.5 years for a man and 17.5 years for a woman). Personal and social attitudes to ageing may conflict. Conversely, an older person who wishes to be working, physically energetic, or sexually active may meet with disapproval from family and friends who expect her to 'retire'.

Psychological therapies

Clinical psychologists have recently begun to show a greater interest in treating elderly people (Woods & Britton 1985, Stokes & Goudie 1990) and have successfully applied behaviour therapy techniques for treating anxiety, phobias, depression and sexual problems. Some fear that learning-based theories may have less value because older people tend to be more rigid psychologically and less inclined to change, but there is no evidence that normal older people cannot learn.

The same is not true of dementia sufferers. Nevertheless, psychology has contributed much to their treatment, from the use of behavioural analysis (Hodge 1984) and specific examples of behaviour modification (Woods & Britton 1985, Ch. 7) to evaluation of more general therapies.

Reality orientation (RO)

This originated as a resocialisation technique in the back wards of American mental hospitals, but became metamorphosed into a treatment for dementia. It was enthusiastically embraced by staff in day care, residential homes and wards, partly because it was optimistic. But the optimism became excessive, RO was used as a universal 'therapy' whether it suited individual patients or not, and eventually got a bad name. Research (Brook et al 1975, Holden & Woods 1988) shows that the principle of encouraging orientation can help some patients in some aspects of their mental state and behaviour. Active involvement of the patient, and learning which makes use of procedural memory, are particularly effective. "Classroom RO' has probably now had its day, but as a '24 hour' technique RO can be useful in dealing with disorientation, mistaken ideas, distorted memories and some disturbed behaviour.

Reminiscence

This is less a specific therapy than a general principle (Butler 1963, Norris 1986, Thornton & Brotchie 1987) that elderly people often gain satisfaction, confidence and a sense of identity from reminiscing. Dementia sufferers may find reminiscence particularly satisfying. Lack of recent memory and helplessness in the present makes them fall back on remote memories in a search for identity and security. Of course their stories may be fragmentary or repetitive, but good reminiscence therapy allows for this and helps the person expand from the merely stereotyped. Photographs, slides and films, old objects, old songs and dances, 'theatre' where the sufferer 'performs' old work or domestic activities, handling old objects, and visits to the person's school, childhood home or other familiar scenes have all been effectively used. However, like reality orientation, reminiscence is not for all. For some, old memories evoke only sadness, regret or bitterness which they would rather avoid and may not be able to work through.

Validation therapy

This technique (Feil 1982) was introduced to escape from some of the impersonal excesses of 'classroom'-style reality orientation. It looks to the emotional state which underlies a patient's disoriented speech and behaviour. If she talks of wanting her mother, is it because she is feeling insecure, and would be helped by reassuring emotional or physical contact? If she wants to go off to work, is it because she is bored, and would benefit from exercise or activity?

Psychopharmacology

The changes in drug absorption, pharmacodynamics and activity with age are complicated. From the practical point of view certain principles are of day-to-day use:

1. Most research in pharmacology and therapeutics has until recently been carried out on younger subjects. Check that any statements about a drug are relevant to elderly people.

2. The body's ability to handle drugs changes in various ways with the process of ageing, but not in any absolute sense. Age is not in itself a contraindication to any drug.

3. The normal interpersonal variation in drug handling and effects is greater in old age. One person may both need and tolerate large doses of a particular drug, while another, apparently similar, person may obtain the same therapeutic effect with a lower dose, and even that low dose may cause harmful side-effects.

4. Because of this great variability, it is important to start any drug at a very small dose and build up gradually, particularly when using drugs with long half-lives or persistent metabolites.

5. Gradual reduction in renal function and reduction in some hepatic enzymes is the norm in old age so drugs which are cleared by these pathways need particular care.

6. Side-effects of drugs may appear at much lower doses than in younger patients, and in some cases at well below the therapeutic dose for that patient. An elderly schizophrenic patient may not tolerate therapeutic doses of any antipsychotic drug without major parkinsonian side-effects.

7. Even simple or mild side-effects may have disastrous consequences. Mild postural hypotension from an antidepressant can lead to a fractured femur, and mild anticholinergic effects can cause severe urinary retention or constipation.

8. Drug interactions are common, partly because of some doctors' penchant for polypharmacy. The assessment of any elderly patient should include a careful listing of all her medications. In many cases cutting or stopping drugs, simplifying schedules or changing to safer equivalents will lead to improvement in some or all of her symptoms (Findlay et al 1989).

9. It may not be clear what drugs the patient is actually taking, and compliance can be a major problem. Again polypharmacy may be responsible. The patient may have a cupboard full of drugs whose purpose she does not understand, or which she has forgotten about. The drug list which the general practitioner has may not be the list of drugs that the patient is taking. Patients who are being treated both at home and in a day hospital or respite ward are in particular danger of mix-up and poor communication about changes.

ORGANIC CONDITIONS

Delirium

Incidence

Delirium as a consequence of physical illness or toxic effects is commoner in elderly people than in younger age groups (see Lindesay et al 1990). It affects between 10 and 25% of patients aged over 65 years admitted to medical wards (Hodkinson 1973, Bergmann & Eastham 1974), and is especially common after hip and cardiac surgery. Unknown numbers suffer delirious states at home. The incidence may be high partly because elderly people are more prone to have one or more physical illnesses, and to be taking one or more drugs. In addition the ageing brain is more susceptible to insult, perhaps involving the cholinergic and noradrenergic systems which are important in cognition and the wake–sleep cycle. Dementing people are especially susceptible to superadded delirium (Hodkinson 1973).

Causes

The causes of delirium are no different in the elderly than in younger people, though some are relatively more important. Common infections and other general illnesses are potent causes and even quite simple conditions like constipation can lead to delirium in susceptible patients. Delirium is also a side-effect of a wide variety of drugs. Delirium tremens and benzodiazepine withdrawal should always be considered, and head injury, with the possibility of subsequent subdural haemorrhage, may not be reported. It is always sensible to consider these common conditions before subjecting the patient to more intensive investigation. Even a move ('translocation') can cause temporary delirium, though this is probably only true of those with an early or latent dementia.

Some patients suffer from more than one potential cause of the delirium. In some cases, particularly of possible stroke or transient ischaemic attack, the cause of the delirium may remain obscure even after scanning. Disentangling possible delirium in a dementia sufferer may be even more difficult. An acute change in mental state, or the emergence of one or more of the characteristic features (Table 31.4) should suggest possible delirium, but may be simply due to further progress in the illness, particularly in multi-infarct dementia. On the other hand, many dementing people will suffer physical illnesses which do not cause delirium or worsening of their mental state. Lipowski (1983) reported no detectable cause for delirium in between 5 and 20% of cases.

Table 31.4 Clinical features which tend to distinguish delirium from dementia. Global mental impairment is common to both conditions.

Delirium	Dementia
Rapid onset	Slowly progressive
Acute medical cause	Slowly progressive cause
Clouding of consciousness	Clear consciousness
Sleep disturbance	Normal sleep pattern, but 'clock' may be wrong
Irregular variability	Tends to be worse towards evening but otherwise stable
Restlessness and unease	Usually settled apart from aimless wandering or searching
Visual perceptual disturbances	Hallucinations uncommon and not usually disturbing
Lability of affect and distress	Lability less common

Clinical features

The characteristic variability of delirium means that a doctor's assessment does not necessarily reflect the patient's mental state over the whole day. Family or nursing reports of delirious symptoms at other times of day or night must be taken seriously.

Delirium is a serious condition and as many as 30 or 40% of delirious medical ward patients die of the underlying cause. However, the rest have a good prognosis and only 5% or less go on to develop dementia. It is important to find the cause quickly and then to be relatively optimistic. The condition may last longer in old age; for example, delirium tremens or delirium after a stroke may last for many weeks. Patients who do not instantly recover after their physical state or investigations have apparently returned to normal should not be prematurely diagnosed as suffering from dementia. At the very least they should be physically well for 2 weeks before any medium- or long-term decisions are made.

Differential diagnosis

Dementia. The classical distinction between delirium and dementia (Table 31.4) is an important but not absolute guide; features of delirium can appear during dementia, particularly if progress is rapid, and many cases of delirium have few or none of the distinguishing features except for the acute course.

Affective disorders and psychosis. The lability of affect common in delirium sometimes becomes pervasive and patients may develop mood congruent ideas or delusions which suggest a diagnosis of primary affective disorder. In a somewhat similar way psychotic symptoms in delirium may suggest a primary psychosis. It is in fact most unlikely that a primary affective disorder or primary psychosis would begin coincidentally with a physical illness.

Management

As at all ages the treatment of delirium is the treatment of the cause. Lindesay et al (1990) rightly emphasise psychological aspects of management, which should aim at:

1. Reducing under-stimulation and maximising the clarity of perceptions, whilst avoiding over-stimulation
2. Minimising the unfamiliarity of the environment
3. Minimising disorientation
4. Reassurance that the illness is physical and temporary, and that any hallucinations are really

being experienced by the patient, but will soon disappear

5. An emotionally calm environment.

Drug treatment should be reserved for those who are severely disturbed, or whose sleep pattern is severely disrupted. Thioridazine should be avoided, since it not uncommonly increases disorientation or restlessness. Cautious use of promazine, haloperidol or droperidol, or a short course of a benzodiazepine or chlormethiazole are among the therapeutic possibilities.

Hospital is not the best environment for an elderly delirious patient, and home treatment should always be considered, though the need for investigation and supervision may make admission necessary. As with dementia, no branch of medicine has sole responsibility for the treatment of delirium. Most patients quite rightly go to medical wards. Liaison psychiatric help is often needed for differential diagnosis and for advice on associated behaviour problems.

Dementia

Epidemiology

Henderson (1986) has pointed to considerable difficulties in conducting community surveys of dementia:

1. Defining the population: are residents in care included or not?
2. Allowing for differing age structures of different populations
3. Differential survival in different populations
4. Using a valid diagnostic test: most simple tests measure impairment at the time of interview, only one of the steps in diagnosis; comprehensive tests are laborious to administer
5. Estimating mild dementia: some surveys give estimates for moderate and severe cases only
6. Differentiating between DAT and other dementias.

Jorm et al (1987; Fig. 31.1) suggest from a meta-analysis of the many epidemiological studies of dementia that the prevalence rises exponentially with age, doubling with each successive period of 5.1 years, as shown by the classic Newcastle study (Kay et al 1964) and a more recent Scottish study (Bond 1987). The median age for suffering from dementia is about 82 years.

Because of the anticipated growth in older age bands the number of sufferers will rise. Though absolute numbers are uncertain, the percentage rise in

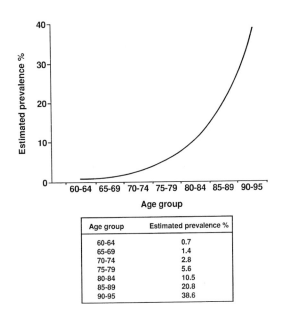

Age group	Estimated prevalence %
60-64	0.7
65-69	1.4
70-74	2.8
75-79	5.6
80-84	10.5
85-89	20.8
90-95	38.6

Fig. 31.1 Prevalence rates of dementia by 5 year age intervals for baseline population, pooled from selected studies (adapted from Jorm et al 1987). The graph can probably be extrapolated to younger age groups, but rates in the over 90s may level out, and almost certainly do not continue to rise exponentially

a particular community can be estimated, using Jorm's formula. In some areas of Britain there will be an increase of nearly 20% in the number of dementia sufferers in the next 10 years. Of course the service *needs* of these extra sufferers and their carers are more important than absolute numbers or percentage increases, but there are few available estimates. The pool of available caring younger people is diminishing because of changes in population structure and social mobility, and because patients' children are increasingly likely to be either working or elderly and frail themselves.

About 70% of elderly dementia sufferers in Britain live in private houses, so the emphasis has always been on community care. About half of those living at home are living with close relatives, who may be coping with a severely disabled or disturbed sufferer. Slightly less than half are on their own and the focus of attention is on the risks of independent living.

Assessment

Identification. O'Connor et al (1988) found that general practitioners knew of roughly 80% of severe dementia sufferers, but they were aware of only 30% of mild sufferers. Regular visits to those aged over 75 years and the use of simple screening instruments such as the MMSE (Iliffe et al 1991b) may improve these figures. It is not yet clear whether early diagnosis helps prevent disability, or helps institute community services which delay admission to costly and unpopular long-stay care. Early diagnosis may bring relatives the help they need to continue caring; or it may 'desensitise' them to outside help, and so speed admission.

Diagnosis of the syndrome. The essential steps in diagnosis are:

1. Demonstrating a global mental impairment compared to that individual's normal performance
2. Showing that this impairment has been gradually progressive over a period of some months
3. Ruling out other causes of a similar clinical picture.

These steps require a clear history, a full mental state examination and at the very least some simple screening investigations. Whilst these are usually carried out if the patient is referred to a psychiatrist, the same cannot be said for all general practitioners and physicians. The commonest mistakes are to rely only on the mental state examination, to use only tests of orientation instead of demonstrating *global* impairment, and to fail to talk to another informant.

In old age neither CT nor MRI are sensitive or specific enough to use for syndrome diagnosis, though combinations of tests increase accuracy to acceptable levels, except in very mild cases (Jacoby & Levy 1980a). In the first few months of dementia a 'wait and see' approach is advisable, asking the patient to return for repeat assessment in 3–6 months.

Differential diagnosis. The differential diagnosis of dementia in an elderly patient includes:

1. Normal old age. A difficult problem for early cases (Henderson & Huppert 1984), and also in people with a lifelong mental impairment, those who are deaf and those with communication problems because of stroke. Attempts to find tests which differentiate very early dementia from normal old age have so far been largely unsuccessful. Bergmann (1977) found that roughly one-third of mild or doubtful cases proved not to have dementia 1 year later and that a further third were still in the doubtful category.

2. Chronic brain damage which is not progressive. This is often quite reasonably called dementia, but the non-progressive nature of the damage following head injury or other insults, and the possibility of some gradual improvement, makes care planning a very different matter in the two conditions, and it is important to differentiate them.

3. Delirium: see above.

4. Korsakov's syndrome. A drinking history is essential in all cases. The restriction of impairment to recent memory, with relative sparing of immediate memory and other intellectual functions should be suggestive.

5. Pseudodementia of depression: see section on affective disorders.

6. Pseudodementia of physical illness. There is some overlap and realistic lack of clarity between this term and the term *reversible dementia*. Is, for example, secondary mental impairment in a hypothyroid patient a true dementia which is reversible or an artefact of the illness? In practice it does not matter, since treatment of the thyroid problems in either case will cure the 'dementia'. Unfortunately, it is commoner for thyroid disorder and dementia to coexist as completely unconnected problems.

Diagnosis of the cause. It is unclear what proportion of the elderly dementing population suffers from each of the many causes of dementia. Clinical and post mortem studies alike are liable to bias, depending on whether they use community or hospital samples and their age structure. Clinical differentiation of DAT from vascular dementia is not reliable, with many apparently mixed cases and even at post mortem there are debates about definitions. It is probable, however, that over 95% of elderly patients suffer from the common forms of dementia — DAT and vascular dementia — and that DAT is commoner, perhaps accounting for 60% of all sufferers.

Roth (1986) and others have noted differences between 'old-old' type 1 and 'young-old' type 2 DAT. Pathological and neurochemical evidence suggests that in older patients damage is more topographically restricted, and more limited to the acetylcholine system. There are less obvious differences between older DAT sufferers and normal people of the same age in their cholinergic systems, in psychological tests, and in their expectation of life (Christie & Train 1984). A concept of *benign senescence* (Kral 1962) has also been proposed, suggesting that very elderly people suffer a much milder form of impairment which is not really dementia. Some have suggested that in young cases there is more parietal lobe damage with a more malignant course (Naguib & Levy 1982), but others disagree (Jorm 1985, O'Carroll et al 1991). It is equally possible to explain the differences between older and younger sufferers using the concept of cerebral reserve. If older people have less reserve then smaller amounts of cerebral damage will emerge earlier and have greater clinical effects.

The prevalence of *multi-infarct dementia* seems to be much less than was previously thought, perhaps representing less than 10% of cases. At the same time other forms of *vascular dementia* have risen in prominence; firstly, *Binswanger's disease* of white matter; latterly, *lacunar dementias*. Furthermore, the borderland between vascular and Alzheimer-type dementia has been complicated by the finding of illnesses related to DAT where the predominant damage is vascular, as in *hereditary haemorrhagic cerebral angiopathy of Dutch type*. Recently, Perry et al (1990) have suggested that *senile dementia of Lewy-body type* may be quite a common cause (up to 15% of elderly cases).

Among rarer causes it is worth noting that *Huntington's chorea* can begin in late life, though dementia is usually less prominent than in younger patients. About 20% of patients with *Parkinson's disease* develop a dementia of subcortical type (Gibb 1989). The relationship of this condition to dementia of Lewy body type without parkinsonism is still not clear. *Syphilis* continues to contribute occasional cases of dementia, usually in a forme fruste of classical general paralysis. Secondary or primary *brain tumours* and non-metastatic effects present more often to neurologists than to psychiatrists. *Metabolic* and other 'medical' causes, often reversible, may be detected by simple screening tests (Table 31.3); but thyroid dysfunction and vitamin B_{12} and folate deficiencies are usually coincidental findings rather than causes of the dementia. *Alcoholic dementia* must always be considered. *Normal pressure hydrocephalus* is worth searching for when early unexplained incontinence, abnormal gait or an atypical pattern of impairment are found. The future contribution of *AIDS dementia* and of *prion-related dementias* is unpredictable, but these diagnoses must be kept in mind.

Estimation of severity. Although there have been many attempts to grade dementia into three or more categories (Hughes et al 1982, Reisberg et al 1982), they have been unsuccessful because of the complexity of the illness. Staging has anyway little practical significance for the sufferer or carers, who are more interested in practical problems. For example, wandering may be severe at mild stages, when the patient is physically fit and partially aware of her situation, and mild at severe stages, when she is frail and unmotivated. Severity is best rated using one of the simpler rating scales. In earlier stages intellectual rating scales are appropriate; later, behaviour rating scales are more useful.

Listing problems. The causes of symptoms in dementia are extremely complicated.

First there are gradual *losses* of function. Some are simple and progressive losses of clearly localised brain functions such as recent memory impairment, agnosias and dyspraxias, the various dysphasias, and, later, more hard neurological signs. Others seem to be due to more generalised damage, such as the impairment of abstract thinking, remote memories, and intelligence.

Secondly there is the *loss of standards*, judgement, conscience, self-control and planning ability commonly found in frontal lobe disorder, and relating to the executive and comparing functions of the brain. Loss of inhibition on cognition, action and feeling can lead to disturbed behaviour, particularly at mild and moderate stages. Similar mechanisms explain loss of control of the bladder and, later, the bowel, emergence of primitive reflexes, some psychotic symptoms and fits.

Third are the *reactions of the patient* to her illness. Insight and emotions decline only gradually and sufferers retain some ability to react into quite late stages, though these reactions become distorted by other impairments and by disinhibition. At early stages depression is reported in 20–40% of cases, anxiety is common, and paranoid reactions and hoarding of possessions may occur. Covering up the embarrassment of the condition and social withdrawal are probably the commonest reactions. As Gilleard has suggested, some sufferers may even sense a frightening disintegration of personality. Later, when insight is lost, the patient may react to what she sees as unnecessary intrusions into her life when she feels entirely competent. Later still she is likely to become more passive and may end her days in a mildly disinhibited euphoria quite out of keeping with the seriousness of her condition.

Fourthly, *family interactions* contribute to the problems of dementia. The family is aware of and remembers all the impairments and disturbances of the patient. They are likely to experience grief for the loss of her mind and personality and be more distressed than she is about her embarrassing behaviour, while simultaneously coping with the burden of her physical and psychological care and arranging services which can feel like an intrusion into family life. Worse still, they are likely to get no thanks from the increasingly withdrawn or egocentric patient. When other relatives and friends desert the patient out of embarrassment, it is no wonder if the now isolated remaining carer is very distressed on occasions, and that the relationship between carer and patient may become disturbed, with effects on the patient's behaviour.

Caring for a dementia sufferer is not usually a role taken on by choice. The research on stress among caring relatives has been well reviewed by Morris et al (1988). The majority of carers are either daughters in middle age or spouses. The burden of caring at home can be enormous. As many as 65% of close carers of day hospital attenders (Gilleard et al 1984a) experience distress at levels equivalent to a psychiatric case. Others, looking perhaps at more willing carers, have found lower levels of distress (Eagles et al 1987).

Whether this strain is tolerable to the carer or not depends somewhat on the patient's symptoms, but more on the nature of the carer's previous relationship with the patient (Gilhooley 1984). Other important factors include the support that the carer feels she receives from her family and others, the services and financial assistance she receives and her methods of coping with stress, some lifelong, some learnt during the experience of caring.

Other factors which may influence the presentation of dementia and which should be assessed are the *environment* in which the patient is living, which can make the difference between a dangerous symptom and a trivial complaint, the *physical health* of the patient and *other disabilities* that she may be suffering from.

Finally, it is important to assess the ability of the patient to understand and make *decisions* on matters such as finances, care and medical treatment.

If all these aspects are covered in discussions with the patient, the caring relatives and others who know her, it is likely that a comprehensive list of problem titles can be prepared (Table 31.5). Estimates of the frequency of individual problems in dementia (e.g. see Burns et al (1990b) on mood disorders, Berrios & Brook (1985) and Burns et al (1990a) on psychotic symptoms) have not been entirely successful since so much depends on which population of sufferers is studied. Of more value are the contributions of Fairburn and colleagues (Morris et al (1989) on eating disorders, Hope et al (1990) on wandering, Ware et al (1990) on aggression) and Stokes (Stokes (1986) on screaming and shouting, Stokes (1987) on aggression) which have looked into the causes of behaviour disturbances, and studies which link problems to the strain they cause (O'Connor et al 1990).

Management

Ideally, treatment should address the cause of the dementia. At present this is a distant hope except in the relatively few cases of reversible dementia. Even in

Table 31.5 A short checklist of potential problems in dementia (Jacques 1988)

Problem	Examples
Memory impairment	Forgets appointments
	Forgets to change clothes, wash, go to toilet
	Forgets to eat, take tablets
	Loses possessions
Disorientation	Time, day or night
	Around house
	Recognising family or other visitors
Needs physical help	Dressing
	Washing, bathing
	Toileting
	Eating
	Housework
	Mobility
Risks in the home	Falls
	Fire from cigarettes, cooker, heating
	Flooding
	Letting strangers in
	Wandering out
Risks outside	Driving, road sense
	Gets lost
Apathy	Little conversation
	Lack of interest
	Poor self-care
Poor communication	Dysphasia
Repetitiveness	Questions or stories
	Actions
Uncontrolled emotion	Distress
	Anger or aggression
	Demands for attention
Uncontrolled behaviour	Restlessness, day or night
	Vulgar table or toilet habits
	Undressing
	Sexual disinhibition
	Shop-lifting
Incontinence	Urine
	Faeces
	Inappropriate excretion
Emotional reactions	Depression
	Anxiety
	Frustration
	Embarrassment or withdrawal
Other reactions	Suspiciousness
	Hoarding
Mistaken beliefs	Still at work
	Parents or spouse still alive
Decision-making	Indecisiveness
	Easily influenced
	Poor judgement
	Refuses help
Burden on family	Disruption of social and family life
	Distress, guilt, rejection
	Family discord

the 'untreatable' cases of DAT and vascular dementia there are signs of hope. In multi-infarct dementia aspirin prophylaxis may prove to be helpful. In vascular dementias with hypertension, maintaining blood pressure in the high normal range may perhaps prevent decline (Meyer et al 1987). For DAT, hopes of a treatment which can boost cholinergic activity remain, though it is likely that such treatments will bring only temporary relief, and eventual therapy will have to address the cause of neuronal damage rather than its effects. Christie & Train's (1984) worry that longer survival times in dementia put a huge burden on services may prove to be prophetic.

In practice, management of most cases of dementia consists of trying to find solutions to the problems on the individual's problem list.

Losses. The sufferer should be encouraged to use her remaining abilities to the full. Where there are gaps in her ability, the task is to fill those gaps so that she is not struggling helplessly. Gap fillers relate to all aspects of daily living, ranging from a phone call to remind her to get up in the morning to full nursing care. The carer's imagination and the experience of other carers are the most helpful guides. Sometimes a modest amount of retraining is possible. A patient who has recently forgotten how to use her cooker may be retrained after the device has been simplified, and so gain a few more months of independence. Patients who are repeatedly distressed by constantly rediscovering the death of their spouse may be helped by repeated but sensitive exposure to the facts of the death.

Disinhibition. Although disinhibited or poorly judged behaviour may have an organic basis, it nevertheless is influenced by environment and circumstances. For this reason encouraging normal behaviour can have dramatic effects on patients who otherwise seem to be uncontrollable. For similar reasons simple behaviour modification techniques, altering the reactions of others rather than trying to alter the patient's behaviour directly, can be effective. The labile aggressive man may be more placid with his wife if she realises that his anger is not intended and so learns to react in an unemotional way. However, relatives or staff often have to act as 'external conscience' for the patient, restraining her in a non-punishing way from unwise actions, like walking into the road or taking her clothes off in public. The fine balance between this reasonable care towards vulnerable brain-damaged people and unreasonable intervention in their lives should be debated in each case.

Traditionally, antipsychotic drugs have been used to control disturbed behaviour in dementia, but there is conflicting evidence about their efficacy (Sunderland & Silver 1988). Sometimes small doses of antipsychotic drugs are both safe and effective, but often, for example in repetitive shouters, such large doses are required to quieten that major side-effects occur. Less toxic tranquillisers such as chlormethiazole have some use. Possible 5-hydroxy-tryptamine mechanisms in repetitive behaviour have led to the use of antidepressants such as trazodone. Carbamazepine is helpful in some cases. The best practice is to avoid drug treatment where other measures or greater tolerance of the behaviour are possible.

Reactions. Patients' emotional reactions to early dementia should not be dismissed as part of the illness, but listened to with empathy. In some early cases, talking directly about the diagnosis will be both possible and reassuring. Later, of course, there is a limit to the usefulness of repeated reassurance of any sort. Sometimes the best response to recurrent distress is to change the subject gently, or engage the patient in other activities. The outraged, insightless patient requires skilful and imaginative handling.

If emotional reactions are severe then drug treatment is appropriate, using therapeutic doses of specific drugs for specific problems such as depression, anxiety or paranoid reactions.

Carers. Support for families is of cardinal importance in the management of dementia. First they need to be clearly informed of the diagnosis. This may bring enormous relief if they are blaming the sufferer for laziness or obstinacy, or themselves for impatience or lack of concern. Then they need to be educated fully about the problems which dementia may bring and the services and benefits which are available using talks and literature (Mace et al 1985, HEC 1986, SHEG 1987). They need moral support, practical advice from others and the feeling that they are not alone in caring. Carers' groups are invaluable, though not for everybody. Stress management techniques may be useful, and counselling may help in coping with grief or with disturbances to family and social life. Most of all, families need regular, planned respite. Finally, when the patient dies the process of grief counselling should not end.

Environment. For patients who live at home it is often necessary to 'treat' the environment. This may mean providing reminders and aids around the house, or reducing risks from gas and electrical appliances. Similar principles apply to the design of homes and wards for dementing residents. Ideally, dementia sufferers should be in an environment which combines homeliness, privacy and individuality with compensation for lost abilities and a reasonable level of stimulation, while allowing freedom to wander under good observation (Norman 1987, Weisman et al 1991).

Physical care. Patients with dementia may forget physical symptoms, be unable to communicate them, or suffer anosagnosia or autotopagnosia. They must be treated in this respect (though not in others) rather like infants. The only outward evidence of illness may be restlessness, a deterioration in mental state or frank delirium. Poor medical care leads to both physical and psychiatric problems.

Decisions. Impairment of comprehension, insight, memory, reasoning, judgement, conscience, motivation, communication make it inevitable that dementing patients are less able to make either day-to-day or major decisions from early in the illness. At first the sufferer will be entirely competent, but gradually her competence to make some decisions or judgements will be more and more doubtful, until she becomes legally incapable.

In Britain the law on incapacity separates financial issues from issues of care and treatment. Most of the common and statute law regarding control of finances, testamentary capacity, guardianship and admission under the Mental Health Act, and consent to treatment was not developed with dementia sufferers in mind. The result is that it is both unwieldy and sometimes quite inappropriate. Law reform is urgently needed (Age Concern 1986, SAD 1988).

In all areas of decision-making the choice for a dementia sufferer is:

- She takes her own decisions
- She arranges to hand them over to others because she feels unable to handle them herself
- Decisions are taken over from her through a legal process, because she is not only unable to manage them herself, but is also unable to direct other people to manage for her.

In addition she may be more or less suggestible as a result of her illness, and the motives of families and financial advisers may not always be entirely altruistic. Her ability to communicate her views will be impaired to some extent. It is nearly impossible to define exactly when the patient becomes unable to understand enough to decide for herself. And it is perfectly possible to be competent in one area, such as whether to accept a home help, and not another, such as whether to sell one's house.

Patient's views are an amalgam of previously held views ('substitute judgement'), presently expressed views and passive 'behavioural consent'. Many cannot express their views even if they hold them or become too apathetic or suggestible. In such a circumstance the views of relatives may be taken as more important. Relatives have no legal right to take decisions for incapable patients, although doctors and others sometimes give them such rights. They are protected by the common law if their actions are in the best interest of the patient. The powers of a mental health guardian, the responsible medical officer, the Court of Protection or a curator bonis are limited by law. So there are decisions which theoretically only the patient herself can ever take but which she may become unable to take.

One example of this is medical treatment. The Mental Health Act does not cover medical treatment unless it can be causally linked to the mental illness. Doctors who prescribe treatment and nurses and others who administer it do so 'in good faith', in accordance with professional expectations, and with the protection of the common law which would consider it neglectful if the treatment is necessary and not given. This is all very well in life-saving treatment in early dementia and where everybody is agreed. If there are disagreements or uncertainties about the importance of the treatment the patient's voice may be missing from the discussion, and a strong relative or a strong doctor can override other views.

Terminal care of dementia sufferers is a particularly sensitive subject. At this stage the patient cannot contribute to discussions about how far investigation or treatment should proceed. Normal practice is to consider any previously expressed wishes of the patient, to consult with relatives and staff caring for her, but to make the decision to treat or not on the basis of her present quality of life, expectation of recovery and level of distress. 'Living wills', by which a person declares that they do not wish to be actively treated under certain conditions, are not binding in Britain, but should be taken into consideration. Active euthanasia for dementing people is difficult even to conceive of, since the patient's request would, to be valid, necessarily have been made before the dementia began, and it is almost impossible for an individual to predict what their own experience of dementia would be. Consent by relatives could hardly be valid, and the suspicion might be that relatives and staff were motivated by impatience at caring, when a more appropriate response would be to try to improve the lot of the vulnerable sufferer.

Research is another controversial and difficult area (Brooke 1988). Here there is rarely the protection of necessity. Even in therapeutic research, it is hard to argue that the patient will necessarily be better off as a result, and the argument that fellow patients may benefit later is difficult to explain. The discussions, explanations and consents which ethics committees rightly demand in all research on patients will be impracticable beyond the early stages. Some have got round this problem by concentrating their efforts on the earliest stages of the illness. The subject deserves wide debate both by psychiatrists and lawyers.

Advocacy. In response to some of the deficiencies of the law and to the risk that vulnerable dementing patients may be exploited, or neglected, or not have their views represented, the concept of advocacy has been introduced. Family and professionals of course act as advocates in many cases but, where the patient is isolated or at particular risk, there is virtue in having someone whose sole function is to represent her in seeking help or benefits, in discussions about decisions, or in commenting on standards of care. The appointment of a lay advocate, perhaps through the Alzheimer Society, may be appropriate. Law reformers need to address the peculiar needs of insightless patients who desperately need advocacy but would reject it if offered.

Conference. In the absence of an adequate legal framework or developed advocacy the best practice, when there is debate about a dementing patient's competence and if she may be at risk in any way, is to hold a case conference involving all concerned. This helps avoid compulsory measures in most cases, whilst encouraging creative thinking about ways of reducing risks or helping her come to rational decisions. Case conferences must never, however, be used to bully vulnerable patients or reluctant carers.

Psychosis

'Old' psychosis — the 'graduate' population

The advent of antipsychotic drugs in the 1950s led to a progressive decrease in the long-stay schizophrenic population of psychiatric hospitals, the so-called 'graduates'. Elderly chronic schizophrenic patients are now more likely to be found in the community, often living alone or in hostel accommodation which cannot offer the physical or psychiatric nursing care which they need. The result has been a slow increase in referrals from this group, often physically frail and living in poor conditions.

'New' psychosis — late life schizophrenia (late paraphrenia) and related disorders

Kraepelin (1919) used the term paraphrenia to describe an illness with delusions and hallucinations but without schizophrenic changes in affect, form of thought and personality. Roth & Morrissey (1952) noted that illnesses of this description were the commonest form of psychosis in old age and called this 'late paraphrenia'. Since that time there has been considerable debate as to whether late paraphrenia is or is not schizophrenia of late onset ('senile schizophrenia' of Fish (1960)).

Old age psychotic disorder is not common. Only 10% of hospital admissions are for psychosis, and population studies, if they locate any cases at all, have shown prevalence rates of less than 1% (Eastwood & Corbin 1985). The peak incidence of schizophrenia in males is between the ages of 15 and 30 years, and male hospital admission rates fall through old age, but for women a later peak has been found and admission rates rise in the eighth and ninth decades. If the figures for late life psychosis are added to those from younger people the lifetime risk is roughly equal between the sexes, but with more of the risk for females occurring in late life.

Aetiology. Some aetiological factors support the link with schizophrenia but others suggest specific environmental factors:

1. Sex. In Kay & Roth's series (1961) the sex ratio for old age schizophrenia was 9:1 for females to males, though others have found it as low as 4:1. Even allowing for the preponderance of elderly women in the community this is a very striking sex difference. Perhaps susceptible women are protected from psychosis in earlier life and need particular environmental stresses for it to emerge later.

2. Genetics. The risk of schizophrenia and paraphrenia in first-degree relatives of late paraphrenics is about half that found in first-degree relatives of younger schizophrenics. Naguib et al (1987) found a relationship between certain HLA types, deafness and old age schizophrenia.

3. Personality. Kay & Roth (1961) found that 45% had lifelong paranoid or schizoid personality traits, and that this factor was independent of genetic and sensory causes.

4. Sensory deprivation. Deafness has been shown to be associated with old age schizophrenia in between 25 and 40% of cases (Post 1966, Kay & Roth 1961, Cooper 1976). Visual impairment is less commonly relevant.

5. Social isolation. All studies have found that the great majority of these patients are socially isolated. They are often unmarried, divorced or separated, or they married late and had few children. Their personality may have also led to isolation, and deafness increases this tendency.

6. Life events. Some studies have shown a preponderance of life events preceding old age schizophrenia. However, in many cases the isolation and suspiciousness of the sufferer delay referral so that events before onset are unclear or modified by paranoid misinterpretation.

7. Organic factors. Naguib & Levy (1987) showed that some patients with old age schizophrenia have CT evidence of organic brain changes. However, these changes do not appear to relate directly to the cognitive impairment which some patients exhibit, or to outcome (Hymas et al 1989), so their significance is unknown.

Clinical features. The onset is usually insidious, and in the past some cases of late-onset delusional disorder have been thought of as personality developments in schizoid or suspicious individuals rather than true psychosis. Resistance to help because of lack of insight may prevent diagnosis for years after the first psychotic experiences.

Paranoid symptoms may include any combination of persecutory, grandiose, erotic and jealous ideas or delusions. Hallucinations are most commonly auditory, but olfactory hallucinations, somatic hallucinations of electricity or rape and visual hallucinations, usually of flashes, also occur. In some patients, perhaps 10–20%, only delusions are present, as in Kraepelin's *paranoia* (1919), or *persistent delusional disorder* (see Ch. 20), though some of these may have had organic brain lesions (Flint et al 1991). Typical first-rank symptoms are found in about 30% of cases. These may include experiences of intrusion into the thoughts or body of the sufferer. Complaints of intrusions into her personal space in the sense of house or property are much more typical. An important consequence of this is that when the patient is admitted to hospital or moves house to escape from her persecutors, the symptoms may temporarily disappear (Post 1966). This can give the impression that the symptoms were exaggerated at home, or that the patient is now cured. However, a return visit home, or time to settle into a new personal space of hospital or a new house brings a resurgence of symptoms. Typical negative symptoms are uncommon, and indeed patients often preserve strong paranoid personality traits, making management difficult.

Evidence of cognitive impairment is found in a small proportion of patients, though estimates vary widely, depending largely on exclusion factors in individual studies. Many patients are proud of their continuing mental alertness and see this as protection against their persecutors. Possibly no more than expected develop dementia in the long run. If dementia does develop, the psychotic symptoms may 'dissolve' and antipsychotic treatment is no longer needed.

Depression secondary to the persecutions is not uncommon, and causes difficulties in differentiating old age schizophrenia from affective or schizoaffective disorders. The more usual reaction is of outrage and anger. The patient retaliates against her persecutors, who are likely to be unsuspecting neighbours. Calling in the police or a solicitor is as likely as calling in the doctor, and lack of insight usually leads the patient to suggest that the neighbours rather than her need treatment.

Treatment. Antipsychotic drugs are effective in old age schizophrenia and delusional disorder (Post 1966, Hymas et al 1989), and long-term treatment is necessary. Christie (1982) has shown the quite dramatic effect on the need for hospital long-stay care by comparing 1970s figures with Roth's figures from the 1940s (Roth 1955). Compliance is a problem and the psychiatrist may have to resort to indirect means to persuade the patient to take drugs. Some patients have a trusted 'ally' who can persuade; a CPN who gradually gets to know her can become such an ally; suggestions that the drug will help her 'cope with the persecution better' or 'will put the problem into the background' may help; few patients have enough insight to feel that treatment is fully justified. Compliance is not helped by the tendency of antipsychotic drugs to produce more side-effects the older the patient. Oral drugs which are relatively free of the common side-effects of antipsychotics, such as sulpiride and pimozide, are more likely to be acceptable. Depot treatment is tolerated by some patients, is easier to monitor over a long period but occasionally leads to intractable side-effects. Relieving isolation and deafness have been proposed as possible treatments. There is as yet no firm evidence that these measures help in the long term even if they do in the short term.

Other conditions with paranoid or hallucinatory symptoms

The differential diagnosis of paranoid symptoms and of hallucinations in old age is complicated and there is considerable overlap between some of the conditions.

Secondary paranoid states. A variety of organic cerebral conditions and treatment with steroids, antiparkinsonian or other drugs can sometimes produce psychotic phenomena without obvious mental impairment. History, and investigation of the patient's physical state, are important in all cases of paranoid psychosis.

Delirium. The psychotic symptoms of delirium may be mistaken for symptoms of a primary paranoid psychosis. The acute time-course, relation to physical illness, evidence of cognitive impairment, and characteristic symptoms of delirium (Table 31.4) should help to distinguish between the disorders. In delirium, visual hallucinations are commoner than auditory hallucinations, whilst the reverse is the case in schizophrenia.

Dementia. Paranoid and other psychotic symptoms are common in dementia (Berrios & Brook 1985). Paranoid ideas may be a reaction to memory impairment in a sensitive individual, or may relate to the basic disease process. Agnosias, receptive dysphasia, impairment of comprehension and other related disorders may explain misinterpretations which lead on to more fixed paranoid beliefs (Flint et al 1991). Visual hallucinations have traditionally been ascribed to delirium occurring in the course of multi-infarct dementia, but Perry (1990) has linked them instead to a diagnosis of Lewy body dementia.

Paranoid ideas and hallucinatory experiences in dementia are usually relatively transient and ill formed. They respond, though often incompletely, to antipsychotic medication. If small doses are not effective it is unlikely that a large dose will work.

Affective disorders. Psychotic symptoms are common in both severe depressive illness and in hypomania in old age. The admixture of symptoms helps to differentiate, as does the affective colouring of the experiences. A curious phenomenon is the persistence of psychotic symptoms between episodes in some patients with a long history of recurrent affective disorder.

Schizoaffective disorder. Post (1971) described a number of cases who did not fit into either the description of psychotic illness or affective illness, but who were intermediate in clinical features, aetiology and outcome.

Hallucinations of sensory deprivation. Berrios & Brook (1984) suggested that visual hallucinations without marked paranoid ideas might be a non-specific phenomenon in elderly patients, linked to visual impairment rather than to any particular diagnosis. The 'visions' are of people, animals or scenes and the patient has a degree of or even complete insight. If there is no other associated psychiatric disorder then the term *Charles–Bonnet syndrome* is appropriate (Damas-Mora et al 1982). Small doses of antipsychotic drugs can be helpful, but

some patients can use reassurance to help them pay less attention to the hallucinations.

The same is true of what is probably the auditory equivalent of this phenomenon, *musical hallucinations* (Berrios 1990) in those with a hearing impairment.

Affective disorders

Epidemiology

Longitudinal studies of the natural history of affective disorder show a general trend for episodes to occur more frequently and to last longer (Zis & Goodwin 1970, Cutter & Post 1982). The incidence of new cases of major affective disorder is at its peak in young adulthood, and probably declines steadily through the rest of life. Possibly less than 10% of new cases emerge in old age, and few of them are bipolar cases. Angst (1973) described a worse prognosis in later-onset cases, but Winokur (1975) found no difference from early onset cases.

A review of several community studies suggested a rate of between 1 and 2.5% for severe or psychotic depression (Eastwood & Corbin 1985) though some (Copeland et al 1987b, Lindesay et al 1989) give rates of 4–5%. Female rates are always higher than male rates, but may fall somewhat in later age groups. On the other hand, less severe depressions are common. Figures of 10–15% are regularly found, though of course the difficulties of defining mild disorders are notorious. Figures for all degrees of depression reach 22–33%.

Aetiology

Genetic factors are much less important causally in affective disorder beginning in late life (Mendlewicz et al 1972), whilst physical illness is significant in between 60 and 75% of cases. In a community study of major depression Murphy (1982) showed the importance of life events, physical illness and lack of a confiding relationship. The relevance of cerebral pathology in late life to the aetiology of major depression is controversial. It is unlikely to be very important since the prevalence of the condition does not rise with increasing age. The many losses to which elderly people are susceptible explain the relatively high prevalence of milder depressions, though sufferers may hesitate to complain because such losses are expected (Parkes 1964).

Shulman & Post (1980), Stone (1989) and Broadhead & Jacoby (1990) have emphasised that new cases of mania are often related, perhaps causally, to brain disease, at least in men. And a link between onset of depressive illness in elderly men and a later diagnosis of abdominal cancer has been postulated, though not all are agreed.

Clinical features

Since the concept of involutional melancholia was abandoned it has been clear that there are few significant differences between early and late-onset depressions. There are cohort period and age differences in, for example, the prevalence of religious delusions, and in the content of hypochondriacal ideas, including the very common fear of dementia.

Atypical presentations of depressive disorder are relatively common. The most debated is *pseudodementia*, or cognitive change in depression. Measurable cognitive impairment is often found during late life depressions, but usually returns to normal after treatment. Jacoby & Levy (1980b) among others have shown brain scan abnormalities in some elderly depressives, and some have shown relationships between these changes and apparent cognitive impairment. But the nature and significance of the changes are disputed, and it is not proven that they have any effect on treatment or prognosis. One possible explanation of pseudodementia is that it represents a crossing of the threshold of dementia in a persons whose cerebral reserve is already compromised. If this were true then depressive illness with pseudodementia would predict the later development of dementia as Kral (1983) has suggested. The following list of clinical features (adapted from Wells 1979) distinguishing pseudodementia from dementia is helpful:

- Past history of depressive illness
- Depressed mood
- Diurnal variation in mood
- Other biological symptoms
- Islands of normality
- Exaggerated presentation of symptoms.

Agitation is much commoner in older depressives, as are *paranoid symptoms*. Hypochondriacal symptoms and other abnormal illness behaviour, pseudo-personality disorder, and *mixed affective disorder* are also quite common.

Hypomania usually occurs in people with a past history of bipolar affective disorder, though there is some evidence that male admission rates rise with age (Eagles & Whalley, 1985). Its first onset in old age should raise the suspicion of a physical illness or cerebral pathology. It is particularly rare to have true mania in old age, and the mental overactivity and elation of hypomania is not always matched by outward signs of overactivity. Indeed, the prevailing affect may be irritability. Delirium is an important and sometimes difficult differential diagnosis, since it can present with some of the features of hypomania, whilst more severe cases of hypomania tend to develop a pseudo- or real delirium.

Treatment

Drug treatment. Age is not in itself a contraindication to any antidepressant, and some patients, particularly those with a long past history, can tolerate large doses of standard tricyclic drugs. However, the likelihood of anticholinergic and cardiovascular side-effects rises with age, and for many the classic drugs are unacceptable. Other tricyclics which may have fewer side-effects are still popular; these include doxepin, dothiepin and lofepramine. Careful supervision is essential when starting these drugs and adjusting doses, with daily lying and standing blood pressure measurement if possible and education of the patient and her family about potential side-effects. Access to blood level monitoring may be helpful, but does not always predict side-effects or efficacy. Newer less toxic drugs are becoming more widely used, including trazodone, fluvoxamine and fluoxetine. Some clinicians use monoamine oxidase inhibitors as second line drugs with good effect, even in major depression, though delayed postural hypotension may be a problem with these otherwise relatively safe drugs. With all antidepressants small starting doses, gradual increases, and prolonged trial periods of up to 2 months are required. Lithium augmentation (Finch & Catona 1989) and other combination treatments are worth trying in intractable cases.

Lithium. Clearance of lithium declines steadily in later life. Equivalent doses lead to higher blood levels and relatively low blood levels can lead to toxic effects. For these reasons lithium must be administered with considerable care, and in lower doses than for younger patients. Blood levels of 0.4–0.7 mmol/l may be effective (Foster et al 1977). Regular thyroid and renal function checks are most important in this age group, and the lithium level should be retested if there is any intercurrent infection, or change in drug treatment, especially diuretics.

Electroconvulsive therapy (ECT). Problems with antidepressant drugs have persuaded many clinicians that ECT has an important part to play in the treatment of late life depression, as a first-line treatment in severe illness, and where drugs are contraindicated, fail or have undesirable side-effects. Benbow (1989) reviewed the literature and concluded that it is a safe and effective treatment for major depressions in old age with a good response in 70–80% of cases. Unfortunately, the failure of a course of ECT to provide prophylaxis leaves a problem, and some clinicians consider maintenance ECT in chronic cases. Benbow also concluded that, provided there is no evidence of a space-occupying lesion, dementia is not a contraindication to ECT if coexisting depression warrants its use.

Prognosis

There has been considerable controversy about the prognosis of depressive illness in elderly people. Post's classical study in 1962 suggested that with treatment most patients had a good outcome, though only 26% showed full recovery at follow-up and 12% were continually ill. Murphy (1983) was pessimistic, finding 35% well but 29% continually ill and 14% dead at 1 year follow-up of a mixed hospital and community group. Psychotic patients did particularly badly. Baldwin & Jolley (1986), however, found a much better prognosis, with 60% well and only 18% continually ill. Perhaps the samples from these and other studies come from rather different populations, but it is also possible that those who obtained better outcomes may have used more active treatments, particularly for severe cases. Murphy and others have found that poor physical health and adverse life events contribute to poor outcome.

Differential diagnosis

Dementia. As well as the problem of pseudodementia, there are often difficulties in distinguishing the social withdrawal, lack of self-care and apathy of early dementia from depression. Depression during dementia causes particular difficulties. If there is doubt a trial of antidepressants is advisable.

Other organic depressive disorder. The diagnosis of affective disturbance after a *stroke* is difficult, most of all in patients with communication problem. Robinson et al (1984) linked lesions in the left frontal cortex to depressive symptoms, but depression may also be due to emotional lability, reactive distress, organic apathy or lack of motivation and side-effects of drugs (House et al 1991). Lability is particularly common and may respond to

antidepressants such as fluoxetine or small doses of antipsychotic drugs.

Differentiating depression and mild *parkinsonism* is sometimes difficult as retardation and a downcast expression occur in both conditions. Poor communication may impede examination. The picture is confused further because the side-effects of antiparkinsonian drugs include delirium, hallucinations, depression, elation and sexual disinhibition, paranoid states and even obsessional symptoms.

Depression is a feature of other physical illnesses common in old age such as infections, hypothyroidism and tumours and it is a side-effect of many drugs used in elderly patients. Every new case of depression requires a full medical history, physical examination and screening investigations.

Suicide and parasuicide

Suicide

In Britain, 20–30% of all suicides are elderly people, despite the fact that only 15% of the population is over 65 years in age. The rate declined in the 1960s due to detoxification of the gas supply and has remained fairly steady since (Shulman 1978, Lindesay 1991). Rates for men are roughly twice those for women, and continue to increase with advancing age, whilst the female rate may gradually fall. The main factors which predict late life suicide include not only age and male sex, but physical illness (estimates range from 35 to 85% of cases), social isolation, widowed or separated status, alcohol abuse and, most especially, depressive illness and a past history of depression (Barraclough's (1971) series included 80% who had depressive illness). Barraclough emphasised that around 80% of suicides had contacted their general practitioner in the 3 months before death, and de Alarcon (1964) stressed the particular relevance of hypochondriacal ideas.

Parasuicide

In contrast, parasuicide is relatively uncommon in older age groups, contributing only about 5% to the total (Kreitman 1976, Hawton & Fagg 1990). The male-to-female ratio is much more even than in younger people. Elderly parasuicides are more likely to represent failed suicide rather than being gestures of distress, or manifestations of relationship difficulties or personality problems. Pierce (1987) found that 90% of attempters had depressive illness (though not necessarily severe), and 50% were admitted to a psychiatric hospital. Over 60% were physically ill. Kreitman found that 8% of parasuicides (and 20 times the expected rate in men) went on to complete suicide within 3 years of the attempt. All suicidal behaviour in the elderly should be taken seriously, and depressive illness should be suspected. Of course, there are also some personality-disordered people who have habitually harmed themselves over many years and continue to do so.

Neurosis

Prevalence

Epidemiological studies of neurosis are beset with methodological difficulties. Arguments about definition of syndromes, the issue of 'caseness', the boundary between personality and neurotic disorders, and the correct classification of 'depressive neurosis' are but some of the pitfalls. Kessell & Shepherd (1962) showed that whilst there was no great decline in community prevalence in neurosis in older people, and general practitioner attendances for neurotic disorders fell little, there was a marked fall in referrals to psychiatrists. Elderly people with neurotic disorders probably accept their complaints more readily, and general practitioners may be reluctant to refer on, perhaps considering such disorder to be 'just old age'. Estimates of prevalence range between 1 and 10% (Eastwood & Corbin 1985). Copeland et al (1987a) found rates of clinical neurosis of 4% but 'subcases' amounted to a further 16%. Male prevalence rates are always lower but may hold with increasing old age, whilst female rates seem to fall somewhat in the 'old-old'. Most studies find 'old' and 'new' cases to be roughly equal in frequency.

Clinical features

Bergmann (1978) examined a group of subjects with late-onset neurosis and found that most had symptoms of anxiety or depression. Anxiety symptoms may be generalised or may present as panic attacks or phobias. A particular phobia, uncommon in younger people but relatively common in the elderly, has been named *space phobia* by Marks (1981). Agoraphobics experience anxiety in crowded places, whilst space phobics become anxious in open spaces where they have no supports to hold on to. They usually have few background neurotic traits, and have had some physical illness or accident which has led them to fear falling or lack confidence in their mobility. They often become housebound. They respond relatively poorly to both physiotherapy and behaviour therapy.

Aetiology

By factor analysis of background variables Bergmann showed that physical illness, a feeling of loneliness (as distinct from actual isolation), impaired self-care and 'anxiety-prone' or 'rigid, insecure' personality traits contributed to the development of new cases of neurosis in old age.

Differential diagnosis

Obsessional disorders, eating disorders, hypochondriasis or abnormal illness behaviour rarely emerge for the first time in late life. New symptoms suggestive of any of these disorders should make the clinician think first of other diagnoses, using a hierarchical approach.

Physical illness. Patients who feel ill but cannot identify clear symptoms may present pseudoneurotic symptoms, or present their symptoms in an exaggerated fashion. An apparent eating disorder is much more likely to be caused by serious physical illness than by a late-onset neurosis. Kay and Bergmann (1966) found that one of the best predictors of mortality in elderly psychiatrically ill patients was a physical complaint.

Acute or chronic brain disease. Disinhibitory mechanisms can lead to the emergence or magnification of neurotic personality traits or symptoms.

Affective disorder. Depressive illness, hypomania or a mixed affective disorder can present in old age with pseudoneurotic symptoms. In particular, the complaint of hypochondriasis, which does rarely begin as a neurotic disorder in later life, is much more likely to be caused by a depressive illness.

Treatment

Given the likely causal factors in late life neurosis, treatment should aim at resolving, or helping the patient come to terms with, problem issues such as physical ill health or loneliness. Unfortunately, older people's tendency to dislike change can make even simple counselling or brief problem-solving psychotherapy hard work. Anxiolytic drugs should in general be avoided, though in severe or intractable cases sedative antidepressants are helpful, especially where there is evidence of a marked change from the person's normal self.

Alcohol problems

Prevalence

There are more elderly abstainers, and those who do drink take on average less than younger people (Dight 1976, Saunders et al 1989, Iliffe et al 1991). The present elderly cohort may simply be continuing lifelong habits, but many elderly people also cut down their alcohol intake. As an individual ages, tolerance to alcohol is likely to decrease, because of reduction in important liver enzymes and changes in the response of the brain to alcohol. The same dose of alcohol produces higher blood levels, more intoxication and more adverse effects. Financial considerations also play a part; elderly people are often relatively poorer than they were when of working age. Furthermore, at present there are social pressures against drink among many but not all elderly groups, and many social activities for older people are not associated with drinking as they would be for younger people.

As might be expected the prevalence of heavy drinking is lower than in younger people (Saunders et al 1989). Defining the numbers who have alcohol problems is difficult, for there is probably considerable under-reporting. Often the relevant questions are simply not asked, in the mistaken belief that older people, and especially older women, rarely drink. In fact, although the female rate of problem drinking remains significantly below the male rate (Edwards et al 1973), it rises in old age, and the highest prevalence among women is in the 80s. Recent changes in the drinking habits of younger women will change this pattern in the future.

New and old cases of alcohol abuse tend to show some differences (Rosin & Glatt 1971). 'New' cases are more neurotic in type, with less evidence of a background personality disorder. Precipitating life events (including sudden access to excess time and money at retirement) and physical ill health are more common. Alcohol abuse may also be a symptom of or a reaction to psychiatric illness. The elderly depressive or the mild dementia sufferer may begin drinking heavily for the first time in their lives, and here cause and effect can be difficult to disentangle. Alcohol-related dementia remains a controversial subject, but in all cases of dementia enquiry about past alcohol consumption is essential. Korsakov's syndrome is, of course, a common finding in 'old' cases.

Treatment

The link between practical problems and recent onset allows greater optimism about treatment, which can focus on the person's circumstances and social milieu. Treatment is assisted by the availability of non-drinking social activities, by the absence of social stigma about abstinence and by a greater tendency among families to control an elderly person's finances in order to control her drinking. Effects of alcohol on the elderly person's physical state and mobility further encourage abstinence.

People who have abused alcohol over many years may also cut down their intake. But it is also quite common for their drinking to continue along the pattern of earlier years, and the associated physical or psychiatric problems continue or intensify. Those in lodgings or a hostel are particularly at risk.

Drug abuse

Drug abuse is not a major problem among elderly people except in relation to prescribed drugs such as benzodiazepines, opiates and other analgesics, occasionally barbiturates and other 'older' drugs, and less obvious drugs of abuse, particularly laxatives.

It is sometimes felt that withdrawal of drugs of dependence from an elderly person is cruel, since they have 'not long to go'. However, the subtle personality and cognitive changes, which can lead to mistaken diagnoses of personality disorder, depression, dementia or a physical illness, are such that abstinence may greatly improve a person's quality of life. The greatest arguments arise over hypnotics in patients who show no obvious adverse effects, but are clearly psychologically dependent.

Sexual problems

It is commonly believed that older people, especially older women, have little sexual interest and limited sexual ability. Many couples continue to have active sex lives and sexual interest continues into advanced old age in most people, though social pressures and lack of opportunity inhibit many. Physiological changes can make intercourse more difficult, especially for women, and slower responses may work for or against a particular couple. Illness and drugs sometimes interfere with sexual activity, and, even though these may be temporary problems for one or other partner, reinstituting sexual relations after a break can be a major problem.

Some dementia sufferers begin to make sexual demands on their partners after years of lack of interest, or show disinhibited sexual interest in other adults or children. Indiscriminate sexual behaviour by a resident in a care home or ward can cause considerable distress among staff and relatives.

Doctors and others may have to overcome a 'counter-transference' difficulty in addressing sexual problems in people who could be their parents or grandparents. This may interfere with questioning and therapy, especially where subjects such as extramarital relationships, cross-generation relationships or homosexuality are concerned.

PERSONALITY

Normal changes of old age

In the past, social gerontology has been divided between those who believed that it was normal for older people to *disengage* from social life and activities, and become more introspective, a process sometimes seen as a preparation for death, and those who stressed the benefits of continued *engagement* in physical and mental activity. Both theories have been replaced by an emphasis on *continuity*, that is, that ageing individuals usually retain the attitudes, interests and styles of relating which make up their personality. However, whether for biological, psychological or social reasons, it is commonly found that cautiousness, introversion and obsessionality do tend to increase with age, but there is great interpersonal variation. Those who had these characteristics as lifelong traits may adjust to old age relatively easily.

People who had disordered personalities in younger years rarely come to psychiatric attention, except as residents in homes and hostels, where their egocentricity, impulsiveness or lack of concern for the consequences of their actions make them less than ideal residents. 'Mellowing' is said to occur in some psychopaths in later life. Those with lesser degrees of personality disorder are only likely to see psychiatrists if they suffer another psychiatric disorder or in response to adverse life events.

During the decades of old age many planned or unplanned changes occur in family and other relationships, social circumstances and housing. It is unlikely that all will be entirely consonant with the individual's personality characteristics. At a time when change is becoming more difficult to cope with major problems can arise. The independent-minded individual who develops parkinsonism or a stroke where outside help becomes essential may be a very 'bad' patient, resenting the dependent position, reacting violently against any hints of infantilisation and so responding poorly to attempts at rehabilitation. They present to the liaison psychiatrist as depressed, but the depression hides an underlying resentment of their predicament.

Personality disorder and illness

Some elderly people present with an exaggeration of previous personality traits, even to the point of caricature. It is frequently assumed that this is a part of the normal ageing process, but it may be a manifestation of frontal lobe or other brain damage, early dementia without obvious global impairment, depressive illness, hypomania or paranoid psychosis. Personality disorder is lifelong by definition, and therefore *personality change* or *exaggeration* in old age demands an explanation. A careful history is essential, concentrating particularly on lifelong traits of personality, the time sequence of changes, their relationship to important life events and other possible symptoms of illness.

'Senile squalor'

Clark et al (1975) and Macmillan & Shaw (1966) described elderly people who seemed to become by choice reclusive and eccentric in old age, and could end up living in squalor. Many seemed oblivious of the conditions they were living in and were very resistant to help. Many of Clark's group were physically ill and half died after admission to hospital. In Macmillan & Shaw's group there was a preponderance of psychiatrically ill people. A variety of names have been used to describe these patients, such as senile squalor syndrome and Diogenes syndrome. A related, probably obsessive problem of compulsive collecting, which can also lead to squalor, is called *syllogomania*. It is likely that elderly people may live in squalor for very varied reasons, including unrecognised physical illness, early dementia, other psychiatric illness and lifelong eccentricity of personality. Old age is not in itself a cause of eccentricity. There is no need to define a syndrome of squalor, but squalor as a symptom merits further investigation.

THE ELDERLY WITH MENTAL RETARDATION

A growing number of people with mental retardation are entering old age. Some of these will suffer dementia, especially those with Down's syndrome, and some will have other psychiatric conditions. The expansion of community care for mental retardation means that most will be living at home or in supported accommodation. The difficult decisions about who should take responsibility for this small but important group need further debate.

LEGAL CONSIDERATIONS

The elderly mentally disordered offender

Police and the courts can be unreasonably lenient to elderly law breakers, due either to an ageist belief that the elderly are inevitably less responsible for their actions or to a protective paternalism. Courts may feel that harrowing trials are not appropriate for relatively frail elderly people. And an elderly person fits uncomfortably into a prison system geared to managing young offenders. This set of attitudes can act against elderly people. It removes their right to answer accusations made against them, and may brand them as sick or incapable when they are in fact perfectly well and responsible for their actions. It also leaves the victims of crime with no redress.

Crime is less common among the elderly than among younger groups, and it is important to emphasise the possible links between crime and psychiatric illness. Elderly people who have traffic accidents, shop-lift, are violent or make disinhibited sexual advances to others require careful assessment for early dementia and other disorders, though unfortunately they may not be referred for reports. The same is true of the elderly who are putting themselves at risk without necessarily committing any crime. Incautious drivers, wanderers, people who make repeated complaints about their neighbours can all come to the attention of police, but no further action is taken.

The same attitude can infect the legal system when the elderly person is the victim of crime. This can relate to violence in the home, bogus workmen or accusations of stealing by home helps. The older person's evidence is taken as less valid than that of a younger person, and investigations are not pursued as vigorously as they might be.

Abuse of and by elderly people

Elderly victims of abuse by family or other carers are the subject of increasing concern (Eastman 1984). Carers' groups often discuss angry and violent feelings when the group has become cohesive. Figures are difficult to interpret, because definitions of abuse vary greatly, and under-reporting is likely. At its broadest, abuse can include irritability and verbal abuse, physical neglect, financial exploitation, sexual abuse as well as direct physical assault. Objective evidence of physical abuse is difficult to assess in elderly people prone to falls, or those who bruise easily. The problem of whom to believe is particularly thorny when the possible victim is dementing. Vulnerable elderly people can also be victims of abuse by those whose job it is to care for them. Financial exploitation by solicitors, neglectful treatment by doctors, undue restraint in institutions, physical aggression and sexual abuse by nursing or other care staff all need considerably more attention than they get at present.

Psychiatrically ill elderly people may also become verbally abusive, or physically or sexually aggressive towards their informal and formal carers. In close relationships carers may find it difficult to discuss such problems openly. Once again, carers' groups are helpful.

Prevention is the best approach to problems of abuse. Better training and support of staff and informal carers is vitally important. The value of regular visits by relatives, senior nursing staff, medical staff and students to long-stay wards should not be underestimated. Openness in discussing the mixed feelings that caring for elderly people induces should be encouraged. Respite from caring is most important of all.

THE FUTURE

Only effective treatments or preventative measures will be able to slow the increase in prevalence of the common forms of dementia which is expected over the next three decades. Even massive programmes of hospital or nursing home building will not cope with this increase. The majority of sufferers will live in their own homes, without much informal support. The public probably has little enthusiasm for community care of dementia sufferers (Wells et al 1984), which has yet to prove its effectiveness. Nevertheless, that is what the future holds for hundreds of thousands of patients. Research must concentrate on finding simple, valid and reliable procedures for early detection and diagnosis of dementia, assessment of these patients' needs and evaluation of community care programmes.

The prevalence of other psychiatric disorders will not rise significantly with demographic changes. But changes in the attitudes of future cohorts of older people are likely to bring minor psychiatric disturbances more to psychiatric attention. Future generations of elderly people may also be less passive, more educated in the facts of ageing, and more aware of their rights. They may expect that effective help, including good-quality institutional care, will be available, and will wish to participate in decisions about their care. Old age psychiatry will be a more varied but even more challenging field of work than it is at present.

REFERENCES

Age Concern 1986 The law and vulnerable elderly people. Age Concern, Mitcham.

Angst J 1973 Classification and predicion of outcome of depression. Schatlauer Verlag, Stuttgart

Arie T, Dunn T 1973 A 'do-it-yourself' psychiatric-geriatric joint patient unit. Lancet ii: 1313–1316

Baldwin R C, Jolley D J 1986 The prognosis of depression in old age. British Journal of Psychiatry 149: 574–583

Barraclough B 1971 Suicide in the elderly. In: Kay D W K, Walk A (eds) Recent developments in psychogeriatrics, Headly, Ashford, pp 87–97

Benbow S M 1989 The role of electroconvulsive therapy in the treatment of depressive illness in old age. British Journal of Psychiatry 155: 147–152

Bergmann K 1977 Prognosis in chronic brain failure. Age and Ageing 6(suppl): 61–66

Bergmann K 1978 Neurosis and personality disorder in old age. In: Isaacs A D, Post F (eds) Studies in geriatric psychiatry. Wiley, Chichester

Bergmann K, Eastham E J 1974 Psychogeriatric ascertainment and assessment for treatment in an acute medical setting. Age and Ageing 3: 174–188

Berrios G E 1990 Musical hallucinations: a historical and clinical study. British Journal of Psychiatry 156: 188–194

Berrios G E, Brook P 1984 Visual hallucinations and sensory delusions in the elderly. British Journal of Psychiatry 144: 652–664

Berrios G E, Brook P 1985 Delusions and the psychopathology of the elderly with dementia. Acta Psychiatrica Scandinavica 72: 296–301

Bond J 1987 Psychiatric illness in later life: a study of prevalence in a Scottish population. International Journal of Geriatric Psychiatry 2: 39–57

Brink T L 1979 Geriatric psychotherapy. Human Sciences Press, New York

Broadhead J, Jacoby R 1990 Mania in old age: a first prospective study. International Journal of Geriatric Psychiatry 5: 215–222

Brook P, Degun G, Mather M 1975 Reality orientation, a therapy for psychogeriatric patients: a controlled study. British Journal of Psychiatry 127: 42–45

Brooke H (1988) Consent to treatment and research. In: Hirsch S R, Harris J (eds) Consent and the incompetent patient. Gaskell/Royal College of Psychiatrists, London

Burns A, Jacoby R, Levy R 1990a Psychiatric phenomena in Alzheimer's disease: I: disorders of thought content. British Journal of Psychiatry 157: 72–75

Burns A, Jacoby R, Levy R 1990b Psychiatric phenomena in Alzheimer's disease: III: disorders of mood. British Journal of Psychiatry 157: 81–85

Butler R N 1963 The life review: an interpretation of reminiscence in the aged. Psychiatry 26: 65–76

Capewell A E, Primrose W R, MacIntyre C 1986 Nursing dependency in registered nursing homes and long term care geriatric wards in Edinburgh. British Medical Journal 291: 1719–1721

Central Statistical Office 1991 CSO annual abstract of statistics, 1991. Her Majesty's Stationery Office, London

Challis D, Davies B 1986 Case management in community care. Gower, Aldershot

Christie A B 1982 Changing patterns in mental illness in the elderly. British Journal of Psychiatry 140: 154–159

Christie A B, Train J D 1984 Changes in the pattern of care for the demented. British Journal of Psychiatry 144: 9–15

Clark A N G, Mankiker G D, Gray I 1975 Diogenes syndrome: a clinical study of gross neglect in old age. Lancet i: 366–373

Cooper A F 1976 Deafness and psychiatric illness. British Journal of Psychiatry 129: 216–226

Copeland J R M, Kelleher M J, Kellett J M, Barron G, Cowan D, Gourlay A J 1975 Evaluation of a psychogeriatric service: the distinction between psychogeriatric and geriatric patients. British Journal of Psychiatry 126: 21–29

Copeland J R M, Dewey M E, Griffiths-Jones H M 1986 Computerized psychiatric diagnostic system and case nomenclature for elderly subjects: GMS and AGECAT. Psychological Medicine 16: 89–99

Copeland J R M, Gurland B J, Kelleher M J, Smith A M R, Davidson I A 1987a Depression and neurosis in elderly men and women in an urban community: assessed using the GMS–AGECAT package. International Journal of Geriatric Psychiatry 3: 177–184

Copeland J R M, Gurland B J, Dewey M E, Kelleher M J, Smith A M R, Davidson I A 1987b Is there more dementia, depression and neurosis in New York? A comparative study of the elderly in New York and London using the computer diagnosis AGECAT. British Journal of Psychiatry 151: 466–473

Cutter N R, Post R M 1982 Life course of illness in untreated manic–depressive illness. Comprehensive Psychiatry 23: 101–115

Damas-Mora J, Skelton-Robinson M, Jenner F A 1982 The Charles Bonnet syndrome in perspective. Psychological Medicine 12: 251–261

de Alarcon R 1964 Hypochondriasis and depression in the aged. Gerontologica Clinica 6: 266–277

de Zoysa A S R, Blessed G 1984 The place of the specialist home for the elderly mentally infirm in the care of mentally disturbed old people. Age and Ageing 13: 218–223

Department of Health 1989 Working for patients. Her Majesty's Stationery Office, London

Department of Health and Social Security 1972 Services for mental illness related to old age. Her Majesty's Stationery Office, London

Department of Health/Department of Social Security, 1989 Caring for people: Community care in the next decade and beyond. Her Majesty's Stationery Office, London

Dight S 1976 Scottish drinking habits: a survey of Scottish drinking habits and attitudes to alcohol. Her Majesty's Stationery Office, London

Eagles J M, Gilleard C J 1984 The functions and effectiveness of a day hospital for the demented elderly. Health Bulletin (Edinburgh) 42: 87–91

Eagles J M, Whalley L J 1985 Ageing and affective disorder: the age of first onset of affective disorders in Scotland 1969–1978. British Journal of Psychiatry 147: 180–187

Eagles J M, Craig A, Robinson F, Restall D B, Beattie D A G, Besson J A O 1987 The psychological well-being of supporters of the demented elderly. British Journal of Psychiatry 150: 293–298

Eastman M 1984 Old age abuse. Age Concern England, London

Eastwood R, Corbin S 1985 Epidemiology of mental disorders in old age. Recent Advances in Psychogeriatrics 1: 17–33

Edwards G, Hawker A, Hensman C, Peto J, Williamson V 1973 Alcoholics known or unknown to agencies: epidemiological studies in a London suburb. British Journal of Psychiatry 123: 169–183

Erikson E 1963 Childhood and society. Triad Granada, London, pp 241–242

Feil N 1982 Validation: the Feil method. Edward Feil Productions. Cleveland, Ohio

Finch E J L, Catona C L E 1989 Lithium augmentation in the treatment of refractory depression in old age. International Journal of Geriatric Psychiatry 4: 41–46

Findlay D J, Shamara J, McEwen J, Ballinger B R, MacLennan W J, McHarg A M 1989 Double-blind controlled withdrawal of thioridazine treatment in elderly female inpatients with senile dementia. International Journal of Geriatric Psychiatry 4: 115–120

Fish F 1960 Senile schizophrenia. Journal of Mental Science 106:938–946

Flint A J, Rifat S L, Eastwood M R 1991 Late-onset paranoia: distinct from paraphrenia? International Journal of Geriatric Psychiatry 6: 103–109

Folstein M F, Folstein S E, McHugh P R 1975 Mini-mental state. Journal of Psychiatric Research 12: 189–198

Foster J R, Gershell W J, Goldfarb A I 1977 Lithium treatment in the elderly. Journal of Gerontology 32: 299–302

Gibb W R G 1989 Dementia and Parkinson's disease. British Journal of Psychiatry 154: 596–614

Gilhooley M L M 1984 The impact of caregiving on caregivers: factors associated with the psychological well-being of people supporting a dementing relative in the community. British Journal of Psychological Medicine 57: 35–44

Gilleard C J 1984 Living with dementia: community care of the elderly mentally infirm. Croom Helm, London

Gilleard C J, Belford H, Gilleard E, Whittick J E, Gledhill K 1984a Emotional distress amongst the supporters of the elderly mentally infirm. British Journal of Psychiatry 145: 172–177

Gilleard C J, Gilleard E, Whittick J E 1984b Impact of psychogeriatric day hospital care on the patient's family. British Journal of Psychiatry 145: 487–492

Greene J G, Timbury G C 1979 A geriatric psychiatry day service: a five year review. Age and Ageing 8: 49–53

Hawton K, Fagg J 1990 Deliberate self-poisoning and self-injury in older people. International Journal of Geriatric Psychiatry 5: 367–373

HEC 1986 Who cares: information and advice for those caring for a confused person. Health Education Council, London

Henderson A S 1986 The epidemiology of Alzheimer's disease. British Medical Bulletin 42: 3–10

Henderson A S, Huppert F A 1984 The problem of mild dementia. Psychological Medicine 14: 5–11

Hodge J 1984 Towards a behavioural analysis of dementia. In: Psychological approaches to the care of the elderly. Croom Helm, London

Hodkinson H M 1973 Mental impairment in the elderly. Journal of the Royal College of Physicians 7: 305–317

Holden U P, Woods R T 1988 Reality orientation: psychological approaches to the 'confused' elderly. Churchill Livingstone, Edinburgh

Hope R A, Fairburn C G 1990 The nature of wandering in dementia: a community based study. International Journal of Geriatric Psychiatry 5: 239–245

House A, Dennis M, Mogridge L, Warlow C, Hawton K, Jones L 1991 Mood disorders in the year after first stroke. British Journal of Psychiatry 158: 83–92

Hughes C P, Berg L, Danziger W L, Coben L A, Martin R L 1982 A new clinical scale for the staging of dementia. British Journal of Psychiatry 140: 566–572

Hymas N, Naguib M, Levy R 1989 Late paraphrenia — a follow-up study. International Journal of Geriatric Psychiatry 4:23–29

Iliffe S, Haines A, Booroff A, Goldenberg E, Morgan P, Gallivan S 1991a Alcohol consumption by elderly people: a general practice survey. Age and Ageing 20: 120–123

Iliffe S, Haines A, Gallivan S, Booroff A, Goldenberg E, Morgan P 1991b Assessment of elderly people in general practice: social circumstances and mental state. British Journal of General Practice 41: 9–12

Ineichin B 1990 The extent of dementia among old people in residential homes. International Journal of Geriatric Psychiatry 5: 327–335

Jacoby R, Levy R 1980a Computerized tomography of the elderly: 2. Dementia: diagnosis and functional impairment. British Journal of Psychiatry 136: 256–259

Jacoby R, Levy R 1980b Computerized tomography of the elderly: 3. Affective disorders. British Journal of Psychiatry 136: 270–275

Jacques A 1988 Understanding dementia. Churchill Livingstone, Edinburgh

Jorm A F 1985 Subtypes of Alzheimer's dementia: a conceptual analysis and critical review. Psychological Medicine 15: 543–553

Jorm A F, Korten A E, Henderson A S 1987 The prevalence of dementia: a quantitative survey of the literature. Acta Psychiatrica Scandinavica 76: 465–479

Kay D W K, Bergmann K 1966 Physical disability and mental health. Psychosomatic Research 10: 3–12

Kay D W K, Roth M 1961 Environmental and hereditary factors in the schizophrenias of old age (late paraphrenia) and their bearing on the general problem of causation in schizophrenia. Journal of Mental Science 107: 649–686

Kay D W K, Beamish P, Roth M 1964 Old age mental disorders in Newcastle upon Tyne. British Journal of Psychiatry 110: 146–158

Kendrick D C 1987 Psychological assessment. In: Pitt B (ed) Dementia. Churchill Livingstone, Edinburgh

Kessell N, Shepherd M 1962 Neurosis in hospital and general practice. Journal of Mental Science 108: 159–166

Kidd C B 1962 Misplacement of the elderly in hospital. British Medical Journal ii: 1491–1495

Kraepelin E 1919 Dementia praecox and paraphrenia. Translated by Barclay R M. Churchill Livingstone, Edinburgh

Kral V 1962 Senescent forgetfulness: benign and malignant. Journal de l'Association Medical Canadien 86: 257–260

Kral V 1983 The relationship between senile dementia (Alzheimer type) and depression. Canadian Journal of Psychiatry 28: 304–306

Kreitman N 1976 Age and parasuicide ('attempted suicide'). Psychological Medicine 6: 113–121

Lindesay J 1991 Suicide in the elderly. International Journal of Geriatric Psychiatry 6: 355–361

Lindesay J, Briggs K, Murphy E 1989 The Guy's/Age Concern survey: prevalence rates of cognitive impairment, depression and anxiety in an urban community. British Journal of Psychiatry 155: 317–329

Lindesay J, MacDonald A, Starke I 1990 Delirium in the

elderly. Oxford University Press, Oxford

Lipowski Z J 1983 Transient cognitive disorders in the elderly. American Journal of Psychiatry 140: 1426–1436

Lodge B, McReynolds S 1985 The use of multidisciplinary assessment by the community dementia team. Age Concern, Leicester

Macmillan D, Shaw P 1966 Senile breakdown in standards of personal and environmental cleanliness. British Medical Journal ii: 1032–1037

Mace N L, Rabins P V, Castleton B, Cloke C, McEwen E 1985 The 36-hour day: caring at home for confused elderly people. Hodder & Stoughton/Age Concern England, London

Mann A H, Graham N, Ashby D 1984 Psychiatric illness in residential homes for the elderly: a survey of one London borough. Age and Ageing 13: 257–265

Marks I 1981 Space phobia: Syndrome or agoraphobic variant? Journal of Neurology, Neurosurgery and Psychiatry 44: 387–390

Meacher M 1972 Taken for a ride. Longmans, London

Mendlewicz S, Fieve R, Rainer J 1972 Manic-depressive illness: a comparative study of patients with and without a family history. British Journal of Psychiatry 120: 523–530

Meyer J S, Rogers R L, Judd B W, Mortel K R, Sims P 1987 Cognition and cerebral blood flow fluctuate together in multi-infarct dementia. Stroke 19: 163–169

Morris C H, Hope R A. Fairburn C G 1989 Eating habits in dementia: a descriptive study. British Journal of Psychiatry 154: 801–806

Morris R G, Morris L W, Britton P G 1988 Factors affecting the emotional wellbeing of the caregivers of dementia sufferers: a review. British Journal of Psychiatry 153: 147–156

Murphy E 1982 Social origins of depression in old age. British Journal of Psychiatry 141: 135–142

Murphy E 1983 The prognosis of depression in old age. British Journal of Psychiatry 142: 111–119

Naguib M, Levy R 1982 Prediction of outcome in senile dementia: a computerized tomography study. British Journal of Psychiatry 140: 267–271

Naguib M, Levy R 1987 Late paraphrenia: neuropsychological impairment and structural brain abnormalities on computed tomography. International Journal of Geriatric Psychiatry 2: 83–90

Naguib M, McGuffin P, Levy R, Festenstein H, Alonso A 1987 Genetic markers in late paraphrenia. British Journal of Psychiatry 150: 124–127

Norman A 1987 Severe dementia: the provision of longstay care. Centre for Policy on Ageing, London

Norris A 1986 Reminiscence. Winslow Press, London

O'Carroll R, Whittick J, Baikie E 1991 Parietal signs and sinister prognosis in dementia: a four year follow-up study. British Journal of Psychiatry 158: 358–361

O'Connor D W, Pollitt P A, Hyde J B, Brook C P B, Reiss B B, Roth M 1988 Do general practitioners miss dementia in elderly patients? British Medical Journal 297: 1107–1110

O'Connor D W, Pollitt P A, Roth M, Brook C P B, Reiss B B 1990 Problems reported by relatives in a community study of dementia. British Journal of Psychiatry 156: 835–841

Parkes C M 1964 The effects of bereavement on physical and mental health: a study of the case records of widows. British Medical Journal ii: 274–279

Pattie A H, Gilleard C J 1976 The Clifton Assessment Schedule: further validation of a psychiatric assessment

schedule. British Journal of Psychiatry 129: 68–72

Perris C 1968 The course of depressive psychosis. Acta Psychiatrica Scandinavica 44: 238–248

Perry E K, Kerwin J, Perry R H, Irving D, Blessed G, Fairbairn A 1990 Cerebral cholinergic activity is related to the incidence of visual hallucinations in senile dementia of Lewy body type. Dementia 1: 2–4

Philpott M P, Levy R 1987 A memory clinic for the early diagnosis of dementia of Alzheimer type. International Journal of Geriatric Psychiatry 2: 195–200

Pierce D 1987 Deliberate self-harm in the elderly. International Journal of Geriatric Psychiatry 2: 105–110

Pitt B, Silver C P 1980 The combined approach to geriatrics and psychiatry: evaluation of a joint unit in a teaching hospital district. Age and Ageing 9: 33–37

Post F 1962 The significance of affective illness in old age. Maudsley monograph 10. Oxford University Press, Oxford

Post F 1966 Persistent persecutory states of the elderly. Pergamon Press, Oxford

Post F 1971 Schizo-affective symptomatology in late life. British Journal of Psychiatry 118: 437–445

Rabins P V 1986 Establishing Alzheimer's disease units in nursing homes: pros and cons. Hospital and Community Psychiatry 37: 120–121

RCPsych 1979 Guidelines for collaboration between geriatric physicians and psychiatrists in the care of the elderly. Bulletin of the Royal College of Psychiatrists 3: 85–86

Reisberg B, Ferris S H, de Leon M J, Crook T 1982 The global deterioration scale for assessment of primary degenerative dementia. American Journal of Psychiatry 139: 1136–1139

Robinson R A 1975 The assessment center. In: Howells G (ed) Modern perspectives in the psychiatry of old age. Churchill Livingstone. Edinburgh

Robinson R G, Kubos K L, Starr L B, Krishna R, Price T R 1984 Mood disorders in stroke patients: importance of location of lesion. Brain 107: 81–94

Rosin A J, Glatt M M 1971 Alcohol excess in the elderly. .Quarterly Journal of Studies on Alcohol 32: 53–59

Roth M 1955 The natural history of mental disorder in old age. Journal of Mental Science 101: 281–301

Roth M 1986 The association of clinical and neurobiological findings and its bearing on the classification and aetiology of Alzheimer's disease. British Medical Bulletin 42: 42–50

Roth M, Morrissey J F 1952 Problems in the diagnosis of mental disorder in old age. Journal of Mental Science 98: 66–80

Roth M, Tym E, Mountjoy C Q et al 1986 CAMDEX: a standardised instrument for the diagnosis of mental disorders in the elderly with special reference to early detection of dementia. British Journal of Psychiatry 149: 698–709

SAD 1988 Dementia and the law: the challenge ahead. Scottish Action on Dementia, Edinburgh

Saunders P A, Copeland J R M, Dewey M E et al 1989 Alcohol use and abuse in the elderly: findings from the Liverpool longitudinal study of continuing health in the community. International Journal of Geriatric Psychiatry 4: 103–108

Scott J, Fairbairn A, Woodhouse K 1988 Referrals to a psychogeriatric consultation-liaison service. International

Journal of Geriatric Psychiatry 3: 131–135

Scottish Home and Health Department 1979 Scottish health authorities priorities for the eighties. Her Majesty's Stationery Office, Edinburgh

Scottish Home and Health Department 1989 Scottish health authorities review of priorities for the eighties and nineties. Her Majesty's Stationery Office, Edinburgh

SHEG 1987 Coping with dementia: a handbook for carers. Scottish Health Education Group, Edinburgh

Shulman K 1978 Suicide and parasuicide in old age. Age and Ageing 7: 201–209

Shulman K, Post F 1980 Bipolar affective disorder in old age. British Journal of Psychiatry 136: 26–32

Shulman K I, Shedletsky R, Silver I L 1986 The challenge of time: clock drawing and cognitive function in the elderly. International Journal of Geriatric Psychiatry 1: 135–140

Stokes G 1986 Screaming and shouting. Winslow Press, London

Stokes G 1987 Aggression. Winslow Press, London

Stokes G, Goudie F 1990 Working with dementia. Winslow Press, London

Stone K 1989 Mania in the elderly. British Journal of Psychiatry 155: 220–224

Sunderland T, Silver M A 1988 Neuroleptics in the treatment of dementia. International Journal of Geriatric Psychiatry 3: 79–88

Thornton S, Brotchie J 1987 Reminiscence: a critical review of the empirical literature. British Journal of Clinical Psychology 26: 93–112

Ware G J G, Fairburn C G, Hope R A 1990 A community-based study of aggressive behaviour in dementia. International Journal of Geriatric Psychiatry 5: 337–342

Weisman G D, Cohen U, Ray K, Day K 1991 Architectural planning and design for dementia care units. In: Coons D H (ed) Specialised dementia care units 83–106. Johns Hopkins University Press, Baltimore

Wells C E 1979 Pseudodementia. American Journal of Psychiatry 136: 895–900

West P, Illsey R, Kelman H 1984 Public preferences for the care of dependency groups. Social Science and Medicine 18: 287–295

WHO 1986 Dementia in later life: research and action. World Health Organization technical report series 730. World Health Organization, Geneva

Wilkin D, Hughes B, Jolley D J 1985 Quality of care in institutions. In: Arie T (ed) Recent advance in psychogeriatrics, Churchill Livingstone, Edinburgh

Winokur G 1975 The Iowa 500: heterogeneity and course in manic–depressive illness. Comprehensive Psychiatry 16: 125–131

Woods R T, Britton P G 1985 Clinical psychology with the elderly. Croom Helm, London

Zis A P, Goodwin F K 1970 Major affective disorder as a recurrent illness. Archives of General Psychiatry 36: 835–839

32. Suicide and parasuicide

N. Kreitman

INTRODUCTION

The psychiatrist is always under an obligation to consider the medical, psychological and social aspects of the phenomena with which he is concerned. The value of this triple approach is nowhere illustrated more clearly than in the study of 'suicidal behaviour', a term generally used to embrace both suicide and so-called 'attempted suicide' or parasuicide. The two forms of suicidal behaviour are best considered quite separately, and will be discussed in turn before the relationship between them is reviewed.

SUICIDE

Definition and basic statistics

The importance of suicide from the public health point of view is persistently under-recognised, even though in most European countries it ranks among the ten most frequent causes of mortality. According to the Registrar-General approximately 5000 suicides are currently recorded annually in the UK, ten times the number of homicides. Such figures of course raise questions concerning the Registrar-General's definition of suicide. Official statistics are based on verdicts reached by coroners (or by the Crown Office in Scotland) and reflect a 'legal' decision in which the key element is that the deceased intended to take his own life. The authorities require unequivocal evidence of such intent before classifying a death as suicidal. Many psychiatrist have commented that such a restrictive definition leads to serious underestimation, arguing that, as with a clinical diagnosis, a decision should be reached on the balance of probabilities. Certainly, studies in which psychiatrists have reviewed the decisions of the legal authorities and have reached their own conclusions suggest that the official figures may represent only half to two-thirds of all suicides (McCarthy & Walsh 1966, Ovenstone 1973). Moreover, all such esti-

mates refer only to deaths brought to the attention of the authorities. It is not possible to say how many further suicides are not reported by the general practitioner or are concealed from him by the patients' families. It is evident that the Registrar-General's estimates are very conservative, but enlarging the figures by adding to the suicide rates various classes of 'undetermined' deaths (most of which are probably suicides) does not alter the relative positions of population subgroups, and the official figures continue to be useful for epidemiological purposes.

Methods for ascertaining the cause of death and the precise legal definitions used vary considerably from country to country. The extent to which official statistics can be employed when comparing the rates from different countries has been much discussed. The general opinion is that comparisons of absolute values are hazardous, but that something can be learned by contrasting the profiles or *patterns* of rates characteristic of different countries, for example by comparing how their rates vary by age. Changes within each country over time can also be fruitfully explored. (See Chapter 11 for discussion of the concept of 'rate'.)

The official suicide rates for recent years, for England and Wales and for Scotland, are given in Table 32.1. They are expressed as rates both for the total population and for adults only; since suicide is very rare in

Table 32.1 Annual suicide rates per 100 000 of the population for England and Wales, and for Scotland (average of 1986–1988)

	Males	Females
England and Wales:		
Total population	11.7	4.2
15 years and over	14.8	5.2
Scotland:		
Total population	16.3	6.0
15 years and over	20.8	7.4

children it is preferable to use the latter if possible, especially for international comparisons.

A fuller picture emerges from consideration of the age–sex-specific rates. Those for England and Wales are shown in Figure 32.1. For men the rates increase between adolescence and early maturity but the curve then reaches a plateau before increasing again in the oldest groups. This is a recent development; the pattern before the mid-1960s was for the male rates to increase steeply and linearly with age. For females the rates are always lower than those for men of comparable age. They peak in later life but actually decline again in the most elderly. For both sexes, however, suicide is predominantly a problem of middle and later life.

The corresponding age–sex-specific rates for Scotland are shown in Figure 32.2. Again the male rates are higher than the female at all ages. For males the contemporary pattern is for suicide to be particularly salient among the young and middle aged, with a peak in the 45–54-year-old age group, and again quite different from what was reported a few decades ago. Even for women the inflection point in the curve for recent years is appreciably earlier in life in Scotland than in England and Wales.

Thus, it is no longer true that Scotland has lower suicide rates than England and Wales, as has traditionally been the case, and in Scotland the rates peak in both sexes at an earlier age. These differences are unlikely to be an artefact of ascertainment procedures, but their explanation is not yet clear, though higher unemployment and alcohol consumption have both been incriminated (see below).

The various rates cited above indicate that in both

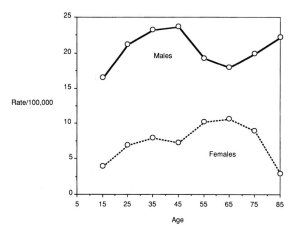

Fig. 32.2 Suicide rates per 100 000 of the population by age and sex for Scotland for the period 1986–1988.

Scotland and in England and Wales the risk for suicide for males is higher than for females. This relationship is one of the most consistent findings in the literature, embracing virtually all countries and all times, although it awaits a convincing explanation. But at least in developed countries the gap is steadily closing; this may come about in various ways but is most often because the female rate has risen to meet a stationary or more slowly increasing male rate. Figure 32.4 illustrates the convergence of the sex-specific rates over the earlier part of this century for England and Wales.

Marital status also has a marked effect upon suicide rates; some Scottish data, which show a pattern very similar to that of other European countries, are shown in Table 32.2. Close inspection will indicate that the effects of marital status vary by age. In general terms, and after standardising by age, the divorced are the group with the highest rates followed by the single and widowed, with married individuals coming lowest. This sequence may reflect differences in personality and psychopathology, but could also be the consequence of the differing satisfactions and stresses of the four civil status categories. In line with the second alternative is the suggestions that childlessness may be of particular importance (Veevers 1973). The effects of bereavement are also important and the raised rate among widows has been shown to be due to an excess of suicides shortly after the death of the spouse (MacMahon & Pugh 1965).

Suicide rates and unemployment are also linked. Swinscow (1951) drew attention to the high ecological correlation between deaths by suicide and unemployment levels in Britain over a 20 year period, and the

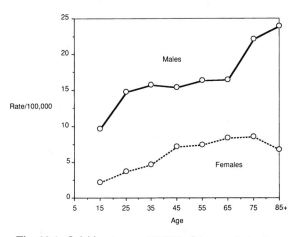

Fig. 32.1 Suicide rates per 100 000 of the population by age and sex for England and Wales for the period 1986–1988.

Table 32.2 Suicide by age and marital status in Scotland: average annual rates per 100 000 of the population for 1972–1983

Age (years)	Males				Females			
	S	M	W	D	S	M	W	D
15–24	8.6	9.3	—	—	3.7	2.9	—	—
25–34	26.8	8.5	(113.2)	35.9	11.8	4.5	(39.8)	20.4
35–44	37.3	13.0	73.9	54.6	12.7	7.4	(13.9)	27.5
45–54	35.1	14.7	45.5	63.0	22.6	9.9	22.6	32.5
55–64	40.4	13.8	37.4	55.7	18.4	9.9	18.1	26.2
65+	25.9	11.8	30.1	62.2	9.1	7.7	10.6	22.3
All groups	16.7	12.1	34.1	48.4	7.8	7.3	13.2	24.6

S, single; M, married; W, widowed; D, divorced. Rates with numerators of less than 5 are not shown; and those based on between 5 and 10 are given in parentheses.(See Kreitman 1988.)

same observation has been made in many other countries (e.g. see Boor 1980). Sainsbury (1955) confirmed that the rates for the unemployed were markedly higher than for those in gainful employment. More recent literature has been summarised by Platt (1984, 1986). In general, this research has upheld the strength of the link between unemployment and suicide. Interpretation of the association must take account of possible selective factors affecting the unemployed, since in times of economic recession the psychologically handicapped are particularly liable to lose their jobs, and to have greater difficulty than the more able members of society in finding new employment. Nevertheless there is much evidence to incriminate unemployment itself as a contributory factor to suicide, especially for those who are on the margins of the labour market. High unemployment among men is also positively associated with a high suicide rate among women, suggesting an indirect effect of unemployment on family life.

The impact of unemployment may also be relevant to the major differences in the suicide rates of the different social classes. Figure 32.3 shows for men (among whom social class can be determined more readily than for women) that the rate varies inversely with social status, and does so dramatically. The risk of being unemployed, especially for a sustained period, is also greater in the lower social classes, but a full exploration of the gradient in suicide rates would need to consider downward social drift as well as the effects of class-specific environmental pressures.

The secular trends in suicide rates as illustrated in Figure 32.4 for England and Wales between 1901 and 1961 show two interesting features. Perhaps the most striking is the marked fall in the rates with the onset of each of the major wars in this century. This effect is clearly visible for both men and women. It can also be

seen that with the cessation of hostilities the rates climbed back to the prewar levels and continued thereafter to follow the overall trends for the century. This pattern has also been reported from countries such as Switzerland which were not actually engaged in fighting but in which there was considerable apprehension that the nation might be involved in armed conflict. This dramatic effect of war might be explained by the fall in unemployment, which is usually a feature of a state of belligerency, but most writers have proposed that it owes more to the increased state of national cohesion, which gives people who might normally lack any clear role for themselves a definite and valued place in their society. The second feature is the convergency between the sexes already mentioned.

Between the later 1950s and the early 1970s a new

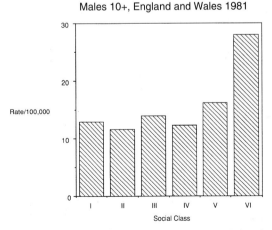

Fig. 32.3 Age-standardised suicide rates by social class (males aged 16 years and over) for England and Wales for 1981.

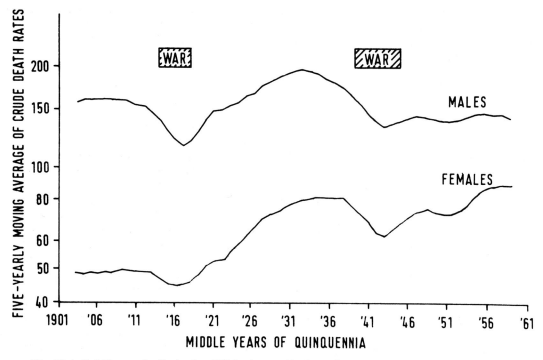

Fig. 32.4 Suicide rates for England and Wales (source: Registrar-General for England and Wales 1961).

feature emerged in the UK. Suicide by domestic gas almost disappeared after a decade in which its carbon monoxide content was steadily reduced. In general there was no compensatory increase in the use of other methods (for exceptions see Kreitman 1976). The net result was a marked decrease in the crude suicide rates for both sexes (the male data are shown in Fig. 32.5). Data from Holland, the only other European country in which domestic gas suicide was at all common, shows a similar if weaker effect. It is intriguing that the removal of one lethal agent had such a dramatic impact. Since 1971 there has been a minor recrudescence of gas suicides by men using car exhaust fumes. Analogous studies in the USA have focused on the availability of handguns, since suicide there among men is most commonly by shooting. Although the evidence for a causal link is not conclusive, states with comparatively stricter gun control laws have a lower overall suicide rate due to fewer suicides by firearms and in spite of a minor 'compensatory' increase in rates for other types of suicide (Lester et al 1980, 1982).

Societies which undergo a marked cultural change often reflect the transition in the pattern of their suicide rates. For example, in Japan before World War II many of the most acute social stresses tended to fall on young people. Age-specific rates for suicides showed a minor peak among individuals in their 20s with a

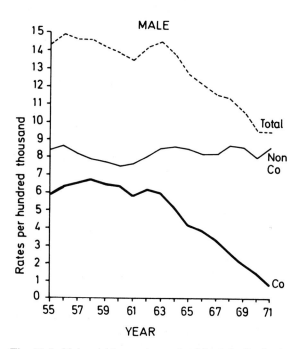

Fig. 32.5 Male suicide rates by mode of death for England and Wales. CO, deaths by carbon monoxide poisoning; non-CO, deaths by other means.

marked decline in middle life and a second peak in the older age groups. However, after the war American occupation of Japan profoundly affected the whole social fabric and many former values and social institutions lost their efficacy. It is of great interest that subsequent suicide rates for that country show an approximation to the American pattern (Kato 1969).

The sensitivity of suicide rates to social influences has for long excited the interest of sociologists, and indeed much of the fundamental work in sociology was done in the context of suicide studies. The problem that sociologists have attempted to answer is that of delineating what kinds of social relationships can explain variations in suicide rates between different social groups. The earliest theories were advanced by Emil Durkheim (1858–1917) whose views still dominate the field and who proposed several varieties of suicide, the most important of which he designated *anomic* and *egoistic*. The former arises in social situations in which the normative values of a community lose their force, and whose members therefore have no standards to guide them in times of stress. The second variety refers to a condition in which individuals become separated from their social group and lose their sense of community involvement, ceasing to feel that social norms have any significance for them. Durkheim's distinction between the two varieties has often been confused by subsequent workers, and indeed his own account (Durkheim 1951) is not always explicit. Nevertheless, his notions concerning the divorce of the individual from normative standards has been a major impetus behind subsequent studies. Sainsbury (1955), for example, was able to show in London the close correlation between suicide and social isolation of various kinds, including that attendant upon old age and the departure of offspring, physical handicap with its limitations of everyday activities, and the loss of family life consequent to divorce. Moreover, though Durkheim himself purported to be discussing processes of a purely sociological nature, the subjective sense of loss of contact and loss of values are salient psychological processes attending many suicidal deaths.

Of the other sociological theories, that of status incongruity (Gibbs 1967) may be briefly mentioned. In this view individuals are particularly susceptible to suicide when, although they are members of a well-defined social group, they deviate from the other members on some salient characteristic. For example, in the southern USA being white is in general also associated with being relatively wealthy and well educated. A white man who is uneducated or poor is at a higher risk for suicide than other white men; similarly, blacks who have risen to higher social levels are also at higher risk than those who have not. The facts are not in dispute — although in the USA and elsewhere the epidemiology of suicide is rapidly changing — but the theory of suicide as deviance has not attracted wide support.

Other aspects

Suicide occurs more commonly in the spring and summer, when the monthly rate is elevated by nearly 10%, in both the northern and southern hemispheres. Various explanations have been proposed. Depressive disorders, as reflected in admissions to mental hospitals, are commoner in spring and summer. Evidence is also being reported of similar seasonal variation in depressive mood among the general population (Nayha 1986). Further, it has been suggested that for the depressed individual the sense of alienation is heightened in the spring, the rebirth of nature jarring with his own feelings of gloom and purposelessness. In line with this view is the fact that the spring peak is more evident in rural than urban communities. It is also true, however, that although unemployment falls in the spring the migration of labour increases and the associated stresses provide an alternative if less poetic explanation. It would be entirely in line with current thinking if the seasonal fluctuation turned out to be linked with both psychosocial stresses *and* depressive affect.

In many but not all countries discrepancies between the high rates for urban areas and low rates for rural districts have also been recognised for a long time, but there is no evidence that the rate of suicide increases with the size of the city (Registrar-General of England and Wales 1961). Possible but unproven hypotheses concerning the urban–rural differences are: (1) that unstable individuals tend to migrate to cities; (2) that the stresses associated with immigrant status in the city are reflected in a raised suicide rate; and (3) that social cohesion is greater in country districts then in the more anonymous style of life in large cities.

Religious affiliation is often quoted as being correlated with suicide, with low rates characterising Catholic communities. But the relationship has little to do with religious doctrine. In Europe the main gradient in suicide rates is from the Protestant north to the more Catholic areas of the south. The same gradient reflects the level of urbanisation, which is least in the areas around the Mediterranean. Economic prosperity also tends to decline towards the south. As a further complication it is quite possible that the declaration of a suicide verdict may be inhibited because of social stigma in Catholic communities. When data from *within* one country are analysed, with appropriate controls for urbanisation and social class, only minor differences have been detected between Catholic and Protestant areas, and such discrepancies as have been found are generally ascribed to the greater social cohesion of the Catholic communities.

Similarly, much has been written alleging an inverse relationship between homicide and suicide. Most of the data supporting a negative correlation are based on cross-cultural comparisons at an ecological level, which in general illustrate a reciprocal pattern, though with numerous exceptions. Cross-cultural data of this kind are rarely a satisfactory basis for firm conclusions (see Ch. 11). Studies of different groups within a single society, and of fluctuations in homicide and suicide over time, show little evidence of any relationship. Insofar as they are related at all, homicide and suicide rates tend to vary over time in parallel (Holinger & Klemen 1982).

Epidemics of suicide have been known since antiquity, and were a problem of some seriousness among the Roman legions in isolated parts of the Empire. Some historians believe that the punitive legal attitudes towards suicide first developed in just that setting. Other epidemic outbreaks have been regularly noted throughout history; one rather striking example was the spate of apparently political suicides by burning that occurred worldwide in the early 1970s. There is always a risk that suicide within an institution such as a prison or a mental hospital may initiate a train of such deaths, and the steps needed to terminate a series of this kind are similar to those required for other acute outbreaks of psychiatric disorder such as mass hysteria.

Recently the role of imitation in suicides occurring outside institutions has received considerable attention. There is increasing evidence that a well-publicised suicide by a famous person can be followed by a wave of suicides using the same method, particularly among individuals who share the characteristics such as age and sex of the 'model'. It appears that this contagion effect can be demonstrated even for the fictional suicides of characters in television series (Phillips 1979, 1982). These imitation suicides apparently represent true additions to the overall numbers, and do not simply occur among individuals who would in any case have killed themselves sooner or later.

Clinical aspects

The undoubted importance of social influences in determining the prevalence of suicide should not obscure the major role played by psychological illness in such deaths. Studies from the UK and Eire suggest that up to half of all suicides have been in contact with psychiatric services at some point in their lives, and the proportion may be expected to rise as increasing numbers of people seek psychiatric attention. Usually the contact has been shortly before their death. Retrospective studies, both British and American, suggest that over 90% of suicides have suffered from a diagnosable mental illness at some time, but this was often not recognised or was inadequately treated (Robins et al 1959, Barraclough et al 1974). The three disorders of greatest importance are affective disorders, alcoholism and psychopathy, in that order.

Affective disorders

Patients treated by psychiatrists for manic–depressive psychosis and reactive depression have approximately 30 times the risk of the general population of dying by suicide (Guze & Robins 1970), and if such cases are followed up for the rest of their lives there is good agreement that 15% will kill themselves. The increased risk is most evident in the months or years following their initial treatment.

It is therefore important to try to identify patients with affective disorders who are at high risk, although the task is difficult because of the low absolute rate of suicide in the short and medium term. Certain predictors can be derived from what is known of the epidemiology of suicide in general; the variables which delineate vulnerable categories in the population at large are equally powerful predictors among depressed patients. Thus, male depressives are traditionally at greater risk than females, and the old rather than the young. However, in line with the changing epidemiological profile of suicide some recent research suggests that age and sex are losing their predictive power (Fawcett et al 1987). Social isolation has already been mentioned, and will often be linked to being widowed, separated or divorced. The personal background of the patient is also relevant; a history of bereavement in childhood or of a broken home from other causes may indicate a heightened risk. Recent bereavements are also important; raised suicide rates have been shown both for those recently bereaved of their spouses and for only sons recently bereaved of their mothers (Bunch et al 1972). Farberow et al (1966) have documented that depressed patients with hostile, passive–dependent relationships with their doctors seem to be another vulnerable subgroup. They persistently complain about their treatment and symptoms yet refuse to cooperate with everything offered. These are very difficult patients to manage, yet they may be precisely those most likely to kill themselves. The risks attached to patients with a history of parasuicide will be discussed more fully later, but here it may be noted that compared to the general population such a history increases the risk of death by suicide about 100 times, and it seems very likely that among the depressive group too a history of self-harm is another indication of high risk (McDowell et al 1968).

As mentioned above, the early months following psychiatric contact seem to be a particularly vulnerable period, which some authors ascribe to a lifting of psychomotor retardation at a time when mood has yet to improve, thereby increasing the risk that suicidal impulses will be put into operation. It is equally likely, however, that these early cases represent relapses after partial remission of the illness. The anticipation, whether realistic or not, of loss of support by the therapist or institution may be a further factor, and one which can easily be overlooked if therapy is defined in narrow pharmacological terms.

The mental state examination sometimes fails to elicit suicidal ideas by a depressed patient who soon afterwards kills himself. This may be due to the patient's own reticence, but is often to be ascribed to reluctance on the part of the physician to probe fully through a misplaced fear that such enquiries may suggest suicide to a patient who has not previously entertained such notions.

Since suicide among depressives is so markedly dependent on social factors it is not too surprising that attempts at prediction based solely on symptoms have had limited success. Nevertheless the clinical features of the illness must also be considered. Depth of depression may be an adverse factor, especially when manifest as hopelessness or severe anhedonia. The expression of marked guilt feelings and ideas of unworthiness also provide a warning, as does painful meditation by the patient about someone who has already died; fantasies of being reunited with departed relatives are a common theme in suicide notes. On the positive side, obsessional features may afford some protection against a suicide outcome, as may hypochondriasis (Stanbeck et al 1965). It has been reported (Roose et al 1983) that the presence of delusions is also an unfavourable risk factor but against this must be set the current consensus that the diagnostic label of endogenous or neurotic type of affective disorder has no prognostic value.

The question is sometimes posed as to why the improved methods of treatment for depression now available have not had a demonstrable impact on the suicide rate. It is not possible, of course, to guess what the suicide rate would have been if modern therapies had not been developed, and without such control

data no one can say whether or not there has been any effect. But two points are worth making. Firstly, most patients with severe affective disorders do not kill themselves; additional determinants appear to be social as well as clinical, as already discussed. It would be difficult to demonstrate the effects of varying only one component (treatment) in such a complex network of causes. Secondly, it is known that the therapy of patients with affective disorder who died by suicide has usually been inadequate as judged by customary clinical standards (see the section on management and prevention below). Advances in therapy can have no effects if they are not applied.

Alcoholism

The risks of eventual death by suicide among alcoholics has been very variably quoted by different workers using different definitions of alcoholism. Many of the classical studies have now been shown to be flawed, and a recent review suggests that the lifetime risk of suicide among hospital-treated alcoholics is probably about 3–4% (Murphy & Wetzel 1990). Since treated alcoholics include many who are young or in middle life, their mortality from suicide is greatly in excess of that of members of the general population of comparable age. A noteworthy feature of follow-up studies on alcoholics is that the maximum risk appears to be within the first few years following contact with psychiatric services. However, attempts to distinguish those who eventually kill themselves from the remainder have not been conspicuously successful, though it has been noted that of the eventual suicides nearly all relapse into heavy drinking after initial improvement (Kessel & Grossman 1961). Loss of a key interpersonal relationship by estrangement or death of the spouse has been well documented for the 6 weeks prior to suicide in many of these patients (Murphy et al 1979). The coexistence of marked depressive symptoms, even many years before death, may also serve as a warning sign (Berglund 1984).

Personality disorder

The association of personality disorder and suicide is difficult to document statistically in view of the notorious unreliability of the diagnosis. Moreover, many individuals with personality disorders present as alcoholics or drug addicts and the effect of these associated factors is impossible to separate. Nevertheless, there seems little doubt that individuals whose lives are fraught with problems of poor employment, inadequate interpersonal relationships, rage reactions, difficulties with the law, and possibly low intelligence are more likely than most to end their days by self-destruction.

Schizophrenia

This diagnosis occurs infrequently in population-based series of suicides, since schizophrenia is not a common condition. However, follow-up studies of schizophrenic patients show that suicide is an important cause of death, though exact figures are difficult to obtain. Many schizophrenic suicides are by unusual and violent means, such as self-immolation or jumping in front of trains. Recent studies of patients treated by modern methods of therapy do not seem to yield very different estimates from those of earlier decades. Schizophrenic patients at risk of suicide may be distinguished by the severity of their depression and more particularly by hopelessness concerning their future (Roy 1982, Drake & Cotton 1986).

Other conditions

Many other psychiatric disorders, including neurosis and drug addiction, are associated with a raised suicide rate, although available data are less extensive for these conditions. A useful review chiefly based on American studies is by Miles (1977). Patients with the acquired immune deficiency syndrome (AIDS) are also at increased risk of suicide (Marzok et al 1988).

Management and prevention

Acutely suicidal patients constitute an important group of psychiatric emergencies. They should be treated as in-patients. This can be offered on an informal basis, which will usually be accepted as many patients are alarmed at their own impulses and are glad to accept help. Of the remainder, the refusal of voluntary admission is often linked to pessimism regarding the possibility of effective help. The most acutely ill and pessimistic are, of course, those who can be treated most satisfactorily, and a firm statement to that effect, but without detailed argument, will sometimes lead to acquiescence with the proposal to enter hospital. For the remainder compulsory detention will be necessary, but in practice is required infrequently.

The ward management of the patient judged to be an acute risk for suicide poses certain difficulties. In former times many hospitals employed a routine whereby the patient was closely supervised by a special nurse round the clock, and who went to great lengths to ensure that there was no conceivable means whereby the patient could harm himself. Such an oppressive regime probably caused more deaths than it prevented. Supervision of acutely suicidal patients should be as unobtrusive as possible, though all staff must, of course, be alerted to the danger. Perhaps the most salient point in the management of the patient is the vigorous therapy of the mental illness. All too often electro-convulsive therapy (ECT) is withheld from depressed patients where indication for its use clearly exist, but instead time is spent in juggling the choice and dosage of anti-depressant drugs. It is equally important to persist in attempts to establish an effective psycho-therapeutic relationship with the patient, even in the face of psychosis, in order to convince him that the therapist cares very much indeed whether he survives. Once the acute episode is past, patients who have been at high risk of suicide should be offered sustained follow-up to maintain the psychotherapeutic relationship and to monitor the course of the illness; frequently, the resolution of a depressive episode takes much longer than either the patient or the therapist appreciates at the time, and a late relapse will sometimes lead to profound pessimism on the patient's part which may in turn prompt a suicidal act.

The association of suicide and social isolation has frequently been mentioned. For some patients, such as the severe psychopath or the chronic alcoholic, the isolation is often in substantial measure a consequence of the patient's own behaviour. With elderly patients, particularly those with affective disorder, it is more likely to be an antecedent to the illness. Whatever the cause, every effort should be made to enhance the patient's social integration. Here a psychiatric social worker with good knowledge of the informal networks in the local community can usually achieve more than the psychiatrist.

Many people who commit suicide communicate their intention to do so. Sometimes this is to a psychiatrist. A further proportion talk to their relatives, their general practitioners, or to some other physician. One cannot deduce from the fact that these individuals subsequently kill themselves that people in general and the medical profession in particular are commonly insensitive to the receipt of such intimations from patients, or that they usually act ineffectively. One can, however, conclude that more effective attention to suicide hints or threats by patients could make an appreciable impact upon the suicide rates of the nation. One of the main priorities in suicide prevention activities must be to increase the teaching of psychiatry to medical students and to general practitioners so that high-risk cases can be recognised and to emphasise that no threat of suicide should ever be dismissed as trivial. The same is true for the education of social workers, lawyers, clergymen and others, who may be the people to whom the future suicide first turns.

In the USA well over 100 suicide prevention centres have by now been established, and in this country the Telephone Samaritan organisation functions in a broadly analogous manner. In both instances the aim is to reduce the frequency of suicide by providing a 24 hour service to which despairing individuals can turn for help. Anonymity is a key feature, and the telephone figures largely as a means of initial contact. The members of the Telephone Samaritan organisation are non-professional volunteers who receive training in a counselling technique termed 'befriending' (Varah 1965). It has been shown that the Samaritan organisation does succeed in attracting the potentially suicidal, since there is evidence that those who are users of the organisation have higher than average suicide rates (Barraclough & Shea 1970). These agencies represent a tremendous investment of energy, but it is not easy to evaluate their efficacy. Most investigations find that the suicide rate in areas in which the Telephone Samaritans or similar services operate is not demonstrably different from the rate in matched control zones.

Lastly, there is the possibility of primary prevention among defined groups of the population known to be particularly at risk for suicide. One such comprises the elderly, especially those who are living alone. The future may see the construction of 'at risk' registers of such people who are, of course, also a hazard for numerous other psychiatric and physical illnesses, and it is possible that by routine attention to such groups by social workers and general practitioners a number of suicides may be prevented. A second obvious group to whom special attention should be directed are those who have survived some form of self-injury or self-poisoning, and these will be considered in the next section.

PARASUICIDE

The first problem that arises in the discussion of non-fatal self-destructive behaviour is that of terminology. Traditionally the term 'attempted suicide' has been used and for decades has led to confusion, especially by general practitioners and general physicians, since most patients are not in fact 'attempting suicide' in the literal sense of trying to kill themselves. Kessel (1965) proposed 'deliberate self-injury and self-poisoning' as an alternative term. The emphasis thus shifts to whether the patient has deliberately initiated an act of self-damage and leaves open the often intangible issue of his ultimate intention. This view is certainly preferable, but the terminology proposed can lead to difficulties if the patient has not poisoned himself in the toxicological sense. Moreover, the term should logically include cases of acute alcoholic poisoning, which are not normally regarded as part of the spectrum of suicidal behaviour, and by abandoning all reference to suicide the opportunity is lost to stress the real danger represented by such actions. For present purposes the term 'parasuicide' (Kreitman et al 1970a) will be employed, as referring to any act deliberately undertaken by a patient who mimics the act of suicide, but which does not result in a fatal outcome. Parasuicide, then, is a self-initiated and deliberate act in which the patient injures himself or takes a substance in a quantity which exceeds the therapeutic dose (if any) or his habitual level of consumption, and which he believes to be pharamacologically active. (The word may also be used, according to context, for the individual who carries out a parasuicidal act.)

Although reliable data on the frequency of parasuicide among the general population is difficult to obtain there is little doubt that the number of patients being seen at hospitals has markedly increased over recent decades, not only in the UK but in most other Western countries as well (Weissman 1974). A sizeable body of epidemiological information is now available and some of the findings will be briefly reviewed, with specific reference to Edinburgh, which is particularly fortunate in its data collection facilities, but which does not appear to have higher parasuicide rates than elsewhere in Britain (Morgan et al 1975, Platt et al 1988). Any description can only be provisional; after a period of rapid increase the rates have stabilised and are now beginning to fall, while in certain details the clinical characteristics of parasuicidal patients have also changed over time (Holding et al 1977).

Epidemiological aspects

Parasuicide is predominantly encountered among young people aged between 15 and 25 years. At all ages women have higher rates than men, although after the age of about 50 years the difference is unimpressive (Fig. 32.6).

Rates for different marital status groups (Table 32.3) show that the divorced are most at risk for parasuicide, despite their relatively greater age. Single men of all ages have higher rates than married men.

Parasuicide rates also vary markedly with social class; among men the rate is currently 15 times higher in

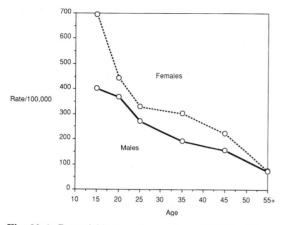

Fig. 32.6 Parasuicide rates (persons) per 100 000 of the population in Edinburgh for the period 1987–1989.

Table 32.4 Parasuicide rates (episodes) per 100 000 of the population in men in Edinburgh 1982, by duration of unemployment

	Incidence of parasuicide	Ratio of risk
Duration of unemployment:		
Less than 4 weeks	1012	8.8
5–26 weeks	615	5.4
27–52 weeks	1193	10.4
More than 52 weeks	2164	18.9
All unemployed men	1345	11.8
All employed men	114	

social class V than in I and II (982 per 100 000 compared to 66 per 100 000 of the population). This may be linked with high rates for two other variables, namely overcrowding and unemployment. In the early 1970s the former was one of the most powerful predictors of parasuicide, especially among women, for whom the rate among the over-crowded was some three times higher than among those not overcrowded, but over subsequent years the difference has lessened. In contrast, unemployment has become increasingly important as a correlate of parasuicide. It has always been the case that the rate among the unemployed has been much higher than among the employed. This difference persists even after standardising for age and social class — an important precaution since unemployment during a recession tends to be particularly likely among young men in the lower social classes. The parasuicide rate increases with the length of time for which the individual has been out of work; Table 32.4 shows that for those unemployed for over a year

the rate is about 19 times that for the employed. Two factors appear to be responsible for this high relative risk. One is the obvious stress of being unemployed, especially on those individuals who at other times would be classified as marginally occupied and whose work pattern tends to be intermittent but who can no longer find temporary work. The second factor is the inability of the less talented and the psychologically less robust to hold a job or to find alternative occupations in times of high competitiveness in the labour market. However, there is evidence that personal vulnerability of this kind has become progressively less relevant as unemployment has become more and more of a mass phenomena (see Platt 1986).

Other social variables associated with parasuicide have been demonstrated by ecological techniques, described in Chapter 13 (Philip & McCulloch 1966). Areas with high rates of parasuicide have been shown to be characterised by high rates for juvenile delinquency and breaches of the peace, housing evictions and rent arrears, road accidents, cruelty to children, venereal disease, and illegitimate births. Such areas tend to be either the central disintegrating zones of the city or other sections prominent for social pathology of diverse kinds (McCulloch & Philip 1970).

Differences between city areas have been found to persist even when due allowance is made for discrepancies in the age–sex characteristics of the sub-population and their differences in marital status, overcrowding, unemployment and social class (Buglass et al 1970). It has been suggested that these high-risk areas might also be characterised by tolerant attitudes which enhance the likelihood of parasuicide. However, direct investigation has shown that the attitudes of residents in such areas are more hostile to parasuicide than in low-risk areas (in contrast to attitudes on other forms of 'deviance' such as delinquency), which may imply that parasuicide is seen as particularly shocking.

Table 32.3 Average annual parasuicide rates (patients per 100 000 of the population) by marital status for the period 1987–1989 (Source: Edinburgh)

	Males	Females
Divorced	597	956
Widowed	245	98
Married:		
Under 35 years	158	257
35 years and over	92	157
Single:		
Under 35 years	535	776
35 years and over	283	140

Individuals who carry out parasuicidal acts tend to be linked together by personal acquaintance with greater frequency than would be expected by chance (Kreitman et al 1970b). This does not mean that most parasuicides are imitative but it does support the view that it is a form of behaviour which is socially recognised within certain groups.

The features of parasuicide discussed so far concern admission to hospital. Studies to determine the extent of the problem as seen at the general practitioner level (Hershon 1968, Kennedy & Kreitman 1973) suggest that a further 20–30% of cases are treated by the general practitioner without hospital admission, though the latest study indicated that most of the non-admitted patients are referred to a psychiatrist sooner or later. It was also shown that the characteristics of patients seen at hospital were identical to those of patients not so referred, with the exception that self-injury appeared to be relatively more frequent in the non-referred cases and constituted approximately 10% of all the cases known to the general practitioners. No one can say how many further cases of self-poisoning or self-injury might occur which are not brought to the notice of primary medical services.

In the UK, poisoning by drugs is by far the commonest mode of parasuicide, with self-injury, domestic gas poisoning and other methods collectively accounting for only about 10% of hospitalised cases. Among the drug group, preference for one or other type of agent appears to vary somewhat according to age, with barbiturates being more popular among older patients. A noticeable trend in the last decade has been the steady increase in the use of the newer psychotropic preparations at the expense of the barbiturates as a means of self-poisoning. This undoubtedly reflects changing prescription practices by general practitioners. At the same time the increase in poisoning by aspirin and paracetamol, which are freely available without prescription, has paralleled that for prescribed drugs. Thus, there is no evidence that the prescribing habits of general practitioners are responsible for the increase in the number of self-poisonings in recent years, although the types of prescriptions issued will clearly be reflected in which drugs are to hand and are consumed.

Psychological aspects

Much has been written concerning the psychological aspects of parasuicide, especially with regard to intent. The main difficulty is that after the act many patients cannot describe clearly what their intentions had been, but it is important to note that this confusion of motive is itself an important characteristic of the majority of patients. Nevertheless, it is possible to recognise a number of themes.

1. Many individuals describe a blind reaction in which some immediate relief from a stressful situation has been sought; they have been described as seeking an 'interruption' (Shneidman 1964) in an unendurable state of tension.

2. Some will reveal explicitly or implicitly that they were trying to secure the attention and solicitude of other people in their immediate environment, often after more conventional means of doing so had failed. Such an account is commonly elicited from patients with marital difficulties or other kinds of family crisis, or may be reported in connection with conflicts with authorities, such as the police or the local housing department. Here the parasuicidal act represents the 'cry for help' lucidly described by Stengel & Cook (1958).

3. Allied, but worth distinguishing, are those patients for whom the act has been coercive, a means of making others around them feel anxious or guilty, and towards whom they may express aggressive feelings. Sometimes this hostility is reflected by the patient's family and friends, who may react angrily, especially if the parasuicidal act is a repetition.

4. Another motive sometimes adduced, though often not very explicitly, is that of testing the benevolence of fate. Here the patient is replicating a primitive 'trial by ordeal' in which he stakes his life in a hazardous enterprise, interpreting survival as evidence that destiny intended him to live. This is sometimes linked with the individual's wishing to test his capacity for taking desperate action, rather analogous to the dangerous pranks of the adolescent.

5. Sometimes it seems that the patient intended to kill himself but was prevented either by his own ignorance of the required dosage or by chance intervention by others. More commonly patients will report an indifference as to whether or not they survive, rather than a clear decision to end their lives.

Thus, it is possible to describe a variety of motives underlying parasuicide; in most patients the motives are multiple, and may be mutually contradictory. Recognition of this has led to the ascription of marked 'ambivalence' to the act, usually an ambivalence between the wish to live and the wish to die. Such a formulation may be useful in describing the mental state of those who actually kill themselves. But with parasuicide the concept of a simple duality of motives is naive. It is also important to appreciate that in over half the male patients and almost the same proportion of women the act occurs under the influence of alcohol. It is scarcely surprising, therefore, that motivations are so often multiple and apparently confused.

Intensity of depressive affect has been shown to be related to the patient's expressed wish to die and the length of time spent contemplating the act. Currently, there is considerable interest in clarifying which aspects of depression are linked with 'suicidality'; it seems that it is pessimism about the future which is of primary importance (Beck et al 1975). There is *no* consistent relationship between depth of depression and the amount of damage the patient inflicts upon himself, as indicated, for example, by the depth of coma (Birtchnell & Alarcon 1971).

Lastly, it must be remembered that whatever the patient's motivation most parasuicides occur in an interpersonal context, and will only be understandable if viewed from a sociocultural as well as an individual viewpoint. The full significance of the act can only be grasped if the psychiatrist has some awareness of the norms and values of the group from which the individual comes and if he has understood the dynamics of the patient's psychosocial situation.

Psychometric studies show that as a group parasuicides contain a high proportion of personality disorders, tend to be hostile to others and to themselves, and have high levels of anxiety (Philip 1970). These characteristics are also found in mixed groups of psychiatric patients, but the parasuicides have more extreme scores. Other tests have demonstrated traits such as impulsiveness, unpredictability and emotional immaturity, with those individuals who make repeated 'attempts' being particularly noteworthy in these respects. However, there is no such thing as a specifically 'parasuicide-prone' personality (Casey 1989).

Psychiatric disorders

Most parasuicides have a recognisable psychiatric abnormality, but there is a danger that the dramatic character of the act may distract the psychiatrist from making a proper diagnosis. Among young people, minor reactive depressions are particularly common, the act often occurring in the context of domestic friction or similar interpersonal stress. States of 'adolescent turmoil' are well represented, as are personality disorders among women and delinquency among young men, many of the latter being in difficulties with the police at the time of the act. Among the middle aged, women show a preponderance of rather more severe depressive reactions, though personality disorders are also commonly encountered. In this age range alcoholism becomes a major factor among men, and in

some series appears to be the commonest diagnosis for parasuicide patients in middle life. Involutional depressions are also seen. The older age groups figure relatively infrequently but among them marked depressive reactions may be conspicuous. Such patients may also have considerable physical disability and be leading isolated lives. At all ages epilepsy and mental defect are represented more commonly than among the population at large.

An appreciable minority of patients show no evident psychopathology apart from their parasuicidal behaviour, and these are best regarded as basically normal individuals subjected to acute situational stresses.

Management and treatment

All parasuicides must be taken seriously. The first consideration is, of course, the treatment of the patient's injuries or toxic state. The latter should be assessed and treated by a physician with a particular interest in toxicology in view of the very large number of drugs now available. The patient's level of consciousness is itself a poor guide to the urgency of medical care; with poisoning by ferrous salts, for example, consciousness may be unimpaired until shortly before death from hepatic coma.

Secondly, all patients should be assessed psychiatrically, preferably when any toxic effects that may have been present have subsided. It is not possible to make any but the crudest provisional diagnosis if any degree of delirium persists.

Close collaboration between physicians and psychiatrists is optimally provided in regional poisoning treatment centres in which specialised resuscitation facilities can be concentrated, interdisciplinary collaboration fostered, and research carried out. Despite official recommendations regarding the establishment of such centres (Hill 1968) few were established, and the more usual arrangement is for the patient to be seen in a general hospital ward or the emergency department. The formidable workload so generated has led to experiments in assessment by non-medical members of the psychiatric multidisciplinary team (Hawton et al 1979) and by junior physicians and surgeons who have been given supplementary training and have an expert opinion readily available (Gardner et al 1978). These arrangements can evidently function well. The important point is that the patient must be assessed psychiatrically by a competent person able to call on the support of an experienced psychiatrist whenever required: for better or worse, official guidelines no longer regard it as mandatory for a psychiatrist to be involved directly in every case. Guidance on the management of parasuicides has been issued by the Royal College of Psychiatrists (1983) and by the Department of Health and Social Security (1984).

Psychiatric judgement should not be influenced by the 'medical seriousness' of the act: there is some association between the amount of injury or of toxicity sustained by the patient and the severity of his psychological illness (Kessel 1965, Rosen 1970) but it is too weak to be depended upon for clinical purposes. A patient with agitated depression and intense morbid preoccupation may be seen after he has taken half-a-dozen aspirins, while a young girl, with no evidence of psychopathology except for the act itself, may be moribund through an overdose taken following a quarrel with her mother.

It is understandable, given the dramatic presentation of parasuicide, that assessment tends to be concentrated on the risks of repetition or of death by suicide in the near future. These are of course important considerations, and are dealt with in the next section, but prognosis is not the sole issue; the majority of parasuicides are suffering from some current psychiatric disability, whether this be a personality disorder or a discrete illness, or both. A diagnostic assessment along orthodox lines should always be carried out and appropriate therapy initiated. A psychosocial formulation should also be made and given equal weight. Most parasuicides are precipitated by a florid social crisis which may be exploited to therapeutic advantage, and the social worker often has a major contribution to make. Other aspects of management have been considered by Kessel (1965) and Kreitman (1979).

Further suicidal activity

One of the outstanding difficulties in the treatment and management of parasuicides is the high repetition rate; various series report between 20 and 30% of patients with further similar acts within 12 months. Conversely, of all parasuicides seen in general hospitals about half will be 'repeaters'. The clinical and epidemiological characteristics of this group have been described (Kreitman & Casey 1988) and items predictive of repetition have been identified and prospectively validated. They are, in order of importance: (1) prior history of parasuicide; (2) personality disorder; (3) habitual heavy consumption of alcohol; (4) prior psychiatric illness; (5) unemployment; (6) social class V; (7) drug abuse; (8) criminal record; (9) recent interpersonal violence; (10) 25–45 years in age; (11) single, separated or divorced. Details are given in Kreitman & Foster (1991). When arranged as a scale they differentiate groups with repetition

rates ranging from near zero to about 50%. It is unlikely that prediction can be refined much further. Parasuicide has been shown to be associated with adverse life events (Paykel & Prusoff 1975) which almost by definition occur haphazardly and hence cannot be predicted from data available at the time of assessment (though unemployment and low social status may reflect both proneness and vulnerability to adverse events). As in other contexts, the 'medical seriousness' of the act itself in terms of the amount of physical damage sustained by the patient is at best a weak predictor of a further attempt (Greer & Lee 1967, Bagley & Greer 1971).

Characteristics which point to a repetition of parasuicide are not consistently those which predict completed suicide. The risk of the latter needs to be assessed separately, but the task is often difficult. Studies of the risk of death by suicide among parasuicidal patients suggest that approximately 1–2% will die from this cause over a 1–2 year follow-up period, and that thereafter the risk continues but at a decreasing level; the period of greatest danger is in the few months following the parasuicidal act itself. These are small proportions of all those at risk, so that it is difficult to amass enough cases for predictive criteria to be easily defined, except perhaps in rather special situations. So far as generalisation can be risked, it seems that (1) male parasuicides are more likely to commit suicide than women. There is a further association with (2) age: Edinburgh data show that the risk of men aged 35–54 years is about 10 times higher than for younger men. Other criteria include (3) being separated, widowed or divorced; (4) unemployment or retirement; (5) living along; (6) being in poor physical health; (7) suffering from a specific mental disorder including alcohol dependence. A useful dictum is that 'the more closely attempted suicides approximate completed suicide in personal and social characteristics, the greater the likelihood of death from a subsequent attempt' (Tuckman & Youngman 1963). Some, but not all, authorities also believe that the risk of ultimate suicide increases with each successive parasuicide in a patient's history. Quite apart from these features any patient who, after recovering from parasuicide, expresses a continuing intention to die should be considered a psychiatric emergency.

To date there is little firm evidence concerning the best way of preventing either repetition or death by suicide among the parasuicidal group. There is some evidence, albeit marginal, that simply being admitted to hospital after parasuicide may have some effect in reducing the likelihood of a further episode (Kennedy 1972). Randomised control studies (Chowdhury et al

1973, Gibbons et al 1978) of intensive aftercare have failed to yield significant differences (although social problems are ameliorated). Nevertheless, routine psychiatric attention certainly has some part to play in secondary prevention. It is noteworthy, for example, that depressed patients are among those with the best prognosis so far as repetition is concerned, presumably because depression is often treatable. For the remainder, prophylactic success may have to wait for the advent of successful treatments for alcoholism and psychopathy. Meanwhile, there is room for vigorous experiment.

A clinical overview

It may be helpful at this point to summarise the considerations to bear in mind when examining a parasuicidal patient. The assessment, which should whenever possible include talking to the relatives and friends — not simply as 'informants' but as part of the patient's interactive environment — should lead to a formulation covering the following questions:

1. What is the patient's physical state?
2. What is the psychiatric diagnosis? Separate decisions are required for formal mental illness and for personality disorder. Both recent and habitual alcohol and drug consumption should also be noted.
3. What were the psychodynamic and interpersonal factors leading to the parasuicide?
4. What is the risk of (a) repetition of parasuicide and (b) suicide, over the next year or two?
5. What treatments or other interventions, immediate or longer term, are required for (a) the physical damage, (b) the psychiatric illness and (c) the patient's social situation, and how are these to be organised?

Some guidance on each of these points has been given in preceding sections. It is worth stressing that the commonest error in clinical assessment is to overlook a psychiatric illness because attention is narrowed to the immediate circumstances which precipitated the act.

PRIMARY PREVENTION

So much suicidal activity occurs in a setting of social pathology that prevalence rates are likely to be influenced primarily by changes in basic social conditions, including both short-term fluctuations, such as unemployment, and more durable changes, such as the norms of marital behaviour or alcohol consumption. Any activities that can be undertaken by the government, local authority social work departments or voluntary agencies to mitigate the consequences of adverse social factors deserve full support for this reason alone.

It has been generally assumed that more direct preventive action is feasible for those individuals who are in distress and who might be influenced to seek assistance from an appropriate agency rather than proceed to parasuicide. Although the role of general practitioners and of social workers is a vitally important one the obvious agency of choice is the Telephone Samaritans. It has been shown, so far as the Samaritans are concerned, that their clientele does in fact approximate more to the population of parasuicides than of suicide. Yet a study in which parasuicides were questioned regarding their choice of action revealed that it was not ignorance of the existence of help-seeking agencies which had dictated their behaviour. Instead, the patients variously cited a need for immediate relief, often coupled with the desire to make a dramatic impact on other family members, disenchantment with the help they had already received from various agencies, or a reluctance to bring to the attention of strangers what seemed to them an essentially personal problem (Kreitman & Chowdhury 1972). These attitudes, when viewed against the foreseeable consequences of their behaviour, may not be logically consistent, but do indicate some of the difficulties which primary prevention encounters, and it has been shown that an increase in the number of Samaritan clients within a city makes no impact on the parasuicide rate (Holding 1974).

Finally, it must be pointed out that, although a proportion of parasuicides can be considered as failures of preventive care, nothing can be learned from such figures regarding the successes, that is to say, those individuals whom general practitioners, social agencies and others have successfully averted from parasuicidal action. It is to be hoped that the increasing dissemination of knowledge through the caring professions will highlight the importance of the early recognition of depressive illness and of alcoholism and increase sensitivity to the risk of parasuicide in these and allied conditions.

Much the same considerations apply to the primary prevention of suicide. Counselling services of the kind already mentioned are generally set up with the chief aim of preventing suicide rather than parasuicide. There is no evidence at an epidemiological level that they succeed. All the same, treatable mental illness, especially affective disorder, is much more salient among suicides than among parasuicides. The early detection of such illnesses among the general population, the early implementation of treatment, and where possible (as with lithium for manic–depressive psychoses) the initiation of secondary preventive regimes should lead to some reduction in suicide; this contention however is based upon reasoning rather than evidence, for so far the gains from improved clinical practice have not been reflected in a demonstrable decrease in suicide mortality.

THE RELATIONSHIP OF SUICIDE AND PARASUICIDE

When individuals who commit suicide are compared and contrasted with parasuicides certain differences and similarities emerge. The only survey in which both forms of behaviour have been studied simultaneously in a single population (Kennedy et al 1974) is now a little dated but is the best available. In view of the changing pattern of suicide over past decades the comparison needs updating, and will continue to require periodic revision.

Prevalence

The first point to note is the relative frequency of the two phenomena. Table 32.5 shows data from Edinburgh for parasuicide based on the total number of hospital-referred cases. Also shown are estimated rates derived from Kennedy's survey of general practice in the city (Kennedy 1973). If these figures are typical of the whole of the UK they can then be compared with the Registrar-General's data for official suicide notifications for the same period. The official figures are certainly minimal but it is evident that parasuicide is approximately 15 times more common for men and 30 times more so for women. Even if the 'true' suicide rate is assumed to be double the official figure (and this is probably an over-correction) parasuicide is still a vastly more frequent phenomenon: if all suicides were saved and reclassified as

Table 32.5 Comparison of annual parasuicide and suicide rates (persons per 100 000 of the population aged 15 years and over)

	Males	Females
Parasuicide (Edinburgh 1970):		
Hospital-referred (a)	179	243
Total known to		
general practitioners (b)	199	277
Suicide (UK 1969; c)	13.8	9.1
Ratio b/c	14.4	30.4

parasuicide it would make little difference to the rate for the latter.

Since age exerts such a marked effect on the rates of both forms of suicidal behaviour, any assessment of their relative frequency based only on crude rates is unsatisfactory. On the same basis of calculation as that used in Table 32.4 the relative excess of parasuicide to suicide among young women can be shown to be of the order of 190 times, while that for older men is about four times, both of these being minimal ratios.

These very approximate indices merely exemplify the relative magnitudes, so far as they can be ascertained, of the two aspects of suicidal behaviour. A more direct link is established by considering the proportion of parasuicides who later kill themselves, and conversely the proportion of suicides who have earlier suffered some form of self-damage. As already noted, in short-term follow-up studies on various samples, mostly from the UK, an estimated 1–2% of parasuicides have been found to kill themselves within a 1–2 year period. This proportion is some 50–100 times the risk of death by suicide among the general population, and may be compared with ratios of 140:1 (Tuckman & Youngman 1963) and of 80–100:1 (Motto 1965) cited from the USA. However, to determine the total contribution of parasuicide to suicide mortality one would need to know the lifetime expectation of suicidal death for parasuicides. This information is not available, although some authors have quoted an estimate of 20% eventual mortality (Dorpat & Ripley 1967).

Conversely, studies of suicide, usually defined on the basis of coroners' verdicts, have reported figures for earlier parasuicide. Excluding investigations based on very special groups, studies which have relied solely on information contained in court records give figures of 10–20% of all suicides having made an earlier 'attempt'. Those which have supplemented official records by more detailed enquiry cite proportions of 20–30%. A study which included deaths judged by psychiatrists to be suicide (as distinct from the narrower legal definition) and also carried out additional enquiries into the deceased's background reported a frequency of 40% (Ovenstone 1973). Such figures relate to a lifetime history, although one may well be sceptical about the completeness of data concerning the years long preceding death: nevertheless they suggest that about half of all suicides are 'first attempts'. Among those with a positive history of parasuicide approximately half occur in the 12 months preceding death; these cases often show chronically unstable lives with frequent episodes of self-poisoning and a history of alcoholism or sociopathy.

Table 32.6 Summary comparison of parasuicides and suicides in the UK

	Parasuicide	Suicide
Secular trend	Now stationary	Increasing in males, stationary in females
Sex	Commoner in females	Commoner in males
Age group	Mostly below 45 years	Mostly above 45 years
Marital status	Highest rates in divorced and single	Highest rates in divorced, single and widowed
Social class	Higher in lower classes	Somewhat higher in lower classes
Urban/rural	Commoner in cities	Commoner in cities
Employment status	Associated with unemployment	Associated with unemployment and retirement
Effects of war	?	Lower in wartime
Seasonal variation	None evident	Spring peak
Broken home in childhood	Common	Common
Physical illness	No obvious association	Probable association
Main psychiatric diagnoses	Situational reaction, depression, alcoholism	Affective disorder, alcoholism
Personality type	Psychopathy common	No special type

Motivational aspects

It is sometimes stated or implied that the two forms of suicidal behaviour can be distinguished by their different motivations. Among suicides it is said that the balance of motives is such that the wish to die emerges stronger than any other desire, and that the patient's primary concern is to terminate his life. Conversely, for parasuicide, the interpersonal aspects are emphasised, with quasi-pejorative terms such as 'manipulative' being put forward.

There may be some truth in this distinction but it is far too simple; the pattern of motivations to be found among both suicides and parasuicides, even within a single individual, is often a highly complex one. It may be true that the suicide wishes solely to withdraw from life, but often he will entertain fantasies of reunion with predeceased loved ones, or may be motivated by a wish to inflict guilt and remorse for his death on other members of his circle. One in five suicides in a Californian study were found to have been carried out in the presence of another person (Andress & Corey 1978) and some writers believe that most suicides are basically interpersonal acts in a wider sense. Conversely, although most parasuicides do not wish to terminate their lives, but rather are concerned to seek an intermission of consciousness and to signal their distress to others, they may be so strongly impelled as to be willing to gamble on survival. These considerations tend to emphasise the overlap rather than the separation of the classes of suicidal behaviour.

Qualitative differences

These have already been presented and are summarised in Table 32.6

REFERENCES

Andress V, Corey D 1978 Survivor-victims: who discovers or witnesses suicide. Psychological Reports 42: 759–764
Bagley C, Greer S 1971 Clinical and social predictors of repeated suicide attempts. British Journal of Psychiatry 119: 515–521
Barraclough B, Shea M 1970 Suicide and Samaritan clients. Lancet ii: 868–870
Barraclough B, Bunch J, Nelson B, Sainsbury P 1974

A hundred cases of suicide: clinical aspects. British Journal of Psychiatry 125: 355–373

Beck A T, Kovacs M, Weissman A 1975 Hopelessness and suicidal behaviour: an overview. Journal of the American Medical Association 234: 1146–1149

Berglund M 1984 Suicide in alcoholism: a prospective study of 88 suicides: 1. The multidimensional diagnosis at first admission. Archives of General Psychiatry 41: 888–891

Birtchnell J, Alarcon J 1971 Depression and attempted suicide: a study of 91 cases seen in a casualty department. British Journal of Psychiatry 118: 289–296

Boor M 1980 Relationship between unemployment rates and suicide rates in eight countries 1962–1976. Psychological Reports 47: 1095–1101

Buglass D, Dugard P, Kreitman N 1970 Multiple standardisation of parasuicide ('attempted suicide') rates in Edinburgh. British Journal of Preventive and Social Medicine 24: 182–186

Bunch J, Barraclough B, Nelson B, Sainsbury P 1972 Suicide following bereavement of parents. Social Psychiatry 6: 193–199

Casey P 1989 Personality disorder and suicidal intent. Acta Psychiatrica Scandinavica 79: 290–295

Chowdhury N, Hicks R, Kreitman N 1973 Evaluation of an aftercare service for parasuicide (attempted suicide) patients. Social Psychiatry 8: 67–81

Department of Health and Social Security 1984 The management of deliberate self-harm. HN(84): 25. Her Majesty's Stationery Office, London

Dorpat T L, Ripley H S 1967 The relationship between attempted suicide and committed suicide. Comprehensive Psychiatry 8: 74–79

Drake R E, Cotton P G 1986 Depression, hopelessness and suicide in chronic schizophrenia. British Journal of Psychiatry 148: 554–559

Durkheim E 1951 Suicide: a study in sociology. Translated by Spaulding J, Simpson G. Free Press, New York

Farberow N, Shneidman E, Neuringer C 1966 Case history and hospitalisation factors in suicides and neuropsychiatric hospital patients. Journal of Nervous and Mental Disease 142: 32–44

Fawcett J, Scheltner W, Clark D, Hedeker D, Gibbons R, Coryell W 1987 Clinical predictors of suicide patients with major affective disorders: a controlled prospective study. American Journal of Psychiatry 144: 35–40

Gardner R, Hanka R, Evison B, Mountford P, O'Brien V, Roberts S 1978 Consultation — liaison scheme for self-poisoned patients in general hospital. British Medical Journal ii: 1392–1394

Gibbs J (ed) 1967 Suicide. Macmillan, New York

Gibbons J, Butler J, Urwin P, Gibbons J 1978 Evaluation of a social work service for self-poisoning patients. British Journal of Psychiatry 133: 111–118

Greer S, Lee H 1967 Subsequent progress of potentially lethal attempted suicide. Acta Psychiatrica et Neurologica Scandinavica 43: 361–371

Guze S, Robins E 1970 Suicide and primary affective disorder. British Journal of Psychiatry 117: 437–438

Hawton K, Gath D, Smith E 1979 Management of attempted suicide in Oxford. British Medical Journal ii: 1040–1042

Hershon H 1968 Attempted suicide in a largely rural area during an eight-year period. British Journal of Psychiatry 114: 279–284

Hill D 1968 Hospital treatment of acute poisoning. SHHD report. Her Majesty's Stationery Office, London

Holding T 1974 The BBC 'Befrienders' series and its effects. British Journal of Psychiatry 124: 470–472

Holding T A, Buglass D, Duffy J C, Kreitman N 1977 Parasuicide in Edinburgh — a seven year review 1968–1974. British Journal of Psychiatry 130: 534–543

Holinger P C, Klemen E H 1982 Violent deaths in the United States 1900–1975: relationships between suicide, homicide and accidental deaths. Social Science and Medicine 16: 1929–1938

Kato N 1969 Self-destruction in Japan. Folia Psychiatrica et Neurologica Japonica 23: 291–307

Kennedy P 1972 Efficacy of a regional poisoning treatment centre in preventing further suicidal behaviour. British Medical Journal iv: 255–257

Kennedy P, Kreitman M 1973 An epidemiological survey of parasuicide ("attempted suicide") in general practice. British Journal of Psychiatry 123: 23–34

Kennedy P F, Kreitman N, Ovenstone I M K 1974 The prevalence of suicide and parasuicide ('attempted suicide') in Edinburgh. British Journal of Psychiatry 124: 36–41

Kessel N 1965 Self-poisoning. British Medical Journal ii: 1265–1270, 1336–1340

Kessel N, Grossman G 1961 Suicide in alcoholics. British Medical Journal ii: 1671–1672

Kreitman N 1976 The coal gas story. British Journal of Preventive and Social Medicine 30: 86–93

Kreitman N 1979 Reflections on the management of parasuicide. British Journal of Psychiatry 135: 275–277

Kreitman N 1988 Suicide, age and marital status. Psychological Medicine 18: 121–128

Kreitman N, Casey P 1988 The repetition of parasuicide: an epidemiological and clinical study. British Journal of Psychiatry 153: 792–800

Kreitman N, Chowdhury N 1972 Distress behaviour: a study of selected Samaritan clients and parasuicides ('attempted suicide') patients. British Journal of Psychiatry 123: 1–8

Kreitman N, Foster J 1991 The construction and selection of predictive scales with special reference to parasuicide. British Journal of Psychiatry 159: 185–192

Kreitman N, Philip A E, Greer S, Bagley C 1970a Parasuicide. British Journal of Psychiatry 116: 460–461

Kreitman N, Smith P, Eng-Seong Tan 1970b Attempted suicide as language: an empirical study. British Journal of Psychiatry 116: 465–473

Lester D, Morrel M 1980 The influence of gun control on suicidal behaviour. American Journal of Psychiatry 137: 121–122

Lester D, Murrel M 1982 The preventive effect of strict gun control laws on suicide and homicide. Suicide and Life Threatening Behaviour 12: 131–140

McCarthy P D, Walsh D 1966 Suicide in Dublin. British Medical Journal i: 1393–1396

McCulloch W, Philip A E 1970 The social prognosis of persons who attempt suicide. Social Psychiatry 5: 177–182

McDowell A, Brooke E, Freeman-Browne D, Robins A 1968 Subsequent suicide in depressed in-patients. British Journal of Psychiatry 114: 749–754

MacMahon B, Pugh T F 1965 Suicide in the widowed. American Journal of Epidemiology 81: 23–31

Marzok P, Tierney H, Tardiff K et al 1988 Increased risk of suicide in persons with AIDS. Journal of the American Medical Association 259: 1333–1337

Miles C P 1977 Conditions predisposing to suicide: a review. Journal of Nervous and Mental Disease

4: 231–246

Morgan H G, Pocock H, Pottle S 1975 The urban distribution of non-fatal deliberate self-harm. British Journal of Psychiatry 126: 319–328

Motto J 1965 Suicide attempts: a longitudinal view. Archives of General Psychiatry 13: 516–520

Murphy G E, Wetzel R 1990 The lifetime risk of suicide in alcoholics. Archives of General Psychiatry 47: 383–392

Murphy G E, Armstrong J W, Hermele S O, Fischer J R, Clendenin W W 1979 Suicide and alcoholism: interpersonal loss confirmed as a predictor. Archives of General Psychiatry 36: 65–69

Nayha S 1986 Seasonal variation in mental depression and its correlation with occupation. Social Psychiatry 21: 72–75

Ovenstone I 1973 A psychiatric approach to the diagnosis of suicide and its effects upon the Edinburgh statistics. British Journal of Psychiatry 123: 15–22

Paykel E S, Prusoff B A 1975 Suicide attempts and recent life events: a controlled comparison. Archives of General Psychiatry 32: 327–333

Philip A E 1970 Traits, attitudes and symptoms in a group of attempted suicides. British Journal of Psychiatry 116: 475–482

Philip A E, McCulloch J W 1966 Use of social indices in psychiatric epidemiology. British Journal of Preventive and Social Medicine 20: 122–126

Phillips D P 1979 Suicide, motor vehicle fatalities, and the mass media: evidence toward a theory of suggestion. American Journal of Sociology 84: 1150–1174

Phillips D P 1982 The impact of fictional television stories on US adult fatalities: new evidence on the effect of the mass media on violence. American Journal of Sociology 87: 1340–1359

Platt S 1984 Unemployment and suicidal behaviour: a review of the literature. Social Science and Medicine 19: 93–115

Platt S 1986 Parasuicide and unemployment. British Journal of Psychiatry 149: 401–405

Platt S, Hawton K, Kreitman N, Fagg J, Foster J 1988 Recent clinical and epidemiological trends in parasuicide in Edinburgh and Oxford. Psychological Medicine 18: 405–418

Registrar-General for England and Wales 1961 Statistical review part III: 240. Her Majesty's Stationery Office, London

Robins E, Murphy G, Wilkinson R H, Gassner S, Kayes J 1959 Some clinical considerations in the prevention of suicide based on a study of 134 successful suicides. American Journal of Public Health 49: 888–899

Roose S P, Glassman A H, Walsh B T, Woodring S, Vital-Herne J 1983 Depression, delusions, and suicide. American Journal of Psychiatry 140: 1159–1162

Rosen D 1970 The serious suicide attempt: epidemiological and follow-up study of 886 patients. American Journal of Psychiatry 127: 764–770

Roy A 1982 Suicide in chronic schizophrenia. British Journal of Psychiatry 141: 171–177

Royal College of Psychiatrists 1983 Guidance on the management of deliberate self-harm. Bulletin I: 210–212

Sainsbury P 1955 Suicide in London. Maudsley monograph 1. Chapman & Hall, London

Shneidman E 1964 Suicide, sleep and death. Journal of Consulting Psychology 28: 95–106

Stanbeck A, Achte K, Romon R 1965 Physical disease, hypochondria and alcohol addiction in suicides committed by mental hospital patients. British Journal of Psychiatry 111: 933–937

Stengel E, Cook N 1958 Attempted suicide. Maudsley monograph 4. Oxford University Press, London

Swinscow D 1951 Some suicide statistics. British Medical Journal i: 1417–1423

Tuckman J, Youngman W 1963 Identifying suicide with groups among attempted suicides. Public Health Reports 78: 763–766

Varah C 1965 The Samaritans. Constable, London

Veevers J E 1973 Parenthood and suicide: an examination of a neglected variable. Social Science and Medicine 7: 135–144

Weissman M 1974 The epidemiology of suicide attempts. Archives of General Psychiatry 30: 737–746

33. Psychiatry in general practice

I. Pullen

INTRODUCTION

It is not always appreciated that it is general practitioners (GPs), rather than psychiatrists, who deal with the majority of psychiatric morbidity in the community. GPs manage 90–95% of identified psychiatric problems themselves, only seeking the help of the psychiatric services with 5–10% of cases. Thus, inevitably, hospital-based psychiatrists gain a distorted view of psychiatric disorders and may even imagine that the patients they look after are the only people who are psychiatrically ill. This chapter is written for the psychiatrist rather than the GP, with the aim of providing a clearer picture of those disorders that occur in the community and the role of the GP in the care of the mentally ill.

THE PATHWAY TO PSYCHIATRIC CARE

Goldberg & Huxley (1980, 1992) describe the selection processes which operate on psychologically disordered individuals which determine which of them will seek care; having sought care, which will have their disturbances detected; having been detected, which will be treated in primary care and which will be referred for psychiatric care. They suggest a simplified model with five levels, each level representing different populations of subjects. In order to pass from one level to another it is necessary to pass through a 'filter' (see Table 33.1).

LEVEL 1 — MORBIDITY IN RANDOM COMMUNITY SAMPLES

The epidemiology of mental disorders in the community has been bedevilled by the difficulty of defining a 'case'. Before the 1970s community surveys rarely defined what was meant by a 'case' and in many instances the definition depended entirely on the whim of the individual research worker. Common sense suggests that if the research worker's criteria are very stringent he will find fewer 'cases' than if his criteria are very broad. This lack of consensus has meant that the reported number of psychiatrically ill in the community has tended to vary considerably between surveys. It has also meant comparisons between different populations and the study of the relationships between possible aetiological factors and psychiatric illness have been impossible. During the 1970s the situation was improved by the use of carefully defined diagnostic criteria in epidemiological surveys. However, although it is clearly important to use a strict definition of a 'case' in such studies, it is by no means clear what the defining characteristics should be. Most diagnostic schemes are derived from patients seen in hospital practice and it is debatable whether or not these same defining characteristics should be applied to individuals in the community. Do we only regard someone as a 'case' if they have the same constellation of symptoms as patients seen in the hospital? Patients seen in general practice sometimes lack the symptoms necessary to fulfil the criteria for a specific diagnostic label.

Some people would argue that these patients are merely distressed by life's circumstances and are not in any way 'ill', and that treating them raises their expectations so that they come to believe that any distress or anxiety is pathological and in need of treatment. However, people who react adversely to stresses like bereavement or the breakup of a marriage often have very real and distressing symptoms and respond well to treatment, be it counselling or drugs. Some diagnostic schemes require that a person must have some disturbance of function before being labelled 'ill' and in that sense anyone who presents himself to the doctor for treatment, no matter what his symptoms, could be regarded as a 'case'.

How then have these issues over 'caseness' been resolved? Recent epidemiological surveys, which have used strict case definitions, have been seeking to

Table 33.1   Five levels and four filters, with estimates of annual period prevalence rates at each level

---

Level 1   The community
260–315/1000 per year
....First filter
(Illness behaviour)

Level 2   Total mental morbidity — attenders in primary care
230/1000 per year
....Second filter
(Ability to detect disorder)

Level 3   Mental disorders identified by doctors ('conspicuous psychiatric morbidity')
101.5/1000 per year
....Third filter
(Referral to mental illness services)

Level 4   Total morbidity — mental illness services
23.5/1000 per year
....Fourth filter
(Admission to psychiatric beds)

Level 5   Psychiatric in-patients
5.71/1000 per year

From Goldberg & Huxley (1992).

identify in the community people whom 'a psychiatrist would not be surprised to see in the out-patient clinic and benefiting from some form of treatment' (Finlay-Jones et al 1980). Hence they have used diagnostic interviews and criteria which would normally be used in the assessment of hospital patients. Several centres have used Wing's Present State Examination (PSE)/Catego/Index of Definition (ID) system (Wing et al 1974) and some have used Spitzer's Research Diagnostic Criteria (RDC) (Spitzer et al 1978). In Edinburgh a survey has been carried out using both of these sets of criteria in the same population and this has allowed comparison between them. This demonstrates that applying different diagnostic criteria to the same population results in different people being identified as cases.

As Table 33.2 shows, the prevalence of minor psychiatric morbidity in the community varies between 9 and 15% in different centres, depending on the criteria used. The equivalent rates for cases of depression vary between 6 and 9% and for cases of anxiety between 3 and 4.5%. These figures are all for women. Rates for total psychiatric morbidity in men are reported as being somewhat lower at 7–12.5%. Other workers have used the Clinical Interview Schedule (Goldberg et al 1970) and General Health Questionnaire (Goldberg 1972), instruments specially designed for use in the community. They obtain a higher annual period prevalence of psychiatric disorder in the community of between 25 and 31.5%

(Goldberg et al 1976, Goldberg & Williams 1988, Goldberg & Huxley 1992).

Despite some variation in the reported rates of psychiatric morbidity between surveys, a consensus does seem to be emerging, with rates of around 15% for women and 10% for men. However, the agreement is not as good as it looks. The Edinburgh study (Dean et al 1983), which compares several diagnostic schemata in the same population, demonstrates that although two different schemata frequently pick out the same people as 'cases' the labels they assign are often very different. For instance, the same 'case' might be labelled 'depression' by one diagnostic schema and 'anxiety' by another. Many community

Table 33.2   Estimates of the prevalence of minor psychiatric disorder in women in different centres

Centre	Method	Rate (%)
London (1981)	PSE–ID–Catego	14.9
Canberra (1979)	GHQ–PSE–ID–Catego	11.0
Edinburgh (1983)	PSE–ID–Catego	8.7
Edinburgh (1983)	RDC	13.7
Newhaven (1978)	SADS-L+RDC	15.0

Based on Bebbington et al (1981), Henderson et al (1979), Weissman & Myers (1980), and Dean et al (1983).
PSE, Present State Examination; RDC, Research Diagnostic Criteria; GHQ, General Health Questionnaire; ID, Index of Definition; SADS-L, Schedule for affective disorders and Schizophrenia—Lifetime version.

'cases' have a mixture of anxiety and depression and their labelling as a 'case' of one or the other is a fairly arbitrary procedure and depends on the precise criteria being used. Some would argue that these problems arise because all of these studies use hospital-derived criteria. A study by Jenkins et al (1985), in which 27 experienced GPs rated a videotaped consultation, demonstrates how poor the diagnostic agreement is between GPs using both the International Classification of Diseases (ICD; World Health Organization (WHO)) and the International Classification of Health Problems in Primary Care (ICHPPC-2; WONCA 1979), a special adaptation of the ICD designed to meet the needs of GPs. Using ICD-9 the GPs produced nine different diagnoses and, with the ICHPPC-2, eight.

A more valid approach would be to study and describe the disorders which do exist in the community and devise operational definitions for these before attempting to assess their prevalence. In order to go some way towards solving these problems the General Practice Research Unit of the Institute of Psychiatry, in cooperation with the WHO and the National Institute of Mental Health in the USA piloted a diagnostic scheme for use in general practice. It comprises a triaxial classification (Regier et al 1982), with physical ill health, psychological ill health and social difficulties as the three axes. The description of the patient's illness is thus based on the symptoms the GP actually encounters in his patients and not on hospital-based diagnostic schemes. It is hoped that this will result in a better understanding of the disorders which occur in the community, their prevalence, who should treat them, their outcome and their response to treatment. Current diagnostic labels do not predict outcome (Mann et al 1981), although the overall severity of symptoms does.

LEVEL 2 — TOTAL MORBIDITY IN PRIMARY CARE

One might imagine that many of these 'cases' picked up in community surveys never seek medical help. However, the available evidence suggests that the majority of patients with psychiatric symptoms of any severity do in fact go to their doctor for help. Goldberg & Huxley (1980) compared a number of prevalence rates derived from community surveys and general practice studies and found, somewhat to their surprise, that they were all very similar, suggesting that patients with psychiatric symptoms almost invariably seek medical help. Consultation rates tend to increase with the severity of symptoms as determined by the General Health Questionnaire (GHQ; Goldberg 1972) score (Burvill & Knuiman 1983). A study by Ingham & Miller (1976) also demonstrates that patients with psychiatric symptoms are less likely to tolerate symptoms without consulting than patients with physical symptoms like backache. They demonstrated that 32% of non-consulters have backache which is just as severe as that of at least 70% of consulters, but that the proportion of non-consulters who were equally depressed was only 9%. Additional evidence is to be found in the community studies mentioned earlier, some of which investigated consultation behaviour. Of Brown & Harris' (1978) Camberwell depressives, 68% had consulted their doctor and Weissman & Myers (1978) found that although only 10% of their community depressives had seen a psychiatrist, 87% had seen a primary care physician for their symptoms.

Having established that many patients with significant psychiatric symptoms do indeed consult their GP, how can we establish the magnitude of the workload that this constitutes for the average doctor? One way is to look at all patient–doctor contacts and another is to examine the percentage of patients who consult the doctor at his surgery with psychiatric symptoms. Investigating the percentage of general practice consulters who consult with psychiatric symptoms has proved difficult and the same problems have arisen as in community studies, in particular the lack of fixed criteria for diagnosing 'psychiatric cases'. It has therefore been impossible to know whether different results represent true differences between different practices or different diagnostic criteria. An early study in the 1950s reported between 6 and 65% of consulters as psychiatrically ill and the Royal College of General Practitioners' Research Committee (1958) found that individual GPs regarded between 26 and 72% of their patients as psychiatrically ill. The same problems arise with national morbidity surveys. In one practice included in the second survey almost 10% of registered patients were diagnosed as suffering from an affective psychosis between 1970 and 1976, compared with 1% in most other practices (Dunn 1985). This led Dunn (1986) to urge that GPs' diagnostic habits should be validated before their records are used to provide data on 'official' estimates of psychiatric morbidity.

A large-scale survey of general practice in west London (Williams et al 1986) examining more than 3 000 consultations found that the presence of minor psychiatric morbidity doubled the probability of contact with primary medical care, and about one fifth of consultations could be attributed to it. This figure is higher than that produced by a national morbidity survey of general practice (HMSO 1979) which relied on GPs' diagnoses. Williams et al (1986) also concluded that health variables exerted much more influence on consulting that the sociodemographic variables.

Shepherd and his colleagues established satisfactorily that most of this variability was due to characteristics of the doctor rather than to different rates of psychiatric morbidity (Shepherd et al 1966). They did this by giving a self-rated questionnaire to the same patients as were assessed by the doctor. The GPs identified between 15 and 72.5% of consulters as being psychiatrically ill, whereas the questionnaire identified a much narrower range, between 20.1 and 35.8% of consulters. This demonstrates that when case detecting is standardised, the percentage of consulters who are identified as psychiatrically ill does not vary greatly between practices and that reported rates are mostly dependent on attributes of the doctor and his personal diagnostic criteria.

There are few studies which help us establish clearly the number of GP consulters who are psychiatrically ill. One good study in a single general practice (replicated by Skuse & Williams 1984) does examine the relationship between those the GP regards as psychiatrically ill and those the psychiatrist would regard as a 'case' (Goldberg & Blackwell 1970). The GP identified 19.5% of consecutive attenders as being psychiatrically ill whereas 30.8% were found to be 'cases' by the psychiatrist, who used a combination of the GHQ and the Clinical Interview Schedule (Goldberg et al 1970) to identify them. The cases 'missed' by the doctor tended to have presented with physical symptoms, and this is presumably why the psychiatric symptoms went unnoticed.

It is difficult, then, to draw any firm conclusions about the percentage of GP consulters who are psychiatrically ill. From the data available it would seem that on average around 20% are regarded by their GP as psychiatrically ill (HMSO 1979), although there is considerable variability between individual GPs. However, some psychiatric cases are probably being 'missed' (i.e. do not pass through Goldberg & Huxley's second filter), so that around 30% would meet the criteria for a psychiatric illness if seen by a psychiatrist.

LEVEL 3 — CONSPICUOUS MORBIDITY IN PRIMARY CARE

The fact that the GP apparently 'misses' some cases of psychiatric morbidity should be set in context. Some of these 'missed' cases will have minor, self-limiting conditions which improve spontaneously. Perhaps of more importance, the studies of GP identification frequently disregard the way in which GPs work. The average duration of a consultation in primary care is about 7 minutes, during which time the GP must select which aspects of the patient's complaints he regards as important. He will often spread diagnostic decisions over several sessions and defer making a firm diagnosis until the patient has presented the same symptoms on several occasions. Thus, testing the diagnostic efficiency of a GP on the basis of a single index consultation may not do justice to GPs (Blacker & Clare 1987).

Nevertheless, attempts have been made to answer the question of whether being identified as a case shortens the course of the disorder. Johnstone & Goldberg (1976) examined the outcome of three groups: those identified by the GP as psychiatrically ill; those he did not initially diagnose as ill but who were revealed to him by the psychiatrist as being so; and those he did not diagnose as a 'case' and did not either know about or treat. They found that the two treated groups had shorter illnesses than the third untreated group, and at 12 month follow-up the only group which did not show improvement was the one which had not been known to or treated by the GP. The ones who suffered most by not having their illnesses diagnosed and treated were those with the most severe illnesses.

Blacker & Clare (1987) in an excellent review of depressive disorder in primary care cite seven studies demonstrating that GPs fail to detect between 33 and 50% of cases of psychiatric disorders presenting to them. In the case of depression, Freeling et al (1985) noted that major depressives missed by their GP were more likely to be suffering from physical illnesses (30%) to which the depression seemed to be related. They were also less obviously depressed and their illnesses had lasted longer. Even though only a few of their recognised depressives had completed even a minimal course of antidepressants, they had all fared better at 3 months' follow-up than the unrecognised group. However, the identified depressives differed from the non-identified in having a shorter illness at the time of diagnosis.

No firm conclusions can yet be drawn from these studies, but the results do suggest that patients get better quicker if their doctor is aware that they have psychiatric symptoms, and hence it would seem to be of benefit to patients if their GP is a skilful psychiatric case detector.

IMPROVING GP CASE DETECTION SKILLS

A number of workers have studied the attributes of GPs who are good case detectors. Marks and his colleagues (1979) find that those who are good at detecting psychiatric cases are empathic, interested in psychiatry and tend to ask questions about the patient's family and home. Their study has been repeated in Charleston (Goldberg et al 1980) with similar findings. In addition, this second study demonstrates that doctors who are good case detectors are self-confident, clarify their patients' complaints, have accurate knowledge and high academic ability. Ten aspects of a family doctor's interview style were identified which improved significantly with training and were related to his accuracy as a case detector:

Outset:
1. Eye contact at outset
2. Clarifies presenting complaint
3. Uses directive questions for physical complaints
4. Uses 'open to closed cones'

Interview style:
5. Empathic style
6. Sensitive to verbal cues
7. Sensitive to non-verbal cues
8. Does not read notes during history
9. Can deal with over-talkativeness
10. Asks fewer questions about past history.

It is possible, therefore, not only to identify the characteristics of the doctor who is an accurate case detector but also to improve accuracy by interview skills training and improving knowledge.

So far we have been dealing with doctor characteristics and the ability to detect psychiatric disorders. Demographic characteristics of patients are also associated with the likelihood of being identified as a case (Marks et al 1979). Unemployment, female sex, separation, divorce and being widowed are associated with an increased likelihood of psychiatric disorders being detected, whereas being male, unmarried, young (between 15 and 24 years old) and educated beyond the age of 23 years are characteristics associated with a lower chance of having their illnesses diagnosed.

ILLNESSES FOUND IN GENERAL PRACTICE

Of patients diagnosed as psychiatrically ill in general practice, 87% have a diagnosis assigned by their GP of neurosis, insomnia, tension headache or physical disase of psychogenic origin, whereas only 5.5% are diagnosed as psychotic (HMSO 1979). Shepherd and his colleagues (1966) compared the distribution of the main diagnostic categories in their survey of 12 London general practices with those found in psychiatric out-patients and in-patients (Table 33.3). This demonstrates that GPs are dealing with a different mix of patients from hospital psychiatrists, with fewer cases of psychosis and personality disorder but an increased number of patients with neurotic disorders. Although the proportions are different, there is considerable overlap, with GPs looking after patients with the same diagnostic label as those seen by the psychiatrist.

However, the general practice group could still be different from the point of view of severity of illness,

Table 33.3 Comparison of the distribution of psychoses, neuroses and character disorders between a survey of 12 London general practices, Maudsley Hospital out-patients, and first admissions to mental hospital in England and Wales for 1957

Category	General practice survey (%)[a]	Maudsley Hospital out-patients (%)[b]	Mental hospital first admissions, England and Wales 1957 (%)
Psychoses	4.2	24.5	72.3
Neuroses	63.4	43.6	18.1
Character disorders	3.9	23.2	4.6
Miscellaneous	28.5	8.9	4.6
Total	2049	6752	48 266

From Shepherd et al (1966).
[a]Shepherd et al (1966).
[b]Hare (1962).

symptom profile, response to treatment or prognosis. It may be that severely ill patients are referred to the psychiatrist, leaving the GP to look after less severe illnesses. Alternatively, hospital and general practice patients who have the same diagnosis might be identical, at least with respect to severity and prognosis.

It is frequently stated that primary care depressives are milder, more 'neurotic', more 'reactive' and less 'biological' than those found in psychiatric settings (Blacker & Clare 1987). Certainly such patients are very well represented in primary care, but the question remains whether depressions in this setting are always of this type, or whether cases of more severe depressive illness also exist but escape referral to the psychiatric services. Sireling et al (1985) compared 'GP depressives' with psychiatric out-patient depressives: the mean Hamilton score and the mean Raskin score were both significantly less in general practice cases with 'shorter illnesses, as well as less primary and less endogenous depression'. However, as patients receiving antidepressants at the time of entry and those who were felt to be so ill as to require psychiatric referral were excluded from the sample, these findings were almost inevitable. 'Exceptionally severe cases of depression are likely to gravitate quickly into psychiatric care, but it is important to bear in mind that depressed patients found within the psychiatric services represent a distillation or 'creaming off of the cases from a comparatively dilute pool of disorders in the community' (Blacker & Clare 1987). After controlling for this, Brown et al (1985) found considerable overlap between the severity of depression in the two populations, but GP decisions about referring are less influenced by severity of the illness than complicating factors such as alcohol abuse, threats of self-harm and personality difficulties.

Therapeutic trials in general practice are another source of data. Blackburn et al (1981) compared the response of depressed patients in hospital and in general practice to a number of treatments. They were able to recruit a cohort of patients in general practice that showed no difference in severity of illness prior to treatment from hospital patients, as measured by the Hamilton Rating Scale and the Beck Depression Inventory, and the depressed patients in general practice were just as likely to fulfil the RDC for primary major depressive disorders (Spitzer et al 1978).

Another way to look at severity of depressive illness in primary care is to consider the impact on individuals. Johnson & Mellor (1977) studied over 200 consecutive cases of depressive disorder in general practice, half of whom were unable to continue with their normal lives.

The next issue is whether or not depressives in general practice differ in prognosis or response to treatment. It could be that the patients the GP does not refer differ in that they respond well to the kind of treatment he provides, whereas the patients referred to the psychiatric services do not. There is some collateral support for this view in that GPs give 'failure to respond to treatment' as one of their main reasons for referring patients to psychiatrists (see below).

In the trial mentioned above (Blackburn et al 1981) the researchers did in fact find a difference in response to treatment between hospital and general practice depressives. The latter responded poorly to drugs and did significantly better with cognitive therapy, either alone, or in combination with drugs. By contrast, the hospital group did best with a combination of cognitive therapy and pharmacotherapy, and there was no difference in outcome between the groups who received drugs alone and cognitive therapy alone. The general practice patients also got better quicker and required fewer treatment sessions. These findings are consistent with the theory that general practice depressives are qualitatively different from those seen in hospital. It could be that depressive illnesses seen and treated in primary care are more environmentally determined and that treatment aimed at helping the patient develop better coping strategies is therefore more effective. There is also a suggestion that the general practice depressives may respond to lower doses and shorter courses of treatment (see below). All these fragments of information suggest that many of the depressive illnesses seen in general practice are qualitatively different and respond to different treatments to those seen in hospital.

There are no data about hospital/general practice differences for other psychiatric illnesses, but as only 5–10% of all psychiatric disorders are referred to the psychiatric services it is likely that the GP manages other severely ill psychiatric patients, apart from depressives, without reference to the psychiatrist. However, most schizophrenic patients are managed by psychiatrists at some time during their illness.

The natural history of neurotic illnesses is covered elsewhere (see Ch. 22) and so will not be considered in detail here. Nonetheless, from the point of view of the GP it is interesting to speculate whether most of his psychiatric work consists of treating a small cohort of patients with chronic relapsing conditions or whether a large percentage of his patients each have short-lived illnesses. Cooper et al (1969) in a 7 year follow-up of patients in primary care found that the mean annual psychiatric prevalence rate for women was 17%, whereas the 7 year prevalence was 52%.

This suggests a considerable change year by year in the identity of those diagnosed as neurotic and refutes the suggestion that it is the same group of patients that the GP sees year in, year out. On the other hand, the same study found that 37% of female patients and 21% of male patients consulting with psychiatric symptoms obtained a psychiatric diagnosis in four out of five succeeding years. Dunn & Skuse (1981) confirmed that the identity of those diagnosed as psychiatrically ill changes from year to year. They report a 20 year study of a single GP's practice. Nearly 75% of the women on the GP's list and 50% of the men consulted at least once over the 20 years with a psychiatric problem. However, a core of patients did have chronic problems; one in six women and one in 20 men received a diagnosis of depression in 10 or more of the 20 years.

These findings, together with those of the other studies, make it clear that there are two subgroups of neurotic patients in primary care: one with an acute onset, usually in response to stress, which recovers quickly (Mann et al (1981) estimated these to constitute about 25% of general practice cases) and another with chronic or recurrent symptoms.

The GP does of course look after patients with a range of psychiatric disorders. Table 33.4 gives some idea of the numbers of patients with a variety of psychiatric problems that an average GP might expect to have on his list. These disorders are discussed in detail in the relevant chapters.

ASSOCIATION WITH PHYSICAL DISORDERS

Another way in which psychiatric disorders in primary care differ from those seen by the psychiatric services is that they are more frequently associated with physical illness or physical symptoms. This could be partly due to the fact that physical symptoms act as an 'admission ticket' to the GP, the patient believing that a physical complaint is more socially acceptable than a psychiatric one. There does, however, seem to be a genuine association between physical and psychiatric illness. This close relationship is demonstrated in a study by Goldberg and Blackwell (1970). They found that the GP identified only one-third of his psychiatric cases as being entirely psychiatric. Twenty per cent had unrelated physical and psychiatric disorders, 40% had psychiatric illness with related somatic symptoms and 8% had physical illness with associated psychiatric disturbance.

Reporting a large series of depressed primary care patients (733), Watts (1970) showed that 'only a small number' presented with symptoms that were 'clearly depressive' in type. The ten symptoms most commonly presented were:

1 Tiredness, shortage of energy, feelings of being weak and run-down
2. Headache
3. Anxiety or tension
4. Depressed mood
5. Backache
6. Insomnia
7. Pains in the chest
8. Dyspepsia
9. Giddiness
10. Pains in the trunk, arms and legs.

Pain was responsible for no less than 35% of the presenting symptoms.

Shepherd et al (1966) found that patients with chronic psychiatric illness had a high incidence of chronic physical illness. It is not possible to decide from these data whether those who are psychiatrically ill have an increased prevalence of physical illness, or whether the increase is an artefact due to higher consultation rates resulting in more physical illness being detected. Eastwood & Trevelyan (1972) report a trial which successfully resolves the issue by assessing patients who were part of a physical screening programme. All the people being screened were also screened for psychiatric disorder and if they were thought to be psychiatrically ill their psychiatric status was confirmed by the Clinical Interview Schedule. They were matched for age, sex, marital status and social class with a control group who were not psychiatrically ill. The patients were all subjected to physical screening tests covering the whole range of body systems and a physical examination. The number of

Table 33.4 Psychiatric disorders and social pathology in a hypothetical average population of 2500

	Cases per annum
Acute major disorders	
Severe depression	12
Suicide attempts	3
Suicide	1 (every 3 years)
Chronic mental illness	55
Severe mental handicap	10
Neurotic disorders	300
Social pathology	
Chronic alcoholism (known cases)	5
Chronic alcoholism (unknown cases)	25
Juvenile delinquency	5–7
Problem families	5–10
Broken homes (one-parent families with children under 15)	60

From RCGP (1981).

psychiatric patients free from physical disease was significantly less than the control (18.5 versus 38.7%) and those who were psychiatrically and physically ill had a larger number of physical diseases per individual than the controls. The results of this study are clear-cut: psychiatric illness and physical illness are associated. Whether this is because some individuals in certain environmental circumstances are prone to develop both emotional and physical disorders is impossible to say.

Whatever explanation we might favour, the fact remains that patients presenting to their GP with psychiatric symptoms often have physical symptoms as well. He therefore has the difficult task of deciding whether or not to investigate and treat a physical or psychiatric disorder. The psychiatrist, because of his different expectations, tends to miss physical illness in his patients (Koranyi 1979) just as the GP tends to miss psychiatric illness.

ASSOCIATION BETWEEN PSYCHIATRIC DISORDERS AND SOCIAL DYSFUNCTION

There is a strong association between psychiatric disorder and social dysfunction. Chronic neurotics in particular have a marked excess of all forms of social difficulty, including material social circumstances and housing difficulties and problems with interpersonal relationships. Cooper (1972) found that the degree of social dysfunction was related to the clinical severity of the illness, as did Wing and his colleagues (1981), who found that out-patient 'cases' had more social dysfunction than community 'cases'. The relationship between neurotic symptoms and social bonding has been examined in more detail in a random sample of an Australian population (Henderson et al 1978). This study demonstrates that there is an inverse relationship between neurotic symptoms and social bonds, particularly close affectionate ties. It is not possible to decide from these data whether a lack of social relationships causes neurotic illness or whether having neurotic symptoms makes social bonding less likely, but there seems little doubt that neurotic disorders and social dysfunction, both material and interpersonal, go hand in hand. A further study by Henderson (1981) indicates that it is the perception of social relationships as being inadequate under conditions of adversity which is associated with neurotic symptoms rather than real deficiencies in social relationships.

There is some evidence to suggest that social factors, both interpersonal and material, do play a part in the aetiology of minor psychiatric disorders. Brown

& Harris (see below) found that rates for psychiatric illness in women were higher in the lower socio-economic groups. They also found that women who lacked a confiding relationship were more likely to become psychiatrically ill in the face of stress. A primary care study (Wright et al 1980) found that the single most important predictor of score on a self-report depression questionnaire was socioeconomic status: the higher the status the less likely it was that the person would rate themselves as depressed.

Where outcome is concerned the patient's material social circumstances have been shown to be the best predictors — better than clinical factors (Huxley et al 1979). It is less clear whether outcome is affected by the quality of social support; Mann and his colleagues (1981) found that a 'good quality of family life' at the time of assessment discriminated between those who improved early and those who did not. Huxley et al (1979) found no association between quality of social support and outcome but this study was of psychiatric out-patients, not general practice patients. They are therefore a highly selected group and we know that patients referred to psychiatric services are less likely to have good social support than those not referred. On the evidence available it seems that good social support does improve outcome, which suggests that improving a patient's social support may also aid recovery.

TREATMENT IN THE PRIMARY CARE SETTING

Just as the classification of mental illnesses is based on psychiatric patients in hospital, so most treatment regimes are based on assessments made on hospital patients, although recently there has been a tendency for more drugs to be evaluated in the primary care setting. As we have seen, some patients treated by GPs have similar characteristics to patients treated by psychiatrists, but many do not.

Shepherd et al (1966) were among the first to examine the treatment actually received by patients diagnosed as 'psychiatric' in general practice. They studied the treatment of those labelled neurotic or psychosomatic and found that 46% received drug treatment, 24% counselling, 2% psychotherapy and 12% symptomatic treatment for physical symptoms. More recently, Watson & Barber (1981) found that 90% of depressed patients in Glasgow were treated with drugs, 2.9% with counselling and drugs, and 2% by psychiatric referral. GPs are often criticised for prescribing drugs instead of counselling their patients, and this study certainly reveals an astonishing lack of counselling and a very widespread use of drugs. However, a GP is responsible for so many patients that if he were to counsel all those on his list who have psychiatric symptoms for 10 minutes a month, he would need to work an extra 14 hours a week (Kessel 1965). A study of consultations in general practice (Buchan & Richardson 1973) underlines how little time the GP has available for those with psychiatric symptoms. Those suffering from a new anxiety state spent 6.3 minutes with the doctor and 84% received tranquillisers; those with a new depressive illness were seen for 5.6 minutes and 50% were given a tranquilliser or an antidepressant. Although GPs seem reluctant to admit to 'counselling' or 'psychotherapy', most doctors do use their relationship with the patient to therapeutic advantage and some doctors have special sessions devoted to patients who require longer interviews.

What therapies have been demonstrated to be useful in general practice patients with psychiatric symptoms? Trials carried out in general practice patients have demonstrated the superiority of both amitriptyline (Blashki et al 1971) and imipramine (Murphy 1976) over placebo. Furthermore, Blashki et al found amitriptyline in a dose of 150 mg/day to be more effective than a dose of 75 mg/day. Unfortunately, the majority of primary care treatment trials are flawed for one reason or another. Nevertheless, two well-designed trials deserve mention. Paykel et al (1988) treated 141 general practice depressives with amitriptyline (median dose 125 mg) or placebo. Amitriptyline was superior to placebo in probable and definite depression (RDC) but not in mild depression. In the second trial conducted in general practice (Thomson et al 1982), although both amitriptyline and tryptophan were found to be superior to placebo, many depressed patients did respond to placebo, 40% having recovered within 12 weeks of starting 'treatment'. Blashki et al (1971) had an even better response to placebo in their drug trial, with 60% of the placebo group well 38 days after starting 'treatment'. Neither trial was able to predict response to placebo. It is tempting to wonder whether placebo should not be the first-line treatment of depression in primary care! However, the Thomson trial demonstrates that not all placebo patients do well; ten patients in all were withdrawn from the trial because of failure to respond to treatment and eight of these were found to have been on placebo. Even the 20% of patients on amitriptyline who had zero blood levels at 4 and 12 weeks did better than those on placebo. Until the characteristics of patients who are likely to respond to

placebo are identified, antidepressants continue to be the treatment of choice for depressives in general practice.

On the whole, psychiatrists tend to prescribe tricyclic antidepressants in higher doses than do GPs who fear that high doses will cause unacceptable side-effects and therefore further reduce patient compliance. Despite the findings of Blashki et al to the contrary, it is also the clinical experience of most GPs that patients get better on low doses and it could be that low doses or short courses of antidepressants are effective in most general practice depressives. The dosage appropriate for depressed patients in general practice certainly seems sufficiently open to question for psychiatrists to be less derogatory about the clinical practice of their general practice colleagues. But GPs should be encouraged to use higher doses of antidepressants where a patient has failed to respond to a low dose.

But does the GP prescribe the appropriate medication? A study by Sireling et al (1985) demonstrates that although GPs do miss some patients with major depressive disorder, they do prescribe antidepressants appropriately. Patients diagnosed as depressed and treated with antidepressants had higher Hamilton scores and were more likely to fulfil the criteria for major depressive disorder (Spitzer et al 1978) than those diagnosed and treated with tranquillisers.

As well as giving tranquillisers to depressives, GPs also tend to diagnose as having an anxiety state patients whom the psychiatrist diagnoses as having a depressive illness (Mann et al 1981). Blacker & Clare (1987) point out that GPs often base their management decisions on the strength of the primary presenting symptoms rather than the patient's membership of a particular diagnostic group, and the degree of 'understandability' of the disorder. Downing & Rickels (1974) found that GPs tend to prescribe, in situations of mixed symptoms, according to the predominance of anxiety or depressive symptoms. Thus, cases in which both symptoms featured equally tended to come off badly in terms of obtaining the appropriate treatment. If GPs equate 'understandable symptoms' with being 'appropriate or normal', then patients will be denied appropriate treatment. Blacker & Clare stress that in general practice a more satisfactory definition of caseness would give greater weight to the form and degree of the ensuing depressive reaction and less to the circumstances against which it arose. There are also patients receiving psychotropic drugs who do not seem to be psychiatrically ill. Murray et al (1981) found that 5%

of male and 10% of female 'probable non-cases' (as determined by a low score on the GHQ) were in receipt of psychotropic drugs. The choice of antidepressant for use in primary care may be different from that used in psychiatric in-patients where medication is rigorously supervised. The fatal toxicity (Cassidy & Hendry 1987) should be known for any antidepressant prescribed to a depressed patient who will be unsupervised at home. The use of drugs relatively safe in overdose may be preferable to the traditional tricyclics.

Johnson (1973) and Thomson et al (1982) graphically demonstrate the problems encountered in treating depressed patients in a primary care setting. Most patients do not comply with treatment. Three-quarters of the patients studied by Johnson had stopped taking medication within a month, and 20% of Thomson's patients had stopped within 3 weeks. The reasons given by Thomson et al were side-effects, worsening symptoms or early recovery. Johnson found that other sources of non-compliance were failure of the GP to warn patients about the delay in therapeutic response, the possibility of side-effects, and the need to continue taking the medication regularly, coupled with a low consultation rate (often once in 6 weeks). Other patients thought medication inappropriate or feared becoming dependent on medication. It is therefore probable that a considerable part of the failure of treatment with antidepressants in general practice is due to basic failures of understanding and communication between doctor and patient.

Lader (1975) criticises the use of medications in situations of stress-related disorder in that they inhibit the patients' own efforts to organise themselves and meet the stresses. While this is sensible on theoretical grounds, it has not been tested experimentally. Although Johnson identified a stress factor in 80% of cases, no doctor attempted to modify precipitating or social factors. He concludes that conditions in an urban general practice are far from ideal for treating depressed patients but that most patients seemed to recover in spite of inadequate treatment. There are no reported investigations of the effect of counselling by GPs of patients with neurotic disorders, but there are some studies which have evaluated the therapeutic benefit of non-medical counsellors and of social workers. Corney (1984) assessed the value of allocating depressed women to a social worker in addition to existing services. Overall, allocation to a social worker did not result in additional improvement in symptoms or social adjustment, not did it result in reduced medical consultation, but there was some benefit in women whose depression was an acute exacerbation of a chronic condition and in those needing practical help with a social problem. This confirms an earlier study by Cooper et al (1975) which demonstrated that social work intervention improved the prognosis of chronic neurotics from both the social and psychiatric point of view. These findings suggest that the attachment of a social worker to the primary care team could result in a better management of this group of patients, who are normally a heavy burden on the medical services, contributing more than their share to the GP's workload and also having high rates of referral to medical and surgical specialists and to hospital for admission. Ashurst (1982) confirms that counselling can be helpful in treating some patients and that patients who have been on tranquillisers for more than 6 months have more chance of getting off drugs if they are being counselled.

All this is at a very preliminary stage but it does suggest that non-medical counselling can benefit selected groups of patients and that it may be particularly useful in those with chronic symptoms who are normally difficult and time-consuming to treat.

Clinical psychologists can make a valuable contribution in the primary care setting and the Trethowan committee (Department of Health and Social Security 1977) recommends that clinical psychologists should be attached to the primary care team. They are not only able to provide counselling skills but also offer a range of cognitive–behavioural treatments useful in primary care: relaxation techniques, treatment of phobias, cognitive treatment for depression and autogenic training for stress-related disorders. Blackburn et al (1981) report a large study comparing cognitive therapy carried out by psychologists and drug therapy for depression, either alone or in combination, in general practice clinics and in out-patients. In general practice, cognitive therapy was superior to drug treatment, although considerably more expensive. It remains to be seen whether a form of cognitive therapy can be devised that might be used within the time constraints imposed by general practice. There is a growing trend for psychologists to work closely with GPs and to receive referrals directly from them without psychiatric involvement.

Community psychiatric nurses are another group of mental health workers who are working more closely with the primary care team, sometimes being based in a health centre or group practice. Patients prefer to be treated by them than go to an out-patient department for follow-up (Paykel et al 1982). As their numbers increase, more of their work is with neurotic patients at the primary care level rather than with chronic psychotic patients (Wooff et al 1986).

A number of general practices are pioneering the use of patient groups in a primary care setting (Zander 1982). These tend to be support groups for chronic neurotic patients of for those who are involved in some crisis, such as bereavement. The GP is usually responsible for selecting the patients and establishing the groups, but after that they are often conducted by health visitors or social workers. I know of no assessment of the value of such groups but it would seem a realistic and cost-effective way of providing support for large numbers of patients and worthy of further evaluation.

THIRD FILTER — REFERRAL TO THE PSYCHIATRIC SERVICES

GPs refer 5.5% of those they identify as psychiatrically ill to the psychiatric services (HMSO 1979). A further 4.4% are referred to other medical services for investigation. There is some evidence that men are more likely to be referred than women, probably reflecting the perceived impact of psychiatric disorder on the traditional breadwinner. Younger patients pass through the filter more readily than older patients, as do those of higher socioeconomic status (perhaps because they request referral themselves), but the role of marital status is unclear. However, the sex difference in the USA is reversed. Illness variables include seriousness, especially psychosis (19.1% referred compared with 5.5% of all diagnoses; HMSO 1979) and those expressing suicidal thoughts.

A recent study of 250 patients newly referred to the mental health services in south Manchester (Gater & Goldberg 1991) shows that almost two-thirds were referred directly by their GPs, non-medical sources accounting for only 2% of new cases.

Since many patients who are psychiatrically ill are not referred, Fahy (1974b) carried out a prospective study to examine the characteristics of those depressed patients who were referred from general practice. The most important characteristics of those who were referred promptly to the psychiatric services were male sex and symptoms of subjective retardation and of hopelessness. Of the depressed patients, 31% were referred to physicians and surgeons and 5% were admitted by them. Those patients were characterised by physical stress or illness coinciding with, or shortly preceding, the onset of depressive symptoms. Those who were actually admitted to medical or surgical beds were all severely depressed and markedly agitated. This study highlights the fact that many patients

with psychiatric illnesses are usually referred to physicians and surgeons because the GP wants to exclude a physical cause for the somatic symptoms with which they present. Shepherd et al (1966) found between 2 and 10%, depending on the psychiatric diagnosis, were referred to a non-psychiatric consultant.

What are the GP variables? Older doctors are more likely to refer than their younger colleagues; those in urban practice more than rural; and those in single-handed practice more than those in group practices. GPs who have a high detection rate for psychiatric morbidity also have high referral rates per 1000 patients at risk, although they all refer about 5% of those they identify.

The availability of psychiatric services plays only a small part in the shaping of referral patterns of minor psychiatric disorders, although where a choice of psychiatric facilities exists there is some evidence that patients with certain diagnoses are differentially referred (Brown et al 1988, Low & Pullen 1988).

Kessel (1963) advised that GPs should refer according to three principles: diagnosis, severity of illness, and failure of treatment. What reasons do GPs give for referral to a psychiatrist? The most common reason given in a study by Kaeser & Cooper (1971) was failure of response to his own treatment (46% of referrals to the consultant clinic and 33% of referrals to the emergency clinic). In 30–40% of cases, pressure from the patient or his relatives was the main reason and in these the GP would not otherwise have referred the patient. Younger GPs report greater pressure from patients for referral than do their older colleagues (Armstrong et al 1991). Behavioural disturbance or serious social difficulties were the reason for referral to the emergency clinic in 50% of cases and the assessment of suicidal risk in 30%. There were few cases where the GP stated that he wanted advice about how best to treat the patient himself (Kaeser & Cooper 1971). In a more recent study (Pullen & Yellowlees 1985), 18% of GPs gave no specific reason for making the referral.

Often, GPs refer patients for behavioural or social reasons and, as psychiatrists, we may feel this is inappropriate. It is sometimes difficult for hospital-based staff to realise how worrying it is for a GP to cope with a patient who is suicidal or violent without being able to provide observation and round-the-clock care as we can in hospital. In fact (see below), the patients with social crises and urgent problems are the ones who appear to benefit most from psychiatric services and yet the ones we feel most reluctant to deal with. As far as the elective non-urgent referrals are concerned the GP frequently does not have a clear idea of what the psychiatrist has to offer, and it is difficult therefore for him to refer patients whom all psychiatrists would consider appropriate. Some psychiatrists are keen to see neurotic patients suitable for psychotherapy while others wish to see only the frankly psychotic. It would seem advisable for individual psychiatrists to work out with their referring GPs the type of cases they would like to be referred and the type of patients with which the GP feels most in need of help. The growth of 'sectorisation' and closer links between individual psychiatrists and GPs (see below) should aid this dialogue.

In fact there is no firm evidence to suggest that referral to a psychiatric out-patient department results in an improvement in prognosis. Davies (cited by Kaeser & Cooper 1971) compared the outcome of referred patients with those treated by the GP himself and found no significant difference. A study in London of the outcome of psychiatric referrals did not produce encouraging results (Hopkins & Cooper 1969); 18% were not seen, 29% subsequently lapsed from treatment and altogether 57% were rated as unimproved at the end of their period of specialist care. The results were most favourable for patients referred because of acute symptoms, social crises or other urgent reasons; least so for patients with chronic problems who had been referred for psychotherapy and long-term readjustment. Such results clearly suggest that referral to a psychiatric out-patient clinic does not result in as much benefit to the patient as we like to imagine, although it may establish new consulting patterns. Curran & Pullen (1990) found that frequent general practice attenders significantly reduced their consultation rate in the 6 months after psychiatric referral.

Given that the outcome of referral is rather disappointing, what do GPs and patients feel about the contribution made by hospital psychiatrists? Kaeser & Cooper (1971) studied consumer satisfaction in those referred to hospital. Just over half the GPs found referral helpful, as did the patients. Gask (1986) studied a cohort of 30 new out-patients who were seen once only by a psychiatrist. The GPs were happy with the single consultation for 22 of the patients; however, only half of the patients had consulted their GP in the 3 months after the hospital visit and most of the treatments recommended by the psychiatrists were not carried out by the GPs.

Very few studies have identified the characteristics of patients who are most likely to benefit from psychiatric referral. One such, by Murphy (1976), compares the outcome of neurotics who were referred to hospital with those who were not. At follow-up 1 year later he found a subgroup of patients who had improved with specialist care and not at all without it; these were introverts who had not taken psychotropics nor had time off work. But really it is not possible to come to any conclusions on the basis of one small study. Research into this area is very limited and more work needs to be done before clear guidelines can be given about which patients are likely to benefit from psychiatric referral and which would do best if looked after by the GP himself. There are disadvantages to the patient in being referred, of being labelled 'ill' and 'psychiatric', and these disadvantages need to be offset by some clear advantage to the patient if referral is to be justified.

The recent implementation of a new contract for GPs in the National Health Service, and the advent of so-called 'budget holding' practices empowered to 'buy' services for their patients may alter referral patterns. Whereas the GP may be charged for an out-patient appointment with a psychiatrist, referral to a community psychiatric nurse will be free. As emergency cases will also attract no fee, there may be a temptation for these GPs to refer a higher proportion of their patients as 'emergencies'.

COMMUNICATION BETWEEN GPS AND PSYCHIATRISTS

In many centres the only contact between psychiatrists and GPs is by letter and many psychiatrists never meet the GPs who refer them patients. The need for clear communication in medicine is often emphasised, but little attention has been given to communication between doctors. Two studies looked at GP referral letters to routine out-patient clinics and an emergency clinic (de Alarcon & Hodson 1964, Birley & Heine 1971) and found that only 23% of letters mentioned current treatment. Williams & Wallace (1974) considered two-way communication between psychiatrists and GPs and concluded that 'the standard of communication in letters needs to be improved on both sides'.

A recent study of two-way communication looked at 120 referral letters sent to psychiatric clinics in 1973 and 1983 and the psychiatrists' replies (Pullen & Yellowlees 1985). The 'key items' that GPs identified as being of greatest importance for the psychiatrist to include in a report on out-patients were: (1) diagnosis; (2) treatment recommended; (3) follow-up arrangements; (4) prognosis; and (5) a concise explanation of the condition (a formulation). The length of psychiatrists' letters ranged from 1–4 sides of A4 paper and consultants' letters were significantly shorter than those written by registrars, although the average score for the inclusion of 'key items' was similar (approximately 3.5 per letter). While over 88% of letters included the first three key items, in 1983 only 27% mentioned prognosis and 60% a concise explanation of the case. A linked study (Yellowlees & Pullen 1984) found that GPs would prefer psychiatrists to write a letter of less than one and a quarter sides of A4 and like headings to be used.

Perhaps the best advice on letter writing comes from a small book on writing and talking about patients. Kessel (1984) sets out five elements of good communication: first, the communicator must himself acquire the information that he has to pass on; second, he must not be too lazy or too busy to convey it; third, he must keep in mind exactly what he needs to tell; fourth, he should always consider what the recipient will want to know; last, the door should always be kept open for further communication.

The psychiatrist needs to understand the realities of general practice. Each GP will receive many letters per day from specialists. These letters will be scanned and then filed, only to be seen again once the patient is in the surgery for his next short (5–7 minute) consultation. Concise letters with important information highlighted by headings will be much more effective than long rambling letters in which key information will be difficult to find.

Another issue that has been studied is the case summary. Often when patients are discharged from hospital, GPs are sent a copy of a case summary that is designed primarily for the hospital casenotes. Most people agree that this is a discourteous form of communication and far from ideal as a means of obtaining the cooperation of a colleague who is sharing the patient's management. Many GPs find the case summary valuable because it acts as such for their own notes, but in addition they do need a letter which contains the same five 'key items' of information mentioned above.

The Access to Health Records Act (1990) which came into operation in 1991 gives patients the right of access to information about themselves recorded in medical casenotes. This means that every letter to a GP, and indeed anything written in the casenotes, must be written in the knowledge that the patient might well wish to read it. Thus, speculative and judgemental comments and jargon must be avoided. It is also a requirement of the Act that information from third parties should not be available to the patient without that person's consent. It is to be hoped that letters will become more comprehensible for both patient and GP. One recent pilot study looked at a record of shared care to be held by the patient (Essex et al 1990). Eighty-four patients in south London in touch with either a community psychiatric nurse or psychiatrist as well as their GP and suffering from a chronic major psychiatric illness held shared care records over an 18 month period. Patients found the records very acceptable and were enthusiastic about their use. They valued being consulted about what was recorded and found the record of their treatment and progress useful. However, most of the local psychiatrists approached regarded the scheme with great misgivings, even those who were already working closely with GPs. The authors concluded, rather sadly, that the obstacles to further development of the shared records related to the attitudes, perceptions and anxieties of the doctors, nurses and managers.

THE RELATIONSHIP BETWEEN PSYCHIATRISTS AND GPS

There is a debate about whether or not psychiatrists should take over the care of a greater proportion of the psychiatrically ill patients at primary care level, that is, make the third filter more permeable. The WHO (1973, 1983) recommended the GP as being the best person to deal with psychiatric illness at primary care level, the reasons being that psychiatric morbidity in primary care is a mixture of psychological symptoms and physical illness, and the GP is in a better position than the psychiatrist to deal with these diverse problems and more able to provide long-term follow-up. It would seem best, therefore, for the role of the primary care physician to be strengthened rather than for the psychiatrist to take over more of his cases.

A number of situations already exist where face-to-face contact could occur, giving opportunity for advice or training. The consultant domiciliary visit provides one such opportunity. Unfortunately, busy GPs and psychiatrists seldom find it easy to meet in a patient's house for such a visit. So the opportunity for the GP to see the psychiatrist at work and to confirm or change his own clinical opinion or style is lost. In some areas psychiatric emergency calls are met by a hospital-based 'crisis intervention' team, which potentially gives the psychiatric staff another opportunity to work hand in hand with the GP. The theory behind this approach is that if an individual is faced with a sudden and severe stress, trained help during the early stages of the 'crisis' may speed resolution and prevent the development of chronic symptoms or the need for hospital admission. The GP welcomes this type of consultation. He is always involved in crisis intervention himself and the visit of the specialist team to his patient's home gives the psychiatrist a better understanding of the complex of social and family problems with which the GP deals and should result in a management plan which is more relevant than that which might be obtained from an out-patient clinic.

Another way in which communication can be improved is by each psychiatrist serving a defined area and getting to know a manageable number of GPs. This is becoming the most common way of organising psychiatric services, with the psychiatrist receiving requests from a group of GPs for domiciliary visits, out-patient consultations, and day hospital and in-patient admissions. A growing number of psychiatrists make regular visits to primary care premises. Strathdee & Williams (1984) conducted a postal questionnaire study of all consultant psychiatrists in England and Wales. They found that 19% spent some time in primary care settings, although there was considerable regional variation. A similar survey in Scotland reported that 56% of consultant psychiatrists work in this way (Pullen & Yellowlees 1988).

Tyrer (1984) reports on a study which investigates the feasibility of replacing hospital out-patient clinics with psychiatrists consulting in primary care. Five clinics were set up to serve a population of 78200. There was a corresponding reduction in out-patient clinic sessions, but despite this there was a net increase of one session per week devoted to the care of this population. The five clinics were visited at varying intervals (once a week to once a month) by the psychiatrist, depending on the size of the catchment area. He found that the patients preferred the service, that the psychiatrist saw a higher proportion of neurotic disorders and adjustment reactions than in the hospital out-patient clinic, and that there was a greater decrease in the number of hospital admissions from the study catchment area than from the rest of the catchment area of Mapperley Hospital (Tyrer et al 1984). Unfortunately, this result is confounded by the fact that a day hospital was opened at Mapperley Hospital during the study period and the admission rate to this day hospital from the study area was greater than the admission rate from the rest of Mapperley's catchment area.

There have been some fears that closer contact with GPs may result in increased numbers of referrals to psychiatric services. If GPs referred 7.5% of their psychiatric cases instead of 5%, which is a fairly small shift of their current practice, the workload of the psychiatric services would increase by 50%! Do GPs refer a different range of problems to clinics in different settings? Two recent studies have addressed this question. A case–register study (Low & Pullen 1988) looked at all new out-patients (12 741) referred to Edinburgh general psychiatrists over a 5 year period. Primary care clinics dealt with a larger proportion of patients receiving the label 'adjustment reaction' and 'no psychiatric illness' when compared with general or psychiatric hospital clinics. The primary care clinics also saw proportionately more neurotic and fewer psychotic cases than the psychiatric hospital clinics, and fewer psychotic patients than the general hospital psychiatric clinics. The domiciliary visits contained a higher proportion of psychotic patients than any of the other settings. Brown et al (1988) compared referrals to primary care and hospital out-patient clinics from two south London general practices. Women in all diagnostic groups were preferentially referred to the primary care clinics where attendence rates on first and subsequent appointments were substantially higher than at the hospital clinics. Most studies suggest that patients are less likely to default from attendance at clinics in primary care. One prospective study has failed to find any difference between a health centre and a psychiatric hospital clinic (Zegleman 1988).

Although there has been an enormous increase in the number of psychiatrists visiting health centres on a regular basis during the past 15 years, Creed & Marks (1989) argue that the specific aims of such visits are not clear from the literature. Most psychiatrists visit health centres to hold conventional out-patient clinics in a setting close to the patient's home (the 'shifted out-patient' model). That is, the psychiatrist aims to improve secondary care by providing it in the primary care setting. Mitchell (1985) has warned that visiting a health centre does not necessarily improve liaison between psychiatrist and GP and is not synonymous with the 'liaison–attachment' model. This model involves regular meetings between psychiatrist and GPs. Patients about to be referred and those recently assessed are discussed, particular clinical problems are explored and the management plans of specific patients may be jointly planned. Creed & Marks conclude that their liaison–attachment scheme is cost effective but that further evaluations are required. Another model described by Mitchell (1985) is the 'conjoint consultation in the health centre' where the psychiatrist joins the patient and GP in the GP's consulting room, by prior agreement of the patient, to facilitate where GP and patient feel 'stuck'.

Even where individual psychiatrists have set out merely to shift their out-patient clinic into a conveniently placed health centre, by sharing facilities with GPs they frequently become involved in other activities such as supporting other primary health care staff, formal teaching sessions and case conferences, and discussing patients that they have not personally seen (Pullen & Yellowlees 1988). The general view, both of psychiatrists and GPs, is that working more closely together could improve the standard of care and reduce hospital admissions (Strathdee 1987). But is there any evidence to support this view? Williams & Balestrieri (1989) used data from the study by Strathdee & Williams (1984) and compared them with figures on psychiatric admissions in England and Wales. Within the limitations of the methodology (the less than perfect response rate to the original questionnaire, the accuracy of admission data and the linearity assumption inherent in their use of regression coefficients), the results are clear: in those parts of the country where there has been a greater increase in general practice-based psychiatry, there has also been a greater decline in admissions of non-psychotic patients.

A final suggestion for improving communication and understanding between psychiatrists and GPs, and thereby improving the care of the mentally ill, is that each should do the other's job for a while during training. A 3 year compulsory vocational training programme has now been established in general practice. In many, but not all, schemes psychiatry is part of the rotation for one of the 6 month training periods. Zander (1982) warns that training in a psychiatric hospital in a post not designed for GPs might be counterproductive, in that it would ill-equip the trainee for the type of disorders he will have to deal with as a GP. This is a valid criticism of the present system where many general practice vocational trainees will occupy posts normally filled by a psychiatric trainee. But in spite of this deficiency the training goes some way towards improving the GP's skills and increasing his understanding of what psychiatric services can provide. It would improve matters further if the psychiatrist in training had to do a mandatory period in general practice, thereby giving him first-hand experience of the GP's role in the community. Two psychiatric training schemes are at present experimenting with such a rotation into general practice.

PREVENTIVE PSYCHIATRY IN GENERAL PRACTICE

The possibility that psychiatric disorders might be prevented by counselling patients at times when they are under stress is a plausible one and there is some evidence to support this idea. Caplan (1981) reports how cognitive guidance and social support of patients can help them tolerate stress without increased risk of physical or mental illness. He cites how surgical patients who received anticipatory guidance and encouragement needed less medication postoperatively and were discharged from hospital significantly earlier than a control group who received no such guidance. Widows and widowers under the age of 45 years who were given the opportunity to anticipate their bereavement were subsequently not as distressed after their spouse's death as those who were not given this opportunity (Glick et al 1974). Translating these findings into practicalities, the Royal College of General Practitioners (1981) has produced a report, *Prevention of Psychiatric Disorders in General Practice*. This recommends that, with the aim of preventing psychiatric illness, the primary care team should provide anticipatory guidance and social support at times of psychosocial change in patients' lives. Although common sense suggests that this approach may prevent psychiatric illness, there is as yet little evidence that it actually does so. Even if such support was shown to be of value, it would be impracticable to provide it for all potential recipients. Every GP has around 2000 patients and stressful life events are common. He could not conceivably counsel and support them all. So before this report could be translated into action, as well as establishing whether or not counselling does prevent psychiatric illness in people under stress, it would also be necessary to have a clear idea of who was most likely to become ill so that a high-risk group could be identified.

Although in our present state of knowledge it is not feasible to set up a prophylactic service, the idea of being able to prevent psychiatric illness is an attractive one and worthy of further investigation.

REFERENCES

Armstrong D, Fry J, Armstrong P 1991 Doctors' perceptions of pressure from patients for referral. British Medical Journal 302: 1186

Ashurst P 1982 Counselling in general practice. In: Clare W A, Lader M (eds) Psychiatry and general practice. Academic Press, London

Bebbington P, Hurry J, Tennant C, Sturt E, Wing J K 1981 Epidemiology of mental disorders in Camberwell. Psychological Medicine 11: 561

Birley J L T, Heine B E 1971 The psychiatric emergency clinic: an inquiry into the process of referral and disposal. Cited by Kaeser A C, Cooper B 1971 The psychiatric patient, the general practitioner, and the outpatient clinic. Psychological Medicine 1: 312

Blacker C V R, Clare A W 1987 Depressive disorder in primary care. British Journal of Psychiatry 150: 737

Blackburn I M, Bishop S, Glen A I M, Whalley L J, Christie J E 1981 The efficacy of cognitive therapy in depression: a treatment trial using cognitive therapy and pharmachotherapy, each alone and in combination. British Journal of Psychiatry 139: 181

Blashki T G, Mowbray R, Davies B 1971 Controlled trial of amitriptyline in general practice. British Medical Journal i: 133

Brown G W, Harris T 1978 Social origins of depression. Tavistock, London

Brown R M A, Strathdee G, Christies-Brown J R W, Robinson P H 1988 A comparison of referrals to primary-care and hospital out-patient clinics. British Journal of Psychiatry 153: 168

Buchan I C, Richardson I M 1973 Time study of consultations in general practice. Scottish Health Service studies 27. Scottish Home and Health Department, Edinburgh

Burvill P W, Knuiman M W 1983 The influence of minor psychiatric morbidity on consulting rates to general practitioners. Psychological Medicine 13: 635

Caplan G 1981 Mastery of stress: psychological aspects. American Journal of Psychiatry 138: 413

Cassidy S, Hendry J 1987 Fatal toxicity of antidepressants in overdose. British Medical Journal 295: 1021

Cooper B 1972 Clinical and social aspects of chronic neurosis. Proceedings of the Royal Society of Medicine 65: 509

Cooper B, Fry J, Kalton G 1969 A longitudinal study of psychiatric morbidity in a general practice population. British Journal of Preventive and Social Medicine 23: 210

Cooper B, Harwin B G, Delpha C, Shepherd M 1975 Mental health care in the community: an evaluative study. Psychological Medicine 5: 372

Corney R H 1984 The effectiveness of attached social workers in the management of depressed female patients in general practice. Psychological Medicine Monograph suppl 6

Creed F, Marks B 1989 Liaison psychiatry in general practice: a comparison of the liaison-attachment scheme and shifted outpatient clinic models. Journal of the Royal College of General Practitioners 39: 514

Curran S M, Pullen I M 1990 Audit of a psychiatric liaison service — the value of general practice casenotes. Psychiatric Bulletin 14: 727

de Alarcon J, Hodson M H 1964 Value of the general practitioner's letter. A further study in medical communication. British Medical Journal ii: 435

Dean C, Surtees P G, Sashidharan S P 1983 Comparison of research diagnostic systems in an Edinburgh community sample. British Journal of Psychiatry 142: 247

Department of Health and Social Security 1977 The role of psychologists in the health services. Report of the sub-committee. Her Majesty's Stationery Office, London

Downing R W, Rickels K 1974 Mixed anxiety and depression: fact or myth? Archives of General Psychiatry 30: 312

Dunn G 1985 Records of psychiatric morbidity in general practice: the national morbidity surveys. Psychological Medicine 15: 223

Dunn G 1986 Patterns of psychiatric diagnosis in general practice: the second national morbidity survey. Psychological Medicine 16: 573

Dunn G, Skuse D 1981 The natural history of depression in general practice: stochastic models. Psychological Medicine 11: 755

Eastwood M R, Trevelyan M H 1972 Relationship between physical and psychiatric disorder. Psychological Medicine 2: 263

Essex B, Doig R, Renshaw J 1990 Pilot study of records of shared care for people with mental illnesses. British Medical Journal 300: 1442

Fahy T J 1974a Pathways of specialist referral of depressed patients from general practice. British Journal of Psychiatry 124: 231

Fahy T J 1974b Depression in hospital and general practice: a direct clinical comparison. British Journal of Psychiatry 124: 240

Finlay-Jones R, Brown G W, Duncan-Jones P, Harris T, Murphy E L, Prudo R 1980 Depression and anxiety in the community: replicating the diagnosis of a case. Psychological Medicine 10: 445.

Freeling P, Rao B M, Paykel E S, Sireling L I, Burton R H 1985 Unrecognised depression in general practice. British Medical Journal 290: 1880

Gask L 1986 What happens when psychiatric out-patients are seen once only? British Journal of Psychiatry 148: 663

Gater R, Goldberg D 1991 Pathways to psychiatric care in South Manchester. British Journal of Psychiatry 159: 90

Glick I O, Weiss R S, Parkes C M 1974 The first year of bereavement. Wiley, New York

Goldberg D P 1972 The detection of psychiatric illness by questionnaire. Maudsley monograph 21. Oxford University Press, London

Goldberg D P, Blackwell B 1970 Psychiatric illness in general practice: a detailed study using a new method of case identification. British Medical Journal 2: 439

Goldberg D P, Huxley P 1980 Mental illness in the community. Tavistock, London

Goldberg D P, Huxley P 1992 Common mental disorders. A bio-social model. Tavistock/Routledge, London

Goldberg D, Williams P 1988 A user's guide to the General Health Questionnaire. NFER, Windsor

Goldberg D P, Cooper B, Eastwood M R, Kedward H B, Shepherd M 1970 A standardized psychiatric interview for use in community surveys. British Journal of Preventive and Social Medicine 24: 18

Goldberg D P, Kay C, Thompson L 1976 Psychiatric morbidity in general practice and the community. Psychological Medicine 6: 565

Goldberg D, Steele J, Smith C, Spivey L 1980 Training family practice residents to recognise psychiatric disturbances. Final report, contract number ADAMHA 278-78-003 (DB). Department of Psychiatry, Biometrics and Family Practice, Medical University of South Carolina

Henderson S 1981 Social relationships, adversity and neurosis: an analysis of prospective observations. British Journal of Psychiatry 138: 391

Henderson S, Byrne D G, Duncan-Jones P, Adcock S, Scott R, Steele D P 1978 Social bonds in the epidemiology of neurosis: a preliminary communication. British Journal of Psychiatry 132: 463

Henderson S, Duncan-Jones P, Byrne D G, Scott R, Adcock S 1979 Psychiatric disorders in Canberra. Acta

Psychiatrica Scandinavica 60: 355

HMSO 1979 Morbidity statistics for general practice — second national study 1971–1972. Studies on medical population subjects 36. Her Majesty's Stationery Office, London

Hopkins P, Cooper B 1969 Psychiatric referral from a general practice. British Journal of Psychiatry 115: 1163

Huxley P J, Goldberg D P, Maguire G P, Kincey V A 1979 The prediction of the course of minor psychiatric disorders. British Journal of Psychiatry 135: 535

Ingham J G, Miller P M 1976 The determinants of illness declaration. Journal of Psychosomatic Research 20: 309

Jenkins R, Smeeton N, Shepherd M 1985 Classification of mental disorder in primary care. Psychological Medicine Monograph suppl 12: 1

Johnson D A W 1973 Treatment of depression in general practice. British Medical Journal 2: 18

Johnson D A W, Mellor V 1977 The severity of depression in patients treated in general practice. Journal of the Royal College of General Practitioners 27: 419

Johnstone A, Goldberg D 1976 Psychiatric screening in general practice: a controlled trial. Lancet i: 605

Kaeser A C, Cooper B 1971 The psychiatric patient, the general practitioner, and the outpatient clinic: an operational study and a review. Psychological Medicine 1: 312

Kessel N 1963 Who ought to see a psychiatrist? Lancet i: 1092

Kessel N 1965 The neurotic in general practice. Practitioner 194: 636

Kessel N 1984 Communication between GPs and hospital doctors: a hospital consultant's view. In: Walton J, McLachlan G (eds) Doctor to doctor. Writing and talking about patients. Nuffield Provincial Hospitals Trust, London

Koranyi E K 1979 Morbidity and rate of undiagnosed physical illnesses in a psychiatric clinic population. Archives of General Psychiatry 36: 414

Lader M 1975 The social implications of psychotropic drugs. Journal of the Royal College of General Practitioners 95(b): 304

Low C P, Pullen I M 1988 Psychiatric clinics in different settings: a case register study. British Journal of Psychiatry 153: 243

Mann A H, Jenkins R, Belsey E 1981 Outcome of neurotic illnesses in general practice. Psychological Medicine 11: 535

Marks J N, Goldberg D P, Hillier V F 1979 Determinants of the ability of general practitioners to detect psychiatric illness. Psychological Medicine 9: 337

Mitchell A R K 1985 Psychiatrists in primary health care settings. British Journal of Psychiatry 147: 371

Murphy H M B 1976 Which neuoses need specialist care? Canadian Medical Association Journal 115: 540

Murray J, Dunn G, Williams P, Tarnopolsky A 1981 Factors affecting the consumption of psychotropic drugs. Psychological Medicine 11: 557

Paykel E S, Mangen S P, Griffith J H et al 1982 Community psychiatric nursing for neurotic patients: a controlled trial. British Journal of Psychiatry 140: 573

Paykel E S, Freeling P, Hollyman J A 1988 Are tricyclic antidepressants useful for mild depression? A placebo controlled trial. Pharmacopsychiatry 21: 15

Pullen I M, Yellowlees A J 1985 Is communication improving between general practitioners and psychiatrists?

British Medical Journal 290: 31

Pullen I M, Yellowlees A J 1988 Scottish psychiatrists in primary health-care settings: a silent majority. British Journal of Psychiatry 153: 663

RCGP 1981 Prevention of psychiatric disorders in general practice. Royal College of General Practitioners, London

Royal College of General Practitioners' Research Committee 1958 The continuing observation and recording of morbidity. Journal of the College of General Practitioners 1: 107

Regier D A, Burns B J, Burke J D et al 1982 A proposed classification of social problems and psychological symptoms for inclusion in a classification of health problems. In: Lipkin M, Gulbinat W, Jupko K (eds) Psychosocial factors affecting health. Praeger, New York

Robertson N C 1979 Variations in referral pattern to the psychiatric services by general practitioners. Psychological Medicine 9: 355

Shepherd M, Cooper B, Brown A C, Kalton G W 1966 Psychiatric illness in general practice. Oxford University Press, Oxford

Sireling L I, Freeling P, Paykel E S, Rao B M 1985 Depression in general practice: clinical features and comparison with outpatients. British Journal of Psychiatry 147: 119

Skuse D, Williams P 1984 Screening for psychiatric disease in general practice. Psychological Medicine 14: 365

Spitzer R L, Endicott J, Robins E 1978 Research diagnostic criteria. Rationale and reliability. Archives of General Psychiatry 35: 773

Strathdee G 1987 Primary care–psychiatric interaction — a British perspective. General Hospital Psychiatry 6: 69

Strathdee G, Williams P 1984 A survey of psychiatrists in primary care: the silent growth of a new service. Journal of the Royal College of General Practitioners 34: 615

Thomson J, Rankin H, Ashcroft G W, Yates C M, McQueen J K, Cummings S W 1982 The treatment of depression in general practice: a comparison of L-tryptophan, amitriptyline and a combination of L-tryptophan and amitriptyline with placebo. Psychological Medicine 12: 741

Tyrer P 1984 Psychiatric clinics in general practice. British Journal of Psychiatry 145: 9

Tyrer P, Seivewright N, Wollerton S 1984 General practice psychiatric clinics: impact on psychiatric services. British Journal of Psychiatry 145: 15

Watson J M, Barber J H 1981 Depressive illness in general practice: a pilot study. Health Bulletin (Scotland) 39: 112

Watts C A 1970 A long term follow-up of mental hospital admissions from a rural community. Journal of the Royal College of General Practitioners 20: 79

Weissman M M, Myers J K 1978 Psychiatric disorders in a US Community. Acta Psychiatrica Scandinavica 62: 99

WHO 1973 Psychiatry and primary medical care. World Health Organization, Copenhagen

WHO 1978 Mental disorders: glossary and guide to their classification in accordance with the ninth revision of the international classification of diseases. World Health Organization, Copenhagen

Williams P Balestrieri 1989 Psychiatric clinics in general practice — do they reduce admissions? British Journal of Psychiatry 154: 67

Williams P, Wallace B B 1974 General practitioners and psychiatrists — do they communicate? British Medical Journal i: 505

Williams P, Tarnopolsky A, Hand D, Shepherd M 1986 Minor pyschiatric morbidity and general practice consultation: the West London survey. Psychological Medicine Monograph Suppl. 9: 1

Wing J K, Cooper J E, Sartorius N 1974 The measurement and classification of psychiatric symptoms. Cambridge University Press, London

Wing J K, Bebbington P, Hurry J, Tennant C 1981 The prevalence in the general population of disorders familiar to psychiatrists in hospital practice. In: Wing J K, Bebbington P, Robins L N (eds) What is a case? Grant McIntyre, London

WONCA (World Organisation of National Colleges, Academies and Academic Associations of General Practitioners/Family Physicians) 1979 International classification of health problems in primary care (1979 revision, ICHPPC-2). Oxford University Press, Oxford

Wooff K, Goldberg D P, Fryers T 1986 Patients in receipt of community psychiatric nursing care in Salford 1976–1982. Psychological Medicine 16: 407

Wright J H, Bell R A, Kuhn C C, Rush E A, Patel N, Redmon J E 1980 Depression in family practice patients. Southern Medical Journal 73: 1031

Yellowlees A J, Pullen I M 1984 Communication between psychiatrists and general practitioners. What sort of letters should psychiatrists write? Health Bulletin (Scotland) 42: 285

Zander L 1982 Management of psychiatric illness in general practice. In: Clare W A, Lader M (eds) Psychiatry and general practice. Academic Press, London

Zegleman F E 1988 Psychiatric clinics in different settings — default rates. Health Bulletin (Scotland) 46: 286

34. Psychiatry in general medicine

G. G. Lloyd

INTRODUCTION

The development of psychiatric units in general hospitals has enabled psychiatry to become more closely integrated with general medicine, thereby ending over a century of geographical and intellectual isolation. More psychiatrists are now able to contribute to the management of patients with those psychiatric disorders which particularly confront clinicians in other medical specialties (Lloyd 1991). Collaborative research studies have shown that there is a high prevalence of psychiatric disorder in medical and surgical patients, much of it unrecognised and therefore untreated. A greater awareness of these problems has increased demands for psychiatric input to clinical care.

This area of practice is usually referred to as liaison psychiatry, an imperfect term but one which emphasises the links which psychiatry has with other specialties. It covers the whole spectrum of psychiatric disorders and employs all the therapeutic approaches available to the general psychiatrist. However, the pattern of presenting symptoms often differs quite strikingly from those encountered in psychiatric hospital practice. There are fewer cases of psychotic illnesses and proportionately more of affective, organic and somatising disorders.

Britain has lagged behind other countries, most notably the USA, in the development of liaison services. American psychiatry has a longer tradition of collaboration with other medical disciplines, much of this arising from the growth of psychosomatic medicine in the 1930s. At that time the aetiology of many physical illnesses was thought to be largely psychological and the concept of a specific group of psychosomatic illnesses was developed. These included peptic ulcer, essential hypertension, bronchial asthma and ulcerative colitis. Psychological methods of treatment, particularly interpretive psychotherapy, were widely regarded as the treatments of choice. Evidence to support the assumptions of psychological causation was never provided and, in retrospect, the aspirations of the psychosomatic movement can be seen to have been overambitious. The view that there is a distinct category of psychosomatic illnesses has now been abandoned. Nevertheless, psychosomatic medicine established a base in the general hospital from which present psychiatry services have developed.

One of the distinctive features of liaison psychiatry is that clinical responsibility usually has to be shared with another clinician. There have been successful examples of jointly run clinics for certain groups of patients, including those with pain and malignant disease. The clinical work of a liaison service should be coordinated by one senior psychiatrist, although several psychiatrists may develop areas of special interest; clinical psychologists, social workers and liaison nurses also have important contributions to make. The service should not be governed by the bureacracy of geographical sectors; nothing irritates a physician more than to be told he cannot make a referral to a particular psychiatrist because the patient does not live at an appropriate address.

A survey of the practice of liaison psychiatry in Britain found that there is considerable clinical, teaching and research activity (Mayou & Lloyd 1985). Most of the clinical work involves ward consultations in response to requests from other clinicians but several respondents claimed to have developed closer links with specific medical and surgical units. However, it seemed clear that services have grown haphazardly and are undertaken by general psychiatrists in addition to their other commitments. Lack of sufficient time means that many aspects of the work cannot be undertaken satisfactorily. Few districts have given any priority to the development of liaison psychiatry and there are only a handful of specifically designated liaison posts.

Descriptive accounts of individual services give an indication of the pattern of referrals. Thomas (1983) noted that approximately 30% of referrals were for the management of psychological reactions to physical illness and a similar number for unexplained physical symptoms. Fewer patients were referred for coincidental psychiatric disorder, cerebral complications of physical illness and abnormal behaviour producing physical illness. In the USA McKegney et al (1983) observed that the commonest diagnostic categories were adjustment disorder, organic mental disorder, alcohol and drug abuse and affective disorder. Depressive disorders and organic brain syndromes were also the commonest diagnoses in the series reported by Lipowski & Wolston (1981), the depressive disorders usually fulfilling DSM-III criteria for dysthymic disorder or adjustment disorder with depressed mood.

PREVALENCE AND RECOGNITION OF PSYCHIATRIC MORBIDITY

The reported prevalence of psychiatric disorder in medical and surgical patients varies widely according to the population studied and the criteria used (Mayou & Hawton 1986). Most studies have assessed patients on a single occasion and therefore do not clarify the evolution of psychological symptoms, nor their relationship to underlying physical illness. They have included patients whose psychiatric disorder accompanies physical illness together with those whose psychiatric disorder presents with somatic symptoms in the absence of organic pathology. These groups are quite different from one another and need to be considered separately. Early studies relied on unstandardised clinical interviews which did not control for interviewers' variability. The introduction of standardised assessments resulted in greater reliability. Studies based on questionnaires have reported much higher prevalence rates than those which have incorporated standardised psychiatric interviews. Almost certainly this reflects the inappropriate nature of some questionnaires for this type of population, largely because they include somatic items which generate many false positive scores. Existing questionnaires have nearly all been developed for use with patients with primary psychiatric illness. They need to be modified and restandardised when applied to medical populations; alternatively, use should be made of newer scales specifically developed for these patients. However, when suitable methods of assessment have been used they have consistently shown that the prevalence of psychiatric disorder in general hospital patients is substantially higher than in the community at large. Psychiatric disorder predisposes to a high utilisation of medical facilities (Fink 1990). This is due to several factors, including increased

susceptibility to physical illness, different forms of illness behaviour and the process of somatisation.

The difficulty encountered in diagnosing psychiatric illness in medical patients is one of the reasons why physicians and surgeons often underestimate all forms of psychiatric disorder in their patients. For example, a study of in-patients with neurological disorders assessed the prevalence of psychiatric morbidity as 39%. Subsequent scrutiny of the medical notes and discharge letters suggested that only just over a quarter of these cases had been recognised by the neurologists (Bridges & Goldberg 1984). Only a minority of patients recalled the neurologists having enquired about their mood and this was no more likely to have occurred in those with psychiatric disorders than in those without. These observations suggest that the neurologists were insensitive to psychological cues or that coexisting psychiatric illness was simply not considered. Several reasons were thought responsible for these omissions. Many patients regarded the neurologist as a doctor who only investigated physical causes for their symptoms; some did not wish to burden the doctor with their emotional problems; but others criticised the lack of privacy on the ward and complained that the doctor had not spent sufficient time with them.

An important implication of these observations is that many patients would benefit if their psychiatric morbidity were recognised and treated accordingly. Few would disagree with this sentiment. Psychiatric disorders are responsible for considerable distress and can be persistent, particularly in patients with a previous psychiatric history. Maguire et al (1980) have demonstrated the value of recognising psychological symptoms in women who have undergone a mastectomy for breast cancer. The women were randomly assigned either to a group receiving routine care or to a group receiving regular counselling from a specially trained nurse. Affective disorders were significantly less common in the counselled group 12–18 months after surgery, largely because the nurse had identified those women who were significantly depressed and had referred them for psychiatric treatment which had been effective.

How might better recognition be achieved? One approach which has been recommended is for the clinician to make use of one of the large number of questionnaires as a screening instrument (Goldberg 1985). None of these makes a psychiatric diagnosis but several provide a profile of scores in addition to a global score indicating the probability that a disorder is present. If a questionnaire is to be used in routine clinical work a validation study should be carried out so that the threshold score is adjusted to give best discrimination between cases and non-cases in the population concerned. The trouble with this approach is that it is mechanistic and it has not been shown to lead to effective intervention (Gater et al 1992). Ideally, psychiatric disorder should be detected on the basis of a clinical interview conducted by a doctor who is familiar with the types of psychiatric disorders likely to be seen in medical patients and sufficiently sensitive to respond to psychological cues and to enquire directly about emotional symptoms. The appropriate interviewing skills should be taught during undergraduate and postgraduate training, thereby enabling the doctor to recognise psychiatric illness more readily. The relevant cues are easier to detect if the interview is conducted in privacy rather than in a large, open medical ward.

PSYCHOPATHOLOGY OF PHYSICAL ILLNESS

There is convincing evidence that psychiatric and physical disorders occur together much more commonly than can be explained by chance. The nature of this relationship is a complicated one and several mechanisms have to be considered to understand the psychiatric morbidity of physically ill patients.

Antecedent psychiatric illness

The first possibility is that psychiatric illness may play a causal role in the development of various physical conditions. Evidence for this comes from observations concerning the mortality rates of psychiatric patients. Over a century ago it was established that patients in psychiatric hospitals had a much higher mortality rate than the general population. Tuberculosis and other infections accounted for much of this excess and almost certainly these illnesses resulted from the insanitary conditions in which the psychiatrically ill were treated rather than from psychiatric illness itself. Subsequent studies have continued to show an increased mortality rate but this has been steadily declining, particularly when reports have included data for out-patients.

Recent observations have shown an increased number of deaths from diseases of the nervous and circulatory systems. Sims (1978) has concluded that the mortality rate is increased two to three times for psychiatric in-patients and up to two-fold for out-patients. Even when suicidal and accidental deaths are excluded the mortality remains increased compared with the rest of the population. Two recent prospective studies have examined the links between psy-

chological symptoms and the development of ischaemic heart disease. Haines et al (1987) observed that phobic anxiety symptoms were predictive of fatal and non-fatal episodes of ischaemic heart disease while Appels & Mulder (1988) found that antecedent symptoms which were associated with subsequent myocardial infarction included low mood, insomnia, tiredness and loss of libido, this constellation being referred to as 'vital exhaustion'.

The premature mortality of psychiatrically ill patients may be explained via a number of indirect links, particularly smoking, alcohol and drug toxicity. It is not clear whether psychiatric illness itself predisposes to physical morbidity. Some evidence to suggest that it does comes from the work of Vaillant (1979), who has shown an association between poor mental health and subsequent physical disease in a cohort of previously healthy men even when the effects of smoking, alcohol, obesity and other factors had been taken into account.

Other psychological factors, apart from psychiatric illness, have been claimed to affect physical health. Unexpected psychological stresses, especially natural disasters, have often been reported to predispose to sudden death. Systematic research in this field has tended to show an excess of stressful life events occurring during the weeks prior to a number of acute physical illnesses (Creed 1985) and Murphy & Brown (1980) have claimed that the association between life events and the onset of physical illness is mediated by an intervening psychiatric illness, usually depression. Life stresses also influence the reporting of symptoms and make it more likely that medical treatment is sought for conditions which would otherwise be endured.

There has been renewed interest in the role of personality factors. The best known work in this area concerns the influence of 'Type A behaviour' on the development of coronary artery disease. This concept, first proposed by the American cardiologists Friedman & Rosenman (1959), applies to a pattern of behaviour characterised by aggressiveness, hostility, a sense of time urgency and a competitive striving for achievement. At least three prospective studies have shown it to be a risk factor for the development of various forms of coronary heart disease, including myocardial infarction, but other studies have failed to support these claims. Subsequent work has shown that modification of type A behaviour using techniques derived from cognitive therapy is followed by a reduction of the re-infarction rate in patients who have already experienced one or more episodes of myocardial infarction (Friedman et al 1984). Evidence has also been presented to suggest that cancer is linked to a particular personality profile, sometimes known as type C, characterised by emotional suppression, compliance, conformity, stoicism and unassertiveness (Cull 1990). Coping style may also influence the prognosis of cancer. Greer et al (1979) have shown that the outcome of treatment for breast cancer was significantly better for women who responded with denial or 'fighting spirit' than for women who adopted an attitude of stoicism or hopelessness.

Psychological consequences of physical illness

Some degree of psychological adjustment is required in all illnesses except the very trivial. Unpleasant somatic symptoms affect the patient's lifestyle, especially the ability to work and enjoy leisure activities. Most people acknowledge the need to modify their lives temporarily in accordance with the demands of their illness and the ensuing changes in behaviour are usually adaptive in the sense that they increase the prospects of recovery and resumption of former activities. Minor mood changes are common but they are not usually distressing in themselves nor do they interfere with overall adjustment. In clinical practice it can be difficult to decide when the psychological reaction to illness is pathological. There is considerable variability between observers and decisions are often influenced by the interviewer's disposition to regard as normal any symptom he considers understandable in the presence of physical disease. This is a highly subjective phenomenon. Studies which have employed quantitative methods of assessment have shown that the severity of symptoms is continuously distributed and there is no clear separation to allow precise case definition. Even in those cases where there is general agreement that the psychological response is pathological there is no consensus about the diagnostic categories to be used. This is largely a result of the fact that psychiatric nosology has been derived from observations on patients with primary psychiatric disorders and only recently have psychiatrists given much thought to the psychological problems of the medically ill. DSM-III introduced a potentially important development with its multiaxial format. This permits the diagnosis of psychiatric illnesses, physical illnesses and psychosocial stresses on separate axes, but there is no consideration of the possible relationships between these axes which might enable the aetiology of psychiatric illness to be understood.

It is soon apparent to anyone who works in a general hospital that patients respond very differently to illnesses which at face value seem similar to one another in nature and severity. The factors which determine the different responses are not fully understood but a useful framework has been proposed in terms of the personal meaning, or subjective significance, which an illness has for the individual. Lipowski (1969) has proposed that this is the key to the psychological response and that it is shaped by several factors including the patient's personality, social circumstances, the nature of the illness and the treatment required.

Adjustment disorders

The commonest affective symptoms secondary to physical illness are those of an undifferentiated neurotic syndrome with a mixture of anxiety and depression. The symptoms are usually transient, tending to subside within a few weeks, particularly if there is resolution of the underlying physical illness. In the case of acute illness, such as myocardial infarction, symptoms develop within 2 or 3 days. Anxiety is the earliest response and is prominent when there is uncertainty about the diagnosis or treatment required. Depression is a later development and can last for weeks. Whatever the prevailing mood, the patient's preoccupations are focused on the implications of the illness and its treatment. Derogatis et al (1983) reported that adjustment disorder was the commonest psychiatric diagnosis made in patients with malignant disease and similar observations have been made on men with human immunodeficiency virus (HIV) infection and acquired immune deficiency syndrome (AIDS) (King 1989).

Adjustment disorders are classified in ICD-10 with the group of neurotic, stress-related and somatoform disorders. They are subdivided according to their duration — brief or prolonged — and to the predominant mood. They can be regarded as a partial syndrome of a specific mood disorder, merging imperceptibly with a healthy adjustment on the one hand and with major affective disorder on the other. The symptoms can be alleviated by reassurance, support and explanation of the nature of the underlying illness; these functions are best undertaken by the clinician in overall charge of the case. Psychotropic medication or skilled psychotherapy are rarely required. Considerable emotional distress often arises because of inadequate or conflicting information. There is now abundant evidence that most patients want their doctors to discuss the nature of their illness frankly, even when the condition carries a poor prognosis.

Many of the criticisms levelled at doctors specifically mention the lack of frankness, and clinical practice is slowly changing in the light of these comments.

Phobic anxiety disorders

Anxiety in response to illness usually forms part of an adjustment disorder and subsides once the acute, life-threatening phase of the illness resolves. Phobic anxiety is induced by specific objects or situations and tends to persist unless appropriate treatment is arranged. Repeated venepuncture or hypodermic injection can lead to a needle phobia which prevents compliance with future treatment. This can have serious implications if it delays treatment of malignant disease or chronic disorders such as diabetes. Conditioned phobic responses can also develop during chemotherapy or radiotherapy, both of which cause unpleasant side-effects, including anorexia, nausea, vomiting and hair loss. The conditioned response takes the form of anticipatory anxiety, nausea and vomiting; these symptoms may be so severe that the patient avoids further treatment for the underlying malignancy. Short-term benzodiazepine therapy may overcome this problem sufficiently to allow treatment to proceed but a more effective solution can be provided by means of systematic desensitisation.

Post-traumatic stress disorder

In general hospital practice this problem is seen in patients who have been admitted with physical injuries following accidents, violence and natural or man-made disasters. The trauma is always of an exceptionally threatening degree, outside the range of everyday human experience and would be markedly stressful to virtually everyone. However, the physical injuries actually sustained may be quite trivial. There is a delay of several weeks or months between the trauma and onset of symptoms. Anxiety is a central feature. It is associated with chronic tension, increased vulnerability and emotional blunting. Flashbacks of the trauma are experienced regularly. They many be evoked by situations which remind the patient of the original incident and which therefore tend to be avoided. Sleep disturbance is common, with vivid nightmares of the trauma. Other symptoms include irritability, poor concentration and guilt at having survived the traumatic event. Cognitive–behavioral techniques and antidepressant medication have been claimed to reduce the intensity of symptoms but attention is now being given to providing immediate psychological support following disasters with the aim of preventing the subsequent development of post-traumatic stress disorder.

Depressive episodes

Psychological symptoms sometimes persist even after the physical illness has resolved. Usually they are depressive in nature and when they reach sufficient intensity they fulfil the diagnostic criteria for a depressive episode of mild, moderate or severe degree. Anorexia, weight loss, constipation and other somatic symptoms of depression cannot be given their usual diagnostic significance because they may all be directly caused by organic pathology. Greater importance should be attached to the psychological symptoms, particularly anhedonia and loss of interest in external affairs. Depression arises from the patient's awareness of the illness and the implications it has for future aspirations and way of life. The concept of secondary depression provides a useful framework to understand these symptoms. The prognosis of secondary affective disorders can be seen from studies of patients following a myocardial infarction. Stern et al (1976) found that 35% had symptoms of anxiety or depression 6 weeks after the attack, this figure falling to 20% by 12 months. Similar observations were made by Mayou (1979), who emphasised that the patient's mental state was also influenced by events independent of the heart attack. Lloyd & Cawley (1983) showed that psychological symptoms precipitated acutely by the infarction were likely to be transient, lasting only a few weeks. However, 19% of patients had developed psychiatric morbidity 4 months later and in 11% this continued at least until 12 months after the infarct (Lloyd 1986). Depression has also been described as a long-term complication in women who have had a mastectomy for breast cancer. Maguire et al (1987) assessed a series of women at intervals up to 12 months after the operation and found that 20% had developed a moderate or severe mood disturbance lasting at least 8 months. Similar figures were reported by Morris et al (1977), who followed their patients for 2 years after surgery, but much lower rates have been obtained when stricter diagnostic criteria were used (Dean 1987).

The persistent nature of these symptoms indicates that active treatment is required. Rehabilitation programmes have been specifically designed for certain illnesses although evaluation studies have not always demonstrated beneficial effects. The same reservation applies to interpretive psychotherapy, which nevertheless is employed by many psychiatrists when the patient's psychological response appears to be a consequence of unresolved conflicts which the illness has uncovered. Speigel et al (1989) have demonstrated the value of supportive group psychotherapy in women with metastatic breast cancer. Psychotherapy consisted of weekly sessions for 12 months during which patients were encouraged to ventilate their feelings about their illness and discuss ways of coping with cancer. They were also taught a self-hypnosis method of pain control. This type of psychological intervention was associated with a prolonged survival time. Cognitive therapy is also being used to modify those attitudes which are considered to have an adverse effect on outcome (Moorey & Greer 1989).

The decision to use antidepressant medication should be based on criteria similar to those employed in treating depressive episodes not associated with physical illness. However, medical patients appear to have a poor tolerance of tricyclic drugs (Popkin et al 1985), so preference should be given to one of the newer antidepressants, such as fluoxetine or paroxetine.

Organic mood disorders

Affective symptoms can also result from structural brain disease and from disturbance of neurotransmitter mechanisms caused by the metabolic effects of the illness or by drugs used in treatment. One of the most important aspects of these disorders is that the mood disorder — either depression or mania — may be the first manifestation of underlying physical pathology and this emphasises the importance of a thorough physical assessment of all patients who develop psychiatric illness. Suspicion of underlying physical illness should be particularly high when there is no obvious psychosocial precipitant, when the first psychiatric episode develops in middle or late life or when there is no family or previous personal disposition to mood disorder (Whitlock 1982).

Observations from the USA and Canada have shown a significant prevalence of undetected physical pathology in patients presenting with various psychiatric syndromes. Hall et al (1978) examined 658 consecutive patients in a psychiatric clinic and found that 9% had a medical disorder which was considered to have caused the psychiatric illness. Nearly half of these were unknown to the patient or physician. Similarly, Koranyi (1979) studied over 2000 consecutive patients at a psychiatric clinic and found that 43% had a major physical illness, in 18% of whom physical illness was considered to be the sole cause of the psychiatric disorder. In both these studies cardiovascular, endocrine and neurological disorders were the predominant medical diagnoses.

Several types of physical disorder can present with affective symptoms. Cerebral disorders are prominent among these. Depression is a well-recognised manifestation of diffuse and localised cerebrovascular disease. Robinson et al (1984) studied patients with strokes and claimed that the site of the lesion has an important influence on the development of affective symptoms, with left anterior infarcts being associated with the greater severity of depression. However, other modifying variables have been identified, including functional disability, intellectual impairment, age and quality of social support. The association between mood disorder and the site of the stroke has not been confirmed by others, so this putative link requires further investigation. Brief episodes of mood disturbance also occur in up to 25% of patients with cerebrovascular disease (House et al 1989). These are described as pathological emotionalism or emotional lability. Their defining characteristics are sudden episodes of crying which are not under normal social control, together with inappropriate laughter.

Depressive symptoms in stroke patients respond to antidepressant medication (Lipsey et at 1984), so it is important not to regard depression as an inevitable and irreversible complication. Depression can be the presenting symptom of a cerebral tumour, multiple sclerosis, parkinsonism, Huntington's chorea and epilepsy.

Endocrine disorders are also well-established causes of affective symptoms, notably hyperthyroidism, hypothyroidism, Cushing's syndrome and Addison's disease. Other conditions which have been associated with an affective presentation include malignant disorders, connective tissue diseases and some infectious diseases, particularly viral infections such as glandular fever, herpes simplex and coxsackie virus infection. Non-viral infections associated with a depressive presentation include brucellosis, typhoid and toxoplasmosis.

The affective symptoms associated with physical disorders may be aggravated or caused by prescribed drugs. There is evidence that drugs account for an increasing incidence of psychiatric disorder, and affective disorders form one of several groups of drug-induced psychiatric syndromes (McClelland 1981). Many classes of drugs have been implicated, the most common being antihypertensive agents such as reserpine and methyldopa, analgesics, L-dopa and corticosteroids.

Mania is a much rarer complication of physical disorders and drug therapy, with the exception of steroids, which are known to precipitate manic symptoms in some patients. Krauthammer & Klerman (1978) have reviewed reported cases of mania accompanying physical illness, grouping the causes into infections, neoplasms, epilepsy, metabolic disturbance and drugs. It was assumed that the mania resulted from direct brain involvement or neurotransmitter imbalance.

Whitlock (1982) has discussed the relative role of genetic and constitutional factors in the aetiology of organic mood disorders. He concluded that in patients with drug-induced conditions there is often a history of previous affective disorder or a positive family history. In these cases the drug merely precipitates the depression, and the patient's mood usually returns to normal when the offending agent is withdrawn. However, in patients who develop affective illness after structural brain damage, Whitlock concluded that there is little genetic predisposition and that the cerebral impairment is directly responsible for the psychiatric symptoms.

An organic anxiety disorder with the essential clinical features of generalised anxiety disorder, panic disorder or a combination of both can develop as a consequence of hyperthyroidism, temporal lobe epilepsy, phaeochromocytoma or hypoglycaemia. Occasionally, a delusional (schizophrenia-like) disorder may be the first manifestation of a physical illness or complicate a long-standing condition such as temporal lobe epilepsy. The delusions may be accompanied by hallucinations and schizophrenic thought disorder. The evidence for such an association is most convincing for epilepsy but many other conditions have been implicated.

Acute and transient psychotic disorders

Acute psychoses are common complications of physical illness. Usually they take the form of an organic syndrome characterised by the typical features of impaired consciousness, memory disturbance, muddled thinking, disturbance of the sleep cycle and perceptual abnormalities, particularly in the visual modality. These are discussed in detail in Chapter 15.

Occasionally, transient psychotic disorders develop in the absence of signs of organic cerebral disturbance. The characteristic picture is that of an acute delusional system, almost always of a persecutory nature, which involves the staff who are treating the patient. There may be aggressive outbursts or the patient may try to leave hospital against advice. These psychotic disorders are probably precipitated by the emotional impact of the

illness and its treatment and by the disruption which the illness causes to the patient's familiar environment. They are usually brief, lasting only a few days, but the associated behavioral disturbances can be very disruptive to clinical management. Neuroleptic drugs are usually required; sometimes the symptoms do not completely resolve until the patient is discharged home to familiar surroundings.

Other behavioral syndromes

Chronic illnesses can lead to widespread changes in behaviour in addition to the specific psychiatric disorders already described. Restrictions on diet, exercise and other habits are difficult for some patients to accept and they may rebel intermittently by not complying with their treatment. This pattern of behaviour is seen in association with ischaemic heart disease, chronic renal failure and, especially, diabetes mellitus. Adolescents find it particularly difficult to come to terms with dietary control, insulin injections and self-monitoring of blood glucose, all of which set them apart from their peer group. Episodes of hypoglycaemia and ketoacidosis are relatively common. In some patients these episodes become recurrent, often in response to stressful life events, and the term 'brittle diabetes' has been used to describe their poor glycaemic control and early development of complications. Eating disorders, both anorexia and bulimia nervosa, have been reported to occur more commonly in diabetics (Steel et al 1987), an understandable association in view of the attention to diet and weight required for smooth glycaemic control.

Functional disability is sometimes greater that would be expected from the extent of physical pathology. Return to work and resumption of leisure activities are delayed and the patient continues to complain of somatic symptoms. There may be varying degrees of depression, anxiety and irritability, but in many cases the only symptoms are physical and the patient becomes progressively more disabled without apparent organic cause. Disability of this nature can be seen after many illnesses but it is particularly likely to occur after traumatic injuries sustained in accidents which are believed to be due to someone else's negligence or incompetence. Claims for compensation appear to prolong the disability further. Once the behavioral pattern becomes established it is reinforced by overprotective behaviour on the part of relatives who take on a new role, reversing the dominance hierarchy within the family (Tarsh & Royston 1985).

If chronic invalidism is to be prevented it is important to establish liability quickly and to settle compensation as soon as possible. Rehabilitation needs to be planned after a careful evaluation of the patient's physical and psychological condition; family therapy is required if relatives' behaviour appears to be contributing to disability.

SOMATIC PRESENTATION OF PSYCHIATRIC ILLNESS

Somatic symptoms occur in all psychiatric illnesses and in some they dominate the clinical picture to such an extent that patients believe themselves to be physically ill. This perception determines the pattern of contact with medical services. Patients consult their general practitioner or hospital doctor and describe their symptoms entirely in physical terms. This presentation has come to be known as somatisation, a term which has been defined in various ways but which essentially refers to the presentation of psychological distress with somatic symptoms which are attributed to organic disease. General practice studies have emphasised how frequently this phenomenon occurs. A study in Manchester found that 50% of patients presenting with a new episode of psychiatric illness satisfied criteria for somatisation (Bridges & Goldberg 1985). In only half the cases were the psychiatric disorders detected, the somatic symptoms appearing to distract the doctor from the correct diagnosis. Several of these patients would be referred to medical clinics and they account for the high proportion of patients attending clinics for neurology, gastroenterology, dermatology and genito-urinary medicine who are psychiatrically ill but who have no physical pathology.

Presenting symptoms

Pain

There is a wide range of presenting symptoms (Lloyd 1983). They include dizziness, fatigue, localised weakness, anorexia and weight loss, but pain is probably the commonest. Pain is a subjective experience which cannot be confirmed or refuted by objective tests. If psychological factors are thought to be important in its aetiology there may be a clear association with stressful life events and the pain may be relieved by alcohol or psychotropic drugs. It is described in indefinite terms and is poorly localised, not conforming to dermatomes or peripheral nerve distribution.

Facial pain has an established association with psychiatric illness. Feinmann et al (1984) studied patients referred to an oral surgery clinic because of atypical facial pain or facial arthromyalgia. Over half were diagnosed as being psychiatrically ill, with neurotic depression being the commonest diagnosis. Bass & Wade (1984) reported similar observations in a series of patients with chest pain who had undergone coronary arteriography. Psychiatric illness was much commoner in those without significant coronary disease. Psychological factors are often invoked to account for pain in the lower back, abdomen, pelvis and external genitalia. The more chronic the pain and the fewer the organic findings, the more likely it is the pain is psychologically determined. In some cases a psychiatric illness such as depressive or anxiety disorder is the sole cause. These conditions may induce pain because of increased muscle tone and faulty posture; they also increase awareness of the minor bodily aches which are part of everyday experience. In other cases the explanation lies in the concept of learned behaviour. The complaint of pain is used to attract sympathy or other rewards, or to avoid undesired responsibilities.

Fatigue

It is not sufficiently recognised that fatigue is a common symptom of psychiatric disorder. Fatigue may be exclusively physical or psychological but is usually a combination of both. The patient complains of poor concentration, exhaustion after minimal mental or physical exertion, muscle tenderness and dizziness. The sleep pattern is altered, with frequent waking or hypersomnia. There may also be various autonomic symptoms affecting the cardiovascular or gastrointestinal systems. This pattern of symptoms may become established after a viral infection and is often referred to as myalgic encephalomyelitis (ME) or postviral fatigue syndrome. In many cases, however, there is no convincing evidence of a viral aetiology, either from the history or viral antibody titres. Nevertheless, patients are often adamant that their symptoms are due to infection, resist any attempt at a psychological explanation and refuse to accept psychiatric treatment (Kendell 1991).

The symptoms of the chronic fatigue syndrome are similar to those of a depressive or anxiety disorder, so there is considerable overlap between patients diagnosed as psychiatrically ill and those diagnosed as having the postviral fatigue syndrome. Most studies which have assessed these patients psychiatrically have found that at least half have a psychiatric disorder when operational criteria are used. The commonest diagnosis is a depressive illness, followed by anxiety disorders and somatisation disorder. For patients who do not fulfil criteria for these syndromes, ICD-10 still retains the terms neurasthenia, which can therefore be diagnosed when chronic fatigue is not associated with any other psychiatric or physical condition

Other presenting symptoms

Psychiatric illness has also been associated with symptoms of hyperventilation, disfigurement, supposed food allergy and irritable bowel. The latter condition is the commonest single diagnosis made in gastroenterology out-patient clinics. Its essential features are abdominal distension, pain relieved by bowel movement, altered bowel habit and a sense of incomplete evacuation. There are a number of non-colonic symptoms which suggest a diffuse smooth muscle disorder; these include nausea, vomiting, dysphagia and frequency of micturition. Approximately 50% have a psychiatric illness; neurotic personality traits and environmental stress have also been implicated (Creed & Guthrie 1987).

Many of these patients will be referred to a liaison psychiatry service, especially if the physician has uncovered evidence of psychological causation. Psychiatric diagnosis requires positive evidence of psychiatric disorder and not merely absence of organic disease. Nevertheless, it is probably wise for the psychiatrist to start by taking a detailed history of the presenting physical complaints to establish confidently that organic pathology has not been missed; it will also convince the patient that the psychiatrist is not dismissing the somatic complaints. The interview should then proceed to enquire about psychological symptoms, family history and personal background in the usual manner. If a psychiatric condition is diagnosed it is necessary to discuss this with the patient so that the links between somatic symptoms and associated emotional factors can be understood.

Psychiatric syndromes

Various types of psychiatric disorder can present in this manner but it has been difficult to categorise them according to any established psychiatric nosology. The commonest conditions are depressive and anxiety disorders, including phobias and panic attacks. The typical psychological symptoms can be uncovered by direct enquiry and the conditions respond to conventional treatment with drugs or psychological therapies.

Somatoform disorders

Other disorders are more difficult to classify. ICD-10 has introduced a specific group of somatoform disorders, the essential features of which are repeated presentation of physical symptoms together with persistent requests for medical investigations, in spite of repeated negative findings and reassurance by doctors that the symptoms have no physical basis. The glossary also states that the degree of understanding that can be achieved about the cause of the symptoms is often disappointing and frustrating for both patient and doctor. The group is subdivided in ICD-10 as shown below:

F45.0	Somatisation disorder
F45.1	Undifferentiated somatoform disorder
F45.2	Hypochondriacal disorder
F45.3	Somatoform autonomic dysfunction
F45.4	Persistent somatoform pain disorder
F45.8	Other
F45.9	Unspecified

Somatisation disorder is similar to the condition previously termed Briquet's syndrome or St Louis hysteria. It is characterised by multiple, recurrent and frequently changing symptoms which involve many organ systems. It is much commoner in women and usually starts in early adult life. In the USA it is said to affect 1% of the female population. Clinical experience suggests that it is much less common in Britain. This may reflect differences in medical practice between the two countries. American patients have ready access to a large number of specialists and this may determine a greater range of symptoms. Thus, it would be easier for them to accumulate the criteria required for somatisation disorder than it would be in countries like Britain where referral to specialists is controlled by a general practitioner. The diagnosis of undifferentiated somatoform disorder is to be used when physical complaints are multiple, varying and persistent but do not fulfil the criteria of somatisation disorder.

Hypochondriacal disorder involves a persistent preoccupation with the possibility of having one or more serious physical illnesses or a preoccupation with some aspect of physical appearance. Cancer, heart disease and AIDS are the conditions with which hypochondriacal patients are most commonly preoccupied. Concern about disfigurement typically involves the nose, ears, eyes or breasts; the condition, sometimes referred to as dysmorphophobia, leads to a demand for cosmetic surgery even when the anatomical part appears completely normal to an objective observer. A high prevalence of severe neurotic illness has been found among patients who have undergone cosmetic rhinoplasty, so careful psychological assessment is necessary for patients whose insistence on plastic surgery appears disproportionate to anatomical deformity. Fixed delusional ideas about disease or deformity should not be classified as a hypochondriacal disorder but as a persistent delusional disorder (see Ch. 20). An example of this condition is the delusion of infestation with skin parasites ('delusional parasitosis') for which patients are usually referred to a dermatologist.

Somatoform autonomic dysfunction is a newly introduced category to cover symptoms resulting from functional disorder of organs which are largely or completely under control of the autonomic nervous system. The symptoms include sweating, hyperventilation, dyspepsia, irritable bowel and dysuria, and the category is subdivided according to the predominant organ system involved. There is clear evidence of psychological stress in many patients but this is not the case in a substantial proportion who fulfil the diagnostic criteria. Persistent somatoform pain disorder applies to chronic pain which cannot be explained fully by physical pathology or a physiological process and which occurs in association with psychosocial problems that are considered to be the main causative influences. It should not be diagnosed if pain is associated with a depressive or anxiety disorder of if it is due to muscle tension.

Dissociative (conversion) disorders

This term includes those disorders previously classified as conversion hysteria. ICD-10 aims to avoid using the term 'hysteria' as far as possible because of its varied meanings, but it is still used in clinical practice, particularly by neurologists. Dissociative symptoms involve loss or distortion of neurological function not adequately explained by organic disease. Loss of memory, or dissociative amnesia, is usually partial and selective for traumatic events. It often involves a loss of personal identity, so the patient cannot recall his name, occupation, age, family or other personal details. Patients with dissociative amnesia may wander from home for several days at a time, sometimes assuming a new identity in the process. This condition, dissociative fugue, often ends with the patient presenting at a casualty department many miles from his home address. Other dissociative symptoms which present to neurologists include motor paralysis, aphonia, pseudoseizures, sensory loss and gait disturbance (Marsden 1986).

Factitious disorders

Patients who repeatedly feign signs or symptoms of illness create enormous diagnostic and management problems and considerable hostility from their doctors once the correct diagnosis is established. Factitious disorder can be subdivided into two main groups. One consists of physical signs or abnormal laboratory results which are fabricated in a subtle and undisclosed manner. They include dermatitis artefacta, self-induced anaemia, hyperthyroidism and hypoglycaemia. The patients are typically young, unmarried women employed in nursing or other careers allied to medicine and they nearly always have unresolved conflicts involving dependency, sexuality or hostility. The other group comprises dramatic symptoms suggesting an acute surgical emergency, pathological lying and a tendency to wander from one hospital to another with a similar presentation each time. This condition, also know as Munchausen's syndrome, is nearly always confined to men from the lower socioeconomic classes who have a long history of social maladjustment. The motivation for this behaviour is obscure. It can best be understood in terms of a morbid attraction to the sick role and pleasure at deceiving doctors. Factitious disorders are distinguished from somatoform and dissociative disorders by the assumption that symptoms and signs are under voluntary control. They also have to be distinguished from malingering, in which there is an obvious goal such as avoiding criminal prosecution or military conscription.

Factors influencing the somatic presentation

The somatic presentation of psychiatric illness has never been adequately explained. Some people are selectively aware of bodily functions and this sensitivity may shape the pattern of their symptoms if they develop a psychiatric illness. Cultural factors appear to play an important part. Somatic symptoms are much commoner in developing countries than they are in Western culture. The limited acceptance and greater stigma of psychiatric illness have been implicated but it is also clear that the native languages of several developing countries lack the vocabulary for emotional expression available in Western languages (Leff 1981). Emotional distress has therefore to be expressed in words which refer to bodily feelings. Somatisation also appears to be associated with advancing age and lower social class, and to be commoner in patients with a previous personal or family history of physical illness. The impaired ability to verbalise emotional distress has been termed alexithymia. This is said to be characterised by reduced symbolic thinking so that inner attitudes, feelings, wishes and drives are not revealed. Taylor

(1984) has claimed that this often underlies the communication of emotional distress through physical complaints, because of a difficulty verbalising feelings and distinguishing between bodily sensations and emotional states.

Managing the somatising patient

Whatever the associated psychiatric disorder, most clinicians believe it is important to alter the patient's attribution of the symptoms so that they come to be recognised as being linked to psychological rather than physical factors. It is helpful to summarise the negative physical findings and laboratory tests. This should be followed by a discussion of the somatic symptoms of depression and anxiety disorders, some of which may become manifest during the consultation. Finally, there should be an explanation of the reasons for linking the patient's symptoms to his mood state or current psychosocial difficulties. This process of reattribution may take several consultations. If it is unsuccessful or incomplete the patient will continue to regard himself as physically ill and demand referral to other doctors in the hope that an organic diagnosis will be made eventually.

It is important to identify the acute-onset conditions underlying the somatic facade. These nearly always involve an anxiety or depressive disorder and they respond to conventional treatment with cognitive–behaviourial therapy or antidepressant drugs. If the diagnosis is overlooked there is a risk that symptoms will become chronic and an abnormal pattern of illness behaviour established. The prospects for effective treatment are greatly reduced once this occurs.

Cognitive and behavioural techniques are now being used in managing persistent somatisers (Mayou 1988). A model used in treating patients with hypochondriasis is based on the assumption that complaints are maintained by avoidance behaviour, such as seeking reassurance and checking bodily status. Treatment involves preventing reassurance and encouraging exposure to situations the patient has avoided because of fears for his health (Salkovskis & Warwick 1986). Cognitive therapy has been shown to reduce symptoms and functional disability in patients with non-cardiac chest pain (Klimes et al 1990). These patients were taught how to anticipate and control pain using relaxation, respiratory control and distraction techniques. They were also discouraged from seeking reassurance, for example repeated pulse checking, and to engage in exercise to counteract avoidance. Cognitive challenge was used to alter residual beliefs about organic illness. Relaxation and

brief dynamic psychotherapy have also been shown to be effective for symptoms of the irritable bowel syndrome which had not responded to standard medical treatment (Guthrie et al 1991). Behavioural treatments have a place in the management of chronic pain; tricyclic antidepressants are a useful adjunct.

Somatisation disorder and factitious disorder are less responsive to treatment and the pattern of behaviour is more likely to change as a result of altered life circumstances than in response to specific psychiatric intervention. However, a psychiatric assessment is important in establishing the diagnosis and preventing unnecessary investigations, thereby reducing the iatrogenic risks to the patient and the financial burden they create for health services.

ALCOHOL- AND DRUG-RELATED PROBLEMS IN MEDICAL PATIENTS

The physical morbidity associated with alcohol abuse is well established and correlates closely with national per capita consumption. Alcohol affects virtually every organ system so the manifestations of excess consumption are diverse. It contributes indirectly to many problems which present in general hospitals, including attempted suicide, obesity, violence and accidents. British studies have consistently shown that just over a quarter of male medical admissions have a current or previous alcohol problem. Figures for women tend to be lower and more variable, reflecting lower consumption and greater reluctance to admit to alcohol abuse.

The medical conditions associated with alcohol abuse are shown in Table 34.1.

Several reports have described patients with advanced complications, particularly liver disease, and have emphasised the need for earlier detection. The failure to detect alcoholism at an earlier stage in its evolution has been attributed to doctors' neglect to ask the appropriate questions about drinking habits. Many patients with alcohol problems are admitted to general hospitals for illnesses not classically related to alcohol abuse and their drinking will not be detected unless specific enquiries are made. Blood tests, including mean corpuscular volume (MCV) and γ-glutamyltranspeptidase (GTT), are not sufficiently sensitive. Problem drinkers are more likely to be detected during a clinical examination and interview if the right questions are asked. A high index of suspicion is essential. During the early stages of a drinking career patients may present repeatedly with ill-defined, multiple symptoms, including dyspepsia, anorexia, nausea, diarrhoea and sexual problems. Physical examination may indicate obesity, a plethoric

Table 34.1 Medical disorders associated with excessive alcohol consumption

System	Disorder
Cardiovascular	Hypertension Cardiomyopathy
Gastrointestinal	Oropharangeal cancer Oesophageal cancer Gastritis Mallory–Weiss syndrome Pancreatitis Malabsorption
Hepatic	Fatty change Acute hepatitis Cirrhosis Primary liver cancer
Neurological	Withdrawal symptoms Alcoholic blackouts (amnesia) Wernicke–Korsakoff syndrome Dementia Cerebral haemorrhage Cerebellar degeneration Peripheral neuropathy
Musculoskeletal	Myopathy Gout Dupuytren's contracture
Respiratory	Pneumonia Tuberculosis
Endocrine and reproductive	Hypoglycaemia Hypogonadism Pseudo-Cushing's syndrome Infertility Fetal alcohol syndrome
Skin	Spider naevi Palmar erythema Acne rosacea

face, poor dental hygiene, hypertension, atrial fibrillation and hepatomegaly. In the nervous system there may be a tremor, ataxia, peripheral neuropathy and minor cognitive impairment.

Screening and early detection have been advocated on the assumption that intervention will give the patient an opportunity to modify his drinking habits before irreversible physical damage has occurred.

Alcoholic patients are often referred to psychiatrists in general hospitals for the management of withdrawal symptoms and for continued treatment of the underlying alcohol dependence. The results are rarely satisfactory but there is now evidence that intervention at an earlier stage might be successful in reducing future alcohol-related problems. Chick et al (1985) have demonstrated the beneficial effects of systematic screening and counselling by a specially trained nurse.

In a controlled study, newly identified problem drinkers were allocated either to an intervention or a control group. Those in the intervention group received a special session of counselling, informing them of the adverse effects of alcohol on their health and advising them to modify their drinking habits or, in some cases, to become completely abstinent. They were given advice on how to avoid situations where drinking was most likely to occur and some were also recommended to contact other treatment agencies. Follow-up interviews 12 months later indicated that the patients who had received the intervention had a better overall outcome, although both groups had reduced their consumption to a similar extent.

Regular monitoring of GGT is a useful adjunct to counselling if the level is already raised. The results should be discussed as soon as possible with the patient and they can prove a strong incentive to reduce consumption or maintain abstinence.

Problems related to drug abuse appear to be increasing in general hospital practice although their frequency is much less than those due to alcohol. Physical complications are associated particularly with intravenous use. Respiratory depression and coma occur after accidental overdoses. Hepatitis, endocarditis and AIDS are frequent complications if needles are shared. In some areas at least half of patients with HIV infection have contracted it through contaminated needles rather than sexual contact.

The treatment of drug-dependent patients in general hospitals chiefly involves managing withdrawal symptoms, which develop soon after the patient has been admitted for either a drug-related or coincidental problem (Lloyd 1991). Long-term management is best undertaken in special treatment centres.

LIAISON WITH OTHER SPECIALISTS

Approximately 2% of in-patients in British teaching hospital are referred to a psychiatrist during their admission. It is likely that far more patients would benefit from referral but there are many reasons why advice is not sought more often. Referral to a psychiatrist is often resented or completely rejected by patients, especially those who somatise their emotional difficulties. Other barriers to referral include failure to recognise psychiatric symptoms, dissatisfaction with the available services and the doctor's antipathy towards psychiatry. Physicians are much more likely than surgeons to be interested in the psychological aspects of their patient's illnesses and to accept responsibility for treating them (Mayou & Smith 1986).

The need for improved liaison between physicians and psychiatrists has been expressed by several writers, most clearly perhaps by Tattersall (1981) in relation to patients with diabetes. But he argued that the role of the psychiatrist should be a subsidiary one and that in most cases it should be the physician who diagnoses and treats emotional disorders. Splitting physical and emotional care, he warned, can create confusion and allow the patient to manipulate one doctor against another.

To improve their contribution to general medical care, psychiatrists need to respond promptly to requests for consultation and to develop harmonious working relationships with their medical colleagues. Much will depend on the level of staffing. A department which is fully integrated within a general hospital is more likely to provide the necessary expertise than a distant mental hospital. But this will not happen if psychiatrists move into the general hospital without adequately changing their mode of practice (Creed 1991).

Providing a better liaison service results in an increased number of referrals (Brown & Cooper 1987). This is obviously to be encouraged if it leads to more effective treatment, improved quality of care and reduced medical costs. An expanding service depends on the availability of psychiatrists who have been properly trained in liaison psychiatry and who have adequate time to devote to this work.

REFERENCES

Appels A, Mulder P 1988 Excess fatigue as a precursor of myocardial infarction. European Heart Journal 9: 758–764

Bass C, Wade C 1984 Chest pain with normal coronary arteries: a comparative study of psychiatric and social morbidity. Psychological Medicine 14: 51–61

Bridges K W, Goldberg D P 1984 Psychiatric illness in in-patients with neurological disorders: patients' views on discussion of emotional problems with neurologists. British Medical Journal 289: 656–658

Bridges K W, Goldberg D P 1985 Somatic presentation of DSM-III psychiatric disorders in primary care. Journal of Psychosomatic Research 29: 563–569

Brown A, Cooper A F 1987 The impact of a liaison psychiatry service on patterns of referral in a general hospital. British Journal of Psychiatry 150: 83–87

Chick J, Lloyd G, Crombie E 1985 Counselling problem drinkers in medical wards: a controlled study. British Medical Journal 290: 265–267

Creed F 1985 Life events and physical illness. Journal of Psychosomatic Research 29: 113–123

Creed F 1991 Liaison psychiatry for the 21st century: a review. Journal of the Royal Society of Medicine 84: 414–417

Creed F, Guthrie E 1987 Psychological factors and the irritable bowel syndrome. Gut 28: 1307–1318

Cull A 1990 Psychological aspects of cancer and chemotherapy. Journal of Psychosomatic Research 34: 616–619

Dean C 1987 Psychiatric morbidity following mastectomy: preoperative predictors and types of illness. Journal of Psychosomatic Research 31: 385–392

Derogatis L R, Morrow G R, Fetting J et al 1983 The prevalence of psychiatric disorders among cancer patients. Journal of the American Medical Association 249: 751–757

Feinmann C, Harris M, Cawley R 1984 Psychogenic facial pain: presentation and treatment. British Medical Journal 288: 436–438

Friedman M, Rosenman R H 1959 Association of specific overt behaviour pattern with blood and cardiovascular findings. Journal of the American Medical Association 169: 1085–1096

Friedman M, Thoresen C E, Gill J J et al 1984 Alternation of Type A behaviour and reduction in cardiac recurrences in post-myocardial infarction patients. American Heart Journal 108: 237–248

Gater R, Goldberg D, Evanson J et al 1992 The detection and treatment of psychiatric illness in a general medical ward: a cost-utility analysis. Journal of Psychosomatic Research (in press)

Goldberg D 1985 Identifying psychiatric illness among general medical patients. British Medical Journal 291: 161–162

Greer S, Morris T, Pettingale K W 1979 Psychological response to breast cancer: effect on outcome. Lancet ii: 785–787

Guthrie E, Creed F, Dawson D, Tomenson B 1991 A controlled trial of psychological treatment for the irritable bowel syndrome. Gastroenterology 100: 450–457

Haines A P, Imeson J D, Meade T W 1987 Phobic anxiety and ischaemic heart disease. British Medical Journal 295: 297–299

Hall R C W, Popkin M K, Devaul R A, Faillace L A, Stickney S K 1978 Physical illness presenting as psychiatric disease. Archives of General Psychiatry 15: 1365–1320

House A, Dennis M, Molyneux A, Warlow C, Hawton K 1989 Emotionalism after stroke. British Medical Journal 298: 991–994

Kendell R E 1991 Chronic fatigue, viruses and depression. Lancet 337: 160–162

King M B 1989 Psychosocial status of 192 outpatients with HIV infection and AIDS. British Journal of Psychiatry 154: 237–242

Klimes I, Mayou R A, Pearce M J, Coles L, Fagg J R 1990 Psychological treatment for atypical non-cardiac chest pain. Psychological Medicine 20: 605–611

Koranyi E K 1979 Morbidity and rate of undiagnosed physical illness in a psychiatric clinic population. Archives of General Psychiatry 36: 414–419

Krauthammer C, Klerman G L 1978 Secondary mania: manic syndromes associated with antecedent physical illness or drugs. Achieves of General Psychiatry 35: 1333–1339

Leff J P 1981 Psychiatry around the globe: a transcultural view. Marcel Dekker, New York.

Lipowski Z J 1969 Psychosocial aspects of disease. Annals of Internal Medicine 71: 1197–1206

Lipowski Z J, Wolston E J 1981 Liaison psychiatry: referral patterns and their stability over time. American Journal of Psychiatry 138: 1608–1611

Lipsey J R, Robinson R G, Pearlson G D, Rao K, Price T R 1984 Nortriptyline treatment of post-stroke depression: a double-blind study. Lancet i: 297–300

Lloyd G G 1983 Medicine without signs. British Medical Journal 287: 539–542

Lloyd G G 1986 Myocardial infarction and mental illness. Journal of the Royal Society of Medicine 80: 101–104

Lloyd G G 1991 Textbook of general hospital psychiatry. Churchill Livingstone, Edinburgh

Lloyd G G, Cawley R H 1983 Distress or illness? A study of psychological symptoms after myocardial infarction. British Journal of Psychiatry 142: 120–125

McClelland H A 1981 Psychiatric disorders. In: Davies D M (ed) Textbook of adverse drug reactions, 2nd edn. Oxford University Press, Oxford pp 479–502

McKegney F P McMahon T, King J 1983 The use of DSM-III in a general hospital consultation-liaison service. General Hospital Psychiatry 5: 115–121

Maguire G P, Lee E G, Bevington D J, Kucheman C S, Crabtree R J, Cornell C F 1978 Psychiatric problems in the first year after mastectomy. British Medical Journal i: 963–965

Maguire G P, Tait A, Brooke M, Thomas C, Sellwood R 1980 The effect of counselling on the psychiatric morbidity associated with mastectomy. British Medical Journal 281: 1454–1455

Marsden C D 1986 Hysteria: a neurologist's view. Psychological Medicine 16: 277–288

Mayou R A 1979 The course and determinants of reactions to myocardial infarction. British Journal of Psychiatry 134: 588–594

Mayou R A 1988 Psychiatric treatment of somatic symptoms. Current Opinion in Psychiatry 1: 150–154

Mayou R A, Hawton K 1986 Psychiatric disorder in the general hospital. British Journal of Psychiatry 149: 172–190

Mayou R A, Lloyd G 1985 A survey of liaison psychiatry in the United Kingdom and Eire. Bulletin of the Royal College of Psychiatrists 9: 214–217

Mayou R A, Smith E B O 1986 Hospital doctors' management of psychological problems. British Journal of Psychiatry 148: 194–197

Moorey S, Greer S 1989 Psychological therapy for patients with cancer: a new approach. Heinemann, Oxford

Morris T, Greer H S, White P 1977 Psychological and social adjustment to mastectomy: a two-year follow-up study. Cancer 40: 3281–3287

Murphy E, Brown G W 1980 Life events, psychiatric disturbances and physical illness. British Journal of Psychiatry 136: 326–338

Popkin M K, Callies A L, Mackenzie T B 1985 The outcome of antidepressant use in the medically ill. Archives of General Psychiatry 42: 1160–1163

Robinson R G, Kubos K L, Starr L B, Rao K, Price T R 1984 Mood disorders in stroke patients: importance of location of lesion. Brain 107: 81–93

Salkovskis P M, Warwick H M C 1986 Morbid preoccupations, health anxiety and reassurance — a cognitive behaviourial approach to hypochondriasis. Behaviour Research and Therapy 24: 597–602

Sims A 1978 Hypotheses linking neuroses with premature mortality. Psychological Medicine 8: 255–263

Spiegel D, Bloom J R, Kraemer H C, Gottheil E 1989 Effect of psychosocial treatment on survival of patients with metastatic breast cancer. Lancet ii: 888–891

Stern M J, Pascale L, McLoone J B 1976. Psychosocial adaptation following an acute myocardial infarction. Journal of Chronic Diseases 29: 513–526

Tarsh M J, Royston C 1985 A follow up study of accident neurosis. British Journal of Psychiatry 146: 18–25

Tattersall R B 1981 Psychiatric aspects of diabetes: a physician's view. British Journal of Psychiatry 139: 485–493

Taylor G J 1984 Alexithymia: concept, measurement and implications for treatment. American Journal of Psychiatry 141: 725–732

Thomas C J 1983 Referrals to a British liaison psychiatry service. Heath Trends 15: 61–64

Vaillant G E 1979 Natural history of male psychological health: effects of mental health on physical health. New England Journal of Medicine 301: 1249–1254

Whitlock F A 1982 Symptomatic affective disorders. Academic Press: London

35. Forensic psychiatry

D. Chiswick

Forensic psychiatry is concerned with the application of the law to psychiatric practice, the relationship between crime and psychiatry and the treatment of mentally abnormal offenders. In this chapter there is discussion of mental health legislation; some legal implications of mental disorder; crime and mental disorder; and the problems of the mentally abnormal offender in the criminal justice system.

MENTAL HEALTH LEGISLATION

Purpose

The rule that treatment proceeds only with the agreement of the patient is a cherished tradition of medical practice, but in clinical psychiatry the use of compulsory measures for admission and treatment is common. Psychiatric disorders may impair the patient's ability to make a rational decision. Where the consequences of the disorder may endanger patient and public, the law is available to protect the interests of both parties. Mental health legislation is neither new nor unique to the Western world. Since the Act for Regulating Madhouses of 1774, Britain has had laws controlling the activities of asylums, and since 1890 there have been laws concerning compulsory admission to hospital (Unsworth 1987). British legislation, in contrast with that of other countries, is complex and sophisticated and it has, over the years, been something of a model for other nations.

Background

Legislation must strike a balance between the loss of liberty for the mentally sick and the rights of the patient, and of society, to be protected from the consequences of his untreated illness. Important themes, with which we may or may not agree, can be identified in current mental health law. First, the legal rights of psychiatric patients as consumers of treatment have

been acknowledged. Second, a series of post-war scandals in psychiatric hospitals has demonstrated the absence of effective monitoring of standards. Third, the public is suspicious about some psychiatric treatments and wishes to exert control over their use. Fourth, in an era of litigation hospital staff are anxious about their legal rights. Finally, the legalism that has dominated American mental health legislation since the early 1970s has arrived in Britain. It was initially articulated largely through the efforts of Larry Gostin, a gifted lawyer, who worked as a legal advisor to MIND (the National Association for Mental Health). He marshalled the arguments against the Mental Health Act 1959 in a way that gained the ear of government. The amendments to the 1959 Act are enshrined in the Mental Health Act 1983.

The law and clinical judgement

There are three elements in the civil commitment of patients to hospital. There must be:

1. The presence of a mental disorder as defined in law
2. An element of risk to the welfare of the patient or of others
3. No alternative to hospital admission as a means of safeguarding that risk.

These are the legal criteria but it cannot be over-emphasised that there is a subjective element to all this. What constitutes a mental disorder and a risk, and the best way of dealing with them, are ultimately matters of clinical judgement. If he acts in good faith, a doctor cannot be guilty of any civil wrong or criminal offence though his decision may be subjected to judicial review (British Medical Journal legal correspondent 1986). Good practice requires a proper attempt at persuasion for informal treatment before resorting to the law.

The Mental Health Act 1983

The emphasis in this chapter is in describing English legislation. The Mental Health (Scotland) Act 1984 and the Mental Health (Northern Ireland) Order 1986 are broadly similar to legislation in England and Wales. The Mental Health Act 1983 introduced:

1. More stringent conditions for compulsory admission and detention
2. More opportunities for appeals against detention
3. Completely new laws relating to consent to treatment for detained patients
4. A Mental Health Act Commission
5. A Code of Practice
6. New measures for admitting offender patients to hospital.

Definition of mental disorder

Mental disorder is defined by statute as 'mental illness, arrested or incomplete development of the mind, psychopathic disorder and any other disorder or disability of mind'. It is important to distinguish those sections of the Act that refer to 'mental disorder' and those that refer to one of the four specific forms of mental disorder. In general, the shorter-term detention orders apply to patients with mental disorder, whereas the longer-term orders require the doctor to identify which of the four specific forms of mental disorder is present. The four categories of mental disorder are:

1. Mental illness
2. Psychopathic disorder
3. Mental impairment
4. Severe mental impairment.

The last two categories have major implications for the compulsory admission to hospital of the mentally retarded. The terms 'mental handicap' or 'mental retardation' do not appear in the definition of mental disorder, although they are within its scope by virtue of the reference to incomplete or arrested development of the mind. Mental retardation may be grounds for admission under a short-term order, but detention for any longer is only possible where the patient suffers from mental impairment or severe mental impairment. These terms are creations of the Act; they do not equate with any specific clinical syndrome. They are forms of mental retardation in which there is significant or severe impairment of intellectual and social functioning in association with abnormally aggressive or seriously irresponsible conduct. Long-term detention of the mentally retarded is therefore only permissible in those patients who manifest antisocial behaviour.

The statutory definition of psychopathic disorder is couched solely in behavioural terms. It is defined as 'a persistent disorder or disability of mind (whether or not including significant impairment of intelligence) which results in abnormally aggressive or seriously irresponsible conduct'. The continued inclusion of psychopathic disorder in mental health legislation is a source of controversy for many reasons: the disorder is defined solely by antisocial behaviour, which is then explained by virtue of the disorder; clear distinction of the behaviour from that shown by many recidivist offenders has not been demonstrated and the bulk of medical evidence suggests that the behaviour is not treatable in medical terms.

Mental illness, the category which accounts for the largest number of admissions under the Act, is undefined. The words used here, as elsewhere in the legislation, are supposed to have the meaning that ordinary, sensible people would ascribe to them.

Compulsory admission under Part II of the Act

Civil admission under Part II may be effected by the routes summarised in Table 35.1. In general, shorter periods of detention are associated with ease of application and limited rights of appeal for the patient. Longer periods of detention require a more elaborate process of application, but include the greatest level of safeguards for the patient. All require the joint involvement of doctor and nearest relative or of doctor and approved social worker.

The clinician has a choice with non-urgent cases whereby he may implement either sections 2 or 3. Where assessment is the principal requirement, or where it is probable that treatment is likely to be effective quickly, then section 2 is appropriate. Patients who are likely to require a longer period of treatment, with a liability to recall to hospital after leaving, should be dealt with by section 3.

Section 3 draws a crucial distinction between the major forms of mental disorder (mental illness and severe mental impairment) and the minor forms (psychopathic disorder and mental impairment). An important innovation of the 1983 Act was the inclusion of a treatability clause for the minor forms of disorder. Thus, for psychopathic disorder and for mental impairment, treatment must be likely to alleviate or prevent a deterioration of the condition.

There is no provision in the Act for compulsory treatment in the community although the use of guardianship goes a little way towards it. A mentally

Table 35.1 Compulsory admission procedures in England and Wales under Part II of the Mental Health Act 1983

Section	Situation	Medical signatories	Applicant	Psychiatric condition specified in the Act	Duration of detention	Manner of termination [a]	Appeal procedures
2	Admission for assessment	Two doctors, one of whom is approved	Nearest relative or an approved social worker	Mental disorder	28 days	1. Patient discharged or remains informally 2. Application for section 3 initiated	Mental Health Review Tribunal on application by patient
3	Admission for treatment	Two doctors, one of whom is approved	Nearest relative or an approved social worker	1. Mental illness or severe mental impairment 2. Psychopathic disorder or mental impairment only if 'treatable'	6 months, renewable for a further 6 months and then at yearly intervals	1. Patient discharged or remains informally 2. Discharged by the nearest relative unless barred by RMO	Mental Health Review Tribunal on application by patient, nearest relative or automatically by hospital managers
4	Emergency admission	Any doctor	Nearest relative or an approved social worker	Mental disorder	72 hours	1. Patient discharged or remains informally 2. Regraded to section 2 or application for section 3 initiated	None
5(2)	Emergency detention of informal patient	The doctor in charge or his nominated deputy	None	None specified	72 hours	1. Patient discharged or remains informally 2. Regraded to section 2 or application for section 3 initiated	None
5(4)	Nurse's holding power for informal patients	A first-level trained nurse	None	Mental disorder	6 hours	1. Patient discharged or remains informally 2. Section 5(2) applied by doctor	None

NB. Patients absconding from hospital and remaining absent for 28 days are deemed to be 'discharged by the process of law' and cannot be recalled to hospital under the same application.

[a] The responsible medical officer (RMO) may terminate any of these compulsory admission authorities *before* the prescribed period of detention.

Table 35.2   Compulsory admission for offenders under Part III of the Mental Health Act 1983

Section	Purpose	Maximum duration	Authority
35	Remand for report	12 weeks	M, C
36	Remand for treatment	12 weeks	C
37	Hospital or guardianship order	6 months, renewable	M, C
38	Interim hospital order	6 months	M, C
41	Restriction on discharge	Without limit of time or for defined period	C
47	Transfer of convicted prisoner	Unlimited	Home Secretary
48	Transfer of untried and other prisoners	Until further action by a court	Home Secretary
49	Restriction on discharge	Lapses on normal date of release from prison	Home Secretary

M, magistrates' court; C, crown court.

disordered person can be made the subject of guardianship under section 7. This gives authority to a guardian to require the patient to reside at a specified place and to attend at any specified centre for the purpose of medical treatment, education or training; medication cannot be administered without the patient's consent. The therapeutic benefit of treating patients compulsorily in the community while on extended leave has been reported (Sensky et al 1991), but it is not legal to use the Act in this way.

In Scotland, applications for admission other than by short-term orders, require the approval of a sheriff — a legally qualified judge.

Compulsory admission under Part III of the Act

Part III provides two routes by which the compulsory admission to hospital of mentally disordered offenders may be effected: a court may order hospitalisation either before trial or after conviction and the Home Secretary may direct the transfer to hospital of both untried and convicted prisoners (see Table 35.2).

Remands to hospital. The examination of an accused person in a prison, for the purpose of preparing a pretrial report, is often unsatisfactory. The psychiatrist does not have the benefit of observing the prisoner over a period of time, and there may be a need for investigations which cannot easily be undertaken in the hospital wing of a prison. Remand to hospital for assessment for defendants unsuitable for bail is provided by section 35. Only one medical report is required and there must be reason to suspect that the accused person is suffering from a mental disorder. A patient remanded under section 35 can only receive treatment to which he has consented. Section 36 provides for treatment, compulsory if appropriate, of remanded patients in hospital, but it cannot be used for defendants charged with murder. The court must be satisfied on the evidence of two doctors that detention in hospital for treatment is appropriate; the mental disorder must be either illness or severe mental impairment. In hospital, the provisions of Part IV of the Act apply to section 36 patients.

Hospital orders. For any offence that is punishable by imprisonment (with the exception of murder where there is a fixed penalty of life imprisonment), the court can set aside punishment and instead order admission to hospital under section 37. The great majority of hospital orders are in the category of mental illness. The grounds are broadly similar to those for admission under section 3 except that the appropriateness of, rather than the necessity for, hospital treatment is specified. Courts must be satisfied, by evidence from the doctor who will be in charge of the patient's care, or from a representative of the hospital managers, that a bed is available for the patient. A patient admitted by hospital order has almost the same rights as those admitted under civil powers. The consultant may send the patient on leave of absence or discharge him whenever he sees fit, irrespective of the length of sentence that the court might have imposed in place of a hospital order.

Restriction orders. Where a crown court (but not a magistrates' court) considers that the offender might commit further offences if at liberty, and that it is necessary to protect the public from serious harm, it may impose a restriction order upon discharge (section 41). This removes from the doctor the authority to order the discharge or leave of absence of the patient; instead, such authority rests with the Home Secretary. Approximately 15% of hospital orders carry restrictions on discharge. The Mental Health Act gives these patients similar rights of appeal to those of hospital order patients.

The discharge of restricted patients is a task not undertaken lightly by the Home Secretary; public protection looms large in his considerations. In 1972 Graham Young was convicted of two charges of murder and two of attempted murder (all by poisoning); these occurred within a few months of his conditional discharge, under a restriction order, from Broadmoor Hospital. The Aarvold Committee (1973), established in the wake of the Graham Young case, recommended that an advisory board on restricted patients should advise the Home Secretary on cases of particular concern. The function of the advisory board is to give advice on the likelihood of dangerousness on release.

Interim hospital orders. Where a patient detained under a hospital order subsequently proves unsuitable for treatment, the case cannot be returned to court for consideration of a penal sentence. A mechanism for assessing suitability for a hospital order is provided by the interim hospital order (section 38). The offender must be suffering from a category of mental disorder for which admission under a hospital order may be appropriate.

Transfer of prisoners to hospital. Prisoners, whether untried or convicted, who become mentally disordered can only receive treatment in prison if they give consent. Untried and convicted prisoners may be transferred to hospital by direction of the Home Secretary. In hospital, the provisions of Part IV of the Act apply to transferred prisoners. For convicted prisoners the requirements for a transfer direction (section 47) are similar to those for a hospital order.

In most cases the Home Secretary also applies a restriction direction (section 49), so that in hospital the patient is in the same situation as any patient under a restriction order. The Home Secretary may direct transfer of the patient back to prison if he is satisfied that treatment in hospital is no longer required or appropriate. Untried and other categories of unconvicted prisoners may be transferred to hospital for urgent treatment under section 48. The mental disorder must be either mental illness or severe mental impairment.

Consent to treatment

The issue of consent to treatment poses particular problems in clinical psychiatry. Some patients, lacking insight into the nature of their illness, may refuse treatment, while others as a consequence of mental disorder may lack the capacity to give consent. The common law, including some recent judicial decisions, governs consent to treatment for all patients except where it is specifically overridden by statute. In particular the provisions of Part IV of the Mental Health Act apply to most detained patients and to specified psychiatric treatments (see Table 35.3).

The general position is the same in psychiatry as elsewhere in medical practice. Any form of physical treatment (e.g. electroconvulsive therapy (ECT) or medication) for mental disorder requires the real consent of the patient. This is 'the voluntary and continuing permission of the patient to receive a particular treatment, based on an adequate knowledge of the purpose, likely effects and risks of that treatment including the likelihood of its success and any alternatives to it' (Department of Health and Welsh Office 1990). Two elements of real consent are of particular significance in psychiatric practice. These are the competence of the patient to give consent and the disclosure of information by the doctor.

Competence. The capacity of a patient to give real consent is a matter for the clinical judgement of the doctor. Some patients, for example those suffering from a mental handicap, or organic brain disease or depression with retardation, may passively accept care in hospital yet not really appear capable of understanding the implications of treatment. Can the doctor treat such patients who are not competent to give consent? If the treatment is for mental disorder, it is usually appropriate to detain the patient under the Mental Health Act and apply Part IV. However, the House of Lords in *F* v *West Berkshire Health Authority* (Gunn 1990) reaffirmed the doctor's duty in common law to provide treatment for an incompetent patient

Table 35.3   Consent to psychiatric treatment by mentally disordered patients

Patient	Treatment	Consent governed by
Informal and competent	Any appropriate psychiatric treatment [a]	Common law requirements for real consent
	Urgently necessary psychiatric treatment	Common law doctrine of necessity
Informal and incompetent	Any appropriate psychiatric treatment [a]	Common law duty of care but it may be appropriate to detain under the MHA and invoke Part IV
	Urgently necessary psychiatric treatment	Common law doctrine of necessity
Detained	Electroconvulsive therapy or medicines for mental disorder for more than 3 months	Consent *or* second opinion under Part IV of the MHA (section 58)
	Psychosurgery or male libido-reducing hormone implant	Consent *and* second opinion under Part IV of the MHA (section 57)
	Immediately necessary psychiatric treatment	Part IV of the MHA (section 62)
	Any other psychiatric treatment	No consent needed

[a] For psychosurgery and male libido-reducing hormone implants the provisions of section 57 of the Mental Health Act (MHA) apply.

so long as such treatment was in the best interests of the patient; the test for the latter being practice according to a responsible body of medical opinion. The case of *F* concerned the sterilisation of a mentally handicapped woman. The House of Lords held that this was a special treatment for which a declaration of the High Court should be sought before proceeding; other special operations may fall into this category.

Disclosure of information by the doctor. The nature of the explanation of the treatment given by the doctor will vary according to the particular patient and the particular treatment. The patient should receive sufficient information to understand in broad terms the nature, likely effects and risks of the treatment and information about any alternatives. The doctor may give additional information according to his professional judgement. The House of Lords in *Sidaway* v. *Bethlem Royal Hospital and Others* concluded that the amount of information disclosed by the doctor must reach the 'reasonable level of care' laid down in *Bolam* v. *Friern Hospital Management Committee* in 1957. The

doctor is not negligent if he discloses information in accordance with a practice rightly accepted as proper by a body of skilled and experienced medical men.

Detained patients. Part IV of the Mental Health Act is of profound importance, providing, as it does, a statutory basis for the implementation of certain treatments for certain patients. It provides safeguards for patients by grading treatments according to their seriousness, and by involving more people in decision-making for the more serious treatments. It affords protection to staff by clarifying the legal circumstances in which treatments may, or may not, be given to psychiatric patients. Its provisions apply without exception to treatment for mental disorders; it has no applicability for physical disorders, except insofar as a mental disorder requiring treatment has a physical cause, e.g. delirium. With one important exception, it only applies to patients detained, or liable to be detained, in hospital for more than a few days.

Section 57 treatments. Treatment under section 57 requires the consent of the patient and a concurring second opinion. The section is unique in Part IV by virtue of its application to all patients, including out-patients and informal in-patients. (In Scotland the provisions of the equivalent section of the Scottish Act apply only to detained patients.) Section 57 applies to the most serious and irreversible forms of psychiatric treatments. At present, these are psychosurgery for mental disorder and the surgical implantation of hormones to reduce male libido. For either of these treatments the patient must give real consent. In addition he must be interviewed by three people (one of whom is an independent doctor) appointed for the purpose by the Mental Health Act Commission. Treatment can only proceed if the three people verify that the patient has given real consent and the doctor agrees that the treatment is appropriate and should be given.

Between 1987 and 1989 there were 52 referrals under section 57 to the Mental Health Act Commission; all but one concerned psychosurgery. The refusal of the Commission to grant a certificate for the administration of goserelin (a hormone antagonist used in the treatment of prostatic cancer) to curb libido in a paedophile was overturned by judicial review. The court ruled that goserelin was not a hormone and it was not administered by surgical implantation; it therefore was not a section 57 treatment.

Section 58 treatments. Here it is necessary to have either the consent of the patient or the opinion of an independent doctor appointed for the purpose by the Mental Health Act Commission. The section only applies to detained patients, and there are only two forms of treatment presently within its provisions: ECT and medication for mental disorder given for more than 3 months during a period of detention. There are nearly 4000 referrals per year under section 58 to the Commission; approximately half for ECT and half for medication. Even for consenting patients, the consultant must complete a certificate of consent for the particular treatment, which contains a statement that the patient is capable of understanding its nature, purpose and effects. Medication given for up to 3 months does not fall within section 58 and can therefore be given without the patient's consent.

Urgent treatment. Where urgent treatment is required, it is possible to dispense with the patient's consent. Normally, the authority for such treatment is derived from the common law duty of care owed by the doctor to his patient and from the doctrine of necessity. There must be an immediate danger to the health or safety of the patient or of others, and the treatment must be reasonable and in proportion to that danger. For detained patients, authority for giving urgent treatment for mental disorder is provided by section 62. This seeks to provide a balance between, on the one hand, the hazards or irreversible consequences of the treatment and, on the other, the degree of danger presented by the patient's mental condition.

Mental Health Review Tribunals

There are 15 Mental Health Review Tribunals in England and Wales established on a regional basis; tribunal members are appointed by the Lord Chancellor. Each region has a lawyer as chairman who convenes a panel of tribunal members to hear applications. A tribunal must consist of three members: a lawyer as chairman, a medical member and a lay member. In the case of patients under restriction orders, the chairman must be a specially approved judge.

Tribunals are governed by the Mental Health Review Tribunal Rules 1983. The right of application to a tribunal is available for nearly all categories of detained patients and, in many cases, for the nearest relatives also. However, many patients do not exercise their right of application and the Act requires automatic referral of such cases by the hospital managers, and by the Home Secretary in the case of restriction order patients.

In essence, the decision of a tribunal to direct discharge hinges upon its being satisfied that either the patient does not have a mental disorder, or that hospital treatment is not appropriate or not necessary. It has absolute authority to direct discharge or a delayed discharge, and it may also recommend leave of absence or transfer of the patient to another hospital or to guardianship. For restricted patients, the options available to a tribunal are different: it may order discharge or conditional discharge (if necessary deferred until suitable arrangements can be made), but it has no other powers. In Scotland, patients may appeal against their detention to a sheriff, whose powers are almost the same as those of a tribunal.

Mental Health Act Commission

An independent inspectorate for mental hospitals, some form of which had existed since 1774, was disbanded in England and Wales in 1960, only to be resurrected in 1983 in the form of the Mental Health Act Commission. By contrast, Scotland took no such action in the 1960s and its Mental Welfare Commission has continued to function for the last 30 years. The principal functions of the Mental Health Act Commission are:

1. To review the powers of detention under the Act by visiting hospitals and nursing homes and interviewing, in private, detained patients
2. To appoint doctors for the purpose of providing second opinions under Part IV of the Act
3. To keep under review the long-term treatment of detained patients
4. To prepare for the Secretary of State a code of practice, for doctors and other staff, on the admission and treatment of patients suffering from mental disorder.

The Commission has a chairman and 91 part-time members, the majority of whom are professionals from the fields of medicine, nursing, social work, psychology and law. There are also academic and lay members. The work of the Commission is described in the biennial reports which it is required to prepare (Mental Health Act Commission 1989). Its draft code of practice, 236 pages in length, met with heavy criticism, and the government has produced a much more reasonable document (Department of Health and Welsh Office 1990).

LEGAL IMPLICATIONS OF MENTAL DISORDER

There are many situations where the presence of a mental disorder may have serious legal implications for a patient. The most important situations are described below.

Voting rights

By application of the common law, 'peers, prisoners and idiots' may not vote at elections. A person who is on the electoral roll and who presents himself at the polling station may cast his vote. Patients who are compulsorily detained in hospital may not register for the electoral roll. However, under the Representation of the People Act 1983 involuntary patients may do so, provided they can complete, in the presence of an authorised member of the staff but without assistance, a patient's declaration.

Marriage and divorce

Marriage is a contract which may be terminated by divorce (commonly) or by annulment (rarely); mental disorder may be relevant in both methods of termination. For the contract to be valid, both partners must understand its nature. Mental disorder is not an automatic indicator of a lack of capacity to consent to

marriage, but a marriage may be annulled if it can be shown that either partner did not consent to the marriage by virtue of unsoundness of mind. A further ground for nullifying a marriage is where either partner, although consenting, was suffering from mental disorder within the meaning of the Act of a nature to render the individual unfitted for marriage. The test is stringent; the person must be incapable, as a result of mental disorder, of living in the married state or of carrying out the duties of marriage.

Since the Matrimonial Causes Act 1973, the sole ground for divorce is that the marriage has irretrievably broken down. This may be based on one of the following five facts: adultery, unreasonable behaviour, desertion, living apart for 2 years where the respondent consents to divorce, and living apart for 5 years whether or not the respondent agrees to divorce. The presence of a mental disorder may be relevant in establishing unreasonable behaviour; it may also affect the capacity of a respondent to give proper consent to divorce after 2 years' separation.

Confidentiality of medical information

Psychiatric patients are likely to have information about them made known to others without their knowledge or consent: they may also be denied access to their medical records by reason of their mental condition. Reports on detained patients are routinely submitted to hospital managers, mental health review tribunals and the Mental Health Act Commission. The Home Office receives detailed information on restricted patients. Sometimes a psychiatrist may feel compelled to disclose to a third party information about a patient whom he considers likely to be violent. The Court of Appeal has ruled that disclosure is lawful where the doctor believes it to be in the public interest (McHale 1990). The Tarasoff case in California has given rise to the duty-to-warn doctrine whereby doctors in America must alert potential victims who are considered to be seriously at risk from patients under their care (Mackay 1990).

The Access to Health Records Act 1990 gave patients right of access to case notes made from 1 November 1991. Psychiatric patients are likely to be frequent users of the Act. It contains a clause that access can be refused where it is likely to cause serious harm to the physical or mental health of the patient.

Driving

It is a requirement of the Road Traffic Act 1972 that an applicant for a driving licence must disclose any relevant disability. A relevant disability is any disability prescribed by the 1972 Act, or any other disability, that is likely to cause the driver of a vehicle to be a source of danger to the public. Where the authorities are satisfied that a relevant disability exists, the licence must be refused. The only mental disorder prescribed in the Act is severe mental handicap. However, depending on the individual case other disorders may be regarded as a relevant disability. The dangers of psychotic patients, or those with depressive illnesses, driving are probably underestimated. The Medical Commission on Accident Prevention recommends that doctors should advise patients with acute psychiatric illness not to drive (Cremona 1986).

Managing property and affairs

There is an assumption that mentally disordered people are capable of managing their affairs until the contrary is proved. In practice, the inability of some patients to deal with their affairs may cause serious problems to relatives, creditors and business associates. On the other hand, patients themselves may worry that, during an episode of illness, their affairs may be taken out of their hands irrevocably.

Power of attorney. Where a person is, for whatever reason, unable to manage his affairs, he may give instructions that someone else may act for him. This instrument, a power of attorney, can only be made by a person who has the capacity to understand what it means and its implications. An ordinary power of attorney ceases to have effect when such capacity is lost. However, under the Enduring Powers of Attorney Act 1985, a person can, when mentally well, make an enduring power of attorney which gives instructions to be implemented in the event of actual or impending incapacity of the donor.

Court of Protection. The Court of Protection is an office of the Supreme Court which has the power to appoint a receiver to manage the property and affairs of a person who, by reason of mental disorder, is incapable of managing them himself. In Scotland an equivalent appointment is that of a curator bonis appointed by the Court of Session or a sheriff court. Part VII of the Mental Health Act 1983 describes the duties and powers of the Court of Protection; its proceedings are governed by the Court of Protection Rules 1984. In effect it exercises sole control over the property and affairs of the mentally disordered person. Application to the court may be made by any person, but is usually by a relative.

The important role for doctors is in assessing the mental condition of the person and his capacity to manage his affairs. A certificate from only one doctor is necessary, and he does not require to be recognised under section 12 of the Act. For this purpose mental disorder is as defined by the broad definition in the Act (which encompasses mental illness, mental retardation, psychopathic disorder and any other disorder or disability of mind). Before examining the patient, the doctor should brief himself with some knowledge of the extent of the patient's property and affairs. It is important to ascertain whether the patient understands the obligations of owning property or assets. The doctor is required to state the grounds upon which he bases his conclusions and he should describe these in simple language.

Making a will

The test of a person's ability to make a will is, as elsewhere, his capacity to understand the nature and effects of the task. This is referred to as testamentary capacity; it depends upon the testator being of sound disposing mind. The validity of a will may be challenged either before or after the death of the testator on the grounds that such capacity was lacking. Doctors may be called upon to assess testamentary capacity in patients who are known to have a mental disorder and who wish to make a will. The crucial questions are:

1. Does he understand the nature and implications of making a will?
2. Does he have some appreciation of the extent of his estate?
3. Does he appreciate which people may reasonably expect to be beneficiaries (even though he may choose to exclude them)?

It is possible for a valid will to be made by a mentally disordered person during a lucid interval, and by a person whose affairs are being managed by the Court of Protection. A careful examination is necessary. The precise nature of any mental disorder is of less importance than the way it may be related to the requirements for testamentary capacity.

CRIME AND PSYCHIATRY

A biological basis for crime

Every year in Britain approximately 2 million people are convicted of criminal offences. Their offences are diverse: from urinating in public and being drunk and disorderly to business fraud and homicide. Theft, in its various forms, accounts for over 80% of indictable crime. We know nothing of the psychological features of the great majority of offenders, who are in any case the convicted and therefore unsuccessful criminals: we know less than nothing of their undetected counterparts, who are responsible for a greater amount of crime.

In spite of the diversity of criminal behaviour, speculation that criminality is an individualised trait has sustained the search for its biological determinant. West (1988) has reviewed the psychobiological approach to criminality which embraces consideration of personality, organic factors, psychodynamic theory and experimental psychology. Certainly an association between lower intelligence and delinquency is supported by empirical research (Rutter and Giller 1983). In the last 40 years attention has shifted to abnormalities in the electrical activity of the temporal lobe, the metabolism of serotonin and psychophysiological responses (Weller 1986).

One reason why this search continues to be pursued with vigour is the evidence from genetic studies of criminals which suggests that something is indeed inherited. Over 60 years ago Lange, in a monograph entitled *Crime as Destiny* found that concordance for criminality was over six times higher in monozygotic twins than in dizygotic twins (Editorial 1983). Further twin studies supported this finding, except when a wider range of offences (e.g. driving offences and treason) were included (Dalgaard and Kringlen 1976). These findings have been reinforced by results from adoption studies. A Scandinavian adoption survey demonstrated a genetic factor in petty criminality (mainly non-violent property offences) in the absence of alcohol abuse, and a further analysis of the same adoption data examined the interaction of genetic and environmental factors. The results suggested that, for male offenders, low social status and unstable preadoptive placement, in combination with genetic predisposition, increased the risk of petty criminality (Cloninger et al 1982).

To summarise, it is tempting to talk of a constitutional propensity for criminal behaviour. If such a propensity exists it may have a genetic component which is modified by environmental, cultural or even economic factors. The interaction of biological and social disadvantage is encapsulated in a disturbing study of 14 juveniles on death row in America (Lewis et al 1988). The youths showed serious central nervous system deficits, low intelligence and multiple psychotic symptoms. Five had been sodomised by a relative and nearly all came from violent families.

Crime and mental disorder

Psychiatrists have a natural interest in criminal behaviour when it is more closely related to mental disorder but the relation between crime and mental disorder is deceptively complex with many unanswered questions. The paucity of research in this topic is due, in part, to major methodological and conceptual problems (Gunn 1977a). The definitions of criminal behaviour and mental disorder lack precision so that analysis of their interdependence is obscure. Criminal behaviour is what society chooses to designate as criminal at any given time. Social attitudes towards crimes, particularly for example sex crimes, change over time; abortion, homosexuality and prostitution have all undergone decriminalisation within the last 30 years.

All criminal acts depend on contributions from the perpetrator, the environment and sometimes from the victim; their interaction is unique on every occasion. Among those factors associated with the perpetrator might be the presence of mental disorder, but this will only be known in those offenders who happen to undergo psychiatric examination. The relationship of the disorder to the offence may range from the coincidental to the causal. It is not possible to make sweeping generalisations about the association between particular psychiatric syndromes and particular crimes.

While acknowledging these caveats, it is convenient to review the relationship between crime and mental disorder by considering the extent of mental disorder among offenders, the criminality of psychiatric populations, and the manner in which specific psychiatric disorders might sometimes be associated with criminal acts.

Mental disorder in offenders

Psychiatric assessments are not routinely conducted on all offenders and there has been no psychiatric survey in Britain of a court cohort of offenders. Such research is difficult to carry out, and not surprisingly most studies are of prison populations. The psychiatry of imprisonment, the psychiatry of criminal prosecution and the psychiatry of offending are all separate issues. Decisions to remand in custody, and to impose a sentence of imprisonment, are highly selective and the resulting population is almost certainly not typical of the generality of offenders for any given crime.

It is in prisoners awaiting trial that the greatest prevalence of psychiatric disorder is found. Such populations, particularly in the prisons serving the major cities, contain large numbers of people with multiple social and medical disabilities, including psychiatric illness. At Brixton Prison in London (the largest remand prison in Europe) Taylor & Gunn (1984) showed that 9% of all receptions were considered to be psychotic (mainly schizophrenic), while a further 9% showed symptoms of withdrawal from alcohol or drugs. Their figure for psychotic illness is markedly higher than that reported in any of the British prison studies comprehensively reviewed by Coid (1984). A recent study (Gunn et al 1991) of 1769 men serving prison sentences identified 2% who were psychotic and warranted transfer to hospital. A further 20% had treatment needs; these were mainly prisoners with substance abuse and with personality disorders. Surprisingly, only seven prisoners were considered to be mentally retarded. Eight suffered from epilepsy.

Among the rootless population to be found in any urban conurbation there are high levels of recidivist offending, sometimes involving crimes of significant violence, and high levels of multiple social and psychiatric pathology. As resources for the shelter and care of such people diminish, the number who find their way into remand prisons charged with offences at all levels of seriousness is likely to increase.

Criminality in psychiatric populations

The rate of offending among psychiatric patients compared with that of the general population is not known with any certainty. There are ethical problems in investigating the topic, and it is difficult to control for socioeconomic factors. Less than 1% of admissions to psychiatric hospitals in England and Wales are accounted for by offender patients under Part III of the Mental Health Act. There is no doubt that mentally ill offenders are more likely to be detected and arrested (Robertson 1988). Attention has been directed to the criminal careers of former psychiatric patients, but results are conflicting. Hafner and Boker (1982) concluded that the rate of violent offending by 533 mentally disordered offenders in West Germany was quantitatively similar to the rate of violence for the population at large. These early views that offending was no more nor less likely among psychiatric patients than in the population generally have been questioned by Mullen (1988). For subgroups of psychiatric patients, particularly those with schizophrenia, the risk of violent offending is at least twice the expected rate.

It is impossible to conclude that one particular form of offence is the hallmark of one particular psychiatric condition. Nonetheless, it is helpful to consider the generality of offending that may be associated with different disorders.

Schizophrenia

Criminal acts committed by schizophrenics may be closely or distantly related to the phenomenology of the illness. Such phenomenology may be florid in form (e.g. delusional mood, paranoid delusions or misinterpretations of the environment), or it may consist of the negative features (e.g. a deterioration in personality and social functioning) which characterise residual schizophrenia (Taylor 1985). In either situation there may be a contribution from the effects of alcohol or drug abuse or from a premorbid antisocial personality or from a highly charged interpersonal relationship. The offence itself may vary from the trivial to the catastrophic and may seem a gross over-reaction to mundane events. Most violence by schizophrenics, as by others, is domestic in nature. The tension and dislocation, which are common features in families caring for a schizophrenic member, may precipitate violence in the emotionally volatile schizophrenic.

The association between violence and schizophrenia has probably been understated: sanguine views that such a relationship was a recognised but insignificant feature have been shaken by research at Brixton Prison. Taylor & Gunn (1984) found that the prevalence of schizophrenia in men convicted of homicides and other crimes of violence was approximately 25 times greater than in the population on which the prison draws. Does this high association tell us something about the illness itself or about the consequences of failing to treat it properly? Many schizophrenics suffering their first episode of illness obtain treatment through a forensic source after experiencing rejections elsewhere (Johnstone et al 1986). Violent behaviour by hospital in-patients is associated with a diagnosis of schizophrenia (Noble and Rodger 1989).

Affective disorder

Affective disorders are common, and only rarely are they associated with the commission of a major crime. Mania and hypomania commonly lead to acts of public disorder, minor violence and fraudulent dishonesty in association with grandiosity, but rarely result in serious offending. Homicidal acts committed during states of depressive illness are classically of the altruistic type. The victim is invariably a family member; there may be more than one victim, and such acts are commonly followed by the suicide or parasuicide of the assailant.

The relationship of other crimes to depressive illness is more contentious. An episode of shoplifting occurring for the first time in a middle-aged person, male or female, should alert the clinician to the possibility of a depressive illness. Impaired concentration and indecisiveness may contribute to the behaviour, and sometimes it may result from the effects of inappropriately prescribed medication such as benzodiazepines. People facing court proceedings are likely to be unhappy and some may even be clinically depressed. It is therefore important to establish the presence or otherwise of depressive symptomatology prior to commission of the offence. The clinical examination should be supplemented by accounts from relatives whenever possible.

Personality disorder

It is not surprising that offending is a common feature among those who attract a diagnosis of antisocial personality disorder, for the diagnosis will have been made on the basis of the offending. There is no convincing evidence that offenders, labelled recidivists by the courts and psychopaths by psychiatrists, are demonstrably different. Even if the diagnosis is accepted as a clinical entity, there remains little of the former optimism that such patients are treatable. Today, the compulsory detention of psychopaths is controversial and the admission of such patients under hospital orders is virtually confined to the special hospitals (Grounds 1987). The likelihood of their offending after discharge from hospital is much greater than it is for mentally ill or mentally handicapped patients (Gibbens & Robertson 1983).

The diagnosis of an offender as psychopathic may have important implications; length of sentence, admission to a special hospital, management in prison and the likelihood of gaining parole may all be affected by the application of such a diagnosis.

Neuroses

Some offenders commit the same minor offence again and again. Often the behaviour is senseless (e.g. petty shoplifting or indecent exposure) and shows a marked resistance to any form of therapeutic intervention. Commonly such offenders have fragile personalities and manifest a range of neurotic behaviour patterns, e.g. phobic symptoms and panic attacks. They are often unhappy people, either socially isolated or in dependent relationships with dominant partners. Their criminal acts may be exciting and rewarding episodes in an otherwise drab and unfulfilled existence.

Mental retardation

Among adult offenders in general it is unlikely that mentally retarded offenders are over-represented, although imprisonment seems to be a more likely outcome for them. Social disadvantage and an unstable home background are associated with offending in mentally retarded people, just as they are for the general population. In recent years, the use of hospital orders for the admission of mentally retarded offenders has fallen drastically.

Sex offences and arson are over-represented among crimes committed by mentally retarded offenders (Turk 1989). Sex offending may range from a trivial episode of indecent exposure to a sexual assault upon a victim, perhaps a child, who is usually a previous acquaintance of the offender. Arson by the mentally retarded probably reflects persistence of the normal childish interest in setting fires. Most vulnerable among the mentally retarded are those with IQs in the borderline range together with a superficial degree of social competence. They may be exploited by more sophisticated offenders and are less likely to escape apprehension by the police.

Substance abuse

There is a strong association between substance abuse and offending. The seriousness of such offending varies from minor acts of public disorder through theft and robbery to assaults and homicide. Chronic drinkers with multiple social handicaps form a large proportion of the short-sentence populations in most prisons. Many receive medical care only at times of imprisonment. Driving offences and crimes of dishonesty, which may include prolonged fraudulent activity, are features of drinkers with less impoverished backgrounds. Intoxication, by drink or drugs, is commonly a feature of a range of offences, including homicides and sex offences (Lindqvist 1991). In a Scottish sample of 400 individuals charged with murder, Gillies (1976) reported that 58% of male accused and 30% of female accused were intoxicated at the time of the offence. Over a third of the victims had also been abusing alcohol. Drink is a common feature of domestic violence between marital partners. Offending may also be associated with the neuropsychiatric sequelae of alcoholism, such as delirium tremens and alcoholic hallucinosis.

More than 10% of men in prison are drug dependent before entering prison. Their management, particularly since the human immunodeficiency virus (HIV) epidemic in drug users, is a major problem.

Organic conditions

Disinhibition and impaired judgement, characteristic of organic brain disease, may lead to minor crimes of dishonesty or sex offences, the latter often involving children befriended by the accused. However, elderly men who offend are more likely to have alcohol and personality problems or a functional psychosis than dementia. In younger men, organic brain damage as a consequence of head injury may lead to disorderly or violent behaviour.

Epilepsy

Serious violence as an ictal phenomenon is exceedingly rare and the utmost caution is required before asserting such a link. Nonetheless, epileptics are over-represented in prison populations, although there is no evidence of a relationship between epilepsy and crimes of violence (Gunn 1977b). The explanation for the increased prevalence of epilepsy among prisoners is uncertain. It may be that some degree of brain damage is responsible for both the epilepsy and antisocial behaviour. However, Whitman et al (1984) concluded that the important socioeconomic correlates of epilepsy account for the association, and not some intrinsic relationship between epilepsy and aggression. Similarly, violence in temporal lobe epilepsy is not simply an ictal phenomenon (Herzberg & Fenwick 1988).

Pathological (morbid) jealousy

The clinical features of this syndrome are described in Chapter 20. It is of forensic importance because of the association with spouse homicide and the malignancy of the condition. Although the classical presentation is readily diagnosed, the distinction between pathological and normal jealousy is rarely clear-cut. Mullen (1990) stresses the importance of taking a global view of the patient's judgement, feelings and behaviour within the context of the relationship with the partner. Jealousy, whether or not pathological, is a common source of violence between partners. In a sample of psychotic homicides at Broadmoor, Mowat (1966) found that 12% had killed as a consequence of morbid jealousy. They were predominantly middle-aged men who had been morbidly jealous for an average period of 4 years before the homicide.

DANGEROUSNESS

The concept

The possibility of offender patients committing acts of serious harm is of particular significance when advising courts (and the Home Office) on the imposition (and removal) of restrictions on discharge under section 41 of the Mental Health Act, and more generally when considering the discharge from hospital, particularly secure hospitals, of offender patients who have committed acts of violence. These decisions require the psychiatrist to consider what is generally referred to as the dangerousness of the offender.

There is no satisfactory definition of the term although the Butler Committee on mentally abnormal offenders (Home Office & DHSS 1975) suggested 'a propensity to cause serious physical injury or lasting psychological harm'. The concept of dangerousness is, however, confounded by the impossibility of its accurate prediction, and by the social and legal responses which nonetheless follow a positive prediction. The identification of dangerousness generally, as a step in protecting the public, is disputed as a justifiable exercise (Floud & Young 1981). Nonetheless, public and political attitudes toward dangerousness have forced psychiatrists, rightly or wrongly, to apply themselves to the task of its prediction (Walker 1991).

The prediction of dangerousness

Hazards

The accuracy of psychiatric predictions of dangerousness, and the method by which they are made, are fiercely disputed. Steadman (1983), an indefatigable critic, argues that the predictions of psychiatrists owe more to magic than they do to science or even art. He suggests that psychiatrists lack any specific skills or technology which enable them to make predictions of any greater accuracy that those that would be obtained by chance. The psychiatric expert, over-awed by the heavy responsibility upon him, is likely to err on the side of caution. Errors resulting in prolonged and pointless detention usually escape public attention. However, a decision to release a patient who subsequently re-offends results in major public concern in which professional reputations may be tarnished. A further problem in predicting the likelihood of future violent behaviour in a selected group of people is that violence will be manifested, in any event, by a proportion of the larger population of whom the group form a part.

Research findings

The relation between dangerousness and mental disorder may be examined in a variety of ways. The important questions for examination are:

1. Is mental abnormality a significant contribution to re-offending on release from custody?
2. What is the extent of offending in discharged psychiatric patients who had been deemed dangerous?
3. Is there a uniform methodology for the psychiatric assessment of dangerousness?

Research provides some limited answers to all these questions. A Home Office study (Home Office & DHSS 1975) showed that male offenders discharged from hospital had lower reconviction rates in general than a comparable group of men released from prison. However, the reconviction rates for violent or sexual crimes were similar at about 6% in both groups. This and other studies suggest that, regardless of mental abnormality, the most reliable guide to future violence by offenders is their previous record. In Britain, about 10% of patients discharged from maximum security hospitals are likely to commit serious crimes of violence (Bowden 1981).

These studies refer to patients whose release had been determined on the basis of clinical judgements. What of those dangerous patients released 'by accident?' A successful appeal by one Johnnie Baxstrom in the US Supreme Court in 1966 brought about release from a maximum security hospital, not only of Baxstrom, but also of 966 similarly detained patients. A follow-up of the criminal careers of these patients provided an opportunity for a natural experiment (Steadman & Cocozza 1974). Of 176 patients discharged to the community, there were 20 re-arrests, but only seven involved violence. For the group as a whole, only 3% were returned to conditions of maximum security.

This research suggests that psychiatric disorder is not a significant contributor towards dangerousness, the existence of which is, in any case, overestimated in psychiatric institutions. Do psychiatrists have special techniques for the assessment of dangerousness, and are their assessments reliable? The short answer to both these questions is 'no'. Psychiatrists reach their conclusions in the same way as other prediction makers do, and agreement between psychiatrists on dangerousness assessments was no greater than that between school teachers (Quinsey & Ambtman 1979) or other professionals (Montandon & Harding 1984). Psychiatrists, in comparison with other groups, seem to over-diagnose dangerousness. Rarely do they question the validity of the concept of dangerousness or their role in its assessment (Harding & Adserballe 1983).

Practical aspects

Given this uncertain theoretical framework, the need for circumspection in the assessment of dangerousness is evident. The task may be impossible; there are certainly no short cuts or tricks by which it can be accomplished. The psychiatrist requires a combination of good clinical skills, common sense and the ability to take a broad and balanced view. The normal task is assessing the likelihood of violent behaviour in a patient with a psychiatric disorder who has shown previous violence. Particular consideration is necessary when transfer to a lesser degree of security is proposed. Detailed reading of casenotes and previous records, discussion with staff and careful examination of the patient are essential. It is important to ask oneself questions concerning the patient, his new environment, any potential victims and the quality of care to be provided.

The patient. What is the nature of the psychiatric disorder and what is its relationship to previous violence? Has it been modified by treatment? Is clinical change a matter of observation or speculation? To what extent does clinical improvement lessen the likelihood of further violent behaviour? Are there complicating factors in the form of premorbid personality, substance abuse or inappropriate sexual behaviour? Does the patient have any explanation for his previous behaviour and can he accept the psychiatrist's conceptual understanding of it? Is his 'inner world' accessible to staff? Do his actions match his words? Does he appreciate the need for continuing treatment? Is he likely to make proper use of people involved in his subsequent care? Is your impression of him similar to those of your colleagues?

Environmental factors. Did situational factors contribute to the original violence? Have they been eliminated in the new environment? Will the new environment provide a standard of care such that changes in the patient's mental state will be noticed? If changes are observed, what action will be taken?

Potential victims. Was the original victim selected by reason of propinquity, or on the basis of the patient's psychopathology, or both? Is it possible to identify potential victims in advance? If so, do they have an awareness of the patient's psychiatric condition? Are they likely themselves to form pathological relationships with the patient, and would they be able to seek advice if the need should arise? If potential victims are living companions are they likely to support the need for continuing treatment?

Aftercare. Circumstances vary in each case. The task of assessing dangerousness is most straightforward when there is a close causal connection between the violent behaviour and psychotic illness. The more tenuous the connection, or indeed the more fragile the diagnosis of psychotic illness, the greater will be the uncertainty of the clinician. Psychotic illnesses run a generally predictable course: the vagaries of human behaviour do not.

The crucial ingredient for the prevention of violence, particularly in the community, is the quality of aftercare provided. This depends on the patient's cooperation in receiving aftercare and an efficient clinical service that can provide it. Responsibility for the care of high-risk patients is accepted by different clinicians with varying degrees of equanimity. It is not work that should be undertaken by those who are constitutionally anxious, or those who are excessively casual.

Offences and offenders

Homicide

Every year approximately 500 homicides are recorded in England and Wales; these include the crimes of murder, manslaughter and infanticide. All defendants charged with murder are examined for the purpose of a psychiatric report. The legal definition of murder is 'the unlawful killing of any reasonable creature under the Queen's peace, with malice aforethought, death occurring within a year and a day of the act'.

For statistical purposes homicide is 'normal' where the outcome is conviction for murder, or for manslaughter other than by reason of diminished responsibility (see below). 'Abnormal' murder comprises convictions for manslaughter due to diminished responsibility, infanticide, homicide in a failed suicide pact and legal findings of insanity. One-third of homicides are abnormal and approximately 8% of all suspects commit suicide before coming to trial. The proportions of murders that are abnormal is high in countries where the homicide rate is low (e.g. in England); as the homicide rate rises, the proportion of abnormal murders falls. More than 75% of victims are known to their killers; family members or a sexual partner of the accused account for 50% of all victims. Death, other than by means of a sharp or blunt instrument, brute force or strangulation is unusual. Quarrels, revenge or a loss of temper account for 50% of killings.

Psychiatric assessment in homicide is usually in respect of a domestic crime with a background of interpersonal strife, jealousy, alcoholism, disability of either victim or suspect, depression or psychosis (Bluglass 1979a). In spouse murder the role of the victim in contributing to her (or his) own death may be substantial. Sometimes the murder may be a 'mercy killing' of a chronically disabled partner.

Infants aged under 1 year are at greatest risk of death by homicide. Some of these are the victims of a mentally ill parent, usually the mother (d'Orban 1979) but other infant homicides by mothers have their origins in situational, relationship and personality problems (Resnick 1969). Some younger child, or infant, victims are killed after chronic ill-treatment, battering or neglect.

The killing of parents or siblings are the rarest forms of family homicide. Patricide is more common than matricide (though both are rare), and was associated in a Scottish study with alcohol intoxication (Gillies 1976). The reported association between matricide and schizophrenia probably owes more to opportunity than it does to any inherent feature of the disease; the usual provider of care for a schizophrenic son is his mother (Chiswick 1981). Matricide by daughters commonly reflects the mutually dependent hostile relationship with a domineering mother that is also characteristic of male matricides (d'Orban & O'Connor 1989). This applies irrespective of any psychiatric disorder.

Where the victim is a stranger, it is unusual to find any evidence of mental illness in the accused; alcohol intoxication is a more probable factor. An exception is the rare instance when a schizophrenic selects a stranger as a victim on the basis of psychotic experiences. The sexual or sadistic murder of a random victim, who may be a child, is rare, although such cases are given prominence by the media.

Sexual offences

Between 1978 and 1988 the number of sexual crimes increased by only 19% compared with an increase of 82% for other crimes of violence; an exception is rape which has more than doubled in frequency. Sexual crimes account for less than 1% of indictable crimes made known to the police but a disproportionate number of accused are remanded for psychiatric reports. Sex offenders are almost exclusively men among whom mental illness is not prevalent.

The offences and offenders are widely heterogeneous. Offences range from a trivial episode of indecent exposure to a sadistic rape. Sexual offences are defined with precision but the same legal offence may conceal a wide range of behaviours. This heterogeneity makes it impossible to arrive at a useful classification; most have been artificially based on one particular facet of the offence or the offender. Few classifications have been tested for reliability; none has any predictive value and most reflect the professional bias of their creators. They are usually based on a confusing mishmash of offence behaviour, imputed motivation, type of victim, personality traits and psychological or psychodynamic theory. The psychiatry of sex offending is a fragile and dubious concept because the bulk of offences are not related to psychiatric disorder. The following is a brief account of the more common sexual offences with emphasis on any psychiatric aspects. West (1987) has produced a broadly based account of sex offending in general, and the reader is also referred to Chapter 25.

Rape. Most rapists are under 25 years old; disinhibition by alcohol is common and, in up to a third of cases, two or more youths are convicted together. A proportion of rapists are seriously antisocial criminals for whom violence is a common feature (Gibbens et al 1977). Sexual psychopathology is most likely in young men who commit solitary rapes, and in attackers who rehearse the act in fantasy, or who select a victim for reasons of sexual attractiveness or who submit the victim to degrading acts. Mental illness in rapists is rare but, when present, mania is as likely as schizophrenia. From a third to a half of rape victims are previously known to their attacker. It is now possible in England and Wales for a man to be convicted of the rape of his wife. Psychological sequelae, including depression, sexual dysfunction and poor social adjustment are common in rape victims (Mezey & Taylor 1988).

Incest. The crime of incest is sexual intercourse (vaginal) within a forbidden relationship. It is grossly under-reported, and father–daughter incest is the most common. It is seen across all social classes but is more likely to result in prosecution in lower socioeconomic groups (Cooper & Cormier 1990). Fathers convicted of incest range from those with no record of criminality or alcohol abuse to heavy drinkers with antisocial personalities. Daughters generally show a lack of striking features, though there are some reports of low intelligence or physical handicap as occasional features. Common situational factors are an absent, incapacitated or unavailable wife and sexual disharmony in the marriage. The wife frequently has a passive or dependent role in the partnership. The behaviour is 'secret' between father and daughter; when it becomes known to the wife there is often a long delay before it is reported. Lengthy prison sentences are generally imposed on fathers convicted of the crime.

Sexual offences against children. Sexual offences against children range from minor indecency to violent sexual activity; the former is more common. Among adolescent boys, the crime is associated with poor social skills, physical unattractiveness and limited intelligence. Adult offenders are more likely to be true paedophiles (West 1987). A few paedophiles are recidivists whose sexual activity is almost exclusively with children, but the majority show low rates of re-offending. Social isolation among the mentally handicapped and elderly is sometimes a factor. Sentences vary with the seriousness of the offence.

Indecent exposure. This is the commonest sexual offence and the one with the best prognosis. Most offenders do not re-offend, and in those that do it is rare for there to be progression to more serious sexual offending. A proportion are exhibitionists and very few have any psychiatric disorder.

Treatment of sex offenders. Public clamour about sex offenders who quickly re-offend after serving their sentence has prompted the Home Office to announce its intention to provide treatment for sex offenders in prison. It is a response based on political expediency rather than clinical experience (see Ch. 25), and begs many questions. Who will be treated, for what condition, by what method and by whom?

At present, sex offenders, fearful for their safety, are usually segregated from other prisoners, and experience the worst regimes and conditions. Their principal concern is survival and they are not psychologically available for treatment, even if it could be provided. Prison reforms recently announced (see below) may be relevant for this group of offenders.

Offences against property

Arson. Arson is a serious crime for which a sentence of life imprisonment can be imposed: the lawful form of the activity is a mark of public celebration. Clear-up and conviction rates for the crime are low. As with other crimes, arson is multifactorial in origin and arsonists are a widely heterogeneous group. There is inevitable overlap between categories in any classification, including the one that follows, which is based on the review by Scott (1978):

1. *Motivated fire-setting.* This is a deliberate action with the aim of collecting insurance money or concealing another crime, e.g. murder, or engineering a change of housing.

2. *Political fire-setting.* This is a group activity common at times of social unrest. Not all the participants may be politically motivated.

3. *Suicide by fire.* An epidemic of self-immolation, as an apparent political gesture, occurred in the late 1960s. It is possible that some of the subjects were mentally disturbed. This is a method of suicide sometimes employed by prisoners.

4. *Psychiatric disorder or organic brain disease.* Fire may be set by schizophrenics in response to psychotic phenomena, by the mentally handicapped for reasons of excitement and by alcoholics in states of intoxication, delirium tremens or alcoholic hallucinosis.

5. *No psychiatric disorder.* Adolescents and young adults may set fires out of boredom, for 'kicks' or as a vague form of protest.

6. *Those with no motive.* Some fire-setters gain satisfaction from watching the subsequent fire; they may act heroically, appearing to help the fire brigade. Such individuals sometimes obtain employment as firemen or security guards. Also in this group are those for whom the fire arouses sexual pleasure.

7. *Female fire-raisers.* Women may set fires as a means of attracting attention, creating excitement or more commonly as an act of revenge against husband or lover.

Shoplifting. Shoplifting is a form of theft which is currently perpetrated on a massive scale with huge financial losses to the retail trade. The extent to which this exercise is associated with mental disorder is tiny. A link between depression and shoplifting has been established, particularly in middle-aged defendants, but Gudjonsson (1990) suggests unitary 'causes' are unusual. Gibbens et al (1971) followed up 532 women who had been convicted of shoplifting in London 10 years earlier. They had subsequent rates of psychiatric hospitalisation that were three times higher than expected for women of their age. One group continued to offend in diverse ways. However, about 10–20% of the cohort had been depressed when originally convicted of shoplifting and these were mainly law-abiding women. They continued to manifest mixed physical and depressive symptoms but the majority of these women did not re-offend.

In the assessment of people charged with shoplifting it is important to establish their state of health prior to the offence. The circumstances of the offence are important; depressed shoplifters typically steal items they do not require and make little effort to conceal their actions. Shoplifting is also seen in people with substance abuse, eating disorders, residual schizophrenia and organic states. Some people may shoplift in a state of absent-mindedness or forgetfulness. A lack of intent might be accepted by the court, resulting in acquittal.

Child stealing (plagium)

Child stealing is a rare offence; the majority of such offences are committed by men in custody disputes between parents or, more rarely, in a sexual abduction. Baby stealing, on the other hand, is predominantly a female offence. The classification by d'Orban (1976) based on 24 cases is helpful. He described three types: comforting offences by deprived girls; manipulative offences by hysterical women in unstable relationships with a boyfriend; impulsive offences by psychiatrically disturbed women. Most stolen babies are found quickly and have usually been well cared for by their abductors.

THE MENTALLY ABNORMAL OFFENDER IN THE CRIMINAL JUSTICE SYSTEM

Arrest and prosecution

The behaviour of a mentally abnormal person in a public place may give rise to what might broadly be called 'a disturbance'. Whether such a disturbance reaches the attention of an agency (police, social work or medical), and, if so, how it is dealt with by them, will be determined largely by chance factors (Chiswick et al 1984). The use of police powers, under section 136 of the Mental Health Act, to apprehend a disturbed person and take him to a hospital is almost confined to the Greater London area. Detention in hospital is allowed for up to 72 hours for the specific purpose of assessment by a doctor and social worker.

A mentally disordered person who is detained at a police station may unwittingly provide information which is unreliable, misleading or self-incriminating. Sometimes the style or content of a confession may raise doubts about its authenticity as a voluntarily made statement. It is necessary to keep an open mind on these matters and to recognise the problem of suggestibility in some defendants. Many factors may affect suggestibility, and the use of a standardised test has been reported (Gudjonsson 1984).

Mental disorder and court proceedings

The inappropriate remand in custody of mentally disturbed offenders is a source of concern. A court-based psychiatric service can bring about a substantial reduction in their number (Joseph 1990, James & Hamilton 1991). Most psychiatric disposals are effected at the post-conviction stage of court proceedings, i.e. after the offender has pleaded, or been found, guilty. In a minority of cases, mental disorder may form the basis of a defence to a criminal charge in one of two ways.

Either the existence of a mental disorder may render the defendant unfit to plead, or it may affect his legal responsibility for his actions. These two situations will be considered in turn, but it must be emphasised that unfitness to plead or a lack of legal responsibility are unusual routes to a psychiatric disposal.

Fitness to plead

It would be unjust to try a person who, by reason of mental disorder, lacks the capacity to defend himself in court. Such a person is said to be unfit to plead or under disability such that he cannot be tried (section 2, Criminal Procedure (Insanity and Unfitness to Plead) Act 1991). Unfitness to plead is a matter for determination by a jury in a crown court. A defendant is fit to plead if he has the capacity to:

1. Understand the charge and its implications
2. Distinguish between a plea of guilty and one of not guilty
3. Challenge a juror to whom he might object
4. Follow the evidence in court
5. Instruct counsel on his behalf.

The psychiatric assessment is of the accused's ability, at the time of his trial, to comprehend his situation and adequately communicate instructions to his counsel. The mental state of a defendant may fluctuate from day-to-day, so a brief re-examination of him, on the day of his appearance in court, is a wise precaution. The psychiatric disorders most likely to impair comprehension and communication to this degree are a functional psychosis, organic brain disease and mental retardation (Grubin 1991).

A defendant who makes no reply when asked to plead to the charge is said to be mute on arraignment. Here the jury is asked to decide if the mutism is due to an unwillingness or an inability to speak. If mutism is the result of an inability to speak, then the jury proceeds to decide the issue of fitness to plead in the usual manner. The most likely example is that of a deaf mute, though some method of communication is usually possible, e.g. sign language, writing or even grunts and nods. When failure in communication is compounded by lack of comprehension, as it might be in severe mental retardation, a meaningful trial is impossible.

The Criminal Procedure (Insanity and Unfitness to Plead) Act 1991 introduced important changes for defendants who are unfit to plead. These include:

1. A trial of the facts of the criminal charge
2. Complete acquittal if the facts are not established

3. Flexibility of sentence by the judge if the facts are proven, except for murder cases where there must be mandatory committal to hospital.

Criminal responsibility

To establish guilt it is necessary to demonstrate for most crimes that not only did the defendant commit or bring about the unlawful act, but also that he possessed the necessary state of mind or *mens rea* for that particular crime. The factors of psychiatric relevance that might negate *mens rea* are:

1. Age
2. Mental disorder
3. The effects of alcohol or drugs
4. Automatism.

Age. Children under the age of 10 years are not criminally responsible; it is assumed that they are incapable of forming a criminal intent. They may, however, be made the subject of a care order in a juvenile court. Between the ages of 10 and 14 years a child may be convicted of a crime if, in addition to proof of *mens rea*, there is evidence that the child knew, either in the legal or the moral sense, that what he was doing was wrong. Psychiatric evidence may be led by the prosecution to help establish this fact; it requires a global consideration of the child's social, intellectual and moral development.

Mental disorder. The defence which rests upon an absence of *mens rea* due to insanity is known as the insanity defence, and if successful it results in a special verdict of not guilty by reason of insanity (section 2, Trial of Lunatics Act 1883). The rarity of this finding cannot be over-emphasised; in indictable cases its use is virtually confined to murder. It results in an acquittal and, until recently, the defendant was automatically committed to a hospital specified by the Home Secretary, where he was detained under the terms of a restriction order. There is a right of appeal against the finding, even though it is an acquittal.

The verdict is governed by the McNaughton Rules, which were established in 1843 by the judges in reply to a request from the House of Lords. Daniel McNaughton's crime and its consequence have been well described (West & Walk 1977); he was acquitted on a charge of murdering William Drummond, private secretary to Sir Robert Peel, then Prime Minister. McNaughton is said to have acted on the basis of paranoid delusions. His crime occurred at a time of intense concern about the vulnerability of public figures to assassination attempts. The Rules established that there was an initial assumption of sanity and legal responsibility in all cases. The essential part for determining the insanity defence is as follows:

To establish a defence on the ground of insanity, it must be clearly proved that at the time of the committing of the act, the party accused was labouring under such a defect of reason, from disease of the mind, as not to know the nature and quality of the act he was doing, or, if he did know it, that he did not know he was doing wrong.

Thus, it is necessary for the defendant to prove three matters: first that he was suffering a disease of the mind at the time of the crime; second that this caused a defect of reason; third that the defect of reason robbed him of the capacity to either know what he was doing or know that it was wrong. The rules present problems for the examining psychiatrist. It may be difficult to establish a retrospective diagnosis with any degree of accuracy, and the requirement to consider what the patient did, or did not, know is an unfamiliar clinical task.

A range of disposal options for defendants who successfully plead insanity is now possible through the Criminal Procedure (Insanity and Unfitness to Plead) Act 1991. However, if the crime is murder, there must be mandatory committal to a hospital. The new legislation has important implications for cases of insane automatism (see below).

The effects of alcohol or drugs. Intoxication by drink or drugs does not in itself constitute a defence to a criminal charge. However, there are three situations where evidence of voluntary intoxication might affect an accused person's criminal responsibility:

1. If a crime requires proof of a specific intent, evidence of intoxication may be used to demonstrate an inability to form that intent.
2. If alcohol or drugs have caused a disease of the mind, an insanity plea under the McNaughton Rules may be possible.
3. If alcohol or drugs have caused an abnormality of the mind, a plea of diminished responsibility (in murder only) may be possible.

Courts have been very cautious for obvious reasons in allowing defendants who claim an absence of intent due to self-intoxication to escape conviction. In crimes requiring a specific intent (e.g. murder), evidence of self-induced intoxication could be used to demonstrate the absence of the necessary mental element. Such a defence would not be possible, however, in crimes which only require a demonstration of basic intent (e.g. manslaughter). The consequences of alcohol abuse will only support an insanity plea where there is evidence that it has produced a disease of the mind which satisfies the McNaughton Rules. Alcohol abuse itself cannot support a plea of diminished responsibility, but abnormalities of mind produced by it, including for example the compulsion to drink in an alcoholic, may well do so (Griew 1991).

Automatism. An act which occurs outside the control of a person's mind is, for legal purposes, referred to as an automatism. It constitutes a defence because the mind does not accompany the body's actions. Criminal acts, performed during episodes of altered consciousness, are recognised as rare events which may occur in an epileptic fit (Gunn 1978), while asleep (Oswald & Evans 1985), in a state of hypoglycaemia or when concussed. The court is concerned with attributing blame and protecting the public. For these reasons it distinguishes automatism due to a disease of the mind (insane automatism) from those where there is no disease of the mind (non-insane automatism). The distinction is legally important but without clinical foundation. Defendants declared to have an insane automatism will be dealt with under the flexible disposals for the insanity defence (see above); non-insane cases automatically walk free from court.

It is difficult to identify a logical thread in the manner by which the courts have determined what is, and what is not, a disease of the mind. Arteriosclerosis and epilepsy were regarded as diseases of the mind, but not organic states associated with a brain tumour and with hypoglycaemia. Absent-mindedness, even in association with a depressive illness, was accepted in support of non-insane automatism in a case of shoplifting. In recent years, important rulings have determined that both epilepsy and sleep-walking are, for legal purposes, diseases of the mind (Fenwick 1991).

Diminished responsibility

It has been emphasised that the two verdicts, unfitness to plead and the insanity defence, although of great legal significance, are less important in practice. For murder only, the legal wrangles associated with insanity can be side-stepped by use of the plea of diminished responsibility. Today, nearly all offenders who escape conviction for murder on psychiatric grounds do so on the basis of diminished responsibility. Until 1957 in England, criminal responsibility was an all-or-none issue; the accused was, or was not, responsible for his actions. Section 2 of the Homicide Act 1957 introduced a halfway stage of diminished responsibility whereby a charge of murder may be reduced to the less serious charge of manslaughter. The relevant section states:

Where a person kills or is party to the killing of another, he shall not be convicted of murder if he was suffering from such abnormality of mind (whether arising from a condition of arrested or retarded development of mind or any inherent causes or induced by disease or injury) as substantially impaired his mental responsibility for his acts and omissions in doing or being a party to the killing.

Whereas a life sentence is mandatory following conviction for murder, the judge has wide discretion in manslaughter; and most cases result either in a determinate prison sentence, or in committal to hospital under a hospital order. However, in some cases, particularly domestic killings by women or by the elderly, there may be a probation order or a deferred prison sentence.

To sustain the defence, proof is required on a balance of probabilities of three matters: first, that the accused was at the time of the crime suffering from an abnormality of mind; second, that the abnormality of mind resulted from one of the causes specified in section 2 of the Homicide Act 1957; third, that the abnormality of mind substantially impaired mental responsibility. Although psychiatrists seem willing to testify that an abnormality of mind exists, the phrase is not one that can be defined in medical terms. It has been given the widest of interpretations by the courts following an authoritative judgement by the then Lord Chief Justice in the case of *Byrne* in 1960. He said an abnormality of mind was 'a state of mind so different from that of ordinary human beings that the reasonable man would term it abnormal'.

Practical aspects. There is no corpus of clinical knowledge that can help a psychiatrist decide what is meant by an abnormality of mind, mental responsibility or substantial impairment. Courts accept what they choose to accept; much depends on the circumstances of the case and the degree of compassion, whether great or little, for the defendant. Without the willingness of psychiatrists to stretch their evidence, diminished responsibility would become unworkable; yet it may represent the only means of securing a compassionate disposal for a defendant who attracts sympathy from the court. Resting as it does on such slender theory, it is not surprising that its use borders on the indiscriminate. Nearly all the major psychiatric syndromes have been accepted under section 2, as have a host of ill-defined conditions such as emotional immaturity, dissociative states and, most recently, the premenstrual syndrome. Diminished responsibility exists solely to circumvent the fixed disposal of life imprisonment for people convicted of murder (Dell 1984). Recently the government overturned a vote by the House of Lords to abolish the fixed penalty for murder.

Infanticide

A forerunner of diminished responsibility was the special provision made for dealing with mothers who killed an infant child of their own. The Infanticide Act 1938 provides that if a woman causes the death of her child, who must be under the age of 12 months, and the court is satisfied that the balance of her mind was disturbed by reason of her not fully having recovered from the effect of giving birth to the child, or by reason of the effect of lactation consequent upon the birth, she is guilty of infanticide and the court disposal is exactly as for manslaughter. In practice, the usual disposal is by way of a probation order with or without a condition of psychiatric treatment. The killing of an infant under the age of 12 months is not in itself sufficient to sustain the charge or defence of infanticide; there must be evidence to demonstrate that the balance of the mind was disturbed. Psychiatrists are required to put their evidence within the framework of the Infanticide Act 1938 and this can cause similar problems to those described for diminished responsibility.

Psychiatric disposals after conviction

After an offender has been convicted, the sentencer may request a psychiatric report to assist him in making an appropriate disposal. This is a clinical task requiring consideration of the nature of any psychiatric disorder, the need for, and likely benefits of, treatment and the legal conditions under which such treatment should be given. It is necessary to couple these clinical considerations with an awareness of the court's probable attitude and expectations, particularly in respect of public protection. Treatment may be provided by one of three methods:

1. As an informal in-patient or out-patient
2. As a condition of probation
3. Under the terms of a hospital, guardianship, restriction or interim hospital order.

Informal treatment is appropriate for well-motivated offenders who have committed minor offences, e.g. a depressed shoplifter. Where there might be value in maintaining some sanction in the event of non-compliance with treatment, a psychiatric probation order (section 3, Powers of Criminal Courts Act 1973) may be useful. The treatment may be as an out-patient or in-patient, in which case the probationer has the status of an informal patient. A crucial element in a psychiatric probation order is the agreement of the probationer to receive treatment and that of the doctor to provide it. Non-compliance with treatment may provide grounds for a breach of probation and a return to court.

The conditions necessary for making hospital, guardianship, restriction and interim hospital orders have been previously described. A recommendation for admission to a special hospital should only be made where it has been indicated, on the Secretary of State's behalf, that a place would be available for the offender.

The preparation of psychiatric reports for the court

In only a small proportion of criminal cases are psychiatric reports requested, but the provision of these reports is of importance to both the accused and the court. Psychiatric recommendations may influence decisions about guilt, responsibility and sentence. The purpose of the report is to provide expert advice to assist the court in its work. In giving his opinion, the psychiatrist advises the court but he does not direct it, and the final decision rests with the court. In practice, recommendations for treatment are the exception rather than the rule (Bowden 1978), and courts are usually only too willing to accept them.

Reports may be provided on defendants detained in prison, in hospital or on bail in the community. The psychiatrist should be certain that he understands why a report has been requested; there may be a hidden agenda. Circumstances vary but he should, firstly, read all the background information, including the statements of witnesses; secondly, examine the accused; thirdly, seek additional information from relatives or prison staff if appropriate; and, fourthly, reflect on the case and on the questions that have been asked before writing his report.

The examination of the accused is unusual in that it does not take place in the setting of the normal doctor–patient relationship (Chiswick 1985). The purpose and non-confidential nature of the interview should be explained to the defendant and his agreement to it sought. History taking and mental state examination follow normal lines, but it is important to obtain an account of the offence from the accused in his own words which should be noted.

The report should address the particular questions asked; usually the chief issue is disposal but sometimes fitness to plead or responsibility may be in doubt. In homicides, it is essential to comment on the question of diminished responsibility. Sound advice on the preparation of reports has been given by Bluglass (1979b). The report is addressed to laymen and should be clear, concise and free of jargon and technical terms. It should be impartial and balanced, and demonstrate sensitivity to the court's needs. It may be read out in court and must be free of moral censure, sarcastic humour and pomposity. Any recommendations should be unambiguous and practicable and be based upon clinical observations contained in the report. Only recommendations that are of a psychiatric nature should be made. The report should state the name of the accused and the charge. It aids clarity and discipline if the report is arranged in sections:

1. A note of when, where and for how long the accused was examined, together with a description of all sources of information.
2. A short sentence giving his age, marital status and living situation.
3. A brief chronological account of his educational, occupational and social history, emphasising any factors of psychiatric relevance.
4. The family history, noting any points of psychiatric importance.
5. The previous medical and psychiatric history.
6. A note of any previous criminal record.
7. A brief note of the circumstances of the offence, as related by the accused, with emphasis on any relevant psychiatric points. (Where the defendant pleads not guilty, the court must ensure that previously undisclosed material is not heard before guilt has been determined).
8. Features found on psychiatric examination.
9. The psychiatrist's opinion, together with discussion, where relevant, on the particular questions that have been asked.
10. A clear statement of conclusions or recommendations.

The report should conclude with the name, designation and qualifications of the psychiatrist.

The psychiatrist appearing in court as an expert witness should be properly prepared; he should answer the questions put to him clearly and he should avoid the temptation to stray beyond his remit. Grounds (1985) has provided sensible words of caution for the prospective psychiatric witness.

Forensic psychiatry in practice

Practical forensic psychiatry consists largely of the assessment and treatment of mentally abnormal offenders. Any catchment area psychiatric service is bound to see patients whose contact with the service is precipitated by an offence. Psychiatric services for offender patients should contain various elements:

1. An effective emergency service to the police and the courts
2. Out-patient clinics for the assessment of 'cold' referrals from courts, probation service, solicitors and other sources
3. Liaison with probation and other community-based services for offenders
4. Liaison with the prison medical service
5. Access to a range of in-patient facilities, from open ward to medium security, for the treatment of patients before trial and after conviction
6. Liaison with the special hospitals for patients returning from, or requiring, treatment under conditions of special security.

In addition to offender patients, certain non-offender patients are likely to be referred to forensic psychiatry services. These are people, usually suffering from chronic functional psychoses (e.g. treatment-resistant schizophrenia) or organic brain disease (e.g. after head injury), who show serious degrees of behavioural disturbance that prove unmanageable in conventional psychiatric units. They probably constitute the most disturbed and difficult patients seen in psychiatric practice (Coid 1991).

Specialists in forensic psychiatry perform a substantial amount of their clinical work in regional secure units, special hospitals and prisons.

Regional secure units

The Butler Report (Home Office & DHSS 1975) was a major factor in setting in motion the development of better facilities for the assessment and treatment of mentally abnormal offenders. In essence the Butler committee recommended, as a matter of urgency, the establishment of secure facilities in each of the regions of England and Wales. Significantly, it was envisaged that the units would be the base for a regional forensic service. Progress has been slow but by 1990 there were approximately 600 places available in regional secure units (Snowden 1990). Length of stay is generally between 12 and 18 months.

Special hospitals

Nearly 2000 patients are detained under relevant mental health legislation in the three special hospitals in England (Ashworth, Broadmoor and Rampton), and in the State Hospital in Scotland. The hospitals are part of the National Health Service. They provide treatment under special security for patients deemed to be of 'dangerous, violent or criminal propensities'. Most patients are offenders but a smaller proportion are civilly detained patients transferred from other hospitals. Length of stay is much greater than in the regional secure units. The function of the special hospitals has been reviewed by Hamilton (1990). They have an unhappy history. Conflicts between requirements for treatment and for security, difficulties in interdisciplinary working and cultural affinities with the prison service have been identified in a series of reports and inquiries (NHS Health Advisory Service 1988). However, they have problems not of their own making; there is particular concern at the long delays in effecting the transfer to other psychiatric services of patients who no longer require treatment in conditions of high security.

Prisons

Given the high level of psychiatric morbidity among prison populations, it is not surprising that psychiatrists have an important clinical function in penal establishments. Prisoners may be examined by a psychiatrist for one of four main reasons:

1. For preparation of a psychiatric court report
2. At the request of a prison medical officer
3. For preparation of a psychiatric report for parole consideration
4. For advice in management of prisoners who are behaviourally disturbed.

Some psychiatrists may provide a psychotherapy service for selected prisoners.

Prisons are currently in crisis. They face problems which particularly affect mentally abnormal prisoners. A series of prison riots has led to a judicial enquiry (Home Office 1991) which has called for fundamental reforms; these include the need for improved conditions for mentally disordered prisoners, sex offenders and prisoners infected with HIV. In recent years the annual number of suicides in prison has doubled (Smith 1991). A radical report by HM Chief Inspector of Prisons for England and Wales (1990) is critical of the squalid conditions for prisoners awaiting trial and the failure to apply proper standards of care for prisoners thought to be at risk of self-harm. Separate reports have called for an overhaul of the prison medical service.

In the face of all these problems it is a sobering thought that many mentally disordered offenders receive their only psychiatric care when in prison. Coid (1988a, 1988b) has described the lack of facilities in many areas for the treatment of offender

patients and, more worryingly, the negative attitude of some psychiatrists to offenders, even those who are clearly suffering from psychotic illnesses.

REFERENCES

Aarvold Committee 1973 Report on the review of procedures for the discharge and supervision of psychiatric patients subject to special restrictions. Cmmnd 5191. Her Majesty's Stationery Office, London

Bluglass R 1979a The psychiatric assessment of homicide. British Journal of Hospital Medicine 22: 366–377

Bluglass R 1979b The psychiatric court report. Medicine Science and the Law 19: 121–129

Bowden P 1978 Men remanded into custody for medical reports: the selection for treatment. British Journal of Psychiatry 132: 320–331.

Bowden P 1981 What happens to patients released from the special hospitals? British Journal of Psychiatry 138: 340–345

British Medical Journal legal correspondent 1986 Legal proceedings by mental patients. British Medical Journal 292: 820

Chiswick D 1981 Matricide. British Medical Journal 238: 1279–1280

Chiswick D 1985 Use and abuse of psychiatric testimony. British Medical Journal 290: 975–977.

Chiswick D, McIsaac M W, McClintock F H 1984 Prosecution of the mentally disturbed: dilemmas of identification and discretion. Aberdeen University Press, Aberdeen

Cloninger C R, Sigvardsson S, Bohman M, von Knorring A 1982 Predisposition to petty criminality in Swedish adoptees. II Cross-fostering analysis of gene–environment interaction. Archives of General Psychiatry 39: 1242–1247

Coid J 1984 How many psychiatric patients in prison? British Journal of Psychiatry 145: 78–86

Coid JW 1988a Mentally abnormal prisoners on remand: I — rejected or accepted by the NHS? British Medical Journal 296: 1779-1782

Coid JW 1988b Mentally abnormal prisoners on remand: II — comparison of services provided by Oxford and Wessex regions. British Medical Journal 296: 1783–1784

Coid JW 1991 "Difficult to place" psychiatric patients. British Medical Journal 302: 603–604

Cooper I, Cormier B 1990 Incest. In: Bluglass R, Bowden P (eds) Principles and practice of forensic psychiatry. Churchill Livingstone, Edinburgh

Cremona A 1986 Mad drivers: psychiatric illness and driving performance. British Journal of Hospital Medicine 35: 193–195

Dalgaard O C, Kringlen E 1976 A Norwegian study of criminality. British Journal of Criminology 16: 213–232

Dell S 1984 Murder into manslaughter: the diminished responsibility defence in practice. Maudsley monograph 27. Oxford University Press, Oxford

Department of Health and Welsh Office 1990 Code of Practice: Mental Health Act 1983. Her Majesty's Stationery Office, London

d'Orban P T 1976 Child stealing: a typology of female offenders. British Journal of Criminology 16: 275–281

d'Orban P T 1979 Women who kill their children. British Journal of Psychiatry 134: 560–571

d'Orban P T, O'Connor A 1989 Women who kill their parents. British Journal of Psychiatry 154: 27–33

Editorial 1983 Crime as destiny? Lancet i: 35–36

Fenwick P B C 1991 Brain, mind, insanity, and the law. British Medical Journal 302: 979–980

Floud J, Young W 1981 Dangerousness and criminal justice. Cambridge studies in criminology 47. Heinemann Educational, London

Gibbens T C N, Robertson G 1983 A survey of the criminal careers of hospital order patients. British Journal of Psychiatry 143: 362–369

Gibbens T C N, Palmer C, Prince J 1971 Mental health aspects of shoplifting. British Medical Journal iii: 612–615

Gibbens T C N, Way C, Soothill K L 1977 Behavioural types of rape. British Journal of Psychiatry 130: 32–42

Gillies H 1976 Homicide in the west of Scotland. British Journal of Psychiatry 128: 105–127

Griew E 1991 Alcoholism and diminished responsibility. Journal of Forensic Psychiatry 2: 79–84

Grounds A 1985 The psychiatrist in court. British Journal of Hospital Medicine 34: 55–58

Grounds A T 1987 Detention of "pyschopathic disorder" patients in special hospitals. Critical issues. British Journal of Psychiatry 151: 474–478

Grubin D H 1991 Unfit to plead in England and Wales 1976–88. British Journal of Psychiatry 158: 540–548

Gudjonsson G H 1984 A new scale of interrogative suggestibility. Personality and Individual Differences 5: 303–314

Gudjonsson G H 1990 Psychological and psychiatric aspects of shoplifting. Medicine, Science and the Law 30: 45–51

Gunn J 1977a Criminal behaviour and mental disorder. British Journal of Psychiatry 130: 317–329

Gunn J 1977b Epileptics in prison. Academic Press, London

Gunn J 1978 Epileptic homicide: a case report. British Journal of Psychiatry 132: 510–513

Gunn J, Maden A, Swinton M 1991 Treatment needs of prisoners with psychiatric disorders. British Medical Journal 303: 338–341

Gunn M 1990 Consent to treatment: Journal of Forensic Psychiatry 1: 81–87

Hafner H, Boker W 1982 Crimes of violence by mentally abnormal offenders. Oxford University Press, London

Hamilton J 1990 Special hospitals and the state hospital. In: Bluglass R, Bowden P (eds) Principles and practice of forensic psychiatry. Churchill Livingstone, Edinburgh

Harding T W, Adserballe H 1983 Assessments of dangerousness: observations in six countries. International Journal of Law and Psychiatry 6: 391–398

Herzberg J L, Fenwick P B C 1988 The aetiology of aggression in temporal lobe epilepsy. British Journal of Psychiatry 153: 50–55

HM Chief Inspector of Prisons for England and Wales 1990 Report of a review of suicide and self-harm in prison service establishments in England and Wales. Her Majesty's Stationery Office, London

Home Office 1991 Prison disturbances April 1990. Report of an inquiry by the Rt. Hon. Lord Justice Woolf and His Honour Judge Stephen Tumim. Her Majesty's Stationery Office, London

Home Office & DHSS 1975 Report of the committee on mentally abnormal offenders. Cmnd 6244. Her Majesty's Stationery Office, London

James D V, Hamilton L W 1991 The Clerkenwell scheme: assessing efficiency and cost of a psychiatric liaison service to a magistrates' court. British Medical Journal 303: 282–285

Johnstone E C, Crow T J, Johnson A L, MacMillan J F 1986 The Northwick Park study of first episodes of schizophrenia: I. Presentation of the illness and problems relating to admission. British Journal of Psychiatry 148: 115–120

Joseph P L 1990 Mentally disordered homeless offenders — diversion from custody. Health Trends 22: 51–53

Lewis D O, Pincus J H, Bard B et al 1988 Neuropsychiatric, psychoeducational, and family characteristics of 14 juveniles condemned to death in the United States. American Journal of Psychiatry 145: 584–589

Lindqvist P 1991 Homicides committed by abusers of alcohol and illicit drugs. British Journal of Addiction 86: 321–326

Mackay RD 1990 Dangerous patients. Third party safety and psychiatrists' duties — walking the Tarasoff tightrope. Medicine, Science and the Law 30: 52–56

McHale JV 1990 The obligation of the psychiatrist to preserve the patient's confidences. Journal of Forensic Psychiatry 1: 91–101

Mental Health Act Commission 1989 Third biennial report 1987–1989. Her Majesty's Stationery Office, London

Mezey G C, Taylor P J 1988 Psychological reactions of women who have been raped: a descriptive and comparative study. British Journal of Psychiatry 152: 330–339

Montandon C, Harding T 1984 The reliability of dangerousness assessments: a decision making exercise. British Journal of Psychiatry 144: 149–155

Mowat RR 1966 Morbid jealousy and murder. Tavistock, London

Mullen P E 1988 Violence and mental disorder. British Journal of Hospital Medicine 40: 460–463

Mullen P 1990 Morbid jealousy and the delusion of infidelity. In: Bluglass R, Bowden P (eds) Principles and practice of forensic psychiatry. Churchill Livingstone, Edinburgh

NHS Health Advisory Service 1988 Report on services provided by Broadmoor Hospital. NHS Health Advisory Service, London

Noble P, Rodger S 1989 Violence by psychiatric in-patients. British Journal of Psychiatry 155: 384–390

Oswald I, Evans J 1985 On serious violence during sleep-walking. British Journal of Psychiatry 147: 688–691

Quinsey V L, Ambtman R 1979 Variables affecting psychiatrists' and teachers' assessments of the dangerousness of mentally ill offenders. Journal of Consulting and Clinical Psychology 47: 353–362

Resnick P J 1969 Child murder by parents. American Journal of Psychiatry 126: 325–334

Robertson G 1988 Arrest patterns among mentally disordered offenders. British Journal of Psychiatry 153: 313–316

Rutter M, Giller H 1983 Juvenile delinquency: trends and perspectives. Penguin, Harmondsworth

Scott D 1978 The problems of malicious fire-raising. British Journal of Hospital Medicine 19: 259–263

Sensky T, Hughes T, Hirsch S 1991 Compulsory psychiatric treatment in the community. I. A controlled study of compulsory community treatment with extended leave under the Mental Health Act: special characteristics of patients treated and impact of treatment. British Journal of Psychiatry 158: 792–799

Smith R 1991 "Taken from this place and hanged by the neck . . . . ." British Medical Journal 302: 64–65

Snowden P 1990 Regional secure units and forensic services in England. In: Bluglass R, Bowden P (eds) Principles and practice of forensic psychiatry. Churchill Livingstone, Edinburgh

Steadman H J 1983 Predicting dangerousness among the mentally ill: art, magic and science. International Journal of Law and Psychiatry 6: 381–390

Steadman H J Cocozza J J 1974 Careers of the criminally insane. Lexington, Toronto

Taylor P 1985 Motives for offending among violent and psychotic men. British Journal of Psychiatry 147: 491–498

Taylor P J, Gunn J 1984 Violence and psychosis I — Risk of violence among psychotic men. British Medical Journal 288: 1945–1949

Turk J 1989 Forensic aspects of mental handicap. British Journal of Psychiatry 155: 591–594

Unsworth C 1987 The politics of mental health legislation. Clarendon Press, Oxford

Walker N 1991 Dangerous mistakes. British Journal of Psychiatry 158: 752–757

Weller M P I 1986 Medical concepts in psychopathy and violence. Medicine, Science and the Law 26: 131–143

West D J 1987 Sexual crimes and confrontations. Cambridge Studies in Criminology 57. Gower, Aldershot

West D J 1988 Psychological contributions to criminology. British Journal of Criminology 28: 77–92

West D J, Walk A (eds) 1977 Daniel McNaughton: his trial and the aftermath. Headley, Ashford

Whitman S, Coleman T E, Patmon C, Desai B T, Cohen R, King L N (1984) Epilepsy in prison: elevated prevalence and no relationship to violence. Neurology (Cleveland) 34: 775–782

36. Drug treatments

J. B. Loudon

INTRODUCTION

In 1918 Jauregg, the first Nobel prizewinner for work in psychiatry, demonstrated that a physical treatment, deliberate infection with malaria, could be used to halt the progress of a neuropsychiatric condition, tertiary syphilis.

Sen and Bose in 1931 suggested the use of *Rauwolfia* alkaloids for the treatment of insanity. Lange, a Dane, had proposed lithium for use in excited states in 1886; Cade noticed the sedating effect of lithium on guinea-pigs, and in 1948 successfully treated a patient suffering from mania with lithium salts. (See Blackwell (1985) for a fuller account.) Two years later in France, in search for a drug to mitigate surgical shock, chlorpromazine was synthesised; it is a member of the phenothiazine group of compounds, which had been known to chemistry for the previous 60 years. Several workers, including Erhlich and Bodoni, had suggested the use of methylene blue, the first phenothiazine, for the treatment of psychosis in the 1890s. Laborit recognised the unique effects of chlorpromazine. Sigwald, Paraire, then Delay and Deniker, all in Paris, were among the first to use the new compound with success in the treatment of psychosis. Within the next 8 years, Yonkman had used the word 'tranquilliser' to describe the clinical effects of reserpine, iproniazid had been found to be both a euphoriant and a monoamine oxidase inhibitor (MAOI); Sternbach had described the sedating effects of chlordiazepoxide, Janssen had synthesised haloperidol and Kuhn had described the antidepressant effect of imipramine. Despite an explosion of expenditure and research effort, no new forms of drug treatment for psychiatric illness have been found since then and activity has been concerned with consolidation and the production of versions of already known compounds, with similar efficacy (Caldwell 1978).

This failure to advance further is a reflection of the absence of any clear understanding of the specific bio-chemical or neurophysiological abnormalities underlying the major psychiatric disorders. The dopamine and monoamine hypotheses derive from the actions of phenothiazines and antidepressants. All drug treatments in psychiatry are empirical. Their use is specific for only a small proportion of the total psychological morbidity present in the community. They are rarely curative in their own right. At best they tip the balance between pathological forces and therapeutic factors in a direction favourable to the patient.

A few general statements can be made about the drugs used in psychiatry. Many have a complex pharmacology, with metabolites which are themselves pharmacologically active and which persist for a long time. Very often there is a considerable delay between the use of a drug and the appearance of the desired clinical effect, despite an immediate pharmacological action. This imposes difficulties of explanation and persuasion for a public used to the more rapid effects of antibiotics and analgesics. Many drugs used in psychiatry have been excessively 'dirty' with respect to side-effects, which frequently require additional treatment, giving rise to the risk of drug interactions. The relatively recent isolation of monoamine receptor sub-types offers the prospect of 'cleaner' compounds, more specific in action. On the other hand, when a drug used in psychiatry is successful its effect can be outstanding. It therefore becomes important that the prescriber understands the nuances of dosage, side-effect and interaction to extract the maximum possible benefit from the compound employed.

There is a popular misconception that psychiatry only emerged from the dark days of the asylum in the 1950s with the introduction of these new drugs. In fact it was the impact of World War II and its aftermath which produced the change in expectation and atmosphere which has proved to be so beneficial to the specialty.

The general public and the media are now much more aware of the limitations of psychotropic drugs and of the dangers of excessive use. In the UK, government exerted control of expenditure on benzodiazepines. Successful treatment of a patient with medication means the education of both him and his relatives about the role of drugs in treatment. Time has to be spent talking about the risks of non-compliance, and about side-effects, and using ingenuity to minimise these as far as possible.

The international drug industry now devotes a considerable amount of money and effort to producing new psychotropic compounds. Despite this effort, no major advances have taken place in the last 25 years. One explanation of this is that, until recently, new compounds were found by the use of a series of screening tests on thousands of newly synthesised compounds, mainly involving animals, in search of a profile similar to those of existing useful drugs. The description of receptor subtypes, elucidation of the molecular structure of receptors, computer modelling, tailoring of drug molecules accordingly, and the development of drugs aimed at specific combinations of receptor sub-types is proceeding apace. Currently, the antidepressant range is as crowded as the β blocker range in general medicine. To become familiar with a few representatives of each class of drugs is as necessary in psychiatry as in general medicine. In deciding which drug to use, a psychiatrist must separate the interest of the drug industry in new patentable compounds of similar efficacy to existing drugs (from the profits of which further research can be financed) from those of the patient in a drug which will expedite recovery without troublesome side-effects and, indirectly, a large tax bill. Fashions in promotion have to be recognised for what they are. For these reasons, and given the financial environment in which most psychiatrists operate in the UK, most psychiatric services will prescribe within the guidelines of a local formulary. Although this is restrictive, it allows for the best use of resources and prevents prescribing independence shading off into idiosyncrasy. Advances in drug treatment can come only from the pharmaceutical industry as it has the required resources. Its promotional activities should be treated with sceptical reserve.

The withdrawal in the last decade of two newer antidepressants (zimelidine and nomifensine) and the problems of benzodiazepines such as triazolam, act as warnings against uncritical acceptance of claims of low toxicity. The 'yellow card' system, operated by the Committee on Safety of Medicines, is as useful in psychiatry as in physical medicine, and was responsible for the detection of severe reactions to nomifensine 7 years after its introduction.

THE CONTROLLED CLINICAL TRIAL

In the development of a new drug treatment, compounds are tested in animals for toxicity and to determine gross pharmacological characteristics. In order to confirm pharmacokinetic and metabolic predictions, human volunteers will then be given single doses. Regular doses will later be given to assess side-effects and possible toxicity. This constitutes phase one of evaluation. Phase two involves 'open' studies of the drug in patients carrying the targeted diagnosis. 'Open' implies that all involved are fully aware of the novel nature of the compound, and that its effect on the illness is a combination of a specific drug action and the non-specific factors mentioned below. In the third phase, strict controls are employed to isolate the non-specific factors from the action of the drug in which the investigator is interested. Such a study is known as the double-blind clinical trial.

Drug treatment in psychiatry is only one of a number of influences which determine the outcome for a patient. Such influences — for example faith, the effect of outside events, and time — are quite as potent. Further, the results of treatment can only be judged on ill-defined criteria. A controlled clinical trial is a device by which treatment is compared with no treatment or with one of known efficacy in a population of patients with defined characteristics, who are so arranged to cancel out the influence of extraneous events.

The expectations by both clinician and patient of a treatment's effect are so potent in altering the apparent outcome that objective assessment requires that both are kept in ignorance of whether the treatment given is the one under test, a dummy or a standard drug. The incidence and nature of side-effects may give a clue to the identity of the treatment; if the morbidity of the condition without treatment is high, placebo tablets may be ethically unjustifiable. If the result of a study is to be intelligible elsewhere, the patients entered must fit recognisable categories. It is now the practice to assess patients entering a study by means of a standardised and thus reliable interview to discover whether the patient possesses symptoms which satisfy accepted diagnostic criteria. Thus, borderline cases are excluded and some homogeneity of the patient population is assured. This is important when assessing a new treatment against one of known effect. On the other hand, a study based on a very tightly defined population will not answer questions about the limits of usefulness of a particular drug across a group of conditions.

Impairment of function caused by a psychiatric disorder derives from many factors, including subjective unease, impairment of intellectual function, disturbance of personal relationships, the presence of alarming symptoms and loss of insight. Although the usefulness of a patient's statement that he feels better can be recognised by the use of simple analogue scales to quantify his improvement, measurement of response requires the use of a variety of rating scales, completed by both patient and observers, which have been previously shown to be sensitive to change in the variable to be measured, and reliable in the hands of investigators.

Shepherd (1975) cites the six questions posed by Hill to which the investigator must have satisfactory answers before proceeding to enter patients in a study. The questions address issues such as the safety and known effectiveness of the treatment, the choice of patients and obtaining consent, the ethics of simulated treatment and the possible hazard resulting from the treating clinician being unaware which treatment his patient is receiving.

It is now mandatory for all clinical research studies to have received consent from a properly constituted ethics of research committee, usually multidisciplinary in composition, with lay representation.

Statistical considerations are of such great importance that a statistician must be involved from the start in the design of a clinical study. He advises on the required size of each group to be studied in order to give a reasonable likelihood of obtaining a statistically significant result. For instance, unless testing against placebo, a comparison will require a patient sample of at least 100 to show a 25% difference in efficacy at the 90% confidence limit. This is costly to achieve; studies ignoring such advice, using smaller samples, deserve little attention. He will arrange randomisation of patients in the treatment groups so that patient variables, such as age, sex, social class and previous history, which might affect the outcome, will be equally distributed. Finally, he will prevent the clinician from peeping prematurely at the results while a study is in progress, thus risking invalidation. This applies even if the treatments are coded, as bias is introduced where it should be excluded.

Other considerations affect the outcome of a trial. Patients, even in hospital, are adept at avoiding taking their medication, and if improvement is to be related reliably to a particular drug treatment, some measure of the quantity of a drug present in patients' tissues must be used. This may be direct, by estimation of plasma level, or indirect, either by measurement of hormones influenced by the drug or by provocation tests. Treatment is but one of a series of influences affecting a patient's well-being and events in the patient's social environment may well have an adverse effect on this, and thus distort the outcome measurements.

AUDIT

Thinking psychiatrists have always wished to maintain a high standard of care by critically evaluating their clinical practice. This process, otherwise known as clinical or medical audit, has been incorporated into the operation of the National Health Service as a result of recent political changes. Thus far the process is the responsibility of the medical profession. Audit is continuing. It involves a group of professional peers, whether at ward, unit, district or national level, meeting in confidence, to set standards of practice in any area of clinical activity, and then measuring to see whether actual practice meets the standard. As a result of the comparison, practice is modified and improved. This is the audit cycle. Further comparison is then made, and so on. No psychiatrist should seek to evade his responsibilities in this. Properly approached, audit should be neither coercive nor threatening.

The area of drug treatment lends itself particularly to audit, whether at the level of appropriate use of drugs, or an examination of the rate of specified side-effects occurring from a particular treatment. The treatment of a cohort of patients suffering from a certain illness can be examined for full use of recommended treatments. Correct dosage, proper use of blood tests, action taken on the results and proper recording are all relevant. The patient and his relatives' understanding of the treatment is also measurable.

THE NEUROLEPTIC DRUGS (ANTIPSYCHOTICS, 'MAJOR TRANQUILLISERS')

These drugs have been differentiated from the purely sedative compounds such as barbiturates and benzodiazepines — 'the minor tranquillisers' — by the term 'major tranquillisers'. In many respects this description is misleading and inadequate to differentiate between the two and therefore should not be used. 'Neuroleptic' refers to the properties of these drugs in producing particular effects by actions on specific systems within the central nervous system (Shepherd 1980).

Structure/activity relationships

Manipulation of side-chains at two positions on the phenothiazine nucleus has considerable effect in altering potency. Substitution at one of these positions by chlorine, thiomethyl or carbon trifluoride groups greatly increases antipsychotic potency. The thioxanthene molecules are similar, except that the nitrogen at a particular point in the phenothiazine molecule is substituted by carbon. The phenothiazines and thioxanthenes are classified by the nature of the side-chain at this point (thioxanthene equivalents in parentheses): aliphatic side-chain, chlorpromazine (chlorprothixene); piperidine side-chain, thioridazine; piperazine side-chain, fluphenazine and trifluoperazine (zuclopenthixol, flupenthixol and thiothixine). Piperazine-substituted phenothiazines and thioxanthenes are highly potent. The first carbon atom of the side-chain is attached by a double bond in the thioxanthenes, giving rise to the existence of two isomers. Of these the *cis* or α compounds are the more potent.

Esterification of piperazine phenothiazines and thioxanthines, as well as of haloperidol, with a fatty acid in the form of decanoate or enanthate gives rise to the injectable depot preparations, where the ester is injected in an oily vehicle to delay absorption.

Haloperidol is the prototypical drug for the group of neuroleptics known as the butyrophenones, of which droperidol is a member. A related group is the diphenylbutylpiperidines which include pimozide (used orally) and fluspirilene (by injection); these are highly potent compounds which, by virtue of their extreme lipid solubility, act as depot preparations in their own right.

There are other neuroleptic drugs available from different classes of molecule, including oxypertine, an indole compound, loxapine, a dibenzoxazepine and two substituted benzamides, sulpiride and remoxipride (metoclopramide, an antiemetic, is also a substituted benzamide). Clozapine, a dibenzodiazepine, after introduction and withdrawal in the 1970s because of haematological toxicity, has recently been reintroduced, with particular safeguards, for therapy-resistant cases of schizophrenia (see below). Reserpine is now very little used because of its limited efficacy compared with other neuroleptics and its undesirable side-effects, including cardiovascular collapse and severe depressive mood changes. In certain movement disorders such as Huntington's chorea and tardive dyskinesia a monoamine-depleting drug may be required. Tetrabenazine has fewer peripheral effects and a shorter duration of action than reserpine, and is given in a dose range of 25–200 mg/day.

Pharmacological actions

Chlorpromazine is still the most widely prescribed of the neuroleptic drugs and is used as a reference.

All clinically effective neuroleptics can be shown by radioligand-binding assays of dopamine receptors to displace such ligands with a facility which parallels their potency as antipsychotic drugs. β-Flupenthixol and promazine, a phenothiazine, which both lack dopamine-blocking activity, are not effective as antipsychotic drugs. It is thought that neuroleptic compounds exert their major effect at or near the dopamine receptor in the central nervous system. It is a facile assumption, and lacks proof, that the basic lesion in schizophrenia is at the dopamine receptor. Side-effects result from dopamine receptor blockade in the hypothalamus and basal ganglia; the therapeutic action is thought to occur in the limbic system. Currently used neuroleptic drugs will inevitably have profound effects on posture and locomotion, and on homeostatic and endocrine functions. Dopamine receptors can be categorised on the basis of the presence (D_1) or absence (D_2) of adenyl cyclase as a second messenger in the postsynaptic membrane.

Other dopamine receptors are being characterised. D_1 receptors are found in the basal ganglia, and blockade presumably leads to extrapyramidal side-effects. D_2 receptors, while appearing elsewhere, are found in the limbic system, and selective D_2 blockers may be effective neuroleptics without causing the side-effects associated with D_1 blockers.

'Atypical' neuroleptics which have a strong anticholinergic effect, such as thioridazine and clozapine, are less likely to produce motor side-effects. The same is true of remoxipride, maybe because of its affinity for D_2 receptors. The distinction of the D_3 receptor, which may be the route by which neuroleptics exert their effect, raises the possibility of more specific treatments, free from side-effects. Clozapine also affects serotonin (5-HT) receptors.

The electroencephalogram (EEG) shows an increase in synchronisation and an increased voltage during neuroleptic administration, and incoming sensory stimulation has less effect in blocking alpha rhythm, e.g. on arousal. The aliphatic-substituted phenothiazines especially lower the seizure threshold, and these drugs must be used with caution in patients in whom the fit threshold may already be low congenitally or during withdrawal states. All drugs in this group have a complex action on the autonomic nervous system due to the production of α blockade, increased adrenergic drive due to re-uptake inhibition and anticholinergic activity. With regard to α-adrenergic blockade, the relative potencies are droperidol > chlorpromazine > thioridazine > fluphenazine > haloperidol > trifluoperazine > pimozide. Chlorpromazine will produce miosis, and thioridazine, the most strongly muscarinic of the neuroleptics, mydriasis. The anticholinergic effects include diminished sweating and salivation, urinary retention, blurring of vision and constipation. Many neuroleptics, with the important exception of thioridazine, diminish the chemoreceptor response in the brain stem, although there is little action on vomiting induced by peripheral mechanisms. Tests of psychological function show impaired vigilance but not impairment of intellectual function.

The effects on the cardiovascular system are also complex. Chlorpromazine and thioridazine especially are prone to produce an orthostatic hypotension which may be troublesome in the elderly. Tolerance may develop and can be accompanied by a compensatory tachycardia. They also have some anti-arrhythmic effect on the heart, displaying a quinidine-like action which may antagonise the effect of digoxin. A variety of electrocardiogram (ECG) changes may be seen, especially with thioridazine and pimozide which produces alterations in the QT interval and the T wave.

Absorption and metabolism

Chlorpromazine appears in blood 30 minutes after ingestion of an oral dose, with the peak concentration being reached in 3 hours. Because of a first-pass phenomenon, determined genetically, whereby as much as 90% of an orally ingested dose may be degraded before access is gained to the systemic circulation, parenteral injection increases bioavailability severalfold. All neuroleptics are highly bound to lipid-containing membranes and plasma proteins; hence, to ensure a rapid onset of action it is necessary to give a loading dose initially to saturate the binding sites. Chlorpromazine has a relatively short half-life in plasma but gives rise to a plethora of active metabolites. Catabolism occurs in the liver, mainly by conjugation, with metabolites excreted in the urine and bile. There is a ten-fold variation in the plasma concentration achieved by a human population for a given dose, but there is little correlation between plasma level and clinical response. This may be because elimination from plasma is faster than from lipid-rich sites such as the brain. On the other hand, the plasma level correlates well with the rise in prolactin secretion, probably because hypothalamic inhibitory control of the hypophysis is outside the blood–brain barrier. The rate of elimination of the drug is decreased in the elderly. Tolerance does not appear to develop with regard to antipsychotic effects but does so regarding sedative and locomotor effects. The phenothiazine drugs have little addictive potential, but some physical dependence develops.

With regard to the depot preparations, active drug appears in the plasma within a few hours of injection. In the first 2–4 days there will be a small peak of plasma level — which may cause extrapyramidal side-effects — followed by a fairly steady plateau for the next 16–20 days. For the properties of other neuroleptics, see Table 36.1.

The butyrophenones have little effect on the cardiovascular system and have little anticholinergic potential.

Table 36.1 Neuroleptic potency and commonly accepted dosage limits of antipsychotic drugs

Drug	Equivalent potency (mg)	Maximum daily dose (mg)	Maximum parenteral dose (mg)
Phenothiazines			
Chlorpromazine	50	1500	150
Thioridazine	50	800	Not available
Trifluoperazine	2.5	30	10
Fluphenazine	1 (depot 25 mg)	10	100[a]
Thioxanthenes			
Fluphenthixol	2 (depot 40 mg)	Not applicable	200[a]
Zuclopenthixol	10 (depot 200 mg)	Not applicable	600[a]
Butyrophenones			
Haloperidol	1 (depot 100 mg)	30	10
Droperidol	2	80	10
Diphenylbutylpiperidines			
Pimozide	1	30	Not available
Fluspirilene	0.5	Not applicable	12[a]

[a] These figures refer to single doses of depot preparations which have been reached incrementally.

Side-effects of neuroleptics

Disorders of movement (Marsden & Jenner 1980)

Pseudoparkinsonism. This syndrome, found particularly in the elderly, usually develops after a few days in the early stages of treatment with neuroleptics and is especially characterised by rigidity and akinesia, with tremor less apparent. Hypersalivation also occurs at times. A proper examination for the presence of this syndrome involves testing function in all four limbs and trunk, in addition to examination of the mouth, gait and facial muscles. The 'rabbit syndrome' — a rapid perioral tremor — seems to be a variant. Dopaminergic blockade in the basal ganglia is the obvious mechanism, although why the syndrome does not develop immediately is not clear.

Acute dystonia. This may range from clenching of jaw muscles or protrusion of the tongue to an oculogyric crisis or opisthotonos, most often occurring early in treatment with the potent neuroleptics. The younger patient seems most at risk, and the syndrome is associated with falling blood levels of neuroleptic. Hypo- or hyperdopaminergic states in the basal ganglia have been hypothesised as the cause.

Akathisia. This is experienced by the patient as a distressing motor restlessness, greatest in or restricted to the lower limbs, which leads to constant movement and shifting of position and an inability to relax. It is so intensely unpleasant that its presence may lead a mildly disturbed patient to become more so. It is important to be constantly aware of the possibility that this syndrome has developed so that relief may be afforded without delay. A β_2 blocker such as propranolol is more use than an anticholinergic. The appearance of acute akathisia soon after treatment starts may predict treatment unresponsiveness and the subsequent development of tardive dyskinesia. The responsible mechanism has not yet been identified, but its appearance most closely fits the time-course of peak blood levels and receptor occupancy. An iron deficiency may predispose. The exact incidence of these motor side-effects is uncertain, as much depends on the readiness with which they are recognised. In the early stages of treatment about one-third of patients taking aliphatic- or piperidine-substituted neuroleptics will develop these syndromes and about two-thirds for piperazine-substituted compounds or haloperidol.

The use of antiparkinsonian drugs

Any patient displaying agitation or posturing shortly after ingestion of neuroleptic drugs is likely to be suffering from a motor side-effect, and this possibility must be excluded before attributing the behaviour to histrionics or to a manifestation of the illness for which treatment is being given. Where conditions allow, this can be done by a reduction in dose, but where the neuroleptic has been given in a depot form or when it is clinically important to know whether an increase in dosage of neuroleptic is necessary, the only practicable way of finding out is by the parenteral administration of procyclidine (5–10 mg) or orphenadrine (20–40 mg). It may be necessary to repeat the dose within 30–40 minutes. Should this produce relief of side-effects, regular oral procyclidine or orphenadrine may be acceptable for a few days. The continuing need for antiparkinsonian treatment should be assessed by a phased withdrawal, and most patients should be off all antiparkinsonian medication within a few weeks.

When a patient suffering from extrapyramidal side-effects is being withdrawn from neuroleptics, antiparkinsonian medication may have to be continued well beyond the apparent end of neuroleptic treatment because tissue stores will continue to release the drug for some weeks (Wistedt et al 1981).

Despite the prevalence of extrapyramidal syndromes in patients taking neuroleptic drugs, it is bad practice to prescribe an anticholinergic automatically at the same time. There are several reasons for this: the first is that antiparkinsonian drugs alter the absorption of neuroleptics by changes in gut motility. They may also have some effect in increasing catabolism of neuroleptic drugs in the liver and it has been shown that their use tends to reduce the therapeutic action of neuroleptic drugs (Johnstone et al 1983).

They may enhance the development, and obscure early stages, of the syndrome known as tardive dyskinesia (see below). There are also several reports that these drugs may be abused for their euphoriant effect. Finally, and most crucially, patients maintained chronically on antiparkinsonian drugs and neuroleptics show little increase in extrapyramidal side-effects when the former are withdrawn (Johnson 1978).

The drugs which are of value in the treatment of neuroleptic-induced extrapyramidal syndromes are all strongly atropinic. Chlorpromazine, and especially thioridazine, are also strongly atropinic; in susceptible patients, the combination of one of each group may therefore give rise to an atropine psychosis, characterised by delirium, restlessness, visual hallucinations and tremor. Unless the possibility of such a development is borne in mind, it will often not be recognised for what it is, and the unfortunate patient may be given more neuroleptics, thus worsening his predicament. The immediate management should be withdrawal of the offending agents. The effect of intravenous physostigmine (1–2 mg) is diagnostic, but rarely necessary in practice.

Other drugs used in the treatment of idiopathic Parkinson's disease, such as L-dopa and bromocriptine, have no place in the management of neuroleptic-induced extrapyramidal syndromes.

Tardive dyskinesia

About 20% of patients chronically ingesting neuroleptic drugs, especially those who are female and elderly, with organic brain damage, suffering from affective disorder and who manifest other extrapyramidal side-effects early on, will develop a syndrome characterised by stereotyped buccolingual masticatory movements or by choreoathetoid and dystonic movements affecting trunk and limbs. In florid form the syndrome is probably not reversible, which makes early detection and prompt action important. It is believed that the syndrome develops as a result of hypersensitivity of dopamine receptors in the basal ganglia to chronic blockade by neuroleptic drugs.

A form of denervation sensitivity can be shown to develop in experimental animals but with a different time-course and requiring provocation for the dyskinesia to be demonstrated. A full understanding of the aetiology of the syndrome in man has not yet been achieved. As Rogers (1985) and others have shown, a similar neurological disorder can be found in psychotic patients treated never or sparingly with neuroleptics, and in those for whom treatment was stopped a long time ago. It is not clear why tardive dyskinesia should particularly affect nervous control of the oral-facial muscles. Animal work suggests that neuroleptics may affect striatal γ-aminobutyric acid (GABA)-containing neurones (Fibiger & Lloyd 1984).

The syndrome is not painful nor disabling physically but in terms of social function it confers considerable handicap. Prevention can only take the form of monitoring of drug intake with the minimum effective dose being employed; antiparkinsonian drugs should only be used when required and neuroleptic drugs should only be used when indicated for the treatment of drug-responsive symptom complexes (Barnes 1990). The concept of 'drug holidays' — periods of a few days or weeks when the patient is free of drugs — punctuating chronic treatment has not been shown to be of any benefit in preventing (and may even enhance) the development of tardive dyskinesia.

No neuroleptic available for general use has been shown to be free of the risk of development of this syndrome (although the substituted benzamides and clozapine may be relatively benign in this respect). There is no clearly effective treatment for tardive dyskinesia.

It is a characteristic of the syndrome that its manifestations will worsen when the responsible neuroleptic is withdrawn and the symptoms can often be suppressed transiently by increasing the dose, though this merely serves to worsen the underlying position. Drugs which enhance cholinergic transmission have been employed with limited success, especially choline hydrochloride 5 g/day (not available commercially). In severe cases any drug such as tetrabenazine which depletes presynaptic dopamine storage granules may be given a trial (Simpson et al 1982). Clonazepam has been used with success in the dystonic form.

Depressive syndromes

A dysphoria is not uncommonly seen in patients treated with neuroleptics. There have been a number of claims over the years that neuroleptics cause depressive syndromes. These are not major depressive illnesses. What is seen is the result of the natural progression of the syndrome being treated (Hirsch 1982, Galdi & Hirsh 1983). Tricyclic antidepressants have nothing to offer in the management of such depressive symptoms (Kramer 1989)

Autonomic and hormonal side-effects

The elderly are particularly prone to develop hypotension when treated with chlorpromazine or thioridazine. The strongly muscarinic nature of thioridazine leads to the frequent development of ejaculatory impotence (Barnes et al 1979). With these compounds in particular, anticholinergic manifestations are frequent, including blurring of vision, dry mouth and constipation. Chlorpromazine has a poikilothermic effect, which is important where elderly people living in poorly heated houses are concerned. Impaired glucose tolerance tests may be found during its administration, and amenorrhoea, breast engorgement and galactorrhoea may occur with any neuroleptic.

Hypersensitivity reactions

In the early days of the phenothiazines, possibly due to impurities in synthesis, a sensitivity-type cholestatic jaundice was relatively common, but is now very rare. About one in 10 000 patients will develop a blood dyscrasia, usually agranulocytosis and usually within the first 3 months of treatment (see below for a discussion of clozapine). Both patients receiving and those handling the drug may develop skin reactions, including rashes, urticaria and dermatitis.

Weight gain

Fluphenazine and flupenthixol, the most commonly used neuroleptics in depot form, are associated with weight gain, probably because of actions unrelated to the antipsychotic. The prevalence of obesity may be as high as 30%, with gross obesity in 50%. The dextro-rotatory isomer of fenfluramine is a potent anorectic (Editorial 1991a), by an action on serotonergic neurones, has little effect on dopaminergic systems, and can be used as an adjunct to dietary restriction in the treatment of drug-induced obesity in schizophrenic patients (Goodall et al 1988).

Cardiotoxic effects

On the basis of reports of sudden death of patients on pimozide, the Committee on Safety of Medicines has recommended (1990) that all patients should have an ECG prior to starting the drug. It is considered that the drug is contraindicated in those with prolongation of the QT interval or a past history of cardiac arrythmia. Treatment should start on a low dose, gradually increased to a maximum of 20 mg/day. Patients on higher doses should have regular check ECGs, and the dosage reviewed if changes occur. Concurrent treatment should be controlled, especially to avoid hypokalaemia.

The neuroleptic malignant syndrome

This disorder consists of hyperthermia, muscle rigidity and autonomic instability and may occur in 0.2% of those receiving neuroleptics, especially men under 40 years of age. Potent dopaminergic blockers like haloperidol seem particularly liable to produce the syndrome, but other drugs affecting central dopaminergic transmission may be responsible (Roseburn & Stewart 1989). Symptoms may appear from a few days to a few weeks after treatment starts, will build up in 2–3 days and subside as the drug clears from the body. Creatine phosphokinase may be markedly elevated. Other factors such as exhaustion and dehydration may also be involved as reintroduction of the drug some weeks later may not be followed by a recurrence of symptoms. In management, recognition of the syndrome is important, as the mortality is 20%. The body temperature must be reduced, respiration may need assistance and infections treated. Combined treatment with bromocriptine (60 mg/day) to enhance

dopaminergic activity and dantrolene (10 mg/kg) to reduce muscle tone has recently been reported to be of help (Abbot & Loizon 1986).

Epidermal and ocular manifestations

Exposure to ultraviolet light of a patient taking chlorpromazine is likely to lead to an allergic response in areas of skin exposed. It can be prevented, using an ultraviolet filtering cream or by a change to thioridazine. Those who have been taking phenothiazines for many years may develop a harmless but unsightly dark slate-grey pigmentation of skin. Corneal and lens opacities are described in those taking neuroleptics chronically, and thioridazine in a daily dose of above 800 mg/day is particularly implicated in causing retinitis pigmentosa. It is therefore best to avoid the long-term use of thioridazine in such amounts.

Interactions with other drugs

By inhibiting the re-uptake of monoamines, neuroleptic drugs will tend to reverse the hypotensive action of guanethidine and similar compounds used in the treatment of hypertension. Thioridazine may reverse the inotropic effect of digitalis by its quinidine-like action. The potential of strongly atropinic phenothiazines for causing a toxic confusional state in interaction with other drugs with an atropinic action is described above. The analgesic effect of morphine and the respiratory depression caused by other opiates such as pethidine are both potentiated by the phenothiazines. All neuroleptic drugs potentiate the cerebral depressant effect of alcohol and sedative drugs of the barbiturate/benzodiazepine type. Because tricyclic antidepressants are degraded along the same catabolic pathway as neuroleptic drugs, the administration of a neuroleptic to a patient already on tricyclic antidepressants is likely to both enhance and prolong activity of both compounds. The simultaneous ingestion of antacids and neuroleptics is likely to reduce absorption and so enhance the first-pass phenomenon.

Indications

Neuroleptics are indicated for the treatment of particular symptom complexes found within diagnostic categories, rather than of the diagnosis itself. An individual presenting without these particular symptom complexes will probably not benefit from these drugs and indeed may suffer unacceptable side-effects. Moreover, many patients improve spontaneously when admitted to hospital.

Active schizophrenic symptoms such as hallucinations and delusional beliefs are responsive to neuroleptic medication. Passive symptoms such as apathy and affective blunting seldom are, despite claims made for newer antipsychotics (although a withdrawn patient made active by akathisia may seem to have improved). The symptoms of other psychoses, as well as agitation and excitement, also respond to neuroleptic medication.

The non-specific tension and complaints of anxiety which frequently accompany less severe syndromes, while responsive to neuroleptic medication, are best not treated with neuroleptics as there are safer alternatives available. Neuroleptic drugs are therefore used primarily in the management of acute schizophrenic episodes and mania. The simultaneous use of sedatives with neuroleptics may sometimes allow a lower dose of the latter to be employed.

The other main indication for neuroleptic treatment is in the long-term maintenance treatment of patients with schizophrenia for whom chronic drug treatment can be shown to be associated with an improved outcome.

Neuroleptic drugs are used in other areas in psychiatric practice, although the indication is much less precise. The treatment of those with organic brain damage will be described later.

It is traditional to treat agitated depressive illnesses with a combination of a neuroleptic and a tricyclic antidepressant. The combination may only serve to increase the effective plasma level of the tricyclic antidepressant, and may give rise to problems of hypotension and accumulation of atropinic side-effects. However, a combination of a tricyclic and a neuroleptic may be required to avoid electroconvulsive therapy (ECT) in certain depressive psychotic illnesses.

It has been claimed for many neuroleptics that on their own, in low doses, they have an antidepressant effect as great as the tricyclics. It is possible that blockade of α_2-adrenergic receptors on the presynaptic neurones is the responsible mechanism. The mixed anxiety/depressive syndromes are more likely to respond than endogenomorphic illness. Such treatment has little potential for abuse, nor should it be lethal in overdose. However, there is a distinct risk of tardive dyskinesia. Fluphenazine 1–2 mg/day is commonly employed.

It is clear from their effect on fit threshold that neuroleptic drugs have little part to play in withdrawal syndromes whether from opiates or the alcohol/barbiturate group. Chlorpromazine is used outside psychiatry as an antiemetic, and to potentiate opiates in the management of intractable pain and in terminal care.

Depot versus oral preparations

Because it has been shown in most branches of medicine that compliance with oral medication is poor, and because in many psychiatrists' experience patients often present in relapse, having stopped taking their medication a few weeks or months before, there is a prevailing view that maintenance with a depot neuroleptic preparation is more secure and more likely to succeed than with an oral preparation. However, studies comparing oral and depot maintenance show little difference of outcome. When set against the 30% expectancy of tardive dyskinesia in 2 years for those receiving depot neuroleptics, the advantage seems slight. The dose should be adjusted to the minimum and the inter-injection interval to the maximum consistent with symptom control. Unless some care is taken, patients receiving monthly injections of a depot neuroleptic for a long time may be given them as a matter of course, with little thought to dosage, side-effects or whether the original indication still exists. A long-lasting oral neuroleptic, such as pimozide, may be given twice or thrice a week effectively, while paying heed to the cardiac risks. A patient attending a day hospital may be managed in this way.

In acute treatment, depot neuroleptics can overcome the apparent resistance of symptoms to oral drugs caused by efficient first-pass metabolism. If the legal circumstances allow, they may also be given to a resistant patient. Once given they cannot be recalled and may cause prolonged side-effects. This occurs mainly in the elderly, possibly causing loss of independence for months. The short-acting drug fluspirilene, which has a half-life of 55–150 hours, is therefore to be preferred.

Management of acute excitement

In addition to the appropriate environmental and behavioural measures, the drug management of acute psychotic excitement demands rapid onset of effect, short duration of action to allow flexible dosing according to response, and adequate control of the symptoms. Intoxication, overdose, intracranial pathology and drug-induced extrapyramidal syndromes must all be excluded. Parenteral benzodiazepines may well fail through uncertain absorption or disinhibition.

Droperidol given every 30 minutes in doses of 5–10 mg intramuscularly, or 5–20 mg orally, affords rapid control of excitement, aggressive behaviour and agitation. The effect lasts for 3–4 hours. Such management allows time for further assessment and allows options to remain open which would otherwise be closed by mounting disturbance. Extrapyramidal side-effects are rare with short-term use. Patients with suspected liver damage require a more cautious dosage schedule. A recently introduced alternative is a depot preparation of zuclopenthixol acetate which lasts for 3 days, given in a dose of 50–100 mg.

Dosage

The neuroleptic to be employed must be given in a dose adequate for control of the particular patient's symptoms. When a patient's past history is known, experience may dictate the dosage at which he is likely to respond. When starting with no previous knowledge the wide variation of plasma level achieved in a population for a given dose must be borne in mind, and the dose increased until control of the relevant symptoms is obtained, always bearing in mind the side-effects and general clinical condition of the patient. Improvement can be expected within 24–36 hours for excitement, within 3–6 weeks for delusions and hallucinations and over 6 months for chronic states. Most adult psychotic patients will need 300 mg or more of chlorpromazine per day. Few are likely to need more than 1 g/day.

A maximum of 200 mg should be given at any one time by mouth, and by injection 150 mg is the upper limit. Even then, care must be taken to ensure that the patient comes to no harm through hypotension or ataxia. Routine measurement of serum antipsychotic drug levels cannot be justified by enhanced response. The theoretical need of a few patients for large doses leads to the concept of 'megadose' treatment. Use of such doses — chlorpromazine 2–3 g/day or haloperidol 150–200 mg/day — disregards possible long-term complications and has not been shown to have any advantage over standard regimes. Table 36.1 shows the potency of other commonly used neuroleptic drugs relative to chlorpromazine. Indeed, there is evidence that doses of haloperidol as low as 10 mg/day should suffice for many patients (Rifkin et al 1991).

Treatment-resistant schizophrenia

Causes of resistance include associated psychosocial tensions, failure to take the medication, its being given in the wrong dose — too much or too little — and then failure of the drug to work. The outlook for certain treatment-resistant patients appears to be improved by the availability of clozapine. The cost of clozapine treatment compared to chlorpromazine may make the pharmacy budget holder blench, but the cost of inpatient care for a chronically disturbed individual is higher. The cost to the patient of a blood dyscrasia is potentially high, but the regular mandatory monitoring of the white cell count through the manufacturer's service reduces this — all those treated in the UK who developed neutropenia to date recovered on drug withdrawal. Treatment resistance could be defined as failure to respond to a full exploration of both the dosage envelope of a standard oral neuroleptic and of a depot neuroleptic, given for 6 months.

When clozapine is introduced, the other neuroleptic treatments should have been withdrawn. Starting with a low dose of clozapine reduces the risk of side-effects, the most troublesome of which are sedation, hypersalivation, weight gain, fever, liver enzyme changes, convulsions and constipation. Benign ECG changes occur.

DRUGS USED IN THE AFFECTIVE DISORDERS

The tricyclic antidepressants, re-uptake inhibitors and receptor antagonists — the 'heterocyclics'

The first member of this class of antidepressants, imipramine, was introduced into clinical practice in 1958. It differs from the phenothiazine promazine only in having the sulphur atom replaced by an ethylene linkage. This confers a different configuration to the tricyclic molecule but its other physicochemical properties are similar. In the same way amitriptyline has a structural relation to the thioxanthines, although there is no isomerism. Clomipramine is the homologue of chlorpromazine. There are many others in this family of drugs.

The last decade has seen many new classes of antidepressants introduced. The tricyclics have a wide range of effects, few being required for the antidepressant effect. Selective re-uptake inhibitors such as maprotilene, trazodone, fluoxetine (plus nomifensine and zimelidine — both now withdrawn) act directly on one neurotransmitter only. Mianserin antagonises α_2 adrenoceptors powerfully but does not inhibit the re-uptake of noradrenaline or 5–HT. Trazodone may produce a mixed agonist/antagonist effect on 5–HT receptors. As noted above, neuroleptics may exert an antidepressant effect by antagonising presynaptic adrenoceptors.

Therapeutic actions

It has been known for two decades that the tricyclic antidepressants affect particular neuronal networks in the central nervous system dependent on 5-HT and noradrenaline as transmitters. Their action is fairly immediate in the brain, but all antidepressant drugs show a delay between first dose and therapeutic response, usually of 10–21 days. All the tricyclic antidepressants block the presynaptic re-uptake of noradrenaline and/or serotonin. This formed the basis for the 'monoamine hypothesis' of depressive illness.

However, there is now doubt as to whether this is a necessary or sufficient explanation for the action of these drugs. Mianserin is an α_2 antagonist and only a weak inhibitor of noradrenaline and serotonin re-uptake but is nonetheless an effective antidepressant. Many antidepressant treatments produce a direct or indirect blockade of postsynaptic β receptors, which suggests that diminished noradrenergic activity may be a prerequisite of antidepressant effectiveness. Alternatively, adrenergic receptors may be supersensitive in depressive illness. Tests of the functional activity of noradrenergic systems, using drugs of known effect on hypophyseal hormone release, before and after antidepressant treatment suggest that, overall, noradrenergic activity is increased in depression. The receptor changes apparently induced take over 2 weeks to occur, i.e. their time-course is comparable to that of clinical improvement. It would appear that intact serotonergic neuronal systems are also necessary for the action of antidepressants affecting noradrenergic neurones (Tyrer & Marsden 1985).

There have been vehement arguments about the respective roles played by deficiencies or excesses of one or other of these two neurotransmitters in the aetiology of depressive illness. It is clear that networks of neurones depending on one or other for synaptic transmission are intimately associated within the brain, together with cholinergic, dopaminergic and other transmitter systems. The possibility of affecting one system without compensatory changes taking place in the others is therefore remote. As with the neuroleptics, the tricyclic antidepressants vary widely in their effect on muscarinic receptors, and in their ability to sedate. Tricyclic antidepressants also block histamine receptors in the central nervous system. There is no convincing evidence that this is other than an unlooked for side-effect and blockade of histamine receptors does not seem a necessary condition for effective antidepressant activity.

Serotonin-selective re-uptake inhibitors

Such is the lag between original identification and commercial launch, new antidepressants which had their origin in interest during the mid 1970s in serotonin metabolism in depressive illness have been introduced only recently. Fluvoxamine (1987), fluoxetine (1990), sertraline (1990) and paroxetine (1991) are all specific re-uptake inhibitors for serotonin and therefore should have a 'cleaner' profile of side-effects. In particular, weight gain and lethality are avoided, at the expense of headache and nausea. All are considerably more expensive than the other antidepressants.

Pharmacology

Tricyclic antidepressants are tertiary amines and are demethylated in the liver to secondary amines which are also biologically active. Thus, a patient taking imipramine will also have desipramine circulating; those taking amitriptyline will show plasma levels of nortriptyline. The secondary amines are available as antidepressant agents but have no advantage clinically over their parent compounds. (A 'pro-drug', lofepramine, is commercially available, inactive as an antidepressant itself. It is metabolised to desipramine, and seems to be an expensive way to prescribe desipramine.) The tertiary amines tend to affect serotoninergic function, the secondary affect noradrenergic function. Of the circulating drug, 90% is bound to plasma protein and some explanation of the delay in onset of the antidepressant effect may be the time taken to saturate available binding sites owing to the convention of initiating treatment with a low dose. For a given dose of drug there is wide variation of the plasma levels achieved within a population. The half-life of the commonly used antidepressants in plasma is commonly 10–20 hours, although this is much increased in the elderly. It must be remembered that fluctuations in drug concentration in the brain may be somewhat different from those seen in plasma. Unless it has been shown in a particular patient that the profile of side-effects experienced requires the daily dose to be split into three or four parts, it is as therapeutically efficient to give the daily dose in a single bolus at night. This will tend to increase compliance because sleep is enhanced.

Some consider intravenous infusion of tricyclics, especially clomipramine, to be beneficial. There is little evidence in favour of this procedure, which seems rather arduous for the recipient, and may not hasten any antidepressant response if that is linked to receptor changes. The newer antidepressants, especially the serotonin-selective ones, tend to be given in a fixed dose, for patients of all ages. The active metabolite of fluoxetine, norfluoxetine, has a half-life of several weeks, necessitating a 5 week gap between stopping fluoxetine and starting an MAOI.

Plasma levels and therapeutic effect

It is difficult to assess the action of a drug on the brain

when markers of its activity can only be identified peripherally. The lack of hard criteria for effectiveness and the need to use soft criteria such as symptoms adds to this difficulty. Variations in patient selection criteria have also added to the inconsistency of the results of studies of the relationship between plasma level of tricyclics and antidepressant effect. Only with respect to nortriptyline has a reasonably consistent result been obtained by different workers. For this drug it would seem that there is a 'therapeutic window', with a good antidepressant response being associated with plasma levels between 50 and 140 mg/ml. Two-thirds of patients will achieve such plasma levels on a dose of nortriptyline of 150 mg/day.

It is suggested that if there is no therapeutic response after 3 weeks the most likely cause is excessive dosage, and the daily intake should be reduced to 75 mg/day. If there is still no effect after a week, 225 mg/day should be employed. It is somewhat confusing that, for amitriptyline, which is metabolised into nortriptyline, no such therapeutic window has been demonstrated. For imipramine there is some indication that, where side-effects permit, some patients may need a daily dosage well in excess of 200 mg/day.

Side-effects and toxicity

In compounds with strong atropinic activity, the expected side-effects of dry mouth, constipation, urinary retention and blurring of vision are common. Hypotension is often experienced, especially by the elderly, and many patients complain of hand tremor and excessive sweating. Patients with an untreated closed-angle glaucoma may suffer severe deterioration of vision, although if pilocarpine drops are used regularly on the eye this can be avoided.

Tolerance does develop to the sedative effects and insomnia will result if the drug is withdrawn abruptly. A few patients, accustomed to a fairly high dose of a tricyclic antidepressant, will experience a withdrawal syndrome if the drug is abruptly discontinued (Annotation 1985). This syndrome is characterised by malaise, headache, nausea, abdominal pain, diarrhoea and restlessness, and is due to cholinergic hyperfunction.

Certain antidepressants have an adverse effect on cardiovascular function. This is in addition to hypotension and tachycardia, which are both more severe in the elderly. Several members of the group, especially amitriptyline and imipramine and their active metabolites, sensitise the myocardium to catecholamines, leading to arrhythmias which are suspected of being the cause of sudden death in patients taking these

drugs. Amitriptyline especially has a quinidine-like effect and may induce T wave changes in the EGG. These effects make ECT somewhat hazardous in patients receiving tricyclic antidepressants who are elderly or suffer from cardiovascular disorder. Myocardial membrane stabilisation by the tricyclics may also contribute to their toxicity.

In those with myocardial damage or who are predisposed to cardiac arrhythmias, the older tricyclic antidepressants may precipitate fatal ventricular arrhythmias. Congestive failure may be worsened and cardiomyopathies exacerbated.

Jaundice, rashes and agranulocytosis may occur rarely. In the light of reported reactions it is advised that patients on mianserin should have a full blood count every 4 weeks for the first 3 months of treatment, and that they should continue to be observed for fever, sore throat and stomatitis thereafter. Such reactions are commoner in the elderly.

Orgasmic impotence is reported for both females and males. There is no evidence of teratogenicity. All antidepressants, new and old, may lower the convulsive threshold and should be used with caution or under anticonvulsant cover in epileptics.

Patients treated with tricyclic antidepressants often show an increased appetite for carbohydrate foods and may develop a pronounced weight gain. Although part of this gain may represent recovery of a previous loss, it may be a serious problem, especially in women. It appears to happen less with drugs with a selective action on 5–HT uptake or receptors, like trazodone or fluoxetine.

Tricyclic poisoning

The tricyclic antidepressants are lethal in overdose (Table 36.2), both for the patient and her children and, given the ever-present risk of suicide in depressive illness, this makes proper and appropriate prescription essential. Such elementary precautions as a conscious assessment of suicidal risk at each interview, only 1 week's supply to be given at a time until the patient is better, and the employment of a relative to supervise tablet storage should be a matter of routine.

The complex variety of effects on the myocardium, including sensitisation to catecholamines, inhibition of vagal activity and quinidine-like effects, make the management of tricyclic poisoning in a specialist poisons treatment unit or intensive care unit essential. In severe poisoning, respiratory depression, hypotension, conduction defects and metabolic acidosis can lead to coma, convulsions and respiratory or cardiac arrest which are quite unresponsive to resuscitation. Because

Table 36.2 Fatal poisoning, prescription data and fatal toxicity indices 1975–1984 for antidepressant drugs for England, Wales and Scotland

Drug	Year introduced	Fatal poisonings		Deaths per million prescriptions
		Observed	Expected	
Tricyclics up to 1970				
Desipramine	1963	13	5.7	80.2[**]
Dothiepin	1969	533	372	50.0[***]
Amitriptyline	1961	1181	886	46.5[***]
Nortriptyline	1963	57	51	39.2
Doxepin	1969	102	114	31.3
Imipramine	1959	278	342	28.4[***]
Clomipramine	1970	51	160	11.1[***]
Tricyclics and other antidepressants 1974 et seq				
Maprotiline	1974	83	77	37.6
Trazodone	1980	6	15	13.6[*]
Mianserin	1976	30	187	5.6[***]
Lofepramine	1983	0	3.7	0.0
Monoamine oxidase inhibitors				
Tranylcypromine	1960	15	9.0	58.1[*]
Phenelzine	1959	24	36.7	22.8[*]
Isocarboxazid	1960	3	8.2	12.8
All antidepressants		2551		34.9

After Cassidy & Henry (1987).
[*]Significantly different from all antidepressants at 5% level ($p < 0.05$).
[**]Significantly different from all antidepressants at 1% level ($p < 0.01$).
[***]Significantly different from all antidepressants at 0.1% level ($p < 0.001$).

the drug is highly protein bound, later dialysis is of no benefit. If the patient's condition permits, gastric lavage is always worthwhile up to 24 hours after ingestion, especially if there is to be a delay in transfer of the patient. There is a risk of cardiac arrest even 4–6 days after the poisoning and cardiac monitoring should be continued until 12 hours after the QRS complex has normalised (Crome 1982).

Interactions with other drugs

Phenytoin, phenylbutazone, aspirin and phenothiazines compete for plasma protein-binding sites. Neuroleptic drugs compete for the catabolic pathway of the tricyclics, and oral contraceptives will delay metabolism. Fluoxetine taken simultaneously with tricyclics will raise the plasma level of the latter considerably. All the uptake inhibitors antagonise the action of hypotensives, such as guanethidine, and the hypotensive effect of clonidine will also be reversed. In combination with other atropinic drugs there is a risk of atropine psychosis developing, which may be difficult to distinguish from symptoms of the depressive syndrome. Tricyclic antidepressants are hazardous in combination with MAOIs and deaths have resulted from the combination. A discussion of the simultaneous use of both

types of antidepressant for therapeutic purposes follows later. Clomipramine and other serotonin-specific drugs are especially dangerous with tranylcypromine. This may have something to do with the latter's strong amphetamine-like effect as amphetamine is potentiated by tricyclics. The administration of direct-acting sympathomimetic amines to patients taking tricyclics may result in a severe hypertensive episode.

The newer antidepressants

There is no doubt that it is incongruous to treat a condition where there is a high risk of self-harm with an agent which is potentially lethal when taken in a dose equivalent to not more than 1 week's supply. There is also little doubt that many patients find the side-effects of the older tricyclic antidepressants unacceptable, particularly weight gain, and that this has an effect on compliance, especially in the long term. The series of new antidepressants produced since 1970 show similar overall efficacy to the tricyclics. Fewer side-effects and lower toxicity in overdose are claimed. These compounds seem to have less effect on the myocardium and may be safer to use in the elderly (see below). Needless to say, they are considerably more expensive than the long-established drugs. In general the new drugs should be used when there is a positive indication in a particular patient. Their long-term effects will have to be known before they can be considered for regular use, particularly as nomofensine was in use for 7 years before its toxicity became apparent.

Indications for antidepressant treatment

Tricyclic antidepressants have a two-fold place in the management of depressive illness: first in the acute treatment of a depressive syndrome, and second to prevent relapse in the short and long term (for details, see Ch. 19).

The time over which a patient may benefit from the regular ingestion of an antidepressant is so long that it is important to bear in mind which stage of treatment is current. The benefits of continuing treatment have been clearly demonstrated. Continuing education and reminders of the rationale for long-term therapy highlight the need for treatment so that regular tablet taking is not seen as a useless, morally suspect activity. It should be noted that all antidepressants may precipitate mania in those with an underlying bipolar disposition. Lithium is to be preferred for those who suffer from a bipolar affective disorder and who require long-term treatment.

Obsessional symptoms which occur in association with depressive mood are particularly likely to respond to clomipramine or one of the newer serotonin-specific drugs. The effect is enhanced by the simultaneous involvement of the patient in a behavioural programme, and is often lost if the drug is withdrawn (Marks et al 1980). Fluoxetine and fluvoxamine have been used with benefit in bulimia nervosa (see Ch. 23).

There is no reliable clinical indicator of which tricyclic antidepressant should be chosen, except a previous response by that patient. It is traditional to use amitriptyline in agitated and imipramine in retarded depressives, but there is little hard evidence to support this practice. Imipramine may need to be used in higher doses than amitriptyline, but otherwise there is little to choose between them. Doxepin and dothiepin are as sedative as amitriptyline, but dose-for-dose are less potent. Desipramine is largely free from anticholinergic and sedative side-effects. Clomipramine appears to act particularly well in combination with L-tryptophan 2 g/day, and thus may be employed if a disappointing result has been obtained with another tricyclic in a patient with an endogenomorphic illness (Walinder et al 1976) (but see below for caveats regarding L–tryptophan). Of the newer serotonin-specific drugs trazodone is more sedative, fluvoxamine less so and

fluoxetine is quite alerting. The latter may make the tense patient temporarily more anxious, requiring the short-term use of benzodiazepines on an as-needed basis.

If antidepressants are withdrawn shortly after a patient has responded, relapse is likely. After a period which may vary from weeks to several months, and which probably depends on the natural history of the condition, relapse does not occur. This 'end-point' can only be found by trial and error, by gradually reducing the daily intake of antidepressant in steps several weeks apart and reviewing the patient's clinical state before making a further reduction. Continuity of care is important in this respect, as the clinician who has known the patient when both ill and well is likely to recognise illness returning.

The monoamine oxidase inhibitors

Isoniazid, used in the chemotherapy of tuberculosis, was found to cause euphoria as a side-effect, and in 1955 was shown to produce inhibition of monoamine oxidase (MAO). Within a few years iproniazid had been shown to be of benefit in the treatment of depressive illness but, owing to its hepatotoxic effect, it was soon abandoned. Although upwards of six other MAOIs have been used clinically, phenelzine, isocarboxazid and tranylcypromine, which illustrate the important points, will be discussed here.

Action

As their name implies, all members of this class of antidepressants inhibit the enzyme MAO, which is present in brain, gut, liver and platelets. Both hydrazine derivatives (such as phenelzine) and tranylcypromine (a non-hydrazine) cause irreversible inhibition. In this way, it was supposed, the MAOIs increased the availability of neurotransmitter at postsynaptic receptors by inhibiting metabolic degradation of the monoamines noradrenaline and 5–HT.

As has been found with tricyclic antidepressants, the antidepressant effect of the MAOI appears to be linked to a down-regulation of adrenoceptors.

Naturally occurring amines such as tyramine and phenolethylamine are found in many foods and have a pharmacological action as indirect sympathomimetics, by producing release of monoamines with a transmitter action from presynaptic storage granules. MAO exists in multiple forms in both the brain and body. MAO-A oxidises noradrenaline, 5–HT and tyramine; MAO-B oxidises phenylethylamine and tyramine, but not noradrenaline or 5–HT. MAOIs exist which preferentially inhibit one or other of these forms of MAO and such selective inhibitors are finding their way into clinical practice. MAO-B inhibitors have found a role in the treatment of Parkinson's disease.

Although no MAO-A inhibitor is available as an antidepressant, moclobemide and brofaromine, which are reversible inhibitors, have performed well in trials and little if any blood pressure rise is detectable after tyramine ingestion; therefore, dietary restrictions could be unnecessary, although will still be recommended.

Some MAOIs, especially tranylcypromine, have a strong amphetamine-like action, and reports exist of dependence on and abuse of these agents for this reason. All MAOIs reduce REM sleep. They have little atropine-like activity, but they exert some action on the autonomic nervous system.

MAO is to be found in the blood platelet and the degree of inhibition of the platelet enzyme can be measured in the laboratory. It has been shown that a therapeutic response to phenelzine occurs when platelet MAO is more than 80% inhibited, and that this usually occurs in a daily dosage range of 60–90 mg. Several studies which have found phenelzine inferior to other antidepressants have used doses of only 45–60 mg/day.

Side-effects and toxicity (Blackwell 1991)

The cheese reaction. As mentioned above, the MAOIs in clinical use produce inhibition of all forms of MAO at all sites in the body. Therefore, naturally occurring monoamines such as tyramine and phenylethylamine which are normally destroyed in the gut and the liver gain access to the systemic circulation, and are able to produce pressor effects on the cardiovascular system. Patients taking MAOIs who ingest certain foodstuffs (see Table 36.3) rich in these two amines frequently suffer from flushing and a pounding headache, and may occasionally develop a cerebrovascular accident owing to a catastrophic rise in blood pressure.

Not only foodstuffs but many proprietary preparations available over the counter also contain pressor amines. Interactions with non-sympathomimetic drugs are described below. Treatment of such an interaction is by an α-adrenergic blocker, such as phentolamine 2–5 mg intravenously. If this is not available, chlorpromazine 200 mg orally or 50 mg given slowly intravenously will do instead. Out-patients may be given 200 mg chlorpromazine tablets for emergencies, but patient education, the automatic issuing of a warning card, and behaviour on part of the prescriber making it clear that he takes the possibility of such an interaction seriously are much more important. Dietary

Table 36.3 Foodstuffs implicated in producing a 'cheese' reaction in association with the MAOIs

Cheese, especially the mature varieties

Degraded protein:
  Chicken liver
  Hung game
  Pickled herrings
  Patè

Yeast and protein extracts:
  Marmite
  Bovril
  Oxo

Alcoholic drinks:
  Beer
  Chianti wine

Certain vegetables and fruit:
  Broad bean pods
  Green banana skins

precautions have to be continued rigorously for as long as the patient is on the MAOI and for at least 10 days thereafter.

Other side-effects. These include those affecting the cardiovascular system, the most common of which is hypotension. This phenomenon is ill-understood, but is clinically quite important as it is often the limiting factor in determining for how long and at what dose the MAOIs may be used. Phenelzine is an offender in this respect and with it gravity-dependent oedema of the ankles may also occur. Retention of urine and failure of ejaculation both occur. Other side-effects occurring during treatment with MAOIs include dry mouth, blurred vision and constipation.

Insomnia may be troublesome, especially with tranylcypromine, though it is sometimes possible to combat this by giving the entire daily dosage in divided amounts before midday.

Iproniazid was dropped from clinical use because of hepatotoxicity. Other hydrazine derivatives, such as phenelzine, also cause jaundice occasionally. They may also cause a systemic lupus erythematosus-like syndrome with the appearance of erythema nodosum. The risk of this is sufficient to require the monitoring of liver function and autoimmune activity every 3–6 months in patients taking these drugs in the long term.

Overdosage with the MAOIs leads to a syndrome characterised by agitation, hallucinations, hyper-reflexia and hyperpyrexia, leading eventually to convulsions with marked instability of blood pressure. The elderly are particularly prone to develop such complications and, if treatment with the MAOIs must be embarked upon in the elderly, monitoring of the clinical effect must be frequent as a toxic confusional state precipitated by these drugs can be very slow to correct itself. Interactions with certain other drugs can produce a similar syndrome to that of overdosage (see below).

Interactions with other drugs

The interactions of the MAOIs with other drugs fall into three categories; those which can be understood on the basis of universal inhibition of MAO, those which occur on the basis of interference with enzymatic degradation pathways in the liver, and those which are ill-understood.

Indirectly acting sympathomimetics such as amphetamine, and to a lesser extent directly acting drugs like ephedrine which are to be found in proprietary cures for allergic or infective rhinitis, are likely to produce a hypertensive crisis. Similarly, precursors of biogenic amines such as L-dopa and 5-HT can produce a similar reaction. In theory, directly acting sympathomimetics should not produce a hypertensive crisis, as they are catabolised by O-methyltransferase within the synaptic cleft, but avoidance of all sympathomimetics during treatment with MAOIs is the best council. Sedative substances such as alcohol, the barbiturates, phenothiazines and benzodiazepines, and also anticholinergics, are potentiated by the MAOIs by competition for degradation pathways.

Certain drugs such as the tricyclic antidepressants and pethidine when given to a patient already taking an MAOI may produce a syndrome similar to that shown by an overdose of MAOI alone. Hyperpyrexia is prominent and the syndrome may be so severe as to be indistinguishable from an encephalopathy. This interaction would appear to be mediated by serotonergic neurones and may be best reversed by cautious use of intravenous chlorpromazine. Tranylcypromine and clomipramine are particularly potent in this respect and are lethal together.

If tricyclic antidepressants and an MAOI are to be used together in the treatment of intractable depressive states, a sedative tricyclic such as amitriptyline or trimipramine and a less amphetamine-like MAOI such as phenelzine are best employed. The patient must be started on both compounds simultaneously after a period on no antidepressant at all. The MAOI should be given in the morning and the tricyclic in the evening in low dosage, and cautiously both increased together.

Because of the irreversible nature of the inhibition of MAO, a period of at least 10 days should elapse after withdrawal of an MAOI before a tricyclic antidepressant of any kind is administered. A similar interval should be allowed before a switch is made from another MAOI to tranylcypromine. A patient should be clear of most tricyclic antidepressants 5 days after withdrawal of the drug, but 5 weeks must elapse between withdrawal of fluoxetine and starting MAOIs.

MAOIs ought to be completely withdrawn before any patient undergoes an anaesthetic for elective surgery. Emergency operative treatment can take place immediately but any resuscitation is more fraught for the anaesthetist. Similarly, a patient can receive modified ECT within 10 days of stopping an MAOI, but it is important to consult with the anaesthetist first.

Indications

It is becoming easier to lay down clear indications for the use of the MAOIs (Nutt & Glue 1989) Their role in the management of depressive illness has been especially clouded by reactions to their apparent ineffectiveness in early trial and the interactions with cheese and other foodstuffs. Trials of phenelzine against placebo which have used a dosage of greater than 60 mg/day and a duration of treatment greater than 6 weeks have tended to show that it is an effective agent. It seems likely that phenelzine is inferior to the tricyclic antidepressants in the management of endogenomorphic depressive illness. There are those who claim that the MAOIs are not true antidepressants and should be referred to as 'psychic energisers'. As the biochemical aetiology of depressive illness is ill-understood, it must be doubted whether the tricyclic drugs can be considered true antidepressants either.

Those who have continued to accept the MAOIs as useful drugs have described an atypical depressive syndrome responsive to them. This is characterised by a relative lack of the biological symptoms of endogenomorphic depressive illness, and a preponderance of anxiety and hypochondriacal symptoms, relatively unresponsive to the tricyclics. A depressive illness marked by excessive intake of food and excessive sleep is said to be particularly likely to respond.

Neurotic depression in out-patients without melancholic features may be another indication for first-line treatment with MAOIs. In melancholia the MAOIs should be kept as a third-line treatment, to be used in those resistant to tricyclic drugs and/or ECT.

Phenelzine appears to be superior to placebo and simple sedation in the management of phobic anxiety, but only if treatment is continued for at least 8 weeks. The relative merits of drug treatment and behaviour therapy in the management of these conditions is uncertain. Much may depend on the particular patient. Panic disorder is another indication for MAOIs.

Monoamine precursor treatment

L-Tryptophan

L-Tryptophan, the precursor of serotonin, is a naturally occurring amino acid, with an average dietary intake of 2 g. Only the laevo isomer of tryptophan is biologically active. Taken in protein, it has to compete with other aromatic and large neutral amino acids to enter the brain. A high-carbohydrate and protein-poor meal elevates brain tryptophan. L-Tryptophan is readily absorbed from the gut, but has a short half-life in plasma, and it is customary to give the total daily dose in four parts.

The first enzyme on the pathway from L-tryptophan to 5-HT is tryptophan-5-hydroxylase, which is normally unsaturated with tryptophan, and appears to be the rate limiter for the synthetic process. Therefore, an increase in available tryptophan leads to an increase in the rate of synthesis of 5-HT.

In man, an oral dose of tryptophan is followed within 30 minutes by an increase of cerebrospinal 5-hydroxyindoleacetic acid, the degradation product of 5-HT. It is not clear that the increase in synthesis of 5-HT brought about by an oral dose of L-tryptophan brings about an increase in functional activity of serotonergic neurones. Although clear-cut as far as control of diet is concerned, the effect on mood is less easily distinguishable (Wurtman 1984). There is a further complication in that administration of daily doses of L-tryptophan in excess of 3 g/day leads to its diversion down alternative metabolic pathways and to no increase in synthesis of 5-HT. At one point it was claimed that L-tryptophan was of equivalent efficacy in the treatment of depressive illness to ECT. These claims have not been substantiated, and the current position would appear to be that L-tryptophan is superior to placebo in the treatment of mild to moderate depressive illness, especially those conditions found in out-patients and in general practice (Thomson et al 1982).

There is also some suggestion that an oral dose of 3 g taken at night may have some hypnotic effect, which would be in keeping with the putative role of 5-HT in regulating sleep activity. L-Tryptophan in divided doses totalling 2 g/day also has something particular to offer in the treatment of therapy-resistant depressive illness, combined with antidepressants which have an effect on serotonergic systems, such as clomipramine and the MAOIs. Excessive L-tryptophan given with an MAOI can give rise to a symptom complex similar in many respects to an overdose of MAOI alone.

For 20 years L-tryptophan taken on its own appeared to be free from dangerous side-effects, and the most common complaint was of a transient nausea. In recent years, especially in the USA but occasionally in the UK, a syndrome consisting of eosinophilia, fever, respiratory symptoms and myalgia has occurred. L-Tryptophan has been available as an over-the-counter drug in the USA, and was used widely. It is possible that an impurity has contaminated the production of a major supplier. L-Tryptophan is still available in the UK on a named-patient basis. The psychiatrist continuing to use it on his patients would be well advised to obtain written consent and to perform a differential white cell count every month. The main favourable feature of L-tryptophan in the treatment of depressive illness is its non-lethality in overdose.

L-Dopa, the precursor of dopamine, does not appear to have any practical use in clinical psychiatry; and, as might be expected, may worsen some psychotic states. Tyrosine, the precursor of noradrenaline, has been reported to have some antidepressant activity, but is not in regular clinical use.

The lithium ion

Lithium belongs to the same column in the periodic table as sodium and potassium, and is an alkali earth metal. Lithium bromide was mentioned a century ago as being particularly useful as a sedative. In the 1940s lithium was used briefly as the chloride to substitute for table salt in the management of hypertension. Severe toxicity resulted, leading to withdrawal of the compound. Although brief, this episode left an impression of dangerousness. The use of lithium carbonate demands the same of doctor and patient as insulin in diabetes mellitus.

Action

Although lithium has been found to have many actions in biological systems, its mode of action in the treatment of affective disorders has not been identified. As there is a putative disorder of sodium metabolism in the affective disorders, lithium might be expected to exert an influence and one postulated mode of action is on the sodium-dependent adenosine triphosphatase (ATPase) in cell membranes. Lithium can stimulate both sodium- and magnesium-dependent ATPase. It also inhibits adenyl cyclase and inositol phosphate intracellular secondary messenger systems throughout the body and in brain by altering the functions of guanosine triphosphate (GTP)-binding proteins (Avissar 1988). Also, it may alter the distribution of calcium and magnesium across excitable membranes (Waldmeier 1990).

None of these changes can be integrated with the predictions of the monoamine hypothesis of the affective disorders. Both noradrenaline and serotonin are affected by lithium; both show an increase in turnover and metabolism in the short term, but a decrease in the long term. The activity of sites on blood platelets which mediate uptake of 5-HT, a process similar to presynaptic uptake by neurones, is also increased by lithium (Coppen et al 1980).

Serum level

For treatment of acute mania, serum levels at 12 hours of 1-1.4 mmol/l are required. Above 1.5 mmol/l side-effects become more troublesome and dangerous and no clinical advantage accrues. For prophylaxis, a 12 hour level above 0.5 mmol/l is required, and somewhere in the range 0.5–0.8 mmol/l should be the target; the elderly should be maintained at the lower end (Coppen et al 1983). Those who have been well on lithium for a number of years should also be maintained at a lower serum level.

Giving the total daily intake as a single dose at night minimises the intake, and also, rather surprisingly, reduces nocturia and the risk of renal damage. The serum level may be measured at any time between 12 and 24 hours after the last dose, as long as the interval is constant, to allow comparison of results. However, anything less than 12 hours is unsatisfactory because of the rapid decline in serum level during the initial phase of excretion.

Absorption and excretion

In the UK, lithium is administered as the carbonate, although the acetate is available elsewhere. Absorption is rapid and serum levels peak at 3–4 hours. Thereafter the serum level shows a biphasic fall, rapidly to 12 hours postingestion and slower for the next 12–24 hours. Lithium exists as the free ion in plasma and is found in the cerebrospinal fluid at about half the serum concentration. It replaces up to 10% of sodium in bone and is concentrated in muscle and thyroid gland. Apart from minimal quantities lost in sweat, the only route of excretion is in the urine. Lithium clearance is about 20% of the glomerular filtration rate, is independent of the plasma level, and diminishes with age. Lithium resorption takes place in the proximal tubule in association with sodium handling, so any alteration in sodium balance will affect lithium balance.

Dosage

Therapeutic levels of lithium are likely to be achieved by a daily dosage of 800–1600 mg. In the early stages of treatment frequent dosage allows more ready access of lithium to the intracellular compartment. In the manic phase a greater proportion of lithium is held intracellularly, and with recovery the daily dose may have to be reduced to avoid excessively high serum levels.

In view of the 10–20 fold peaks of concentration in the distal renal tubule, it used to be assumed that the daily dosage should be divided to lessen renal side-effects. The current view is that the interpeak troughs are more important, and that the longer the tubule is in contact with low urinary concentrations of lithium the less likely are side-effects such as polyuria. On this basis, some have advocated alternate-day lithium ingestion. This demands a lot from the patient and may be reserved for the educated and disciplined.

Slow-release tablets of lithium carbonate are available but some doubt remains whether the absorption pattern in vivo is actually much different with these preparations, so soluble is lithium carbonate; they may alleviate gastric side-effects. Lithium is now available in 250, 300 and 400 mg standard and 400 mg slow-release preparations. There is much to be said for a particular hospital standardising on one preparation, if only to avoid potentially dangerous confusion over tablet strength. Lithium tablets are not pleasant to swallow and the stronger tablets can reduce the number which needs to be taken.

Preliminaries to lithium treatment

In view of the chronic nature of lithium treatment it is essential to establish baseline renal, cardiac, and thyroid function, plus body weight. For this purpose, a full blood count, plasma electrolyte and urea levels, creatinine clearance, ECG and serum thyroxine level suffice. In a manic patient, a 24 hour urine collection may be out of the question, but should not prevent lithium treatment. The serum level 24 hours after a single 600 mg dose gives some idea of renal function — a level above 0.25 mmol/l indicates renal impairment and the need for caution in dosage. Alternatively, serum creatinine or lithium renal clearance can be measured, although the latter requires accurate collection of urine.

Monitoring lithium treatment

It is essential to continue to estimate serum lithium as long as the patient continues on the drug, no matter how long and no matter how stable the serum level has been. If lithium is to be withdrawn for any reason, it should be done in stages over 3 or 4 months, as there is a lithium withdrawal syndrome, a manic relapse manifesting at about day 21 after lithium is stopped (Mander & Loudon 1988). Initially, weekly estimations suffice unless lithium is being used in the treatment of mania, when more frequent checks are advisable in view of the likelihood of fluctuating fluid and electrolyte balance. An estimation should be performed 5–7 days after any dosage change. If stable serum levels have been achieved after a month the interval may be increased to 4 weeks, and thereafter estimations should be carried out not less than every 2 months. Thyroid function should be checked every 6 months and a raised thyroid-stimulating hormone (TSH) level on two occasions suggests hypothyroidism. This is not an indication to end lithium treatment. Thyroxine should be added gradually until the TSH level falls to within normal limits. A 24 hour urine volume should be measured, and an ECG should be performed each year.

Side-effects and toxicity (Ghose 1977)

Patients starting on lithium treatment commonly complain of some nausea, looseness of bowels, and thirst. Later they may experience fatigue, muscle weakness, some polyuria and hand tremor. These symptoms often disappear and their reappearance should be taken seriously (see below). During established treatment, tremor, weight gain, polydipsia and polyuria, mild memory impairment, oedema and goitre are common. On investigation leucocytosis is frequent, and hypothyroidism may occur quite suddenly in 10–15% of females above 50 years of age; this is associated with the presence of thyroid antibodies prior to treatment. ECG changes, including T wave inversion and QRS widening, also occur and seem both harmless and reversible when treatment is ended. Lithium tremor exists in two forms, one constant and one episodic, during periods of stress or excitement. The latter can be improved by the addition of small quantities of a β blocker such as propranolol 10–20 mg four times per day.

Concomitant ingestion of alcohol, phenothiazines or tricyclic antidepressants will worsen the tremor. The weight gain may be up to 10 kg, and any attempt to diet should be carefully supervised in case of excessive sodium loss. Increased intake of sweetened soft drinks as a result of polydipsia may be partially responsible. Two-thirds of patients with relatively low serum levels of lithium complain of thirst, which is not due to other drugs. Impending toxicity is heralded by anorexia, vomiting and diarrhoea (which compound the problem by inducing

sodium loss), coarse tremor, ataxia, dysarthria, confusion and sleepiness. These are associated with a serum lithium level of 1.5–2.0 mmol/l. Above 2 mmol/l consciousness is impaired and neurological manifestations, such as fasciculation, nystagmus, hyperreflexia and convulsions, become apparent. Eventually, coma and death supervene when the serum level rises above 4 mmol/l. Brain damage may occur with serum levels over 3 mmol/l. If a patient presents with such symptoms and a lower than expected serum level it may be that the intracellular level is still high, as the serum level precedes the intracellular level in falling after intoxication. Treatment is by saline and osmotic diuresis (not by tubular diuretics), or sometimes dialysis (Goddard et al 1991).

Both the thyroid and renal side-effects are caused by inhibition of adenyl cyclase, in the kidney rendering the tubule insensitive to vasopressin. Some lithium patients develop a quite heroic diuresis of 4–6 litres per day. They require to be identified by screening all patients for polyuria. Initially, this is reversible if lithium is stopped, but a few patients develop permanent polyuria. When identified, careful consideration should be given to the need for continued lithium treatment, once a day dosage, and the minimum plasma level which can be employed (Hetmer et al 1991). The reversibility of the tubular dysfunction can be assessed by withdrawing the patient temporarily from lithium and measuring urine osmolality after synthetic vasopressin (Editorial 1979).

Chronically high serum levels undetected because monitoring is inadequate may dispose to the development of renal damage. This means that if a general practitioner takes over the regular monitoring of lithium treatment from the psychiatric clinic there is a case for an annual return to the latter for review.

A thiazide diuretic can be used to ameliorate polyuria as it shifts the site of sodium resorption, and the daily intake of lithium must be cut accordingly. Amiloride is also of benefit (Battle et al 1985), with less risk of toxicity. Lithium can aggravate established or expose latent Parkinson's disease, again by an effect on adenyl cyclase (Tyrer et al 1980).

Interactions with other drugs

Lithium is relatively safe in combination with most psychotropic agents. Tremor can be a problem (see above). Haloperidol, or perhaps any potent neuroleptic, given in heavy doses to a patient with high serum concentrations of lithium may produce a picture of toxicity, involving severe, treatment-resistant, extrapyramidal syndromes. Unless recognised quickly this may have permanent sequelae. As long as such extremes are avoided or remedied early the combination may be safely used, for instance in the management of manic illnesses.

Any drug affecting renal function will influence lithium balance adversely. Such drugs include diuretics, tetracyclines, non-steroidal anti-inflammatory agents and phenylbutazone. The combination of lithium, a thiazide and digoxin is particularly hazardous, being likely to cause severe digoxin toxicity by producing hypokalaemia.

Indications

Lithium may be used in the treatment of acutely ill manic patients whose overactivity and irritability are manageable without neuroleptics. It is widely used in the prevention of recurrent manic–depressive (bipolar) and more recently recurrent depressive (unipolar) affective disorders (Souza et al 1990). In the bipolar group, trials demonstrate a considerable reduction of morbidity. In practice results are less dramatic (Markar & Mander 1989). For unipolar depressives it is as effective as tricyclic antidepressants. There are benefits for those having a subsequent delivery following puerperal psychosis when started immediately post partum (Stewart et al 1991). Other indications are less clear. Lithium has something to offer in schizoaffective and cyclothymic disorders, and, despite suggestions, little to offer in the management of Huntington's chorea, tardive dyskinesia, alcoholism or aggressive personality disorders. The status of lithium as a drug in the treatment of a depressive episode as opposed to prevention of relapse is uncertain.

It is a matter of clinical judgment as to who should be given lithium treatment chronically. The ill-effects of recurrent illness on an emerging personality in adolescence and the likelihood of relapse are one indication for long-term lithium treatment. Recurrent affective disorders at any age with an interval of less than 2 or 3 years is another indication. There is no certainty that, even after a number of years spent taking lithium, further relapses will not occur if the drug is stopped. If lithium is used chronically after the first illness episode it may be reasonable to withdraw it gradually after 5 years free of relapse. Otherwise, the clinician has to weigh the inconvenience and long-term hazards of lithium treatment — which are few, for patients do not die as a result of lithium prophylaxis, nor is there an equivalent of tardive dyskinesia — against the likelihood of further relapses with their attendant risk of damage to marriages and careers, and of suicide.

Lithium treatment failures

In recurrent illness, lithium may take up to a year to exert its full effect. That apart, failure of lithium prophylaxis may be summed up as: first, failure to take medication; second, failure to take enough, and only then, failure to act. Education improves the patient's attitude to lithium treatment (Peet & Harvey 1991) and compliance. Regular plasma level estimations should ensure compliance and an adequate plasma level. Rapid cyclers, that is, those with more than four mood swings per year, tend to respond only partially to lithium prophylaxis.

A patient who is taking his tablets and with a therapeutic plasma level for long enough who remains unwell or whose mood is unstable may benefit from the addition of an MAOI, a tricyclic antidepressant or a neuroleptic. However, tricyclics and MAOIs do tend a destabilise bipolar manic–depressives and should only be used in brief courses. Methyl folate supplements may enhance prophylaxis for some patients (Godfrey et al 1990).

Anticonvulsants

In the last 40 years there have been occasional reports that anticonvulsants had an antimanic effect. In 1973 Okuma, using carbamazepine, observed acute antimanic — as well as prophylactic — effects. More recently, sodium valproate has also been shown to have similar properties in manic–depressive illness.

Carbamazepine is structurally not dissimilar to imipramine, but has no effect on monoamine reuptake, nor is it a neuroleptic. It is a GABA agonist, and is also effective in inhibiting seizures kindled from repeated stimulation of limbic structures. As well as being an anticonvulsant it has beneficial effects on behavioural disorders associated with epilepsy. Valproate mediates its anticonvulsant effect through indirect effects on GABAergic systems.

Carbamazepine is slightly less effective in the treatment of acute mania but appears to be of equivalent efficacy to lithium in the prophylaxis of relapse in bipolar illness (Luszuat et al 1988). Rapid-cycling bipolar illness, comparatively resistant to lithium, is considered a particular indication for carbamazepine (Psychological Medicine 1982). Unipolar illness is less amenable to anticonvulsant treatment, although it is better than a placebo. In small-scale studies, valproate can be shown to have an antimanic effect and to enhance the effectiveness of lithium (McElroy et al 1989).

Carbamazepine has some advantages over lithium in that weight gain is not a common side-effect and it is a less toxic compound. As it induces its own catabolism the half-life falls with chronic use from 25 to 15 hours. Generally, an effect results from a daily dose of 400–1200 mg, less in the elderly, although serum levels — 12 hours after the last dose — should be below 50 μmol/l. Regular plasma level estimation at 6 month intervals suffices. It is better to start with a small dose and build up the daily intake.

Common initial side-effects include drowsiness, unsteadiness, lassitude, headache, rashes, nausea and vomiting. Up to 15% of patients may develop hyponatraemia, but it is seldom symptomatic. Regular monitoring of serum sodium is not justified. However, where side-effects seem excessive the possibility should be borne in mind (Mucklow 1991). The appearance of a rash should raise the possibility of a haematological disturbance. Although the risk is slight, it is sufficient to require checks more frequently early in treatment. Lithium may enhance the neurological toxicity, although neuroleptics seem quite safe in combination. Valproate is clearly teratogenic, and carbamazepine probably is (Editorial 1991b).

Therapy-resistant depressive illness

Up to 20% of a depressed population will still be unwell 2 years later. Those with psychotic symptoms, recurrent illnesses, and medical disorders, females and disordered personalities are at risk. Covert reasons include poor compliance, hidden endocrinopathies, adverse domestic environments, especially a lack of intimacy and previous sexual abuse. Sometimes the clinician will have failed to fully explore the dosage envelope of both tricyclics and MAOIs, or ECT has been given only once (Scott 1988). Treatment manoeuvres available include combining all physical treatments with cognitive–behaviour therapy. A conventional antidepressant should be given to maximal doses (imipramine at 250 mg/day) and then lithium added. A selective serotonin re-uptake inhibitor could be added, after removal of lithium and reduction in dose of the tricyclic. MAOIs should be tried next with or without lithium and L-tryptophan. Having been withdrawn from all drugs, MAOIs and tricyclics can be used together — phenelzine 15 mg in the morning and amitriptyline 25 mg at night — not tranylcypromine or clomipramine. The dose of each can be doubled or trebled. Triiodothyronine and imipramine has its adherents. Much time must be spent supporting the patient through all this.

SEDATIVE DRUGS

Several classes of sedative drugs have been used in the last century; bromides, paraldehyde, barbiturates, glutethimide, meprobamate and methaquolone are obsolete and sometimes dangerous. To all intents and purposes, the benzodiazepines are the only sedative drugs appropriately in use in clinical psychiatry at the present time.

The benzodiazepines

Chlordiazepoxide was introduced in 1960 and diazepam in 1963. Since then a large number of clinically active benzodiazepine compounds have been synthesised, and it is likely that further generations of benzodiazepines will emerge in the future. Diazepam is the most commonly prescribed of all psychotropic compounds, and it has been estimated that one in 10 adults in the UK regularly consumes a sedative drug. Alprazolam, not prescribable on the National Health Service in the UK, is widely used in the USA to treat panic disorder.

Mechanism of action

The pharmacological actions of the benzodiazepines, like the barbiturates, require the presence of GABA, an inhibitory neutrotransmitter. There are two types of specific receptor site for benzodiazepines in close association with the GABA receptor. There is a possibility of a separate sedative and anxiolytic action based on these two types. Such receptor sites are found in great density in the cerebral cortex, and to a lesser extent in the limbic system and spinal cord. The benzodiazepine receptor is not identical with the GABA receptor, but is in such close relationship that benzodiazepine activity enhances GABA activity when GABA is in low concentrations at receptors. An endogenous ligand for the benzodiazepine receptor is still being sought, after several candidates have been rejected. The position is further complicated by the existence of agonists, antagonists and inverse agonists for the benzodiazepine receptor.

Benzodiazepines enhance the inhibitory action of GABA on its receptors, situated presynaptically on neurones releasing noradrenaline and serotonin among others: some anxiolytic and sedative effects may be thus mediated.

The activity of spinal reflexes and the duration of after-discharge of neurones in the limbic system are also depressed. In addition, benzodiazepines block the cortical arousal which occurs after stimulation of the midbrain reticular activating system. In the EEG, the benzodiazepines cause an increase in fast (i.e. beta) activity and the seizure threshold is raised. This parallels their clinical use as anticonvulsants. With regard to sleep, both REM and stage 4 sleep are suppressed. With continued ingestion of benzodiazepines, REM sleep begins to reappear after a latency of a few days and, if the sedative is then withdrawn, a period of disturbed sleep with a much greater REM sleep content ('REM rebound') ensues. This sequence is indicative of the development of tolerance, and the presence of rebound hyperexcitability parallels cerebral adaptive mechanisms.

All benzodiazepines available for clinical use have sedative, anxiolytic, and anticonvulsant properties.

Absorption, metabolism and excretion

The relative usefulness of various members of the benzodiazepine family clinically depends mainly on their widely varying properties with respect to absorption and duration of activity (see Table 36.4). Some benzodiazepines are absorbed relatively slowly, for example oxazepam which takes about 3 hours to reach its peak plasma concentration following oral administration. Others, such as diazepam, are rapidly absorbed and reach their peak concentration in an hour, while lorazepam and chlordiazepoxide are somewhere in between, reaching their peak concentration at 1–2 hours. The rapid onset of action which can be expected with diazepam may explain its popularity as a drug of abuse. In contrast, given by the intramuscular route diazepam is very poorly absorbed, whereas lorazepam is quickly and easily absorbed.

Another area of major difference between benzodiazepines is in their metabolic fate. Some, for example oxazepam, lorazepam and temazepam, are inactivated in a one-stage metabolism by conjugation

with glucuronic acid. Others, such as diazepam and chlordiazepoxide, are metabolised by hepatic microsomes to an active compound, desmethyldiazepam, which has a half-life of over 60 hours even in a young healthy adult. In the neonate and in the elderly, and also in those with liver damage, this half-life and that of the parent compounds may be considerably increased. The longer the half-life, the more liable the compound is to accumulate when given regularly, especially in those with poor excretory capacity.

As a general principle, drugs which have a short half-life require to be given more often and a swifter onset of effect can be expected. Drugs with a longer half-life will take time to exert their effect, but may be given less often. Therefore, it can be expected that diazepam need only be taken once a day, but preferably at night, to avoid potentially dangerous sedation at the time of peak concentration. On the other hand, for swift onset of action, as in an exacerbation of anxiety or a withdrawal state, a drug such as lorazepam would be preferable.

Tolerance, dependence and withdrawal

As mentioned above, exposure to the benzodiazepines leads to a fairly rapid development of tolerance to the sedative effects, which also include hypnotic effects. On the other hand, there is less tolerance to the anti-anxiety effects and to effects on muscular activity.

Because the earlier benzodiazepines and their metabolites had such a long half-life, withdrawal effects and evidence of physical dependence were rare. Moreover, such reactions were usually not recognised for what they were because they tended to occur 7–10 days after withdrawal. However, the shorter-acting one-step-metabolised compounds do produce a withdrawal syndrome confirming the development of physical dependence.

Table 36.4   Half-lives and metabolites of some benzodiazepines in adults

Compound	Comparative dose (mg)	Half-life (hours)	Active metabolites	Half-life (hours)
Alprazolam	0.5	9–20	None	—
Lorazepam	1.0	8–24	None	—
Oxazepam	15	3–25	None	—
Temazepam	10	3–25	None	—
Triazolam[a]	0.25	1.5–5	Hydroxytriazolam	7
Diazepam[a]	5	14–70	Desmethyldiazepam	30–200
Chlordiazepoxide[a]	25	4–29	Desmethylchlordiazepoxide	28–100
Nitrazepam[a]	2.5	15–30	None	—
Clonazepam[a]	0.25	19–60	None	—

[a] Metabolism by oxidation.

Withdrawal convulsions have been reported more often following the abrupt ending of a course of lorazepam, and in the USA alprazolam. Further evidence of a physical dependence syndrome is provided by the proportion (said to be 15–40%) of all those exposed to benzodiazepines who develop a specific withdrawal syndrome characterised by sensory hypersensitivity, including hyperacusis and tinnitus, false perceptions and agitation or confusion. These symptoms appear to be qualitatively different from re-emerging symptoms of anxiety and may last anything from 3 months to over a year. Dependence may become a problem after as little as 6 weeks of regular use. Withdrawal can generally be carried out without hospital admission although those on high doses, at risk of suicide or in whom previous attempts at withdrawal have failed may need to be admitted.

Personality factors, especially passivity and dependence, predict a poor outcome (Tyrer et al 1983). Abrupt withdrawal should be avoided; it is subjectively highly unpleasant and potentially dangerous. Gradual reduction over a period between 4 and 16 weeks is far better; one rule of thumb is 4 weeks for every year on the drug. Over this time, the daily intake should be reduced in steps of 5 mg for diazepam — equivalent to lorazepam 0.5 mg and temazepam 5 mg — every week until withdrawal symptoms appear, when the interval may have to be increased to allow the patient to come to terms with existence at that dosage. The decrements may have to be smaller towards the end of withdrawal.

Some other drugs may assist the process, including the substitution of longer-acting benzodiazepines, carbamazepine (Schweizer et al 1991) and sedative antidepressants (although an effect on the fit threshold may be anticipated from the latter). It is unrealistic to expect someone whose sole technique for coping with stress was pharmacological to manage withdrawal without something to replace the drug. Education, counselling, anxiety management training, cognitive therapy, self-help groups and family support all have a role to play.

The outcome for a third of patients is quite good; another third may require anti-depressant treatment and a third are left with many problems which often result in resumption of benzodiazepine use (Higgitt et al 1985).

Side-effects and toxicity

Impairment of consciousness as a side-effect would be expected with this group of drugs. Some interference with muscle activity is also reported, and respiratory depression may be caused during a too rapid infusion of diazepam intravenously. It has been reported anecdotally that the benzodiazepines, like alcohol, may increase the expression of aggression and hostility. It is difficult, though, to disentangle specific benzodiazepine effects from non-specific factors associated with the personality and situation of the individual. Menstrual dysfunction and interference with male sexual function are occasionally reported.

A more serious syndrome of toxicity appears with excessive prescription of these compounds in the elderly. A toxic confusional state characterised by clouding of consciousness, ataxia, double incontinence and loss of personal function is frequently seen in old people who are exposed to the longer-acting benzodiazepines in doses which are without risk in the young adult. Iatrogenic poisoning of the elderly by diazepam and nitrazepam is a common experience to any specialist in geriatrics and is a major cause of unnecessary hospitalisation, fractures and domestic breakdown. In 1979, shortly after the introduction of triazolam to Holland, the drug was withdrawn after an outcry in the press over alleged psychotogenic effects. Elsewhere it was difficult to believe a member of a family of drugs so benign in general could be so troublesome. In recent years, it has become apparent that triazolam can indeed induce psychotic experiences in those not otherwise thus disposed — it also causes anterograde amnesia. Finally, because of its short duration of action it shares alcohol's disadvantage as a hypnotic — rebound anxiety and agitation can catch the patient at a low ebb in the early hours of the morning (Oswald 1990, Bixler et al 1991). The product licence for triazolam in the UK was withdrawn in 1991 pending a reassessment.

One of the main appeals of the benzodiazepines is their complete safety in acute overdose. Deaths have been reported following benzodiazepine overdosage, but usually as a result of falls, inhalation of vomit or combination with alcohol. Extremely large amounts can be taken and little more than prolonged sleepiness produced.

Interactions with other drugs

Apart from producing a cumulative sedative effect when combined with other central nervous system depressants, such as alcohol or the neuroleptics, benzodiazepines show few troublesome interactions. The benzodiazepines are not inducers of hepatic enzymatic activity in man and thus do not increase the destruction of other drugs to any appreciable extent. The metabolism of digoxin is decreased. Allopurinol, cimetidine, disulfiram and oestrogen decrease the metabolism of those benzodiazepines which are oxidated.

Indications

The main indication is in the short-term treatment of anxiety. Anxiety occurring in the context of a major psychotic illness is best dealt with by treating the psychosis, though it is possible that smaller quantities of neuroleptics may be required if benzodiazepines are used simultaneously. Chronic anxiety states or characterological anxiety are best treated by other means such as behavioural programmes of varying kinds, and all sedative drugs must be used with caution because of the risks of long-term dependence and misuse (Tyrer 1989). On the other hand, even in such conditions, when the patient has 'earned' his prescription by continuing severe distress, a judgment based on a misplaced sense of moral superiority over the patient must not be allowed to deny him significant relief from what is a very safe type of drug. Unless the syndrome being treated is severe and continuous, irregular use at the lowest possible dose as indicated by the occurrence of symptoms is to be preferred, and the duration of treated should be made clear to the patient in advance.

There is no pharmacological difference between a drug which is sedative by day, and one which is a hypnotic when taken at night. It is quite senseless, therefore, for a patient to be given one compound during the day and a closely related compound at night to induce sleep in the belief that different pharmacological actions are involved. In the short term the benzodiazepines induce sleep very effectively and a decision has to be made whether this action is to be accompanied by daytime sedation, in which case a longer-acting compound may be chosen, or not, in which case a shorter-acting one-step-metabolised drug is appropriate (with attention to morning anxiety). There is little point in using a benzodiazepine in the treatment of insomnia in the context of a functional psychosis since either a neuroleptic or an antidepressant taken in a single dose at night an hour or two before bedtime will act quite effectively.

It must be understood that the hypnotic effect of benzodiazepines is relatively short lived and within a few weeks most users will have become completely habituated. However, as a result of cerebral adaptive changes, such chronic users are in a pharmacological trap, for withdrawal from the hypnotic involves up to 6 weeks of broken sleep and disturbing dreams, a disinclination to suffer which probably led to the original prescription. Compounds such as nitrazepam which continue to affect the patient the next day should not be used, as they cause impaired psychomotor performance which is not apparent to the subject.

The benzodiazepines are frequently used for treating withdrawal states from alcohol and other sedative compounds. In acute withdrawal reactions, a compound which can be expected to exert a rapid effect is to be preferred. It should be noted in this context, and in the context of anticonvulsant activity, that intramuscular diazepam is poorly absorbed and, if diazepam is to be used, slow intravenous injection is preferable.

Chlormethiazole

Chlormethiazole is a sedative drug derived from the thiazole moiety of thiamine, vitamin B_1. It is readily absorbed when taken by mouth, and can be given in an intravenous infusion. It has weak anticonvulsant effects and produces a strong sedative effect. Its half-life is relatively short — 6–8 hours — following fairly rapid absorption. There are no active metabolites and accumulation does not occur with regular use.

Side-effects include tingling of the nose, conjunctival irritation and gastrointestinal upsets. The drug potentiates phenothiazines and butyrophenones, and has an additive effect with barbiturates and alcohol which may be lethal.

Chlormethiazole infusions are sometimes used in status epilepticus and in toxaemia of pregnancy. In psychiatry it is frequently used as a hypnotic in the elderly, and in the management of senile confusion. It has enjoyed some popularity as a cover for alcohol withdrawal, tempered in recent years by reports of deaths occurring when the drug is taken chronically in combination with alcohol. If chlormethiazole is to be used in the management of alcohol withdrawal, this should be on an in-patient basis only and the patient should be off all chlormethiazole by the seventh day of withdrawal. It is convenient to start the withdrawing patient on a dose sufficient to suppress all manifestations of withdrawal (commonly 2–4 g in 24 hours) and then reduce the dose by half every 24 hours.

Propranolol

In small doses (20–80 mg/day), propranolol has a role in the treatment of anxiety states dominated by autonomic symptoms such as tachycardia, tachypnoea, flushing and sweating. It may also afford relief to those with severe performance anxiety, especially when physical symptoms are the main manifestations (Editorial 1985). Certain lithium-induced tremors (see above) respond to small doses of propranolol.

Propranolol may also be combined with other anxiolytic drugs, especially in the treatment of chronic anxiety, and it has been used with success in alcohol and benzodiazepine withdrawal. Neuroleptic-induced akathisia sometimes responds to propranolol in small doses (Lipinski et al 1983). For 20 years reports have appeared of the effectiveness of large (2 g/day) doses of propranolol in the treatment of schizophrenia and, recently, there have been reports that propranolol added to neuroleptic treatment improves the response of treatment-resistant schizophrenia. This effect may be mediated by interference with the degradation of the neuroleptic in the liver, thus raising its plasma level (cf. neuroleptics in tricyclic treatment). The availability of *d*-propranolol, which is not a β blocker, has allowed examination of possible additional properties which might be antipsychotic. One recent study (Manchanda & Hirsh 1986) suggests that while propranolol is less effective than conventional neuroleptics in schizophrenia it is significantly better than placebo.

Buspirone

This drug is unrelated to any existing psychotropic agent and does not exhibit any cross-tolerance with benzodiazepines, barbiturates or alcohol. It has no effect on benzodiazepine receptors. Its action appears to be mediated through 5-HT_{1A} receptors, where it is a partial agonist, and D_2 receptors, to which it weakly binds. It is not sedative, nor is it a muscle relaxant. There is no withdrawal syndrome. In anxiety disorder the starting daily dosage is 5 mg t.i.d. rising to 10 mg t.i.d. with a maximum per day of 60 mg. It is not effective on a 'p.r.n.' basis. Mild agitation is sometimes reported initially. Onset of action is gradual, over 3 or 4 weeks. Side-effects included dizziness, nausea, headache and nervousness. Concomitant prescription of MAOIs is not advised. The drug does not substitute for benzodiazepines, which must be tailed off gradually (as described above) as buspirone is introduced. It is not lethal in overdose.

WITHDRAWAL OF OPIATES FROM DEPENDENT PATIENTS

Physical dependence on a drug involves a state of adaptation to acquired tolerance of that drug. Consequently, if the drug is suddenly withdrawn or antagonised there is a period of rebound hyperactivity of previously suppressed functions while the organism adjusts to this unfamiliar drug-free state, for example rebound REM sleep after hypnotics, fits after sedatives, 'cold turkey' after opiates. The object of drug substitution is to allow gradual withdrawal of a substituted longer-acting compound to mask this rebound hyperactivity and counteract its subjectively unpleasant consequences. In opiate withdrawal, there is a rebound hyperactivity of the catecholaminergic and serotonergic system, which is directly or indirectly responsible for most of the subjectively unpleasant experiences of withdrawal.

Methadone provides an effective means of covering withdrawal from opiates but it has several disadvantages. It is itself a drug of dependence which other addicts will gladly buy, and it is difficult to be sure one is not giving the drug user more than he needs to prevent withdrawal symptoms, or to be sure that while professing a wish to withdraw from opiates he is not merely seeking to cover a temporary hiatus in his normal supply of heroin.

Clonidine, an α agonist drug, can modify opiate withdrawal symptoms to a clinically useful extent at a dose of 0.3–1.2 mg/day (Gold et al 1978). Mild dizziness from hypotension is a common side-effect, and insomnia can be treated with an occasional dose of a benzodiazepine. By the fourth day of treatment clonidine can be tailed off. The efficacy of this treatment is shown by the failure of parenteral naloxone, a specific opiate antagonist which will immediately cause a severe withdrawal reaction in someone who is dependent on opiates, to produce such a reaction. This rapid control of rebound hyperexcitability allows for early transition to an opiate antagonist, given on an out-patient basis, which will block entirely the euphoriant and other additive effects of opiate drugs used illicitly.

Naloxone itself has a very short duration of action but its longer-acting analogue naltrexone is used for this purpose. Using clonidine and naltrexone together appears to be very effective and allows for a very short in-patient stay (Brewer et al 1988).

DRUGS USED IN THE MANAGEMENT OF ALCOHOL PROBLEMS

The role of various cerebral monoaminergic systems in prolonging problem drinking is being clarified. As with opiate and cocaine dependence, it is apparent that there is a prolonged abstinence syndrome following alcohol withdrawal, due to the length of time various disordered cerebral mechanisms take to return to normal function. Various classes of compounds, including tiapride (Shaw et al 1987), specific serotoninergic re-uptake inhibitors, dopaminergic blockers and GABAergic drugs (Lhuintre 1990) have shown promise in decreasing the relapse rate, perhaps by suppressing the chronic abstinence syndrome (Meyer 1989). As yet these treatments cannot be generally recommended.

However, one splint to the resolve of a newly abstinent problem drinker has been available for many years, and not enough use may be made of it (Chick 1989). Disulfiram in a dose of 300–600 mg/day is an irreversible inhibitor of acetaldehyde dehydrogenase — for up to 14 days. Acetaldehyde is an intermediate step in the destruction of alcohol, and treatment with disulfiram causes a five- to ten-fold rise in acetaldehyde if alcohol is consumed (metronidazole and sulfonylurea hypoglycaemics have the same effect). A marked flushing of face and body, a throbbing headache, nausea, vomiting, sweating, dizziness and malaise are experienced. This experience may last between 30 minutes and 4 hours. Side-effects in the absence of alcohol include skin disorders, sexual dysfunction, a metallic taste and hepatotoxicity. The drug facilitates the accumulation of nickel and lead. It is teratogenic. All alcoholic vehicles may provoke a reaction, including lotions and medicinal syrups. There is no case for provoking a 'test' reaction in a patient starting on the drug. Disulfiram use in the treatment of alcohol problems has to be integrated with other approaches.

DRUG THERAPY AND THE ELDERLY

Although the elderly are as variable in their reactions to drugs as younger members of the population, they tend to be more susceptible to the toxic effect of psychotropic drugs. Because their social circumstances are often unfavourable, this frequently results in unnecessary hospital admission, which imperils their place in the community. As a large proportion of psychiatric practice is concerned with the elderly it is important to be aware of the following factors affecting their response to drugs.

The reduced cardiac output and cardiac reserve of the elderly leads to impaired perfusion of the gut, which in turn will tend to hamper the absorption of orally administered drugs. The number of absorbing cells in gut epithelium and the surface area available for absorption are both decreased and an alteration in gastric pH as a result of decreased acid production may reduce absorption still further. The composition of the blood changes because the elderly patient has less body water and a lower plasma albumen. Many psychotropic drugs are strongly protein bound, and a lower plasma albumen leads to a reduced number of binding sites and hence an increased ratio of free to bound drug. This will effect benzodiazepines, tricyclics and phenothiazines.

The ageing person effectively contains a greater proportion of lipid in both body and brain and many psychotropic drugs are strongly lipophilic. Administration of these drugs will therefore have less initial effect as they are drawn into lipid-rich sites but, once given, their duration of action will be considerably enhanced.

The central nervous system suffers loss of neurones with ageing and in communication language there is an increase of 'noise'. The ageing brain is thus vulnerable to insults which would have been insignificant a few decades previously. This applies particularly to hypoxia. It is likely that the amount of brain tissue affected by psychotropic agents is also decreased, thus increasing local concentrations.

Most psychotropic agents are inactivated in the liver, the metabolic capacity of which is also decreased with age. Lipophilic drugs are poorly excreted by the kidney and so have to be transformed by conjugation with glucuronide, the larger part of which takes place in the liver.

Many psychotropic agents have unwanted side-effects involving the cardiovascular system. The homeostatic ability of the elderly is diminished and they are often unable to withstand hypotensive and dysrhythmic side-effects.

Inappropriate prescription of psychotropic agents is a major cause of iatrogenic disorder in the elderly. Mention has already been made of the vulnerability of the elderly to long-acting benzodiazepines. Some elderly patients will be extremely sensitive to the cardiovascular side-effects of tricyclic antidepressants and neuroleptics; others will be surprisingly tolerant.

Because of reduced creatinine clearance, the daily requirement for lithium carbonate is unlikely to be over 600 mg in the over 70s and may be as low as 125 mg. The propensity of psychotropics to produce confusion must be borne in mind, as must the need for as simple a schedule of administration as possible to minimise misunderstandings. It should become a matter of habit for any person supervising drug treatment in the elderly to reassess the dosage of the agent being used at frequent intervals as it is commonly possible to achieve reductions. This is of special relevance with neuroleptics, especially of the depot variety, and sedative drugs. Pseudoparkinsonism can be both insidious and debilitating. Because many elderly patients suffer from a multiplicity of physical pathologies, interactions with other compounds may occur.

Many demented patients display signs of agitation, paranoid ideation, frequent aggressive behaviours and a reversal of day and night activity. Such behaviours make home care a difficult task and are not easy to deal with even in a day unit or long-stay ward. The temptation to sedate is therefore considerable, but it should not be forgotten that an over-sedated patient may be even more of a problem for the nurse or carer. It is important to gain experience with as few representatives of each type of drug as possible so that by familiarity the potential problems with each can be recognised swiftly.

In the management of behavioural disorder a hierarchy of drugs should be adopted, with mild short-acting sedatives at one end and the potent neuroleptics at the other. A patient should only move towards the more potent and more dangerous drugs after full exploration of the dosage range of the mildest compound. Such a hierarchy might extend from chlormethiazole to oxazepam to promazine to thioridazine to trifluoperazine to droperidol. Depressive reactions may develop semi-covertly, responding to antidepressant medication. The reported benefits of trazodone in senile agitation may derive from this. It cannot be emphasised enough that it is important to reassess the need for any such drug frequently and to keep the dosage as low as is consistent with the desired action. Dosage may be tailored to exacerbations occurring at a particular time of day. Extrapyramidal side-effects must be recognised quickly, otherwise severe semi-irreversible extrapyramidal syndromes may result. Although they may seem obvious choices, D_2-selective blockers have yet to prove their usefulness in this area. Depot neuroleptics are particularly hazardous in this respect. It may be quite adequate for many oral neuroleptics to be given every second or third day. For a more detailed discussion see Crome & Roy (1984).

Drugs are still being promoted with claims that they enhance cerebral metabolism and increase cerebral blood flow by vasodilatation. On the basis of the central deficit in cholinergic transmission in Alzheimer's disease, various precursors, anticholinesterases and muscarinic antagonists have been tried out (Whalley 1989). A recent study of tetrahydroaminoacridine (tacrine), a central cholinesterase inhibitor, suggests some effect on Alzheimer's disease, but at the expense of considerable toxicity (Eagger et al 1991).

DRUG TREATMENT IN THE MENTALLY HANDICAPPED

Four factors affect the use of drug treatments in the mentally handicapped. First, one-third will suffer from cerebral dysrhythmia and anticonvulsants will be required for the resulting behavioural disturbance. Second, the drugs will be acting on immature brains, and may give rise to paradoxical (e.g. sedatives causing overactivity) or idiosyncratic (e.g. neuroleptics in minute doses causing severe dystonias) effects. Third, many handicapped patients suffer from the same mental illnesses as are treated in general psychiatric units. Fourth, communication about side-effects will be impaired.

The symptom complexes specific for neuroleptic treatment are rare in the handicap field and these drugs are more usually employed as non-specific 'behaviour control agents'. This is not ideal, as the patients suffer the usual long- and short-term side effects. Other less toxic alternatives may not be available, however, as the benzodiazepines are not benign in their effect on the handicapped. Because of family dynamics, oral neuroleptics may be given parsimoniously or excessively and depot preparations have the advantage of allowing the drug to be given as the clinician wishes, in as small a dose as is consistent with the desired effect. Environmental manipulation may be more potent than any drug, however.

The handicapped suffer much affective disorder, both episodic and phasic, and the tricyclics and lithium are often highly effective. Management of a drug as toxic as lithium requires special care but may improve the patient's lot considerably and allow the caring relative much relief.

Anticonvulsants need their dose to be carefully adjusted and the patient should be on as small a dose as possible. Low-grade toxicity from anticonvulsants often mimics behaviour disorder, and regular assessment of anticonvulsant dosage by plasma level estimation is important, partly to avoid unnecessary prescription of neuroleptics (Collacott et al 1989).

DRUG TREATMENT IN PREGNANCY AND THE PUERPERIUM (Loudon 1992)

Most common psychotropic drugs have not been shown to have a teratogenic effect, despite previous concern about benzodiazepines and tricyclics. Lithium use in the first 3 months of pregnancy is, however, associated with congenital malformation of the atrioventricular valves and septa, though the increased risk is not great enough to justify termination of pregnancy after inadvertent exposure. Kallen & Tandberg (1983) found that nine out of 59 infants were malformed or died in the neonatal period when their mothers had taken lithium during pregnancy, compared to one out of 38 children born to manic–depressives who had taken other drugs. Though rare, neonates may show side-effects commonly associated with the psychotropic drug taken during pregnancy by their mothers, including extrapyramidal syndromes, the 'floppy infant' syndrome from benzodiazepines, cardiovascular dysfunction and withdrawal phenomena from tricyclics, hypothyroidism from lithium, over-sedation and signs of opiate withdrawal.

Many psychotropic drugs are found in breast milk in small but detectable quantities. Although the total daily dose per kilogram of body weight for the suckling child may be well below the conventional therapeutic dose, because of immature hepatic function and both reduced body lipids and binding sites the drug effect may be appreciable. The pressures on such a mother — in need of treatment but determined to do the best for her child and guilty that her own needs may prejudice her baby's welfare — are considerable. Rather than make a rigid distinction between breast-feeding and drug treatment it may be wiser to give the drug in divided doses and monitor the child's well-being carefully, in collaboration with the health visitor. The exceptions to this rule are the benzodiazepines and lithium, both of which enter breast milk in quantity. Treatment with lithium is a contraindication to continued breast-feeding. A healthy baby may tolerate its mother taking diazepam up to 20 mg/day, but a sick or premature child will not. Oxazepam in intermittent doses is to be preferred (Kanto 1982).

DRUG TREATMENT IN CHILDREN

Because children are continuously developing, firm rules for drug treatment are not possible. Liquid preparations tend to be absorbed faster and may be more palatable for the younger child. However, faster absorption can lead to wider fluctuations in the plasma level and a more uncertain therapeutic effect. Suspensions of drugs, such as phenytoin, need vigorous shaking at each administration as the drug tends to settle to the bottom of the container; chronic use of sugar-based preparations promotes dental decay. In the convulsing child, rectal administration of a diazepam solution by a syringe and soft plastic tube is practical for parental

as well as professional use. (Lorazepam is probably better for intramuscular administration.) Because of more efficient hepatic metabolism, half-lives of drugs are shortened in older children. If wide fluctuations in plasma levels are to be avoided, more frequent administration is required. Where an attempt is being made to match dosage to size of child, surface area is to be preferred as the criterion of size, as it relates most closely to the volume of distribution. There is an implication that the dose may thus vary greatly for children of the same age.

For certain drugs, especially the anticonvulsants, plasma ranges for maximum effectiveness are established; appropriate fine tuning of dosage can improve control and reduce the need for polypharmacy. The possibility of paradoxical effects of drugs (e.g. amphetamine) in children which are in common use in adults must be borne in mind. The role of psychotropic medication in the treatment of psychiatric disorders in children is so limited that there is little excuse for experimentation with new compounds. It is better to be familiar with possible side-effects so that their unforeseen or unrecognised occurrence does not lead to non-compliance. The prescribing doctor must realise that drug treatment in children touches on sensitive areas in the relationship between child and parent. They must not be used for trivial or self-limiting disturbances, nor as a sop to parents. The doctor must be aware of the placebo effect for himself as well as the family; if he is to use a drug in a particular situation, he must possess evidence of its effectiveness. There is no room for eccentric practice in this area (Black 1991). This implies that accurate assessment is a necessary precondition for all prescribing. The variation in diagnosis and prescription of stimulants for hyperactivity in different countries serves as a warning against loose practice in this respect. As in the rest of psychiatry, drug treatment on its own is of little value and rarely curative. Support, behaviour modification and counselling are crucial.

REFERENCES

Abbott R J, Loizon L A 1986 Neuroleptic malignant syndrome. British Journal of Psychiatry 148: 47–51

Annotation 1985 Problems when withdrawing antidepressives. Drugs and Therapeutics Bulletin 24: 29–31

Avissar 1988 Lithium inhibits adrenergic and cholinergic increases in GTP binding in rat cortex. Nature 331: 440–452

Ayd F 1980 Parenteral droperidol for acutely disturbed behaviour. International Drug Therapy Newsletter 15: 3

Barnes T R E, Bamber R W K, Watson J P 1979 Psychotropic drugs and sexual behaviour. British Journal of Hospital Medicine 21: 594–600

Barnes T R E 1990 Tardive dyskinesia: can it be prevented? In: Hawton K, Cowen P (eds) Dilemmas and difficulties in the management of psychiatric patients. Oxford University Press, Oxford

Battle D C, von Riotte A, Gavira M, Grupp M 1985 Amelioration of polyuria by amiloride in patients receiving long term lithium therapy. New England Journal of Medicine 312: 408–414

Bixler E O, Kales A, Manfred R L et al 1991 Next day memory impairment with triazolam use. Lancet 337: 827–831

Black D 1991 Psychotropic drugs for problem children. British Medical Journal 302: 190–191

Blackwell B 1985 Book review. Psychological Medicine 15: 695

Blackwell B 1991 MAOI interactions with other drugs. Journal of Clinical Neuropharmacology 11: 55–59

Brewer C, Rezae H, Bailey C 1988 Opioid withdrawal and naltrexone induction. British Journal of Psychiatry 153: 340–343

Caldwell A E 1978 History of psychopharmacology. In: Clark W G, Del Giudice J (eds) Principles of psychopharmacology, 2nd edn. Academic Press, New York

Chick J 1990 Alcohol dependence: what treatment works? In: Hawton K, Cowlen P (eds) Dilemmas and difficulties in the management of psychiatric patients. Oxford University Press, Oxford

Collacott R A, Dignon A, Hauck A, Ward J W 1989 Clinical and therapeutic monitoring of epilepsy in a mental handicap unit. British Journal of Psychiatry 155: 522–525

Committee on Safety of Medicines 1990 Cardiotoxic effects of pimozide. Current Problems 29

Coppen A, Swade C, Wood L 1980 Lithium restores abnormal platelets 5-HT transport in patients with affective disorders. British Journal of Psychiatry 136: 235

Coppen A, Abou Saleh P, Millin P, Bailey J, Wood K 1983 Decreasing lithium dosage reduces morbidity and side effects during prophylaxis. Journal of Affective Disorders 5: 353–362

Crome P 1982 Anti-depressant overdosage. Drugs 23: 431–461

Crome P, Roy D H 1984 Drug treatment in the elderly. In: Gaind R N (ed) Current themes in psychiatry. Spectrum New York

CSM update 1985 Adverse reactions to anti-depressants. British Medical Journal 291: 1638

de Montigny C, Cournoyer G, Morisette R, Langlois R, Caille G 1983 Lithium carbonate and tricyclic antidepressants in resistant unipolar illness. Archives of General Psychiatry 40: 1327–1334

Eagger S A, Levy R Sahakian B J 1991 Tacrine in Alzheimers disease. Lancet 337: 989–992

Editorial 1979 Lithium and the kidney — grounds for cautious optimism. Lancet ii: 1056–1057

Editorial 1985 Betablockers in situational anxiety. Lancet ii: 193

Editorial 1991a Dexflenfluramine. Lancet 337: 1315–1316

Editorial 1991b Teratogenesis with carbamazepine. Lancet 337: 1316–1317

Emrich H M, Dose M, von Zerssen D 1985 The use of sodium valproate, carbamazepine and oxcarbazepine in patients with affective disorders. Journal of Affective Disorders 8: 243–250

Fibiger H C, Lloyd K G 1984 Neurobiological substrates of tardive dyskinesia; the GABA hypothesis. Trends in Neurological Sciences, Dec: 462–464

Galdi J, Hirsch S R 1983 The causality of depression in schizophrenia. British Journal of Psychiatry 142: 621–625

Ghose K 1977 Lithium salts — therapeutic and unwanted effects. British Journal of Hospital Medicine 18: 578–583

Glen A I M, Johnson A C, Shepherd M 1981 Continuation therapy with lithium and amitriptyline in unipolar depressive illness — a controlled clinical trial. Psychological Medicine 11: 409–416

Goddard B, Bloom S R, Frackowiak R S J, Pusey C D, McDermott J, Liddle P F 1991 Lithium intoxication. British Medical Journal 302: 1267–1269

Godfrey P S A, Toone B K, Carney M W P et al 1990 Enhancement of recovery from psychiatric illness by methylfolate. Lancet 336: 392–395

Gold M S, Redmonde D E, Kleber H D 1978 Clonidine in opiate withdrawal. Lancet i: 929–930

Goodall E, Ostoby C, Richards R, Watkinson G, Brown D, Silverstone T 1988 A clinical trial of the efficacy and acceptability of d-fenfluramine in the treatment of neuroleptic induced obesity. British Journal of Psychiatry 158: 208–213

Higgitt A C, Lader M, Fonagy P 1985 Clinical management of benzodiazepine dependence. British Medical Journal 291: 688–690

Hetmer O, Juul Povlsen U, Ladefoged J, Bolwig T G 1991 Lithium: long term effects on the kidney. British Journal of Psychiatry 158: 53–58

Hirsch S 1982 Depression 'revealed' in schizophrenia. British Journal of Psychiatry 140: 421–423

Johnson D 1978 The prevalence and treatment of drug induced extrapyramidal symptoms. British Journal of Psychiatry 132: 27–30

Johnstone E C, Crow T J, Ferrier N et al 1983 Adverse effects of anticholinergic medication on positive schizophrenic symptoms. Psychological Medicine 13: 513–527

Lusznat R M, Murphy D P, Nimn C M H 1988 Carbamazepine vs lithium in the treatment and prophylaxis of mania. British Journal of Psychiatry 153: 198–204

Kallen B, Tandberg A 1983 Lithium and pregnancy — a cohort study on manic depressive women. Acta Psychiatrica Scandinavica 68: 134–139

Kanto J H 1982 Use of benzodiazepines during pregnancy, labour and lactation with particular reference to pharmacokinetic considerations. Drugs 23: 354

Kramer M S, Vogel W H, DiJohnson C et al 1989 Antidepressants in "depressed" schizophrenic patients. Archives of General Psychiatry 46: 922–929

Lhuintre J P, Moore N, Trang et al 1990 Acamprosate appears to decrease alcohol intake in weaned alcoholics. Alcohol and Alcoholism 25: 613–622

Lipinski J F, Zubenko G S, Barreira P, Cohen B M 1983 Propranolol in the treatment of neuroleptic induced akathisia. Lancet ii: 685–686

Loudon J B 1992 Psychotropic drugs in pregnancy. Current Obstetrics and Gynaecology 2: ii

McElroy S L, Doch Jr P E, Pope H G, Hudson J I 1988 Journal of Cinical Psychiatry 50(suppl): 23–29

Manchanda R, Hirsch S R 1986 Does propranolol have an anti-psychotic effect? A placebo controlled study in acute schizophrenia. British Journal of Psychiatry 148: 701–707

Mander A, Loudon J B 1988 Rapid recurrence of mania following abrupt discontinuation of lithium. Lancet ii: 15–17

Markar H R, Mander A J 1989 Efficacy of lithium prophylaxis in clinical practice. British Journal of Psychiatry 155: 496–500

Marks I M, Stern R S, Mawson D, Cobb J, MacDonald K 1980 Clomipramine and exposure of obsessive compulsive rituals. British Journal of Psychiatry 136: 1–25

Marsden C D, Jenner P 1980 The pathophysiology of extrapyramidal side effects of neuroleptic drugs. Psychological Medicine 10: 55–72

Meyer R E 1989 Prospects for a rational pharmacotherapy of alcoholism. Journal of Clinical Psychiatry 50: 403–412

Mucklow J 1991 Carbamazepine and hyponatraemia. Prescribers Journal 31: 61–64

Nutt D, Glue P 1989 Monoamine oxidase inhibitors: rehabilitation from recent research. British Journal of Psychiatry 154: 287–291

Peet M, Harvey N S 1991 Lithium maintenance — a standard education programme for patients. British Journal of Psychiatry 158: 197–204

Psychological Medicine 1982 Use of the anticonvulsant carbamazepine in primary and secondary affective illness. Psychological Medicine 12: 701–704

Rifkin A, Doddi S, Karajgi B, Borenstein M, Wackspress 1991 Dosage of haloperidol for schizophrenia. Archives of General Psychiatry 48: 166–170

Robertson M M, Trimble M R 1982 Major tranqillisers used as anti-depressants. Journal of Affective Disorders 4: 173–193

Rogers D 1985 The motor disorders of severe psychiatric illness: a conflict of paradigms. British Journal of Psychiatry 147: 221–232

Roseburn P, Stewart T 1989 A prospective analysis of twenty four episodes of neuroleptic malignant syndrome. American Journal of Psychiatry 146: 717–725

Schwizer E, Richets K, Case W G, Greenblatt D J 1991 Archives of General Psychiatry 48: 448–452

Scott J 1988 Chronic depression. British Journal of Psychiatry 153: 287–297

Shepherd M 1975 The evaluation of treatment in psychiatry. In: Sainsbury P, Kreitman K (eds) Methods of psychiatric research, 2nd edn. Oxford Medical Publications, Oxford

Shepherd M 1980 Psychotropic drugs and taxomic systems. Psychological Medicine 10: 25–33

Simpson G M, Pi E H, Swannell J J 1982 Management of tardive dyskinesia. Drugs 23: 381–383

Souza F G M, Mander A J, Goodwin G M 1990 The efficacy of lithium in prophylaxis of unipolar depression. British Journal of Psychiatry 157: 718–722

Stewart D E, Klonpeahouwer J L, Kendell R E, van Hulst

A M 1991 Prophylactic lithium in puerperal psychosis. The experience of three centres. British Journal of Psychiatry 158: 393–397

Thomson J, Rankin H, Ashcroft G W, Yates C M, McQueen J K, Cummings S W 1982 The treatment of depression in general practice: a comparison of L-tryptophan amitriptyline, and a combination of L-tryptophan and amitriptyline with placebo. Psychological Medicine 12: 741–751

Tyrer P 1989 Risks of dependence on benzodiazepine drugs — the importance of patient selection. British Medical Journal 298: 102–104

Tyrer P, Marsden C 1985 New anti-depressant drugs: is there anything new they tell us about depression? Trends in Neurological Sciences, Oct: 427–431

Tyrer P, Alexander M S, Rogan A, Lee I 1980 An extrapyramidal syndrome after lithium therapy. British Journal of Psychiatry 136: 191–194

Tyrer P, Owen R, Dawling S 1983 Gradual withdrawal of diazepam after long-term therapy. Lancet i: 1402–1406

Waldmaer P C 1990 Mechanisms of action of lithium in affective disorders; a status report. Pharmacology and Toxicology 66 (suppl S): 121–132

Walinder J, Skott A, Carlsson A, Aagy A, Ross B E 1976 Potentiation of the antidepressant action of clomipramine by tryptophan. Archives of General Psychiatry 33: 1384–1389

Whalley L J 1989 Drug treatments of dementia. British Journal of Psychiatry 155: 595–611

Whitford G M 1978 Acetylator phenotype in relation to MAOI anti-depressant drug therapy. International Pharmacopsychiatry 13: 126–127

Wistedt B, Wiles D, Kolakowska T 1981 Slow decline of plasma drug and prolactin levels after discontinuation of chronic treatment with depot neuroleptics. Lancet i: 1163

Wurtman R J 1984 Behavioural effect of nutrients. Lancet i: 1145–1147

37. ECT and other physical therapies

C. P. L. Freeman

ELECTROCONVULSIVE THERAPY (ECT)

Introduction

Since the last edition of this textbook, both the American Psychiatric Association (1989) and the Royal College of Psychiatrists (1990) have published guidelines on the use of ECT. Both documents set out clearly what can be regarded as good practice for ECT though there are important differences between them. It is now over 10 years since the original Pippard & Ellam (1981) report, and Pippard has recently presented (1991) a follow-up report. This shows that although anaesthetic and nursing practice have improved and ECT suites and machines are now of a higher standard, psychiatric practice has really not changed. It seems that although psychiatrists continue to prescribe ECT they take little interest in its conduct. It is as if they were to write tricyclic antidepressant on the drug Kardex and then leave the type of drug, route of administration and so on for someone else to decide upon. With the above guidelines, the information is readily available for psychiatrists. The question has to be asked: are psychiatrists fit to give ECT?

History

As early as 1785 an account was published by Dr W. Oliver describing the results of administering camphor in a case of melancholia. The camphor was given orally and induced an epileptic seizure which relieved the symptoms. The patient relapsed some weeks later but, when given a second camphor-induced seizure, responded well. This was probably the first recorded case of seizure therapy for depression. Throughout the 19th century there was some interest in camphor-induced fits for a variety of conditions, but it was not until the early 1930s that a more reliable way of inducing epileptic seizures was

found. Laszlo Meduna commented on the apparent biological antagonism between schizophrenia and epilepsy. He noted that the two conditions rarely occurred together and that, if they did, the epileptic fits appeared to have an ameliorating effect on the course of the schizophrenia. Meduna, a Hungarian psychiatrist, first used the traditional 25% camphor in olive oil but then introduced Metrazol (Cardiazol) convulsion as a treatment for schizophrenia. Metrazol is a synthetic soluble derivative of camphor which when given intravenously produces epileptic fits. Also in the 1930s two Italians, Cerletti and Bini, were working on inducing epileptic fits in dogs by the passage of a brief electrical stimulus. They were attempting to produce sclerosis in Ammon's horn and then to see if it was the cause of temporal lobe epilepsy. Cerletti was able to establish that there was a large difference between a convulsant and a lethal dose of electricity. He therefore wondered whether his technique could be safely applied to humans and might provide a more reliable way of inducing fits than Metrazol injections. Cerletti and Bini induced the first electroconvulsion in man in 1938, in a schizophrenic patient, using a stimulus of 110 V for half a second. Electricity proved to be a safe, reliable and simple way of producing fits.

ECT was given in the 1940s and 1950s without anaesthetic, so-called unmodified or straight ECT. However, the development of drugs such as gallamine and suxamethonium, capable of briefly paralysing muscles, and of short-acting anaesthetic agents such as thiopentone and methohexitone, led to the introduction of modified ECT. This resulted in the virtual elimination of one of the main side-effects of early treatment, bony fractures, particularly spinal fractures, caused by the massive muscle spasms that occurred at the time of seizure.

Since 1938 a number of other methods of inducing seizures have been proposed, such as photoconvulsion and the inhalation of the convulsant ether flurothyl; neither of these treatments are as reliable or safe as ECT. More recently there has been the introduction of unilateral ECT (U/ECT), which markedly reduces the side-effects of the treatment.

We now know that Meduna's observations about epilepsy and schizophrenia were wrong and it would appear that ECT was introduced as a treatment for the wrong illness and for the wrong reasons. Even so it has proved to be an enduring treatment and it is estimated that some 200 000 individual applications are performed in the UK each year (Pippard & Ellam 1981). The number of ECT treatments fell during the early 1980s but have now levelled out. Pippard's most recent report (1991) described 12-fold differences in rates of ECT per 100 000 of the population between adjacent regions in south-east England.

Developments in recent years include the introduction of constant-current brief-pulse ECT machines, attempts to monitor fitting more accurately with electroencephalograms (EEGs) and a growing evidence of definite differences between bilateral and unilateral treatment (Fig. 37.1).

Evidence for the efficacy of ECT in various disorders

Depressive illness

There is a overwhelming evidence that ECT is an effective treatment for severe depressive illness, particularly psychotic depressions for which it is the most effective and rapidly acting treatment available. In the 1960s there were several large studies which compared ECT with different antidepressant drugs and with placebo tablets. These studies were double blind as far as the drug treatments were concerned but not for the comparison between ECT and drug. Weschler et al (1965) reviewed 153 studies on a total of nearly 6000 patients where drugs and ECT had been compared. Percentage figures for overall improvement with different treatments were as follows: ECT 72%; tricyclics 65%; monoamine oxidase inhibitors 50%; and placebo tablets 23%. Two large multicentre trials were published in the mid-1960s. In the USA Greenblatt et al (1964) reported a trial on depressed patients admitted to three state hospitals in Greater Boston. Assessment was made at the end of 8 weeks and ECT was significantly more effective than all other treatments. In the UK the Medical Research Council trial (Medical Research Council Clinical Psychiatry Committee 1965) of the treatment of depressive illness compared ECT with imipramine,

phenelzine and placebo. Percentages of patients with no or only slight symptoms were as follows: ECT 71%, imipramine 52%; phenelzine 30%; and placebo 39%. An interesting finding in this study was the sex difference between treatments. ECT was clearly more effective than all drug treatments in women, but in men ECT and imipramine were equally effective and both superior to phenelzine and placebo. When the patients were followed up for a further 6 months it was found that about half the imipramine non-responders recovered completely when given a course of ECT.

There have been six such studies in the last 15 years, all carried out in the UK. The results are summarised in Table 37.1. Five of these studies showed a clearly positive result in favour of real ECT, thus refuting the argument that ECT works because it is a powerful placebo. The one study that showed no difference was on a small number of patients and a unilateral brief pulse stimulus was used.

What is also clear from these studies is that improvement does occur with "sham" or simulated ECT, at least in the short term. Unfortunately, none of the studies have included a rigorously controlled follow-up period and subjects have gone on to have further ECT and/or antidepressant drugs so that comparisons of the relative efficacy of real versus sham ECT several weeks after the end of treatment cannot be drawn.

The study by Brill et al (1959) is often quoted as evidence that repeated induction of unconsciousness is as effective as ECT. What is less often quoted is that only 16 of the 97 subjects in that trial were depressed, the rest being schizophrenic or schizoaffective, and most were chronically ill.

There is no evidence of a synergistic effect between ECT and tricyclic antidepressants in the treatment of depressive illness. Studies which have compared ECT plus placebo drugs with ECT plus imipramine 150 mg daily show no difference in outcome, but do show that the combination of ECT and imipramine produces fewer relapses at 6 month follow-up.

Predictors of response to ECT in depression. Although a number of trials were carried out in the 1960s looking for clinical features which might be associated with a good response to ECT, it is not possible to say with any certainty that there are particular symptoms that predict good response and others that predict poor response. As a general rule, the more symptoms of classical 'endogenous' depression the depressed patient has, the more likely he is to respond (Table 37.2); so that a cluster of symptoms such as severe depression, diurnal variation

1933 Insulin coma *Sakel* Vienna

1940s Deep insulin therapy (DIT) clinics in all mental hospitals

1956 *Boardman* Controlled trial shows chlorpromazine superior

1957 *Ackner* publishes first controlled trial showing insulin to be no more effective than barbiturate anaesthesia

Phenothiazines replace insulin as treatment of choice for schizophrenia

1956 *Ulett* trial of photoconvulsion

1957 Indoklon (flurothyl) introduced. *Krantz* (1970) trial of flurothyl vs ECT

1966 Multiple monitored ECT *Blachly*

1934 Camphor shock therapy *Meduna* Budapest

1935 Cardiazol shock therapy *Meduna* Budapest

1937 *Kennedy* reports on 1000 cases of convulsive therapy in schizophrenia

1937 First ECT *Cerletti* and *Bini* Rome

1940 First ECT in USA *Gonda* Chicago

1940 Curare used as a muscle relaxant *Bennett*

1950 *Meschan* reports 35% incidence of spinal fractures with ECT

1951 Succinyl choline introduced

1954 *Jarvie* reports on use of ECT in depression

1958 First unilateral vs bilateral controlled trial *Lancaster*

1959 Controlled trials of modified vs straight ECT *Seager*

Bilateral ECT remains dominant treatment mode in USA

Unilateral ECT becomes dominant treatment mode in Scandinavia

1970s Introduction of brief-pulse stimulation and 'constant-current' machines and beginning of EEG monitoring of fits

1980s Increasing evidence of bilateral vs unilateral ECT differences favouring bilateral

1990s? ECT remains most effective treatment of melancholia. Increasing evidence of its general anti-psychotic properties ??

1936 Prefrontal leucotomy *Moniz* and *Lima* Lisbon

1940 Modified leucotomy *Freeman* and *Watts* Georgetown, USA

1943 *Moniz* shot in spine by leucotomised patient

1949 *Moniz* and Hess receive Nobel Prize in physiology and medicine

1949 Freeman describes transorbital leucotomy

1960s to present. Variety of modified operations introduced. Still no controlled trials. Number of leucotomies gradually fall

1990s ?

Fig. 37.1 The development of physical treatments in psychiatry.

Table 37.1   Recent trials of real versus simulated ECT

Reference	Number of patients	Groups compared	Stimulus	Rate of ECT	Outcome
Freeman et al (1978)	20 + 20	Bilateral temporal versus simulated for first two treatments then real for both groups	Sine wave	6 (2/week)	Significantly more rapid onset of response noted in simulated group, who also needed more treatments
Lambourn & Gill (1978)	16 + 16	Unilateral temporal versus simulated	Brief pulse	6 (3/week)	No difference between groups, both improved
West (1981)	11 + 11	Bilateral temporal versus simulated	Sine wave	6 (2/week)	Clear differences in favour of real ECT
Johnstone et al (1980)	35 + 35	Bilateral frontal versus simulated	Sine wave	8 (2/week)	Both groups showed steady improvement. Real group significantly greater improvement but accounted for mainly by deluded depressives. No difference between groups at 1 month follow-up
Brandon et al (1984)	42 + 53	Bilateral temporal versus simulated	Sine wave	8 (2/week)	Clear superiority of real ECT
Gregory et al (1985)	23 + 23 + 23	Bilateral temporal versus (Lancaster) versus simulated	Sine wave	Varied (2/week)	Bilateral superior to unilateral. Both superior to simulated

of mood, early morning wakening, loss of weight, loss of appetite and libido would indicate a likely good response. Two particular symptoms, retardation and depressive delusions, respond well to ECT and there is good evidence that patients with depressive delusions are more likely to fail to respond to tricyclic drugs. In the Northwick Park trial (Johnstone et al 1980), delusions were the most consistent predictor of response and, in those patients who had both delusions and retardation, retardation by itself did not predict response when this overlap was allowed for. Those features of illness which are said to predict poor response to the treatment such as hypochondriacal symptoms, ill-adjusted personality, neurotic traits and a fluctuating course to the illness may be associated with a poor response to all physical methods of treatment rather than to ECT in particular. A recent study by Abrams & Vedak (1991) reported on 47 men given ECT for melancholia. No clinical predictors were found, suggesting that once patients with non-melancholic depression are excluded the ability to predict response from clinical features is lost. There was still sufficient variability in outcome to allow predictors to emerge but none of the core features of melancholia either alone or in clusters did so.

Mania

Butyrophenones such as haloperidol and droperidol, phenothiazines and lithium represent the mainstay of treatment for manic illness. Though McCabe (1976) showed that ECT-treated manics fared significantly better than untreated manics in terms of mortality, time spent in hospital, and social recovery, this was a retrospective study. A study comparing ECT and lithium (Small 1986) shows both treatments to be

Table 37.2   Indications for ECT in depressive illness

1. Failure to respond to an adequate course of a tricyclic or second-generation antidepressant, with continuing moderate to severe symptoms of depression
2. Severe depression where a rapid response is needed because of suicidal risk or because the patient is not eating or drinking
3. Depressive stupor
4. Depressive illness with nihilistic or paranoid delusions
5. Depressive illness with marked retardation
6. Patients with mixed depression and schizophrenic symptoms
7. Severe puerperal depression
8. In the elderly where ECT may be safer than tricyclic antidepressants
9. Inability to tolerate side-effects of antidepressants

effective but suggest that ECT may have advantages in producing greater and more rapid symptom relief. The ECT-treated group had a mean of 10.6 seizures. Interpretation of the results is difficult because of the large doses of neuroleptics that were used in both groups, and because many patients had relapsed on lithium treatment; so the trial may be biased against lithium.

Acute schizophrenia

Clinical opinion in the UK appears to be about equally divided between those who think that ECT is occasionally an appropriate treatment in acute schizophrenia and those who think it is not (Pippard & Ellam 1981). From the results of open trials, mainly carried out in America, it appears that ECT does not produce greater symptomatic relief than pheno-thiazine drugs, and does not reduce the length of stay in hospital or affect relapse rates. In a large study (May 1968) in California, drugs plus psychotherapy or drugs alone gave the best results, psychotherapy and milieu therapy produced the worst response and ECT was in the mid range. A small but well-designed study (Taylor & Fleminger 1980) found that when phenothiazines plus ECT were compared with phenothiazines plus stimulated ECT in young male schizophrenics, the former group showed significantly greater improvement up to 8 weeks but at 16 weeks from the start of treatment the phenothiazine plus simulated treatment group had caught up. Interestingly, improvement occurred not just in depressive symptoms within the schizophrenic illness but across the range of all psychotic symptoms. Abraham & Kulhara (1987) and Brandon et al (1985) have shown that the combination of ECT and

phenothiazines is superior to sham ECT plus phenothiazines in the short term. Both studies showed that real-ECT-treated patients did better for the first 6–8 weeks of treatment, but by week 12 of follow-up the sham ECT plus drug group had caught up. At present it is not possible to say what type of patients are likely to respond. The three studies described above were on predominantly young, relatively recent-onset schizophrenic patients. There is some evidence then that ECT may be an adjunct to phenothiazine drug treatment, producing a more rapid antipsychotic effect than drugs alone, though Janakiramaian & Channabasavanna (1982) found an advantage only for ECT and low-dosage chlorpromazine (less than 300 mg/day) and not for ECT and high-dosage chlorpromazine (more than 500 mg/day).

These studies raise the possibility that ECT has a more general antipsychotic effect rather than a specific antidepressant one. In contrast, Kochler & Saver (1983) found that a group of first-admission schizophrenic patients without Schneider first-rank symptoms responded significantly better to ECT than those patients with such symptoms.

It is a commonly held clinical view that certain specific features of schizophrenia such as catatonic excitement or stupor respond to ECT. Again there is little evidence apart from clinical observation for this. It is certainly possible that brief anaesthesia producing a break in consciousness may help to relieve such symptoms without markedly affecting the underlying schizophrenic process.

Chronic schizophrenia

There is powerful evidence from a number of studies that ECT is not an effective treatment in this condition, even when given in a fairly long course of 12–20 treatments. Schizophrenic patients may occasionally develop additional marked depressive symptoms warranting treatment with an anti-depressant or ECT.

Neuroleptic malignant syndrome (NMS)

There is an increasing number of case reports of the use of ECT in the NMS. In nearly all cases neuroleptics have been discontinued and ECT has been only one of a variety of treatments that have been initiated. It is therefore difficult to evaluate the part played by ECT in these cases. ECT may be a treatment option when conservative treatment and/or drug treatment with dopamine agonists such as dantrolene have failed. In contrast, there have been one or two reports of the recurrence of NMS after it has largely resolved with conservative treatment when ECT has been instituted.

Refractory Parkinson's disease

Recently, there have been many reports of the use of ECT in this condition when affective symptoms are absent. On/off phenomena, old age and extensive previous use of dopamine agonist drugs, particularly in high doses, all appear to be good predictors of response to ECT. Usually, only 3–5 treatments are needed to produce improvements and there is little advantage in giving long courses. Dopamine agonist medication should be reduced during ECT as there are reports of marked organic brain syndrome.

When high-dose medication and ECT are given together, relapse after ECT is frequent, and Zervas & Fink (1991) have used maintenance ECT at 4–6 weekly intervals to control this. The treatment has been reviewed by Abrams (1989).

ECT may have a place in the treatment of Parkinson's disease which has become refractory to medication. It is not known if resistance develops to ECT in the same way as occurs with drugs. No controlled trails have been published.

ECT in other disorders

There is no evidence that ECT is an effective treatment in obsessive–compulsive disorder, anorexia nervosa, organic confusional states or as an aid to narcotic drug withdrawal. There may be occasions when there are good grounds for suspecting an underlying depressive illness such as in a patient with hypochondriacal symptoms or atypical facial pain. In these circumstances the presenting complaints may be symptomatic of a depressive illness and ECT is used to treat the depressive illness rather than as a specific treatment for the presenting symptoms. There is some evidence that ECT is effective in the termination of severe delirious states where the underlying disorder is being treated and where other means of treatment for the delirium such as tranquillizers have proved ineffective.

ECT should not be used as a treatment of last resort when all other treatments have failed and when a psychiatrist simply does not know what to prescribe next. Nor should it be used as a sort of screening instrument across the range of depressive disorders, on the basis that at least all ECT responders will be given the treatment and non-responders will not come to any great harm. This is poor practice.

ECT does seem to be an effective treatment in puerperal psychosis and in some schizoaffective disorders. This probably reflects the basically affective nature of a large proportion of these two illnesses. Although ECT is not a treatment for dementia it is sometimes helpful in mildly demented patients with depressive symptoms. Scandinavian psychiatrists use ECT for delirious states, but these are not organic in origin. The Danish term *delirium acutum* refers to what Anglo-American psychiatrists would call florid acute schizophrenia. ECT should not be used as a treatment to control aggressive violent behaviour.

Physiological changes with ECT

ECT causes marked changes in many systems and it is important to have some knowledge of these to be able to assess the possible risks and the clinical contraindications.

EEG changes after a single ECT treatment consist usually of a brief period of episodic delta activity (0.5–3.5 Hz). As a course of ECT continues, delta activity may become continuous with some theta (4–7.5 Hz) activity. The EEG usually returns to normal within 3 months of the last treatment. It should not be assumed that an EEG is a totally useless investigation after a course of ECT. Some studies, particularly after U/ECT, have shown that the EEG becomes normal within a few days. A normal EEG may therefore be a helpful result in excluding certain pathologies but an abnormal EEG would be difficult if not impossible to interpret. In the sleep EEG, ECT appears to increase rapid eye movement (REM) sleep, to decrease REM latency and reduce total sleep time.

ECT produces a number of important cardiovascular changes, the magnitude of which depend to some extent on whether effective vagal blockade has been achieved with atropine. In the absence of atropine there is an initial bradycardia during the passage of current and subsequent seizure. This is due to vagal stimulation of the heart. There follows a tachycardia which subsides over the next 2 or 3 minutes. With good vagal blockade the initial bradycardia is abolished and the subsequent tachycardia is less pronounced. Changes in blood pressure mirror changes in pulse rate. Cerebral circulation increases dramatically during either spontaneous or electrically induced epileptic seizures. Animal studies using ECS (electroconvulsive shock) have shown increased permeability of the blood–brain barrier to a number of substances during this rise. Work in Edinburgh (Mander 1986) on magnetic resonance imaging (MRI) before and after ECT supports the view that

ECT produces a large increase in blood–brain barrier permeability.

ECT has a number of endocrine effects. The adrenal cortex responds rapidly and plasma cortisol levels are increased after a single treatment, the rise lasting for 2–4 hours. Rises also occur in adreno-corticotrophic hormone (ACTH), growth hormone and prolactin levels. The clinical significance of these changes has yet to be determined. These neuro-endocrine changes are discussed more fully in Chapter 7.

Mode of action of ECT

ECT is a complex package of interventions consisting of:

1. The repeated rapid induction of unconsciousness
2. The administration of an anaesthetic drug, a muscle relaxant and sometimes atropine
3. The passage of electricity across the brain
4. The induction of a bilateral grand mal epileptic seizure
5. Considerable medical and nursing attention
6. A varied set of attitudes and expectations on the part of the patient and his family

The studies comparing sham with real ECT show that the electricity and/or the epileptic fit are necessary for ECT to exert its full effect but that, in non-deluded depressed patients, other factors such as 1, 5 or 6 above may play a part. Studies carried out on unmodified ECT clearly demonstrate that the anaesthetic and muscle relaxant drugs are not essential and that they probably do not diminish the antidepressant effect of ECT. Ottosson (1960) showed that more powerful electrical stimulation did not have any increased effect and that an electrical stimulus that elicited no fit or a very limited fit was less effective. He also produced some tentative evidence that the cumulative length of fitting as measured in seconds through the course of treatment was positively correlated with clinical outcome.

Because it was thought that supraliminal stimulation did not enhance therapeutic effect but merely increased the degree of the retrograde and anterograde dysmnesia, the clinical aim in the early 1980s was to induce generalised seizure activity with a minimum of electrical energy. However, recent studies have suggested that the amount of electrical energy may be an important variable. Low-dosage bilateral ECT (B/ECT) with the amount of current titrated to just produce a seizure appears to be highly effective whereas right U/ECT using the same procedure is therapeutically weak although generalised seizures of equivalent length are produced.

There is clear evidence that, at least for U/ECT, the amount of electrical energy is important, and that one needs to administer more than the minimum required to just produce a seizure. There is increasing evidence that the same may apply to B/ECT, though applied energy may not need to exceed threshold by as much.

The relationship between ECT and changes in hormone-releasing factors and neurotransmitters is discussed more fully in Chapter 7.

There is no evidence that ECT works by fear, by punishing the patient in accordance with his depressive view of himself or by the memory impairment that it produces.

Mortality, morbidity and side-effects

Death associated with ECT is an extremely rare event. The Registrar General's figures for England and Wales show that there has been a gradual fall in deaths due to ECT; there were eight in 1959, three in 1962 and one in 1966. Heshe & Roeder (1976) studied all ECT given in Denmark in one year and found one death in over 22 000 treatments. This figure is similar to Barker & Baker's (1959) study in England and Wales which showed one death per 28 000 treatments. Up to date figures indicate that the overall rate of death within 6 days of surgery is one in 200, but that the risk of dying as a direct result of anaesthesia is very small. Anaesthesia is entirely responsible at the rate of around one in 10000 (Scott 1986), with approximately half of the deaths occurring within 24 hours and sudden cardiovascular collapse in the postoperative period being the commonest cause of death.

The risk of death would seem to be no greater than when anaesthetics are used for other brief procedures. We must, however, remember that ECT is given in a course of treatments which increases the risk to the individual patient. When death does occur it is usually due to a cardiovascular cause such as myocardial infarction or ventricular arrhythmia. There is thus a very small but definite mortality associated with the treatment. This must be set against the overall decrease in mortality observed in ECT-treated patients compared with those treated by small doses of tricyclic drugs or psychotherapy (Avery & Winokur 1976).

Orthopaedic complications such as spinal midthoracic fractures, fractures of long bones, jaw dislocations and fat emboli secondary to long bone fracture were almost exclusively associated with unmodified ECT and are now virtually never seen. Clinically, this means that conditions such as osteoporosis or ankylosing spondylitis are no longer contraindications. Other major complications are all rare, occurring in less than one in 500 treatments. They include myocardial infarction, congestive cardiac failure, cardiac arrhythmias, pulmonary embolism, aspiration pneumonia, prolonged apnoea, cerebrovascular accidents, status epilepticus, bladder rupture, bleeding from peptic ulcers and sub-conjunctival or nasal haemorrhages. Epilepsy occurring after ECT is rare, though occasional tardive grand mal seizures have been reported. When they do occur they are usually single or occasional fits and persistent epilepsy does not occur. In fact ECT is an anticonvulsant and fit threshold rises as a course of ECT progresses.

Effects of ECT on memory

Does ECT cause brain damage? This topic has been extensively reviewed Weiner (1984). There is no evidence from animal work in monkeys, cats or rats that ECT even though given in an unmodified form and at a frequency and number greater than customary in clinical practice causes any neuropathological changes.

Selective brain damage including actual neuronal loss and gliosis can occur in the hippocampus but only following sustained generalised seizure activity lasting more than 90 minutes, multiple brief recurrent seizures (more than 26 in 8 hours) or sustained continuous limbic seizures (lasting longer than 3–5 hours). None of these conditions is likely to occur in clinically given ECT. Some early studies did show petechial haemorrhages but these were a consequence of the increase in arterial and central venous pressure associated with unmodified seizures. A recent description of the normal post mortem findings of a patient who had had 1250 treatments underlines these conclusions. There is, however, an important distinction between gross structural damage as revealed by routine neuropathology, computerised tomography (CT) or MRI and functional change of a more subtle kind. It is certainly not possible at this time to say that neurochemical and/or neuro-physiological changes such as alteration in protein synthesis do not occur. Such changes might well form the basis of the enduring cognitive impairment that some patients experience.

Memory impairment is by far the most important undesirable effect of ECT. The interaction between depression, which also causes cognitive impairment,

and ECT is complex and it is convenient to consider impairment of memory in four areas separately:

1. Short-term retrograde amnesia (0–3 months)
2. Retrograde amnesia for remote events
3. Short-term anterograde amnesia (0–3 months)
4. Long-term or permanent anterograde amnesia.

Short-term retrograde amnesia. Some patients experience a retrograde amnesia for events leading up to and during a course of ECT. There may be complete amnesia for a few minutes or hours before each treatment, though many patients can remember events right up until the anaesthetic quite clearly. Patchy amnesia may stretch back in time for several weeks, but it should be remembered that such forgetfulness is also very common in severely depressed patients who do not receive ECT.

Such retrograde impairment is not usually distressing and may be welcomed by the patient for helping him to forget the painful experience of his illness.

Retrograde amnesia for remote events. Testing personal remote memories is extremely difficult as each individual's experience is unique and standardised tests are impossible to construct. Some patients certainly do complain of gaps or holes in their memory stretching back several years. Squire & Chase (1981) have shown that B/ECT in particular may effect memory over the previous decade and that patchy loss of memory for some personal events, television programmes or major news items may occur.

Weiner (1986) has shown that B/ECT can produce long-term impairment of personal memories irre-spective of whether a sine wave or pulsed stimulus is used, but that the combination of bilateral electrode placement with high-energy sine wave stimuli produced the greatest impairment.

Short-term anterograde amnesia. There is usually some degree of anterograde amnesia, especially if the patient is confused after treatment. More importantly, some patients show difficulty in retaining new learning for a few days or even a few weeks after the course of ECT finishes. Clinicians should be aware of this and appreciate that some patients may find it hard to remember phone numbers, messages, shopping lists, etc., for a few weeks after a course of ECT. There have been two large studies, by Weeks et al (1980) and Johnstone et al (1980), which have studied the magnitude and dura-tion of cognitive impairment. Both are in agreement that such impairment is common but short lived. After 3 months of ECT treatment there is no impairment whatsoever. It must be remembered that depressive illness itself has a profound effect on cognitive function. Thus, patients' subjective complaints may be related as much to the memory impairment caused by depression as to that caused by ECT. Secondly, studies which show that patients do as well on cognitive tests after ECT as they did before do not necessarily show that ECT does not cause impairment. It may be that, as treatment progresses and depression lifts, cognitive impairment due to depression is replaced by cognitive impairment due to ECT. Both studies quoted above had control groups of either non-ECT treated depressives or depressives treated by simulated ECT to control for this factor.

There is overwhelming evidence that U/ECT given to the non-dominant hemisphere causes fewer side-effects, particularly less memory impairment and less post-ECT confusion. It is also clear that U/ECT must be given to the non-dominant hemisphere. When Halliday et al (1968) gave dominant-hemisphere ECT they found greater impairment on tests of verbal learning than occurred with B/ECT.

Long-term permanent anterograde amnesia. The studies discussed so far compare groups of patients and show no permanent changes in memory and cognitive function due to ECT when treated and untreated groups are compared. It is more difficult to demonstrate that ECT does not cause impairment in an occasional individual. It is almost impossible to know in an individual patient who complains of permanent memory impairment after ECT whether the treatment really was responsible. It may be that because ECT affects memory in the short term it sensitises patients to further lapses in memory which would otherwise go unnoticed. Freeman et al (1980) examined a group of self-selected patients who were convinced their memories had been impaired by ECT. Some impairment was indeed found and there was no evidence of faking. Much of this impairment could be accounted for by continuing psychiatric symptomatology, drug and alcohol use. However, there remained some residual impairment which may have been due to ECT. All patients had had B/ECT, some of them many years previously. The degree of impairment was not related to the number of ECT treatments.

The question of long-term memory impairment must for the time being remain an open one. If it does occur it appears to be mild and infrequent. The sort of complaints that patients have are of holes in their memory going back several years before ECT and/or a decreased ability to retain new learning over a period of several years after ECT. There is no evidence at present to implicate U/ECT in such a way.

The work of Ottosson (1960) suggests that when memory impairment does occur it is mainly due to the amount of electrical energy delivered to the patient's brain rather than to the magnitude or duration of the epileptic fit. Hamilton et al (1979) claimed that the degree of memory impairment following ECT is positively correlated with the magnitude of the associated rise in blood pressure and postulate that it may be the increased permeability of the blood–brain barrier which mediates this effect.

Other side-effects

The most common other side-effects are headache, post-ECT confusion and muscle aches and pains (Table 37.3). Although headache is quite common it is rarely troublesome and is well tolerated by patients.

Contraindications to ECT

There is no absolute medical contraindications to ECT. Each case must be assessed on its merits and the clinical question asked: which will cause the greater risk to this patient, continuation of their depressive illness or ECT? Wherever possible ECT should not be given to someone with raised intracranial pressure, cerebral aneurysm or a history of cerebral haemorrhage. Recent myocardial infarction (within 3 months), aortic aneurysm and acute respiratory infection are also relative contraindications.

ECT can safely be given to women during any stage of pregnancy, to patients with cardiac pacemakers, and to epileptics, providing the epilepsy is well controlled. Since the introduction of modified ECT there are no orthopaedic contraindications to the treatment. Most anaesthetists now agree that monoamineoxidase inhibitors do not need to be stopped before general anaesthesia. Finally, old age is not a

Table 37.3 Side-effects related to ECT (subjective complaints of patients) [a]

Symptom	Total reported symptoms (%)	Severe	Mild
Memory impairment	64	27	37
Headache	48	19	29
Confusion	27	9	18
Clumsiness	9	4	5
Nausea/vomiting	5	3	2
Other side-effects	12		

From Freeman et al (1980).
[a] Only 20% reported no side-effects at all.

contraindication and it may well be that ECT is safer than leaving the patient untreated or prescribing tricyclic antidepressants.

The administration of ECT

The Royal College of Psychiatrists' survey (Pippard & Ellam 1981) showed that although ECT is practised with care and consideration for patients' feelings and safety in many centres in Britain, this is by no means universal. Out of a representative sample of 100 clinics they examined, only 43% met or nearly met the standards laid down by the Royal College of Psychiatrists. Of these, 16% were considered to be largely or totally unsuitable for administering ECT at all, and 41% had important shortcomings and a generally low standard of practise.

ECT is a major and effective treatment in psychiatry. It should be properly administered and supervised, and a senior psychiatrist should take a continuing interest in the treatment in each hospital. It should not be given in side rooms off wards or in open wards with only screens pulled round to shield the patient. The minimum requirement is a suite of three rooms: a pleasant and comfortable waiting room with sound insulation between it and a large properly equipped treatment room, and a comfortable recovery room.

Explanation to the patient

As full an explanation as possible should be given. Fears and fantasies about the treatment are often allayed by the facts and rarely made worse. An explanation should include a description of the purpose of the treatment, and procedure involved. The patient should be reassured, told that the treatment takes only a few minutes, is not painful, that there is no need to undress, and that sleep is induced by an injection before the treatment starts. Freeman (1980) found that the majority of patients felt unhappy with the explanation they had been given, not because it was misleading, but because it was either absent or not full enough. Because of the short-term memory impairment associated with ECT many patients forget the explanation they have been given and it is useful to repeat it at the end of a treatment course.

Consent

Informed or real consent requires an understanding of the nature, purpose and likely consequences of a treatment. This should be sought from every patient about to undergo a course of ECT. Many consent forms require the patient to sign that he agrees to have treatment. There should also be wording indicating that the patient has been given an explanation of ECT and its benefits and dangers. Both the doctor and patient should sign this. Consent is usually given to a course of treatment but it may be withdrawn by the patient at any stage.

Further details about consent to treatment and the Mental Health Act are given in Chapter 35.

Testing for cerebral dominance

This should be carried out routinely on all patients who are to receive U/ECT. Right-handed patients are nearly all left hemisphere dominant for language. Less than 1% of right-handed writers have their main language function in the right hemisphere. The left-handed population is heterogenous for lateral specialisation, a substantial proportion of left-handers being left hemisphere dominant for language. So in left-handers careful assessment is required to establish the dominant hemisphere. Unfortunately, there is no simple clinical test which allows accurate determination of language dominance. In cases where there is doubt, or where mixed dominance appears to be present, it is sometimes worthwhile giving the first ECT stimulus to one hemisphere and the second to the opposite. The nurse from the ward who accompanies the patient to the ECT department should be asked to time the period from application of the electrodes to recovery of orientation of time, place and person. This will normally be markedly longer for treatment given on one side rather than the other. Treatment should then continue on the side on which orientation was most rapid.

Premedication and anaesthetic

The patient should empty their bladder before going to the ECT suite. Bladder rupture is an occasional severe complication, particularly in the elderly. Atropine should not be given routinely by subcutaneous or intramuscular injection as a premedication unless there has been a previous problem with excess salivation and bronchial secretions. It is an unnecessary injection which leaves the patient with a dry mouth and adds to the overall stress of the procedure. The main reason why atropine is given is to block the vagus nerve and so protect the heart from bradycardia and arrhythmias. Vagal blockade can be achieved quite successfully with intravenous injection of atropine at the same time as the anaesthetic, though there is some doubt whether a dose of 0.6 mg achieves adequate blockade. Bradycardia is a rare complication and it may be that it is not necessary to give atropine at all during ECT. Glycopyrrolate is an alternative to atropine and may have advantages. It only acts peripherally, not crossing the blood–brain barrier. Doses of atropine are 0.3–0.6 mg s.c. or 0.4–1.0 mg i.v. and for glycopyrrolate 0.2–0.4 mg i.m., s.c. or i.v.

Methohexitone sodium (Brietal) is the drug of choice for ECT anaesthesia. Pitts (1972) showed that methohexitone gives quicker induction and recovery and produces fewer postictal ECG abnormalities, particularly atrial and ventricular ectopic beats. The only advantage of thiopentone (Pentothal) is that recovery is slower and post-ECT confusion is often masked by sleep. A muscle relaxant such as suxamethonium chloride (Scoline) should always be given. It can be given through the same needle as the anaesthetic but from a different syringe. The dose should be adjusted so as to relax the patient as completely as possible without abolishing all signs of convulsion. Oxygen should be given through a face mask both before and after the period of suxamethonium-induced apnoea. The oxygen (100%) should be administered for 20–30 ventilations using positive-pressure ventilation. If this is done adequately, cerebral hypoxia does not occur during ECT. It has the added advantage of reducing fit threshold. U/ECT introduced by Friedman & Wilcox (1942) was first used by Thenon (1956) to reduce memory disturbance. This it does partly because less electrical energy is delivered to the brain and partly because current does not pass through the dominant hemisphere.

The unilateral–bilateral ECT controversy

The standard conclusion that without qualification B/ECT and U/ECT of the right hemisphere are equal in therapeutic properties is no longer tenable.

In their influential paper, d'Elia & Raotha (1975) found 29 studies where U/ECT and B/ECT had been compared. Fifteen studies reported the two methods to be equally effective, 13 reported an advantage for B/ECT and one for U/ECT. The general impression was that in well-controlled clinical trials U/ECT and B/ECT were equally effective, with U/ECT producing much less cognitive impairment. In contrast, the clinical experience and practice of many clinicians was that B/ECT was more effective.

The subject was reviewed again by Abrams in 1986. There has been a consistent trend for published studies over the past 10 years to show differential effects on brain functioning. These results are summarised in Table 37.4.

Conclusions. Most of the U/ECT–B/ECT comparisons have been reported in terms of depressive rating scale scores rather than using definitions of recovery. As yet we do not know if there are specific U/ECT or B/ECT responders. It is no longer possible to recommend unequivocally either U/ECT or B/ECT. A careful cost/benefit analysis has to be applied to each patient. Both types of treatment are effective but B/ECT is more potent. It is, however, associated with greater memory impairment, and persistent amnesia has been recently demonstrated by Weiner (1986) and Squire (1986).

It has been argued that U/ECT could be made as effective as B/ECT if ECT technique was meticulous, benzodiazepines reduced and a wide interelectrode distance used along with a markedly suprathreshold current. This is unproved. Such factors might equally increase the therapeutic power of B/ECT and increase the side-effects for U/ECT.

The Royal College of Psychiatrists' and American Psychiatric Association's recommendations. The Royal College of Psychiatrists (1989) endorses the use of B/ECT as the treatment of choice for severe depressive illness, especially where speed of action is important; but agrees there is still a place for U/ECT where speed of action is less important and minimizing side effects is the primary consideration. In contrast, the American Psychiatric Association Task Force (1990) leaves the decision to the practitioner: 'The individual psychiatrist in each case should decide whether unilateral or bilateral treatment is the best for each particular patient'.

The majority of clinics in the UK and USA use both treatments, and have always used more B/ECT than U/ECT even when 'experts' were recommending U/ECT in the late 1970s and early 1980s. In Scandinavia U/ECT has always been the treatment of choice, and workers in that country appear to have no problems with effectiveness.

Types of ECT machines and electrodes

ECT should never be given with a machine which delivers an untimed stimulus and where the duration of the stimulus depends on how long the operator presses the treatment button. The amount of electrical energy that the patient receives depends on the duration and type of stimulus and the resistance across the patient's head. The advantages of a

Table 37.4   A comparison of U/ECT and B/ECT

Variable	Comparison
Diagnosis of 'melancholic depression'	Greater improvement with B/ECT
Diagnosis 'minor depression'	No difference between U/ECT and B/ECT
Age	Older patients have a higher fit threshold and may respond better to B/ECT
Sex	Seizure threshold is 50–100% higher in men than women, no one has so far demonstrated a specific sex-related difference (though note MRC trial in 1965[a])
Electrical stimulation	B/ECT may produce greater electrical stimulation to diencephalic (specifically hypothalamic) structures
Technique	In clinical practice it is likely that more, missed, shortened or abortive seizures occur with U/ECT, but in several recent studies these were carefully controlled for and do not explain observed differences
EEG	Post-ECT slow wave activity is greater with B/ECT and markedly lateralised to treatment side with U/ECT. EEG returns to normal much more rapidly with U/ECT
Memory	All studies agree that memory impairment is substantially less with U/ECT and in many patients is absent. (See discussion in text)
Other side-effects	Headache with post-ECT confusion less with U/ECT
Prolactin release	Increased with B/ECT more than with U/ECT, suggesting greater hypothalamic stimulation with B/ECT
Cerebral metabolic activity	Both cerebral blood flow and brain electrical mapping data show large difference between B/ECT and U/ECT
Number of treatments required	One study shows 40% U/ECT patients requiring more than ten treatments compared with 17% of B/ECT patients
Degree of response in depression	80% reduction in Hamilton Scale score after six B/ECT treatments compared with 56% reduction after six U/ECT treatments
Percentage of non-responders in depression	70% response rate 3 months after B/ECT, 30% with U/ECT

[a] Medical Research Council Clinical Psychiatry Committee (1965).

constant-current machine is that, no matter how low this resistance, the machine will not deliver more than a certain preset amount of energy. Thus, if the patient happens to have a particularly thin skull, or the electrodes are placed by chance over an emissary vein, there is no danger of an excessive amount of electrical energy being delivered. Two separate electrodes should be used, one in each hand. The commonly used bilateral headset is unsuitable because it does not allow sufficient pressure to be applied and therefore electrical contact can be poor. All the currently available unilateral handsets where both electrodes join onto a single stem have the electrodes placed far too close together. Recommended electrode placements for U/ECT and B/ECT are shown in Figure 37.2.

There should be at least 18–20 cm between the two electrodes in U/ECT. The actual position of the second electrode is less critical.

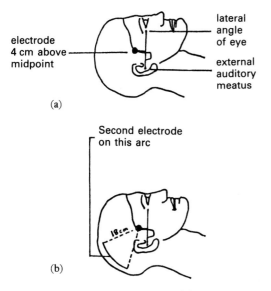

electrode
4 cm above
midpoint

lateral
angle
of eye

external
auditory
meatus

(a)

Second electrode
on this arc

18cm

(b)

Fig. 37.2   (a) Bilateral electrode position.
(b) Unilateral electrode position.

The electrical stimulus

Most older ECT machines deliver a biphasic sinusoidal wave form with a frequency of 50 or 60 Hz, which is very little different from alternating current mains. This is not a particularly physiological stimulus and all the more recent machines deliver a string of high-voltage very brief direct current pulses, each pulse lasting between 1 and 2 ms, with 60–70 pulses being given per second. With this technique much less electrical energy is passed across the brain and Valentine et al (1968) and Weaver et al (1977) have shown that fits can be as reliably induced as with conventional sine wave stimuli. Some of the more flexible American machines retain the ability to give sine wave ECT.

The amount of electrical energy delivered to the brain varies considerably with different wave forms. The ranges given by manufacturers are only approximate as the interelectrode resistance (mainly the resistance of the patient's head) varies considerably.

Most of the electrical energy is dissipated in a series of shunts through skin, connective tissue and blood vessels and only a fraction passes through grey and white matter.

Stimulus dosing

The seizure threshold varies from patient to patient over a 40-fold range and stimulus dosing is a recently introduced technique to try and determine this threshold. This is important because stimuli marginally above the seizure threshold may be less effective than those at a higher intensity, particularly if brief-pulse U/ECT is used. The technique involves starting with what will almost certainly be a subthreshold stimulus and then at the same session increasing the stimulus intensity in stages until a seizure occurs. The technique does not appear to cause greater cognitive impairment or a higher rate of abortive or inadequate seizures. Stimulus dosing is usually only required at the first treatment. If missed seizures occur during a course, restimulation is applied as described below.

How to tell if a fit has occurred

The most reliable way is to use EEG monitor, and most of the currently produced American machines have this facility. These machines have a simple one- or two-channel electroencephalograph which is automatically disconnected when the treatment stimulus is applied and can accurately measure the number of seconds of fitting that the treatment induces. There is some doubt that such single-channel recording is adequate, especially when electrodes are placed frontally, as there is much interference from frontalis muscle activity. Simple observation of the patient is probably unreliable in some cases though several studies have shown high correlations between careful clinical observation and EEG measures. The former tend to give fit length about 10 seconds shorter. The American Psychiatric Association has recommended that EEG monitoring should be routine. The author considers this unnecessary, but the facility for monitoring should be available for occasional patients. Unfortunately, no European-made machines have this facility. The muscle twitching that occurs with suxamethonium depolarisation can be mistaken for the clonic phase of a fit and occasionally the patient is completely paralysed so that no external evidence of fitting can be seen. A simple technique can be used to overcome this problem. This involves isolating one forearm by inflating a blood pressure cuff to above systolic pressure before the muscle relaxant is given. The isolated forearm does not become paralysed and fitting can easily be observed in that limb. This has the advantage that, in the elderly or frail, the dose of muscle relaxant becomes less critical and patients can be completely paralysed yet fitting can still be observed. When U/ECT is given, the cuff should be applied to the ipsilateral forearm. It is thus possible to check that bilateral fitting has occurred.

What to do if no fitting ensues

Occasionally during the course of administering ECT a stimulus is applied but no fit is observed. The psychiatrist then has just a few seconds to decide whether to give a further stimulus before the patient comes round from the anaesthetic. The following routine should be employed:

1. Check with all members of the ECT team that no signs of a fit occurred. If a unilateral or localised fit was induced you may have missed it but it may have been seen by other observers. Because the fit threshold rises after a fit, there is no point in trying to induce a maximal seizure with a second stimulus.

2. Ask the anaesthetist to ventilate the patient with pure oxygen. This lowers the fit threshold. This should be for at least 20–30 inhalations.

3. Check that the electrode sites are well prepared, especially if the patient's hair is covered in insulating hair lacquer.

4. Check that the interelectrode space is dry and that the electrodes were spaced sufficiently far apart.

5. Increase the machine's settings by 25%.

6. Apply a second stimulus using very firm pressure on the electrodes.

7. If there is still no fit, do not repeat the stimulus; make a clear note in the ECT record that no fit has occurred.

8. Ask the doctor in charge to check the patient's medication. Although many psychiatric drugs are epileptogenic, some such as chlordiazepoxide, diazepam and the rest of the benzodiazepines are antiepileptic. Stop all such medication before the next ECT session.

9. At the next session make sure that the patient is well oxygenated, use a higher setting if available on the ECT machine and use the tourniquet technique to check if a fit has occurred.

10. Premedication with caffeine may be suitable for some patients or switch to different anaesthetic agent such as ketamine or etomidate.

A very small proportion of patients will not fit during ECT unless a very large or prolonged stimulus is given. If this is the case it is worth checking the thickness of the skull table with lateral skull radiography and placing the electrodes over the thinnest area. It may also be worth prescribing a small dose of a phenothiazine several hours before ECT in an attempt to lower the fit threshold.

The use of caffeine

Caffeine is a powerful stimulant of the xanthine class and several studies have shown that it can lengthen ECT-induced seizures. The American Psychiatric Association Task Force recommends 250–1000 mg of pure caffeine as 500–2000 mg of caffeine sodium benzoate. Few other seizure-enhancing agents are available. Unfortunately, caffeine is both a central and peripheral stimulant. It should be used with caution in patients who are elderly and/or have cardiac disease as dysrhythmias are particularly likely to occur with this group.

What is an adequate fit?

The figure of 25 seconds is often quoted as the minimum length for an effective seizure. There is little or no evidence for this. In general, seizure length is not correlated with outcome but it may be that a fit of 25 seconds or greater is some rough guide that sufficient current has been passed or that deep structures have been stimulated. In routine clinical practice it seems reasonable to restimulate if a short fit occurs. If a fit lasts longer than 120 seconds, preparation should be made to terminate it before it goes over 180 seconds using either a further dose of barbiturate anaesthesia or intravenous diazepam. Long fits may be associated with cerebral hypoxia and marked cognitive impairment.

Number and frequency of treatments

A set number of treatments should not be prescribed. The patient should be assessed after each treatment to see if further ECT is necessary. A few patients respond dramatically to one or two applications of ECT and further treatments are unnecessary; some patients need as many as 10–12, though most respond to a course between four and eight. There is some evidence that older patients require more treatments and that response to the initial two treatments is highly correlated with overall change at the end of the course. Barton (1973) showed there was no prophylactic value in giving extra ECT after symptomatic improvement in the hope of preventing relapse. He also showed that if relapses do occur they tend to occur early, 69% developing within 2 weeks. Clinically then it is important to monitor a patient's condition carefully for 2 or 3 weeks, but only to give additional treatments if symptoms recur. The most difficult clinical decision is what stage to abandon ECT if it is not relieving symptoms. If there has been no change at all in the patient's depressive symptoms after six to eight treatments, the course should be stopped. Some patients appear to show a brief response early in a course but relapse quickly. In such patients it is worth giving a course of up to 10 ECT treatments.

Treatment should be given two or three times a week. At present there is no convincing evidence that giving daily ECT produces more rapid recovery, and memory impairment is more severe. Once-weekly ECT may be indicated for elderly patients with marked post-treatment confusion or for patients who have brief hypomanic episodes during treatment. If a sustained hypomanic mood change is induced, the course should be stopped. Stromgren (1975) has reported that giving four unilateral treatments per week as compared with two unilateral treatments per week reduced the total treatment time by a mean of 11 days, though one or two more treatment applications were required. Memory impairment and other side-effects were not increased.

Other types of ECT

Unmodified ECT

The author can envisage only two situations in which such treatment would be justified. In some developing countries where anaesthetists are unavailable it may be safer for ECT to be given unmodified than to have a psychiatrist regularly giving anaesthetics. The only physical condition in which it might be safer to give unmodified rather than modified ECT would be severe liver damage where the administration of anaesthetic drugs could be hazardous. If a patient is too disturbed or too aggressive to be safely approached and anaesthetised, he is too disturbed and aggressive to be given ECT.

Multiple monitored ECT (MMECT)

In this treatment a number of ECT stimulations are given consecutively in the same treatment session. The patient is anaesthetised and then over a period of $1-1\frac{1}{2}$ hours given a course of four to six stimulations. There is little evidence that it is more rapidly effective or that the effects are more enduring. It certainly produces more post-treatment confusion and therefore should not be used.

Maintenance ECT (main/ECT)

There has been renewed interest in main/ECT in the last few years. There have still been no controlled trials but there are numerous descriptive reports. Several studies have compared main/ECT with main/ECT refusers and all show marked reduction in relapse rates with main/ECT. A number of studies have shown that relapse rates after acute treatment with ECT are high even when adequate antidepressant medication is maintained. Godber (1987) followed up 163 elderly depressed patients (mean age 76 years) treated with ECT. Follow-up was up to 3 years and in that time 73% of patients experienced one or more relapses. Main/ECT may be indicated particularly in depressed elderly patients in whom other types of prophylactic treatment have failed or when drug treatment cannot be used because of adverse effects. All 12 of the reports that the author has found in the literature, ranging from 1949 to 1990, have shown advantages for main/ECT in terms of fewer episodes of depression, greater improvement and fewer relapses. There would now appear to be sufficient evidence for a properly controlled clinical trial.

Patients' attitudes to ECT

Systematic studies of patients' attitudes to ECT indicate that most people find the treatment beneficial and would therefore consent to have it again (Freeman & Cheshire 1986). Most of the anxiety that ECT arouses in patients is due to fear of side-effects. Although a few patients do continue to complain of unwanted effects even years after the conclusion of treatment, the question of side-effects must be kept in perspective. Patients frequently suffer temporary discomfort or impairment of function following many medical and minor surgical interventions. It is quite likely that attitude studies to treatments such as appendectomy and cholecystectomy would reveal substantial rates of patients' complaints and negative attitudes. What is important is that the benefit to the patient clearly outweighs the cost in terms of side-effects, apprehension, discomfort and stigma. Even though the benefit from ECT seems clear, it is far from clear that psychiatrists have done all they should to reduce the cost to the patient in terms of the factors noted above. Reports by genuine, concerned individuals about side-effects from ECT must not be summarily dismissed by the professional without proper investigation.

Conclusion

The Royal College of Psychiatrists' survey (Pippard & Ellam 1981) found that in different areas of the country there was considerable variation in the amount of ECT given. Some hospitals in Yorkshire gave as many as 13 treatments per 1000 of the population per annum whereas the Oxford region as a whole gave only 1.64 treatments per 1000 per annum. The national average was approximately three per 1000 per annum. Pippard's most recent study (1991) has shown similar differences between areas in south England. It is clear from both reports that, although standards are high in many centres, there are areas of the country where ECT is being given in totally unsuitable clinics by poorly trained or bored psychiatrists with obsolete machines. These are not reasons for abandoning ECT or placing tighter controls on its use. When administered properly it is an extremely effective and safe treatment, and is likely to remain the treatment of choice for severe depression for the foreseeable future.

PSYCHOSURGERY

Definition

The term is used here to mean the surgical treatment of patients who have a psychiatric disturbance by means of surgical removal or destruction of nerve pathways within the brain. It does not include patients who have a recognisable pathological lesions in their brain which is producing psychiatric symptoms, e.g. patients with benign or malignant tumours or epilepsy. Nor does it include the many surgical interventions that have been developed for treatment of chronic pain.

History

The origins of modern psychosurgery go well back into the 19th century. Most medical students are told about the case of the American railway worker Phineas Gage (Harlow 1868) who suffered a penetrating injury to his frontal lobe from an iron bar following an explosion, leaving him with a 3.5 inch channel running through his frontal lobe and emerging from his left cheek. Although beforehand he had been a conscientious and capable foreman, he became irresponsible, irreverent and incapable of planned activity, showing that massive frontal lobe damage, though compatible with survival, produced definite behavioural changes. World War I resulted in a great number of soldiers with head injuries and often localised brain damage. Several authors drew attention to the fact that frontal lobe lesions often left soldiers without motor, sensory or intellectual impairment but with symptoms of euphoria, loss of judgment, disinhibition of instincts and sometimes deficits in attention.

Modern psychosurgery owes its origins to experiments on chimpanzees carried out in the USA in the 1930s. Two workers at Yale, Jacobson and Fulton, showed that destruction of the frontal lobes produced profound and permanent changes in adaptive behaviour. They found that whereas the normal chimpanzee when given a frustrating task to perform may become excited, cry or have tantrums, the chimpanzee without frontal lobes seems quite impervious to frustrating stimuli or to the errors that it makes. They concluded that even the most ferocious chimpanzees could be transformed into a state of friendly docility by such surgical intervention. A Portugese neurologist, Egaz Moniz, excited by these findings, decided to test their applicability to psychiatric patients suffering from severe anxiety and other psychiatric symptoms. In collaboration with Almeida Lima he performed the first series of 20 psychosurgical operations in 1936 (see Fig. 37.1). At first they used alcohol injections and then a knife (leucotome) to sever fibres connecting the frontal lobes with subcortical areas of the brain. Moniz, with another colleague, Hesse, later received the Nobel prize in physiology and medicine for his work.

However, it was not in Europe but in America that enthusiasm for psychosurgery blossomed. Two surgeons from Washington, Walter Freeman and James Watts, modified Moniz' operation and devised the standard prefrontal leucotomy. This was a bilateral operation and consisted of making a burr hole in each temporal region through which a leucotomy knife was inserted and swept up and down in an arc in the coronal plain in an attempt to divide frontal lobe white matter from the rest of the brain completely, whilst leaving cortical grey matter intact (Fig. 37.3). It is estimated that by the mid-1950s some 50 000 such operations had been carried out in the USA and some 10 500 in England and Wales. Freeman later modified his technique and instead of a lateral used a transorbital approach, inserting his famous 'ice-pick' instrument upwards under the eyebrow ridge on each side. Freeman estimated that he personally performed 3500 operations.

The treatment was initially received with great enthusiasm in the pre-phenothiazine era but by the end of the 1950s the operation had fallen into disrepute, partly because of the introduction of phenothaizines, but more importantly because it became increasingly clear that standard prefrontal leucotomy was not an effective treatment in deteriorated schizophrenics and that morbidity from the operation was high. Mortality for early operations varied from 2 to 6%, epilepsy from 10–50%, and between a third and a half of patients developed personality changes involving euphoria, apathy and lack of initiative, and leaving them more rather than less handicapped.

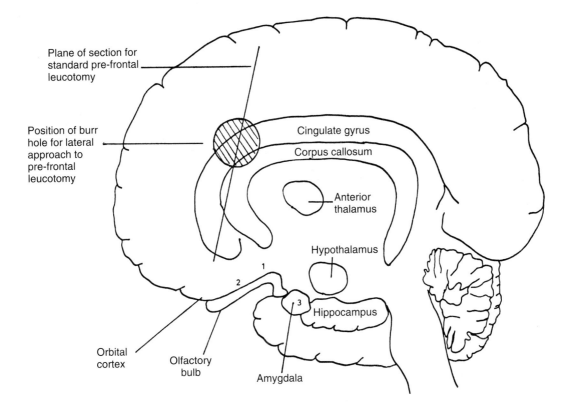

Fig. 37.3   Approximate sites of current psychosurgical lesions (with standard prefrontal leucotomy incision for comparison). 1, Stereotactic limbic leucotomy (lesions in cingulate gyrus and lower medical quadrant of frontal lobe); 2, Stereotactic tractotomy; 3, Amygdalotomy.

Modern psychosurgical operations

It is now generally agreed that there are no indications for standard bilateral prefrontal leucotomy as described by Freeman and Watts and the technique should never be used.

Two main factor stimulated a resurgence of interest in psychosurgery in the 1960s and 1970s. Firstly, the development of stereotactic techniques in neurosurgery. This involves fixing the patient's head in a metal frame and inserting probes through burr holes under X-ray guidance using the frame as a reference point to indicate the depth and angle of the probe. A target site can therefore be more precisely located and destruction of brain tissue can be achieved by heat, cold, surgical resection, or implantation of yttrium-90 radioactive seeds. The second factor has been the clarification of the role of the limbic system and its connections with the frontal lobes (see Ch 6). The limbic system is thought to be intimately involved with

feelings of emotions such as aggression, flight and fight responses and depression and is connected with the frontal lobes in three main areas. Projections run directly into the cingulate gyrus and two pathways pass through the lower medial quadrant of the frontal lobe, terminating in the hypothalamus. In theory then it may be possible to interrupt these pathways selectively and produce enduring effects on emotions such as anger and depression and on the behaviour associated with them.

Modern psychosurgical operations have concentrated on either interrupting the integrity of the limbic system or selectively severing frontal lobe limbic tracts (see Fig. 37.3). It has to be said that the chosen sites of lesions are often based on extremely scanty evidence and on a model of brain function which is naive and crude. In the UK operation sites have been concentrated mainly on frontolimbic connections or on the amygdala. In centres in America, Finland and Japan selective lesions in the cingulate gyrus have been more popular. A large number of different operations are practised around the world and many different methods are used for destroying brain tissue. The three operations currently in use in the UK will be described.

Contemporary operations in the UK

Subcaudate tractotomy. This is a stereotactic technique also known as stereotactic tractotomy. The target site is the lower medial quadrant of the frontal lobe (see Fig. 37.3), the aim being to sever connections between the supraorbital part of the frontal lobe and the limbic system. The technique involves placing yttrium-90 seeds bilaterally at this site.

Stereotactic limbic leucotomy. This operation aims to interrupt two frontolimbic pathways. The first target site is again in the lower medial quadrant and the second is the anterior part of the cingulate gyrus. Electrical stimulation of the target areas is often carried out during the operation and the operation site finally determined by destroying that area which produces the most marked autonomic changes in the patient.

Amygdalotomy. Bilateral lesions are made in the amygdala. Again electrical stimulation is carried out during the operation, which in this technique is either performed under local anaesthetic or involves waking the patient during the course of the operation. Emotional responses, which may be verbal or physical aggression, aid target location.

Multifocal leucocoagulation. Although this technique is no longer used, a recent report by Bird & Crow (1990) is of interest. The technique involves implantation of sheaves of small gold wires (up to 72) in the orbital and paracingulate regions of the frontal lobes. The electrodes are left implanted for up to 10 months and gradually electrocoagulation is progressively carried out. The above authors reported on a 15–20 year follow-up on 142 operations carried out in Bristol. Ninety of these patients had obsessive–compulsive disorder (OCD) and 94% of them showed some improvement with 68% showing complete or marked recovery. There was no operative morbidity and only two patients developed personality change, and this was probably due to other factors.

Indications for psychosurgery

Chronic unremitting depression, chronic severe anxiety and severe obsessional neurosis are the three main indications. The appendix of one published paper (Bartlett et al 1981) summarises what the neurosurgeons and psychiatrists currently involved in psychosurgical treatment in the UK think are the main indications. Depression should be severe, either chronic or persistently recurring and unresponsive or only partly responsive to treatment such as drugs and ECT. Of all conditions there is now the best evidence for OCD. OCD is only an indication if severe and if extensive behaviour therapy and all other treatments have failed. Chronic or recurrent episodes of anxiety or tension or intractable phobic anxiety state may be indications. One centre, the Midland Centre for Neurosurgery and Neurology in Birmingham, carries out amygdalotomy for cases of severe and uncontrollable aggressiveness associated either with a psychiatric condition or with conditions such as temporal lobe epilepsy. No adequate assessments of the technique have been published so it is not possible to say if it is effective.

Outcome after psychosurgery

There have been no properly designed and well-controlled trials of this treatment. Most research consists of collections of cases, sometimes with retrospective matched controls included. Percentage figures are usually given for overall improvement scored on global rating scales. For example, 80% of severe obsessional disorders are claimed to be improved after stereotactic limbic leucotomy, while 50% of similar patients are symptom-free after stereotactic tractotomy; 66% of patients with chronic anxiety and 68% of patients with depression were improved after subcaudate tractotomy. None of these percentage figures have been compared with more active and recently described behavioural treatments for obsessional neurosis.

In the same paper (Bartlett et al 1981) the authors indicate that occasionally they are prepared to accept depressed patients for operation less than 1 year after the illness begins. To the writer this seems unjustified. Treatment-resistant depressions of that duration are not uncommon and spontaneous remission does occur. In the author's opinion psychosurgery should only be considered as a last resort after other treatments have been tried.

The mortality of modern operation is virtually zero and the incidence of postoperative epilepsy around 1%. It seems unlikely that modern operations cause the major changes in personality and functioning that were found after prefrontal leucotomy. As an example of one of the better follow-up studies, Strom Olsen & Carlisle (1971) followed up 210 patients who had had stereotactic tractotomy between 1961 and 1967. Of these, 150 were interviewed at a variable time after operation, 29 had died and in 29 information was only available indirectly from other psychiatrists. Of the

150 who were personally followed up, 75 were depressives, 46 anxiety states, 20 obsessional neurotics and nine schizophrenics or other diagnoses. Of depressives, 56% were rated as recovered or much improved, compared with 50% of obsessional neurotics and 41% of anxiety states. None of the schizophrenics did well. The prevalence of epilepsy was less than 1% and there were no gross frontal lobe changes. Moderate but lasting personality changes occurred in 2.6% and minor or trivial changes in 12.4%. None of the 29 deaths could be attributed to the operation.

Conclusions

Pleas have been made for the past 20 years for properly controlled trials of this treatment and these still need to be carried out. Merely to quote percentage rates of improvement using crude global rating scales in essentially uncontrolled studies provides virtually no scientific support for the efficacy of the treatment at all. Even if full double-blind studies cannot be undertaken, a prospective open study with subjects randomly allocated to psychosurgery or other treatment would be valuable, provided that standardised and reliable diagnostic interviews and outcome measures were used. There is no doubt that a few patients appear to have responded dramatically to psychosurgical intervention, but the evidence for its efficacy remains essentially anecdotal. In obsessional neurosis the treatment should be compared with behaviour therapy, where improvement rates up to 75% have been reported even with seriously handicapped patients, and in depression with continuing treatment with antidepressant regimes and courses of ECT.

The more recent psychosurgical techniques were being developed around the time that the second generation of antidepressants were beginning to come on the market. If the same stringent criteria had been applied to psychosurgery as were applied to these new drugs before they could be licensed, all psychosurgery all over the world would be banned. Although psychosurgery is essentially a surgical technique, it is psychiatric patients on whom it is performed and psychiatrists who refer them. Psychiatrists therefore must be seen to be actively evaluating the treatment they use.

ELECTROSLEEP (SYNONYMS: ELECTRONARCOSIS, CEREBRAL ELECTROTHERAPY (CET))

This technique involves the use of a low-amplitude pulsating direct current which is applied to the forehead and/or mastoid area. No drugs or anaesthesia are used. The current produces a tingling sensation in the skin and appears to induce a state of relaxation lasting 30 minutes to an hour. Usually a series of such treatments is given on a daily, twice weekly or weekly basis. Electrosleep appears to be safe without unpleasant or distressing side-effects and is well tolerated by patients.

Enthusiasm for the technique has been particularly marked in the former Soviet Union and eastern Europe. A number of different machines for applying the treatment are available throughout the world, but in the UK the Somlec machine produced by Ectron Ltd is the only one easily available.

The main indication for the treatment is anxiety, particularly chronic unremitting anxiety. Controlled studies which have compared electrosleep with simulated treatment in the treatment of anxiety show contradictory results. There are four such studies which have compared electrosleep with placebo. In none of these studies did the placebo, which involved the application of electrodes but the passage of no current, control for the tingling effects produced in the skin. When this was done (Von Richthofen 1979) by applying two closely placed frontal electrodes, so that the subjects in the simulated group felt skin tingling as a small amount of current passed through the skin, but none through the brain then no difference could be demonstrated between real and simulated electrosleep. Both treatments produced significant reductions in anxiety as measured by self- and observer ratings but there was no difference between them. This study confirmed previous work indicating that it is the non-specific elements of the treatment such as suggestion, the treatment setting, increased attention and cutaneous stimulation which are responsible for the effect of electrosleep rather than any direct action of electrical current upon neurones.

However, there seems little doubt that electrosleep is an effective way of relaxing patients and the fact that some subjects fall asleep is probably due to that relaxing effect.

There have been recent and well-publicised claims that similar sorts of treatment involving low-voltage direct-current stimulation are effective in overcoming the withdrawal syndrome from opiate drugs. Treatment has involved either conventional electrosleep or electrical stimulation applied to the earlobes, often from a portable stimulator. Such claims have yet to be systematically evaluated. In one study using conventional electrosleep Gomez et al (1979) compared real and simulated electrosleep in opiate addicts undergoing methadone withdrawal.

They found electrosleep a useful additional treatment in relieving anxiety and those subjects receiving real electrosleep were prepared to allow their methadone dosage to be reduced more rapidly.

INSULIN TREATMENT

Insulin coma treatment

This was introduced by Manfred Sakel in 1933 for the treatment of schizophrenia. It is now only historic interest. Sakel was struck by the resemblance between the features of hyperthyroidism and the withdrawal symptoms of opiate addicts and wondered if the latter could be due to thyroid overactivity. He therefore began using insulin as a thyroid antagonist in patients undergoing opiate withdrawal and was surprised to find it helpful. Sakel became convinced that insulin might be useful in other states of excitement and found schizophrenic patients responded to it. During the 1940s and early 1950s insulin coma treatment became the treatment of choice for severe schizophrenic psychoses. The patient was fasted overnight and a coma induced with an early morning injection of insulin. The process was reversed 2 or 3 hours later, either with a nasogastric or an intravenous infusion of glucose. One of the complications of the treatment was spontaneous hypoglycaemic fits and it is possible that these fits were the main reason for any improvement that patients showed. The treatment fell into disuse with the advent of phenothiazines in the mid-1950s and to a lesser extent because of a well-conducted double-blind trial which showed it not to be superior to placebo (Ackner 1957).

Modified insulin treatment

More recently, small doses of insulin have been used on a regular basis to stimulate appetite in psychiatric patients, particularly anorexics. The treatment is often combined with chlorpromazine to sedate the patient and reduce activity. There is no evidence that such a treatment adds anything to good nursing and medical care. As one of the objectives in the treatment of anorexia nervosa is to teach the patient to eat regularly and normally again, the use of appetite stimulants is probably contraindicated.

REFERENCES

Ackner B, Harris A, Oldham A T 1957 Insulin treatment of schizophrenia: a controlled study. Lancet i: 607

Abraham K R, Kulhara P 1987 The efficacy of electroconvulsive therapy in the treatment of schizophrenia: a comparative study. British Journal of Psychiatry. British Journal of Psychiatry 157: 152–155

Abrams R 1986 Is unilateral electroconvulsive therapy really the treatment of choice in endogenous depression? Annals of the New York Academy of Sciences 462: 50–54

Abrams R 1989 ECT for Parkinson's disease. American Journal of Psychiatry 146: 1391–1393

Abrams R. Vedak C 1991 Prediction of ECT response in melancholia. Convulsive Therapy 7(2): 81

Aronson T A, Shukla S. Hoff A 1987 Continuation therapy after ECT for delusion depression: a naturalistic study of prophylactic treatments and relapse. Convulsive Therapy 3: 251–259

Avery D. Winokur G 1976 Mortality in depressed patients treated with electroconvulsive therapy and antidepressants. Archives of General Psychiatry 33: 1029–1037

Barker J C, Baker A A 1959 Deaths associated with electroplexy. Journal of Mental Science 105: 339–348

Bartlett J. Bridges P, Kelly D 1981 Contemporary indications of psychosurgery. British Journal of Psychiatry 138: 507–511

Barton J L, Mehta S, Snaith R P 1973 The prophylactic value of ECT in depressive illness. Acta Psychiatrica Scandinavica 49: 386–392

Bird J M. Crow C D 1990 Psychosurgery in obsessive compulsive disorder. In Montgomery S A, Goodman W K, Goeting N (eds) Obsessive compulsive disorder. Duphar Medical, pp 82–92

Brandon S, Cowley P, McDonald C, Neville P, Palmer R, Wellstood-Eason S 1984 Electroconvulsive therapy: results in depressive illness from the Leicestershire trial. British Medical Journal 288: 23–25

Brandon S, Cowley P, McDonald C, Neville P, Palmer R, Wellstood-Eason S 1985 Leicester ECT trial: results in schizophrenia. British Journal of Psychiatry 146: 177–183

Brill N W, Crumpton E, Eiduson S, Grayson H M, Hellman L I, Richards R A 1959 Relative effectiveness of various components of electro-convulsive therapy. Archives of Neurology and Psychiatry 81: 627–635

d'Elia G, Raotha H 1975 Is unilateral ECT less effective than bilateral ECT? British Journal of Psychiatry 126: 83–89

Freeman C P L, Cheshire K E 1986 Attitude studies on electroconvulsive therapy. Convulsive Therapy 2(1): 31–42

Freeman C P L, Basson J V, Crichton A 1978 Double-blind controlled trial of electroconvulsive therapy (ECT) and simulated ECT in depressive illness. Lancet 1: 738–740

Freeman C P L. Weeks D, Kendell R E 1980 ECT: patients who complain. British Journal of Psychiatry 137: 17–25

Friedman E, Wilcox P H 1942 Electrostimulated convulsion doses in intact humans by means of unidirection currents. Journal of Nervous and Mental Disease 96: 56–63

Godber C, Rosenvinge H, Wilkinson D et al 1987 Depression in old age: prognosis after ECT. Geriatric Psychiatry 2: 19

Gomez E, Mikhail A R 1979 Treatment of methadone withdrawal with cerebral electrotherapy (electrosleep). British Journal of Psychiatry 134: 111–113

Gregory S, Shawcross C R, Gill D 1985 The Nottingham ECT study: a double blind comparison of bilateral, unilateral and simulated ECT in depressive illness. British Journal of Psychiatry 146: 520–524

Greenblatt M, Grosser G H, Wechsler H 1964 Differential response of hospitalised depressed patients to somatic therapy. American Journal of Psychiatry 120: 935–943

Halliday A M, Davison K, Browne M W, Kreeger L C 1968 A comparison of the effects on depression and memory of bilateral ECT and unilateral ECT to the dominant and non-dominant hemispheres. British Journal of Psychiatry 114: 997–1012

Hamilton M, Stocker M,J. Spencer C M 1979 Post ECT cognitive defect and elevation of blood pressure. British Journal of Psychiatry 135: 77–78

Harlow J M 1868 Recovery from the passage of iron bar through the head. Massachusetts Medical and Social Publication 2: 329–347

Heshe J, Roeder E 1976 Electroconvulsive therapy in Denmark. British Journal of Psychiatry 128: 241–245

Janakiramaian N, Channabasavanna S M 1982 ECT and chlorpromazine combined versus chlorpromazine alone in acute psychiatric patients. Acta Psychiatrica Scandinavica 66: 464–470

Johnstone E C, Deakin J F W, Lawley P, Frith C D, Stevens M, McPherson K, Crow T J 1980 The Northwick Park ECT trial. Lancet ii: 1317–1320

Kochler K,. Saver H 1983 First rank symptoms as predictors of ECT response in schizophrenia. British Journal of Psychiatry 142: 280–283

Kramer B A 1990 Maintenance ECT in clinical practice. Convulsive Therapy 6(4): 279–286

Lambourn J, Gill D 1978 A controlled comparison of simulated and real ECT. British Journal of Psychiatry 133: 514–519

Lippman S and selected staff of the University of Louisville School of Medicine 1985 1,250 Electroconvulsive treatments without evidence of brain injury. British Journal of Psychiatry 147: 203–204

McCabe M S 1976 ECT in the treatment of mania: a controlled study. American Journal of Psychiatry 133: 688–691

Mander A 1986 NMR changes in ECT. British Journal of Psychiatry (in press)

May P R A 1968 Treatment of schizophrenia. Science House, New York

Medical Research Council Clinical Psychiatry Committee 1965 Clinical trial of the treatment of depressive illness. British Medical Journal i: 881–886

Oliver W 1785 Account of the effect of camphor on a case of insanity. London Medical Journal 6: 120–130

Ottosson J O 1960 Experimental studies of the mode of action of electroconvulsive therapy. Acta Psychiatrica et Neurologica Scandinavica suppl 145

Pippard J, Ellam L 1981 Electroconvulsive treatment in Great Britain, 1980. A report to the Royal College of Psychiatrists. Gaskell Books, London

Pitts F N 1972 Medical aspects of ECT. Seminars in Psychiatry 4: 27–32

Price T R P, Mackenzie T B, Tucker G J, Culver C 1978 The dose–response ratio in electroconvulsive therapy. Archives of General Psychiatry 35: 1131–1136

Royal College of Psychiatrists 1989 The practical administration of electroconvulsive therapy (ECT). Royal College of Psychiatrists, London

Scott D B 1986 Mortality related to anaesthesia in Scotland. Health Bulletin 44/1: 43–58.

Small J G, Milstein V, Klapper M H, Kellams J J, Miller, Small I F 1986 Electroconvulsive therapy in the treatment of manic episodes. Annals of the New York Academy of Sciences 462: 37–49

Squire L R 1986 Memory functions as affected by electroconvulsive therapy. Annals of the New York Academy of Sciences 462: 307–314

Squire L R, Miller P L 1981 Retrograde amnesia and bilateral electroconvulsive therapy. Archives of General Psychiatry 38: 89–95

Stromgren L S 1975 Therapeutic results in brief interval unilateral ECT. Acta Psychiatrica Scandinavica 52: 246

Strom–Olsen R, Carlisle S 1971 Bifrontal stereotactic tractotomy. British Journal of Psychiatry 110: 609–640

Taylor P J, Fleminger J J 1980 ECT for schizophrenia. Lancet i: 1380–1382

Thenon J 1956 Electrochoque monolateral. Acta Neuropsiquiatrica Argentina 2: 292–296

Valentine M, Keddie K M G, Dunne D 1968 A comparison of techniques in electroconvulsive therapy. British Journal of Psychiatry 114: 989–996

Von Richthofen C L, Mellor C S 1979 Cerebral electrotherapy: methodological problems in assessing its therapeutic effectiveness. Psychological Bulletin 86: 1264–1271

Weaver L A, Ives J D, Williams R, Nies A 1977 A comparison of standard alternating current and low energy brief pulse electrotherapy. Biological Psychiatry 12: 525–543

Weiner R D 1984 Does electroconvulsive therapy cause brain damage? Behaviour and Brain Science 7: 1–54

Weiner R D, Rodgers H J, Davidson J R T, Squire L R 1986 Effects of stimulus parameters on cognitive side effects. Annals of the New York Academy of Sciences 462

Weschler H, Grosser G H, Greenblatt M 1965 Research evaluating antidepressant medications on hospitalised mental patients: a survey of published reports during a five year period. Journal of Nervous and Mental Disease 141: 231–239

West E 1981 Electro-convulsion therapy in depression: a double-blind controlled trial. British Medical Journal 282: 355–357

Zervas I M, Fink M 1991 ECT for refractory Parkinson's disease. Convulsive Therapy 7(3): 222–223

38. Counselling and crisis intervention

Judy Greenwood   J. Bancroft

When someone seeks help in dealing with life's problems, the choice of agency usually depends more on familiarity rather than any rational selection of the most appropriate for the problem. Some might turn to agony columnists in a woman's magazine or telephone the Samaritan service, some to voluntary counselling such as Marriage Guidance or Cruse, whilst others might turn to more professional sources such as the minister of the church, social worker, general practitioner, psychiatrist or health visitor.

Having made contact, the help received is more often determined by the helper's professional background than by a careful appraisal of the individual's needs. Hence some psychiatrists, faced with a person in distress, give priority to deciding whether or not psychiatric treatment is indicated rather than providing whatever help is appropriate. Although most caring professionals have specialist skills which are useful for certain types of problem, each should be able to provide the non-specialist skills that counselling requires. The psychiatrist should have these skills no less than other professionals, for many patients referred to out-patient clinics and seen as emergencies in the evening and at weekends are likely to be in distress rather than psychiatrically ill. And as a more community-oriented approach to psychiatric management develops, the psychiatrist's role in multidisciplinary team may well evolve into supporting volunteer and semiprofessional counsellors, for example in a mental health clinic.

This chapter therefore deals with such non-specialist aspects of counselling and the additional considerations that are required when an individual is 'in crisis'. It is written in an eclectic spirit but with a behavioural bias. Whilst it does not deal with all clinical contingencies, it does aim to provide a practical framework for counselling which can be built upon and adapted. The approach we describe was developed in a general hospital psychiatric service dealing predominantly with patients who had attempted suicide. Such patients presented with a wide range of different stresses and symptoms but shared in common their particular way of reacting to them, i.e. with an overdose.

Not only has this approach evolved to deal with a variety of stresses, it has evolved within a multidisciplinary team, and therefore is appropriate for a variety of professions. We also believe that it can be used in a number of different settings. Much of it involves the application of common sense, for which we make no apology.

COMMON PROBLEMS

The determinants of reactions to stress are variable, involving not only the nature of the immediate problem faced, but also the personality and previous experiences of the individual which make him more or less able to cope with such circumstances and more or less distressed by them. The common causes of distress can be divided into four categories, each of which is associated with a typical emotional reaction.

1. *Loss problems.* Although bereavement is the most obvious loss, other losses such as separation or divorce, loss of self-esteem, loss of body functions following major surgery, and loss of resources such as wealth or employment are also important and share many features. Such loss leads to a pattern of reaction similar to the bereavement reactions described by Lindemann (1944) and Parkes (1975). To begin with the person is in a state of shock, which may be followed by anger or guilt, and over-identification with the lost object, giving way to feelings of grief and depression. As the grief declines, the person gradually attempts to restructure his or her life and fill the gap that has been created. Variation in the timing and importance of the different phases obviously varies according to circumstance.

869

2. *Change problems.* Here the stress or challenge is the arrival of a new condition in addition to loss of the previous situation. Taking on a new work role, getting married, becoming a parent, or passing through a transitional or maturational crisis, as described by Erikson (1969), are typical examples. Although the challenge in a new situation might eventually be positive and potentially rewarding, for some individuals it can nevertheless be very threatening, producing marked anxiety symptoms.

3. *Interpersonal problems.* Conflict within marriages or families is an extremely important cause of distress. It is probably the commonest reason for non-fatal suicide attempts (Bancroft et al 1977). A poor or unhappy relationship has been shown to increase the susceptibility of a woman to depression when faced with other stressful life events (Brown et al 1975). When such interpersonal problems are involved, the most important role for the helping professional may be to facilitate communication within the relationship in the hope of resolving some of the associated hostility and anger. Distress sometimes stems from an apparently impossible choice between alternatives. Thus, with interpersonal problems, the main problem may be deciding whether to stay or leave, or choosing between two possible partners.

4. *Problems from the past.* Some, who have suffered emotional, physical or sexual abuse in childhood, continue to experience emotional problems as an adult. Painful past experiences may need to be reprocessed from an adult perspective in order to gain a sympathetic and understanding view of what happened to the child victim. Once unresolved anger towards the perpetrator, and family members who failed to rescue, has been dealt with a gradual building of trust in intimacy and self-esteem needs to be developed, replacing the defensiveness and self-disgust often prevalent in such patients.

5. *Environmental factors.* These might be many and various, from noisy neighbours to poor housing, lack of resources in the neighbourhood, loneliness or lack of privacy, noise or vandalism, or difficulties at work.

Whilst most individuals who seek counselling are experiencing emotional reactions such as depression, anger or anxiety, some may have additional problems, having attempted to alleviate their distress in maladaptive ways, e.g. overeating, excessive alcohol intake, gambling or tranquilliser abuse. There may be uncharacteristic shoplifting, signs of violence or an overdose. It may in fact be the behavioural rather than the affective disturbance that brings the individual to the attention of the counsellor.

PRINCIPLES OF SIMPLE COUNSELLING

The aims and objectives of the counsellor should be to enable the client to cope more effectively with his current problems of living. The process, in terms of transactional analysis, requires an adult–adult relationship, involving cooperation from the client rather than dependence or regression. Initially, such counselling may be anxiety-provoking as the client is persuaded to confront his current problems and look for new ways of dealing with them rather than relying on his traditional defences or avoidance mechanisms. The patient may have been hoping for a more dependent 'sick role' with the therapist but should be encouraged to accept principal responsibility for what occurs during counselling. It may be necessary to explain why a dependent relationship in such circumstances makes it more difficult to cope with life's problems. Inability to avoid such dependency may be an indication for more long-term psychotherapy rather than goal-oriented counselling.

To begin with, the counsellor should make clear how much time can be given and how regularly they should attempt to meet. Such decisions will be determined not only by the nature and extent of the particular stresses and presenting symptoms but also by the characteristics and resources of the particular patient (and inevitably the time available to the counsellor.) The initial objectives may simply be to define the problems before deciding what further steps to take.

The underlying assumption about the counselling relationship is that, by facilitating the expression of affect and thereby reducing emotional tension, the patient can begin to think more clearly and, encouraged by the counsellor, can achieve a better understanding of his problems and find new ways of tackling them.

For clarification we have broken down the counselling procedures into relatively discrete steps. In clinical practice, these may be combined in various ways. But as a general rule it is usually necessary to focus on establishing rapport and expressing affect before passing on to more cognitive processes such as problem-solving.

Facilitation of the expression of affect

In the context of a trusting and confidential relationship, with the therapist showing genuine non-judgemental interest, with plenty of eye contact and empathy, the patient is encouraged both to give an outline of his problems and in the course of this to express how he is feeling about his current situation.

Common emotions may be grief or anger. In either case, cultural, family or personality factors may have inhibited appropriate emotional expression. Emotional reactions to stress can become a major problem in their own right. Unexpressed anger, often showing itself as sulking, withdrawn or generally negative behaviour, can have a profoundly destructive effect both on the patient and on his close relationships. Similarly, immobilisation by unexpressed grief may prevent someone from beginning to reorganise his life and fill the gaps caused by bereavement.

In each case the counsellor should judge whether it is appropriate to encourage the expression of feelings, as this tactic should not be used indiscriminately. There are instances when affect may be a feature of a seriously disturbed mental state such as an agitated depression or morbid jealousy, where encouraging further expression is likely to aggravate rather than help the problem. But in general, if feelings are perceived by the counsellor as an understandable reaction to the stress and have not been appropriately or sufficiently ventilated, then their expression is likely to be beneficial.

The counsellor can facilitate the expression of affect by first acknowledging its existence, then encouraging or giving permission for the patient to talk about and express feelings. Facilitating the expression of feelings between a patient and his close relatives may also be useful.

The therapist, whilst showing appropriate understanding and empathy for the patient's emotions, must at the same time strive to remain reasonably calm himself, thus encouraging the patient to trust him and have confidence that it is safe to allow such cathartic ventilation of his feelings.

Reflection, clarification and reassurance

Having listened attentively and empathically to the patient's outline of his problems and expression of feelings, the therapist should reflect back what he has heard, both to check that he has understood correctly and to allow the patient to hear his situation redefined by someone outside the problem. Most important, at this early stage, is to attempt to reassure and bolster the patient's self-esteem. This is often difficult when he is surrounded by failure and distress, but it is nevertheless often overlooked by counsellors. Assessment of the patient's past life, together with observations about his current behaviour during the counselling session, may provide the therapist with evidence of strengths and resources and past successes at coping that can be used as

reassurance. Relating to the patient in an adult–adult fashion will increase his self-respect and dignity but it may also be appropriate to use professional authority and experience of other people's problems to assert that the situation will improve and change over time.

By reorganising the patient's problem, aiding the cathartic expression of emotions and boosting morale, the counsellor should have calmed the patient sufficiently to be able to move on to the more cognitive problem-solving stages.

Facilitation of the patient's understanding of his problems and feelings

Whatever the cause, distress is much increased if an individual does not understand why the situation has come about. Aiding understanding is therefore therapeutic and distress-reducing in its own right, and also contributes to the identification of underlying problems and their possible solutions. Similarly, it may be important to point out that, as a result of the distress, the patient's coping mechanisms may have further worsened his basic situation. For example, turning to alcohol, tranquillisers, overeating or violence may have exacerbated the original problem of loss, conflict or change.

Other defence mechanisms may have been used, such as regression (resorting to behaviours learnt at an earlier stage of development) or denial when by an unconscious distortion the problem is no longer seen to be important. Such behaviour succeeds only in postponing a solution and often aggravates the problem it is attempting to avoid. Some individuals, concluding that nothing effective or useful can be done, develop a state of inertia. Such a state of hopelessness inhibits the patient from attempting to cope appropriately. This is the essence of depression and needs psychiatric assessment, which will be discussed later. Others may overwork or show other forms of displacement to avoid facing their obvious distress. In presenting such interpretations the counsellor's role is primarily an educational one, reflecting back perceptions of the patient's current coping style.

Where appropriate, the patient's insight may be further strengthened by examining precipitating factors and their meaning to the patient, for example earlier experiences which have left the individual more vulnerable (e.g. childhood bereavement), current family dynamics and psychosocial circumstances, and factors that may be maintaining the problem (e.g. 'secondary gain'). The patient should be encouraged to examine powerful beliefs and attitudes which may be destructive.

Even if external circumstances cannot be changed, perceptions and internal reactions can be altered, e.g. a person can stop judging themselves harshly, face fear, and learn to accept themselves as they are.

Facilitating problem-solving behaviour

This is a fundamental aspect of counselling for which the adult–adult nature of the counselling relationship is crucial. Problem-solving and the associated decision-making should be done by the patient, not the counsellor, although the counsellor can take an active part in the process.

Common sense steps towards solving problems are:

1. Identify the problem; helping the patient to define the problems appropriately (i.e. in terms that suggest realistic methods of resolution)
2. Identify alternative or new methods of coping with that problem; suggesting additional methods of coping not considered by the patient, i.e. adding to the list of alternatives
3. Cognitively rehearse each alternative and think realistically through its practical implications
4. Choose one alternative to follow, reminding the patient of his strengths and weaknesses so that he will more clearly see which alternative is likely to succeed
5. Define the behavioural steps required to carry out that alternative; helping the patient to break down the chosen method of coping into small manageable steps
6. Carry out these steps one by one; negotiating a 'behavioural contract' with the patient, i.e. getting his agreement and commitment to carry out the steps in a specified sequence and helping him to check the effectiveness or otherwise of his endeavours.
7. Check the consequences to ensure that the choice of alternative has been a suitable one.

Goldfried & Goldfried (1975) pointed out that 'there may exist many good problem-solvers who do not utilise the exact seven-step process (but) the essential point is that poor problem-solvers can be taught to increase the effectiveness of their decision-making process by following this strategy'. It should also be pointed out that choosing from the alternatives does not necessarily follow logically from these steps; it may still be an intuitive process. But the ability to 'feel' the right choice is often enhanced by going through these preliminary stages.

There is also scope for the use of more psychotherapeutic skills. By setting behavioural goals in this way and by analysing in detail the difficulties that the patient has in carrying them out, the counsellor can effectively and quickly identify key attitudes, resistances or defence mechanisms serving to obstruct the behaviour. Various types of psychotherapeutic strategy can then be used to help the patient overcome these resistances, but these are beyond the scope of this chapter.

Other tactics

There are two other things that the counsellor can do which deserve consideration. These are 'giving expert advice' and prescribing psychotropic drugs. We mention these reluctantly because they are often in the forefront of the medically trained counsellor's mind and are more likely to need discouragement than encouragement. Obviously there are occasions when it is appropriate for the doctor to use both of these tactics. But it is seldom so in counselling. There may, of course, be a need for specialist advice, which may be medical, legal or financial. It is usually preferable, however, for this advice to come from some specialist agency which is not involved in the counselling process. In this way, the giving of such advice will not complicate the adult–adult relationship that the counsellor needs and it can be given much more on a 'take it or leave it' basis, without undermining the patient's need to take responsibility for his decisions and action. If in spite of this the counsellor decides to offer advice of this kind then it is important to have considered the consequences first.

When psychotropic drugs are combined with counselling, it becomes necessary to counteract the implication that 'prescription of drugs' equals 'illness' and hence transfer of responsibility to the therapist (see below). It thus needs to be stressed that drugs are being used only as an adjunct to other methods, and as an aid to the patient's own problem-solving efforts. Indications for medication in such circumstances can be summarised briefly as follows:

1. To lower arousal in a patient where it is seriously impairing his ability to adopt problem-solving behaviour or make decisions, and where psychological methods have failed. The aim of such medication, usually a minor tranquilliser, is to reduce arousal only to the point at which effective coping behaviour can be resumed. Such use should be short term or intermittent to avoid risks of dependency.

2. To elevate mood in a patient whose depression is of such severity that he is unable to initiate or carry out any problem-solving behaviour. He is, in other words, immobilised by inertia. The antidepressant

should be prescribed to improve mood sufficiently to allow the patient to participate actively in problem-solving and it should be stressed that the drug is not intended or expected to solve the basic problems.

3. To improve a patient's sleep. Insomnia needs special attention because of its powerful effect in impairing coping. Again, care must be taken to avoid the development of dependency and such drugs should be taken only intermittently (e.g. only two or three nights in succession).

HIV COUNSELLING

Patients should never be tested for human immuno-deficiency virus (HIV) without giving their consent, or before pretest counselling. Some may be obsessionally preoccupied with HIV infection, when frequent testing may be unhelpful and psychiatric intervention more relevant.

The counsellor needs to assess the degree of risk, how the patient will feel about either result, whom they would tell and what implications it would have for their life.

Pretest counselling enables the patient to make an informed decision and offers opportunities for health education and can prepare a patient for a positive result. Advantages of testing include reassurance if the result is negative, improved treatment options if diagnosed positive early, help with decision-making if pregnant. Testing may be disadvantageous if the timing is emotionally bad, if the test might affect insurance or mortgage, or if the risk behaviour occurred in the last 3 months.

PATIENT–THERAPIST CONSIDERATIONS IN COUNSELLING

In order to maximise the counselling relationship, the counsellor uses both empathy and awareness of his own feelings to understand what is involved with the patient's experiences and to formulate his problems effectively. But it is important that the counsellor is cautious about over-identification with the patient's problems, particularly if he has experienced similar conflicts or losses himself. Should his own vulner-abilities become uppermost, the therapist may with-draw from the patient to deal with his own anxiety or may feel a need to take control, especially if the patient provokes feelings of anger or helplessness in the therapist. By being sensitive to their own reactions, therapists can not only avoid these pitfalls, but also avoid being judgemental or taking sides in joint or family counselling. Dealing with feelings of impotence and inadequacy are crucial. Many counselling cases concern bereavement or other irretrievable losses, and the therapist must recognise that simply being able to listen sympathetically is far more therapeutic and helpful to a distressed patient than flight into seeking practical or concrete supports by a therapist needing to do something constructive.

Inexperienced counsellors often fail to give appropriate priority to the simple process of listening. They may also find silences difficult to tolerate, yet such pauses may be crucial, giving the patient both time to reflect within himself and permission to be less hurried with the interview. Many patients feel they must medicalise their problems if talking to a doctor, and many doctors collude with this to avoid their own anxiety and uncertainty how to proceed once the patient begins to reveal feelings rather than facts.

Counsellors should also be aware of colluding with dependency and taking control in the interview. It may make the counsellor feel better, but will not help the patient to cope more effectively. Similarly, prolonging the number of sessions of counselling reinforces the covert message that the patient is not yet able to cope alone. It is sometimes better to terminate a course of counselling earlier and leave 'open access' for further contact if necessary, perhaps expressing confidence in the patient's new coping skills and recognising that he is en route to solutions, rather than has reached his final goal. In other circumstances patients may need to be encouraged to continue contact over a period of time. For example, a relative of a slowly dying person may need such regular contact with the counsellor, as well as the reassurance that it is sensible and responsible to share his problems with someone.

Involvement with other agencies may also be encouraged, e.g. self-help groups, voluntary agencies such as gay organisations, Cruse for the recently bereaved and Women's Aid. Often working in tandem with such an organisation is helpful for the patient, confirming that the problem is not simply medical.

Finally, from the counsellor's point of view, being available and listening sympathetically to other people's distress can itself be distressing. The potential for build-up of tension is considerable and it is important that counsellors themselves can gain support and cathartic ventilation of their feelings by sharing some of their anxieties about their counselling with a supportive person or group.

CRISIS INTERVENTION

Crises occur when people are faced with problems which for them are insurmountable by ordinary methods of coping. Abortive attempts to overcome the problems lead to a state of disorganisation and distress, further undermining the individual's ability to cope. Unless some new problem-solving approach is used, the situation is likely to get progressively worse. Such a novel or changed approach may involve help from other people and that is what is meant by crisis intervention. The basic counselling skills that we have already described play a crucial part in such intervention, but there is an additional and special need in these circumstances to decide whether, before such counselling is offered, a phase of taking over responsibility for the patient is required. As we shall see this phase requires a fundamentally different approach, and the judgement of which course to follow initially presents us with some of the most difficult decisions in crisis intervention.

First let us look more closely at what we mean by crisis and the factors that may lead to it. A basic concept is that 'decompensation' occurs when a person in crisis is overwhelmed. Caplan (1961) described four phases of crisis.

The phases of crisis

Phase 1. Arousal and attempts at problem-solving increase.

Phase 2. Arousal or 'tension' increases further with some impairment of function and resulting disorganisation and distress. Whereas some arousal is necessary for effective coping, if excessive it hinders rather than promotes coping behaviour; the subject becomes too anxious or angry, and too aroused to sleep properly so that fatigue adds to the problem.

Phase 3. Emergency steps are taken and novel methods of coping are tried.

Phase 4. Continuing failure to resolve the problem leads to a state of progressive deterioration, exhaustion and *decompensation* — a vicious spiral downwards.

There are a variety of reasons why attempting to cope sometimes fails. The problems may simply be too great, too numerous or too unfamiliar. The individual may have limited coping resources which are overwhelmed. Such limitations may be constitutional or reflect some temporary or recent factor such as physical illness or ageing. Support that is usually available from family or friends may be lacking at a particularly crucial time.

It is particularly when we are confronted with the affect that accompanies crisis that we find ourselves considering the role of psychiatric factors. For many people in crisis, emotional reactions such as fear, anger or grief are understandable given their circumstances. But in some cases, not only the intensity but also the form of the emotional reaction is incomprehensible and cannot be accounted for by the circumstances. It is then that we consider the possibility of a psychotic illness, possibly triggered by some traumatic experience. Sometimes what initially appears to be incomprehensible becomes less so as we gain further insight into the individual's personality and the special significance of the circumstances to him. But in any case, in between these two extremes of understandable and non-understandable emotional reactions, we have a 'grey area' where it is difficult to judge the appropriateness of the affective response. We may consider the possibility of emotional over-reactivity, sometimes known as neurotic disposition, which can push what should be a manageable problem into a crisis. Such over-reactivity may be of a general kind, or specifically involve certain kinds of threat when a person has been 'sensitised' by earlier experiences of a specific nature. Appraising such factors is seldom easy and usually takes time, not only for getting to know the patient better but also for obtaining information from other sources or informants. Unfortunately there is a tendency for many psychiatrists to reach premature conclusions in deeming the emotional reaction to be psychologically inappropriate and hence indicative of psychiatric illness. This often leads to pharmacological methods of treatment which, for reasons that have already been discussed, further confound the issue. Although in many cases it may be somewhat arbitrary whether the condition is regarded as a psychiatric illness in diagnostic terms, the implications of using the 'illness' label are considerable, as we shall see, and should always be taken into consideration.

Initial assessment

Obviously the initial contact with someone presenting in crisis is used first for assessment. This aims to establish as clearly as possible what recent events have affected the person and in particular those that have persuaded him to seek help. A detailed enquiry of what has been happening in the previous 2 or 3 days can be very informative. This usually points to the principal current problems, though it may be some time before their precise nature or full extent are recognised. It is important to identify what demands the person is facing at this time and what practical steps he is required to take. Throughout the interview, attention should be paid to the person's mental state; the presence of suicidal ideas, the degree of anxiety, agitation or distress, and in particular whether he is capable of carrying out the practical steps that are immediately called for. An assessment should also be made of the support that the patient can obtain from family or friends and whether the home situation is helpful or supportive. But in addition to establishing more about the background and development of the *current* problems, it is also necessary to determine how the person has coped with problems in the past. This may have to wait until his mental state permits or until another informant can be interviewed.

The patient–therapist relationship

Faced with a person in crisis one of the first decisions that the therapist should make is whether there is evidence of 'decompensation' that requires responsibility for the patient's affairs temporarily to be taken over. If so, then a form of crisis intervention is required which we call *intensive care*; care because the patient has to be looked after for a short time and intensive because he will require concentrated personal contact during that time. If such taking over is not necessary or appropriate, then counselling of the kind already described may be offered. The distinction between these two types of help is crucial and concerns the nature of the patient–therapist relationship. Using the concepts of transactional analysis, the relationship involved in intensive care is comparable to that between parent and child or doctor and sick patient. That involved in counselling, as we have already emphasised, is between adult and adult. Even when intensive care is indicated, however, it does not necessarily follow that the patient should be treated or encouraged to see himself as sick. The concept of the 'sick role' was formulated by Talcott Parsons (1951), who pointed out that in our society the 'ill' person is not held responsible for his incapacity and, even more important, is exempted from responsibility for his normal obligations, on the understanding that he seeks appropriate medical help and places himself in a position of dependency on others. But the term 'sick' or 'ill' also implies that the person's state results from a morbid or pathological process. A person in crisis may have been overcome by 'natural disasters' or, simply lacking adequate coping resources, overwhelmed by circumstances that would have been met by most people. Do we in such cases want to encourage a 'sick' role? On occasions the answer is a clear 'yes' because the illness label serves to protect the individual's self-esteem, or allows him to hand over responsibility when he would otherwise insist on retaining it. In other cases, the answer is no because it may discourage the individual from seeking out and learning new coping skills that would place him in better stead to handle similar stresses in the future.

Unfortunately, most psychiatrists receive little training in the concept of illness, except as a diagnostic category whose function has more to do with classification than management. The clinical significance of the illness label is often overlooked, or alternatively more attention is paid to the implications for the psychiatrist than for the patient, e.g. 'if this patient is not psychiatrically ill, I have no business to be treating him'. We believe that proper consideration of the use of the 'illness' label is as important in clinical management as distinguishing between one psychiatric condition and another.

Thus, the early decision which should be reached by the end of the initial assessment is in two parts. First, is this person in or about to be in a decompensated state requiring urgent intervention and intensive care, or can counselling begin straight away? And, secondly, is it appropriate or helpful to label him ill? These important decisions are based on clinical judgement. This is made difficult by the fact that some individuals present themselves in a state of decompensation as a regressive method of coping. It may be difficult to recognise with confidence that this is the case unless one has knowledge of the individual's past history or evidence that he has reacted similarly on previous occasions.

Intensive care

The objective in intensive care is to reverse the patient's decompensation by lowering the level of distress, restoring him to a more normal coping state as quickly as possible so that he can resume some responsibility and the counselling process can begin. The following steps are therefore taken:

1. *Responsibility is explicitly transferred.* The patient is told that, for a short time, his normal responsibilities and obligations will be taken over by others and that he should allow himself to be taken care of. Whether this is justified to him on grounds of illness is decided at this time, after carefully considering the implications of doing so.

2. *The immediate tasks of this take-over are organised.* The therapist should ensure that the patient's current obligations are not only dealt with but are seen to be so by the patient. Children may need to be sent to relatives or taken into care, employers contacted, houses locked, pets fed. Some task which may seem very trivial to the therapist may be of particular importance to the patient and should be dealt with

appropriately. The help of family and friends is mobilised as far as possible, though social services, and community agencies may need to be involved.

3. *The patient is removed from a stressful environment.* This is not always necessary and depends on the extent of support that can be expected from the immediate family and whether the patient's home environment is aggravating the problems. Staying with friends or relatives may suffice. Admission to a hospital or a crisis unit is a further alternative which permits closer and continuing contact with the therapist and hence facilitates the objectives listed below. Admission to a psychiatric hospital can produce its own problems, however, and these will be discussed further (see below)

4. *Arousal and distress are lowered.* Commonly the patient in need of intensive care is distressed, over-aroused and often exhausted. Whenever possible, this should be dealt with psychologically, which involves spending time in the presence of and talking to the patient in a reassuring and concerned manner. Psychotropic drugs have a place, particularly if arousal is very high and unresponsive to psychological methods, and also to ensure adequate sleep.

5. *Appropriate communication is reinforced.* The patient in severe crisis may present as exhausted or distressed, as described above, or less often in a state of shock, perhaps of sudden onset, becoming almost mute and immobile. In either case, an important objective is to re-establish normal communication: to reinforce any normal and relevant conversation by paying more attention to it and to discourage agitated, perseverative or non-communicative forms of behaviour by ignoring them.

6. *Concern and warmth are shown and hope is encouraged.* Underlying the two previous tactics is a need to convey to the patient that the therapist cares, to demonstrate empathy, and to instil hope for a positive resolution of the crisis.

The crisis counselling phase

The key difference between intensive care and counselling in crisis is that in the latter the patient is not being treated as sick or dependent but as an adult with problems who is asking for help. This may be the situation from the outset or it may become so as the person emerges from the state of decompensation, able to resume responsibility for his own affairs. Obviously this transition is a gradual process. The person who breaks a leg needs the 'sick role' to allow healing to occur, as well as the expertise of the medical and nursing professions. After a time,

responsibility is gradually handed back to the patient, who during recovery is no longer 'sick' but expected to take on responsibility for his active rehabilitation. Unfortunately, this transfer of responsibility from the patient and back again is seldom made explicit, and for reasons that we have already mentioned, often not even recognised by either the patient or doctor. Consequently, it not infrequently goes wrong. The sick role is accepted for too long by both doctor and patient, or the latter remains in that role whilst the doctor is acting as if he had left it. It is therefore necessary to be explicit, not only about the take-over of responsibility during intensive care, but also about its being handed back, whether it is done gradually or not. The principles of counselling then to be used have been outlined in the first half of the chapter.

The settings for crisis intervention and counselling

As emphasised earlier, help-giving is not confined to the professional. Intensive care can be provided by a caring neighbour, counselling by a good friend. But these basic principles are, we believe, just as appropriate for the professional and can be applied in a wide variety of settings. One of the main constraints is the limitation of time. Thus, working with patients in their own homes may have particular advantages in some cases, but is expensive in time by comparison with hospital-based help (Hawton et al 1981). In some circumstances, e.g. with family crises, these costs may be justified.

The provision of intensive care often requires special resources. Mobilisation of family and friends will often suffice and be most appropriate, but this is not always possible or desirable. For the psychiatrist, the use of psychiatric in-patient or day patient facilities is an obvious alternative but careful consideration is required to ensure that the advantages are not outweighed by the disadvantages. Most psychiatric hospitals are not oriented to brief admissions. Patients, once admitted, are expected to stay for several weeks and the tempo of intervention is geared accordingly, often with early resort to pharmacological methods. It is therefore difficult to avoid the 'illness label' in these circumstances, or to move readily from it to the 'responsible adult' when the time comes. Also, the 'psychiatric label' may produce undesirable consequences in the patient's peer group or social environment.

These more traditional uses of hospitalisation are being increasingly challenged (Braun et al 1981) and Kennedy & Hird (1980) recently demonstrated the advantages of an in-patient regime geared to short stays. But as yet such changes in psychiatric and nursing practice are not widespread. For this reason, units specifically designed to deal with patients in crisis are of special interest. Cooper (1979) visited a number of such units in Europe and reviewed their activities. They varied from those which were hardly distinguishable from traditional psychiatric wards to those which were clearly designed to provide the type of intensive care and counselling described in this chapter. The Amsterdam Crisis Centre is probably the best example of the latter. In summarising his impressions, Cooper commented on the relative shortage of people who fitted neatly into the stereotype of the person in crisis, i.e. the previously well-adjusted person needing help at the point of crisis, and showing the discrete phases of crisis before returning to normal adjustment. That is not to say, of course, that such people do not occur, but rather that they seldom seek or need help from such agencies. Those who do are more likely to have a chronic personality problem and to experience repeated crises, often of their own making. The 'attempted suicide' population is a good cross-section of such people.

Nevertheless the rapid action, problem definition, short-term planning and emphasis on the 'here and now' that characterises crisis intervention was found to be effective and appropriate, or the only approach suitable for a rapid turnover of patients. It is, however, of particular importance to control problems of dependence in such settings, which is why we have laid so much emphasis in this chapter on the distinction between intensive care and crisis counselling.

Most units using such an approach involve multidisciplinary teams and the following components were commonly observed by Cooper (1979):

1. Frequent meetings of the multidisciplinary teams; two a day is a common frequency with additional contacts between team members or subteams between the regular meetings.

2. Frequent interviews and contacts by individual team members with patients, their families and outside agencies between the team meetings. Again, more than once a day is not uncommon.

3. Rapid decision-making on the basis of early accessible information about the current situation. Case records are correspondingly brief, in contrast to more traditional psychiatric history taking with its extensive notes.

4. Responsibility is usually shared and conventional professional roles become blurred or overlapping.

5. A rapid turnover of patients and a correspondingly short period of involvement and follow-up. The initial intense involvement is often just a few days, with less frequent contact spreading over a few weeks before contact ceases.

As yet, attempts to evaluate the methods of intervention described in this chapter have been extremely limited (e.g. Catalan et al 1980, Hawton et al 1981). Although there are no grounds for believing that such approaches provide a panacea for all problems, we believe that their careful use, evaluation and subsequent modification will not only benefit many people in crisis but will have a salutary effect on the mainstream of psychiatric care.

REFERENCES

Bancroft J, Skrimshire A, Casson J, Harvard-Watts O, Reynolds F 1977 People who deliberately poison or injure themselves: their problems and their contacts with helping agencies. Psychological Medicine 7: 289

Braun P, Kochansky G, Shapiro R et al 1981 Overview: deinstitutionalisation of psychiatric patients, a critical review of outcome studies. American Journal of Psychiatry 138: 736

Brown G W, Bhrolchain M N, Harris T 1975 Social class and psychiatric disturbances among women in an urban population. Sociology 9: 255

Caplan G 1961 An approach to community mental health. Tavistock, London

Catalan J, Marsack P, Hawton K E, Whitwell D, Fagg J, Bancroft J 1980 Comparison of doctors and nurses in the assessment of deliberate self-poisoning patients. Psychological Medicine 10: 483

Cooper J E 1979 Crisis admission units and emergency psychiatric services. Public health in Europe 11. WHO Regional Office for Europe, Copenhagen

Erikson E H 1969 Childhood and society. Penguin, Harmondsworth

Goldfried M R, Goldfried A P 1975 Cognitive change methods. In: Kanfer F R, Goldstein A P (eds) Helping people change. Pergamon Press, New York

Hawton K, Bancroft J, Catalan J, Kingston B, Stedeford A, Welch N 1981 Domiciliary and out-patient treatment of self-poisoning patients by medical and non-medical staff. Psychological Medicine 11: 169

Kennedy P, Hird F 1980 Description and evaluation of a short-stay admission ward. British Journal of Psychiatry 136: 205

Lindemann E 1944 Symptomatology and management of acute grief. American Journal of Psychiatry 101: 101

Parkes C M 1975 Bereavement: studies of grief in adult life. Penguin, Harmondsworth

Parsons T 1951 The social system. Free Press, Glencoe

39. Interpretative psychotherapies

A. W. Clare

INTRODUCTION

The roots of modern psychotherapy lie buried deep in primitive medicine, shamanism, religion, faith-healing and hypnotism. As Ellenberger's magisterial work on the history of dynamic psychiatry has reminded us, historical and anthropological research have brought forth important documents and revealed evidence of the use among primitive people of many of the methods used by modern psychotherapy (Ellenberger 1970). However, it was not until the middle of the 18th century, with the emergence of Mesmer's theories on animal magnetism, that the interpersonal relationship was made the subject of scientific investigation. Mesmer attributed his influence upon his patient's mental state to a physical fluid filling the universe and forming a connecting medium between man, the earth and the heavenly bodies, an explanation favoured to a less dogmatic degree by the Marquis de Puysegur, who in 1784 discovered that he could induce a somnabulistic state during which a genuine dialogue between doctor and patient could be established. In the middle of the 19th century, James Braid, a Manchester surgeon, introduced the term 'hypnosis', which he saw as a purely mechanical process occurring in the brain, and dismissed psychological explanations, but by this time the notion of the unconscious had become well established. Over the latter half of the 19th century, the works of Charcot, Bernheim and Janet introduced the concepts of unconscious motivation to psychiatry and psychology and Freud developed the notion of the unconscious as part of an overall description of 'mental layers' or 'provinces' of the mind.

But it was Freud's theory of the *transference* which changed the direction of thinking concerning unconscious processes, hypnotism and the manipulation of physical and psychological distress by psychological means. Freud himself related how he became aware of what he saw to be the libidinal character of the hypnotic relationship:

And one day I had an experience which showed me in the crudest light what I had long suspected. It related to one of the most acquiescent patients, with whom hypnotism had enabled me to bring about the most marvellous results, and whom I was engaged in relieving of her suffering by tracing back her attacks of pain to their origins. As she woke up on one occasion, she threw her arms round my neck. The unexpected entrance of a servant relieved us from a painful discussion, but from that time onward there was a tacit understanding between us that the hypnotic treatment should be discontinued. I was modest enough not to attribute the event to my own irresistible personal attraction and I felt that I had now grasped the nature of the mysterious element that was at work behind hypnotism. In order to exclude it, or at all events to isolate it, it was necessary to abandon hypnotism (Freud 1925)

For Freud, suggestion worked by virtue of the influencing of a person by means of the so-called transference. It is the transference, or more accurately its recognition and the subjecting of it to the analytical working-through and verbalisation, that forms the very essence of psychoanalysis. By means of the transference, the patient transfers his past emotional attachments, usually involving parental and sibling figures, to the psychoanalyst. The analyst becomes a substitute for the parental figure. Transference may be either positive or negative; in positive transference, the patient loves the analyst and wishes to obtain love and satisfaction from him, whereas in negative transference the patient views the analyst as unfair, unloving, rejecting. Interpretations of transference make the patient aware of the fact that his infatuation with the analyst is not related to the analyst as a person but is simply a reflection of previous emotional entanglements. Interpretation is necessary for modification of behaviour. In the psychoanalytic situation, regression to childhood is necessary for the resolution of conflicts rooted in the past. Thus, Otto Kernberg and his colleagues in their final report on the Menninger Foundation's Psychotherapy Research Project provided the following terse yet comprehensive definition of psychoanalysis as: 'a technique employed by a neutral analyst resulting in the development of a regressive transference neurosis. The ultimate resolution of this neurosis is achieved by techniques of interpretation alone' (Kernberg et al 1972).

It is traditional to regard Freud as the father of modern psychotherapy and classical psychoanalysis as the pure, undiluted, most demanding and most complicated of the many forms that have developed in this century. However, whereas there is in general agreement as to what constitutes psychoanalysis, whether it be of the Freudian, Jungian, Kleinian or Adlerian persuasion, there is much less consistency when it comes to arriving at an acceptable definition of psychotherapy itself. The term is loosely employed to mean helping, treating, advising, guiding, reassuring, educating and even influencing. Contemporary definitions lay particular emphasis on the general relief of suffering through psychological means (Frank 1978), employed by a trained professional (Strupp 1978), involving the setting up in a deliberate fashion of a relationship between therapist and patient (Wolberg 1977) and primarily employing the use of words (Storr 1979). Such key elements come together in the definition of psychotherapy proposed by Meltzoff & Kornreich (1970) as:

the informed and planful application of techniques derived from established psychological principles, by persons qualified through training and experience to understand these principles and to apply these techniques with the intention of assisting individuals to modify such personal characteristics as feeling, values, attitudes and behaviours which are judged by the therapist to be maladaptive.

TYPES OF PSYCHOTHERAPY

Features which appear common to all forms of psychotherapy include: (1) an intense, confiding relationship, which is (2) occurring in a healing setting, (3) is founded on some rationale of therapy and (4) involves a therapeutic procedure. Wolberg (1977) grouped the psychotherapies into those which provide support, guidance, advice and reassurance — the *supportive psychotherapies*, those which attempt to teach the individual new patterns of behaviour and social functioning — the *re-educational psychotherapies*, and those which aim to dismantle and rebuild a new personality — the *reconstructive psychotherapies*. A modified schema of this classification is shown in Table 39.1.

Supportive

This form of psychotherapy is as variously defined as it is widely used. Bloch (1978) describes it as a form

Table 39.1 Types of psychotherapy

Supportive	Re-educative	Reconstructive
Guidance	Behaviour therapy	Freudian analysis
Milieu therapy	Cognitive therapy	Kleinian analysis
Occupational therapy	Interpersonal therapy	Ego analysis
Music therapy	Client-centred therapy	Neo-Freudian therapy
Reassurance	Gestalt therapy	Adlerian therapy
Ventilation	Emotive release	Reichian analysis
	Psychodrama	Brief dynamic therapy
	Transactional analysis	

After Wolberg (1977).

of psychological treatment given to patients with chronic and disabling psychiatric conditions 'for whom basic change is not seen as a realistic goal'. This definition emphasises the notion of therapy as a prop or crutch and envisages the objectives of such an approach as the promotion of the patient's best possible psychological and social functioning, the bolstering of his self-esteem and self-confidence, the cultivation of the patient's sense of and contact with reality, the prevention of relapse and, in certain instances, the transfer of the source of support from professional to family or friends.

However, other definitions of supportive psychotherapy stress its role in enabling individuals to cope with and overcome psychological difficulties presenting more acutely. For example, a Royal College of General Practitioners' Report on prevention of psychiatric disorders in general practice (RCGP 1981) emphasised the importance of supportive intervention in enabling individuals to negotiate 'psychosocial transitions', i.e. particular life-events and challenges which produce psychological reactions, symptoms and disorders commonly seen in patients presenting to general practitioners, health visitors and social workers. The objectives of such supportive psychotherapy include the minimising of the impact of the threatening event, the provision of protection and relief from responsibilities during the crisis or transition, the encouragement of the expression of emotions and talking through the difficulties, and support for the individual in his attempts to seek out new directions in life.

Supportive psychotherapy is also conceived of as the use of psychological means to build individuals up to a point where they can devote themselves to more profound, time-consuming and complex reconstructive psychotherapeutic interventions and as a temporary expedient to contain individuals who are acutely ill and who are awaiting the therapeutic impact of other forms of psychiatric treatment, most notably pharmacological.

There is much more general agreement as to what constitute the key elements of the supportive forms of psychotherapy (Table 39.2). It is now recognised that the interview itself can exercise a psychotherapeutic effect — that the mere act of a doctor listening carefully to what the patient is saying, picking up verbal and non-verbal cues, and enabling the patient to give a full account of his situation and problems can result in a significant improvement. This realisation has led in turn to attempts to dissect out those characteristics of the interview which may exercise particularly beneficial effect. To date, the bulk of the effort has been directed at identifying interview techniques which facilitate case detection but the implications for the facilitation of therapy seem clear. Amongst the interview techniques which appear important are the therapist's ability to note verbal and non-verbal cues, to ask questions in a sequence from open to closed, to avoid using too many direct questions and to emphasise the importance of understanding the here-and-now situation (Marks et al 1979).

Reassurance provided by a therapist equipped to use the therapeutic relationship constructively, able to be both detached and compassionate, and skilled in listening and providing information simply and comprehensively is one of the basic elements of the supportive form of psychotherapy. Reassurance can be used to good effect to relieve fears, boost self-confidence and promote hope. But it is not without its problems. To promote a patient's hopes unreasonably by providing false reassurance, or to intervene prematurely before the patient has explained his situation fully, may be effective initially but will eventually prove useless. However, as Kessel has pointed out in a thoughtful essay on the subject, such a view reflects the perspective of the specialist psychotherapist concerned with the exploration rather than the alleviation of worry (Kessel 1979). The harmful effect of absolving a patient from his responsibilities and of getting between a patient and his recognition of underlying causes can be avoided once it is recognised.

Table 39.2 Elements of supportive psychotherapy

1. The interview
2. Reassurance
3. Explanation
4. Guidance and suggestion
5. Ventilation

Explanation is likewise an important element in psychotherapeutic support. Whereas reconstructive forms of psychotherapy emphasise non-directiveness, a degree of therapeutic passivity and active therapeutic interventions limited to the provision of interpretation, the supportive forms encourage the provision of explanations by the therapist of such diverse matters as the nature of the patient's symptoms, the choice of treatment, and the likely outcome. Explaining to a patient quite why certain symptoms are being experienced and the extent to which they are common can itself be reassuring and therapeutically effective. The goal is not so much deepening of self-understanding as enhancement of the patient's ability to cope by clarifying the nature of the problem faced, the symptoms experienced and/or the treatment recommended.

Guidance and suggestion involve the provision of direct and indirect advice. In general, therapists are encouraged to refrain from advising patients, yet in supportive therapy teaching a patient how and when to ask for help is often a crucial component. Advice may be necessary with regard to particular problems, such as optimal ways of relating to a particularly difficult relative or handling a job interview or to general issues such as making contact with members of the opposite sex. Occasionally advice is ineffective, and persuasion, involving the therapist in a more direct, controlling posture, is required. Suggestion involves the therapist using such techniques as the showing or withholding of approval in attempts to modify a patient's situation. Suggestion operates in all forms of psychotherapy and it has even been postulated that the suitability of an individual for treatment is dependent on his potential openness to the suggestive influence (Strupp 1978). Variables which appear to regulate the forcefulness of suggestion include the significance of the therapist to the patient, the degree to which the patient is or can become dependent and the depth of the patient's anxiety or depression. Individuals whose coping strategies have been overwhelmed are believed to be particularly prone to cling with desperation to any potential helping resource and to respond dramatically to proffered advice, reassurance and guidance.

In recent years, the value of *ventilation* of feelings within the psychotherapeutic setting has received support, and interest has been stimulated in the old notion of catharsis by the rise of the so-called 'emotive release (body) therapies' (see below). It does seem useful for patients to be able to express emotions such as anger, frustration and despair openly. Unfortunately, the amount and quality of emotional expression has rarely been assessed independently and related to outcome, so its value has received little direct experimental verification.

Supportive psychotherapy is widely used in psychiatric settings, in general practice and in settings in which patients with short-lived yet intense emotional crises are seen.

Re-educative

In these forms of psychotherapy deliberate efforts are made, aimed at readjustment, the modification of goals, the relearning of habits and unlearning of habits and attitudes without a direct effort being made to achieve insight into conscious or so-called unconscious conflicts. Such approaches involve an actual remodelling of the patient's attitudes and behaviour. There is less emphasis on searching for causes than on promoting new and more adaptive forms of behaviour. The objective is the modification of behaviour directly through positive and negative reinforcers, with deliberate efforts at environmental readjustment, the liberation of the patient's own creative potentialities and the promotion of self-development. A fundamental assumption made in these forms of psychotherapy is that if the individual can alter a significant pattern in his life he will derive an enhanced sense of self-mastery which will generalise over a wide spectrum of behaviour. Such therapy is in general conducted through, firstly, a variety of techniques aimed at reconditioning behaviour (the so-called behaviour and cognitive therapies) and, secondly, an examination by patient and therapist of ways in which the patient relates to people and to himself.

The various forms of behaviour therapy, group, marital and family therapy, are discussed elsewhere (see below and Chs 38, 40 and 41). In this chapter, some of the newer forms of psychotherapy, which emphasise re-education but which turn away from more orthodox notions derived from classical psychodynamic or behavioural theory, will be examined. These newer forms, while many and varied in form, tend to endorse a number of common assumptions and values. Ideas of self-love and self-acceptance are strongly favoured and are, in turn, derived from a somewhat overdeveloped notion of self-awareness.

The humanistic ideas of Abraham Maslow, Rollo May and Carl Rogers have been especially influential. Initially, client-centred approaches associated with Rogers were thought of as a mode of psychotherapy and were termed 'non-directive'. The term 'client' rather than 'patient' had been adopted to indicate that

this was not a manipulative nor a medically prescriptive model, and the term 'client-centred therapy' was adopted to emphasise the fact that the focus was on the internal phenomenological world of the client. By the end of the 1960s it was clear that this particular approach was not simply a mode of psychotherapy but was an approach attractive to educationalists, psychologists and pastoral workers.

The main characteristic of these newer forms of therapy are re-educative although supportive and even reconstructive elements can be detected, at least in some of the claims made on behalf of this or that approach. While there is a veritable miscellany of approaches, the majority have much in common. Accordingly, only the main therapies are discussed below.

Client-centred psychotherapy

Many of the new approaches to psychotherapy shamelessly borrow from the ideas of Carl Rogers. In the development of client-centred psychotherapy a number of characteristics have emerged which merit mention. The most important and distinctive element is the idea that certain attitudes in the therapist constitute the necessary and sufficient conditions of therapeutic effectiveness. The therapeutic process is marked by a change in the client's manner of experiencing with a corresponding increase in his ability to live more fully in the here-and-now. There is much emphasis on what is termed the *self-actualising* quality of the human organism as the motivational force in therapy and there is concern with the process of personality change rather than with the underlying structure of the personality itself.

Three conditions or attitudes are deemed to be most important for the success of client-centred therapy. First there is the therapist's *genuineness* or congruence, whereby what the therapist is experiencing at an affective or visceral level is clearly present in his awareness and is available for direct communication to his client when appropriate. In Roger's view, genuineness means that the therapist is *being himself*, not denying himself. The second primary attitude is the therapist's *caring*, that is to say his complete acceptance of or unconditional positive regard for his client. Rogers had used the term 'prizing' to convey the intensity of the therapeutic regard involved (Rogers 1978). The third important attitude is the therapist's ability, accurately and sensitively, to understand the experiences and feelings of the client and the meanings they have for him. This *empathy* refers to the therapist's ability to enter into the private, inner world of the client rather than merely understanding what he is saying.

Interpersonal psychotherapy

In the treatment study undertaken by the National Institute of Mental Health (NIMH), interpersonal psychotherapy was one of two forms of psychotherapy (the other was cognitive therapy) which were compared for efficacy in the treatment of depression with imipramine plus clinical management and placebo plus clinical management (Elkin et al 1989). Interpersonal psychotherapy has been designed by Gerald Klerman, Myrna Weissman and their colleagues in the New Haven–Boston Collaborative Depression Project. It differs from psychodynamic psychotherapy in that it is not interpretative and does not involve transference analysis. It differs from cognitive therapy because it does not utilise cognitive-behavioural strategies. Rather, it is based on the premise that depressed persons have difficulties in their social relationships. Depression may result from or aggravate these difficulties. Interpersonal psychotherapy is designed to help depressed persons to improve their social relationships and so reduce the depression.

In interpersonal psychotherapy there is little attempt to explore unconscious motivation. Instead of being preoccupied with early childhood experience therapy is focused unashamedly at the 'here-and-now'. The approach is practical rather than theoretical and a manual detailing procedures and strategies was published in 1984 (Klerman et al 1984).

In the NIMH depression study 250 patients were randomly allocated to each of the four treatment groups. Comparing the two psychotherapies with the placebo plus clinical management approach, there was limited evidence of the specific effectiveness of interpersonal psychotherapy and none for cognitive therapy. Significant differences among treatments were present only for the subgroup of patients who were more severely depressed and functionally impaired; here, there was some evidence of the effectiveness of interpersonal psychotherapy with these patients and strong evidence of the effectiveness of imipramine plus clinical management. In contrast there were no significant differences among treatments, including placebo plus clinical management, for the less severely depressed and functionally impaired patients. Earlier studies by the New Haven–Boston group have suggested that interpersonal psychotherapy plus antidepressant medication is more effective than either treatment alone in the treatment of depression (Weissman et al 1979).

Gestalt therapy

Fritz Perls popularised this approach during the latter part of his life when he was working as a therapist at the Esalen Institute in California. It draws on gestalt psychology, psychodrama, existentialism and psycho-analysis for its ideas. In addition to stressing the immediacy and importance of experience in the 'here-and-now', the approach emphasises psychological *homeostasis*, a concept which suggests a self-regulating balance between the human organism and its physical and social boundaries. Through the observation of an individual's gestures and bodily movements, gestalt therapists claim to discern aspects that reflect unconscious feelings. The object of therapy is to expand the patient's self-awareness, bring him into close contact with his bodily sensations and processes, and improve his relationship with the outside world.

As practised by Perls and orthodox gestalt practitioners, therapy is conducted in a group situation, although there is a 'hot seat', next to the therapist, which the group members occupy in sequence to work closely with him. Great stress is placed on the importance of understanding the body's wisdom by way of its posture, and its sensory, visceral, skeletal and muscular messages as well as by the content of its dreams. Acting out is encouraged and a variety of techniques to assist the ventilation of feelings, including techniques borrowed from psychodrama (see below), are used in the bringing about of the desired end state of therapy, namely the mature co-ordination of the human organism and the full assumption of responsibility by the individual for his own life. In therapy sessions, clients are encouraged to express unresolved feelings, assert views which hitherto have frightened or offended them, role-play and examine personal tendencies to detach, project, split, and deny feelings and attitudes. Gestalt techniques have been freely applied in many of the other new approaches to psychotherapy and in particular to what have been termed the emotive release therapies.

Emotive release (body) therapies

In recent years, gestalt approaches have been supplemented by a colourful variety of so-called emotive release therapies. At the heart of such approaches is the idea of *catharsis*, a notion which anticipated by many centuries the first systematic attempt by Breuer and Freud in the 1890s to turn it into a therapeutic procedure. The theory behind the so-called cathartic method was that neurosis develops as a consequence of some psychical trauma or traumas, evoking fright, shame, pain or anxiety in circumstances in which adequate discharge of the affect was impossible. This undischarged emotion could only be expressed covertly in the form of symptoms. Ultimately, cure could occur only through revival of the memory of the traumatic event and the release of the constrained emotion. The therapist's task, therefore, was to break down the patient's defence or resistance and facilitate the curative discharge of affect through abreaction.

Such ideas are to be found at the core of a miscellany of new approaches in psychotherapy ranging from body therapies such as Rolfing to primal therapy and psychodrama. Similar ideas are to be found in *bioenergetic therapy*, itself a modification of orthodox Reichian therapy (Reich 1942). Wilhelm Reich argued that body tension, and particularly muscular tension, represents actual emotional or psychic energy. The way we stand, walk, gesticulate and express ourselves facially reveals our underlying tensions and conflicts. Reich developed the idea of 'muscular armour' which in the form of chronically fixed muscular attitudes and physical rigidity shields us from an awareness of deeper sexual and emotional conflicts. By combinations of massage, breathing exercises, and postural manipulations, conscious awareness of painful vegetative sensations is said to occur, the flow of psychic energy is facilitated and health is restored. Newer developments place less emphasis on muscular manipulations by skilled therapists and more reliance on the client's own muscle activity exercises and verbalisations.

Psychodrama

A somewhat more sophisticated approach to the release of emotion which also makes therapeutic use of verbal exploration, suggestion and interpretation, and of experiential relieving of earlier traumatic experiences and events, is psychodrama. The elements that make up a psychodrama session are the 'director' or therapist, the protagonist or central subject of the psychodrama, the other 'players' or 'auxiliary egos', the audience and the stage (Moreno 1946). The protagonist is the group member who becomes the focus of the session and whose life provides the situations which are re-enacted. Auxiliary egos are other group members or trained assistants of the director who play roles in the protagonist's life. The audience may be patients, professional workers or even a family. After what is called a warm-up session in which the participants get to know each other a little, an incident is chosen and the protagonist takes the centre of the stage. For example, the protagonist

may complain that he has difficulty handling his boss. Psychodrama has a number of techniques whereby such a difficulty can be re-enacted, including role reversal, role substitution and the use of props.

Psychodramatic techniques and theories have given rise to a number of methods of role-playing which are currently being applied in education, industry and related fields. Psychodrama combines the experiential emphasis of the emotive release therapies with some of the learning theories of orthodox behavioural theory and the interpretative concepts of classical analysis. Role-playing of a less formal kind is also employed in family and marital therapy, with adolescents and in the treatment of social phobias and behavioural problems. Another form of therapy which has developed in recent years and which derives concepts from a number of theoretical positions is transactional analysis.

Transactional analysis

Transactional analysis was founded by Eric Berne (1964) who popularised it in a book entitled *Games People Play*. Whereas Freud divided mental functions into ego, id and superego, Berne took the ego and modified it in a striking fashion. Looking at people's behaviour (which for Berne was the ego), he noticed that sometimes people behave like children, sometimes like adults and sometimes like parents. In analysing interactions or transactions between people, it is necessary to know in which particular ego state the participants are located. What causes problems in life is a lack of congruence between the respective ego states of participants in interactions, i.e. if one participant is in an adult ego state whereas the other is rooted firmly in the role of a child when the appropriate relationship between the two is adult–adult or child–child. Some people go through life being pompous, overbearing 'parents', some are totally locked into an 'adult', rational way of being, while others travel through life as helpless 'children', always asking for things to be done for them that they could well do for themselves.

In therapy, these three ego states are explored and interpreted to the client in individual or group therapy. The traditional defences employed by the client to justify his use of child and parent states as adult states are explored, so that ultimately the adult becomes stronger and displaces the child and the parent from all situations save for those relatively few ones in which they remain appropriate.

Another important idea in transactional analysis is the notion that we are motivated in our daily lives by a desire for physical and mental stimulation of various kinds, so-called 'strokes'. A stroke is defined as a unit of social interaction and there are positive and negative varieties. A positive stroke is basically a loving, supportive statement, whereas a negative stroke is hateful and critical. People seek strokes and if they cannot obtain positive ones they will settle for the negative variety in preference to none at all. In order to obtain the desired amount of strokes, people engage in repetitive and recurrent patterns of behaviour or 'games'. Berne defines a game as a sequence of transactions with an ulterior motive and a 'pay-off'.

Transactional analysis is an attractive therapy with a sharp, gritty style, a blunt, abrasive approach, and a striking ability to make people take a fresh look at the way they manipulate each other. However, the extent to which it produces results superior to more orthodox forms of therapy in the wide variety of conditions and problems for which it is offered by its practitioners as the definitive therapy is questionable.

A number of the newer therapies do not possess a well-defined theoretical framework but function as loose mixtures of analytical concepts, gestalt theories and psychodramatic techniques spiced with philosophical speculations, often of an eastern, semi-mystical kind. The respective contributions of medicine, religion, mysticism and magic, which are present in most forms of psychotherapy, alter in importance as one moves along the road from the classical forms to the more unorthodox. Thus, for example, the charismatic appeal of the therapist, disregarded in classical Freudian analysis save as an aspect of the transference relationship, becomes a central tenet in Rogerian psychotherapy and dominates the relationship in the more dramatic emotive release approaches. Then again, whereas classical analysis rests on a substantial foundation of complex theory and demands from its practitioners an extensive training and time-consuming exposure to its ideas, the newer therapies represent a shift away from the notions of knowledge and expertise and towards a belief in the value of immediacy, non-rational experience and instinctive feelings. There is also the question of the doubtful applicability of some of the newer approaches to mental disorders such as the psychoses and the more severe forms of neurosis.

The *efficacy* of psychotherapy is discussed below but here it is worth emphasising the difficulty of evaluating the claims of such approaches posed by the shift away from notions of treatment and cure to ideas of self-growth, increased awareness and transformation. Asking the question: 'Do these approaches work?' seems as appropriate as trying to evaluate prayer or the effectiveness of good works. There is a fairly extensive literature which supports the Rogerian view of the importance of empathy, genuineness and caring in the therapist (Truax & Carkhuff 1967) but it is still far from clear whether such attributes are sufficient in their own right or are merely supplementary to additional attributes such as professional skill, theoretical knowledge and specific techniques. The more demanding the problem, be it schizophrenia or a highly disorganised family relationship, the more impotent such attributes on their own appear to be.

Reconstructive

The ultimate goal of the reconstructive forms of psychotherapy is to reduce the force of irrational impulses and strivings and bring them under control and to increase the range and flexibility of the various forms of psychological defences. Most forms of reconstructive psychotherapy are rooted in the theoretical framework of a constitutional–dynamic model of personality. This holds that past negative experiences and conditionings have retarded the normal psychological processes of development and serve in adult life to promote immature impulses and desires resulting in conflict between reality and the patient's own system of ideals, values and standards. The resulting tensions, feelings of helplessness and depression, and expectations of failure in turn invoke protective mechanisms, the commonest being *repression*, by means of which an unacceptable idea, impulse or memory is sealed within the unconscious. However, such repression rarely succeeds and the filtering of the repressed idea into conscious life provokes episodes of anxiety and other symptoms. Reactions develop which are opposed to judgement and mature common sense and the individual, while assuming that he is acting as an adult, behaves emotionally as a child. Other defence mechanisms employed include projection, reaction formation, and introjection.

To undertake reconstructive psychotherapy, the therapist must have received special training, which usually includes a personal psychoanalysis and the successful treatment of a number of patients under the supervision of an experienced psychoanalyst. There are four main types of psychotherapy with reconstructive goals, namely Freudian analysis, ego analysis, neo-Freudian analysis and psychoanalytically oriented psychotherapy. While all of these aim at reconstruction, they differ in their methods. Freudian psychoanalysis is, with some modifications, the original technique of Sigmund Freud. Ego analysis retains the classical therapeutic form but focuses on the adaptive functions of the ego. Neo-Freudian psychoanalysis includes the approaches of Rank, Jung, Adler, Horney and Sullivan, and is a modified and active technique. Psychoanalytically oriented psychotherapy derives its theoretical foundation from classical analysis but utilises supportive and re-educative approaches in active therapy.

Psychoanalysis

The key defining concepts of the form of psychological treatment elaborated by Freud in the 1890s are: (1) *free association*, which replaced hypnosis; (2) *interpretation*, which replaced suggestion, and (3) *transference*. Psychoanalytical technique consists essentially in instructing and helping the patient to associate freely, in interpreting both his association and the obstacles encountered by the analysis and as he tries to associate, and in interpreting the analysand's feelings and attitudes towards the analyst. The therapy rests on the psychological theories of the origin of the neuroses and of general mental development formulated by Freud and his followers. Crucial concepts in Freudian theory are: (1) *the unconscious*, the idea that there exists mental activity of which the subject is unaware but which nonetheless exerts a dynamic effect on his behaviour; (2) *resistance*, the idea that consciousness resists the emergence of unconscious tendencies into consciousness and does so by the use of defence mechanisms; and (3) *transference*.

In addition, Freud postulated that the mind can be conceptualised as a psychic apparatus in three parts, namely the *id*, which contains unorganised, unconscious instinctual impulses; the *ego*, which is that part of id which has been modified by the direct influence of the outside world and represents rationality, and the *superego*, which is part of the ego from which self-criticism, self-control, self-hatred and self-recrimination arise. Freudian theory envisages the ego using various defence mechanisms to control the impulses of the id unacceptable to the superego.

Jung's divergence from Freud was due in part to the former's idea of neurosis as a one-sided development of the individual and to the Jungian concept that the unconscious compensated for this imbalance. For Jung, neurotic symptoms were not always residues of childhood experience as Freud insisted but could be understood as attempts on the part of the mind to correct its own lack of balance. In Jung's view, the search for balance, integration and wholeness characterises the second half of life and, not surprisingly, it is in dealing with the problems of older people that Jungian psychoanalysis has been most involved.

Jungian therapy often is concerned with successful people who do not fall into the categories of conventional illness but who complain that life possesses no meaning. In such circumstances, Jungian therapy overlaps with so-called existential therapy and frank pastoral counselling.

Jungian therapy emphasises the value of patients pursuing the products of unconscious fantasy through dreams, reveries, and artistic creativity. In the course of analysis, patients encounter various typical 'primordial' images or *archetypes*, which are familiar in myth, fable and fairy stories. In order to attain balance and integration, the individual must recognise and differentiate himself from the immensely powerful influence of such archetypal images which are, in many instances, projected upon actual people in the external world. Jungian therapy facilitates this process of individuation.

Adlerian psychology reflects its founder's view that aggression, in the sense of self-assertion and the will to power, takes precedence over sex as the prime mover of human behaviour. Adler conceived the infant and child as feeling weak and inferior and driven to achieve in order to overcome such feelings. Adler popularised the concept of striving and modified it into something akin to self-actualising, a goal of completion aspired to but never attained. His view of 'organ inferiority', whereby infantile weakness could be expressed through deficiencies and dysfunctions in particular organs of the body provided a psychological foundation for the development of psychosomatic medicine.

While psychosexual development and the psychology of the ego and its defences against anxiety represent the theoretical foundations of classical psychoanalysis, a development of analytic theory, known as object–relations theory, has been a feature of the development of postwar psychoanalysis, particularly in Britain. The theory, associated with the name of Melanie Klein, focuses on the relationships of the developing infant with other people. Klein emphasised the importance of fantasy in the first 2 years of life. The infant's love and hate are initially directed towards the mother who represents the child's whole world. The lack of cohesion of the infantile ego results in the splitting of impulses into good and bad and one consequence is that the infant views the mother as split into good and bad parts, hereby adopting the so-called *paranoid schizoid position*. As the ego matures and becomes more integrated, this splitting decreases and the mother's good and bad parts and the baby's internalised image of her can be synthesised. Now the child fears that his aggressive and destructive wishes towards his mother may be damaging to her, a realisation which leads to sadness, guilt and concern, the *depressive position*. This is slowly worked through as the child grows but these depressive and persecutory anxieties can return when internal and external pressures become intense. The essential difference of Kleinian from Freudian theory is that, in contrast to the Freudian emphasis on the satisfaction of instincts, the object–relations theorists focus on early object seeking and relating.

These forms of psychoanalytic therapy are time-consuming, involving the subject in 2 years or more of therapy, conducted on a 5-days-a-week, 1-hour-a-day basis, and demanding in terms of money and commitment. Not surprisingly, psychoanalytic forms of psychotherapy are not well represented in centrally funded systems of health care but tend to flourish in situations where the patient exercises his consumer choice directly and by means of personal finance. One consequence is that the sociodemographic make-up of the clients of psychoanalysis is greatly skewed towards the higher social classes and those with appropriate time and money. Critics have continually raised doubts concerning the cost-effectiveness of analytic approaches and the relevance of such therapies to the predicament of the great majority of psychiatric patients. Such doubts have contributed to the momentum behind the development of psychotherapies which, while rooted for the most part in psychodynamic concepts derived from Freud and his followers, are briefer and less expensive.

Brief dynamic psychotherapies

As Marmor (1979) has pointed out, many of Freud's earliest psychoanalytical treatments were of relatively short duration. Bruno Walter, the celebrated conductor, describes in his autobiography how he underwent a six-session therapeutic programme with Freud in 1906 (Walter 1940), while Ernest Jones (1957) recalls how in 1908 in a single 4-hour session Freud was apparently able to elucidate the psychodynamic origins of the composer Gustav Mahler's sexual impotence with his wife and relieve it. In recent years, as pressure has grown for the development of less expensive and less time-consuming therapies, a number of modified approaches associated with Malan in London, Davanloo in Montreal and Sifneos in Harvard have emerged. Davanloo (1979) has described the basic characteristics of short-term dynamic psychotherapy. The patient is seen once weekly, each session lasting an hour. Therapy lasts from five to 15 sessions for those with Oedipal conflicts and up to 25 sessions when there are additional dynamic problems. For particularly disturbed patients, a programme of up to 30 sessions may be indicated. Common to all kinds of brief psychotherapy is the utilisation by the therapist of transference, transference clarification and interpretation. The therapist actively works through any manifestation of what is thought to be transference resistance, and dream analysis and the analysis of defence are used. Therapy ends when evidence is obtained that the 'central neurotic structure' at the core of the patient's difficulty has been resolved.

By about the sixth or seventh session, psychotherapeutic effects become apparent, but the therapy is not successful unless the patient is free of symptoms and all his maladaptive behaviour has changed. In a successful outcome, the patient almost universally refers to himself as a 'free' person, a 'new' person. Termination apparently comes without obvious difficulty. The aim of every session is to put the patient in touch with as much of his true feelings as he can bear (Malan 1979). The therapist needs to judge:

1. The degree to which the patient is already in touch with his true feelings — i.e. the depth of rapport
2. The nature of the hidden feelings of which he is not aware
3. How close these feelings are to the surface
4. The degree of anxiety or pain with which they are invested
5. The patient's capacity to bear it.

The precise status of these brief forms of psychoanalytically derived psychotherapy vis-à-vis classical psychoanalysis is unclear. Some insist that they are in no sense a degradation of the 'pure gold' of psychoanalysis but constitute innovative techniques and approaches that open the way to new objectives and potentialities for psychoanalysis. But the use of words such as 'deep', 'brief', 'supportive' and 'classical' do tend to carry connotations which suggest that the treatment of choice if all else were equal would be psychoanalysis and that other forms of psychotherapy are in some sense watered-down approaches, altered to take account of such external limitations as shortage of time, money or commitment on the part of the individual patient. Such a view helps foster the notion that psychoanalysis would be the preferred psychiatric treatment were facilities, staff, time and money unfettered. However, the question of the efficacy of these various approaches and of the indications for therapy affect their relative standing. Consequently, in practice supportive psychotherapy assumes considerable importance and the precise relevance of psychoanalysis to psychiatric treatment remains the subject of controversy.

Group psychotherapy

This approach enables psychotherapists to use their specialised skills and techniques to the benefit of individual patients who form a group. The underlying rationale is that the very dynamics of group inter-action facilitate the process of helping individuals to develop greater self-awareness, appropriate sensitivity and social skills.

Various different forms of group activity occur in psychiatric settings — activities groups, ward meet-ings, industrial therapy groups, etc. Group-therapeutic approaches can be classified as:

1. Didactic groups, in which educational material and information are presented by the group leader as a basis for guided discussion by group members.

2. Therapeutic social clubs, which are run along organised democratic lines in which patients arrange their programmes while a staff member (psychiatric nurse, social worker, registrar, etc.) remains discreetly in the background.

3. Inspirational groups, which lay particular stress on building and enhancing morale and self-esteem through strong group identification and the arousal of positive group emotions. Such groups include Alcoholics Anonymous meetings and some gestalt therapy approaches.

4. Free interaction groups, which include sup-portive group psychotherapy, intensive group therapy and group analysis. The approach taken to conduct these groups and the content emphasised within them very according to the therapists' theoretical orien-tation. For example, psychoanalytically oriented group therapy sessions pay particular attention to the unconscious meanings of the behaviour of individual patients and of their interactions within the group. Such interactions are explored and analysed by both therapist and patients with a view to exposing neurotic attitudes and achieving a more mature level of personal and social functioning.

Some groups operate as open groups from which improved patients leave and into which new members enter during the life of the group. Closed groups — a characteristic feature of analytic group therapy and psychodynamic group therapy — consist of a parti-cular group of patients who stay in therapy for the life of the group. Some groups may be composed of patients with the same type of problem such as alcohol abuse, drug abuse or poor social functioning, or may be heterogeneous and made up of patients suffering from a variety of conditions. While there is no agreed ideal group size for group therapy, in practice most groups number between six and 12 members. Likewise, the average lifetime of a group varies greatly. Closed groups by definition end when patients begin to leave, which may be after 1–2 years. Open groups continue indefinitely for as long as the therapist is prepared to be involved. Recently, brief psychothera-peutic approaches have developed, and these are limited to 18 months. Some groups are very short term indeed, consisting of intensive marathons in which 16–30 or so hours of therapy are packed into a weekend. Currently, group therapy approaches are used in a wide variety of conditions and settings in psychiatry.

INDICATIONS FOR PSYCHOTHERAPY

What sorts of patients are suitable for the three main forms of psychotherapy? Starting with psychoanalysis as the paradigm of the reconstructive therapies, it is noteworthy that many contemporary analysts insist that Freud was always cautious concerning the therapeutic potential of his creation. In support of this argument Freud's somewhat pessimistic views during the later years of his life are quoted, but it is important to remember that at no time did Freud ever unequivocally disavow a role, and an important role at that, for psychoanalysis in the elucidation and treat-ment of the psychoneuroses and character disorders. It is true that on a number of occasions Freud expressed greater interest in the theory of psycho-analysis than in its application but from the outset he made substantial claims. In 1910, in an address on the future prospects of psychoanalytic therapy, he observed that there was hardly anything like his therapy in medicine 'although in fairy tales you hear of evil spirits whose power is broken as soon as you can tell their name — the name they have kept secret' (Freud 1910) and 6 years later he opened the first of a series of introductory lectures on the subject with the stirring declaration that 'psychoanalysis is a procedure for the medical treatment of neurosis' (Freud 1916). In the sixth lecture on the technique of interpretation he pointed out that the whole purpose of psycho-analysis is what is sought in all scientific work, namely 'to understand the phenomena, to establish a correlation between them and, in the latter end, to enlarge our power over them.' In the 16th lecture, he acknowledged the possibility of therapeutic failure with analysis but then ended the lecture with a characteristically defiant declaration to the effect that there are extensive groups of nervous disorders in which the transformation of our better understanding into therapeutic power had actually taken place, and that in these illnesses, which are difficult of access by any other means, we achieve under favourable conditions successes which are second to no others in the field of internal medicine' (Freud 1916).

What sort of patients did the founder of psychoanalysis regard as suitable? As early as 1905 he laid down a series of restrictive criteria which indicated that the most suitable patient would be a young adult of good intelligence, reasonably educated, well motivated and of reliable character. He expressed the view then, which he was to repeat thereafter, that certain disorders, most notably serious psychotic illness including schizophrenia and manic–depressive illness, organic psychoses and confusional states, were unsuitable, and in 1930 he prophetically argued in a letter to Marie Bonaparte that the main hope for sufferers from severe mental illnesses lay in organic chemistry and endocrinology. He constantly drew attention to the difficulties of practising psychoanalysis and relied on an analogy with surgery, pointing out that just as the surgeon needs a suitable room, good lighting, properly trained assistants and the exclusion of relatives from the scene of the action, so too the analyst needs to practise his art in optimum circumstances and, in particular, free from the potentially intrusive and distorting influences of the patient's relatives.

But Freud never quite withdrew the claim for therapeutic efficacy, as is clear from his comments in one of the second series of introductory lectures which he wrote in 1932–1933. While acknowledging that he had never been a therapeutic enthusiast and that psychoanalysis, like any other treatment, has 'its triumphs and its defeats, its limitations, its indications', compared with other psychotherapeutic procedures, 'psychoanalysis is beyond doubt the most powerful'. As a method of treatment, 'it is one among many, though, to be sure, *primus inter pares*' (Freud 1933).

In the years since Freud, what can be said of the clientele of psychoanalysis? The Menninger Psychotherapy Research Project (Kernberg et al 1972) is still regarded as one of the most important studies of psychoanalytical psychotherapy ever undertaken. The great majority of the 42 cases making up the sample were either professional colleagues family members of professional psychiatrists; overtly psychotic patients and the elderly were excluded, and the diagnostic breakdown revealed a marked predominance of neurotic and personality problems of modest degrees of severity. Freud's dictum 'not too old, not too sick' is very pertinent. In a classic study undertaken by Luborsky et al (1980), a total of 73 patients were treated in 'psychoanalytically oriented psychotherapy', the average number of sessions per patient being 44. Again, the bulk of the sample was made up of young white college-educated individuals, the majority of whom in this case were female and single.

On the basis of the findings from the Menninger Clinic study, the authors derived some indicators concerning the selection of patients for psychoanalytic therapy. They concluded that for patients with what they termed 'high ego strength, high motivation, high anxiety tolerance and high quality of interpersonal relationships', psychoanalysis is the treatment of choice. 'Ego strength' was defined as a combination of the degree of integration, stability and flexibility of the personality, the degree to which relationships with others were 'adaptive, deep and gratifying of normal instinctual needs' and the degree to which the individual's disturbance was manifested by symptoms. Stripped of the technical jargon, what this study revealed was that psychoanalysis is indeed useful for patients who are already reasonably healthy, well-motivated, socially functioning and generally personable. More recent studies, conducted in the main by researchers favourably disposed towards psychoanalysis, have demonstrated similar findings.

The recommended patient clientele for the less pure forms of psychodynamic psychotherapy is not easy to identify but such evidence as there is suggests a similar selection process. The abortive Maudsley–Tavistock trial is interesting in this respect (Candy et al 1972). Now it is true that what doctors accept into a treatment trial is invariably more exclusive than that which they accept for treatment on a daily basis. Nevertheless, they reveal in their selectivity for trials their view concerning the most appropriate subjects for the therapy in question. In the Maudsley–Tavistock study it was agreed from the outset that the aim should be to include only those patients 'who appeared to be highly suitable for the particular form of psychotherapy to be used'. Selection of patients took place in three stages. First, psychiatrists working within reasonable distance of the two centres referred patients who appeared to them to fulfil the selection criteria (Table 39.3). A total of 113 patients were referred. Of these, 23 failed to return the screening questionnaire (which asked for details of the individual's difficulties, family circumstances and history, sexual experience, and occupation). On the basis of Tavistock psychotherapists' assessments of the questionnaire responses of the remaining 90, only 27

Table 39.3 Selection criteria for the Maudsley–Tavistock psychotherapy study (Candy et al 1972)

1. No evidence of serious physical or psychotic illness
2. No serious drug addiction, sexual deviation or sociopathic disorder
3. Discernible and lasting problems in personal relationships
4. No evidence suggesting the need for hospital admission
5. At least average intelligence
6. No previous formal psychotherapy
7. Active motivation for treatment
8. Willingness to participate in a research programme
9. Age between 18 and 45 years
10. Willing for a relative to be seen

were accepted to pass on to the third stage of selection. Each of the 27 was given an interview with one of the four Tavistock participants, the interview being tape-recorded and lasting 90 minutes. The Tavistock participants then met and discussed each interview and agreed to accept eight individuals. These eight represented approximately 9% of those who had completed the questionnaire and 7% of the patients identified as likely candidates for psychotherapy by referring psychiatrists. It may well be that in practice psychotherapists are less selective and the outcome studies reviewed later may well contain less exclusive samples, but it is worth noting that the Menninger Clinic study conducted in the 1960s opened the way for psychotherapists to choose the 'best' patients by underwriting as selection criteria those very features which appear to be indicators of particularly good prognosis. It is also worth noting that patient drop-out is also a feature of psychotherapy; rates in excess of 60% in the first 6 months are commonly reported.

Most psychotherapeutic interventions, whether or not they were intended to be so, are actually brief in form. Garfield (1978) reported that the median length of therapy from a wide variety of settings is six sessions with about two-thirds of the cases terminating prior to the tenth interview. In their meta-analysis of 375 published studies of psychotherapy, representing an evaluation of 25 000 control and 25 000 experimental subjects, Smith & Glass (1977) reported that the average number of sessions was 17 — a figure which many investigators and therapists would consider within the range of brief psychotherapy.

Yet not all patients are regarded as suitable for brief forms of psychotherapy. Davanloo (1979) has argued that selection criteria based on severity and duration of symptoms are not of much value. Rather, some of the most important criteria of selection are:

1. The quality of the patient's human relationships; the presence of some meaningful relationship in the patient's past.

2. The patient's ability to experience and tolerate anxiety, guilt and depression.

3. Is the patient psychologically minded?

4. The patient's motivation to look at himself and go through the uncovering process; wanting to solve his problems by achieving insight into the central neurotic structure underlying his difficulties.

5. One of the most important criteria is the patient's ability to respond to interpretation. This might be a transference interpretation, an interpretation which might be partial or total and which would be related to the psychotherapeutic focus.

From the diagnostic point of view a wide range of patients are accepted for short-term psychotherapeutic treatment, including anxious and depressed patients, patients suffering from long-standing obsessional and phobic symptoms, and patients manifesting clear-cut personality disorders.

Supportive psychotherapy, once considered a stop-gap treatment or a treatment given in lieu of something more profound and effective, has become a major treatment of choice for many patients in specialised psychiatric settings as well as in primary care, general medical and community settings. The recommended patient clientele ranges from quite severely incapacitated, chronically ill, psychotic patients in long-term contact with psychiatric services to mildly ill patients experiencing stress in crisis situations, presenting to general practitioners and requiring support while they struggle to mobilise their own resources and overcome the challenge. For example, Bloch (1979) enumerates chronic schizophrenia, recurrent and chronic depression, hypochondriasis and severe personality disorders as some of the conditions warranting and benefiting from supportive forms of psychotherapy. In contrast, Weissman et al (1974) endorse the value of supportive psychotherapy in the treatment of moderately depressed women attending as psychiatric outpatients. The psychotherapy in this study was described as supportive, emphasised the 'here-and-now', was oriented around the patients' current problems and interpersonal relationships and was directed towards assisting the patients to identify maladaptive patterns and to attain 'better levels of adaptive response'.

In contrast, therefore, with the situation in general medicine — where the more time-consuming, expensive, specialised and complex treatments are usually reserved for the more seriously ill while the simpler, less expensive and more general treatments are applied to the less seriously affected patients — the more demanding and expensive the psychotherapy, the less generally applicable it seems to be. Psychoanalysis is unarguably the most intricate and demanding psychological treatment thus far devised, yet the indications for its use reveal that it is only applicable to a small, select group of patients on the borderline of illness. Supportive psychotherapy, on the other hand, is applicable across the broad spectrum of psychiatric ill health. Whereas psychoanalytic therapy can only be practised by therapists who themselves have undergone intensive training, the supportive forms of psychotherapy can be and are applied by a wide range of professional therapists including psychiatrists, psychologists, general practitioners, social workers, health visitors and counsellors. The implications of such a state of affairs for such issues as psychotherapy training, the reimbursement of psychotherapy fees and the deployment of trained psychoanalytically oriented psychotherapists are currently amongst the more controversial aspects of the field under debate.

ASSESSING OUTCOME OF PSYCHOTHERAPY

The first serious attempt at establishing the efficacy of psychoanalysis was made by Fenichel in 1930 and based on published data on over 700 cases seen at the Berlin Psychoanalytic Institute over a period of 10 years (Fenichel 1930). For the next 20 years (the heyday of psychoanalysis) the quality of the research literature remained poor and Eysenck's famous attack on the therapeutic claims of Freudian analysis exposed this weakness (Eysenck 1952). Eysenck charged that many patients in therapy recovered spontaneously, that there were no grounds for claiming therapeutic effectiveness, that follow-up studies were biased, sampling was skewed and outcome criteria imprecisely stated. Despite energetic rebuttals of Eysenck's claims (Bergin 1963, Meltzoff & Kornreich 1970), little progress was made and the majority of studies conducted during the 1950s and 1960s appeared inconclusive. Over the past decade, outcome research has continued but at the same time there has developed an animated discussion concerning the methodological problems surrounding the evaluation of outcome following psychotherapy. The major problems concern the type of therapy being evaluated, the sampling used, the rating procedures adopted, the levels of skill possessed by participating therapists, the criteria of satisfactory outcome employed in any study of effectiveness, the use of an appropriate control group for comparative purposes and the elimination of the contribution to outcome made by spontaneous recovery.

Type of therapy

Defenders of psychotherapy insist that evaluating psychotherapeutic treatments raises problems of a different order compared with the problems of evaluating a specific drug. Definitions of what precisely constitutes classical psychoanalysis, brief psychoanalytically derived psychotherapy or encounter therapy vary between therapists. It has been shown that therapists from very different theoretical standpoints in practice share many techniques and behaviours (Sloane et al 1975). Discussing the efficacy of psychotherapy in general masks the fact that within the rubric of psychotherapy can be found a bewildering array of approaches, some demanding substantial commitment in terms of training, time and money, others differing little from non-specific counselling and peer support. If progress is to be made in establishing the efficacy or otherwise of psychotherapy, the precise nature of the therapy employed needs to be specified in some detail.

Sampling

Obtaining a sample size sufficient for statistical analysis of the many variables involved in an outcome study has proved difficult. In the abortive Maudsley–Tavistock study, less than 10% of the original referred sample ended up accepted for study. The Menninger Clinic study involved only 42 patients. The extent to which such samples are representative of the ordinary mass of psychiatrically ill patients must remain highly doubtful. The impact too of sampling bias on motivation, a factor believed by many to be of fundamental importance in psychotherapy, can be gauged by recalling that many of the participants in the Menninger Clinic study had actually moved home to be near the clinic in order to obtain treatment, and that few studies take account of the impact of drop-out on the final make-up of the sample under scrutiny. Many studies are biased by virtue of the fact that the participants are not comparable with psychiatric patients, being volunteers, college students, relatives of psychologists and psychiatrists recruited for treatment, or therapists in training. Participants in the Menninger and Pennsylvania psychotherapy projects, for example, were almost certainly derived from the milder end of the psychiatric spectrum.

Rating procedures

Research into the outcome of psychotherapy has involved a wide range of criteria of outcome measured by a variety of test instruments. Outcome criteria have included patient ratings of symptom relief, patient satisfaction ratings, therapist ratings of global improvement, family observations of improvement, ratings of interpersonal behaviour, judgements by skilled and independent raters, personality test scores, and external indices such as job performance, scholastic achievement etc. (Butcher & Kolotrin 1979). Such a variety of rating approaches has made it difficult for researchers to compare results across studies. In recent years, efforts have been made to generate more comparable studies of outcome by providing information on a set of measuring instruments that might serve to standardise assessment techniques (Waskow & Parloff 1975, Parloff 1982, Andrews 1989).

A particular weakness has been the persistent use of crude measures of global change. Global measures are vague and provide little information on specific aspects of an individual's subjective state and behaviour. Ratings made from different perspectives (therapist, patient, independent rater, etc.) correlate moderately with each other at best (Mintz et al 1973); patients' ratings of improvement may be inflated as a consequence of the patients' desire to please, while therapists' ratings have been affected by the degree to which the therapist likes his or her patient (Martin & Sterne 1976).

Levels of skill

While it is generally accepted that the personal characteristics of psychotherapists may well affect patient response, conclusive evidence in support of such a view has been difficult to establish. Much emphasis is laid within classical analysis on the need for any intending analyst to obtain a personal training analysis, but there is scant evidence that receipt of such a training has any impact on patient response. A variety of studies (Holt & Luborsky 1958, Strupp et al 1969) have shown no significant outcome differences between patients seen by analysed and non-analysed therapists. Strupp conducted his study with two therapist groups: experienced analysts conducting private, open-ended therapy and psychiatric residents (none of whom had completed their training) conducting therapy in a clinic setting. The patients in both groups had severe psychiatric problems. Based on questionnaire responses, Strupp found it 'noteworthy' that the patients seen by both groups

were equally satisfied with their treatment 1–2 years post-treatment.

Indeed, a negative relationship between personal therapy and patient improvement has been suggested for situations where therapists are inexperienced and undergoing therapy at the same time as they are treating others. Garfield & Bergin (1971) reported a trend showing that inexperienced therapists achieved better results with patients if they were not undergoing personal therapy. In fact they found that those who had had the most personal therapy achieved the worst results, while those with least personal therapy achieved the best results. Greenberg & Staller (1981), reviewing the available literature on the impact of therapist training on patient outcome, concede that there is no evidence to indicate that psychotherapists who have undergone psychotherapy themselves have more successful careers as therapists than their colleagues who have not had therapy. 'In view of the paucity of reported research evidence', they conclude, 'it is surprising that the value of personal training in psychotherapy is generally accepted.'

Outcome criteria

The specification of outcome after a particular form of psychotherapy poses particular problems. The effectiveness of a treatment method should be measured by the extent to which it meets its objectives, but many of the stated objectives are ill-defined. This is particularly true in the case of the newer forms of psychotherapy which state grandly that the objective of therapy is 'transformation', 'personal growth' or 'self-actualisation', without ever indicating how such objectives might be measured and how their attainment might be recorded. An additional problem is that outcome can be viewed from several perspectives. That is to say, it can be conceived of in terms of psychodynamic change, symptom relief, social adaptation or a combination of any or all available outcome measures.

The issue of dynamic versus symptomatic improvements illustrates the point neatly. Malan et al (1968) make this distinction in their evaluation of the efficacy of their form of brief dynamically derived psychotherapy. In a 2–8 year follow-up of 45 patients assessed but not treated, 23 (51%) were found to be at least symptomatically improved, of whom nine were regarded as symptomatically recovered. However, only one patient was regarded as 'dynamically' recovered. The difficulty and subjectivity of the distinction is revealed by one of the case examples provided, that of a 'symptomatically recovered' but 'dynamically' doubtful 33-year-old man who originally attended for impotence, doubts about his masculinity, difficulties relating to women and related anxieties. At follow-up 4 years later, he was married, potent and happy with his wife. However, the doubts about his dynamic recovery were due to the fact that in the follow-up interview he made two slips of the tongue, and revealed that on the rare occasions during foreplay that his wife made an inappropriate remark, his penis 'would go down just like that', and occasionally found himself unable to urinate in a public lavatory when other men were present.

Only through the use of the psychodynamic hypothetical structure, Malan argues, can one identify all the known manifestations of the original disturbance and thus formulate explicit measures of intervention and outcome. The Tavistock group (Malan et al 1968) makes a very vigorous attack on what is referred to as 'piecemeal survey methods' of assessment, referring to the widely used approach of administering batteries of tests covering various important areas such as symptoms, interpersonal relations, social functioning and so on. Dynamic assessment, Malan argues, must be based on an understanding of the underlying pathological condition and not on behavioural manifestations alone.

Mintz (1981) has subjected the Tavistock approach to a detailed and largely sympathetic analysis, focusing on the crucial issue: even if we do accept the importance of dynamic understanding and assessment, how much does it add to the simpler process of symptom-change evaluation? Mintz concluded, firstly, that if a patient's initial symptoms do not improve there will in general be a reasonable consensus that treatment has not been successful, and, secondly, when the initial symptoms do improve, dynamic and symptomatic assessments converge. However, this does not confront the problem of what one is to make of the situation, which occurred in the Malan study quoted above, in which dynamic and symptomatic improvement do not occur together. Symptomatic improvement is relatively simple to assess and agreement between patient, therapist and independent assessor can be achieved. Dynamic assessment depends on the judgement of an expert clinician and the formulation of dynamically based measures of improvement and change that can be independently rated. Without a study examining and comparing the complex Tavistock dynamic assessment method with simpler measures of change, it is difficult to comment on its reliability and validity.

Rosser et al (1983) reported on an outcome study of psychotherapy in elderly patients disabled by chronic obstructive airways disease. A group of 43 men and 22 women with the disease were randomly allocated for 8 weeks to one of three types of psychotherapy or to an untreated control group and were followed up 6 months later. The group treated by a nurse without training in psychotherapy experienced sustained relief of dyspnoea but tended to undergo 'less psychodynamic change' as measured on the 100-point Health Sickness Rating Scale (Luborsky & Bachrach 1974) and by a rating of the resolution of focal conflict on a four-point ordinal scale (Malan 1963). Psychiatric symptoms were reduced in the group receiving supportive but not analytic therapy. This study did not indicate the superiority of psychodynamic measures of change or of therapy but, as the authors were at pains to point out, eight sessions of psychodynamic analytic therapy would not be regarded by analysts as long enough even though, as we have seen, it is close to the average number of sessions that patients in this form of treatment actually receive. However, the gains achieved by the nurse and the supportive groups once again raise the question of how much can be achieved by the appropriate mobilisation of more basic skills of psychological intervention and support. The patients in this study were elderly, struggling with adverse conditions and chronically materially and emotionally deprived. They felt overwhelmed by a progressive, life-threatening disease and grief and fear of death were central therapeutic themes. Both the nurse and the supportive techniques 'demanded an active concentration on the person as a patient'. 'In contrast, the analytic technique based on interpretation of the transference and transference-childhood links seemed too objective and dispassionate. It proved to be less suitable for very brief therapy and for this symbolically impoverished, physically ill population' (Rosser et al 1983).

Yet, despite the failure to show any obvious impact of dynamic interventions after a most thorough and careful attempt, the authors concluded their paper with a familiar suggestion to the effect that 'for more introspective patients and those prone to severe depression, there may be a role within the medical team for the newly emerging liaison psychotherapist'. There may indeed be such a role, but this study and others in the literature fail to show why a liaison psychotherapist should be so identified, given that in so far as psychotherapy has been shown to be useful it is the supportive form rather than the dynamic one which holds out hope. The implication that dynamically trained psychotherapists are required to teach and supervise supportive psychotherapy is one regularly made but poorly supported by data.

Control patients

Because patients undergoing psychotherapy can improve for reasons other than the therapy (e. g. the mere passage of time), and because they may improve because of so-called non-specific aspects of psychotherapy (e.g. the empathy or involvement of the therapist rather than the Freudian interpretations he makes), it is necessary to control for such potential biases in any study of the efficacy of the various forms of psychotherapeutic intervention. Two main methods are used. The first, or 'wait-list' method, involves randomly assigning patients to the experimental treatment or to remaining on a waiting-list and assessing them after a given period. One such study, comparing a brief form of psychoanalytically derived psychotherapy and behaviour therapy, was that conducted by Sloane and his colleagues in Philadelphia (Sloane et al 1975). A total of 94 patients presenting at a psychiatric outpatient department and diagnosed as suffering from moderately severe neurotic disturbances or personality disorders were randomly assigned to treatment by psychoanalytically trained psychotherapists; treatment by experienced behaviour therapists or to a waiting-list. The three groups were assessed at 4, 12 and 24 months. Measures of outcome included alterations in target symptoms, an assessment of global change and ratings of social adjustment. Virtually all the patients, including those on the waiting-list, improved. The results, as Marmor pointed out in his introduction to the report, 'offer little comfort to those adherents of either group (psychoanalytically derived psychotherapy and behaviour therapy) who are involved in passionately proclaiming the inherent superiority of this particular brand of therapy over all others'.

How does one explain the waiting-list effect? One explanation is that the psychological assessment which preceded assignment to the treatment and waiting-list groups, combined with the information conveyed by the researchers that wait-listed patients could receive therapy in an emergency, was sufficient to create the therapeutic benefits in the wait-list control subjects. Other objections to the use of wait-list controls are that it may lead to outcomes that are more negative than would have occurred merely through the passage of time. Individuals who seek treatment and who end up on a waiting-list may feel disappointed. They may also experience an unintended reverse placebo effect, for on being told that they are being placed on a waiting-list they are in effect being told that they should not expect to improve since no therapy is being provided for them.

The second and alternative approach is to compare psychotherapy with a placebo treatment, i.e. to use a standard research design. Such an approach would appear essential given the fact that there is substantial evidence to show that individuals who believe that they are receiving treatment will improve as a result even if there is no other theoretical reason for the treatment to be effective (Shapiro & Morris 1978). In addition, there are results in the literature which suggest that the outcomes of psychotherapy may, in part at least, be attributable to the influence of placebos. For example, duration of treatment appears unrelated to efficacy. If brief treatment and extended treatment produce equivalent results, there is certainly a suggestion that the particular therapeutic elements are irrelevant to the outcome. Secondly, there is the lack of correlation between experience and training in psychotherapy and the magnitude of therapeutic effect. Thirdly, there is the argument that some of the variance of outcome of psychotherapy is due not to the treatment but to characteristics of the patient (Bergin & Lambert 1978). Patients who are articulate and intelligent and inclined to interpret their problems as being of psychological origin are said to have a higher probability of favourable outcome than patients without these characteristics.

For a therapy to be regarded as a placebo it is necessary that the patient is led to believe that the treatment is efficacious and that the treatment does not contain any other therapeutic components. The problem of the comparison of psychotherapy with placebo treatments is that many placebo treatments include a variety of elements in addition to an attempt to manipulate the belief that one is receiving an efficacious treatment (Prioleau et al 1983). Some studies have used placebo treatments that involve discussion groups in which a therapist explicitly attempts to direct the group's conversation towards topics that are assumed to be irrelevant to the psychological problems which led the patients to be selected for psychotherapy. Such a placebo treatment attempts to control for such variables as duration of treatment, meeting with fellow patients and having the opportunity to engage in conversation in a quasi-therapeutic setting. But the belief that discussions that do not focus on specific problems are not therapeutically effective is an act of faith. It could be that the essential features of psychotherapy which account for such effectiveness as it has are well-reproduced by this kind of treatment. To date, the construction of the perfect form of placebo for use in outcome studies of psychotherapy remains a controversial area.

THE EFFICACY OF PSYCHOTHERAPY

There is remarkably little evidence to indicate that the classical psychoanalytic forms of psychotherapy are significantly more effective than briefer forms of psychotherapy, supportive psychotherapy or the so-called 'new' psychotherapies and counselling. Many reviewers of the literature, disappointed by the minimal superiority of treatment over placebo or non-treatment, have fallen back on identifying research deficiencies and suggesting conceptual frameworks for future and better research (Strupp & Bergin 1969, Luborsky et al 1975).

More recently, a new statistical approach to the analysis of outcome data has been applied with controversial results. Meta-analysis is 'the statistical analysis of a large collection of analysis results from individual studies for the purpose of integrating findings' (Glass 1976). Such an analysis is in contradistinction to casual, narrative discussions of research studies which usually suffer from significant methodological difficulties. Smith & Glass (1977) inspected more than 1000 studies, retained 500 as appropriate and fully analysed the results of 375 controlled investigations into psychotherapy. To be selected, a study had to have at least one treatment group compared with an untreated group or a different therapy group. The most important feature of any outcome study is the magnitude of the effect of therapy. The definition of the magnitude of effect or 'effect size' was the mean difference between the treated and control subjects divided by the standard deviation of the control group. Thus an effect size of +1 indicates that a person at the mean of the control group would be expected to rise to the 84th percentile of the control group after treatment. The effect size was calculated on any outcome variable the researcher chose to measure. The most striking finding was that the average treated patient appeared to be better off than 83% of those untreated with respect to the symptoms of fear, anxiety and lowered self-esteem. The second most striking finding was that there did not seem to be a great deal to choose between the various therapies. Freudian-style psychodynamic therapy achieved an effect size of 0.6 compared with effect sizes of 0.7 for Adlerian therapy, 0.6 for transactional analysis, 0.5 for verbal and non-behavioural cognitive therapies and 0.9 for systematic desensitisation. Correlations between duration of therapy, experience of therapists, group versus individual therapy and effect size were negligible.

Andrews & Harvey (1981) re-examined these data and restricted their meta-analysis to the 81 controlled studies of patients suffering from neurotic disorders and who had sought treatment. Their findings provided further support for the efficacy of psychotherapy. The condition of the typical patient after treatment was better than that of 77% of controls measured at the same time. The verbal psychotherapies had a mean effect size of 0.74, the behavioural 0.97 and the developmental 0.35. However, these groupings were somewhat broad. For example, 'verbal psychotherapies' included psychodynamic and eclectic therapies, hypnotherapy, cognitive therapy and transactional analysis; 'behavioural' included the whole gamut of behavioural techniques; and 'developmental' covered client-centred and vocational therapies and undifferentiated counselling.

More recently, Prioleau and his colleagues undertook an even more restrictive analysis, limiting its scope to psychotherapy rather than behaviour therapy and to studies that included a placebo treatment. Their criteria were met by 32 studies and effect sizes were calculated using a somewhat different method than that of Smith & Glass. They concluded that there was no evidence that for psychiatric patients the benefits of psychotherapy were greater than those of placebo treatment:

Thirty years after Eysenck (1952) first raised the issue of the effectiveness of psychotherapy, 28 years after Meehl (1955) called for the use of placebo controls in psychotherapy, 18 years after Brill et al (1964) demonstrated in a reasonably well-done study that the psychotherapy effect may be equivalent to the placebo effect, and after about 500 outcome studies have been reviewed — we are still not aware of a single convincing demonstration that the benefits of psychotherapy exceed those of placebos for real patients.
(Prioleau et al 1983)

This conclusion provoked a lively debate and peer commentary in the same issue of the journal (*Behavioural and Brain Sciences*) and the argument concerning the efficacy of psychotherapy in general and of specific forms in particular continues. In so far as any consensus of opinion exists it would appear to be that summed up by Frank when he asserts that psychotherapeutic effectiveness is bound up with the fact that 'a helping person listens to a patient's complaints and offers a procedure to relieve them, thereby inspiring the patent's hopes and combating demoralisation' (Frank 1983). However, a number of practical implications follow from that fairly uncontentious declaration of faith. For example, it would appear unnecessary to provide more than simple, inexpensive and straightforward therapeutic interventions, such as are involved in certain forms of supportive psychotherapy. The justification for insisting on psychiatric professionals undergoing expensive and time-consuming psychotherapeutic training would appear to be questionable. More importantly, the whole basis of expanding the specialised psychotherapeutic services would come under scrutiny and an alternative strategy of ensuring that therapists in a wide variety of settings receive training in relatively uncomplicated, structured and goal-oriented forms of therapy would become a better-recognised option. Already, there are signs of a move towards such an emphasis in training. Finally, it is increasingly doubtful whether what Freud termed

'the pure gold of analysis' (Freud 1918) is the high point of psychotherapeutic theory and practice. He felt certain that whatever the elements of 'psychotherapy for the people', the most effective and important ingredients would remain those borrowed from 'strict and untendentious psychoanalysis'. In fact, the current consensus is closer to Storr's view that as research discloses the common factors which lead to a successful outcome in psychotherapy these will turn out to be 'largely independent of the school to which the psychotherapist belongs' (Storr 1979).

REFERENCES

Andrews G 1989 Evaluating treatment effectiveness. Australian and New Zealand Journal of Psychiatry 23: 181

Andrews G, Harvey R 1981 Does psychotherapy benefit neurotic patients? Archives of General Psychiatry 38: 1203

Bergin A E 1963 The effects of psychotherapy: negative results revisited. Journal of Counselling Psychology 10: 244

Bergin A E, Lambert M J 1978 The evaluation of therapeutic outcomes. In: Garfield S L, Bergin A E (eds) Handbook of psychotherapy and behavior change. Wiley, New York

Berne E 1964 Games people play. Grove Press, New York

Bloch S 1979 Supportive psychotherapy. In: Bloch S (ed) An introduction to the psychotherapies. Oxford University Press, London

Brill N Q, Koegler R R, Epstein L J, Forgy E W 1964 Controlled study of psychiatric outpatient treatment. Archives of General Psychiatry 10: 581

Butcher J N, Kolotrin R L 1979 Evaluation of outcome in brief psychotherapy. Psychiatric Clinics of North America 2: 157

Candy J, Balfour F H G, Cawley R H et al 1972 A feasibility study for a controlled trial of formal psychotherapy. Psychological Medicine 2: 345

Davanloo H 1979 Techniques of short-term dynamic psychotherapy. Psychiatric Clinics of North America 2: 11

Elkin I, Shea T, Watkins J T et al 1989 National Institute of Mental Health Treatment of depression collaborative research program: general effectiveness of treatments. Archives of General Psychiatry 46: 971

Ellenberger H F 1970 The discovery of the unconscious. Allen Lane, London

Eysenck H J 1952 The effects of psychotherapy: an evaluation. Journal of Consultative Psychology 16: 319

Fenichel P 1930 Ten years of the Berlin Psychoanalytic Association. German Psychoanalytic Association, Berlin

Frank J D 1978 General psychotherapy: the restoration of morale. In: Arieti S (ed) American handbook of psychiatry, 2nd edn. Basic Books, New York

Frank J D 1983 The placebo is psychotherapy. Behavioural and Brain Sciences 6: 291

Freud A 1925 An autobiographical study. Standard edn

Freud S 1910 The future prospects of psychoanalytic therapy. Standard edn, vol XI (1957)

Freud S 1916 Introductory lectures on psychoanalysis. Standard edn, vol XV (1957)

Freud S 1933 New introductory lectures on psychoanalysis. Standard edn, vol XXII (1957)

Garfield S L 1978 Research on client variables in psychotherapy. In: Garfield S L, Bergin A E (eds) Handbook of psychotherapy and behaviour change. Wiley, New York

Garfield S L, Bergin A E 1971 Personal therapy: outcome and some therapist variables. Psychotherapy: Theory, Research and Practice 8: 251

Glass G V 1976 Primary, secondary and meta-analysis of research. Paper presented as Presidential Address to the 1976 annual meeting of the American Educational Research Association. San Francisco, 21 April 1976

Greenberg R P, Staller J 1981 Personal therapy for therapists. American Journal of Psychiatry 138: 1467

Holt R R, Luborsky L 1958 Personality patterns of psychiatrists, vol II. Edwards, Ann Arbor, MI

Jones E 1957 The life and work of Sigmund Freud, vol 2. Basic Books, New York

Kernberg O F, Burstein E D, Ciyne L et al 1972 Psychotherapy and psychoanalysis: final report of the Menninger Foundation's psychotherapy research project. Bulletin of the Menninger Clinic 36: 1

Kessel N 1979 Reassurance. Lancet i: 1128

Klerman G K, Weissman M M, Rounsaville B J, Chevron E S 1984 Interpersonal psychotherapy of depression. Basic Books, New York

Luborsky L, Bachrach H M 1974 Factors influencing clinicians' judgements of mental health. Eighteen experiences with the health sickness rating scale. Archives of General Psychiatry 31: 292

Luborsky L, Singer B, Luborsky L 1975 Comparative studies of psychotherapies: is it true that 'everyone has won and all must have prizes'? Archives of General Psychiatry 32: 995

Luborsky L, Mintz J, Averback A et al 1980 Predicting the outcome of psychotherapy. Archives of General Psychiatry 37: 471

Malan D H 1963 A study of brief psychotherapy. Plenum Press, New York

Malan D H 1979 Individual psychotherapy and the science of psychodynamics. Butterworths, London

Malan D H, Bacal H A, Heath E S, Balfour F H G 1968 A study of psychodynamic changes in untreated neurotic patients. British Journal of Psychiatry 114: 525

Marks J, Goldberg D P, Hillier V F 1979 Determinants of the ability of general practitioners to detect psychiatric illness. Psychological Medicine 9: 337

Marmor J 1979 Historical aspects of short-term dynamic psychotherapy. Psychiatric Clinics of North America 2: 3

Martin P J, Sterne A L 1976 Subjective objectivity: therapists' effect and successful psychotherapy. Psychological Report 38: 1163

Meehl P E 1955 Psychotherapy. Annual Review of Psychotherapy 6: 357

Meltzoff J, Kornreich M 1970 Research in psychotherapy. Atherton, New York

Mintz J 1981 Measuring outcome in psychodynamic psychotherapy. Archives of General Psychiatry 38: 503

Mintz J, Auerbach A H, Luborsky L et al 1973 Patient's, therapist's and observer's view of psychotherapy: a 'Rashomon' experience or a reasonable consensus? British Journal of Medical Psychology 46: 83

Moreno J 1946 Psychodrama, vol I. Beacon House, New York

Parloff M B 1982 Psychotherapy research evidence and reimbursement decisions: Bambi meets Godzilla. American Journal of Psychiatry 139: 718

Prioleau L, Murdock M, Brody N 1983 An analysis of psychotherapy versus placebo studies. Behavioural and Brain Sciences 6: 275

Royal College of General Practitioners RCGP 1981 Prevention of psychiatric disorders in general practice. London

Reich W 1942 Character analysis. Orgone Institute Press, New York

Rosser R M, Denford J, Guz A et al 1983 Breathlessness and psychiatric morbidity in chronic bronchitis and emphysema: a study of psychotherapeutic management. Psychological Medicine 13: 93

Shapiro A K, Morris L A 1978 Placebo effects in medical and psychological therapies. In: Garfield S L, Bergin A E (eds) Handbook of psychotherapy and behaviour change: an empirical analysis. Wiley, New York

Sloane R B, Staples F R, Cristox A H et al 1975 Psychotherapy versus behaviour treatment. Harvard University Press, Boston

Smith M L, Glass G V 1977 Meta-analysis of psychotherapy outcome studies. American Psychologist 32: 752

Storr A 1979 The art of psychotherapy. Secker & Warburg/Heinemann, London

Strupp H H 1978 Psychotherapy research and practice: an overview. In: Garfield S L, Bergin A E (eds) Handbook of psychotherapy and behaviour change. Wiley, New York

Strupp H H, Bergin A E 1969 Some empirical and conceptual bases for coordinated research in psychotherapy. A critical review of issues, trends and evidence. International Journal of Psychiatry 7: 18

Strupp H, Fox R, Lessler K 1969 Patients view their psychotherapy. Johns Hopkins Press, Baltimore

Truax C B, Carkhuff R F 1967 Towards effective counselling and psychotherapy. Aldine Press, Chicago

Walter B 1940 Theme and variation. Knorf, New York

Waskow I E, Parloff M B 1975 Psychotherapy change measures: a report of the clinical research branch outcome measures project. US Department of Health, Education and Welfare, Washington, DC

Weissman M M, Klerman G L, Paykel E S et al 1974 Treatment effects on the social adjustment of depressed patients. Archives of General Psychiatry 30: 771

Weissman M M, Prusoff B A, Dimascio A, Neu C, Goklaney M, Klerman G L 1979 The efficacy of drugs and psychotherapy in the treatment of acute depressive episodes. American Journal of Psychiatry 136: 555

Wolberg L R 1977 The technique of psychotherapy. Grune & Stratton, New York

40. Therapy with couples and families

J. D. Haldane   Una McCluskey

INTRODUCTION

This chapter is concerned with assessment and treatment when the index patient is a spouse or member of a family and when the focus is on the couple or family rather than on the individual. Its emphasis is on the problems which affect systems of persons in relationship and on the contribution to marital and family therapy of psychiatrists, recognising that other colleagues, e.g. nurses, clinical psychologists and social workers, may have either a primary or a collaborative role in assessment or therapy.

In the UK, marriage counselling began to be provided throughout the country by the Marriage Guidance Councils in the late 1940s, while therapy with families did not begin to develop until the 1960s. Among psychiatrists, those concerned with children or adolescents or with the elderly, share an interest in family dynamics and in enabling the use of family resources in management and treatment; but only the former offer family therapy as a standard response (see also Chs 29, 30 and 31). Psychotherapy for couples was also initiated in the late 1940s; many general psychiatrists have concern for the spouses of their patients; the usefulness and limitations of therapy for sexual disorders are well recognised (see Ch. 25), but clinical services specifically for the treatment of marital problems are available only in a few centres.

PATTERNS OF MARRIAGE AND FAMILY LIFE

Changes and transitions

The majority of adults in our society marry and, of these, the majority remain married to their spouse for a lifetime. But the proportion doing so has been greatly reduced during the past 25 years, no doubt partly because of changes in the laws and procedures relating to divorce. Young people are living together before marriage to a greater extent than in the past; for both men and women the age at first marriage becomes later; and the period between marriage and the birth of the first child has been increasing. Increased divorce and remarriage rates mean that there are more couples in transition between marriages, more single-parent families (most such parents being women) and more step-families. Thus, there are not only more adults but more children who have experience of more than one marriage. There are also more homosexual and lesbian couples, some of whom are caring for the children of one of the partners, or fostering or adopting children. Marital and family life has also been affected by changing practices in family limitation and fertility control; by the steadily increasing employment of women and adversely by the increasing unemployment of men (Mattinson 1988, Clark & Haldane 1990). Many therapists operate as if behaviour such as assertiveness, confidence, ability to express anger in a straightforward way, being clear about needs and wishes, and planning in a strategic way are normal (even desirable) male attributes, but if expressed by a woman are seen as unhealthy, negative, deviant and even destructive (Broverman 1970, Walters et al 1988). All adult members of a family do not have equal access to resources or equal authority in decision-making (McCluskey 1990, Perelberg & Miller 1990). Women usually bear much more than their share of responsibility, but much less than their share of power, so that any shift towards empowering women often involves helping them to be less accommodating and less responsible for family well-being, while at the same time helping men to be more so (McGoldrick et al 1989). To what extent the increase in human immunodeficiency virus (HIV) infection has affected relationships between heterosexual couples is not yet accurately known, but it is more rather than less likely that psychiatrists will need to be competent in working with the consequences of these conditions for both adults and young people. To the increasing awareness of child physical and sexual abuse and their consequences has to be added the revelation by older women of abuse in their childhood. Just as illness or dependency from whatever cause in those over 60 years of age may be a source of major stress in marital and family life, so attention may have to be paid to neglect, deprivation and abuse of the elderly by those who were formerly their dependants.

These changes have taken place within the time-span of a generation, accompanied by: developments in services for counselling, conciliation and mediation (Walker 1989, Lewis et at 1992); an increasing emphasis on the consequences for children of divorce (Clulow & Vincent 1987) and on legislation which more clearly defines children's rights; and by an increasing sensitivity to the potentially long-term, adverse effects of marital discord. There can therefore be less reliance on traditional structures and mores to provide models for marital and family life. Marriage may be construed as the primary, paradigmatic, adult pair relationship or as a subsystem of continuing family relationships over time; as the best form of adult pair relationship or as but one. Information from sociological research and from central government statistics, as illustrated in Chapter 2, shows that the 'nuclear family' represents a steadily decreasing proportion of households in our society; and must not without qualification, be presented as that which is to be regarded as 'normal'. Therefore, throughout this chapter we use the terms 'marriage' and 'family' as a convenient (and so potentially flawed) shorthand description of a wide range of relationships and not as an endorsement of such forms of institutionalised relationship as alone worthy of interest and concern.

Purpose and functions of marriage and the family

Marriage and family living are for some a baleful influence, the cause of ill health and limitation of personal potential; for others the best conceivable system for the promotion of individual well-being and optimal functioning. They may be regarded as the necessary bedrook of a stable society and changes in their patterns seen as a threat to the stability of society. No statement about purpose or functions would be acceptable to all the racial or ethnic groups in a society, nor to all religious denominations. Women and men do not have the same expectations of marriage (Mansfield & Collard 1988), nor once married, do they experience the relationship in the same way. So too, when their relationship becomes problematic, they have different expectations and aims when they seek help (Brannen & Collard 1982). As an expression

of the observations and concepts developed by Menzies (1960), one may define marriage as 'the primary social system of defence against anxiety; that which is sought and found by most adults, as a defence against isolation and alienation from others, and from the self; against loss, emptiness and abandonment, as a container for hope' (Haldane 1991). Here is offered what might be called a minimalist description of purposes and functions. For marriage these can be defined as: (1) the mutual care and nurture of each spouse for the other, expressed in the general organisation of their life, their patterns of work and leisure and in their sexual relationship; (2) the opportunity for, and support in, working through problems, conflicts and difficulties insufficiently resolved earlier in their lives, within such a mutually caring relationship; (3) the promotion of a fuller realisation of the potential of each spouse, particularly in personal relationships; (4) the promotion of a clear ssense of identity, autonomy and independence within the context of bonds of affectionate attachment; (5) the encouragement and maintenance of the capacity to adapt to change, e.g. having children, illness, ageing, death, adverse external circumstances, in some cases the dissolution of the marriage. Whether or not in any marriage these purposes and problems can be maintained, will depend on a number of factors: (1) the cultural, class, occupational and educational background of the couple; (2) their preceptions and experiences of the marriages of their parents and of other adults; (3) their relationships with their parents as individuals and as couples; (4) their personality development, particularly with regard to their ability to make and sustain close, interdependent relationships; (5) the duration and circumstances of their premarital relationship and their age at marriage (Clark & Haldane 1990). The purpose and functions of the family may be expressed in similar ways, including: (1) the mutual care, nurturing and comfort of its members — at first this will be the responsibility of the parental couple, but at a later stage it may be the parents who are most in need of care and protection, by their now adult offspring; (2) learning, education and training — initially the responsibility of the parents, but as the children go to school, relate to their peers and other adults and find work, they also have something to teach and parents have something to learn; (3) the creation of optimum conditions for the promotion of personal learning and integration — if this process is satisfactory, the young persons can assist the continuation of the same process in their parents; (4) the promotion of a process by which individual members can achieve a sufficient degree of autonomy and independence while having a capacity to develop mutually satisfying relationships with individuals and beyond the family.

Frude (1990) reviews the question of health in relation to marital and family life. The evidence may seem equivocal: the rising rate of divorce may indicate dissatisfaction with the marital state, but the rate of remarriage and the formation of step-families may counter the generality of that view. In general, studies of physical and mental health in those who are married compared with those who are single, separated, divorced or widowed lend support to the view that marriage and family life are on the whole beneficent institutionalised relationships, though less so for women than for men.

Practitioners have a responsibility to be adequately informed on what may be considered 'normal' or 'average' in relation to the conditions presented to them. But with regard to marital and family life, there is another dimension, that which is regarded as 'acceptable', which cannot be sufficiently derived from clinical studies alone, but is dependent on information provided, e.g. in sociological studies or in the public and political debates which accompany legislative changes in regard to marital and family life. Not to pay sufficient regard to such dimensions is to risk being out of touch with what persons in other social classes and different economic circumstances consider relevant to their lives and future.

A CLINICAL PERSPECTIVE ON COUPLES AND FAMILIES

Common to most psychiatric practice is the view that an individual, the index patient, is central to the psychiatrist's concern and responsibility, with the corollary that spouse or other family members are peripheral. Assessment with those who present marital or family problems must take account of the fact that the experience, feelings and behaviour of any one person are affected by and influence those of all the others. So also in exploring facilities required or planning treatment; family members wish to be actively involved in this process — a view which will need to be taken increasingly seriously as the shift towards community care gathers pace (Perring et al 1990).

Both index patients and their spouses or families may adopt (consciously or unconsciously), or be cast in, a number of roles in the course of assessment and treatment. They may be willing or reluctant informants, thus helping or hindering the psychiatrist's tasks. They may be willing cooperators or unrelenting saboteurs, neither motivation nor intentions being always clear.

They may be victims or aggressors. Success in treating one person's condition may have unanticipated effects on others and the process of treatment, especially if it involves hospital care, may be stressful for relatives. The well-known situation of the referral of spouse or family member after a patient's discharge home from hospital may represent a delayed reaction to such stress: the patient's illness may have acted as a precipitant, or the equilibrium of the earlier relationship may have been disturbed by admission and separation or by recovery and discharge.

ASSESSMENT

Problems presented by couples and families

The term 'problem' is used in its dictionary meaning of bone of contention, subject of dispute, puzzle, mystery, dilemma, predicament, quandary; it is the term often used by spouses and parents when they first seek help. By 'presented' is meant that individuals, couples or families bring a problem and offer it for attention and scrutiny, a first statement, an introduction to something possibly deeper and more complex. Other terms such as breakdown, dysfunction, disorder and disharmony are no more precise and carry connotations about conceptual frameworks which can be limiting; but 'symptoms' may be appropriate, in that one or more individuals may come with evidence of an illness.

It may be helpful to summarise some of the ways in which distress in marital and family relationships may present:

1. A somatic symptom or complaint may be the first signal that all is not well: a discomfort, an ache or a pain, possibly affecting more than one person.

2. The complaint, anxiety or criticism may be about spouse or child or elderly parent: their health, behaviour, perceived neglectfulness, abuse of another member, relationship (particularly extramarital) with another person.

3. A marital problem may develop as a result of disagreement about response to a family member's expectations. (Should the woman give up her employment to care for the daughter's illegitimate child if her boyfriend does decide to leave her?)

4. Psychosexual difficulties in one or both partners may present overtly, or more covertly in one or both, by other physical or psychological symptoms.

5. The apparently increasing incidence of child physical and sexual abuse reflects problems in parenting and in the marital relationship.

6. Marital conflict, especially when prolonged, can be a precipitant of psychiatric disorder, e.g. schizophrenic episodes, depressive conditions; but it may also be a reaction to such a condition in the spouse or offspring.

7. The contribution to marital and family discord of physical or mental handicap, illness or death, whether of children or of elderly parents, should not be minimised.

8. Parasuicide in young people is frequently indicative of marital discord in their parents or evidence of family pathology, and in a spouse may indicate the potential dissolution of the marriage.

9. Many disorders in children or adolescents, e.g. conduct disorder, psychosomatic conditions and impairment of learning, may be caused by couples in conflict about their relationship or their parenting roles.

Initial consultation

Setting and preparation

There is no reliable information on the prevalence and incidence of marital and family problems, on the proportion of the persons so affected who seek help, or the proportion of those who find themselves referred by a non-psychiatric professional to the psychiatric services. Even if so-called community services develop to the extent anticipated or hoped, it is not yet clear to what further degree the work of psychiatrists will move beyond hospital and clinic settings. Given the potential for the application of marital and family therapy, it is to be hoped that psychiatrists can be flexible about where they are willing to meet couples and families and that in response to crises they will be ready to visit patients in their homes. Rooms organised for one-to-one work are rarely adequate for work with couples and families, especially where there are young children, who need sufficient space for sitting and moving around the room, together with uninterrupted peace and quiet. Some assessments will be undertaken when a spouse or family member is in hospital and day centre provisions may allow interaction with a family over more than the usual consultation time. The writers regret that there has not been a more extensive development of residential settings for the assessment and treatment of families (Haldane et al 1980).

The often claimed difficulties of persuading spouses and family members to attend for consultation can be minimised by attention to administrative details. The first engagement is *not* the first meeting with staff of the psychiatric service; spouse, parent or family will already have been seen by another practitioner and before meeting with the psychiatrist will already have ideas and fantasies about the forthcoming experience. Routine appointment cards sent out from a records office or telephone messages conveyed by someone other than the psychiatrist are less likely to stimulate a positive response than a letter or telephone call from the psychiatrist explaining the purpose and likely duration of appointment and the possibility of negotiation in relation to future appointments.

Consulting with more than one person

The first meeting offers the possibility of actively involving the couple or family in the process, so that they can contribute to a developing understanding of their problem, how this might best be ameliorated and what aims for change or improvement would be realistic. The techniques for and problems in meeting with more than one person are different from those in a one-to-one interview, or when a spouse or family member accompanies the index patient primarily as information giver or receiver. With a family the issues are more complex than with a couple, not only because there are more people in the room, but also because age differences may mean differences in ways of communicating. The complexity is increased if one or more members are in some way disabled or handicapped, especially if this affects speech or language; and if couple or family are accompanied by other persons in roles such as referring agent, advocate or interpreter. The psychiatrist needs to use both a wide-angled and a telescopic perspective, paying attention to whoever is speaking, while remaining aware of others' responses; deciding who is to be given priority of attention and ensuring that this is maintained without interruption. Non-verbal as well as verbal responses must be attended to, because the non-verbal may be more eloquent expressions of important issues than words. The attention of husband, wife, children, has to be drawn to what is being communicated, as evidence of behaviour, experience or relationship. Each individual has the right to be engaged with, taken seriously and presumed to have a valid contribution to make, if the psychiatrist is to have their attentive participation and collaboration. To do all this the practitioner has to feel and be in charge of the process, controlling it in the interests of gaining information which is relevant to the assessment and formulation of the problem. The response to each individual and to their interactions acts as a model and will influence the process and purpose of the consultation.

THERAPY WITH COUPLES AND FAMILIES   903

To take or not to take a history

Whether or not at the first meeting to take a standard personal and family history remains an area of debate among marital and family therapists. If it is thought appropriate, then with a couple a minimum would be: a history from each spouse of the presenting problem and of their relationship; their individual opinions and experiences of their past and current relationship; their views on the nature and causes of the problem and how it might be dealt with. The same is true of history taking with a family, with weight given to what is said by the young people as well as the parents (and possibly grandparents). It is not enough to seek information about verifiable facts: one needs to seek common and separate recollections and an understanding of the meaning for the individuals of events, experiences and their recollections of them. An alternative is to focus on the immediate present: on the current behaviour, experience and relationship of those involved; on their views of the current problem and the potential resolution; on the interaction of the persons in the room. This is not to deny the past but to give priority to immediacy rather than to antecedents. There is as yet no evidence to show which of these approaches is more effective in reaching an assessment which will help in formulating action.

Formulating the problem

Couples and families have the right to conclude the first meeting having reached a sufficient understanding with the psychiatrist about the nature of their problem, identified at least some aspects which can be worked on with a realistic expectation of success and established a possible range of outcomes. This is a minimum if they are to be actively and responsibly involved in shaping the outcome, in ways which do not involve inappropriate dependency. It may not be possible to achieve this kind of agreement and clarification in the first session. To have more than one assessment session may be considered cost ineffective but that view carries the assumption that all that needs to be learned and understood can be achieved in one meeting. For many husbands and wives, parents and children, such an initial assessment may be the first occasion for a long time when they have paid attention to each other and listened and talked to each other. They may never have had the experience of contentious issues being explored in the presence of someone who has not been party to the development of these. Before coming they may have felt hopeless and helpless when confronted with their difficulties. They may never before have had the

opportunity of talking to and hearing each other in the presence of someone who is non-judgmental and encourages them to work on their own without further, or only occasional, assistance.

Most spouses and family members have views about causation: not so much ideas as convictions about what, perhaps more often who, is the cause, or at fault, or to blame, or who is primarily responsible for change of the nature desired. The search for some kind of causative explanation can be not only informative but itself therapeutic, as it tries to separate fact from fantasy, myth from reality; identify vulnerabilities; and clarify the sequence of events and seek to match current experiences against earlier hopes and expectations of the marriage or of parenting roles.

One of the dangers of focusing on the current situation of a family, the 'here-and-now' of the first consultation, is that formal, systematic assessment may be neglected, thus risking the possibility that subsequent therapy has an inadequate base of informed understanding. A number of such systems have been developed: e.g. a structured interview technique which aims to define a focal hypothesis for therapy (Glaser et al 1984); the combined use of interview, rating scales and self-report measures (Wilkinson 1991); the repertory grid, which provides a setting for the elaboration of meaning, the way individuals and groups — therapists, couples and families — construe themselves and each other and the world of events which surround them (Solas 1991). An excellent survey of marital and family problems and their understanding from a psychological perspective is provided by Frude (1990).

THERAPY

Structure and organisation

Sessions: number, frequency and duration

The number of sessions required is affected by the expectations and aims of the work, the therapist's views on the process, and whether the objectives are seen as limited or as a contribution to resolving problems in a phase in the life of a couple or family. For all concerned there is much advantage at the beginning in agreeing on whether the programme is to be open ended, without limit of time, or whether there is to be an agreed number of sessions subject to review. The advantage in agreeing on a fixed number of sessions is that all concerned are aware from the beginning of closure and limitation in time, thus reducing the likelihood of drifting into an inappropriate long-term commitment or dependency (a risk which also affects the therapist). The experience of most marital and family therapists is that, for some benefit to be gained, fewer sessions, at longer intervals, are required than in therapy with individuals. The pace of the work tends to be faster for a number of reasons: (1) the use of relatively more activist, more interventionist techniques, with their focus on existential, 'here-and-now' situations; (2) the focus not primarily on the couple–therapist or family–therapist relationship but on spouses, parents and children in interaction with each other in the present reality as well as in the variously remembered past; (3) the likelihood that something of what happens in the sessions will continue at home. The optimum duration of sessions may vary: much depends on the stamina and tolerance of everyone present, but the preferred duration is 60–90 minutes. (There is much evidence that a pause, a break, an interval, in the session may be helpful to all concerned.)

Creating boundaries for therapy: beginnings and endings

The possibilities for each phase of treatment are set with each beginning: the initial contact, the assessment sessions and each subsequent session; and for continuity, with the way each session ends. These boundary occasions, which define the time, place and experience of the therapeutic encounter, can be free of any formal agenda, the couple or family being free to deal with this as they need to at the time. Another approach is that each session begins with the practitioner asking for a report on tasks agreed at the end of the previous session, and on the couple's or family's experience in undertaking these. Yet again, the therapist may, after the 'settling in' preliminaries, move quickly to a focus on the interactions occurring between the persons in the room, their speech and language, their behaviour, their emotions. Just as it may require both time and sensitive effort to create between family and therapist a working alliance, a collaborative milieu, and, just as such a relationship will be constantly at risk of conflict or sabotage, so endings require preparation and care. Towards the end of each session the therapist must acknowledge its forthcoming closure and the reality of the space before the next meeting. Especially towards the anticipated end of the programme of treatment, the therapist should attend to issues of parting and separation, the experiences of endings. This can assist couples and families to explore, cope with and resolve problems in relation to these experiences within their own relationships and free them to continue whatever work remains to be done on their problems.

Who is to be seen and by whom

There is a developing consensus that couple and family problems are best responded to by *conjoint therapy*, spouses or parents and children together meeting the therapist(s) in the same session (Burnham 1986, Haldane 1988). This is not to say that for such problems no effective help can be given to individuals who for some reason cannot be accompanied by spouse or family; but the focus has to remain on the relationship, not on the individual's private, personal, reality. In *group therapy* the therapist(s) meet with a number of couples or families, in the expectation that each will learn from others and contribute to changes in their relationship in the group setting (Barker 1986, Coche & Coche 1990). In some centres there is *team participation*: while the therapist(s) and couple or family are together in one room, colleagues observe through a one-way screen and are available for, or initiate, support, consultation or supervision during and outside the session. The term 'therapist(s)' is used to indicate that the therapist may function as a singleton or as a member of a *co-therapy pair*. In this mode the therapists can be mutually supportive in what can be stressful work; their way of working together can be a model for spouses or parents; they can learn from each other, and it may be a training experience. (On the other hand, such co-work can be highly stressful, especially when the pair are left unsupported or unsupervised.) In *collateral therapy* one therapist sees one spouse or subsystem of the family (parents, or children), while another at the same time or on a different occasion sees the other spouse or subsystem. This arrangement is now not common as an agreed arrangement for therapies though separate and uncoordinated contributions by different professionals to the management of marital and family problems remain a feature of our health–social service– educational system. It is still common in the work of the psychiatric services that most couples or families meet for therapy with one person, from whatever profession — psychiatry, psychology, nursing, social work — so throughout the greater part of this chapter the therapist is defined in the singular.

Expectations, aims and objectives

Neither the husband and wife in a marriage, nor the parents and children in a family, can each be assumed to have the same expectations or hopes for treatment; and whatever is decided about the aims of therapy should be based on the understanding and agreement of all concerned. From studies such as those of Brannen & Collard (1982) and of Hunt (1985) it is known that while wives tend to hope for help which will be emotionally supportive, husbands look for advice and programmes of action; wives want to explore feelings, while husbands seek decisions. (Do they seek from the therapist what they have not found in their own relationship?) The behaviour of young people, or parental concern about their condition, may be a major factor in the process of seeking help, but the expectations of a child or adolescent rarely match those of their parents. There is a growing awareness that therapist style is gender linked and that in family work the emphasis on rearranging structure, task setting and problem-solving has been promoted by male therapists in contrast to the more process-oriented work of female therapists (McGoldrick et al 1989).

An essential part of the process is the negotiation between therapist and couple or family about the problems they wish to work on and the kind of help *they* seek. This acknowledges both their right and responsibility to explore and define their own expectations and aims and also emphasises professional help as a contribution to a collaborative endeavour. One advantage about agreement on aims is that these can be reviewed from time to time as a basis for evaluating progress and outcome. Some practitioners think it helpful to formulate a written contract of agreement as a basis for therapy; others would see this as potentially restricting. Conceivably as couples and families come to be seen as customers entitled to a 'best buy', such contracts might become mandatory.

It is as important for families as for couples, that aims 'should be specific rather than general; potentially attainable and realistic rather than the expression of a vague, benign hope; within the capacity of the therapist as well as the spouses. They should be partial rather than global, short-term rather than long-term and subject to review as incremental gains are made' (Haldane 1988, p 19).

The range of aims includes the following: (1) for one or more individuals, an increased capacity to communicate what they think, feel and want, with the expectation that their communications will be listened to attentively and responded to; (2) an increased capacity to identify and explore problems and appreciate the contribution of themselves and others to both the cause and the resolution of conflicts and problems; (3) a greater openness and flexibility in relationships, which is dependent at least on respect for differences; (4) changes in roles and responsibilities which take account, for example, of gender differences between husbands and wives and generational differences between parents and children; (5) perhaps most important is the possibility that

individuals might find the degree of psychological 'space' necessary for their sense of identity, their development and their independence, within the constraints of intimate relationships. It will be a *bonus* to most programmes of intervention that couples and families enhance the resources available to them in coping with the inevitability of change and its accompanying pain, distress and opportunity.

Criteria for therapy

For an offer of treatment to be realistic there must be: agreement by the couple or family that there is a problem requiring resolution; a willingness to commit themselves to attend, or be available for, sessions; and the likelihood that they will remain together during the planned course of treatment. It is preferable that spouses, and family members capable of making such a decision, recognise that more than the index patient have contributed to and are affected by the problem and must contribute to its resolution. Given these qualifications, the problems listed earlier are amenable to therapy.

Conditions which are not contraindications

1. Those suitable for therapy are not confined to the class described as 'intelligent and verbally articulate'. Socially disadvantaged, poorly educated, verbally inarticulate, multiproblem couples or families are not, in terms of such categories, unsuitable. Therapy can extend their capacity to articulate their needs to each other, to persons beyond the family and to statutory and voluntary agencies.

2. In a white, multiracial and multicultural society, where the majority of adult couples living together are men and women, there is a risk that some groups will be disadvantaged in their search for help with their relationship problems because of prejudice. Such people include gay and lesbian couples and spouses and families with severe physical or cognitive disabilities or from ethnic minorities: membership of such groups is not of itself a contraindication (O'Brian 1990, Ussher 1990)

3. Age is also not a contraindication. A child's disturbed behaviour or the form of parental concern may be an indicator of parental disharmony: parents may not be able to accept marital therapy but they may be willing to attend with their child(ren). Older couples are no less liable to stress and they can be as responsive to appropriate help as younger couples.

4. Psychiatric conditions need not be a barrier. The opportunity for spouses or family to explore the complexities of cause and effect of the illness of any one

member, and to work through the difficulties posed by the illness and the patient's response to treatment, can enhance the treatment, improve the prognosis and reduce the possibility of adverse effects on family members. (This is not to deny that some patients, e.g. in particular phases of a schizophrenic illness, may be adversely affected by family tensions and conflicts, from which they require protection, and that therapy which opens such experiences to further exploration is contraindicated.)

Contraindications to therapy

There are few unequivocal contraindications to therapy:

1. Some individuals have been so deprived in terms of socioemotional development and are so limited in their capacity to make satisfying and enduring relationships, that couple or family work offers no realistic possibility of change.

2. There are couples and families who, despite making sincere pleas for help, are so entrenched in their relationships to each other that their commitment to making use of help is accompanied by a need to resist change. They may attend for many sessions, or return regularly to review therapy, but persistently resist or sabotage attempts at change. Of course, such an experience may reflect the therapist's attitude and failure, but it is unrealistic to pretend that such deeply rooted avoidance of change does not exist. Others who may appear to resist change are trying to cope with 'an overdose' of it and need someone who will help them manage the change they are already experiencing.

3. Child physical and sexual abuse are conditions increasingly being responded to by a family-oriented approach, but the degree of denial or violence may be such that separation, rather than remaining together, should be the aim; and similarly for some instances of marital violence.

4. When spouses are clearly determined to separate (and possibly take action to divorce) an attempt at therapy may be not only inappropriate, but disabling to the successful resolution of their problems. Conciliation and mediation (Walker 1989) may be a much more appropriate response to the concern of husband and wife (and children if any) but are not likely to be within the remit of the psychiatric services.

Models and conceptual frameworks

Range and variety

Marriage counselling for most of its history has been

strongly influenced by the humanistic psychology of Rogers (1961) and the skills training programme of Egan (1975). Dicks' (1967) text develops the psychodynamic (particularly object relations) model in theory, practice and social context; Crowe & Ridley (1990) integrate the behavioural and systems approaches to therapy with couples; and to these Dryden (1985) adds the rational emotive. In their useful overviews of principles and practices in family therapy, Barker (1986) and Street & Dryden (1988) discuss the psychodynamic, behavioural and systems models, recognising the subdivision of the last into structural, strategic and systemic approaches. Both texts attend to the importance of overlap between or integration of approaches; Barker looks also at group therapy, experiential and extended family systems ways of working and Street & Dryden consider also brief therapy. Others focus on problem-solving in marital and family work (Haley 1976, Will & Wrate 1986, Carpenter & Treacher 1988). In the writers' view, Bowlby's development of attachment theory will be increasingly applied to marital and family therapy (Heard 1978, 1982, Mattinson & Sinclair 1979, Byng-Hall 1990).

Comparisons and contrasts

The *psychodynamic model*, derived from a range of analytic theories, is concerned with: (1) the intrapsychic life of the individuals; (2) the influence of the past, personal and family histories (fact and myth) on present relationships and functioning; (3) the development of insight as the basis for change in behaviour and relationships; (4) the generalising to other circumstances and situations of what happens in the therapy sessions; (5) confrontation, reflection and interpretation as means of mobilising understanding and change; (6) the understanding and interpreting of transference phenomena as essential to the process of change. Such an approach is essentially: (1) historical, concerned with the influences of more than one generation; (2) developmental, considering the life course and critical phases in the development of relationships; (3) concerned with the unconscious factors which influence self in relation to others.

The *behavioural model* is based on the view that changes in selected and monitored behaviour in specific situations can be generalised, will influence the internal experience of individuals and will affect their relationships. Based on detailed history taking and observation of the couple or family, it seeks to define those behaviours which: (1) are dysfunctional for the persons concerned; (2) can be altered, given an adequate definition of, and programme for, tasks and achievement of goals; (3) can be regularly monitored, reviewed and evaluated. The behaviour therapist seeks to achieve agreement on: (1) a contract between the therapist and couple or family, and between the individuals, about what is to be done or not done and what is to be rewarded; (2) how that contract is to be implemented, e.g. in the tasks set and in communication between individuals; (3) the regular monitoring and evaluating of progress.

While the psychodynamic and behaviour models are the approaches most generally used in therapy with couples, developments in family therapy have in various ways been influenced by conceptual frameworks and techniques derived from a systems view of the family (von Bertalanffy 1973). This *systems model* includes a range of problem-solving, change-inducing, activist, interventionist approaches, involving a variety and range of methods of communication and interaction and seeking to modify the change-resisting dynamics of family relationships. It includes many of the major developments in family therapy which are referred to in the texts already mentioned and which have stimulated so much of the excitement in the field of family therapy: therapists have a sense of being engaged in activities which have real potential for change within relatively short, intensive programmes.

Choices and common ground

These models differ in the degree and nature of their emphasis on past or present, feelings or behaviour, insight or other ways of inducing change, reflectiveness or action, and in the process of defining and specifying objectives. They represent different perspectives on personal relationships, different ways of construing meaning, different approaches to change and how best to achieve it. Practitioners' descriptions of their work seem rarely derived from one particular conceptual framework or from formal research, but much more from accumulated experience.

In the development of practice there seems now to be some common ground, such as: (1) reaching agreement with the couple or family about the nature and aims of the work to be done together; (2) defining, in the assessment session(s) and perhaps at intervals thereafter, objectives and aims which are practicable and attainable within a foreseeable period of time; (3) improving communication, i.e. not talking *about* people or issues, but helping spouses, parents and children to listen to and talk *to* each other; (4) finding new ways to resolve conflicts and problems

and rewarding success to mutual satisfaction; (5) being clear about the boundaries and limitations of therapy; (6) recognising that all of these are dependent on assessment and therapy focusing on the relationship, the interactions, the mutual and shared experiences of husbands and wives, parents and children.

Therapy with couples and families focuses on the existential realities of close intimate relationships. These include: the potential for alienation, loneliness and loss; the tension between love and hate, especially when experienced towards the same person(s); the reality and inevitability of conflict; the struggle for a comfortable identity and for personal autonomy; issues of freedom, responsibility and power and the importance of remaining alive to changes in self and others. A significant aim of therapy is to arrive at a state of personal authenticity and truth to self, within the reality of the constraints and opportunities of marital and family relationships; and to develop towards a full realisation of potential, within settings which have to acknowledge the legitimate and changing needs and expectations of others. These perspectives and aims seem universally relevant to therapy, whichever model is being applied. They are elaborated elsewhere (Haldane & McCluskey 1982).

In developing a model for marital and family therapy there is a need to pay particular attention to the dynamics of persons in a relationship within the wider context of their family and social life. However much the external world is mirrored in the personal experiences of spouses and families (so that the focus of therapy may never need to move beyond such realities), changes in employment, the economics of family life, legislation affecting marital and parenting relationships, affect these more private relationships. The great majority of those capable of responding to marital and family therapy are not by any definition ill, or sick, and the term 'patient' may be quite inappropriate. A model which recognises these factors and which makes use of the learning from work with groups and institutions (Menzies 1960, Bridger 1981) has been termed by the writers a *consultative model* and explored at greater length elsewhere (Haldane 1988, Clark & Haldane 1990). The need to relate practice and organisation (and with these, research) has been shown by Mattinson & Sinclair (1979), Haldane (1988) and Woodhouse & Pengelly (1991). If there is not a sufficient congruence between the structures and dynamics of the organisation and the models and practice of face-to-face work, couples and families will receive an inadequate service.

Ethical issues in practice

This work raises many complex ethical dilemmas (Haley 1976, Skynner 1976, Walrond-Skinner & Watson 1987, Clark & Haldane 1990) which can only briefly be summarised here. They include: (1) how to differentiate between the use of therapist power necessary to manage the sessions and its use against the best interest of the family or of individual members; (2) how best to cope with issues of confidentiality and record keeping when much of marital and family work is about revealing what has been hidden and when more and more personnel, have (or claim) the right to obtain information from records; (3) how to be even-handed and non-judgemental when one has strong feelings against one spouse or family member; (4) how to obtain the informed consent of all members of a family, i.e. including children and adolescents; (5) how to articulate the responsibility for change of the therapist and of the couple or family; (6) how to define, or allocate, responsibility and accountability in team-based assessment or therapy, especially when the team is multidisciplinary and its individual members may each be accountable administratively to different systems and ethically to different professional organisations (some of which may not have any form of ethical code or guidelines); (7) how to be experienced by others and by oneself as trustworthy. Several of these issues will in day-to-day practice be regarded as technical, administrative, legal or organisational questions but all have an ethical component.

The therapist

Role, function and responsibility

The therapist is responsible for making available time and space and lack of interruption, i.e. for managing the boundaries of sessions; he is also responsible for defining the minimum rules about the nature and content of the encounter. The practitioner must be simultaneously separate from the system of persons constituted by couple or family, yet also part of the total system involved in the task of assessment or change in order to share in or empathise with the experience of others, while maintaining a sufficient distance to be aware of the total situation. Whether functioning as interpreter, reactor or conductor, the therapist is not the ultimate arbiter of meaning and, while a referee in terms of maintaining minimum rules about what is acceptable behaviour in the session, is not there to promote or encourage a fight. There are a number of senses in which the term 'enabler' may be

used of therapists: in marital and family therapy such a role needs particularly to be focused on identifying and utilising the resources and resilience which are within the individuals and in their relatedness, their strengths as well as their limitations. Successful treatment is a learning process, so that the therapist also has a teaching function: as someone who can help people be better informed, enable them to learn from experience, and from whom they can learn as a model. All models have as one aim the improvement of communications between spouses or between mother, father and children: crucial, therefore, is the *therapist's* capacity to communicate, informed by the knowledge that communication is affected by the gender, age, class, and ethnic group of the participants.

Methods and techniques

There is a wide range of methods and techniques available for maintaining the focus and encouraging the process of therapy. Here are offered some examples:

1. Individuals are encouraged to listen to each other and to talk to each other rather than to or, as it were, through the therapist: this may mean interrupting a third person, so that two can talk.

2. Nothing should be taken for granted or accepted at its face value by speaker or listener, so elaboration, explanation and exploration of what is being communicated is a mode which the therapist encourages.

3. Individuals can be asked to change places, the more readily to talk to each other, e.g. mother and father from opposite ends of the family group to sit face to face, or to help focus the working through of a generational conflict, e.g. a moving around so that parents sit together, facing the children, with granny placed ... where, might be the task for all concerned to explore and decide.

4. Simulation or role-playing are ways of expressing, acting out and working through conflicts which may be too difficult to reveal in direct interaction.

5. Drawing or constructing diagrams are, for some, helpful ways of understanding or clarifying. The individual or joint preparation of a family history in the form of a family tree may be helpful for step-families, or in mediation work, or where family myths and secrets are burdensome.

6. The sculpting of a problem or interaction, a non-verbal, physical demonstration, when sensitively undertaken can stimulate profound (and often disturbing) feelings, a new level of awareness and real potential for change.

7. Paradoxical injunction seeks to induce change by

upsetting an unhealthy, inappropriate, defensive balance and collusive resistance to giving up the presenting symptom. It is most appropriately used for families who show long-term, repetitive patterns of disturbing interaction which do not respond to more direct methods.

8. Circular questioning, in which one member is asked to report on what another might say if the question were addressed to that person.

9. Video recording, used mainly in the service of training, can also be useful in therapy, because recorded behaviour can be played back to family or couple and used as information or focus for discussion, or as a step in promoting changes in interaction.

Medication and other physical treatments

The approaches already described have not included any mention of treatments such as anxiolytics or antidepressants for the relief of anxiety or depression, or prophylactic medication for the control of a mood disorder. This should not be taken to mean that such treatments are seen as antagonistic to, or inconsistent with, the approach described in this chapter. These forms of 'physical treatment' may be an essential first step before therapy with couple or family can begin; or they may accompany and be part of an approach which focuses on relationships and interactions. Deciding on priorities in these matters may be difficult. But with respect to any limitations imposed by the condition of a defined index patient (who remains, legally and contractually, the psychiatrist's primary responsibility), there is no reason why the approaches described in this chapter cannot be applied in such circumstances and much to suggest that they can promote progress.

Evaluation and outcome

Resistance to change

By definition, a closed couple or family system is one which is relatively unaffected by factors outside its system boundary; maintains itself in balance, however distressing to one or more members (any shift being perceived, or less consciously experienced, as threatening), and is resistant to change. This dynamic is as fundamental to systems of persons in relationship as it is to individuals. Marital and family therapy is not primarily concerned with the analysis and interpretation of resistance, but the recognition of its occurrence underlines many of the more activist, interventionist approaches already described. Carpenter

& Treacher (1989), who explore the issue in a positive and helpful way, proposed that the term 'resistance' be replaced by 'stuckness', emphasising the immobility, the non-changingness of the couple/family–therapist system rather than focusing on the couple/family motivation or dynamic. The couple or family may be justified in their resistance to some aspect of treatment: too much may be expected of them too soon, or the treatment may be inappropriate, even harmful. Therapists may also resist change, reflecting their lack of competence, their anxiety, their rigidity of approach, their inability to learn from those they are treating, or their own personal problems.

Evaluating outcome

The participation of couples and families in evaluating the results of therapy is as important as their contribution to a definition of, and agreement about, aims. This practice makes it more likely that outcome of therapy will have meaning and relevance for them than if it is simply matched with a set of standards defined by therapists and professionals. It is a process which should not be confined to the last minutes of a session, or to a part of the last session in a programme of treatment. It is a way of helping people, together, to think about and examine their therapy, to identify what they have done and learned together, to consider how to maintain the process if it has been helpful or find new possibilities if it has not.

Potentially harmful effects

It is as unrealistic to claim of this form of therapy as it is of any other that no harm can be done to individuals or to relationships. It may well be a positive result of working with a husband and wife that they decide to separate or divorce, disengaging from a mutually intolerable relationship; but this is not to guarantee that one or both will be in a better state after the parting than before. The process of therapy may reveal that a problem in a relationship had been a form of defence against a more serious disturbance in the mental health of one or more individuals and such illness may be much more difficult to treat than might have at first been anticipated. For a child or adolescent it may be of benefit to be separated temporarily or permanently from parents, but this does not mean that siblings or parents will not suffer as a result. A willingness to explore and negotiate aims and possible outcomes will go some way to reducing the possibility of harmful effects on couples and families. It must also be acknowledged that for therapists this work can be demanding and stressful, exacerbate personal and relationship problems, and have a destabilising effect on marital and family life. These risks can be minimised by adequate training and continuing support.

RESEARCH

There have been overviews of research in marital work by Hooper (1985), Haldane (1988) and Wilson & James (1991) and by Barker (1986) and Vetere (1988) in family therapy, while Gurman et al (1986) consider both fields of work. There has been some shift (developed most by those who adopt a behavioural model of practice) towards greater specificity in research topics — what method of therapy is most appropriate for particular kinds of problem and under what conditions; and an increasing awareness that research into practice must take account of its organisational and social context. There remains, however, a great need for research which: matches the real everyday concerns of patients and practitioners; takes account of research being undertaken by those who are not primarily clinical practitioners; keeps pace with society's changing realities and perspectives on marital and family life; and brings together the concerns, priorities and expertise of different disciplines.

TRAINING

During the last decade there has been a steady increase in training available for marital and family therapy. Courses vary in content and aims; they are not everywhere monitored by an external institution; a formal qualification is not always granted, but some now lead to a diploma or degree. There is a growing willingness to seek agreement on standards, but not yet a sufficient general evaluation of the training programmes. The number of training programmes for marital therapy is limited, much the greater part of training for work with couples being undertaken by the nationally organised marriage counselling agencies. It would be a contribution to the development of competence if these agencies were to offer appropriately adapted training to medical practitioners, especially general practitioners and psychiatrists. Programmes for training in family therapy tend to be more multidisciplinary in their staffing and membership and are available in a greater variety of locations and institutions than training for marital therapy.

No one should embark on this kind of work without

at least having available regular consultation or supervision. By *consultation* is meant the process of exploring with a colleague (preferably more experienced and senior) problems current in practice and attempting to resolve these. It is not a formal training experience unless the practitioner and senior can give it the priority of regularly setting aside time, recognising that it is not a substitute for supervision. *Supervision* requires a mutual acknowledgement by supervisor and trainee that the former accepts a degree of responsibility for promoting the learning of the therapist; and that the latter sees the purpose as personal and professional development in relation to the task (Mattinson 1975).

Developments which have influenced training in family therapy include recording of sessions on videotape (or on audiotape if video is not available) so that supervisor and therapist have available an account which is likely to be less biased than a verbal account and a range of techniques for live supervision. Such forms of consultation and supervision raise important issues of confidentiality and of privacy versus public scrutiny; and, when several colleagues are involved (i.e. a team supervisory role), of individual, as opposed to shared and collective, responsibility and accountability. Those which involve recording and play-back of sessions increase the exposure of therapists to scrutiny and are likely to increase anxiety.

The knowledge and skills necessary for therapy with couples and families and for effective interdisciplinary collaboration have virtually no place in the undergraduate medical curriculum and though encouraged in postgraduate psychiatric training are available to only a limited number of psychiatrists. Yet psychiatrists are assumed to be competent leaders of multidisciplinary or multiagency teams and, by virtue of completing their postgraduate training, competent consultants or supervisors to others. That consultancy to members of other organisations is not a matter of expertise in prescription is well illustrated by Bridger (1981), and the complex problems, tensions and conflicts inherent in interdisciplinary work are described by Woodhouse & Pengelly (1991). If psychiatrists are to be effective teachers in the field, they must have the training to prepare them for such responsibilities.

THE FUTURE

Whether there is to be any future for the contribution of psychiatrists to therapy with couples and families depends on several factors, only some of which are within their responsibility or control: (1) an acceptance of the role of interpersonal and social factors in both the causation and management of disabling conflict between spouses and within families; (2) a recognition that other professionals and the staff of a number of voluntary agencies are not only competent in marital and family work but have much to teach psychiatrists; (3) a willingness to move from working within hospital and clinic boundaries to other settings of which they may not be in charge; (4) a willingness to recognise that within the interpersonal systems of persons in conflict there lie also resources for change and improvement, provided that any help offered recognises this potential; and (5) an appreciation of the need for training appropriate to these tasks.

REFERENCES

Barker P 1986 Basic family therapy, 2nd edn. Collins, London

Brannen J, Collard J 1982 Marriages in trouble. Tavistock, London

Bridger H 1981 Consultative work with communities and organisations: towards a psychodynamic image of man. The Malcolm Millar Lecture 1980. Aberdeen University Press, Aberdeen

Broverman J, Broverman D M, Clarkson F E 1970 Sex role stereotypes and clinical judgements of mental health. Journal of Consulting and Clinical Psychology 34: 1–7

Burnham J 1986 First steps towards a systemic approach. Tavistock, London

Byng-Hall J 1990 Attachment theory and family therapy: a clinical view. Infant Mental Health Journal 2: 228–236

Carpenter J, Treacher A 1989 Problems and solutions in marital and family therapy. Blackwell, Oxford

Clark D, Haldane D 1990 Wedlocked? Intervention and research in marriage. Polity Press, Cambridge

Clulow C, Vincent C 1987 In the child's best interests? Divorce court welfare and the search for settlement. Tavistock/Sweet & Maxwell, London

Coche J, Coche E 1990 Couples group psychotherapy. Brunner/Mazel, New York

Crowe M, Ridley J 1990 Therapy with couples. Blackwell, Oxford

Dicks H V 1967 Marital tensions. Routledge & Kegan Paul, London

Dryden W 1985 Marital therapy in Britain (2 vols). Harper and Row, London

Egan G 1975 The skilled helper. A model for systematic helping and interpersonal relating. Brooks/Cole, Monterey, CA

Frude N 1990 Understanding family problems. A psychological approach. Wiley, London

Glaser D, Furniss T, Bingley I 1984 Focal family therapy: the assessment stage. Journal of Family Therapy 6: 265–274

Gurman A S, Kniskern D P, Pinsof W M 1986 Research on marital and family therapy. In: Garfield S L, Bergin A E (eds) Handbook of psychotherapy and behavior change, 3rd edn. Wiley, New York

Haldane J D 1988 Marital therapy: research, practice and organisation. The Malcolm Millar Lecture 1987. Aberdeen University Press, Aberdeen

Haldane D 1991 Holding hope in trust: a review of the publications of the Tavistock Institute of Marital Studies 1955—1991. Journal of Social Work Practice 4: 3–4

Haldane D, McCluskey U 1982 Existentialism and family therapy: a neglected perspective. Journal of Family Therapy 4: 117–132

Haldane J D, McCluskey U, Peacey M 1980 Development of a residential facility for families in Scotland: prospect and retrospect. International Journal of Family Psychiatry 1: 357–371

Haley J 1976 Problem-solving therapy. Jossey Bass, San Francisco

Heard D 1978 From object relations to attachment theory: a basis for family therapy. British Journal of Medical Psychology 51: 67–76

Heard D 1982 Family systems and the attachment dynamic. Journal of Family Therapy 4: 99–116

Hooper D 1985 Marital therapy: an overview of research. In: Dryden W (ed) Marital therapy in Britain, vol 2. Harper & Row, London

Hunt P 1985 Clients' responses to marriage counselling. Research report 3. National Marriage Guidance Council, Rugby

Lewis J, Clark D, Morgan D 1992 Whom God hath joined together: the work of marriage guidance. Tavistock/Routledge, London

McCluskey U 1990 Money in marriage. Feminism: explorations in theory and practice. Journal of Social Work Practice 4: 16–28

McGoldrick M, Anderson C, Walsh F 1989 Women in families: a framework for family therapy. Norton, New York

Mansfield P, Collard J 1988 The beginning of the rest of your life? Macmillan, London

Mattinson J 1975 The reflection process in casework supervision. Institute of Marital Studies, London

Mattinson J 1988 Work, love and marriage: the impact of unemployment. Duckworth, London

Mattinson J, Sinclair I 1979 Mate and stalemate: working with marital problems in a social services department. Blackwells, Oxford

Menzies I 1960 A case-study in the functioning of social systems as a defence against anxiety. A report on a study of the nursing service of a general hospital. Human Relations 13: 95–121

O'Brian C 1990 Family therapy with black families. Journal of Family Therapy 12: 3–16

Perelberg R J, Miller A C (eds) 1990 Gender and power in families. Routledge/Tavistock, London

Perring C, Twigg J, Atkin K 1990 Families caring for people diagnosed as mentally ill: the literature re-examined. Her Majesty's Stationery Office, London

Rogers C 1961 On becoming a person. Constable, London

Skynner R 1976 One flesh: separate persons. Constable, London

Solas J 1991 A constructive alternative to family assessment. Journal of Family Therapy 13: 149–169

Street E, Dryden W (eds) 1988 Family therapy in Britain. Open University Press, Milton Keynes

Ussher J L 1991 Family and couples therapy with gay and

lesbian clients: acknowledging the forgotten minority. Journal of Family Therapy 13: 131–148

Vetere A 1988 Family therapy research. In: Street E, Dryden W (eds) Family therapy in Britain. Open University Press, Milton Keynes

Von Bertalanffy L 1973 General systems theory. Penguin, Harmondsworth

Walker J 1989 Report to the Lord Chancellor on the costs and effectiveness of conciliation in England and Wales. University of Newcastle upon Tyne, Newcastle upon Tyne

Walrond-Skinner S, Watson D 1987 (eds) Ethical issues in family therapy. Routledge & Kegan Paul, London

Walters M, Carter B, Papp P, Silverstein O 1988 The invisible web: gender patterns in family relationships. Guilford, New York

Wilkinson I 1991 Family assessment: a basic manual. Gardner, New York

Wills D W, Wrate R M 1986 Integrated family therapy: a problem-centred psychodynamic approach. Tavistock, London

Wilson K, James A 1991 Research in therapy with couples: an overview. In: Hooper D, Dryden W (eds) Handbook of therapy with couples. Open University Press, Milton Keynes

Woodhouse D, Pengelly P 1991 Anxiety and the dynamics of collaboration. Aberdeen University Press, Aberdeen

41. Behavioural and cognitive therapies

Ivy-Marie Blackburn   D. F. Peck

INTRODUCTION

Behaviour(al) therapy, behaviour modification, cognitive therapy and cognitive–behavioural therapy are various terms used to describe the most widely used and the most systematically tested short-term therapies currently used to treat a variety of psychiatric disorders. In this chapter, the theoretical background, development and application of these therapies will be described.

Historically, behaviour therapy predates cognitive therapy, having been developed in the early part of this century (Watson 1924) from conditioning experiments in animals as a reaction against introspection and the 'mentalistic' concepts of psychoanalysis. Thus, learning rather than thinking, according to classical conditioning (Pavlov 1849–1936) or to operant conditioning principles (Thorndike 1874–1949), became the focus for understanding normal and abnormal behaviour. The early 'radical' behaviourists such as Watson did not consider the mind or mental activities to be amenable to scientific study and restricted their analyses and therapeutic operations strictly to observable phenomena, that is, to behaviour.

However, accepted models in science change, and what has been called the 'cognitive revolution' began in the late 1950s and early 1960s. Blackburn (1986) described the changes which have occurred in the learning approach to therapy as an 'evolution' rather than a 'revolution'. The seeds of the cognitive–behavioural movement were sown by a leading behaviourist, Skinner (1963), who in *Behaviourism at Fifty* stated: 'It is particularly important that a science of behaviour face the problem of privacy .... An adequate science of behaviour must consider events taking place within the skin of the organism ... as part of behaviour itself' (p 953).

The evolution, therefore, was away from metaphysical or radical behaviourism, when the young science of behaviourism had to go to great lengths to avoid all reference to private or unobservable events (as being 'soft', unscientific and unparsimonious), to methodological behaviourism when the same scientific principles could be applied to thoughts, attitudes, feelings, etc., as to behaviours. These methodological principles include: an assumption of determinism (that is, that certain classes of events are systematically related); observability; measurement; falsifiability or testability of hypotheses; controlled experimentation; replication and generalisability. Bandura's influential *Principles of Behaviour Modification* (1969) helped to sensitise behaviourists further to the role and importance of cognitive mediational factors in the maintenance and treatment of behavioural disorders. Concurrently, from a different camp, disenchanted clinicians and researchers from the psychoanalytic school, for example Ellis (1962) and Beck (1963), were developing theoretical and therapeutic approaches which stressed the importance of the once taboo mentalistic terms such as cognitions and emotions. They operationalised treatment techniques which became known under the generic term of cognitive therapy.

The essence of a cognitive–behavioural approach lies in systematic specification and measurement of the individual's problems before, during and after treatment, with the method of intervention being closely tied to the individual patient's circumstances. Emphasis is placed not on diagnosing syndromes but on discovering current factors related to the problem, and treatment is only given after a detailed examination of the precise circumstances surrounding the problem — a functional analysis. It has been argued that a less intensive assessment cannot do justice to the complexities of human problems and that without a functional analysis one cannot accurately pinpoint their determining features and cannot therefore devise effective treatment strategies. Ideally, a full functional analysis should be carried out with all patients. In practice, however, a 'cookbook' approach occurs more frequently than might be admitted. Most patients with phobic anxiety will end up receiving systematic desensitisation or flooding, with apparent success. Practising behaviour therapists will probably accept that their experience has taught them that certain techniques tend to be effective with certain problems and, having checked that there are no obvious interfering factors, they will apply the appropriate treatment. They will, of course, monitor results, because the core of a behavioural approach is that behaviour is being changed. Should the treatment not achieve the expected results they will alter the approach. A full functional analysis might have ensured a more efficient initial formulation of the problem, but it would have been more time-consuming.

Kanfer & Saslow (1969) described the main areas of enquiry for history taking relevant to a functional analysis:

1. *Problem situation.* Major complaints are analysed, including the frequency, intensity, duration and precise eliciting conditions.
2. *Problem clarification.* The people and circumstances which tend to maintain the problem and the consequences of the problem to the patient and to others are considered.
3. *Motivational analysis.* A list of possible reinforcers specific to the patient is drawn up.
4. *Developmental analysis.* The history of the present complaint is taken and major life changes are examined.
5. *Self-control.* The patient's attempts to change his own behaviour and other sources of influence are explored.
6. *Social relationships.* The patient's social network is examined, perhaps getting significant others involved in the treatment programme.
7. *Norms of the patient's environment.* Pressures from the patient's social environment are discussed to see how far they are important in formulating treatment goals.

In addition, a full functional analysis should include some of the observational techniques outlined in Chapter 3. A good example of a functional analysis of alcohol abuse is contained in Sobell & Sobell (1973).

BEHAVIOURAL METHODS

In many early descriptions of behavioural approaches, emphasis was placed on the role of learning in the aetiology, maintenance and treatment of psychiatric problems. It was generally held that learning was a crucial concept in three main ways. First, some disorders were associated with lack of learning, e.g. enuresis, or psychopathic behaviour. Second, some disorders were associated with over-learning, e.g. obsessional rituals and phobias. Third, some disorders were associated with loss of previous learning, by neurological dysfunction, e.g. aphasia, or through insufficient or inappropriate reinforcement as in institutionalisation. These notions provided the rationale for the application of learning theory to the amelioration of psychiatric problems. The links between behavioural approaches and learning theory have gradually become less direct, and methods of behaviour change have been sought from wider experimental psychology and other areas.

Systematic desensitisation (SD)

The original technique developed by Wolpe (1958) involved three stages:

1. Training the patient to relax (see next section)
2. Constructing with the patient a hierarchy of anxiety-arousing situations
3. Presenting phobic items from the hierarchy in a graded way, whilst the patient inhibits the anxiety by relaxation.

In this way, the patient, while never experiencing intolerable anxiety, proceeded from mildly frightening situations to previously terrifying ones.

Progress up the hierarchy can be made in imagination, in real life (in vivo) or by a combination of both, depending on such factors as the availability of the feared object or situation and how easily the graded steps can be reproduced in real life. Films, slides and recordings can also be used. The balance of evidence suggests that in vivo SD is more effective, possibly because the treatment setting is more like the real-life situation, thus facilitating generalisation.

When SD is being conducted in imagination the length of the session is generally about 40 minutes, depending on how long it takes to get the patient relaxed; moving up steps in the hierarchy rarely extends beyond 30 minutes. The number of sessions required varies (anything from 10–100 being possible), depending on the complexity of the problem and on the number of hierarchies to be worked through, for it is seldom that a patient presents with a single well-defined phobia. Patients are expected to practise at home what they have learned in the clinical session.

The following illustrates a section of a typical hierarchy for a patient with a phobia of shopping:

1. Entering a quiet shop to purchase one article, e.g. a newspaper, with the exact purchase money in hand
2. Waiting behind one person, otherwise as 1
3. Purchasing more than one article, as 1;
4. As 3, but having to wait for change
5. Asking to see an article before purchasing
6. As 4, but waiting in a queue of several people.

When SD is carried out in vivo, the patient is instructed how to relax and how and when to use relaxation in the clinic, but the actual desensitisation is done in the real situation. Often this 'homework' can be done while the patient is accompanied by a relative, and the presence of such a companion can act as an extra way of breaking down the hierarchy into smaller steps.

SD is one of the most intensively investigated of all kinds of psychological therapy, with over 100 studies looking simply at the relative importance of the various elements involved. There is little doubt about its effectiveness, and as a treatment for phobic anxiety it is extensively used.

Relaxation

Behaviour therapists are not the only practitioners of relaxation, other therapists having used it extensively. Nevertheless, since Wolpe (1958) advocated Jacobson's (1938) technique for SD it has earned a firm place in the behavioural armamentarium. Its role has also gradually extended. Formerly, when used alone, it was regarded as a control procedure, lacking the essential conditioning elements of SD; but gradually evidence accumulated showing that it was often at least as effective as the treatment with which it was compared. This was particularly striking when it was being used as a control procedure with which to compare biofeedback (see below). It has now earned a place in its own right as an effective treatment for anxiety management, headaches, chronic pain, hypertension and other problems. A useful review of relaxation procedures has been provided by Lichstein (1988).

Flooding

Flooding involves exposing patients to a phobic object in a non-graded manner with no attempt to reduce anxiety beforehand. As with SD, flooding can be conducted in vivo or in imagination. In the latter case it is often referred to as implosive therapy, and as such was originally put forward as a psychoanalytic technique, with some similarity to abreaction. A recent application of imaginal flooding is to post-traumatic stress disorder (Cooper & Clum, 1989).

Typically the patient is placed alone in a room with the phobic object, say a cat, and is required to stay there until the fear has diminished. It is argued that fear is maintained by the patient's avoidance of the phobic object or situation, and that if avoidance is not allowed the fear will diminish. The flooding session must be of long duration, normally an hour or more, to be effective. In general, the patient should stay in contact until there are clear indications of marked fear reduction; some reduction is normally seen after 15 minutes. Ending before this may represent another avoidance and could exacerbate the problem. This brings out a resemblance to SD which may not be obvious at first sight. In the initial stages of flooding the anxiety is very high but, due to emotional exhaustion or habituation, after a time it starts to decline so that each recurrence of the frightening stimuli, e.g. a movement of the cat towards the patient, no longer leads to increased anxiety and the stimulus–response link between the cat and the fear has been weakened. Another likely reason for success is the subjects's 'reality testing' of the situation, whereby he discovers that he is less afraid of the phobic object than he had expected to be.

Several studies have compared flooding with SD in the treatment of phobias. Most have shown that there are no major differences in outcome. Flooding seems to be more effective with obsessive-compulsive patients when combined with response prevention (see below).

The decision whether to use flooding or not is by mutual agreement of patient and therapist. Most patients find it less frightening than they had imagined and it is usually much quicker acting than SD.

Breathing techniques

Tense patients often complain about difficulty or disturbance in their breathing. Hyperventilation has an important role in causing and maintaining symptoms among many patients, particularly those who complain of panic attacks. Overbreathing for 1 or 2 minutes can produce a range of symptoms arising from carbon dioxide depletion and hypocapnia. These include dizziness, palpitations, muscular spasms, tingling sensations in the extremities, feelings of unreality and various pains. The overbreathing itself may be identified by the patient as a symptom (i.e. as difficulty in breathing) rather than as a possible cause. Hyperventilation is not a consequence of the panic since it commonly comes first. Training in diaphragmatic breathing and cognitive reinterpretation of symptoms have been shown to be effective in reducing panic (Salkovskis et al 1986).

A recent integration and extension of behavioural approaches to anxiety reduction, anxiety management training, has been described by Suinn (1990). It places great stress on active coping, homework, paced progress, and prevention; its theoretical underpinnings are derived more from skills training than from extinction models. It is also recommended for anger management.

Response prevention

Although SD is often used for the treatment of obsessive–compulsive disorders where there is a phobic element, a combination of flooding and response prevention is now the behavioural treatment of choice for reducing rituals. Controlled studies suggest a success rate of around 70%, which is impressive for a previously intractable condition. The technique involves exposing the patient to a contaminating object, such as a soiled towel, and subsequently preventing them from carrying out their usual cleansing ritual. A useful supplementary procedure is for the therapist to model normal behaviour by, for example, touching the contaminated object and eating something immediately afterwards, and then requiring the patient to do the same.

Obsessional ruminations are amongst the most difficult neurotic symptoms to remove, although certain treatments are claimed to be useful for some patients; for example habituation, in which the patients are exposed to a continuous-loop tape recording of their own voice providing a commentary of their thoughts (Salkovskis & Westbrook 1989). Some success has also been claimed for thought-stopping, where the patient has to try to dismiss immediately the ruminative thoughts. This may be helped by establishing a 'worrying time' in which patients set aside part of each day when they can indulge in their intrusive ruminations. If the thoughts occur at other times, the patient has to try to put them aside with the intention of dealing with them at the assigned time. It is interesting that, during the assigned time, patients often report difficulty in attending to the thought which had previously been so pressing.

Reducing undesirable behaviour

A common goal in therapy is the removal of undesirable behaviour, such as rituals, addictions and aggression. One method, now rarely used, is aversion therapy, which involves producing an unpleasant or painful sensation in association with a stimulus or pattern of behaviour. Its use has been attacked on theoretical and ethical grounds: under some circumstances it may increase the undesirable behaviour, cause emotional conflict, or result in feelings of aggression towards the therapist. More benign aversive stimuli which avoid the infliction of pain have been reported such as unpleasant smells or rapid smoking.

One alternative to such aversion is the withdrawal of reinforcement or removal of the patient from all possible sources of reinforcement. These procedures are most commonly used when the behaviour may be hazardous to the patient or to other patients or staff. 'Time-out', for example, involves the withdrawal of patients from the situation where the undesirable behaviours have occurred and placing them in a bare, empty room for a short period of time, until the behaviours have disappeared. It seems to be the non-reinforcement rather than the isolation which is crucial. Cullen et al (1981) make the point that eliminating undesirable behaviour may be a short-sighted goal and describe a 'constructional' approach, in which the facilitation of desirable behaviour which can produce the same level of reinforcement is advocated.

Aversion therapy may be considered when the patient's behaviour has serious consequences for himself or for others and when it cannot be tolerated even for a short period, for example severely self-injuring behaviour. A recent example is the self-injurious behaviour-inhibiting system (SIBIS) described by Linscheid et al (1990). Other problems may be suitable for covert sensitisation whereby patients are encouraged to conjure up fantasies of their undesirable behaviour and simultaneously to imagine a highly unpleasant experience (e.g. an exhibitionist being caught by the police); this can be supplemented by the patient's snapping an elastic band worn round the wrist.

Although its originators do not explicitly categorise it as such, overcorrection is an aversive technique used to eliminate grossly inappropriate behaviour, mainly in people with a mental handicap, by requiring them to carry out extensive or tedious activities which more than correct for damage done by their actions. It is described in some detail by Foxx & Azrin (1972).

Modelling

Modelling refers to the acquisition of new behaviours by imitation, and its therapeutic use derives from the work of Bandura and his colleagues (e.g. see Bandura

1969). In this form of treatment the patient observes someone else carrying out an action which the patient currently finds difficult to perform. Results are better if the patient can realistically identify with the person serving as the model; because of role differences the therapist is not likely to be the most effective model. Modelling is often used in conjunction with other techniques such as flooding and role-playing, particularly in the treatment of phobic and obsessive-compulsive disorders, but it is also widely used to develop social skills.

Applied-behaviour analysis

Broadly speaking, this approach is more explicitly based on operant conditioning, and assumes that behaviour is maintained by its reinforcing consequences. If the consequences are changed the behaviour will also change. Of all methods of behaviour therapy, these procedures are the most difficult to describe since there is a particularly strong emphasis on tailoring methods for individual patients. There are many procedures or techniques which the therapist may select and adapt according to clinical requirements. The approach lays great emphasis on precise and frequent measurements of problems, specific tightly defined targets, detailed descriptions of dependent and independent variables and, above all, on empirical demonstrations of the relationship between treatment strategy and changes in the therapeutic goals.

Operant-conditioning techniques have been applied to the full range of psychological problems, usually in a single-case experimental design. Some examples are stuttering, obesity, anorexia nervosa, depression, academic achievement, classroom behaviour, drug and alcohol abuse, asthmatic attacks and low back pain.

A major area of application is to the problems of long-term hospitalised groups, such as mentally handicapped, chronic schizophrenic and psychogeriatric patients. There are many studies describing successful applications to such problems as refusal to speak, self-injury, violence, hyperactivity, hoarding, social withdrawal, failure of self-feeding and self-dressing, urinary and faecal incontinence, apathy, and stereotyped movements. Such problems may be commonplace in some settings and this has stimulated the development of detailed procedural manuals and special materials, particularly for people with a mental handicap, which are successful and widely applicable. The Portage project is perhaps the best known, with manuals and materials for infant stimulation, socialisation, self-help, language, cognition and motor development (Weber et al 1975). Even with such packages, however, programmes are tailored to fit the particular needs of each patient.

Berkowitz et al (1971) provided a good example of an operant programme, for teaching severely handicapped children to feed themselves:

1. Nurse, holding child's hand with spoon in it, makes the entire feeding cycle, from plate (scooping food) to mouth and back to plate
2. As 1, but nurse partially releases child's hand 5–7 cm below his mouth, so that he lifts the spoon the last few centimetres himself
3. As 2, but increased to 15 cm
4. Nurse scoops food but releases child's hand at plate level
5. Nurse brings child's hand to plate, but then leaves the child to scoop food and lift the spoon to his mouth
6. Child executes entire self-feeding cycle by himself.

Successful completion of each step is followed by praise, pats on the back and other reinforcers. Progression from one step to the next is made when the child has been successful for at least one entire meal. Retracing is sometimes necessary. The authors reported that all 14 boys trained in this way were successfully taught to feed themselves in periods ranging from 2 to 60 days and that 10 of the 14 were still feeding themselves $3\frac{1}{2}$ years later.

Reinforcement techniques have also been applied to groups of patients in a 'token economy' system. Originally developed as a means of rehabilitating older long-term psychiatric patients, such systems have been extended to several other areas. Token economies share the following characteristics: behaviours necessary for effective day-to-day functioning are specified; a unit of exchange (the token) is selected and its presentation to a patient is made contingent upon the occurrence of the desired behaviour. Finally, an exchange system is devised, by which a specified number of tokens is required to purchase objects or privileges. Thus, the token economy is intended to replicate the conditions of life for people in the general community, in which they benefit or suffer from the consequences of their own actions. The token economy is one of the most effective ways of rehabilitating long-term patients. An excellent account is given by Paul & Lentz (1977).

Bell and pad technique

One of the oldest and most successful of behavioural approaches is in the treatment of enuresis. The patient sleeps on a special pad which when wetted by urine completes an electric circuit. This causes a bell to ring, wakening the patient and interrupting urination. The patient rises, completes urination and remakes the bed. The alarm is reset before going to sleep again. The training is improved by overlearning; that is, in the early stages of treatment the patient is encouraged to drink a lot before going to bed, thus ensuring that many learning trials occur. A useful modification is the use of a vibrating pillow instead of the bell so that others in the family are not disturbed. More complex but reputedly more effective approaches to this problem have been described by Azrin & Foxx (1974). Generally, these techniques are effective in more than 60% of cases, and factors related to effectiveness have been described by Fielding (1985).

Self-control techniques

Analysing and modifying the reinforcing consequences of a response are often not enough in themselves to produce changes in undesirable behaviour; it may be necessary to manipulate the stimuli which elicit it. This is typified by self-control methods, where patients are helped to identify the stimuli which produce the behaviour to be changed, to monitor their own behaviour, and to dispense reinforcers to themselves contingent upon improvements. A patient trying to give up smoking may realise that the greatest temptation occurs while having a cup of coffee after a meal. A decision might then be made to give up the coffee and to substitute a different activity, such as listening to favourite records.

Self-control is often applied to those problems where the patient's behaviour is governed by the immediate consequences, which in the short-term are gratifying but are undesirable or harmful in the long-term. These frequently occur in normal living: 'Shall I read this journal article or watch television?' or 'Shall I eat this cake or shall I stick to my diet?' These techniques have been widely used in the treatment of such problems as obesity, smoking, marital difficulties, gambling and obsessional thoughts.

Stuart (1967) devised a treatment for obesity. Patients are advised:

1. To eat only in one room
2. To do nothing else while eating
3. To buy only food that requires cooking (if precooked food is required by the rest of the family it should be kept in an inaccessible place)
4. To change from favourite brands
5. To slow the pace of eating
6. To develop alternative habits not involving food

7. To indulge themselves, e.g. to buy a new coat or go on an outing, if they have achieved their goals.

Enduring weight loss has been reported with the use of this method, especially when combined with exercise programmes and basic dietary advice. Espie et al (1989) described a similar method for the treatment of insomnia.

Self-control techniques have proved particularly useful in the treatment of alcohol abuse, either alone or as an ingredient of a behavioural 'package'. After a functional analysis of all drinking occasions over at least a week, advice on how to reduce consumption is given. This may include taking smaller sips, not buying drinks in rounds, eating a full meal before drinking, avoiding favourite brands and keeping under specified limits per drinking occasion. Social and other skills are developed as alternatives to drinking. Useful reviews of behavioural approaches to alcohol and other substance abuse are contained in Nirenberg & Maisto (1987). Behavioural approaches have added weight to the evidence that some alcohol-dependent patients may be able to resume social drinking without disastrous consequences (Heather & Robertson 1983).

Biofeedback

Biofeedback can be defined as the use of electronic instruments to monitor small and otherwise undetectable changes in the biological state of subjects and to inform them of these changes so that they can gradually learn to alter and control them. Operant conditioning played a major part in the early development of biofeedback techniques, but it is a matter of debate whether the appropriate theoretical framework is operant conditioning, information processing or skill learning. Notwithstanding such issues, laboratory work has produced some very unexpected and interesting findings with both animals and humans. It has proved possible to train subjects to gain control over such functions as heart rate, blood pressure, skin temperature, single motor unit firing, electroencephalographic activity, pulse amplitude and muscle tension. These techniques have been applied to clinical problems by training patients to gain control over pathophysiological responses. However, it has gradually become apparent that although clinically valuable results can be obtained with the elaborate technology required in biofeedback, for many purposes training in progressive muscle relaxation or meditation are at least as effective (Patel & North 1975), especially when the target response is consistent with reduced autonomic arousal, which is typically the aim with psychiatric problems.

Nevertheless, there are some problem areas where useful results have been achieved, especially with the use of electromyographic feedback to treat neuro-muscular disorders and faecal incontinence. Evidence is available that electromyographic feedback is useful in a variety of problems involving muscular control, such as muscular coordination during labour, treating tics and spasms and training blind people to adopt appropriate facial expressions.

Electroencephalographic feedback has proved to be effective in treating insomnia and some forms of epilepsy. Further useful applications may well emerge from carefully controlled and adequately evaluated research. Meanwhile, despite some extravagant claims to the contrary, a wide role for biofeedback in the treatment of psychiatric disorders has still to be demonstrated. For a review of its clinical applications, see Marcer (1986).

Social skills training

Social skills training is provided for patients who have deficits in forming and/or maintaining relationships with other people. There are three main groups for whom it can be particularly helpful: those with gross and incapacitating interpersonal difficulties but who are not psychotic; patients successfully treated for disorders such as depression or agoraphobia where social skills may have been lost; and long-term psychiatric patients as part of a rehabilitation programme. All such patients may be said to have an inadequate social repertoire and to give and obtain little reinforcement in social encounters. The techniques used are essentially the same for all groups, although there may be differences in the targets.

A major stimulus in social skills training is the work of Argyle (1977) and other social psychologists, demonstrating the importance of non-verbal communication in effective social interaction. Argyle emphasised the importance of meshing channels of non-verbal communication, so that consistent messages are transmitted. An example of an inconsistent message (common in neurotic disorders) would be trying to express anger, but doing so in a slow voice with little facial expression and no eye contact. A number of ways have been documented in which depressed patients show deficit in social skills, in particular in the range, timing and overall rate of their social responses.

Social skills training involves the use of modelling, social reinforcement and shaping, together with elements of role-playing and modification of expectancies. Trower et al (1978) have outlined a basic programme mainly for neurotic adults which can be modified according to the particular needs of each patient, and they demonstrated its effectiveness relative to psychotherapy. Usually the training is done in groups as this provides a ready made social situation and patients feel less intimidated because other group members have similar problems. However, the use of groups involves a risk that inappropriate behaviour may also be modelled.

Targets are arranged in a graded hierarchy, practised in the group and then applied to everyday situations, with patients reporting back their successes and failures at the next meeting. The whole programme is conducted at an unhurried pace as some patients need to accommodate slowly to unaccustomed ways of behaving. No ideal way of handling social situations is taught; rather, patients are encouraged to generate and practise their own selected styles and tactics. Simple coping, rather than slick performance, is the goal.

Goldstein (1973) developed a programme specifically for rehabilitating long-term patients, and a controlled study by Liberman et al (1986) has shown that schizophrenics who have received social skills training function better socially, spend less time in hospital and have fewer symptomatic relapses. Bellack et al (1983) have demonstrated that social skills training can also be useful in severe depression. Finally, social skills training has been used in highly specific situations, such as training alcohol abusers how to refuse a drink, and how to behave in job interviews.

Contracts

In clinical practice it is often useful to draw up a formal written contract in which goals are made explicit and the signatories have clear obligations. A contract is drawn up after a frank discussion of exactly what each party wants from the other and a suitable trade-off of duties and rewards is worked out. The therapist may act as a neutral arbitrator at this stage, and when there are difficulties about its imple-mentation. A contract of this sort is commonly used with marital partners. Contracts may also be drawn up between the individual patient and therapist which specify the roles and expectations of each. Within the contract, goals are never imposed on patients but are mutually agreed after extensive discussion. Contracts should not be broken lightly, but at the same time it may be useful to renegotiate them if they prove too hard to sustain or if early goals have been achieved. Seidner & Kirschenbaum (1980) have indicated that the use of contracts, particularly when they give detailed information about treatment strategy, produces greater participation and more behaviour change.

COGNITIVE THERAPY

Cognitive or cognitive–behavioural therapy refers to a method of therapy based on a theory of the emotional disorders (Ellis 1962, Beck 1967), a body of experimental and clinical studies (Blackburn 1988) and well-defined therapy techniques (Beck et al 1979, Beck & Emery 1985, Hawton et al 1989, Blackburn & Davidson 1990). Theoretically, the emphasis is on information processing; that is, individuals react, feel and behave according to how they process the information contained in their environment.

Cognitive approaches to treatment were first developed for the management of depressive illness and labelled as cognitive therapy (Beck 1964) or as rational–emotive therapy (RET; Ellis 1962). The theoretical underpinning and experimental studies were criticised (e.g. see Ledwidge 1978, Coyne & Gotlib 1983), but generally there has been a positive reaction which has resulted in a mushrooming of basic research and of therapeutic applications to other disorders than depression. The general principles of cognitive therapy will be described, followed by its specific applications.

General principles

Cognitive therapy, like behaviour therapy, is problem oriented. It is aimed at correcting psychological problems (emotional, cognitive and behavioural) and at improving coping skills (dealing with problem situations) to alleviate patients' distress. The main characteristics of cognitive therapy are that it is time limited, structured, and problem oriented; it follows an explicit agenda, deals with the 'here-and-now', and adopts a learning rather than psychodynamic model. It is a scientific method, involving the setting up and testing of hypotheses. Patients are given regular homework assignments and a collaborative relationship between therapist and patient is developed.

Patients are provided with a rationale for understanding their problems, a vocabulary for expressing themselves, and with training in techniques for overcoming distressing affects and for solving problems. In addition to cognitive methods, cognitive therapy uses the whole gamut of behavioural techniques described earlier in the chapter. This is done not only to change behaviour but also to change interpretations, expectations and self-concept. These changes are not taken for granted, but put forward as hypotheses, and discussed after the behavioural experiments, which are replicated until both the therapist and patient are satisfied that cognitive changes have taken place.

Cognitive therapy is more than the routine application of a series of techniques. In addition to mastering the basic therapeutic skills (Truax & Carkhuff 1967), the therapist must conceptualise each case within a cognitive therapy framework following a functional analysis which is similar to that described earlier in this chapter. The focus is on the cognitive factors which maintain dysphoric mood and maladaptive behaviour. Blackburn & Davidson (1990) described the main areas of enquiry to reach a formulation in cognitive therapy. These are:

1. Definition of the problem: what are the major complaints? Which particular functions are affected?
2. Objective factors: what are the current stresses, main past traumatic events and current living situation?
3. Internal vulnerability factors: what are the main attitudes and beliefs which the patient holds about himself and his world? What types of events does he appear to be sensitive to?
4. Mediational cognitive factors: what are the typical automatic thoughts which are expressed and which processing errors do they contain? (See next section for a definition.)
5. Current themes: the recurring theme, for example, failure, loss of control, loss of love or low self-image, will indicate particular vulnerabilities and help the therapist to hypothesise about basic schemata.
6. Coping skills: what are the typical methods of dealing with problems? In what way are these helpful or unhelpful?
7. Emotions: what are the predominant emotions and what situations trigger them?

Specific techniques

The techniques first described for the treatment of depression (Beck et al 1979) are applicable, with some modifications and additions, to many different disorders (Hawton et al 1989); for example, anxiety, obsessional–compulsive disorder, eating disorders, phobic disorders, somatic problems, sexual dysfunction and chronic psychiatric handicaps. Beck (1987) has described the cognitive dysfunctions which maintain depression. These are seen at three levels of thinking, and cognitive therapy techniques are aimed at modifying each of these levels. An example is given below:

STIMULUS
A friend does not telephone
↓

COGNITIVE STRUCTURE
Long and short-term memory of past rejections/loneliness
↓

SCHEMATA
I don't have the necessary qualities to be loved
Life is not worth living if one is not loved
↓

COGNITIVE PRODUCTS   COGNITIVE PROCESSES
She never calls   Selective abstraction
She does not care   Arbitrary inference
Nobody cares ◄——————— Overgeneralisation
It's awful   Magnification
I'm too boring   Personalisation
↓

EMOTIONS
Depression
Anger
↓

BEHAVIOUR
Crying
Ruminations
Avoidance of social contacts

The general aims of cognitive therapy are: to monitor negative automatic thoughts; to recognise connections between cognitions, affect and behaviour; to examine evidence for and against distorted automatic thoughts; to substitute more reality-oriented interpretations; and to learn to identify and alter dysfunctional schemata.

The automatic thoughts (so called because they are the habitual and reflexive commentaries that we make to ourselves and of which we are not necessarily fully conscious) are the basic data of cognitive therapy. Several techniques have been described to help the therapist elicit and modify these thoughts which maintain low or anxious or angry moods and dysfunctional behaviour (e.g. inactivity, ruminating, checking, binging, avoiding, etc.). The patient can be helped to access these thoughts through direct questioning, inductive questioning (a series of questions which guide the patient to discover the related automatic thought), using moments of strong emotion, re-enacting situations in role-plays, using mental imagery to recreate situations or using behavioural tasks to trigger the thoughts. The patient is asked to keep a diary (the 'daily record of dysfunctional thoughts'), using changes in emotions as cues to monitor thinking. These records are also used to practise challenging the automatic interpretations and substituting alternative

interpretations which may lead to less distressing emotions. A variety of other techniques can also be used to modify automatic thoughts; for example, examining the evidence for and against, listing probabilities and collecting information which may invalidate the original interpretation. The basic principle in all these techniques is that the patient is taught to consider his thoughts not as facts but as interpretations which may be more or less accurate and which may be more or less functional in terms of the feelings and the behaviour that they trigger.

Identifying the basic schemata or beliefs which lead the patient to process information in idiosyncratic ways typically occurs later on in therapy and is, generally, more difficult and abstract than identifying automatic thoughts. It is also more difficult to modify the schemata, particularly in the personality disorders described in Axis II of DSM-IIIR (Beck et al 1990).

The schemata are inferred from the implicit or explicit rules which are exemplified in the automatic thoughts. The therapist and the patient, in collaboration, must look for common themes, for the 'shoulds' which are applied to the self and to others, and for the logical implications of automatic thoughts, by, for example, the 'downward arrow technique', of which an example (from Blackburn & Davidson 1990) is given below:

Situation: Starting work again Monday.

Emotion: Anxious (60%).

Automatic thought: What will I say if people ask what was wrong? They will probably think that I am not genuine, just lazy.

Therapist: Suppose they do think that. Why is this so upsetting to you?
                    ↓

Patient: People will be criticising me or laughing at me.
                    ↓

Therapist: Suppose this were true. What would it mean to you?
                    ↓

Patient: They would think I'm no good, just a fake.
                    ↓

Therapist: Suppose that were true. What would that mean to you?
                    ↓

Patient: It would mean that people will look down on me and not respect me. I would be a nobody.
                    ↓

Therapist: Does that indicate that your worth
depends on the approval of various
people? If somebody disapproves or
thinks badly of you, it means that you
are worthless?

As with the automatic thoughts, modifying the
schemata is done through collaborative discussion and
the use of behavioural tasks. Thus, the patient may be
asked to weigh up the advantages and disadvantages of
holding the belief, to examine the evidence for and
against the belief, to question the validity of the
personal contract, to consider the short- and long-
term utility of the personal rule, to disobey the rule in
a behavioural assignment and test the consequences.
The latter technique is similar to response prevention
in behaviour therapy.

Rational–emotive therapy (RET)

RET, developed by Ellis (1962), holds that 'neurotic'
behaviour derives from about 12 irrational beliefs which
put impossible demands on people, for example:

- The idea that it is mandatory for an adult to be
loved by everyone for everything he does — instead of
his concentrating on his own self-respect, on winning
approval for practical purposes, and on loving rather
than being loved.
- The idea that certain acts are awful or wicked, and
that people who perform such acts should be severely
punished — instead of the idea that certain acts are
inappropriate or antisocial, and that people who
perform such acts are behaving stupidly, ignorantly or
neurotically and would be helped to change.
- The idea that it is horrible when things are not
the way one would like them to be — instead of the
idea that it is too bad, that one ought to try to change
or control conditions so that they become more
satisfactory, and, if that is not possible, one had better
temporarily accept their existence.

(See Ellis (1970) for the full list and Dryden (1984)
for more recent developments in RET.)

GENERAL ISSUES

Differential response and generalisation

Symptom substitution, or the re-emergence of a
treated problem in a different guise, seldom occurs in
practice. (However successful treatment will
necessitate adaptation to the clinical changes,
particularly on the part of a spouse, and this may
prove stressful.) Patients typically improve over a
whole range of problems while having treatment for
only a few. This may be because the therapist
incidentally gives advice and support relevant to the
other problems, or because the patient develops a self-
confidence which generalises to other situations.
However, generalisation across problems and situations does not automatically occur. Clinicians should
therefore remember to deal explicitly with all of a
patient's problems and to ensure that success has been
achieved in all situations which are part of the
patient's normal experience. Explicit procedures may
need to be incorporated into the treatment to ensure
that generalisation does occur.

Home practice and spouse involvement

The patient's involvement in treatment is also
emphasised by the extensive use of homework
assignments, as in relaxation practice or in carrying
out a real-life task previously avoided. In addition to
considerations of efficiency and self-dependence,
home practice is helpful in gathering information,
testing hypotheses, and ensuring that treatment
discussed or carried out in the clinic generalises to
everyday situations. Close involvement of the patient's
family has also been shown to enhance effectiveness;
for example, in the treatment of obesity (Brownell et
al 1978) and of agoraphobia (Mathews et al 1981).

Teaching behavioural and cognitive techniques

Although devising a treatment programme for a
particular patient may be a complex procedure
demanding a high level of professional expertise,
programmes can be devised to be administered by
other professional staff, relatives or friends. Several
books have been written specifically for psychiatric
nurses, general nurses, social workers, parents and
teachers, amongst others.

Manuals have been written to help patients to alter
their own problem behaviour, whether it be smoking,
overeating, alcohol abuse or even depression; some are
designed to supplement therapist-administered treatment whereas others are intended for unsupervised
use. A danger of such 'bibliotherapy' is that if the
manuals are applied inappropriately this might
exacerbate problems. (Any technique, whether it be
behaviour therapy, interpretive psychotherapy or
drugs, which has a powerful therapeutic effect is likely
to have an equally harmful effect if misused.)
However, with professional guidance some patients
will undoubtedly find such texts helpful and therapists
will be able to help a correspondingly greater number

of people. A useful review of self-help books has been provided by Turvey (1985).

Several studies have shown that extensive face-to-face therapist contact may not be a sine qua non of clinical improvement. McNamee et al (1989) reported impressive gains in agoraphobics using telephone contact; and Agras et al (1990) found that computer-assisted treatment can be as effective as therapist contact for treating obesity.

Non-psychiatric applications

This chapter describes behavioural approaches applied to psychiatric disorders. Applications to more general medical problems of value in liaison psychiatry have been reviewed by Pearce & Wardle (1989). Increasingly, behavioural approaches are applied at levels other than to individual patients, and in everyday environments. Brownell et al (1980) increased the amount of physical exercise in the general public by placing posters in several buildings extolling the benefits of exercise and suggesting that stairs should be used rather than the lift. Diners have been persuaded to select more low-calorie foods in a cafeteria by the use of calorific labelling. Behavioural programmes have also been implemented at the worksite for a range of problems, including hypertension, obesity, cardiovascular risk reduction, smoking and accident prevention. Such methods may produce only small changes in individuals, but the changes often occur across large numbers of subjects, with a major total benefit.

Interactions with drugs

Although behavioural approaches emphasise the role of environmental events in changing behaviour, there is no incompatibility in combining drugs and behaviour therapy. For example: methohexitone sodium has been used to induce relaxation during systematic desensitisation (Silverstone & Turner 1974); Blackburn et al (1981) have demonstrated the increased efficacy of combining cognitive therapy and antidepressant medication; and Marks et al (1980) advocated the combined use of clomipramine and flooding in the treatment of obsessional rituals. Marks (1982) has given an interesting review of this area.

Efficacy

Evaluating the efficacy of a treatment approach, particularly when comparing a number of treatments, is a complex and awesome task (Candy et al 1972) and

this has understandably deterred many researchers. However, a few studies have been conducted comparing behavioural and other approaches and some consistent trends have emerged. Generally, when global behavioural approaches have been compared with global psychotherapeutic approaches, few systematic differences have been found (Di Loreto 1971, Sloane et al 1975). However, the more precisely defined the targets and the more controlled the procedures, the more experimental findings tend to favour behaviour and cognitive therapy. Compared with psychodynamic approaches, the evidence suggests that behaviour therapy is probably more effective in the treatment of alcohol abuse, social anxieties and phobic disorders. In the treatment of depression, eight well-controlled studies have shown that cognitive therapy is at least as effective as chemotherapy (Blackburn & Davidson 1990). Controlled studies of cognitive therapy for general anxiety disorder, panic disorder, eating disorders and obsessive–compulsive disorder are slowly accumulating. Furthermore, there are few serious rivals to behaviour therapy in the treatment of sexual dysfunction, in the inculcation of self-care skills in the mentally handicapped and in the rehabilitation of long-term patients.

At the risk of oversimplification, the success rate for patients who complete treatment for these kinds of problems is 70–80%. There is, however, no place for complacency since this means that up to 30% of patients are not helped. A further problem is that in many treatment studies the follow-up period has been unduly short, often less than 6 weeks, and long-term effectiveness frequently remains to be established. The exception is the follow-up studies of cognitive therapy for depression. Studies of 1–2 years follow-up post-treatment have indicated that cognitive therapy may have a longer prophylactic effect than medication (e.g. Blackburn et al 1986). These studies were naturalistic in design, however, and need replication in controlled trials.

The main behavioural and cognitive approaches have been described here and it is encouraging that in a period of only just over 20 years techniques have been produced for dealing with most psychiatric problems. One of the main reasons for these promising developments may be that an integral part of the cognitive–behavioural approach is a strong component of self-evaluation. Although the interplay between clinical research and clinical practice is by no means perfect, many behavioural techniques have been considerably refined and modified since they were first described, with a corresponding improvement in efficiency and outcome in clinical practice. Many hopes have not been fulfilled; in particular, the hope that improvement would be rapid and thus demand little therapist time has proved illusory. Equally, many fears have not been realised, in particular that symptom substitution would be a serious problem.

New techniques and conceptual advances appear regularly. Perhaps more than any other factor, it is the self-critical component which assures a successful and fruitful future for cognitive–behavioural approaches in psychiatry.

REFERENCES

Agras WS, Taylor CB, Feldman DE, Losch M, Burnett KF 1990 Developing computer assisted therapy for the treatment of obesity. Behavior Therapy 21: 99–109

Argyle M 1977 The psychology of interpersonal behaviour, 2nd edn. Penguin, Harmondsworth

Azrin N H, Foxx R M 1974 Toilet training in less than a day. S & S, Austin

Bandura A 1969 Principles of behaviour modification. Holt, Rinehart & Winston, New York

Beck A T 1963 Thinking and depression: I. Idiosyncratic content and cognitive distortions. Archives of General Psychiatry 9: 324–333

Beck A T 1964 Thinking and depression: II. Theory and therapy. Archives of General Psychiatry 10: 561–571

Beck A T 1967 Depression: clinical, experimental and theoretical aspects. Harper & Row, New York

Beck A T 1987 Cognitive models of depression. Journal of Cognitive Psychotherapy 1: 5–37

Beck A T, Emery G 1985 Anxiety disorders and phobias: a cognitive perspective. Basic Books, New York

Beck A T, Rush A J, Shaw B F, Emery G 1979 Cognitive therapy of depression. Guilford Press, New York

Beck A T, Freeman A et al 1990 Cognitive therapy of personality disorders. Guilford Press, New York

Bellack A S, Hersen M, Himmelhoch J M 1983 A comparison of social skills training, pharmacotherapy and psychotherapy for depression. Behaviour Research and Therapy 21: 101–107

Berkowitz S, Sherry P J, Davis B A 1971 Teaching self-feeding skills to profound retardates using reinforcement and fading procedures. Behaviour Therapy 2: 62–67

Blackburn I M 1986 The cognitive revolution: an ongoing evolution. Behavioural Psychotherapy 14: 274–277

Blackburn I M 1988 An appraisal of comparative trials of cognitive therapy. In: Perris C, Blackburn I M & Perris H (eds) Cognitive psychotherapy. Theory and practice. Springer-Verlag, Heidelberg

Blackburn I M, Davidson K M 1990 Cognitive therapy for depression and anxiety. A practitioner's guide. Blackwell Scientific, Oxford

Blackburn I M, Bishop S, Glen A I M, Whalley L J, Christie J E 1981 The efficacy of cognitive therapy in depression: a treatment trial using cognitive therapy and pharmacotherapy, each alone and in combination. British Journal of Psychiatry 139: 181–189

Blackburn I M, Eunson K M, Bishop S 1986 A two year naturalistic follow-up of depressed patients treated with cognitive therapy, pharmacotherapy and a combination of both. Journal of Affective Disorders 19: 65–75

Brownell K D, Heckerman C L, Westlake R J, Hayes S C, Monti P M 1978 The effect of couples training and partner cooperativeness in the behaviour treatment of obesity. Behaviour Research and Therapy 16: 323–333

Brownell K D, Stunkard A J, Albaun J N 1980 Evaluation and modification of exercise patterns in the natural environment. American Journal of Psychiatry 137: 1540–1545

Candy J, Balfour F, Cawley R H, Hildebrand H P, Marks I M, Wilson J 1972 A feasibility study for a controlled trial of formal psychotherapy. Psychological Medicine 2: 345–362

Cooper N A, Clum G A 1989 Imaginal flooding as a supplementary treatment for post traumatic stress disorder in combat veterans: a controlled study. Behavior Therapy 20: 281–291

Coyne J, Gottlib I 1983 The role of cognition in depression: a critical appraisal. Psychological Bulletin 94: 472–505

Cullen C, Hattersley J, Tennant L 1981 Establishing behaviour, the constructional approach. In: Davey G (ed) Applications of conditioning theory. Methuen, London

Di Loreto A O 1971 Comparative psychotherapy: an experimental analysis. Aldine-Atherton, Chicago

Dryden W 1984 Rational–emotive therapy: fundamentals and innovations. Croom Helm, London

Ellis A 1962 Reason and emotion in psychotherapy. Citadel Press: Secaucus, NJ

Ellis A 1970 The essence of rational psychotherapy: a comprehensive approach to treatment. Institute for Rational Living, New York

Espie C A, Lindsay W R, Brooks D N, Hood E M, Turvey T 1989 A controlled comparative investigation of psychological treatments for chronic sleep-onset insomnia. Behaviour Research and Therapy 27: 79–88

Fielding D 1985 Factors associated with drop-out, relapse and failure in the conditioning treatment of nocturnal enuresis. Behavioural Psychotherapy 13: 174–185

Foxx R M, Azrin N H 1972 Restitution: a method of eliminating aggressive–disruptive behaviour of retarded and brain-damaged individuals. Behaviour Research and Therapy 10: 15–27

Goldstein A P 1973 Structured learning therapy: towards a psychotherapy for the poor. Academic Press, New York

Hawton K, Salkovskis P M, Kirk J, Clark D M 1989 Cognitive behaviour therapy for psychiatric problems: a practical guide. Oxford University Press, Oxford

Heather N, Robertson I 1983 Controlled drinking. Methuen, London

Jacobson E 1938 Progressive relaxation. University of Chicago Press, Chicago

Kanfer F H, Saslow G 1969 Behavioural diagnosis. In: Franks C M (ed) Behaviour therapy: appraisal and status. McGraw-Hill, New York

Ledwidge B 1978 Cognitive behaviour modification: a step in the wrong direction? Psychological Bulletin 85: 353–375

Liberman R P, Mueser K T, Wallace C J 1986 Social skills training for schizophrenic individuals at risk for relapse. American Journal of Psychiatry 143: 523–526

Lichstein, K L 1988 Clinical relaxation strategies Wiley, New York

Linscheid T R, Iwata B A, Ricketts R W, Williams D E, Griffin J C 1990 Clinical evaluations of self injurious behavior inhibiting system (SIBIS). Journal of Applied Behavior Analysis 23: 53–78

McNamee G, O'Sullivan G, Lelliott P, Marks I 1989 Telephone-guided treatment for housebound agoraphobics with panic disorder: exposure vs. relaxation. Behavior Therapy 20: 490–497

Marcer D 1986 Biofeedback and related therapies in clinical practice. Croom Helm, London

Marks I M 1982 Drugs combined with behavioural psychotherapy. In: Bellack A S, Hersen M, Kazdin A E (eds) International handbook of behaviour modification and therapy. Plenum Press, New York

Marks I M, Stern R, Mawson D, Cobb J, McDonald R 1980 Clomipramine and exposure for obsessive-compulsive rituals: 1. British Journal of Psychiatry 136: 1–25

Mathews A M, Gelder M G, Johnston D W 1981 Agoraphobia: nature and treatment. Tavistock, London

Nirenberg T D, Maisto S A 1987 Developments in the assessment and treatment of addictive behaviors. Ablex, Norwood, NJ

Patel C, North W R S 1975 Randomised controlled trial of yoga and biofeedback in management of hypertension. Lancet ii: 93–95

Paul G L, Lentz R J 1977 Psychosocial treatment of chronic mental patients. Harvard University Press, Cambridge, MA

Pearce S, Wardle J 1989 The practice of behavioural medicine. Oxford University Press, Oxford

Salkovskis P, Jones D, Clark D 1986 Respiratory control in the treatment of panic attacks: replication and extension with concurrent measurement of behaviour and pCO_2 British Journal of Psychiatry 148: 526–532

Salkovskis P M, Westbrook D 1989 Behaviour therapy and obsessional ruminations: can failure be turned into success? Behaviour Research and Therapy 27: 149–160

Seidner M L, Kirschenbaum D S 1980 Behavioural contracts: effects of pretreatment information and intention statements. Behaviour Therapy 11: 689–698

Silverstone T, Turner P 1974 Drug treatment in psychiatry. Routledge & Kegan Paul, London

Skinner B F 1963 Behaviourism at fifty. Science 140: 951–958

Sloane R B, Stephen P R, Cristal A M, Yorkeston N J, Whipple K 1975 Psychotherapy vs behavior therapy. Harvard University Press, Cambridge, MA

Sobell M B, Sobell L C 1973 Individual behavior therapy for alcoholics. Behaviour Therapy 4: 49–72

Stuart R B 1967 Behavioural control of overeating. Behaviour Research and Therapy 5: 357–365

Suinn R M 1990 Anxiety management training: a behavior therapy. Plenum Press, New York

Trower P, Bryant B, Argyle M 1978 Social skills and mental health. Methuen, London

Truax C B, Carkhuff R R 1967 Toward effective counselling and psychotherapy: training and practice. Aldine, Chicago

Turvey A 1985 Treatment manuals. In: Watts F N (ed) New developments in clinical psychology. Wiley, Chichester

Watson J B 1924 Behaviourism. University of Chicago Press, Chicago

Weber S, Jesien G, Shearer D et al 1975 The Portage guide to home teaching. Co-operative educational service agency 12, Portage, WI

Wolpe J 1958 Psychotherapy by reciprocal inhibition. Stanford University Press, Stanford

42. Rehabilitation and community care

J. A. T. Dyer

INTRODUCTION

Serious psychiatric illness may be associated with various kinds of disability which make it difficult or impossible for the individual to fulfil normally expected social roles. This is also true of physical illnesses, as the decline in importance of acute infectious disorders reveals many conditions with chronic morbidity, like stroke or chronic bronchitis. It may be argued, however, that in psychiatry the intimate interaction between biological and social factors in producing disability and handicap is particularly complex and important.

Rehabilitation works at the core of psychiatry, seeking to help those most severely disabled by the most serious psychiatric disorders. This chapter will use schizophrenia as the typical disorder most commonly encountered in rehabilitation services, though these often also contain patients with severe manic–depressive illness, organic brain disease, mild mental subnormality and perhaps severe neurosis and personality disorder as well. Rehabilitation for those with substance abuse and psychogeriatric patients tends to be provided separately as part of the relevant services (see Chs 17 and 31). Rehabilitation services for head-injured patients are seriously deficient and sometimes gear themselves to physical, at the expense of behavioural, problems. As a result psychiatric services, which have a limited contribution to make to head injury management (e.g. in those with severe behaviour disorder), can be used inappropriately.

Rehabilitation has been described by Wing as having two components, enabling and caring: enabling, in the sense of helping the individual to lead as normal a life as possible in spite of his limitations; caring, in helping to create various kinds of protected or supported environments adapted to these limitations. (An expanded definition will be given later). It covers a wide range, from relatively short-term work over a few months restoring an individual

to full functioning, to the provision of long-term support where no onward progress is seen but where the individual's quality of life would collapse if no such service were provided. It is not an area where quick results may be expected. Progress, where it occurs, is often slow (a period of 1–3 years would not be unusual in a transitional facility) and may be interrupted by relapses of illness. Given the interaction between biological and psychosocial factors, however, the rehabilitation psychiatrist is ideally placed to practise 'whole-person' medicine in a multidisciplinary setting and faces the challenge of trying to provide an integrated service from disparate parts.

Rehabilitation is also at the centre of the current policy debate on ways of providing mental health services and the increasing movement in the direction of community care. For various reasons, described below, over the last three to four decades in the UK there has been increasingly an attempt to move away from mental hospitals as the main location for the treatment and care of those with major long-term mental illness and to find alternative ways of providing services in more informal, local and domestic settings. Rehabilitation aids the successful discharge from hospital of those who have been there for some time but is increasingly used in non-in-patient settings to improve or maintain the functioning of people with major psychiatric disability. It is then synonymous with 'community care of the long-term mentally ill', though the latter will not always be provided by specialist rehabilitation teams, who concentrate on the more complex cases.

The term 'community care' is unsatisfactory as a description of extra-hospital services. It is used here because of its wide currency, and because it is now enshrined in the NHS and Community Care Act 1990. It implies a clear boundary between hospital and community (it should be unclear) and also that a sense of community exists outside hospital and not within it. A patient is not automatically part of a richer community marooned in a seaside boarding house or a city group home than in a traditional mental hospital, which might have had a strong community with meaningful roles for patients, albeit with little contact with life outside.

The House of Commons Social Services Committee report on community care (1985) shares these doubts:

The phrase 'community care' means little in itself. It is a phrase used by some descriptively and others prescriptively: that is, by some as a shorthand way of describing certain specific services provided in certain ways and in certain places: by others as an ideal or principle in the light of which existing services are to be judged and new ones developed. It has in fact come to have such general reference as to be virtually meaningless. It has become a slogan with all the weakness that that implies.

It is more helpful to consider 'caring for a community', rather than 'community care', i.e. providing comprehensive and integrated services for a local area and within that deciding the correct balance between hospital and other ways of delivering care, applying principles of accessibility, acceptability, efficiency and effectiveness.

DEVELOPMENT OF REHABILITATION AND COMMUNITY CARE

Rehabilitation is not a new concept. In its modern form its history extends from World War II. Rehabilitation in general, like some other developments in health care, such as blood transfusion and group psychotherapy, acquired a paradoxical impetus from warfare, in which the need to restore role functioning is evidently felt more acutely. Rehabilitation methods were developed by the wartime Emergency Medical Service and special centres for service casualties. There was then, however, as there still is today, an unhelpful administrative dichotomy between medical services and other agencies involved in rehabilitation. Psychiatric rehabilitation was one of the earliest and best developed examples of rehabilitation services. In 1980 the Royal College of Psychiatrists published a report entitled 'Psychiatric Rehabilitation in the 1980s', and this was updated in 1987 (Royal College of Psychiatrists 1980, 1987). These documents set out principles, describe the necessary elements of practice and make recommendations on staff training and on coordination in planning and service provision. They call for one consultant to have a designated responsibility for rehabilitation in each health district, which should also have a multidisciplinary rehabilitation committee.

The current shift towards community care can be traced to a reforming movement in mental hospitals which acquired momentum during the 1950s and 1960s. It was boosted by the introduction of phenothiazine drugs but represented a change of orientation which predated this, in the context of the postwar National Health Service (NHS) and 'welfare state'. Pioneering psychiatrists and superintendents — Bennett, Macmillan, Early, Clark, Affleck, Jones — and others, with their staff, began to try to improve the quality of life for patients in hospital and to prepare for more independent living those deemed capable of it.

The 1957 'Royal Commission on the Law Relating to Mental Illness and Mental Deficiency' (Department of Health and Social Security 1957) recommended that 'No patient should be retained as a hospital in-patient when he has reached the stage at which he could return home if he had a reasonably good home to go to. At that stage the provision of residential care becomes the responsibility of the local authority.' This principle was incorporated in the subsequent Mental Health Acts of 1959 (England and Wales) and 1960 (Scotland).

Considerable optimism was generated by the time of the 1962 Hospital Plan for England and Wales (Ministry of Health 1962) which boldly predicted the abolition of mental hospital beds being half-way achieved by 1975 and their replacement by district general hospital units and local authority provision. The trumpeting rhetoric of Enoch Powell, then Minister of Health, might well have caused the walls to fall down by themselves: 'There they stand, isolated, majestic, imperious, brooded over by the gigantic water tower and chimney combined, rising unmistakably and daunting out of the countryside — the asylums which our forefathers built with such solidity.' The utopian plan to solve mental hospital problems by abolition was also by now being informed by political and economic concerns. The dilapidated hospitals would be expensive to repair and properly staff, with the government's poor husbandry highly visible, as was to be painfully illustrated during the 1970s by a sad series of hospital inquiries into abuse of long-term patients (Martin 1984). Scotland, with smaller and less remote mental hospitals, never adopted a policy of abolition and pursued a slower approach to discharge of long-stay patients, whether through government department inertia or healthy scepticism about the provision of alternative services, or both.

The Hospital Plan proved overoptimistic. Previous arithmetic extrapolations of the fall in mental hospital beds, which began in 1955 in England and Wales (Tooth & Brooke 1961), turned out to have been misleading. Places vacated by long-term schizophrenic patients were occupied by the growing number of elderly people with dementia. Some anti-institutional social campaigners, fuelled by uncritical reading of Goffman's (1961) description of the 'total institution', had encouraged the naive belief that disability would drop away as the patient left through the hospital gates. Early success in discharging patients whose disability was indeed more social than psychiatric ('institutionalism') could not be maintained once those with more intrinsic psychiatric disability were tackled. Furthermore, costs of hospitals did not fall in proportion to their reducing size, because overheads remained and also the residual population became a relatively more disabled one, with greater costs per patient.

The number of residents in mental hospital and psychiatric units in England dropped from 106 900 to 60 300 between 1970 and 1986, while the numbers of admissions increased from 172 900 to 197 300. The increase in admissions was in re-admissions, not first admissions. (Many chronically ill patients who would formerly have experienced a long stay in hospital now experience intermittent hospitalisation via the 'revolving door' and develop 'cumulative chronicity'.) It is hard to obtain accurate information, but it appears that 30 mental hospitals closed between 1980 and 1989 and a further 32 are earmarked for closure before 1995. The reduction in residents in Scotland has been less, from 18 300 in 1970 to 13 500 in 1989, and the rise in admissions (again only re-admissions) proportionately greater, from 22 200 in 1970 to 29 200 in 1989. These trends are shown in diagrammatic form expressed as rates per 100 000 of the population in Figure 42.1. The reduction in residents with functional psychosis is actually greater than these figures would suggest because their decline has been partially offset by increases in psychogeriatric residents. In Scotland over 15 years from 1976 to 1990, for example, the fall by one-quarter in occupied beds conceals the fact that non-psychogeriatric beds fell by more than one half while psychogeriatric beds more than tripled. The proportion of residents aged 75+ years has increased from 24% in 1970 to 46% in 1989.

While beds were being dismantled, the looked-for expansion in alternative community facilities did not materialise to anything like the necessary degree (House of Commons Social Services Committee 1985). Local authorities, who in 1989 gave only about 3% of their social services departments' expenditure

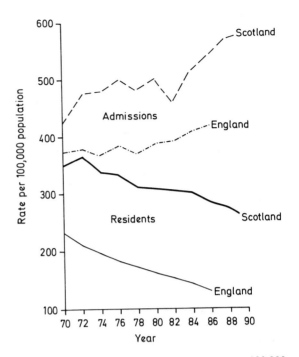

Fig. 42.1 All admissions and residents as rates per 100 000 of the population for mental illness hospitals and psychiatric units, from 1970 onwards; rates for England and Scotland are shown separately. (Source: Scottish Health Statistics and Health and Personal Social Services Statistics, England.)

specifically to the mentally ill (Secretaries of State for Health, Social Security, Wales and Scotland 1989), found themselves with more pressing commitments to children, the elderly and the mentally subnormal and increasingly financially restricted by a government dedicated to reducing public expenditure and mistrustful of local authorities. A report on mental health services for adults in Scotland (Scottish Home and Health Department, Scottish Education Department 1985), for example, noted that local authority day place provision was 2840 places short of the 3000 recommended by Department of Health and Social Security guidelines. Similarly, while 1700 places were required in hostels and other supported accommodation, current provision was 500 places. The report concluded that 'There is at present such a serious shortfall ... of community alternatives to in-patient mental health care, that it has not proved possible to develop the comprehensive locally-based mental health service which is required if care in the community is to become a reality'.

In the 1980s, public concern switched from hospital abuse to community neglect. Critics pointed out an increase in mentally ill 'rootless wanderers' in reception centres, common lodging houses, prisons, park benches and cardboard boxes as well as to the hard to measure burden on unsupported caring relatives (Fadden et al 1987). They warned of the cyclical nature of mental health policy and that the conditions which has been a stimulus to the building of the 19th century hospitals — the languishing of the mentally ill in private madhouses and local authority neglect — might soon be recreated.

Faced with mounting criticism — but also concerned at the steeply escalating cost of social security expenditure on independent residential and nursing home care, which rose from £10 million in 1979 to over £1000 million in 1989 — the government acted. In November 1989 it produced a white paper entitled 'Caring for People: Community Care in the Next Decade and Beyond' (Secretaries of State for Health, Social Security, Wales and Scotland 1989) and there has been subsequent legislation in the NHS and Community Care Act 1990.

These measures give responsibility for the social aspects of community care of the mentally ill (along with the mentally handicapped, physically disabled and elderly mentally infirm) to local authorities, who are, however, directed to become increasingly purchasers rather than providers of services. Voluntary and private providers are to be encouraged. Local authorities are required to produce and publish community care plans for their area, jointly or in concert with plans produced by health authorities. They must also provide assessments of people likely to require community care services and set up care management systems.

A central feature is a change in the method of funding. Whereas the costs of independent and nursing home residential care were previously paid via social security benefit, that money, plus an 'adequate' supplement from the Treasury, is to be transferred to local authorities, who will then provide or purchase services. This has the potential advantage of removing the 'perverse incentive', whereby it can be easier to obtain (perhaps unnecessary) residential care for a person than to provide services in their home; but replacing a system of benefit entitlement with one of a cash-limited fund to local authorities *which is not earmarked specifically for community care* has serious drawbacks. If insufficient money for community care is provided by government, or allocated by local authorities, or both, long-stay patients able to leave hospital will have to compete and queue up for available funds. At the time of writing there is a degree of scepticism as to whether the Conservative government will fully follow through these plans. Ideological difficulties over giving money and responsibility to local authorities are compounded by major political problems over local taxation. Shortly after the Act was passed, implementation was delayed, and the change in the funding mechanism is not due to occur till 1993.

'Caring for People' recognises that these plans will not in any way reduce the necessary NHS provision for community care and also that there will be a continuing need for NHS long-term residential care, preferably in small, more domestic units. It acknowledges that 'there are legitimate concerns that in some places hospital beds have been closed before better, alternative facilities were fully in place' and promises that 'Ministers will not approve the closure of any mental hospital unless it can be demonstrated that adequate alternatives have been developed'. In view of the particularly poor provision of community facilities for the mentally ill to date, some earmarked money, a specific grant for mental illness, is to be paid to local authorities, via health authorities in England and directly in Scotland, to accelerate provision. This is on a project basis, at less than 100% of costs and for a limited number of years.

As well as concerns over whether social services departments will be given financial resources equal to the task, doubts have been expressed about whether these departments have the necessary managerial and professional expertise in relation to services for the mentally ill. Criticisms also refer to an insufficiently focused central leadership and accountability in relation to community care. At the same time, within the NHS, managers are under increasing pressure to hasten to community care for financial reasons: to raise capital from sales of land and buildings and reduce revenue costs by transferring patients to other agencies. An uninformed strand of thinking in the government's NHS 'reforms' appears to see the NHS of the future as an acute 'white-coat' service unencumbered by responsibility for continuing care of chronic illnesses.

A remarkable feature of these changes over the last few decades has been the paucity of studies comparing the benefits and costs of hospital versus community care (Wright 1987). A major study is being conducted by the Team for Assessment of Psychiatric Services (TAPS) in relation to the closure by North East Thames Regional Health Authority (NETRHA) of Claybury and Friern Hospitals, but will not be completed until at least 1994. Preliminary results after 2 years of follow-up show no significant differences before and after discharge in symptom and social behaviour scores. In simple money terms, costs were less in the community than in hospital but undoubtedly the most able and least expensive were selected to leave first. The patients expressed favourable attitudes about the less restrictive conditions they found in the community. It must be noted, however, that the NHS was meeting over 40% of the accommodation costs in the community, and the researchers acknowledge that NETRHA is unusually generous in dowries (annual revenue that leaves hospital with the patient), capital funding and bridging finance (Team for the Assessment of Psychiatric Services 1990).

Although such studies will be important guides, efficacy in one particular set of services does not necessarily mean that a policy is effective in the country as a whole, as is well illustrated in Italy (Jones 1988). Chapter 2 gives accounts of the national experiments in Italy, where mental hospital admission was declared illegal in 1978, and the USA, where the population of the public mental hospitals fell by over 70% in the two decades to 1977. It seems clear overall that the cost of adequate community care is not less than that of the inadequate hospital care provided in the past, and it is higher in the initial overlap period (Thornicroft & Bebbington 1989).

NATURE OF DISABLEMENT

Confusion over terminology has been reduced by the World Health Organization's *International Classification of Impairments, Disabilities and Handicaps* (WHO 1980). Impairment is loss of normal function at the organ level. Disability operates at the level of the person and describes disturbance, due to impairments, in performing normal actions or functions. Handicap refers to disadvantages suffered by an individual as a result of impairments and disabilities; it reflects interaction with, and adaptation to, the environment. For example, cutting motor nerves at the wrist causes impairment in hand muscle function. The individual is then disabled in relation to tasks requiring manual dexterity, but such disability would be more of a handicap to a surgeon than to a psychiatrist. Disability associated with schizophrenia will produce varying amounts of handicap in different settings and types of society.

Wing & Morris (1981) have grouped factors which contribute to disability and handicap in schizophrenia into three categories: psychiatric impairments, social disadvantages and adverse personal reactions to impairments and disadvantages.

Psychiatric impairments

These are features or symptoms associated with the illness itself and are fully described in Chapter 18. Positive symptoms such as delusions, hallucinations and incoherence of speech, and behaviour associated with them, as well as disrupting normal functioning, may be puzzling or frightening to others and lead to social rejection. More problematic in rehabilitation are negative symptoms which form the 'clinical poverty syndrome' (Wing & Brown 1970). These include social withdrawal, poverty of thought and speech, self-neglect, reduced motivation, blunting of affect and difficulty in verbal and non-verbal communication.

It is worth emphasising again here the intimate links between biological and social factors in schizophrenia. The symptoms, despite a presumed biological basis, are responsive to changes in the social environment. Wing & Brown's (1970) classic three-hospital study, for example, showed that the 'clinical poverty syndrome' is closely related to the quality of the hospital social environment. Decreasing the amount of time spent doing nothing and replacing it with work or occupational therapy was associated with a reduction in negative symptoms. But it is possible to go too far or too fast. A social environment which is too stressful may result in a reappearance of florid symptoms. Vaughn & Leff (1976) and others have shown that the risk of relapse in schizophrenia is greater with certain kinds of emotional atmosphere in the home and that it can be reduced by decreasing the amount of time spent in face-to-face contact with key relatives and by medication. Recent evidence, reviewed by Tarrier (1990), also suggests that therapeutic intervention with such families is effective in reducing the risk of relapse. Rehabilitation involves constantly walking the dividing line between under- and over-stimulation.

Although negative symptoms are responsive to social factors, it is important to realise that they are an integral feature of the illness rather than entirely social artefacts as some theories of institutionalism have suggested. This realisation cautions against the naive view that all discharged chronic patients will be able in time to take up normal 'independent' living in the community, a view which can lead to excessive stress (loss of protective asylum) and to failure to provide necessary supports. The evidence that they are integral to the illness includes neuroimaging studies which find morphological brain abnormalities in some schizophrenic patients that are associated with cognitive impairment and with negative symptoms (see Ch. 21) and also from follow-up studies of discharged patients. Johnstone et al (1981) found that a large group of discharged patients who had been out of hospital for 5–9 years did not differ in prevalence of negative symptoms from those still in hospital.

Other impairments may be present, e.g. blindness, deafness, mental subnormality or epilepsy, which compound the handicap and add to the difficulties in rehabilitation. Pushing relevant treatment to the limit is an essential prerequisite and accompaniment to rehabilitation.

Social disadvantages

People who suffer from serious psychiatric illness may have various kinds of social disadvantages. Some of these may have existed before the onset of illness, as with poor educational attainment or lack of occupational skills, and many others follow in the wake of illness, such as increased likelihood of unemployment and poverty. All too often, the 'chains of the asylum' have been replaced by the social straitjacket of poverty, still restricting social and recreational activities. Candidates for rehabilitation tend to lack social supports: they are often effectively single and may be homeless. People with schizophrenia marry less often than other people, and those who do more frequently get divorced and have fewer children.

These social disadvantages have a sad tendency to build up over time. A major challenge of rehabilitation is to prevent this accumulation of disablement.

Adverse personal reactions

Various kinds of adverse personal reactions may form a further barrier between the sufferer from schizophrenia and social integration. They may be his own reactions — the effects on self-image and self-esteem of being ill, not normal, different. They may be the reactions of relatives who have particular difficulty in understanding or coping with the changed behaviour or altered potential of their sick family member, and who may overprotect or reject him. Or they may be reactions of wider society, potential landlords, potential employers and others who may discriminate against the mentally ill, partly through ignorance. It follows, therefore, that rehabilitation should not simply be a process applied to a sick individual but should have as an essential component education of the general public about mental illness and the disabilities and needs of its sufferers. Staff of the rehabilitation team should be involved in this process.

Wing & Morris (1981) include as an extreme example of the disabling effect of adverse personal reactions the phenomenon of 'institutionalism' with its lack of self-direction and reduced self-esteem brought about by impersonal, neglectful and stigmatising environments, *whether in or out of hospital.* (I have more than once admitted patients to a hospital rehabilitation unit in order to reverse institutionalism induced at home.)

DEFINITION OF REHABILITATION

We are now in a position to say what rehabilitation is. As Wing (1980) defined it, it is 'the process of minimising psychiatric impairments, social disadvantages and adverse personal reactions, so that the disabled person is helped to use his or her talents and to acquire confidence and self-esteem through experiencing success in social roles'. Note the emphasis on using positive attributes as well as attacking disabilities and on the importance of 'social roles' as opposed to cruder concepts such as return to work or hospital discharge.

Rehabilitation should be distinguished from resettlement. Resettlement is a simpler concept meaning just what it says — replacing a person into a particular setting, usually from hospital back to community or perhaps from sheltered day facilities to work. It is possible, though far from desirable, to have resettlement of long-stay patients without rehabilitation. Rehabilitation makes resettlement, where it is desirable, more possible and more likely to succeed.

Confusion may also arise over the scope of the term rehabilitation. Sometimes it is restricted to services which seek to change people to a more independent level of functioning and therefore only engage them for a transitional period. Alternatively, it is used in a broader way to include long-term supportive care in or out of hospital which seeks to maintain the optimum level of functioning of the disabled individual and prevent deterioration. Problems can arise, for example, when long-stay wards use the description 'rehabilitation' in order to enjoy the unfortunately greater status which seems to adhere to the narrower, more active meaning of the word, only to experience frustration and disappointment when they find that resettlement and change do not occur. This problem would be diminished if long-term support or maintenance rehabilitation, rather than having a tinge of failure about it, was treated as being as worthy and respectable a pursuit — for those who need it — as is the more active or transitional rehabilitation for those who are less disabled.

PRINCIPLES OF REHABILITATION

Different rehabilitation schemes in varying settings rely on a few basic principles:

1. A programme is devised which is tailored as much as possible to the individual. The programme involves a series of steps, the early ones being small and designed so that success is readily achieved. Continuity of commitment to the individual patient is required.

2. The programme is based on a thorough initial assessment of the individual, taking into account strengths as well as disabilities. Important areas are likely to include the following:

a. Self-care: personal hygiene, care of clothes, cooking, housework, management of money; adequacy of these and need for prompting/supervision

b. Social relationships: interaction skills, socially embarrassing behaviour, contacts with family and friends, needs of carers for support/advice, emotional atmosphere in the home

c. Work history, current ability, use of leisure time

d. Symptoms and medication: whether optimum stabilisation has been reached.

e. The individual's own motivation, goals and talents.

Following on from this assessment, overall aims are formulated, preferably in discussion with the individual, and carers if relevant, and intermediate goals decided upon. Periodic reassessment is undertaken and the aims and goals may require readjustment in the light of progress or altered circumstances.

3. A comprehensive approach is required, remembering again that biological and social factors are bonded together and cannot (properly) be treated separately despite artificial administrative hurdles. Multidisciplinary teamwork and interagency cooperation is of the essence.

PRACTICE OF REHABILITATION

Rehabilitation services around the country show patchy development and different stages of evolution. At the beginning they are often most concerned with helping long-stay patients out of hospital. At first, this is relatively easy and encouraging as the less disabled patients are tackled first (the 'rehabilitation honeymoon'). Things get more difficult when a residue of more disabled patients is reached. By this stage there is also a need to give greater attention to maintaining those patients already discharged from hospital and supporting community care. Appropriate new facilities have to be developed to care for those who would previously have become long-stay in hospital.

It has been customary to talk about two parallel rehabilitation 'ladders' — domestic and occupational — on which patients might make differential progress. Changes in employment conditions have now put an unpleasant snake in beside the ladders and things have become more complicated. This point will be expanded below. One result is that there is less separation between domestic and occupational rehabilitation than there used to be. For example, occupational therapists who formerly set out to prepare patients for re-entry into employment may see this as leading the patient to disillusionment if he cannot get a job, and concentrate instead on training in social skills and productive use of leisure time; the housework and cooking learned in domestic rehabilitation may become important occupational activities in themselves rather than tasks to be fitted round employment. For ease of exposition, occupational and domestic rehabilitation will be described separately here, but the increasing overlap should be borne in mind.

Occupational rehabilitation

The comments above relating to changes in employment conditions cover two main factors. The obvious one is the increased prevailing rate of unemployment. Unemployment in the UK rose sharply from 1979 to a peak of over 3 million (over 13%) in 1986. It then declined somewhat but at the time of writing has risen again to over 2 million. Changes in the method of calculating the figures have led to an underestimation of the problem. There is regional variation, with the problem being worst in Northern Ireland, Scotland and the north of England and least in the south-east of England. Given that those disabled by serious mental illness have diminished competitive power in the job market anyway, a high unemployment rate tends to push jobs almost beyond their reach. Morgan & Cheadle (1975) found that, above an unemployment level of 6%, resettlement in employment was virtually impossible. Below 2% it was easy. The whole community suffers as a result of high unemployment, but the mentally ill suffer disproportionately.

A less obvious adverse change is in the nature of employment itself. Previously, many disabled mentally ill people were able to sustain fairly simple manual jobs from which poor concentration or intolerance of stress did not disqualify them. Factors such as automation and the shrinkage of manufacturing industry mean that these types of jobs have selectively disappeared.

Sadly, the patients in contact with psychiatric rehabilitation services have little prospect of moving on to open employment under recent socioeconomic conditions. Rehabilitation services face the difficult challenge of responding to this fact. Traditionally, they stressed the importance of work, not only for its value in society generally but also because it was held to be a crucial component of the process of rehabilitation itself. Wing & Brown (1970) showed that reducing time spent doing nothing in hospital and replacing it with work and occupational therapy was associated with reduction in negative symptoms. Participating in work settings encouraged a certain amount of social interaction and cooperation without being too socially stressful. Ability to work was shown in a number of studies to be an important predictor of success in rehabilitation.

It is sometimes now suggested that the inclusion of work in rehabilitation programmes is only preparation for disillusionment; that work should be abandoned and replaced by training for unemployment through enhancing social interaction skills and the productive use of leisure time. In the writer's view this would be a mistake. The primary role of work in rehabilitation was never re-entry into employment, even when this was easier: work had intrinsic value both as a means in rehabilitation and as an end in itself. (Work and employment are not the same thing. Employment is one kind of work, i.e. paid work. There are other kinds, such as housework, studying and voluntary work.)

Work is important to mental health in general. Jahoda (1982), from her work in the 1930s, has listed the benefits, over and above financial reward, which work provides to people:

It imposes a time structure on the working day; it enlarges the scope of social relations beyond the often emotionally highly charged family relations and those in the immediate neighbourhood; by virtue of the division of labour it demonstrates that purposes and achievements of a collectivity transcend those for which an individual can aim; it assigns social status and clarifies personal identity; it requires regularity.

Warr (1987) adds that the unemployed lose the 'traction' effect of work (relating to how it pulls you along, how you achieve more when you're busy or how the unemployed man looks out on an untended garden). They have smaller scope for making big decisions and less chance of developing new skills, they suffer frequent humiliations and they lose social status.

There is also evidence, reviewed by Smith (1987), of the adverse consequences of unemployment on mental health. A number of longitudinal studies show that in men (who are easier to classify) unemployment leads to a deterioration in mental health, and re-employment to an improvement. Warr (1987) considers poverty likely to be the most important stress linking unemployment to its adverse health effects. Unemployment, especially long-term unemployment, is also associated with increased risk of both suicide and parasuicide, though here there is less confidence about causality (Smith 1987).

Despite high unemployment, it is still 'normal' to go to work. Although it might take a second thought to agree with Noel Coward that 'Work is more fun than fun', being unemployed is rarely much fun. Those disabled by mental illness, often already poor and with few other sources of social status, should not be condemned to a life of permanent leisure. With their damaged personal resources they are ill-equipped for a role as involuntary pioneers of the leisure age.

Every effort should be made to provide those disabled by mental illness with work opportunities. If paid employment is not attainable, then other ways have to be found of gaining the benefits of work listed above. Increasing use of voluntary work is being made in this respect, as is engaging in further education, perhaps making good prior educational under-attainment, and part-time work is sometimes possible where full-time work would be too demanding. Employers and the general public still need to be educated about mental illness, and various kinds of special or 'sheltered' work situations are needed where full productivity is not expected and/or extra support is required. Work training for the most able candidates needs to be reoriented towards service and clerical rather than manufacturing work and to assimilate new technologies. Wider changes at a national level which would be likely to have mental health benefits include facilitating the creation of more jobs, sharing work out more fairly and decreasing the poverty of the unemployed (Smith 1987).

This defence of the role of work in no way undervalues the new efforts which are being made to help patients to cope with the amount of leisure time which they will have either through their age, their disability or lack of proper provision of work opportunities. It could be argued that rehabilitation services are ahead of society in offering such preparation. Attention is increasingly being given to furthering social interaction skills, interest in current affairs and use of local recreational and educational facilities. While the vulnerability of the schizophrenic

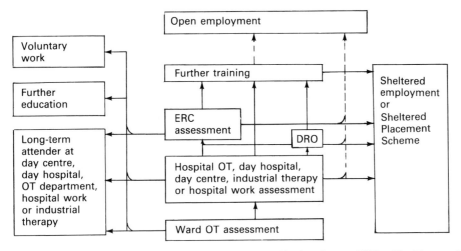

OT = Occupational therapy; ERC = Employment Rehabilitation Centre; DRO = Disablement Resettlement Officer.

Fig. 42.2   Occupational rehabilitation.

patient to social stress has to be borne in mind by enthusiasts in, for example, group interaction techniques, there is little lament for the decline of the more purposeless, repetitive contract type of work such as tying labels.

Figure 42.2 gives an outline of occupational rehabilitation. Traditionally this starts in hospital with an assessment in which the occupational therapist plays a major part and this assessment may be extended in the various settings listed in the figure. Beyond this there are assessment, training and sheltered work opportunities provided by the Department of Employment. The disablement resettlement officer (DRO) is employed in Job Centres to give special attention to employment problems of those with disability. Employment Rehabilitation Centres (ERCs) are scattered throughout the country. These provide assessment in differing work skills over a month or two, but with some exceptions have tended to be geared to physical rather psychiatric disability. Some candidates after ERC assessment are recommended for Skills Training Centres, also open to non-disabled people, where they can obtain training in specific occupations.

The Employment Training scheme is geared towards enhancing the employability of those who have been out of work for 6 months or more and offers work training and an allowance of £10 over benefit for a period of 12 months, and some schemes cater especially for the mentally ill, with a rehabilitative approach. Employment Training is currently run by local Training and Enterprise

Councils in England and Wales (Local Enterprise Companies in Scotland) which are composed predominantly of local private sector employers. The more market forces are allowed free rein, the more the mentally disabled are forced out of these schemes. There is also a Disablement Advisory Service to advise and encourage employers in relation to engaging disabled people.

Sheltered employment is greatly underprovided. A promising recent development is the concept of the Sheltered Placement Scheme, but in the UK at present under 4% of available places are occupied by the mentally ill. Under this scheme a sponsoring organisation supports disabled workers (singly or in a group) in a normal industrial or commercial setting. The employer pays only for the work done, while the sponsor, who pays the actual wages, can be recompensed by the Department of Employment for the shortfall in productivity associated with disability, as well as for costs of training and supervision. This gives those with disability the opportunity to become integrated in normal work settings and perhaps exposes employers to experiential education about disability. Other sources of sheltered employment are local authorities, voluntary organisations and industry itself. Newer approaches include worker cooperatives and co-ownership schemes. Early pioneered the development of independent industrial therapy organisations in Bristol (Early & Magnus 1968), forging links between the hospital and local industrialists, trade unions and charitable organisations. The Bristol organisation developed to provide

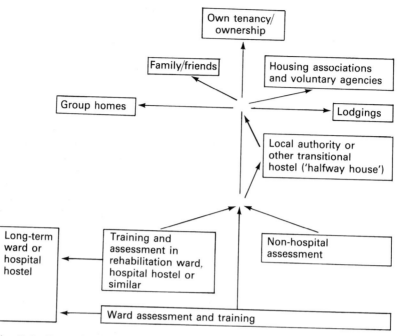

Fig. 42.3 Domestic rehabilitation.

a range of opportunities from a contract factory to sheltered groups in open industry. In the past, some hospital patients benefited from work placements with porters, gardeners, etc., either as incentive pay or sometimes in paid employment. Competitive tendering of ancillary services appears to have been associated with a reduction in such opportunities, though there is no good reason why such possibilities could not be written into the tendering process.

Domestic rehabilitation

Here again (see Fig. 42.3) the traditional path originates in hospital with attempts to promote more individual responsibility in self-care and to provide training. Often special transitional facilities are organised, making use of whatever facilities are offered by the local situation, e.g. turning hospital buildings and staff houses into hostels (Affleck 1981). The most disabled patients need continuous staff availability and perhaps also the benefits of 'asylum', which Wing (1990) describes as having two components, recuperation as well as refuge. They either remain in long-stay wards or in newer forms of care such as 'hostel wards' which provide an equivalent degree of care in a more domestic setting, the latter being especially necessary in localities whose hospital provision is in a

district general hospital (Garety & Morris 1984, Goldberg et al 1985).

Beyond the hospital and hospital hostels, there is a need for accommodation with varying degrees of staff support, both transitional and permanent. Group homes are constituted when small numbers of discharged patients move into what is usually a local authority house or flat and are supported to a varying degree by visiting workers — social worker, community psychiatric nurse (CPN) or volunteer workers or a mixture of these (Ryan 1979). Group homes best suit older patients who want to put down roots. Some patients are accommodated by family or friends, while others are able to sustain their own tenancy or have their own property. Voluntary organisations and housing associations (which acquire government funds to buy and renovate property) are increasingly important sources of supported accommodation for the mentally ill and they produce innovative forms of support. Younger patients prefer flats and bedsits, which can be in cluster arrangements with communal day space. Lodgings with landladies are another important resource — especially for those, usually men, with a disinclination to cook, and some holiday resorts with this type of accommodation available have provided a destination for discharged patients. The provision of support and discreet supervision for the landladies is an important feature not always present. The private sector is not an important provider at present but is receiving political encouragement to become so, including private nursing homes for more disabled patients.

The problem sometimes arises in this field too of the more transitional work being apparently more prestigious, and relative underprovision of permanent accommodation with an adequate degree of support outside hospital can result in some of the more disabled patients remaining in hospital unnecessarily. Mann & Cree (1976) found in a survey of new long-stay patients in hospital that about 40% of those aged under 65 years were suitable for non-hospital residential units. In a later Scottish survey, McCreadie et al (1983) found an almost identical proportion of new chronic patients 'misplaced' in hospital.

Social skills training

Both occupational and domestic aspects of rehabilitation need to be complemented by attention to abilities required for normal social interaction. Social skills training (Trower et al 1979) pays attention to such factors as making conversation, interview behaviour and other employment skills, expressing feelings, appropriate self-assertion, restaurant and pub behaviour, management of money and reduction of socially embarrassing behaviour such as intrusiveness and poor hygiene. It is often linked to education about the use of local recreational facilities and telephones, public transport, post offices, etc.

Rehabilitation resources

Staff

The basic NHS rehabilitation team consists of psychiatrist, nursing staff including CPNs, psychologist, occupational therapist and social worker. Multidisciplinary work is essential, and there may be considerable overlap in the function of team members as well as individual professional strengths. It is helpful if each individual client/patient is allocated a key worker (Royal College of Psychiatrists 1980) who is a regular point of contact, counsellor and organiser of other services for that individual. The psychiatrist is usually accorded a coordinating role though this may be taken by other members. Most psychiatrists involved are general psychiatrists with a special interest in rehabilitation. Nursing staff carry responsibility for much of the basic work of rehabilitation, especially the domestic aspects and supervision of medication. They spend most time with the patient, and have an

important observational role. Unless nurses have aptitude and training for rehabilitation, however, the caring emphasis in their role may sometimes operate at the expense of the enabling. CPNs supervise and support patients out of hospital where their medical knowledge of symptoms, drugs and side-effects helps to differentiate their role from that of the social worker. They have also made liaison with primary care staff a particular feature.

The social worker, while overlapping in supportive and resocialising functions with the CPN and other team members, has special responsibility for family and other important relationships and should prevent the rest of the team from neglecting these essential aspects (Kuipers & Bebbington 1985). There is now sufficient evidence of the benefit of family intervention in reducing risk of relapse in schizophrenia (involving family or relative group work with a problem-solving approach, in selected cases where a patient lives at home in a high 'expressed emotion' setting) to justify some staff specialising in these approaches (Tarrier 1990). Research is continuing to try to tease out what are the essential components of such approaches and how results from special studies can best be translated into everyday practice. So far, it appears that education alone is not enough, and, while family therapy intervention and relatives groups are equally effective, compliance is much better with the former. The social worker also has expert knowledge of welfare administration, and is often the main link with other non-NHS agencies.

The clinical psychologist contributes to overall policy and individual programmes from a psychological viewpoint and can contribute expertise in analysing and alleviating problematic behaviour as well as encouraging other team members to be suitably rigorous in planning and evaluating their work. The training of occupational therapists emphasises the enabling aspect, and they are the experts in assessing occupational capabilities and problems and in organising activities which contribute to occupational rehabilitation.

Two other types of personnel require mention. One is the service manager. It is important that the manager is in sympathy with the work of the rehabilitation team because administrative practices often cut across rehabilitation principles, e.g. contract buying of 'institutional' furniture for hostels, or wishing to avoid any possible risk to patients in activities like decorating or wiring plugs. Overprotective or restrictive attitudes of NHS ancillary staff can also hinder patients from learning to do jobs for themselves while still in hospital while private sector ancillary services may not feel much connection with therapeutic aims. In the increasingly commercial atmosphere in the NHS, managers (on short-term contracts) have to be encouraged not to downgrade services for the long-term mentally ill in favour of services with more 'market' appeal.

The general practitioner and the primary care team also deserve mention here. Although the general practitioner's psychiatric work is predominantly with neurotic and personality disorders he also helps to support and provide medication for psychotic patients out of hospital and is involved in crises. Attention should be given to good communication with general practitioners. The CPN has been mentioned as a particular link between primary care and the specialist team. It is important that as CPNs are attracted towards involvement with the less serious disorders in the primary care setting their traditional supportive function with discharged psychotic patients is not lost. Priorities may have to be set for use of limited CPN resource. (Wooff et al 1986).

Collaboration with non-NHS agencies

A successful rehabilitation service has to overcome artificial administrative barriers. The separate administrative structures of health and social work in England, Wales and Scotland (they are united in Northern Ireland) is particularly regrettable. Patients/clients have to cross the boundary from one service to another, catchment areas may not coincide and inaction may be excused by projecting blame on to the other agency. The document 'Caring for People' (Secretaries of State for Health, Social Security, Wales and Scotland 1989) does nothing fundamental to improve this situation, relying mainly on the largely discredited approach of exhortation towards collaboration in planning and service provision. It does promote the concept of the care manager: 'to take responsibility for ensuring that individuals' needs are regularly reviewed, resources are managed effectively, and that each service user has a single point of contact. The care manager will often be employed by the social services authority, but this need not always be so'. Local authorities are encouraged to link care management with delegated responsibility for budgetary management. Care management lacks a clear definition and can be pursued by a number of different models (Renshaw 1988). It is right that there should be flexibility in implementation, because different client groups in different local services may require different solutions. An important distinction is how much care management

is organisation centred, rationing out resources, and how much it is person centred, more akin to the key worker, making sure the individual gets the services he needs. In terms of collaboration between services, there have been some attempts to set up community teams, which can include local authority staff, to address the problems of the long-term mentally ill in the community.

Joint planning and provision of rehabilitation services includes other agencies also. The housing and education departments of the local authority are important, and mention has already been made of work training and employment agencies and housing associations. Voluntary bodies have an increasingly important part to play. National and local mental health associations have a campaigning and educative role as well as stimulating innovation in and sometimes running local services. Organisations like the National Schizophrenia Fellowship give patients and caring relatives a necessary and important voice and a vehicle for improving services. Unfortunately, the funding of voluntary bodies is not always secure and sometimes projects are funded only on a year-to-year basis so that community care does not have the secure foundation that it deserves.

The rehabilitation consultant still has to play a leading role in trying to ensure that all the necessary ingredients of a comprehensive service are assembled and in stimulating other agencies to attend to the needs of the mentally ill.

Facilities

Bennett wisely cautions against a preoccupation with means rather than ends. The important thing is the overall shape and purpose of the service and tying the different bits together. Particular facilities are often dictated by local history and geography, with their ideology arising as later rationalisation. The range of material elements required by a rehabilitation service include, however:

1. Psychiatric beds — for long-term care and acute relapses and crises
2. Day hospitals, day centres and social clubs
3. Continued care clinic, or other follow-up system for vulnerable patients
4. Supported accommodation, both transitional and permanent
5. Facilities for occupational therapy, work rehabilitation and training, and sheltered work.

Most of the above elements have been discussed already, but some further points may be made here.

In-patient beds for different purposes can be provided in a variety of settings. A major area of debate still is whether there is a continuing role for the mental hospital and, if not, how the 'asylum' function of the hospital can be recreated in other settings (Wing 1990). An interesting report in Scotland from a working party of the National Medical Consultative Committee (Scottish Home and Health Department and Scottish Health Service Planning Council 1989) points out that for some patients in-patient care requires to provide tolerance, security and protection (of the individual from society as well as vice versa) and advocates the development of the 'mental health campus' consisting of various functional modules, on redeveloped mental hospital or new sites, linked to peripheral units and forming a basis for community services. Among the functional modules would be domestic-scale long-stay in-patient units.

Day hospitals and day centres overlap a good deal in practical function (Carter 1981) despite their different names and parentage. Day hospitals, of which there are more, are NHS facilities with medical and nursing input. They cater for various ranges of patients from the acute, through transitional rehabilitation, to long-term support: in practice it is hard to stick to these neat classifications. Day centres are usually run by local authorities or voluntary organisations and may cover the same range, though usually tending more towards long-term support. Day facilities are considered very important in facilitating a move away from in-patient stay (partial hospitalisation), in sometimes averting the need for in-patient admission, and in permitting patients and relatives not to be stuck in unrelieved stressful contact with each other, as well as providing a setting for rehabilitative activities in general. Discharged patients might otherwise suffer a poorer quality of life without the social, recreational and therapeutic opportunities provided in good hospitals. Some form of social club for patients is also found desirable for informal meeting and inexpensive recreation. Some services have followed the American model of community mental health centres, often on a more limited scale, providing a local base for a variety of mental health agencies and activities. These are also sometimes referred to as mental health resource centres. The original American model included in-patient beds (Huxley 1990).

Continued care clinics were set up to aid the supervision and support of chronic patients discharged from hospital. Supervising maintenance medication was a particular function, often by depot injection, and the clinics are often known by the name of the first popular depot preparation. Such clinics help to ensure that this vulnerable group of patients do not get overlooked by services as well as giving patients the benefit of prolonged contact with the same personnel. They also permit expert monitoring of medication which can have troublesome short and long-term side effects and facilitate research. Medication is usually kept at a minimum maintenance level once acute treatment is completed, but may require increase in active phases of rehabilitation to help reduce the risk of acute relapse associated with greater stress.

Continued care clinics are becoming rather less popular and are being replaced by less formal systems of follow-up. These emphasise the need for (and are in turn permitted by) careful monitoring systems for vulnerable and long-term mentally ill people in the community. A computerised register of such people, as developed in York, is one solution (Harborne & Henderson 1989). Such moves are to date hampered by lack of agreed definitions of 'vulnerable' and 'long-term mentally ill'.

Measurement and outcome

If knowledge is to be advanced, it is clearly important that progress, outcome and other variables can be measured in a standardised way. Some useful tools have been developed (see also Ch. 9).

Moos (1974) has devised scales which permit a comparison of the 'atmosphere' of wards and other rehabilitation settings. Rating scales have been produced which summarise relevant behaviours and attributes in patients, many of which have been designed for use by nursing staff, such as Wing's ward behaviour rating scale (Wing 1961), NOSIE (the Nurses' Observational Scale for In-Patient Evaluation) (Honigfeld & Klett 1965) and REHAB (Rehabilitation Evaluation, Hall and Baker) (Baker 1983). Scales also exist specifically for assessing the social behaviour of patients and others (Platt et al 1980).

The difficult question of outcome is discussed by Affleck & McGuire (1984). It is too complex and individual a thing to be measured satisfactorily by crude criteria such as re-entry into work or avoiding hospital admission. Affleck & McGuire's MRSS (Morningside Rehabilitation Status Scale) gives a score for each patient on four dimensions relevant to rehabilitation: dependency on staff and services, activity (work and leisure), social integration and symptoms. The concept of 'qualify of life' is as crucial to outcome as it is difficult to measure. It is a rather individual thing, multifactorial, hard to pin down and laden with value judgements (Jones 1988). In practice, success should be individual and not absolute. While complete separation from services might be success for one candidate, achieving greater independent self-care in a long-term setting might be equal success for another who is more disabled.

The overall success of our current efforts will ultimately be judged by future generations. Shepherd (1990) suggests that to date change has been more in setting than in substance:

The scene is subtly shifting in rehabilitation. The main 'actors' are all familiar, but the 'backdrops' are now different. The scene is now no longer the mental hospital; it is the community hostel, the group home, the day centre, family homes, and, in some cases, the streets. But the patients remain as ever: lonely, poor, unemployed, often confused, sometimes angry about a world that does not seem prepared to meet their — apparently simple — needs.

I am inclined to agree with the conclusion of the House of Commons Social Services Committee report on community care (1985): 'in the final analysis, the outcome will be judged next century, neither by the location of care, nor by the nature of the agency providing care, nor even by the category of staff concerned, but by the quality of care available and the extent to which individual needs are catered for'.

REFERENCES

Affleck J W 1981 The Edinburgh progressive care system. In: Wing J K, Morris B (eds) Handbook of psychiatric rehabilitation practice. Oxford University Press, Oxford

Affleck J W, McGuire R J 1984 The measurement of psychiatric rehabilitation status: a review of the needs and a new scale. British Journal of Psychiatry 145: 517–525

Baker R 1983 A rating scale for long stay patients. Paper presented at the World Congress on Behaviour Therapy, Washington, DC

Carter J 1981 Day services for adults: somewhere to go. Allen & Unwin, London

Department of Health and Social Security 1957 Royal Commission on the law relating to mental illness and mental deficiency. Cmnd 169, Her Majesty's Stationery Office, London

Early D F, Magnus R V 1968 Industrial therapy organization (Bristol) 1960–65. British Journal of Psychiatry 114: 335–336

Fadden G, Bebbington P, Kuipers L 1987 The burden of care: the impact of functional psychiatric illness on the patient's family. British Journal of Psychiatry 150: 285-292

Garety P A, Morris I 1984 A new unit for long-stay psychiatric patients: organization, attitudes and quality of care. Psychological Medicine 14: 183–192

Goffman E 1961 Asylums: essays on the social situation of mental patients and other inmates. Doubleday, New York. 1968 Penguin, London

Goldberg D P, Bridges K, Cooper W, Hyde C, Sterling C, Wyatt R 1985 Douglas House: a new type of hostel ward for chronic psychotic patients. British Journal of Psychiatry 147: 383–388

Harborne G, Henderson A 1989 Monitoring community care in York. Bulletin of the Royal College of Psychiatrists 13: 140–144

Honigfeld G, Klett C J 1965 The Nurses' Observational Scale for In-Patient Evaluation. Journal of Clinical Psychology 21: 65–71

House of Commons Social Services Committee 1985 Community care, with special reference to mentally ill and mentally handicapped people. Her Majesty's Stationery Office, London

Huxley P 1990 Effective community mental health services. Avebury, Aldershot

Jahoda M 1982 Employment and unemployment. Cambridge University Press, Cambridge

Johnstone E C, Owens D G C, Gold A, Crow T J, Macmillan J F 1981 Institutionalization and the defects of schizophrenia. British Journal of Psychiatry 139: 195–203

Jones K 1988 Experience in Mental Health: community care and social policy. Sage, London

Kuipers L, Bebbington P 1985 Relatives as a resource in the management of functional illness. British Journal of Psychiatry 147: 465–470

McCreadie R G, Oliver A, Wilson A, Burton L L 1983 The Scottish survey of 'new chronic' inpatients. British Journal of Psychiatry 143: 564–571

Mann S A, Cree W 1976 'New' long-stay psychiatric patients: a national sample survey of 15 mental hospitals in England and Wales 1972/3. Psychological Medicine 6: 603–616

Martin J P 1984 Hospitals in trouble. Basil Blackwell, Oxford

Ministry of Health 1962 A Hospital Plan for England and Wales. Cmnd 1604. Her Majesty's Stationary Office, London

Moos R 1974 Evaluating treatment environments. Wiley, New York

Morgan R, Cheadle J 1975 Unemployment impedes resettlement. Social Psychiatry 10: 63–67

Platt S, Weyman A, Hirsch S R, Hewett S 1980 The Social Behaviour Assessment Schedule (SBAS): rationale, contents, scoring and reliability of a new interview schedule. Social Psychiatry 15: 43–55

Renshaw J 1988 Care in the community: individual care planning and case management. British Journal of Social Work 18: 79–106

Royal College of Psychiatrists 1980 Psychiatric rehabilitation in the 1980s. Report of the working party on rehabilitation of the social and community psychiatry section

Royal College of Psychiatrists 1987 Psychiatric rehabilitation updated. Bulletin of the Royal College of Psychiatrists 11:71

Ryan P 1979 Residential care for the mentally disabled. In: Wing J K, Olsen R (eds) Community care for the mentally disabled. Oxford University Press, Oxford

Scottish Home and Health Department, Scottish Education Department 1985 Mental Health in Focus. Report on the mental health services for adults in Scotland. Her Majesty's Stationery Office, Edinburgh

Scottish Home and Health Department, Scottish Health

Service Planning Council 1989 Mental hospitals in focus. Her Majesty's Stationery Office, Edinburgh

Secretaries of State for Health, Social Security, Wales and Scotland 1989 Caring for People: community care in the next decade and beyond. Cmnd 849. Her Majesty's Stationery Office, London

Shepherd G 1990 Rehabilitation and the long term mentally ill. Current Opinion in Psychiatry 3: 278–283

Smith R 1987 Unemployment and health: a disaster and a challenge. Oxford Paperbacks, Oxford

Tarrier N 1990 Familial factors in psychiatry. Current Opinion in Psychiatry 3: 269–272

Team for the Assessment of Psychiatric Services 1990 Better out than in? North East Thames Regional Health Authority, London

Thornicroft G, Bebbington P 1989 Deinstitutionalization — from hospital closure to service development. British Journal of Psychiatry 55: 739–753

Tooth G C, Brooke E M 1961 Trends in the mental hospital population and their effect on future planning. Lancet i: 710–713

Trower P, Bryant B, Argyle M 1979 Social skills and mental health. Methuen, London

Vaughn C E, Leff J P 1976 The influence of family life and social factors on the course of psychiatric illness. A comparison of schizophrenic and depressed neurotic patients. British Journal of Psychiatry 129: 125–137

Warr P B 1987 Work unemployment and mental health. Clarendon Press, Oxford

WHO 1980 International classification of impairments, disabilities and handicaps. World Health Organization, Geneva

Wing J K 1961 a simple and reliable sub-classification of chronic schizophrenia. Journal of Mental Science 107: 862–875

Wing J K 1980 Innovations in social psychiatry. Psychological Medicine 10: 219–230

Wing J K 1990 The functions of asylum. British Journal of Psychiatry 157: 822–827

Wing J K, Brown G W 1970 Institutionalism and schizophrenia: a comparative study of three mental hospitals 1960–1968. Cambridge University Press, Cambridge

Wing J K, Morris B (eds) 1981 Handbook of psychiatric rehabilitation practice. Oxford University Press, Oxford

Wooff K, Goldberg D P, Fryers T 1986 Patients in receipt of community psychiatric nursing care in Salford, 1976–1982. Psychological Medicine 16: 407–414

Wright K 1987 Cost-effectiveness in community care. CHE discussion paper 33. Centre for Health Economics, University of York, York

Index